DeJong's

The Neurologic Examination

EIGHTH EDITION

William W. Campbell, MD, MSHA, COL, MC, USA (Ret)
Professor Emeritus
Department of Neurology
Uniformed Services University of Health Sciences
Bethesda, Maryland

Richard J. Barohn, MD, Lt Col, USAFR, MC (Ret)
Gertrude and Dewey Ziegler Professor of Neurology
University Distinguished Professor
Vice Chancellor for Research
University of Kansas Medical Center
Kansas City, Kansas

Wolters Kluwer

Philadelphia • Baltimore • New York • London
Buenos Aires • Hong Kong • Sydney • Tokyo

Acquisitions Editor: Chris Teja
Development Editor: Ariel S. Winter
Editorial Coordinator: Kerry McShane
Marketing Manager: Rachel Mante Leung
Production Project Manager: Linda Van Pelt
Design Coordinator: Joan Wendt
Manufacturing Coordinator: Beth Welsh
Prepress Vendor: Spi Global

Eighth edition

Printed in China

Library of Congress Cataloging-in-Publication Data
Names: Campbell, William W., Jr. (William Wesley), author. | Barohn, Richard J., author.
Title: DeJong's the neurologic examination / William W. Campbell, Richard J. Barohn.
Other titles: Neurologic examination
Description: Eighth edition. | Philadelphia : Wolters Kluwer, [2020] | Includes bibliographical references and index.
Identifiers: LCCN 2018059855 | ISBN 9781496386168 (hardback)
Subjects: | MESH: Neurologic Examination—methods | Nervous System Diseases—diagnosis
Classification: LCC RC348 | NLM WL 141 | DDC 616.8/0475—dc23 LC record available at https://lccn.loc.gov/2018059855

shop.lww.com

CCS0920

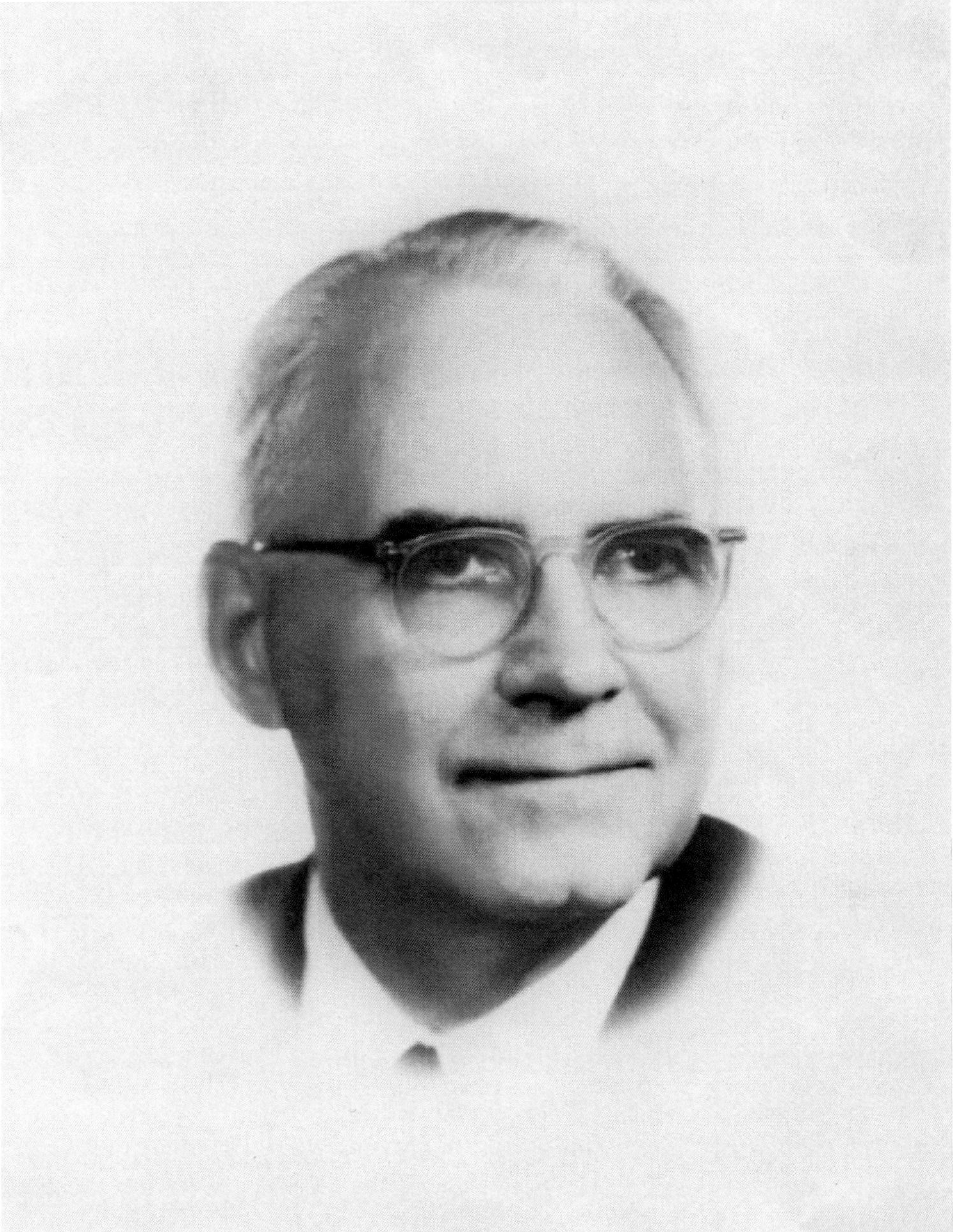

RUSSELL N. DeJONG, MD
1907–1990

Dedication

To Rhonda, Robbie, Wes, Matt, Shannon, Ella, and Will. And to all our former residents and fellows, for all they taught us.

FOREWORD

Standard textbooks of neurology commonly include an introductory chapter on the clinical examination but otherwise provide little guidance as to how this is best performed. The exception is *De Jong's The Neurologic Examination*, first published in 1950, which was intended to present in detail the information necessary to perform a complete and clinically useful examination, accompanied by limited descriptions of the findings in common neurologic entities or disorders. If anything, the need for such an account has increased with the passing years. The art of the neurologic examination is being lost as clinical medicine becomes depersonalized and as new diagnostic and monitoring techniques are used in its place. Moreover, little time is left to learn the intricacies of the physical examination in today's crowded medical school curriculum. The publication of this new (eighth) edition of De Jong's classic text, authored by William Campbell and Richard Barohn, is therefore timely and to be welcomed. It is a pleasure to introduce the book and its authors to another generation of readers.

Dr. Campbell is professor emeritus and former chair of the neurology department at the Uniformed Services University of the Health Sciences in Bethesda, Maryland. I have known him since he was a resident in San Francisco more than 40 years ago. He has had an illustrious career and is well known for his clinical skills and diagnostic acumen. He has authored a number of clinical studies on different aspects of neuromuscular disorders and received the Distinguished Physician Award of the American Association of Neuromuscular and Electrodiagnostic Medicine in 2011. Almost 20 years ago, he took over DeJong's book—the fortunes of which had declined as technologic advances came to influence the practice of neurology—and single-handedly rewrote and revived it. The sixth edition, the first that he authored, was published in 2005 and soon restored the reputation of the book, earning for it a well-deserved place on the bookshelf of many neurologists. He remained the sole author for the seventh edition, published in 2012, but now has been joined by Richard Barohn in preparing this eighth edition.

Dr. Barohn, professor and former chair of the department of neurology at University of Kansas Medical Center, is another accomplished neuromuscular clinician and investigator. In 2013, he received the Distinguished Researcher Award of the American Association of Neuromuscular and Electrodiagnostic Medicine and was named a University Distinguished Professor at the University of Kansas for his achievements.

The book that Campbell and Barohn have authored serves an important need as a guide to both trainees and established physicians. The neurologic examination can be lengthy, often requires much attention to detail, is sometimes performed in difficult or unpleasant circumstances, and may be overwhelming to trainees. Its importance, however, cannot be overemphasized. The findings obtained thereby help to confirm a suspected diagnosis, determine whether any further investigations are needed, indicate the clinical relevance of any laboratory or imaging abnormalities, and suggest the extent and prognosis of many disorders. The competently performed examination also helps to establish a bond between patient and physician that is essential to the welfare of the former and professionally satisfying to the latter.

The neurologic findings become especially meaningful as their relationship to changes in the structure and function of the nervous system comes to be understood. One of the goals of the present volume is to emphasize such a relationship, and the authors have achieved this aim admirably. The text in this new edition has been shortened slightly by reducing discussions of various disease entities to focus on the clinical findings and their significance. Numerous illustrations—most in color—increase the breadth of the book. Several of the older figures from earlier editions have been replaced, and new figures have been added. A number of videos are embedded in the text, with links to many more, as well as to Dr. Campbell's instructive neurosigns.org Web site. In consequence, readers of this book will be able to learn more easily the intricacies of the examination and what to seek when examining patients with different neurologic disorders. They will come to understand the nature and importance of different neurologic signs and will be able to learn from expert clinicians how best to elicit them. Earlier editions have previously received wide recognition and are deservedly familiar to many clinicians. This new edition, which is both scholarly and practical, is even better. It is a mine of information and will be an important resource for many years to come.

Perhaps remarkably in this 21st century but following in the tradition of its predecessors, this new edition is written in its entirety by these two eminent physicians and thus has a uniformity of style that is pleasing. The various chapters fit seamlessly together to produce an integrated and well-rounded account that is based on the accumulated experience and wisdom of its authors. I believe that the book will become an indispensable resource for trainees and practitioners involved in the care of patients with neurologic disorders. I am delighted at its publication, am privileged to introduce it to its intended readership, and congratulate Dr. Campbell and Dr. Barohn for producing such an outstanding volume.

Michael J. Aminoff, MD, DSc, FRCP
Distinguished Professor of Neurology
University of California, San Francisco

PREFACE

The struggle between technology and bedside medicine is nothing new. In his preface to Robert Wartenberg's 1953 *Diagnostic Tests in Neurology*, Sir Gordon Holmes lamented, "There has been within recent years an increasing tendency to rely more and more on laboratory, mechanical and other such methods of investigation of patients suffering with symptoms of nervous disorder at the expense of careful clinical observation." (1) In his introduction to the book, Wartenberg devoted five pages to a section titled *Clinic versus Laboratory*, in which he observed, "There is a growing and deplorable tendency to overload neurological diagnostics with mechanical, technical and laboratory procedures and to overemphasize their importance ... the art of diagnosing with the eyes, ears and fingertips is steadily losing ground." Some of the technology Wartenberg was exhorting against included: EEG, pneumoencephalography, myelography, EMG, and chronaximetry. Wartenberg quoted Moritz Romberg, who wrote of "the great aim which we must seek to achieve, the emancipation of medical science from the trammels of mere mechanical technicalities." Romberg wrote this in 1840.

These pioneering clinicians could not begin to imagine the technology of today and the clinicians of today would undoubtedly stand just as amazed at the technology yet to come, assuming humankind survives to see it. The career span of the authors has witnessed the evolution from radioisotope brain scans, pneumoencephalography, and chromosomal analysis to 3T MRI, PET scans, and next-generation sequencing. But the neurologic examination has been an anchor during the evolution of this technology. The clinical encounter has provided the foundation on which all else is built. Without it, all this wondrous technology might never have escaped the lab.

The examination too has evolved to a degree. We have learned that certain things are not very useful, such as provocative testing for thoracic outlet syndrome, while other things are more useful than once thought, such as olfactory testing, since it became clear that olfactory deficits can signal neurodegenerative disorders. Some things have fallen by the wayside, such as the red lens test and the Wartenberg pinwheel. New, useful things have been described, developed, or rediscovered, such as the head impulse test, the PanOptic ophthalmoscope, the finger rolling test, and the Rydel-Seiffer quantitative tuning fork. The exam done by the 21st century neurologist has become more streamlined and focused. There is less need for a detailed coma exam when the CT done in the ER is already known to show a brainstem hemorrhage.

But the examination remains a central pillar of clinical practice. There are certainly areas where it contributes relatively little. This is not a point of argument and never has been. The neurologist seeing mostly headache patients, or seizure patients, or sleep disorder patients, can certainly get by with minimal exam most of the time. But imaging is of little use in these areas as well. The history is paramount. In other areas of clinical practice, such as neuro-ophthalmology, movement disorders, and neuromuscular disease, the exam is indispensable. Perhaps the academic epileptologist will not suffer much from forgetting how to examine patients, until challenged to keep his or her dignity as the ward attending.

The appropriate use of the history and the clinical examination is to focus and utilize the technology to its fullest potential to solve problems in the service of patient care. The effective clinical neurologist knows what the technology is capable of and how to exploit it to answer a question. The history and examination pose the question. Without the examination and clinical correlation, the technology is blind, as a few recent real-life examples show. It does no good to image the lumbosacral spine for a complaint of leg weakness when the exam shows limb girdle weakness. It does no good to image the lumbosacral spine for a complaint of leg numbness when the exam shows pain and temperature loss in one leg and hyperreflexia in the other. It does no good to order a next generation sequencing panel for a limb girdle syndrome when the exam shows a scapuloperoneal syndrome. It does no good to order an EMG when the exam shows a spastic paraparesis. You cannot believe the imaging report that says the bilateral parieto-occipital signal abnormalities are infarcts when the exam and clinical setting shout PML.

In one astounding case, the only thing gained by imaging the lumbosacral spine and ordering an EMG in an elderly black man with leg weakness was that the electromyographers found the ice-cold feet, absent distal pulses, and subtle margin of gangrene snaking across the toes that led to the diagnosis of distal aortic occlusion. The patient who undergoes total body MRI and whole genome sequencing will be lost in a sea of incidental findings and variants of unknown significance without a clinician to correlate what the technology has unveiled.

Lack of clinical acumen can have lamentable social as well as medical consequences. In one recent case, a woman admitted to the hospital with a hemiparesis was judged by both a neurologist and a neurosurgeon to have a functional deficit after a normal MRI. In fact, she had suffered an episode of hemiplegic migraine. Her insurance company refused to pay for the hospitalization because of the diagnosis of functional hemiparesis.

This edition of *The Neurologic Examination* continues the tradition begun by Dr. Russell DeJong in 1950 of discussing the examination in detail and providing supporting elaboration on some of the underlying neuroanatomy and neurophysiology. Several years ago, the author of the sixth and seventh editions (WWC), recognizing that the size of the book makes it intimidating, undertook to make the material more approachable by reorganizing it alphabetically, making the focus strictly clinical, stripping all but the essence and exploiting the new publishing technology. The result was *Clinical Signs in Neurology: A Compendium.* (2) *Clinical Signs* has numerous embedded videos, as well as links to outside videos, which can be viewed on its Web site or on portable devices such as iPad, iPhone, and Android. This version of *DeJong* shares that technology. There are videos, some of which are medleys, consisting of several examples of such things as abnormal gaits or abnormal plantar responses. The book also contains links to outside videos. The University of Utah library is a national treasure for neurologists. It hosts the Neuro-ophthalmology Virtual Education Library (NOVEL) as well as an extensive collection of videos on the general neurologic examination.

After completion of *Clinical Signs*, the video habit stuck and led to the launch of a Web site, www.neurosigns.org. The Web site now has 72 entries, each with a photo or video and a one or two paragraph description of a sign and its relevance. Because of limits to the number of videos that could be embedded in the text, this edition of *DeJong* contains frequent links to www.neurosigns.org. Others are welcome to contribute to the site.

And all to what end? The end is to preserve the culture of bedside neurology and to preserve the neurologic examination. In our nearly 20-year journey in the footsteps of Russell DeJong, we discovered the Stanford 25, an initiative developed by the Stanford University School of Medicine, whose motto is "Promoting the Culture of Bedside Medicine." They identified 25 core aspects of the physical examination every student should master, and much of it is neurology. They believe, as do we, that caring for the patient starts at the bedside with observing, examining, and connecting with our patients.

We owe our gratitude to the many individuals who contributed to this work. Apologies to anyone inadvertently left out. Thanks are especially due to Stephen Reich, Jason Hawley, Robert Laureno, Sanjeev Nandedkar, Richard Dubinsky, Gary Gronseth, Amanda Sebok, Kent Allen, David Roach, Cheryl Lamp, Timothy Horton, and Kimberly Braxton. Expert advice and support was provided by the team at Wolters Kluwer Health, including Chris Teja, Kerry McShane, Ariel Winter, La Porscha Rogers, Anne Malcolm, Joan Wendt, and Shenbagakutti Arunmozhivarman.

William W. Campbell, MD, MSHA, FAAN, FAANEM
Richmond, Virginia
Richard J. Barohn, MD, FAAN, FAANEM
Kansas City, Kansas

REFERENCES

1. Wartenberg R. *Diagnostic Tests in Neurology: A Selection for Office Use.* Chicago: Year Book Medical Publishers, 1953.
2. Campbell WW. *Clinical Signs in Neurology: A Compendium.* Philadelphia: Wolters Kluwer Health, 2016.

CONTENTS

VIDEOS

The following videos, marked in the book with the video icon, can be found in the companion eBook edition.

Chapter 8

Video 8.1 Demonstration of incorporation of the mental status examination into the physical examination using the Blessed Orientation Memory Concentration test. (Courtesy Nandedkar Productions, LLC, EMG on DVD Series: Volume XIII.)

Chapter 9

Video 9.1 A patient with Broca's aphasia due to a middle cerebral artery stroke.

Chapter 16

Video 16.1 Facial synkinesis following Bell's palsy and after attempted surgical reanimation.

Video 16.2 Hemifacial spasm. (Courtesy Dr. Stephen Reich.)

Chapter 27

Video 27.1 The MRC scale. (Courtesy Nandedkar Productions, LLC, EMG on DVD Series: Volume XIII.)

Video 27.2 Discussion of the examination for pronator drift and its underlying pathophysiology.

Video 27.3 Other subtle signs of hemiparesis, including forearm and finger rolling.

Video 27.4 Abnormal forearm rolling in a patient with a left hemiparesis.

Chapter 28

Video 28.1 Video demonstrating grip and percussion myotonia in a patient with myotonic dystrophy, followed by eyelid, grip, and percussion myotonia with paradoxical myotonia in two patients with paramyotonia congenita. Paradoxical myotonia worsens with successive contractions. (Courtesy Dr. Richard Barohn.)

Chapter 30

Video 30.1 Examples of parkinsonian and essential tremor. The parkinsonian tremor is prominent at rest and dampens with the arm outstretched. Essential tremor is an action tremor, usually not evident at rest but appearing with the hands outstretched; it often involves the head and the voice. (Courtesy Dr. Stephen G. Reich.)

Video 30.2 The first segment of the video demonstrates typical features of a parkinsonian gait with a stooped, flexed posture; short steps; en bloc turning; tremor; reduced arm swing; and impaired postural reflexes. The second segment shows two patients with a festinating gait and the third shows a patient with severe, frequent freezing of gait. (Courtesy Dr. Stephen G. Reich.)

Video 30.3 Evolution of Parkinson's disease over 12 years. (Courtesy Dr. Stephen G. Reich.)

Video 30.4 Chorea in a patient with Huntington's disease.

Video 30.5 Examples of blepharospasm and Meige's syndrome (blepharospasm with oromandibular dystonia). (Courtesy Dr. Stephen G. Reich.)

Video 30.6 Hemiballismus. The movements were unremitting and medically intractable but resolved after pallidotomy. (From Suarez JI, Metman LV, Reich SG, et al. Pallidotomy for hemiballismus: efficacy and characteristics of neuronal activity. *Ann Neurol* 1997;42:807–811.) (Courtesy Dr. Stephen G. Reich.)

Video 30.7 Palatal myoclonus (microtremor). (Courtesy Dr. Jason Hawley.)

Video 30.8 Asterixis. The first segment shows asterixis of the hands, the second segment of the feet. (Courtesy Dr. Robert Laureno.)

Video 30.9 Fasciculations in a patient with end-stage amyotrophic lateral sclerosis.

Chapter 32

Video 32.1 Demonstration of sensory testing with nylon monofilaments.

Chapter 38

Video 38.1 The commonly elicited reflexes.

Video 38.2 Some of the occasionally useful reflexes.

Chapter 40

Video 40.1 Extensor plantar responses, including the Babinski, Chaddock, and Oppenheim. The first segment also demonstrates Rossolimo's sign.

Video 40.2 Ankle clonus.

Chapter 42

Video 42.1 Wartenberg's thumb adduction sign.

Chapter 43

Video 43.1 Cerebellar ataxia with titubation and severe appendicular ataxia causing intention tremor on finger to nose and heel to shin testing.

Video 43.2 Vestibular and cerebellar past pointing and the stepping test.

Chapter 44

Video 44.1 Composite video demonstrating cerebellar ataxia, sensory ataxia in a patient with sensory neuropathy, spastic gait with pronounced scissoring in siblings with hereditary spastic paraplegia, gait apraxia in a patient with normal pressure hydrocephalus, steppage gait due to dense bilateral foot drops in a patient with Charcot-Marie-Tooth disease, and hemiparetic gait following stroke. (Cerebellar ataxia video courtesy John C. Pearson, PhD, and Thomas Mathews, MD, Neurological Teaching Videos, Wright State University Boonshoft School of Medicine.)

Chapter 47

Video 47.1 Physical examination for cervical radiculopathy.

Video 47.2 Segment one, straight leg raising, segment two, Waddell signs.

SECTION A Introduction

CHAPTER 1

Introduction

The importance of the neurologic examination in the diagnosis of diseases of the nervous system cannot be overemphasized. In no other branch of medicine is it possible to build up a clinical picture so exact—with regard to localization and pathologic anatomy—as it is in neurology. This requires not only diagnostic acumen but also a thorough knowledge of the underlying anatomy and physiology of the nervous system, vascular supply, neuropathology, psychology, psychiatry, neuropharmacology, and related disciplines. In addition, neurologic practice demands knowledge of neuroradiology, electroencephalography, electromyography, neurochemistry, microbiology, genetics, neuroendocrinology, neurotransmitters, immunology, oncology, epidemiology, and an understanding of the neuromuscular system.

Neurologic diagnosis is a correlation of data in the study of the human nervous system in health and disease—a synthesis of all the details obtained from the history, examination, and ancillary studies. Nervous tissue makes up about 2% of the human body, and yet it is supplied to all portions of the body. Should the rest of the body tissues be dissolved, there remains an immense network of fibers in addition to the brain, brainstem, and spinal cord. This network is the great receptor, effector, and correlating mechanism of the body. It acts in response to stimuli, acclimates the individual to the environment, and aids in defense against pathologic changes. To understand people, one must first understand the nervous system. Because the nervous system governs the mind and cognitive processes, one cannot study psychology without knowledge of it. Because the nervous system regulates and controls all bodily functions, one cannot study disease of any organ or system of the body without a comprehension of neural function. We are interested, however, not in studying the nervous system and related disease alone but in studying the person whose nervous system is diseased. The formulation of a case in terms of the relationship of the individual to the disease and the relationship of the patient to his or her associates and the environment is as important as providing a precise diagnosis. If we bear this in mind, we can most effectively aid our patients, treat their illnesses, restore them to health, and aid them in regaining their place in society.

Neurologic diagnosis is often considered difficult by the physician who does not specialize in clinical neurology. Most parts of the nervous system are inaccessible to direct examination. Gowers observed "The nervous system is almost entirely inaccessible to direct examination. The exceptions to this are trifling." Many practitioners feel that all neurologic matters belong to the realm of the specialist and make little attempt at neurologic diagnosis. However, many neurologic disorders come within the everyday experience of most practitioners; they should know how to examine the nervous system, when additional studies might be helpful, and how to use the data collected. Furthermore, neurologic dysfunction is the first manifestation of many systemic diseases. Medical diagnosis cannot be made without some knowledge of neurologic diagnosis. True, there are certain rare conditions and diagnostic problems that require long experience in the field of diseases of the nervous system for adequate appraisal. Neurophobia has been prevalent among medical students and nonneurologists for decades, and the explosion of knowledge in neuroscience has if anything made it worse. However, the majority of the more common neurologic entities could and should be diagnosed and treated by the primary care physician.

The neurologic examination requires skill, intelligence, and patience. It requires accurate and trained observation, performed—in most instances—with the help and cooperation of the patient. The examination should be carried out in an orderly manner, and adequate time and attention are necessary to appreciate the details. Each clinician eventually works out a personal method based on experience, but the trainee should follow a fixed and systematic routine until he or she is very familiar with the subject. Premature attempts to abbreviate the examination may result in costly errors of omission. A systematic approach is more essential in neurology than in any other field of medicine, because the multiplicity of signs and variations in interpretation may prove confusing. The specific order that is followed in the examination is not as important as the persistence with which one adheres to this order.

It may be necessary on occasion to vary the routine or to modify the examination according to the state of the patient and the nature of his or her illness. O'Brien emphasized a focused examination driven by the history. If the investigation is long, the patient's interest may flag. Or, he or she may fail to understand the significance of the diagnostic procedures and the need to cooperate. The purpose of the procedures may not be apparent, and he or she may view them as unrelated to his or her presenting complaints. It may help to explain the significance of the tests or their results or to use other means to stimulate interest and cooperation. If fatigue and lack of attention interfere with testing, it may be advisable to change the order of the examination or to complete it at a later date. It is important to bear in mind that slight deviations from the normal may be as significant as more pronounced changes and that the absence of certain signs may be as significant as their presence. On occasion, clues may be obtained merely by watching the patient perform normal, routine, or "casual" actions—such as dressing or undressing, tying shoelaces, looking about the room, or walking into the examining room. Abnormalities in carrying out these actions may point to disorders that might be missed in the more formal examination. The patient's attitude, facial expression, mode of reaction to questions, motor activity, and speech should all be noted.

Interpretation and judgment are important. The ability to interpret neurologic signs can be gained only by carrying out repeated, thorough, and detailed examinations, as well as through keen and accurate observation. In the interpretation of a reflex, for instance—or in the appraisal of tone or of changes in sensation—there may be differences of opinion. The only way the observer may become sure of his or her judgment is through experience. However, the personal equation may enter into any situation, and conclusions may vary. The important factor is not a seemingly quantitative evaluation of the findings but an interpretation or appraisal of the situation as a whole.

The use of a printed outline or form with a checklist for recording the essentials of both the history and the neurologic examination is advocated by some authorities and in some clinics. With such an outline, various items can be underlined, circled, or checked as being either positive or negative. Numerical designations can be used to record such factors as reflex activity or motor strength. Such forms may serve as teaching exercises for the student or novice and as time-saving devices for the clinician, but they cannot replace a careful narrative description of the results of the examination. An outline of the major divisions of the neurologic examination is given in Chapter 5.

No other branch of medicine lends itself so well to the correlation of signs and symptoms with diseased structure as neurology does. However, it is only by means of a systematic examination and an accurate appraisal that one can elicit and properly interpret the findings. Some individuals have a keen intuitive diagnostic sense and can reach correct conclusions by shorter routes, but in most instances, the recognition of disease states can be accomplished only through a scientific discipline based on repeated practical examinations. Diagnosis alone should not be considered the ultimate objective of the examination, but the first step toward treatment and attempts to help the patient. The old saw that neurology is long on diagnosis and short on therapy is outdated. The currently available spectrum of neurologic therapeutics is overwhelming. In cerebrovascular disease, for example, we have gone from "if he can swallow, send him home" to the intra-arterial injection of tissue plasminogen activator. So many agents are now available for the treatment of Parkinson's disease and multiple sclerosis that it almost requires subspecialist expertise to optimally manage these common disorders. There is now even reason for optimism in such previously hopeless situations as spinal muscular atrophy and amyotrophic lateral sclerosis.

This revision of Dr. DeJong's classic text begins with an overview of neuroanatomy, including some of the underlying neuroembryology. The overview provides broad perspective and an opportunity to cover certain topics that do not conveniently fit into other sections. Chapters 3 to 44 are organized as the neurologic clinical encounter typically evolves: history and the general physical examination, followed by the elements of the neurologic examination as commonly performed—including mental status, cranial nerves, motor, sensory, reflexes, cerebellar function, and gait. Early editions covered the sensory examination first, Dr. DeJong's argument being that it required the most attentiveness and cooperation from the patient and should be done early in the encounter. The countervailing argument is that the sensory examination is the most subjective and usually the least helpful part of the examination, and it should be done last. We are more inclined toward the latter view and hope Dr. DeJong would forgive the demotion of the sensory examination. The neuroscientific underpinnings of the neurologic examination are discussed before the clinical aspects. Dr. DeJong's original concept for his textbook was to incorporate the fundamentals of neuroanatomy and neurophysiology and to highlight pertinent relationships to the examination. With the explosion in basic neuroscience knowledge, these efforts, continued in this edition, appear increasingly inadequate. The bibliography lists several excellent textbooks that cover basic neuroscience in the kind of exhaustive detail not possible here. Chapter 53 consists of a discussion of neurologic epistemology, diagnostic reasoning, and differential diagnosis.

There are a number of other textbooks on the neurologic examination. These range from the very brief *The Four-Minute Neurologic Examination* to more comprehensive works intended for neurologic trainees and practitioners. Dr. William DeMyer's textbook is unfailingly entertaining and informative. *Mayo Clinic Examinations in Neurology* continues to be a standard in the field. Dr. Sid Gilman's *Clinical Examination of the Nervous System* includes a discussion of the underlying neuroanatomy. Dr. Robert Laureno's *Foundations for Clinical Neurology* provides unique perspective on the clinical encounter. Dr. Robert Schwartzman's *Neurologic Examination* is excellent; likewise the short textbooks by Ross and Fuller. *Bickerstaff's Neurological Examination in Clinical Practice* was recently revised. *The Neurologic Examination: Scientific Basis for Clinical Diagnosis* by Shibasaki and Hallett examines the scientific underpinnings of the examination. Dr. DeJong's text has long been the most encyclopedic; the tradition is continued in this edition. In this revision, we have included more illustrations, and now, there are embedded videos as well as links to relevant outside videos.

There is a wealth of online information about the neurologic examination. Neurosciences on the Internet (**Web Link 1.1**) is a valuable resource and includes an excellent demonstration of the cutaneous fields of the peripheral nerves. The site Neuroexam.com (**Web Link 1.2**) has numerous videos and is by the author of the popular *Neuroanatomy Through Clinical Cases*. There are numerous links throughout the text to Neurosigns (**Web Link 1.3**), a collection of photos and videos of neurologic examination findings; there is an associated youtube channel, (**Web Link 1.4**). The library at the University of Utah houses a rich repository of neurologic examination videos (**Web Link 1.5**). The Neuro-ophthalmology Virtual Education Library, NOVEL, also at the University of Utah, has an amazing collection of videos (**Web Link 1.6**). NOVEL includes collections by such luminaries as David Cogan, Robert Daroff, William Hoyt, J. Lawton Smith, and Shirley Wray. The Canadian Neuro-Ophthalmology Group maintains an extensive collection of videos, fundus photos and other resources (**Web Link 1.7**). A series of examination videos is available on the EMG on DVD Series: Volume XIII, Practical Neurologic Examination, by Nandedkar Productions, LLC (**Web Link 1.8**).

Ancillary diagnostic techniques have, through the years, played important roles in neurologic diagnosis. The original electrodiagnostic techniques of Duchenne, Erb, and others were introduced in the latter part of the 19th century. Later, neurologic diagnosis was aided by the introduction of pneumoencephalography, ventriculography, myelography, electroencephalography, ultrasonography, angiography, electromyography, evoked potential studies, nerve conduction studies, radioisotope scanning, computed tomography, magnetic resonance imaging (MRI), blood flow studies by single photon emission computed tomography and inhalation methods, positron emission tomography (PET), and others. In previous editions, space was devoted to many of these topics. Some of these techniques have been abandoned. The modern neurodiagnostic armamentarium has become complex and highly specialized. We have moved from the era of air studies to an era of functional MRI, diffusion weighted imaging, and PET. There can only be conjecture about what new technologies may be in use before this textbook is next revised. The reader is referred to the many excellent textbooks and other sources that cover ancillary neurodiagnostic techniques. The focus of this book is on neuroanatomy and neurophysiology, the clinical neurologic examination, clinical reasoning, and differential diagnosis. Current techniques of imaging, electrodiagnosis, and other laboratory studies have revolutionized the practice of neurology. However, their use must be integrated with the findings of the history and neurologic examination. The practice of "shotgunning" with multiple tests is to be discouraged. Such studies do not replace the examination. Not only is it poor clinical practice but also the resource consumption is enormous.

The development of ever more sophisticated imaging studies of the nervous system along with many other sensitive laboratory techniques has raised questions about the continued need and utility of the neurologic examination. In a provocative paper, *I've stopped examining patients!*, Hawkes pointed out that the examination adds little in some common conditions, such as migraine and epilepsy. A flurry of correspondence followed. But in many other common conditions, the examination is indispensable. In such common conditions as Parkinson's disease and amyotrophic lateral sclerosis, the physical examination is essential to the diagnosis. In many other common conditions, the examination is the key to proper diagnosis and management, such as optic neuropathy, benign positional vertigo, Bell's palsy, Alzheimer's disease, and virtually all neuromuscular disorders. In a recent case, extensive evaluations for gait difficulties by a family physician, including lumbosacral MRI and CSF examination, were unrevealing. Only when examination disclosed, spasticity was the problem solved by imaging the neck. The examination determines where to point the scanner. Just as a normal EKG does not exclude myocardial infarction, normal imaging does not necessarily exclude neurologic disease. The clinician relinquishes examination skills at his/her peril.

The neurologic examination will not become obsolete. It will not be replaced by mechanical evaluations; rather, a more precise and more directed neurologic examination will be needed in the future. The neurologic history and examination will remain to hold important in clinical evaluation. Neurodiagnostic technology should supplement clinical evaluation, not replace it. Nicholl and Appleton recently reviewed the role of the clinical examination in neurologic evaluation and emphasized that investigation should follow clinical assessment, not precede it. Aminoff reminds us that it is important the art of the clinical examination is not lost in the era of precision medicine. The neurologist will have to be the final judge of the significance of his or her own findings and those of special studies.

Web Links

Web Link 1.1. Neurosciences on the Internet. http://www.neuroguide.com

Web Link 1.2. Neuroexam.com. http://www.neuroexam.com/neuroexam/

Web Link 1.3. Neurosigns. www.neurosigns.org

Web Link 1.4. Neurosigns on YouTube. https://www.youtube.com/channel/UC7JOrAlJruTYA-aZdSeK7bQ

Web Link 1.5. NeuroLogic Exam at The University of Utah. https://library.med.utah.edu/neurologicexam/html/home_exam.html

Web Link 1.6. The Neuro-ophthalmology Virtual Education Library, NOVEL. https://novel.utah.edu/

Web Link 1.7. The Canadian Neuro-Ophthalmology Group. http://www.neuroophthalmology.ca/

Web Link 1.8. EMG on DVD Series: Volume XIII, Practical Neurologic Examination, by Nandedkar Productions, LLC. https://www.nandedkarproductions.com/productdetail.php?id=21

BIBLIOGRAPHY

Aminoff MJ. The future of the neurologic examination. *JAMA Neurol* 2017;74:1291–1292.

Benarroch EE, Cutsforth-Gregory JK, Flemming KD. *Mayo Clinic Medical Neurosciences: Organized by Neurologic Systems and Levels*. 6th ed. Rochester/New York: Mayo Clinic Scientific Press/Oxford University Press, 2017.

Biller J, Gruener G, Brazis PW. *DeMyer's The Neurologic Examination: A Programmed Text*. 7th ed. New York: McGraw-Hill Education, 2017.

Blumenfeld H. *Neuroanatomy Through Clinical Cases*. 2nd ed. Sunderland: Sinauer Associates, 2010.

Brazis PW, Masdeu JC, Biller J. *Localization in Clinical Neurology*. 7th ed. Philadelphia: Wolters Kluwer/Lippincott Williams & Wilkins, 2017.

Campbell WW. *Clinical Signs in Neurology: A Compendium*. Philadelphia: Wolters Kluwer Health, 2016.

Campbell WW. *Pocket Guide and Toolkit to DeJong's Neurologic Examination*. Philadelphia: Lippincott Williams & Wilkins, 2008.

Caplan LC, Hollander J. *The Effective Clinical Neurologist*. 3rd ed. Shelton: People's Medical Publishing House, 2010.

DeMyer W. Pointers and pitfalls in the neurologic examination. *Semin Neurol* 1998;18:161–168.

Fuller G. *Neurological Examination Made Easy*. 5th ed. New York: Churchill Livingstone, 2013.

Gilman S. *Clinical Examination of the Nervous System*. New York: McGraw-Hill, 2000.

Goldberg S. *The Four-Minute Neurologic Exam*. 2nd ed. Miami: MedMaster, Inc., 2017.

Hawkes CH. I've stopped examining patients! *Pract Neurol* 2009;9:192–194.

Hirtz D, Thurman DJ, Gwinn-Hardy K, et al. How common are the "common" neurologic disorders? *Neurology* 2007;68:326–337.

Johnston SC, Hauser SL. The beautiful and ethereal neurological exam: an appeal for research. *Ann Neurol* 2011;70:A9–A10.

Kandel ER. *Principles of Neural Science*. 5th ed. New York: McGraw-Hill Medical, 2013.

Lim EC, Ong BK, Seet RC. Using videotaped vignettes to teach medical students to perform the neurologic examination. *J Gen Intern Med* 2006;21:101.

Louis ED, Pascuzzi RM, Roos KL, eds. The neurological examination (with an emphasis on its historical underpinnings). *Semin Neurol* 2002;22:335–418.

Massey EW, Pleet AB, Scherokman BJ. *Diagnostic Tests in Neurology: A Photographic Guide to Bedside Techniques*. Chicago: Year Book Medical Publishers, Inc., 1985.

Nicholl DJ, Appleton JP. Clinical neurology: why this still matters in the 21st century. *J Neurol Neurosurg Psychiatry* 2015;86:229–233.

O'Brien MD. Use and abuse of physical signs in neurology. *J R Soc Med* 2014;107:416–421.

Pryse-Phillips W. *Companion to Clinical Neurology*. 3rd ed. Oxford: Oxford University Press, 2009.

Ross RT. *How to Examine the Nervous System*. 4th ed. Totowa: Humana Press, 2006.

Sanders RD, Keshavan MS. The neurologic examination in adult psychiatry: from soft signs to hard science. *J Neuropsychiatry Clin Neurosci* 1998;10:395–404.

Schwartzman RJ. *Neurologic Examination*. Malden: Blackwell Publishing, 2006.

Warlow C. Why I have not stopped examining patients. *Pract Neurol* 2010;10:126–128.

Wartenberg R. *The Examination of Reflexes: A Simplification*. Chicago: Year Book Medical Publishers, 1945.

Wartenberg R. *Diagnostic Tests in Neurology: A Selection for Office Use*. Chicago: Year Book Medical Publishers, 1953.

Weibers DO, Dale AJD, Kokmen E, et al., eds. *Mayo Clinic Examinations in Neurology*. 7th ed. St. Louis: Mosby, 1998.

Ziegler DK. Is the neurologic examination becoming obsolete? *Neurology* 1985;35:559.

SECTION B History, Physical Examination, and Overview of the Neurologic Examination

CHAPTER 2

Overview of the Nervous System

The nervous system consists of the central nervous system (CNS) and the peripheral nervous system (PNS). The nerve roots of the spinal cord connect the CNS to the PNS. The CNS is made up of the brain (encephalon), which lies rostral to the foramen magnum, and the spinal cord (myelon), which lies caudal. The brain is made up of the cerebrum, diencephalon, brainstem, and cerebellum (Figure 2.1). The cerebrum (telencephalon) is the largest component of the CNS. It consists of two cerebral hemispheres connected by the corpus callosum. The diencephalon (L. "between brain," "interbrain") lies between the telencephalon and the midbrain. The brainstem connects the diencephalon with the spinal cord. It consists, from rostral to caudal, of the midbrain, pons, and medulla oblongata. The cerebellum (Latin diminutive of *cerebrum*) is a large, fissured structure that lies posterior to the brainstem. It is composed of a narrow midline strip (vermis) and paired lateral hemispheres and is connected to the brainstem by the superior, middle, and inferior cerebellar peduncles. The spinal cord extends from the cervicomedullary junction to the conus medullaris.

NEUROEMBRYOLOGY

In the embryo, development of the nervous system begins when ectodermal cells start to form the neural tube. The sonic hedgehog gene is vital for normal CNS development. It mediates a number of processes in development, including differentiation of the neuroectoderm. The neural tube begins to form in the 3rd week and is completed by the 4th week of embryonic life. The first stage in neural tube development is a thickening of ectoderm, forming the neural plate. A longitudinal fissure develops in the neural plate and progressively enlarges to form the neural groove. Differentiation of the cephalic from the caudal end of the neural groove is controlled by a signaling molecule called noggin. As the groove deepens, its edges become more prominent and become the neural folds. The folds eventually meet, fuse, and complete the transformation into a tubular structure. The neural tube lies between the ectoderm on the surface and the notochord below. The cranial part of the neural tube evolves into the brain, and the caudal part becomes the spinal cord. With closure of the neural tube, the neural crest—neuroectoderm not incorporated into the neural tube—lies between the neural tube and the surface. Neural crest cells give rise to the PNS. Cells that lie ventral in the neural tube develop into motor cells, and those that lie dorsal develop into sensory cells. Sonic hedgehog is involved in this differentiation. Retinoic acid is also important at this stage, and the use of retinoic acid derivatives for acne treatment in early pregnancy may have catastrophic effects on the developing nervous system.

Neuroepithelial cells in the wall of the neural tube form neuroblasts, which develop into neurons, and glioblasts, which develop into macroglial and ependymal cells. With further maturation, the neural tube wall develops three layers: an innermost ventricular

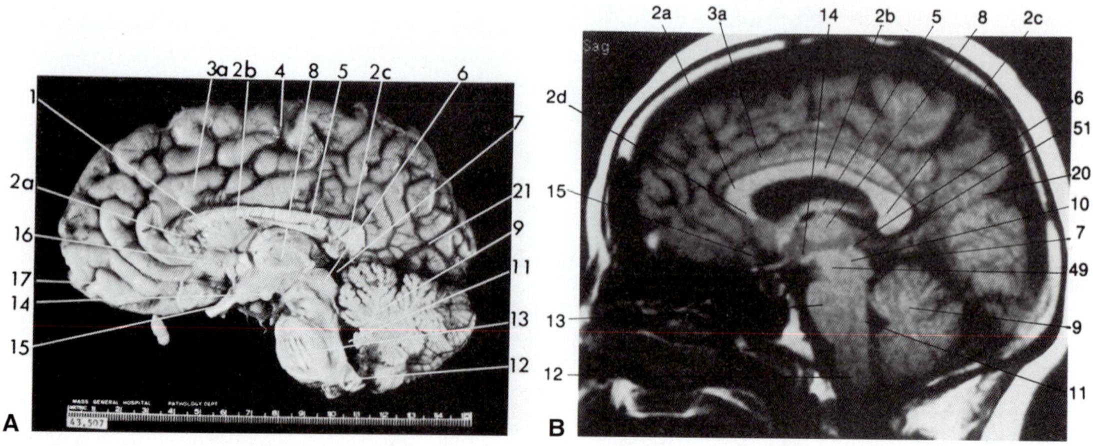

FIGURE 2.1 **A.** Gross brain. **B.** T1-weighted MR image. Approximately matched midline sagittal sections. Sagittal T1-weighted MRI of the brain and upper cervical spinal cord. Labels: *1*, septum pellucidum; *2*, corpus callosum (*a*, genu; *b*, body; *c*, splenium; *d*, rostrum); *3*, cingulate gyrus; *4*, central sulcus; *5*, column of fornix; *6*, quadrigeminal plate; *7*, quadrigeminal cistern; *8*, thalamus; *9*, cerebellum; *10*, aqueduct of Sylvius; *11*, fourth ventricle; *12*, medulla; *13*, pons; *14*, mammillary body; *15*, optic tract; *16*, olfactory area; *17*, gyrus rectus; *20*, parietal-occipital fissure; *21*, calcarine fissure; *49*, midbrain; *51*, pineal gland. (Reprinted with permission from Barboriak DP, Taveras JM. Normal cerebral anatomy with magnetic resonance imaging. In: Ferrucci JT, ed. *Taveras and Ferrucci's Radiology on CD-ROM*. Philadelphia: Lippincott Williams & Wilkins, 2003.)

layer composed of ependymal cells, a mantle (intermediate) layer consisting of neurons and macroglia, and an outer marginal layer, which contains the nerve fibers of the neuroblasts in the mantle layer. The ventricular layer eventually forms the lining of the ventricles and central canal of the spinal cord, the mantle layer becomes the central gray matter, and the marginal layer becomes the white matter. Closure of the tube (neurulation) separates the developing nervous system from the surface ectoderm, forming the neurula (the embryo at 19 to 26 days after fertilization). Neurulation begins near the midpoint of the neural tube and advances toward the anterior (cephalic) and posterior (caudal) neuropores at either end; the anterior and posterior neuropores are the last sites to close. Neurulation is complete by 4 weeks; afterward, the CNS is a long, fluid-filled, tubular structure, and this basic configuration is maintained throughout life. Defective neurulation is common. Neural tube defects (NTDs) are common congenital malformations that result from failure of normal neural tube closure during early embryogenesis (Box 2.1). Neural tube closure is complete by the end of the first month; NTDs happen before a mother knows she is pregnant.

The brain develops from the region of the anterior neuropore, forming three and then five vesicles. First, there is segmentation into three parts: forebrain (prosencephalon), midbrain (mesencephalon), and hindbrain (rhombencephalon) (Table 2.1). The forebrain then divides into the telencephalon, which becomes the cerebrum, and the diencephalon. The hindbrain divides into the metencephalon, which becomes the pons and cerebellum, and the myelencephalon, which becomes the medulla. The five-vesicle stage is complete by 6 weeks of embryonic life. The telencephalon then undergoes midline cleavage into a pair of side-by-side vesicles—primordial hemispheres. Regions of the telencephalon expand (evaginate) to form the cerebral hemispheres. The neural tube lumen continues into the evaginations, forming the ventricular system.

Failure of normal cleavage into two hemispheres results in distinctive anomalies. Milder forms include arrhinencephaly, in which there is absence of the olfactory bulbs and tracts, and agenesis of the corpus callosum. Severe cleavage failure results in holoprosencephaly, in which there is only a single "hemisphere" (alobar prosencephaly), or a partial attempt at division (lobar and semilobar prosencephaly). Prenatal diagnosis is possible using sonography. The genes that control segmentation are also important in development of the face, and some anomalies involve both the face and the brain, particularly holoprosencephaly. Certain patterns of midline facial abnormality predict a severe brain malformation.

Following the segmentation and cleavage stages of neuroembryogenesis, the developing nervous system enters a stage of cellular proliferation and

BOX 2.1

Neural Tube Defects

Neural tube defects (NTDs) are very common. They may be divided into an upper type (anencephaly, encephalocele) and a lower type (spinal dysraphism). Anencephaly is a lethal malformation that results from failure of closure of the anterior neuropore. The brain fails to develop. The face develops, but the cranial vault does not, and the brain may consist of only a tangled knot of primordial central nervous system tissue. Anencephaly is a common cause of stillbirth. There may be enough brainstem present to support vegetative life for a brief period. Failure of the posterior neuropore to close normally causes congenital malformations affecting the lumbosacral region. The most severe of these is myelomeningocele, essentially the posterior neuropore equivalent of anencephaly. The posterior elements of the lumbosacral vertebra fail to develop, the spinal canal is open posteriorly, and the spinal cord and cauda equina are herniated dorsally into a sac that lies over the surface of the lower back. The patients have severe neurologic deficits involving the lower extremities, bowel, and bladder. When the defect is less severe, the sac contains only meninges (meningocele). A mild defect of posterior neuropore closure results only in failure of normal fusion of the posterior arches of the lumbosacral vertebra. Patients are neurologically normal, and the defect is seen only on imaging studies (spina bifida occulta). Spina bifida occulta is quite common, affecting up to 10% of the population. Incomplete defects of anterior neuropore closure cause similar defects affecting the head and neck. An encephalocele is herniation of brain tissue through a bony defect in the skull. Encephaloceles most commonly occur in the occipitocervical region and are clinically obvious. When they involve the base of the skull (basal encephalocele), they may not be obvious. Cranium bifidum is dysraphism limited to the bony elements of the skull, most often the occipital bone; it is the cephalic analogue of spina bifida occulta. Arnold-Chiari malformations may involve defects in closure of both the anterior and posterior neuropore; these complex anomalies are discussed further in Chapter 21.

The pathogenesis of NTDs is multifactorial; both genetic and environmental factors are important, and the pattern of occurrence suggests a multifactorial polygenic or oligogenic etiology. Overactivation of sonic hedgehog signaling has been implicated. There are significant geographic differences, for example, NTDs are very common in Ireland. Folic acid plays a pivotal role in neuroembryogenesis. Genetic defects of the folate and homocysteine pathways have been implicated in the etiology of NTDs; periconceptional folate supplementation reduces the risk, and mothers of affected children may have elevated plasma homocysteine levels. A group at particular risk for having children with NTDs is women receiving certain antiepileptic medications during pregnancy.

migration that is not complete until after birth. Neurons in the germinal matrix proliferate intensely and then migrate to different parts of the nervous system. Cells destined to populate a specific brain region arise from a specific part of the germinal matrix. Processes that interfere with normal proliferation and migration cause another set of congenital malformations that includes microcephaly, megalencephaly, cortical heterotopia (band heterotopia, double cortex), agenesis of the corpus callosum, and schizencephaly. Three major callosal abnormalities have been identified: hypoplasia, hypoplasia with dysplasia, and complete agenesis. Finally, the brain develops its pattern of gyri and sulci. Defects at this stage of neocortical formation produce lissencephaly, in which the sulci and gyri fail to develop (smooth brain); pachygyria, in which the gyri are thicker than normal; and polymicrogyria, in which there are an excessive number of small gyri. These abnormalities may affect all or only part of the brain. Typically, children with these malformations have developmental delay and seizures. Other systems may be involved in these neuronal migration disorders, including eye and muscle (muscle-eye-brain disease, Walker-Warburg syndrome, and Fukuyama congenital muscular dystrophy). Modern imaging, including prenatal magnetic resonance imaging (MRI), may identify some of these disorders.

Even after normal formation, the nervous system may be affected by intrauterine processes. In

TABLE 2.1 The Derivatives of the Anterior Neuropore

Prosencephalon (forebrain)
Telencephalon (cerebral hemispheres)
Pallium (cortical mantle)
Neopallium
Rhinencephalon
Paleopallium (piriform lobe)
Archipallium (hippocampal formation)
Hemispheric white matter
Association fibers
Commissural fibers
Projection fibers
Basal ganglia
Caudate
Putamen
Globus pallidus
Diencephalon
Thalamus
Metathalamus
Epithalamus
Subthalamus
Hypothalamus
Mesencephalon (midbrain)
Rhombencephalon (hindbrain)
Metencephalon
Pons
Cerebellum
Myelencephalon (medulla)

hydranencephaly, the hemispheres are destroyed and the remnants lie in a sac of meninges. This is to be distinguished from hydrocephalus, where the ventricles are markedly expanded. In hydranencephaly, the skull is normal but devoid of meaningful contents, in contrast to anencephaly, in which the skull is malformed along with the brain. In porencephaly, a cyst forms in a region where developing brain has been destroyed or has developed abnormally. Transillumination of the skull with a strong light may help detect these disorders early. The diagnosis may be confirmed by computed tomography, MRI, or sonography, and the diagnosis can be made with sonography in the prenatal period. Numerous conditions may affect the neonatal brain, including germinal matrix hemorrhage, hypoxic-ischemic encephalopathy, cerebral infarction, and infection. Many of these disorders produce "cerebral palsy," an umbrella term with little neurologic meaning.

BONY ANATOMY

The skull is fashioned of several large bones and myriad complexly articulated smaller bones. The major bones are the frontal, temporal, parietal, occipital, and sphenoid; all are joined by suture lines. The major sutures are the sagittal and coronal, but there are numerous others. Sometimes sutures close prematurely (craniostenosis, craniosynostosis), before the skull has completed growth, producing malformed and misshapen skulls (Box 2.2; Figure 2.2). Noggin plays a role in the regulation of cranial suture fusion,

BOX 2.2

Craniosynostosis

The primary clinical manifestation of craniosynostosis is an abnormally shaped skull; the configuration depends on which suture(s) have fused prematurely. The skull is unable to expand in a direction perpendicular to the fused suture line. With synostosis of a major suture, the skull compensates by expanding in a direction perpendicular to the uninvolved sutures. Premature closure of the sagittal suture, the most common form of craniosynostosis, produces a skull that is abnormally elongated (scaphocephaly, dolichocephaly). Synostosis of both coronal sutures causes a skull that is abnormally wide (brachycephaly). When the coronal and lambdoid sutures are involved, the skull is tall and narrow (turricephaly, tower skull). Synostosis of the sagittal and both coronal sutures causes oxycephaly (acrocephaly), a pointed, conical skull. Plagiocephaly refers to a flattened spot on one side of the head; it is due to premature unilateral fusion of one coronal or lambdoid suture. Synostosis involving the metopic suture causes trigonocephaly, a narrow, triangular forehead with lateral constriction of the temples. Synostosis of the posterior sagittal and both lambdoidal sutures produces the "Mercedes Benz pattern." Severe craniosynostosis involving multiple sutures may cause increased intracranial pressure. Craniosynostosis usually occurs as an isolated condition, but there are numerous syndromes in which craniosynostosis occurs in conjunction with other anomalies, particularly malformations of the face and the digits, for example, Crouzon's, Apert's, and Carpenter's syndromes. Several genetic mutations may cause craniosynostosis. There are many potential causes of nonsyndromic craniosynostosis, including environmental, hormonal, and biomechanical factors.

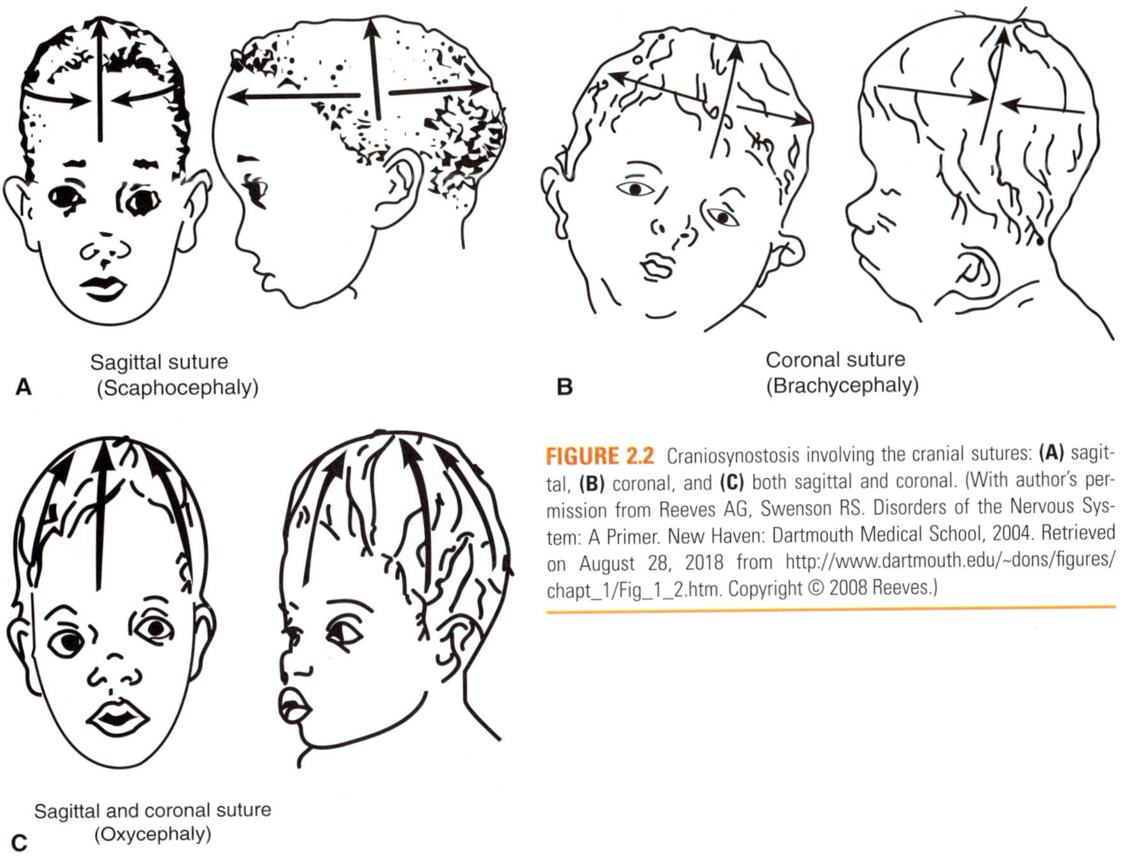

FIGURE 2.2 Craniosynostosis involving the cranial sutures: **(A)** sagittal, **(B)** coronal, and **(C)** both sagittal and coronal. (With author's permission from Reeves AG, Swenson RS. Disorders of the Nervous System: A Primer. New Haven: Dartmouth Medical School, 2004. Retrieved on August 28, 2018 from http://www.dartmouth.edu/~dons/figures/chapt_1/Fig_1_2.htm. Copyright © 2008 Reeves.)

and craniosynostosis may be the result of inappropriate down-regulation of noggin expression.

The interior of the skull is divided into compartments, or fossae. The anterior fossa contains the frontal lobes, which rest on the orbital plates. The cribriform plate lies far anteriorly, between the orbital roofs; when fractured during head injury, cerebrospinal fluid (CSF) rhinorrhea may ensue. The middle fossa primarily contains the temporal lobes, and several major cranial nerves (CNs) run through the area. The posterior fossa contains the brainstem, cerebellum, and vertebrobasilar vessels. Except for CNs I and II, all the CNs run through or exit from the posterior fossa.

The frontal bone contains the frontal sinuses. The temporal bone has two parts: the thin squamous portion forms the temple; the thick petrous part forms the floor of the middle fossa. The squamous part contains the groove of the middle meningeal artery and may be easily fractured, sometimes producing epidural hematoma. The petrous pyramids have their apices pointed medially and their thick bases pointed laterally; deep within are the middle and inner ear structures, the internal auditory meatus, the facial canal with its genu, and the air cells of the mastoid sinus. Fractures through the petrous bone may cause hemotympanum (blood in the middle ear cavity), hearing loss, or facial nerve palsy.

The sphenoid bone has greater and lesser wings and contains the sella turcica. The greater wings form the anterior wall of the middle fossa; the lesser wings form part of the floor of the anterior fossa. The greater and lesser wings attach to the body of the sphenoid, buried within which is the sphenoid sinus cavity. The best way to appreciate the anatomy of the sphenoid bone is to look at it in disarticulated isolation, when the "wings" become obvious. The sella turcica makes up a saddle-shaped depression in the body of the sphenoid; alongside the sella lie the cavernous sinuses. The pituitary gland lies within the sella, and neoplasms of the pituitary may enlarge the sella and push upward out of the sella onto the optic chiasm. Enlargement of the sella is a nonspecific finding in increased intracranial pressure.

The occipital bone makes up the posterior fossa. The clivus forms the anterior wall of the posterior

TABLE 2.2 Major Skull Base Foramina and Their Contents

Foramen	Contents
Cribriform plate	Olfactory nerves
Optic canal	Optic nerve, ophthalmic artery
Superior orbital fissure	III, IV, VI, ophthalmic V, superior ophthalmic vein
Foramen rotundum	Maxillary V
Foramen spinosum	Middle meningeal artery
Foramen ovale	Mandibular V
Internal auditory meatus	VII, VIII, internal auditory artery
Jugular foramen	IX, X, XI, internal jugular vein
Hypoglossal foramen	XII
Carotid canal	Carotid artery

Roman numerals refer to cranial nerves III through XII.

fossa; it ends superiorly in the dorsum sellae and posterior clinoid processes. The basilar artery and brainstem lie along the clivus. Tumors, most often chordomas, may erode the clivus and produce multiple CN palsies. Various structures pass into or out of the skull through the numerous foramina that pierce its base (Table 2.2). Pathologic processes may involve different foramina; the resultant combination of CN abnormalities permits localization (see Chapter 21).

MENINGES

The meninges are composed of the dura mater, pia mater, and arachnoid (Figure 2.2). The pia is thin, filmy, and closely adherent to the brain and its blood vessels, extending down into the sulci and perivascular spaces. The dura mater is thick and tough (the pachymeninges; Gr. *pachys* "thick") and provides the substantive protective covering for the CNS. The dura has an inner, meningeal layer and an outer periosteal layer that is continuous with the periosteum of the inner calvarium. The two leaves of dura separate to enclose the cerebral venous sinuses. The dura closely adheres to the bone at the suture lines and around the foramen magnum. Sheaths of dura cover the cranial and spinal nerves as they exit and then fuse with the epineurium. The vaginal sheath of the optic nerve is a layer of meninges that follows the optic nerve; ultimately the dura fuses with the sclera of the eyeball. Folds of dura separate the two hemispheres (the falx cerebri) and the middle fossa from the posterior fossa structures (the tentorium cerebelli). A diminutive fold (the falx cerebelli) separates the cerebellar hemispheres. The cranial dura is, for the most part, a single layer, distinguishable as two sheets only at the venous sinuses and in the orbit. In contrast, the layers of the spinal dura are separate. The outer, periosteal layer forms the periosteum of the vertebral canal, and the meningeal layer closely covers the spinal cord. This separation creates a wide epidural space in the spinal canal that is not present in the head. The spinal epidural space is a frequent site for metastatic disease. The cranial and spinal dura fuse at the foramen magnum.

The arachnoid abuts the inner surface of the dura, and a web of fine, diaphanous trabeculae crosses the subarachnoid space to connect the arachnoid to the pia (Figure 2.3). Over the surface of the brain and spinal cord, the pia and the arachnoid are closely adherent and virtually inseparable, forming essentially one membrane: the pia-arachnoid, or leptomeninges (Gr. *leptos* "slender"). The subdural space is the space between the dura and the arachnoid. Normally, the space is more potential than real, but under some circumstances, fluid may accumulate in the subdural space. The subarachnoid space lies beneath the arachnoid membrane. Bleeding into the subarachnoid space is a common complication of craniocerebral trauma and the rupture of aneurysms or vascular malformations. The CSF flows through the subarachnoid space. Focal enlargements of the subarachnoid space (cisterns) develop in areas where the dura and arachnoid do not closely follow the contour of the brain, creating a wide space between the arachnoid and the pia. The cisterna magna (cerebellomedullary cistern) is a CSF reservoir posterior to the medulla and beneath the inferior part of the cerebellum (Figure 2.4). Other important cisterns include the perimesencephalic (ambient), interpeduncular (basal), prepontine, and chiasmatic. The term basal cisterns is sometimes used to include all the subarachnoid cisterns at the base of the brain. Focal enlargements of the subarachnoid space produce arachnoid cysts, which may rarely compress the brain or spinal cord.

The lateral ventricles are made up of a body and an atrium (common space), from which extend the horns (Figure 2.4). The temporal horn extends forward into the temporal lobe; the occipital horn extends backward into the occipital lobe. Within the atrium of each ventricle lies CSF-forming choroid plexus. The two lateral ventricles come together in the midline, where they join the third ventricle. The foramen of Monro is the passageway between the lateral and third ventricles. The third ventricle is a thin slit lying in the midline between and just below

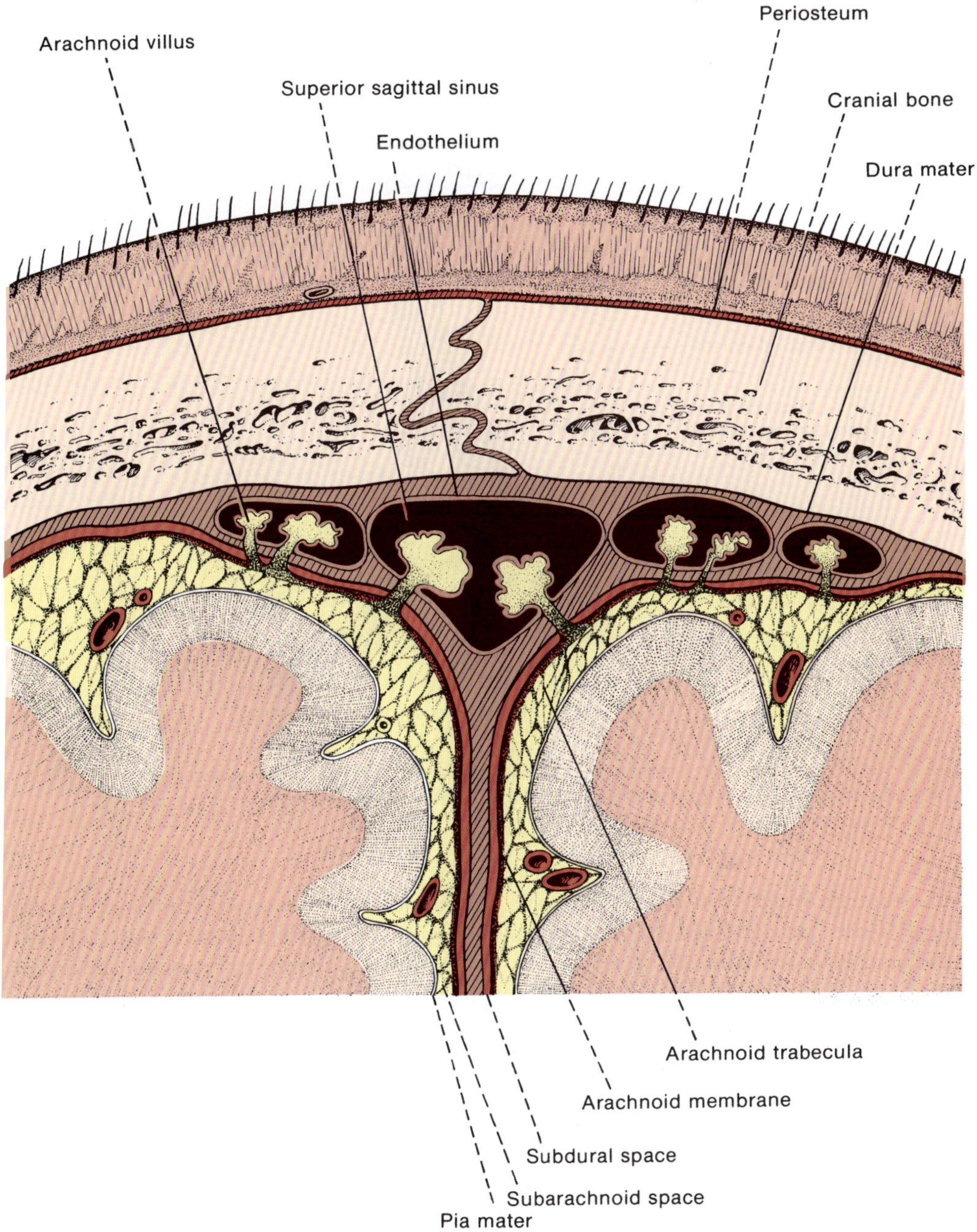

FIGURE 2.3 Schematic diagram of a coronal section of the meninges and cerebral cortex, showing the relationship of the arachnoid villus to the subarachnoid space and superior sagittal sinus. (Modified from Weed LH. The absorption of cerebrospinal fluid into the venous system. *Am J Anat* 1923;31:191–207.)

the lateral ventricles. Anteriorly it forms spaces, or recesses, above and below the pituitary; posteriorly it creates a recess above the pineal gland. The third ventricle ends at the cerebral aqueduct (of Sylvius), which conveys CSF down to the fourth ventricle. The fourth ventricle is also a midline structure that has superior, inferior, and lateral extensions like narrow cul-de-sacs. The inferior extension of the fourth ventricle ends at the cervicomedullary junction; at the obex, it becomes continuous with the central canal of the spinal cord. The lateral recesses of the fourth ventricle contain small apertures—the foramina

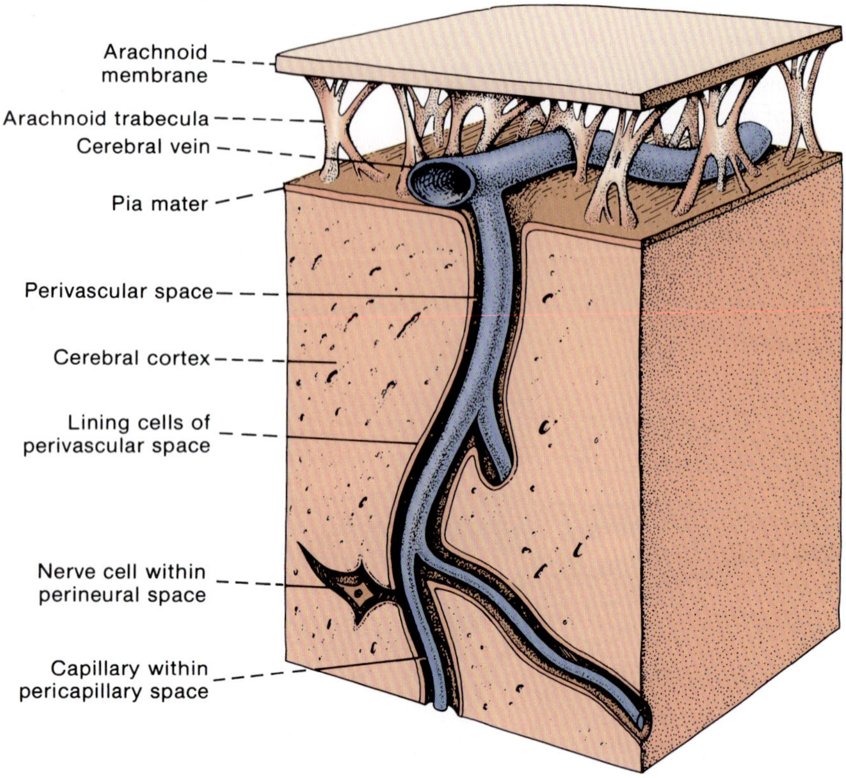

FIGURE 2.4 Schematic diagram of the leptomeninges and nervous tissue, showing the relationship of the subarachnoid space, perivascular channels, and nerve cells. (Modified from Weed LH. The absorption of cerebrospinal fluid into the venous system. *Am J Anat* 1923;31:191–207.)

of Luschka—through which CSF empties into the subarachnoid space surrounding the brainstem. A midline aperture in the roof of the fourth ventricle—the foramen of Magendie—joins the fourth ventricle with the cisterna magna. Choroid plexus lies in the roof of the fourth ventricle. Obstruction to the flow of CSF through this system may cause hydrocephalus (see Chapter 50).

THE CEREBRAL HEMISPHERES

The cerebrum is composed of two hemispheres that are covered by a layer of gray matter, the cerebral cortex. Underneath the cortex is the white matter, which consists of projection, commissural, and association fibers. Deep in the midline of each hemisphere are masses of gray matter: the basal ganglia and the diencephalon. The diencephalon is made up of the thalamus, metathalamus, epithalamus, subthalamus, and hypothalamus.

The cerebral cortex along with its underlying white matter is the pallium, or cerebral mantle. The pallium consists of the phylogenetically recent neopallium, which makes up the majority of the hemispheres, and the paleopallium and archipallium, more primitive areas that are small in humans. The paleopallium is the piriform lobe, and the archipallium is the hippocampal formation. The paleopallium and archipallium constitute the rhinencephalon, which is connected structurally and functionally with the limbic lobe.

The cerebral mantle is intricately folded and traversed by fissures and sulci (Figures 6.1 and 6.2). The cortex is arranged in layers of cells and fibers. Differences in the anatomy of the layers form the basis for cytoarchitectonic maps of the brain. The best-known and most widely used map is that of Brodmann, which divides the brain into 52 identifiable areas (Figures 6.3, 25.1, and 25.2). In primates, especially humans, a huge number of neurons are able to occupy the relatively small intracranial space because of layering of the cortex and the folding that vastly increases the surface area of the brain. The more important fissures divide the hemispheres into lobes, and these in turn are subdivided by the sulci into gyri, or convolutions. A fissure and a sulcus are different, but the terms are not used consistently. Lissencephaly is a congenital malformation in which the normal pattern of sulci fails to develop. A normally sulcated brain is gyrencephalic. Separation of the parts of the brain by surface landmarks is practical anatomically, but the divisions are morphologic; the individual lobes are not necessarily functional units.

The hemispheres are incompletely separated by the median longitudinal (interhemispheric) fissure, within which lies the falx cerebri (Figure 6.4). Deep in the fissure run branches of the anterior cerebral artery. Two major surface landmarks are visible on the lateral hemispheric surface: the lateral (sylvian) fissure and the central (rolandic) sulcus (Figure 6.1). The sylvian fissure begins at the vallecula on the basal surface between the frontal and temporal lobes and runs laterally, posteriorly, and superiorly. It divides the frontal and parietal lobes above from the temporal lobe below. In the depths of the sylvian fissure lies the insula (island of Reil), surrounded by the limiting, or circular, sulcus. The frontal, parietal, and temporal opercula are overhanging aprons of cerebrum that cover the insula. More superficially in the sylvian fissure run branches of the middle cerebral artery. The central sulcus runs obliquely from posterior to anterior, at an angle of about 70 degrees, from about the midpoint of the dorsal surface of the hemisphere nearly to the sylvian fissure, separating the frontal lobe from the parietal. The anatomy of the cerebral hemispheres is discussed further in Chapter 6.

BASAL GANGLIA

Basal ganglia terminology can be confusing, and usage is inconsistent. The caudate, putamen, and globus pallidus (GP) are all intimately related from an anatomical and functional standpoint. The term basal ganglia includes these plus other related structures such as the subthalamic nucleus and substantia nigra. The caudate and putamen are actually two parts of a single nucleus connected by gray matter strands and separated from each other by fibers of the anterior limb of the internal capsule. The heavily myelinated capsular fibers passing between and intermingling with the gray matter bridges cause the caudate-putamen junction to look striped, hence the term corpus striatum or striatum (L. "striped body") to refer to the caudate and putamen. The term corpus striatum is sometimes used to include the GP as well. The caudate and putamen are the neostriatum; the GP is the archi- or paleostriatum. The putamen and GP together are shaped like a lens, hence the term lenticular or lentiform nuclei. The claustrum, amygdala, and substantia innominata are sometimes included as basal ganglia; they are indeed gray matter masses lying at the base of the hemispheres but bear little functional relationship to the other basal ganglia.

The caudate (L. "tail") nucleus is composed of a head, body, and tail. The body and progressively thinner tail extend backward from the head and arch along just outside the wall of the lateral ventricle, ultimately following the curve of the temporal horn and ending in the medial temporal lobe in close approximation to the amygdala. The caudate is thus a long, C-shaped structure with bulbous ends. The putamen lies just lateral to the GP. The GP lies medial to the putamen and just lateral to the third ventricle, separated from the caudate by the anterior limb and from the thalamus by the posterior limb of the internal capsule. The GP (L. "pale body") or pallidum is traversed by myelinated fibers, making it look lighter than the putamen, hence the name. The substantia nigra lies in the midbrain just posterior to the cerebral peduncle. It is divided into pars compacta and pars reticulata portions. In the pars compacta lie the prominent melanin-containing neurons that give the region its dark color and its name.

The basal ganglia are part of the extrapyramidal motor system. The caudate and putamen serve as the central receiving area of the basal ganglia; they send efferent fibers primarily to the GP. The GP is then responsible for most of the output of the basal ganglia. Fahr's disease is a rare inherited disorder causing calcification and cell loss in the basal ganglia.

The basal ganglia generally serve to suppress activity in thalamocortical motor neurons. Hypokinetic movement disorders are characterized by reduced motor function because of higher than normal basal ganglia output, for example, Parkinson's disease. Hyperkinetic movement disorders are characterized by excessive motor activity because of lower than normal basal ganglia output, for example, Huntington's disease. Dysfunction of nonmotor circuits of the basal ganglia has been implicated in Tourette's syndrome and obsessive-compulsive disorder. The basal ganglia are discussed further in Chapters 26 and 30.

THALAMUS

The thalamus is a large, paired, ovoid structure that lies deep in the midline of each cerebral hemisphere, sitting atop the brainstem. The third ventricle lies between the two thalami, which are joined together by the massa intermedia. The dorsal aspect of the thalamus forms the floor of the lateral ventricle, and its medial aspect forms the wall of the third ventricle. It is bounded laterally by the internal capsule and basal ganglia; ventrally it is continuous with the subthalamus. The thalamus is connected with the cerebral cortex by the thalamic peduncles. The anterior thalamic peduncle consists of frontothalamic, thalamofrontal, striothalamic, and thalamostriatal fibers that run in the anterior limb of the internal capsule. The superior thalamic peduncle consists of thalamoparietal sensory fibers from the thalamus to the cortex; these fibers run in the posterior limb of the internal capsule. The posterior thalamic peduncle contains the optic radiations from the lateral geniculate body to the occipital cortex, and the inferior thalamic peduncle carries auditory radiations from the medial geniculate body to the temporal cortex. The thalamic syndrome (Dejerine-Roussy) is characterized by contralateral hemianesthesia and pain due to infarction of the thalamus. The thalamus is discussed further in Chapter 6.

BRAINSTEM

The brainstem extends caudally from the diencephalon to the spinal cord. Rostrally, the midbrain is continuous with the subthalamus and thalamus; caudally, the medulla is continuous with the spinal cord. The rostral limit of the midbrain is an imaginary line between the posterior commissure and mammillary bodies; the caudal limit is defined by a line between the pontomesencephalic sulcus and the inferior colliculi. The pons extends from this point caudally to the pontomedullary sulcus and the medulla from that point to the cervicomedullary junction at the foramen magnum.

The dominant feature of the ventral midbrain is the paired crus cerebri, which contain the cerebral peduncles. Dorsally, the dominant feature is the quadrigeminal plate, made up of the superior and inferior colliculi. The superior colliculus is connected to the lateral geniculate body by the brachium of the superior colliculus; the inferior colliculus is connected to the medial geniculate body in similar fashion. The pulvinar, the most caudal portion of the thalamus, overlies the rostral midbrain laterally. The cerebral peduncles connect the midbrain to the cerebrum above. The superior cerebellar peduncle (brachium conjunctivum) connects the midbrain to the cerebellum behind. The ventral pons is a massive, bulging structure because of the underlying transverse pontocerebellar fibers. Of the brainstem segments, the pons lies closest to the clivus and dorsum sellae. The pons is connected to the cerebellum posteriorly by the middle cerebellar peduncle (brachium pontis). Posteriorly, the cerebellum overlies the pons, separated from it by the fourth ventricle. The cerebellopontine angle is the space formed by the junction of the pons, medulla, and overlying cerebellar hemisphere. Neoplasms may form in the cerebellopontine angle, most often acoustic neuromas. The dorsal aspect of the pons consists of the structures that make up the floor of the ventricular cavity.

The medulla oblongata is the most caudal segment of the brainstem, lying just above the foramen magnum, continuous with the pons above and spinal cord below. The transition to spinal cord is marked by three features: the foramen magnum, the decussation of the pyramids, and the appearance of the anterior rootlets of C1. The inferior olives form a prominent anterolateral bulge on the ventral medulla. Between the two olives lie the midline medullary pyramids. Posteriorly, the cerebellum overlies the medulla, connected to it by the inferior cerebellar peduncle (restiform body). The gracile and cuneate tubercles are prominences on the posterior aspect of the medulla at the cervicomedullary junction.

CNs III through XII emerge from the brainstem. The third nerve exits through the interpeduncular fossa, the fourth nerve through the tectal plate posteriorly. CN V enters the pons laterally, and CNs VI, VII, and VIII all emerge at the pontomedullary junction (VI anteriorly, VII and VIII laterally through the cerebellopontine angle). CNs IX, X, and XI emerge from the groove posterior to the inferior olive. CN XII exits anterolaterally in the sulcus between the inferior olive and the medullary pyramid.

The brainstem is a conduit for conduction of information. All signaling between the body and the cerebrum traverses the brainstem. Information to and from the cerebellum also traverses the brainstem. The brainstem is also the location of CN nuclei III through XII. In addition, the brainstem reticular formation controls vital visceral functions, such as cardiovascular and respiratory function and consciousness.

Many disorders may affect the brainstem. These characteristically produce CN abnormalities on the side of the lesion and long tract motor or sensory abnormalities contralaterally, that is, crossed syndromes. A mnemonic called the "rule of 4" helps recall the anatomy and the brainstem syndromes. The anatomy of the brainstem is discussed further in Chapter 11.

CEREBELLUM

The cerebellum is the largest portion of the rhombencephalon, about one-tenth as large as the cerebrum. The cerebellum is deeply fissured; its surface is broken into a number of folia. If unfolded, the surface area would be about half that of the cerebral cortex. The cerebellar cortex overlies a medullary core of white matter. The cortex is densely packed with neurons, primarily granule cells; in fact, the cerebellum contains more neurons than the cerebral cortex. The branching of the white matter into the cortical mantle and the structure of the folia lends a treelike appearance (arbor vitae). The cerebellum lies in the posterior part of the posterior fossa, behind the brainstem and connected to it by the three cerebellar peduncles (Figure 2.5). It forms the roof of the fourth ventricle and is separated from the occipital lobe above by the tentorium cerebelli. The cerebellar tonsils are small, rounded masses of tissue

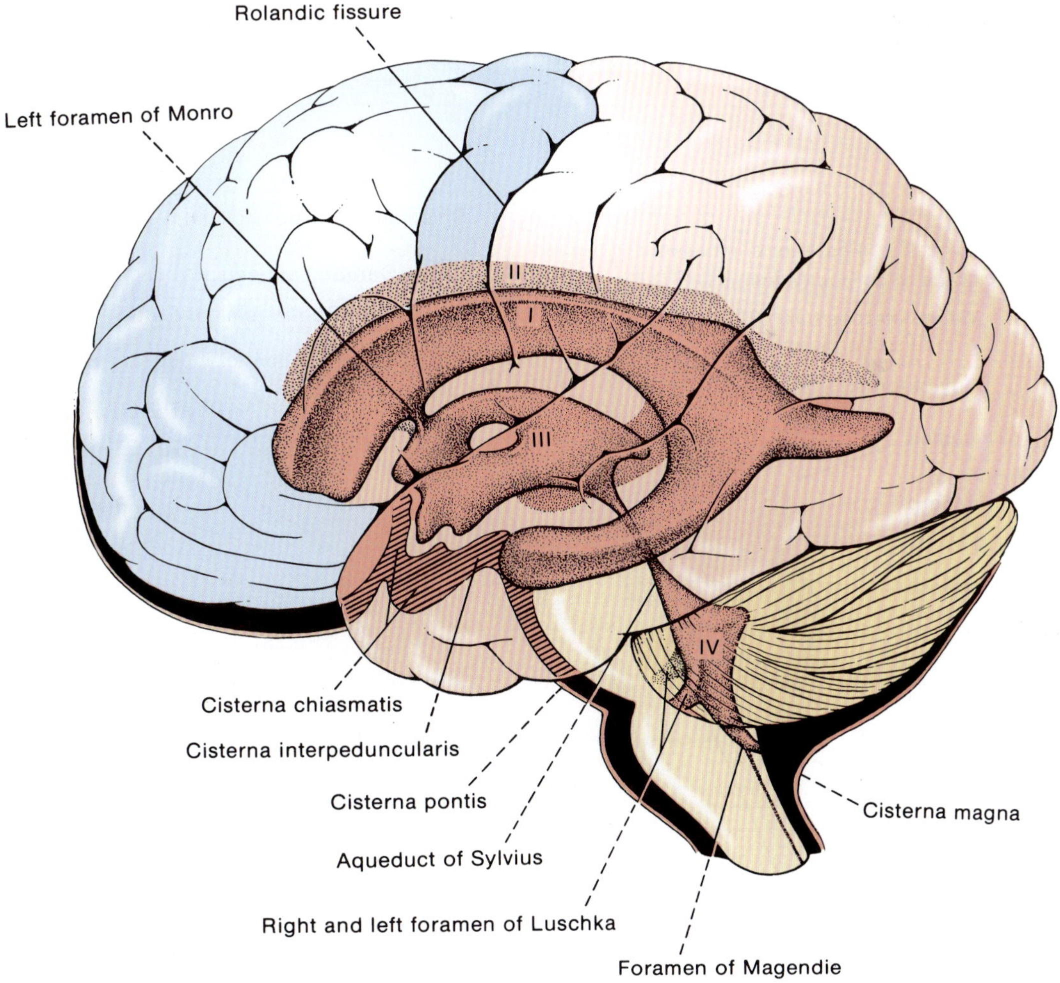

FIGURE 2.5 Diagram of the cerebrospinal fluid spaces, showing lateral, third, and fourth ventricles; foraminal connections with the subarachnoid space; and some of the major subarachnoid cisterns. *I* and *II*, lateral ventricles; *III*, third ventricle; *IV*, fourth ventricle. (Modified from Dandy WE. *Bull Johns Hopkins Hosp* 1921;32:67–123.)

on the most inferior part of each cerebellar hemisphere, just above the foramen magnum. Increased intracranial pressure may cause tonsillar herniation: the tonsils move through the foramen magnum into the upper cervical spinal canal. In Arnold-Chiari malformation, the tonsils are also herniated below the foramen magnum, but this is a congenital anomaly and is not due to increased intracranial pressure.

The cerebellum can be divided into three lobes: anterior, posterior, and flocculonodular, each of which has a vermis and hemisphere portion. There are three major fissures: primary, horizontal, and posterolateral. The anterior lobe lies anterior to the primary fissure; the posterior lobe, by far the largest, lies between the primary fissure and the posterolateral fissure; and the flocculonodular lobe lies posterior to the posterolateral fissure. Anatomists have further divided the cerebellum into a number of lobules and given them arcane names that are not clinically useful. From a physiologic and clinical standpoint, the cerebellum can be viewed as having three components: the flocculonodular lobe, the vermis, and the hemispheres. The flocculonodular lobe is phylogenetically the oldest and is referred to as the archicerebellum. It has extensive connections with the vestibular nuclei and is concerned primarily with eye movement and gross balance. The vermis is the paleocerebellum, or spinocerebellum. It has extensive connections with spinal cord pathways and is concerned primarily with gait and locomotion. The most phylogenetically recent part of the cerebellum is the neocerebellum, or the cerebellar hemispheres, which make up the bulk of the cerebellum. These are concerned with coordinating movement and providing fine motor control and precise movement to the extremities (Figure 2.6). Numerous disorders may affect the cerebellum (see Chapter 43).

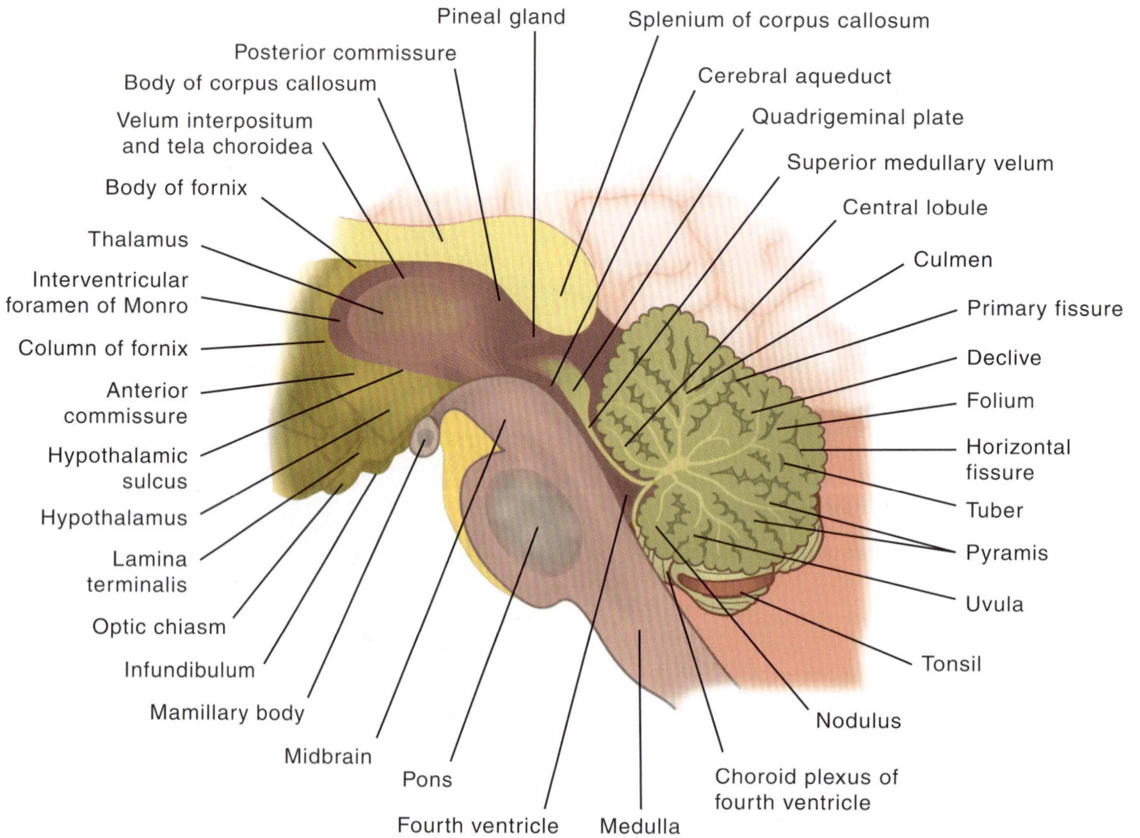

FIGURE 2.6 Midline sagittal section of the brainstem and cerebellum with the third ventricle retouched.

SPINAL CORD

The spinal cord is elongated and nearly cylindrical, continuous with the medulla above and ending in a conical tip, the conus medullaris (Figures 2.7 and 2.8). The spinal cord occupies approximately the upper two-thirds of the vertebral canal, extending from the foramen magnum to a level that varies slightly from individual to individual but in adults lies between the lower border of L1 and the upper border of L2. The filum terminale is a delicate filament of connective tissue that descends from the apex of the conus medullaris to the periosteum of the posterior surface of the first segment of the coccyx (Figure 2.8). The dentate ligaments extend along the lateral surface of the spinal cord, between the anterior and posterior nerve roots, from the pia to the dura mater. They suspend the spinal cord in the vertebral

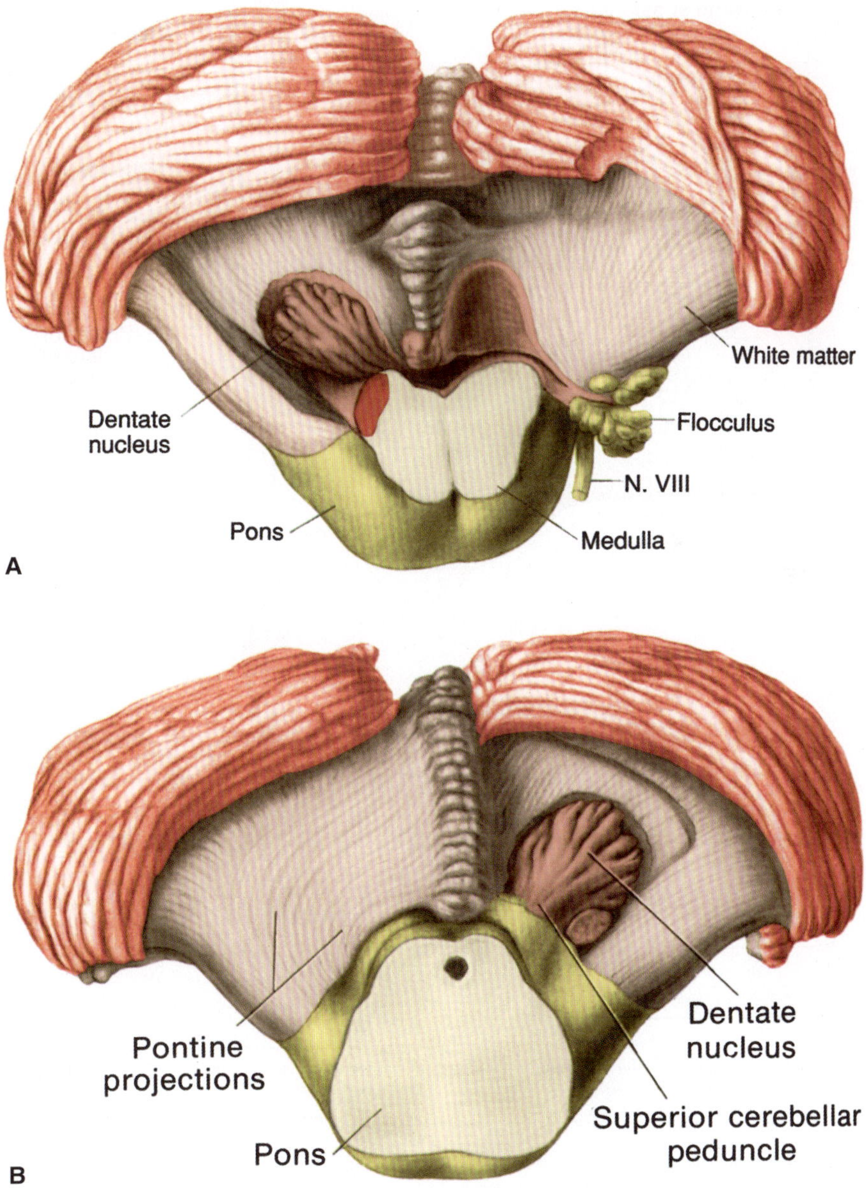

FIGURE 2.7 Drawings of dissections of the left dentate nucleus with portions of the cerebellar cortex and vermis intact. **A.** Dissection of the posterior surface of the cerebellum exposing the dentate nucleus. **B.** Dissection of the superior surface of the cerebellum from above showing the left dentate nucleus in relationship to the isthmus of the pons. (From Mettler FA. *Neuroanatomy*. St. Louis: Mosby, 1948.)

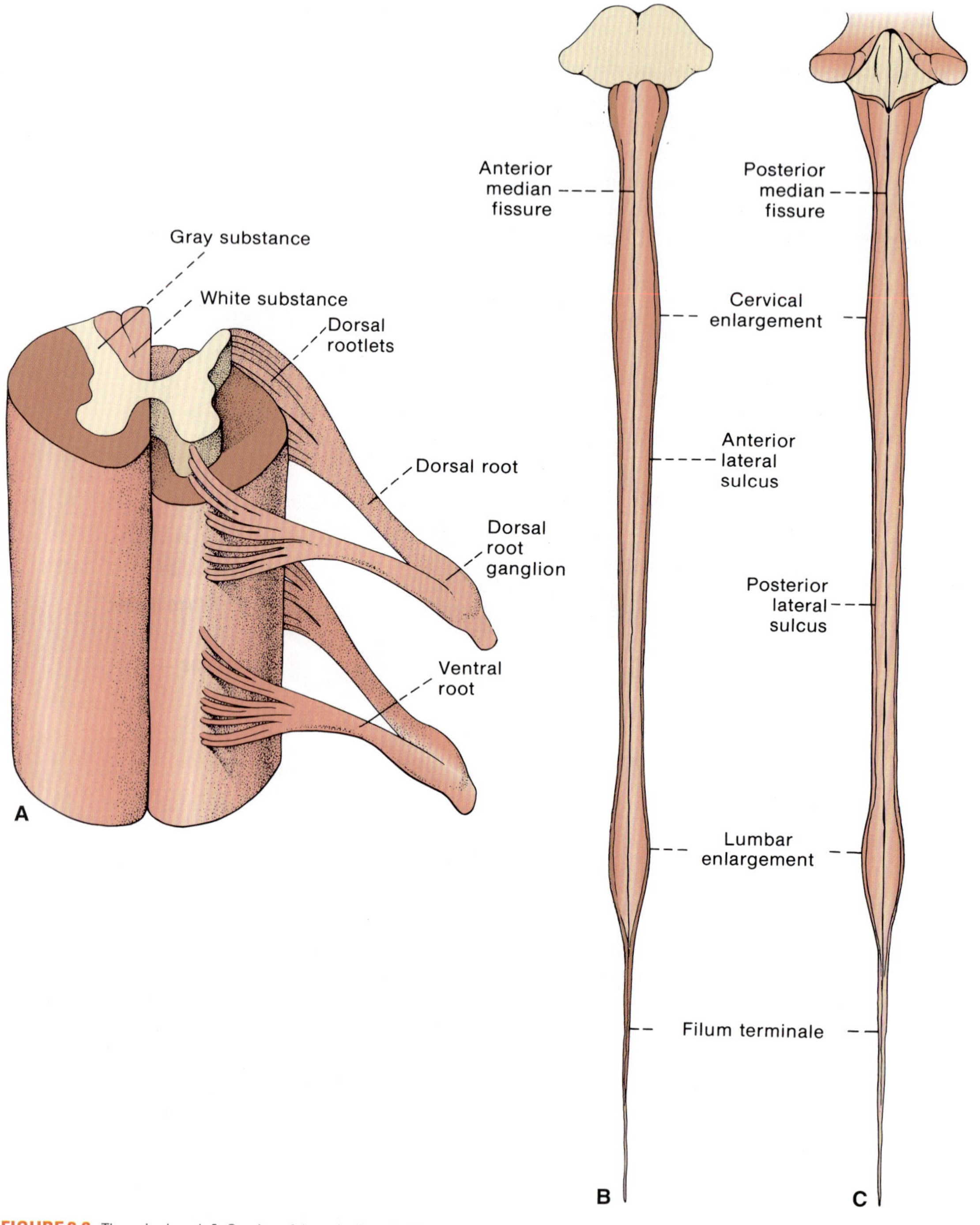

FIGURE 2.8 The spinal cord. **A.** Section of the spinal cord with anterior and posterior nerve roots attached. **B.** Anterior view of the spinal cord. **C.** Posterior view of the spinal cord.

canal. The general organization is the same throughout, but there is some variability in detail at different segmental levels. The cord and vertebral column are of different lengths because of different fetal growth rates, so there is not absolute concordance between cord levels and vertebral levels; this discrepancy grows more significant at more caudal levels. Each spinal cord segment has anterior and posterior roots. The anterior roots convey motor and autonomic fibers into the peripheral nerve. Posterior roots bear ganglia

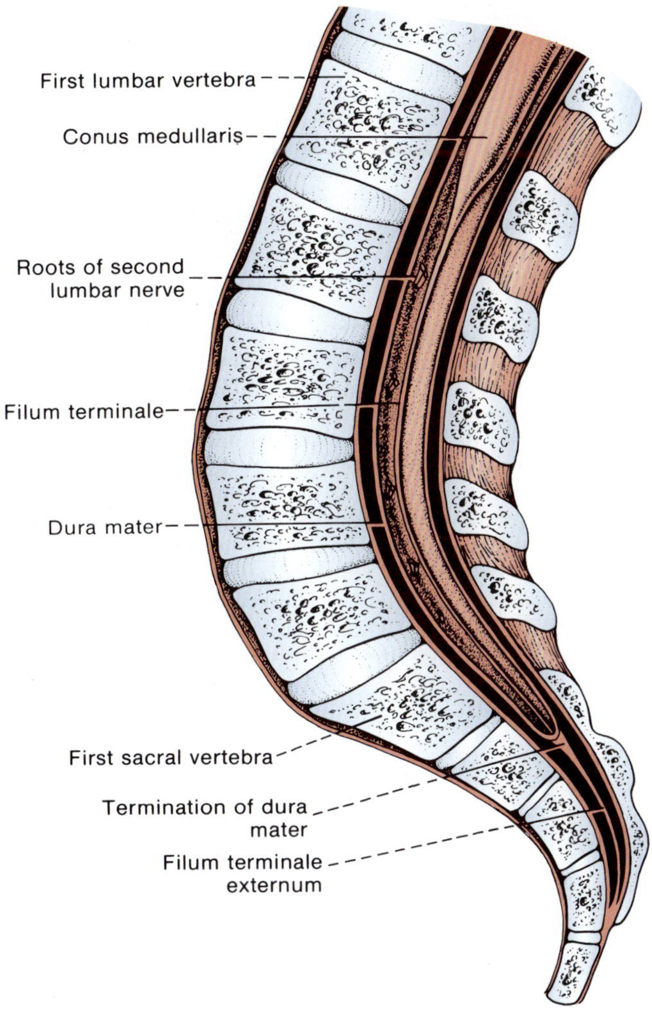

FIGURE 2.9 Sagittal section of the vertebral canal, showing the lower end of the spinal cord, filum terminale, and subarachnoid space. (Modified from Larsell O. *Anatomy of the Nervous System*. New York: D Appleton-Century, 1939.)

composed of unipolar neurons, and the roots are made up of the central processes of these neurons. The ganglion lies in the intervertebral foramen in close proximity to the anterior root. The anterior and posterior roots join just distal to the dorsal root ganglion to form the mixed spinal nerve. In the thoracolumbar region, white and gray rami connect the spinal nerve to the paravertebral sympathetic chain. The spinal cord ends in the conus medullaris. Roots from the lower cord segments descend to their exit foramina, forming the cauda equina (Figure 2.9).

CENTRAL NERVOUS SYSTEM BLOOD SUPPLY

The brain receives its blood supply from the internal carotid arteries (anterior circulation) and the vertebrobasilar system (posterior circulation). The anterior circulation supplies the frontal, parietal, and most of the temporal lobes. The posterior circulation supplies the occipital lobes, brainstem, and cerebellum. Vascular anatomy is discussed in more detail in Chapter 49.

BIBLIOGRAPHY

Bekdache GN, Begam M, Al Safi W, et al. Prenatal diagnosis of triploidy associated with holoprosencephaly: a case report and review of the literature. *Am J Perinatol* 2009;26:479–483.

Biller J, Gruener G, Brazis PW. *DeMyer's The Neurologic Examination: A Programmed Text*. 7th ed. New York: McGraw-Hill Education, 2017.

Copp AJ, Greene ND. Genetics and development of neural tube defects. *J Pathol* 2010;220:217–230.

Dávila-Gutiérrez G. Agenesis and dysgenesis of the corpus callosum. *Semin Pediatr Neurol* 2002;9:292–301.

DeMyer W. The median cleft face syndrome. Differential diagnosis of cranium bifidum occultum, hypertelorism, and median cleft nose, lip, and palate. *Neurology* 1967;17:961–971.

DeMyer W. Median facial malformations and their implications for brain malformations. *Birth Defects Orig Artic Ser* 1975;11:155–181.

DeMyer WE. *Technique of the Neurological Examination*. 6th ed. New York: McGraw-Hill, 2011.

Finnell RH, Gould A, Spiegelstein O. Pathobiology and genetics of neural tube defects. *Epilepsia* 2003;44(Suppl 3):14–23.

Fix JD. *Neuroanatomy*. 4th ed. Philadelphia: Wolters Kluwer/ Lippincott Williams & Wilkins, 2009.

Garabedian BH, Fraser FC. Upper and lower neural tube defects: an alternate hypothesis. *J Med Genet* 1993;30:849–851.

Gates P. The rule of 4 of the brainstem: a simplified method for understanding brainstem anatomy and brainstem vascular syndromes for the non-neurologist. *Intern Med J* 2005;35:263–266.

Hanna RM, Marsh SE, Swistun D, et al. Distinguishing 3 classes of corpus callosal abnormalities in consanguineous families. *Neurology* 2011;76:373–382.

Kaaja E, Kaaja R, Hiilesmaa V. Major malformations in offspring of women with epilepsy. *Neurology* 2003;60:575–579.

Kopell BH, Greenberg BD. Anatomy and physiology of the basal ganglia: implications for DBS in psychiatry. *Neurosci Biobehav Rev* 2008;32:408–422.

Mahalik SK, Vaze D, Lyngdoh TS, et al. Embryogenesis of triple neural tube defects: sonic hedgehog—a key? *J Pediatr Surg* 2011;46:e5–e8.

Millichap JJ, Nguyen T, Ryan ME. Teaching neuroimages: prenatal MRI of muscle-eye-brain disease. *Neurology* 2010;74:e101.

Northrup H, Volcik KA. Spina bifida and other neural tube defects. *Curr Probl Pediatr* 2000;30:313–332.

Pradilla G, Jallo G. Arachnoid cysts: case series and review of the literature. *Neurosurg Focus* 2007;22:E7.

Raghavan N, Barkovich AJ, Edwards M, et al. MR imaging in the tethered spinal cord syndrome. *AJR Am J Roentgenol* 1989;152:843–852.

Richter B, Stegmann K, Roper B, et al. Interaction of folate and homocysteine pathway genotypes evaluated in susceptibility to neural tube defects (NTD) in a German population. *J Hum Genet* 2001;46:105–109.

Simpson JL, Mills J, Rhoads GG, et al. Genetic heterogeneity in neural tube defects. *Ann Genet* 1991;34:279–286.

Slater BJ, Lenton KA, Kwan MD, et al. Cranial sutures: a brief review. *Plast Reconstr Surg* 2008;121:170e–178e.

Standring S, ed. *Gray's Anatomy: The Anatomical Basis of Clinical Practice*. 41st ed. New York: Elsevier Limited, 2016.

Wilson DA, Prince JR. John Caffey award. MR imaging determination of the location of the normal conus medullaris throughout childhood. *AJR Am J Roentgenol* 1989;152:1029–1032.

CHAPTER 3

The Neurologic History

Introductory textbooks of physical diagnosis cover the basic aspects of medical interviewing. This chapter addresses some aspects of history taking of particular relevance to neurologic patients. Important historical points to be explored as they relate to some common neurologic conditions are summarized in the tables.

The history is the cornerstone of medical diagnosis; neurologic diagnosis is no exception. In many instances, the physician can learn more from what the patient says and how he says it than from any other avenue of inquiry. A skillfully taken history will frequently indicate the probable diagnosis, even before physical, neurologic, and neurodiagnostic examinations are carried out. Conversely, many errors in diagnosis are due to incomplete or inaccurate histories. In many common neurologic disorders, the diagnosis rests almost entirely on the history. Most patients with recurring headaches fall into this category, as do some patients with dizziness, sleep disorders, and episodic loss of consciousness. Often the only disease manifestations are subjective, without demonstrable physical signs of disease; we can learn of their nature and course only by description.

The most important aspect of history taking is attentive listening. Ask open-ended questions and avoid suggesting possible responses. Although patients are frequently accused of being "poor historians," there are in fact as many poor history takers as there are poor history givers. Although the principal objective of taking the history is to acquire pertinent clinical data that will lead to correct diagnosis, the information obtained in the history is also valuable in understanding the patient as an individual, his relationship to others, and his reactions to his disease.

Taking a good history is not simple. It may require more skill and experience than performing a good neurologic examination. Time, diplomacy, kindness, patience, reserve, and a manner that conveys interest, understanding, and sympathy are all essential. The physician should present a friendly and courteous attitude, center all his attention on the patient, appear anxious to help, word questions tactfully, and ask them in a conversational tone. At the beginning of the interview, it is worthwhile to attempt to put the patient at ease. Avoid any appearance of haste. Engage in some small talk. Inquiring as to where the patient is from and what he does for a living not only helps make the encounter less rigid and formal, but it often reveals very interesting things about the patient as a person. History taking is an opportunity to establish a favorable patient-physician relationship; the physician may acquire empathy for the patient, establish rapport, and instill confidence. The patient's manner of presenting his history reflects intelligence, powers of observation, attention, and memory. The examiner should avoid forming a judgment about the patient's illness too quickly; some individuals easily sense and resent a physician's preconceived ideas about their symptoms. Repeating key points of the history back to the patient helps ensure accuracy, and it assures the patient that the physician has heard and assimilated the story. At the end of the history, the patient should always feel as if he has been listened to. The importance of the clinical history cannot be overemphasized. History taking is an art. It can be learned partly through reading and study, but it is honed only through experience and practice.

The mode of questioning may vary with the patient's age, education, and cultural background. The physician should meet the patient on a common ground of language and vocabulary—resorting to the vernacular if necessary—but without talking down to the patient. This is sometimes a fine line. The history is best taken in private, with the patient comfortable and at ease.

The history should be recorded clearly and concisely, in a logical, well-organized manner. It is important to focus on the more important aspects and keep irrelevancies to a minimum; the essential factual material must be separated from the extraneous. Diagnosis involves the careful sifting of evidence; the art of selecting and emphasizing the pertinent data may make it possible to arrive at a correct conclusion in a seemingly complicated case. Recording negative as well as positive statements assures later examiners that the historian inquired into and did not overlook certain aspects of the disease.

Several different types of information may be obtained during the initial encounter. There is direct information from the patient describing symptoms, information from the patient regarding what previous physicians may have thought, and information from medical records or previous caregivers. All of these are potentially important. Usually, the most essential is the patient's direct description of the symptoms. Always work from information obtained firsthand from the patient when possible, as forming one's own opinion from primary data is critical. Steer the patient away from a description of what previous doctors have thought, at least initially. Many patients tend to jump quickly to describing encounters with caregivers, glossing over the details of the present illness. Patients often misunderstand much or most of what they have been told in the past, so information from the patient about past evaluations and treatment must be analyzed cautiously. Patient recollections may be flawed because of faulty memory, misunderstanding, or other factors. Sir William Jenner declared, "Never believe what a patient tells you his doctor said." Encourage the patient to focus on symptoms instead, giving a detailed account of the illness in his own words.

In general, the interviewer should intervene as little as possible. However, it is often necessary to lead the conversation away from obviously irrelevant material, to obtain amplification on vague or incomplete statements, or to lead the story in directions likely to yield useful information. Allow the patient to use his own words as much as possible, but it is important to determine the precise meaning of words the patient uses. Clarify any ambiguity that could lead to misinterpretation. Have the patient clarify what he means by lay terms like kidney trouble or dizziness.

Deciding whether the physician or the patient should control the pace and content of the interview is a frequent problem. Patients do not practice history giving. Some are naturally much better at relating the pertinent information than others. Many patients frequently digress into extraneous detail. The physician adopting an overly passive role under such circumstances often prolongs the interview unnecessarily. When possible, let the patient give the initial part of the history without interruption. In a primary care setting, the average patient tells his story in about 5 minutes. The average doctor interrupts the average patient after only about 18 seconds. In 44% of interviews done by medical interns, the patient was not allowed to complete the opening statement of concerns. Avoid interrogation, but keeping the patient on track with focused questions is entirely appropriate. If the patient pauses to remember some irrelevancy, gently encourage him not to dwell on it. A reasonable method is to let the patient run as long as he is giving a decent account, and then take more control to clarify necessary details. Some patients may need to relinquish more control than others. Experienced clinicians generally make a diagnosis through a process of hypothesis testing (see Chapter 53). At some point in the interview, the physician must assume greater control and query the patient regarding specific details of his symptomatology—in order to test hypotheses and to help rule in or to rule out diagnostic possibilities.

History taking in certain types of patients may require special techniques. The timid or worried patient may require prompting with sympathetic questions or reassuring comments. The garrulous person may need to be stopped before getting lost in a mass of irrelevant detail. The evasive or undependable patient may have to be queried more searchingly, and the fearful, antagonistic, or paranoid patient questioned guardedly to avoid arousing fears or suspicions. In the patient with multiple or vague complaints, insist on specifics. The euphoric patient may minimize or neglect his symptoms; the depressed or anxious patient may exaggerate, and the excitable or hypochondriacal patient may be overly concerned and recount his complaints at length. The range of individual variations is wide, and this must be taken into account in appraising symptoms. What is pain to the anxious or depressed patient may be but a minor discomfort to another. A blasé attitude or seeming indifference may indicate pathologic euphoria in one individual, but it could be a defense reaction in another. One person may take offense at questions that another would consider commonplace. Even in a single individual such factors as fatigue, pain, emotional conflicts, or diurnal fluctuations in mood or temperament may cause a wide range of variation in response to questions. Patients may occasionally conceal important information. In some cases, they may not realize the information is important; in other cases, they may be too embarrassed to reveal certain details.

The interview provides an opportunity to study the patient's manner, attitude, behavior, and emotional reactions. The tone of voice, bearing, expression of the eyes, swift play of facial muscles, and the appearance of weeping or smiling—or the presence of pallor, blushing, sweating, patches of erythema on the neck, furrowing of the brows, drawing of the lips, clenching of the teeth, pupillary dilation, or muscle rigidity—may give important information. Gesticulations, restlessness, delay, hesitancy, and the relation of demeanor and emotional responses to descriptions of symptoms or to details in the family or marital history should be noted and recorded. These and the mode of response to the questions are valuable in judging character, personality, and emotional state.

The patient's story may not be entirely correct or complete. He may not possess full or detailed information regarding his illness; he may misinterpret his symptoms or give someone else's interpretation of them; he may wishfully alter or withhold information; or he may even deliberately prevaricate for some purpose. The patient may be a phlegmatic, insensitive individual who does not comprehend the significance of his symptoms, a garrulous person who cannot give a relevant or coherent story, or someone with multiple or vague complaints that cannot be readily articulated. Infants, young children, comatose, or confused patients may be unable to give any history. Patients who are in pain or distress, have difficulty with speech or expression, have intellectual disabilities, or do not speak the examiner's language are often unable to give a satisfactory history for themselves. Patients with nondominant parietal lesions are often not fully aware of the extent of their deficit. It may be necessary to corroborate or supplement the history given by the patient by talking with an observer, relative, or friend, or even to obtain the entire history from someone else. Family members may be able to give important information about changes in behavior, memory, hearing, vision, speech, or coordination of which the patient may not be aware. It is frequently necessary to question both the patient and others in order to obtain a complete account of the illness. Family members and significant others sometimes accompany the patient during the interview. They can frequently provide important supplementary information. However, the family member must not be permitted to dominate the patient's account of the illness unless the patient is incapable of giving a history.

It is usually best to see the patient de novo with minimal prior review of the medical records. Too much information in advance of the patient encounter may bias one's opinion. If it later turns out that previous providers reached similar conclusions based on primary information, this reinforces the likelihood of a correct diagnosis. So, see the patient first, and review old records later.

There are three approaches to utilizing information from past providers, whether from medical records or as relayed by the patient. In the first instance, the physician takes too much at face value and assumes that previous diagnoses must be correct. An opposite approach, actually used by some, is to assume all previous providers were incompetent, and their conclusions could not possibly be correct. This approach sometimes forces the extreme skeptic into a position of having to make some other diagnosis, even when the preponderance of the evidence indicates that previous physicians were correct. The logical middle ground is to make no assumptions regarding the opinions of previous providers. Use the information appropriately, matching it against what the patient relates and whatever other information is available. Do not unquestioningly believe it all, but do not perfunctorily dismiss it either. Discourage patients from grousing about their past medical care and avoid disparaging remarks about other physicians the patient may have seen. An accurate and detailed record of events in cases involving compensation and medicolegal problems is particularly important.

One efficient way to work is to combine reviewing past notes with talking directly with the patient. If the records contain a reasonably complete history, review it with the patient for accuracy. For instance, read from the records and say to the patient, "Dr. Payne says here that you have been having pain in the left leg for the past 6 months. Is that correct?" The patient might verify that information, or he may say, "No, it's the right leg and it's more like 6 years." Such an approach can save considerable time when dealing with a patient who carries extensive previous records. A very useful method for summarizing a past workup is to make a table with two vertical columns, listing all tests that were done—with those that were normal in one column and those that were abnormal in the other column.

Many physicians find it useful to take notes during the interview. Contemporaneous note taking helps ensure accuracy of the final report. A useful approach is simply to take dictation as the patient talks, particularly in the early stages of the encounter. A note sprinkled with patient quotations is often very illuminating. However, one must not be fixated on note taking. The trick is to interact with the patient and take notes unobtrusively. The patient must not be left with the impression that the physician is paying attention to the note taking and not to him. Such notes are typically used for later transcription into some final format. Sometimes the patient comes armed with notes. The patient who has multiple complaints written on a scrap of paper is said to have *la maladie du petit papier*; tech-savvy patients may come with computer printouts detailing their medical histories.

THE PRESENTING COMPLAINT AND THE PRESENT ILLNESS

The neurologic history usually starts with obtaining the usual demographic data, but it must also include handedness. The traditional approach to history taking begins with the chief complaint and present illness. In fact, many experienced clinicians begin with the pertinent past history, identifying major underlying past or chronic medical illnesses at the outset. This does not mean going into detail about unrelated past surgical procedures and the like. It does mean identifying major comorbidities that might have a direct or indirect bearing on the present illness. This technique helps to put the present illness in context and to prompt early consideration about whether the neurologic problem is a complication of some underlying condition or whether it is an independent process. It is inefficient to go through a long and laborious history in a patient with peripheral neuropathy, only to subsequently find out in the past history that the patient has known, long-standing diabetes.

Although a complete database is important, it is counterproductive to give short shrift to the details of the present illness. History taking should concentrate on the details of the presenting complaint. The majority of the time spent with a new patient should be devoted to the history, and the majority of the history-taking time should be devoted to the symptoms of the present illness. The answer most often lies in the details of the presenting problem. Begin with an open-ended question, such as, "What sort of problems are you having?" Asking, "What brought you here today?" often produces responses regarding a mode of transportation. And asking, "What is wrong with you?" only invites wisecracks. After establishing the chief complaint or reason for the referral, make the patient start at the beginning of the story and go through it more or less chronologically. Many patients will not do this unless so directed. The period of time leading up to the onset of symptoms should be dissected to uncover such things as the immunization that precipitated an episode of neuralgic amyotrophy, the diarrheal illness prior to an episode of Guillain-Barré syndrome, or the camping trip that led to the tick bite. Patients are quick to assume that some recent event is the cause for their current difficulty. The physician must avoid the trap of assuming that temporal relationships prove etiologic relationships (the *post hoc ergo propter hoc* fallacy).

Record the chief complaint in the patient's own words. Sir William Osler said, "Give the patient's own words in the complaint." It is important to clarify important elements of the history that the patient is unlikely to spontaneously describe. Each symptom of the present illness should be analyzed systematically by asking the patient a series of questions to clear up any ambiguities. Determine exactly when the symptoms began, whether they are present constantly or intermittently; if intermittently, determine the character, duration, frequency, severity, and relationship to external factors. Determine the progression or regression of each symptom—whether there is any seasonal, diurnal, or nocturnal variability—and the response to treatment. In patients whose primary complaint is pain, determine the location; character or quality; severity; associated symptoms; and, if episodic, frequency, duration, and any specific precipitating or relieving factors. Some patients have difficulty describing such things as the character of a pain. Although spontaneous descriptions have more value—and leading questions should in general be avoided—it is perfectly permissible when necessary to offer possible choices, such as "dull like a toothache" or "sharp like a knife."

In neurologic patients, particular attention should be paid to determining the time course of the illness, as this is often instrumental in determining the etiology. An illness might be static, remittent, intermittent, progressive, or improving. Abrupt onset followed by improvement with variable degrees of recovery is characteristic of trauma and vascular events. Degenerative diseases have a gradual onset of symptoms and a variable rate of progression. Tumors have a gradual onset and steady progression of symptoms, with the rate of progression depending on the tumor type. With some neoplasms, hemorrhage or spontaneous necrosis may cause sudden onset or worsening. Multiple sclerosis is most often characterized by remissions and exacerbations, with a progressive increase in the severity of symptoms. Stationary, intermittent, and chronic progressive forms also occur. Infections usually have a relatively sudden, but not precipitous, onset. They are generally followed by gradual improvement and either complete or incomplete recovery. In many conditions, symptoms appear sometime before striking physical signs of disease are evident—and before neurodiagnostic testing detects significant abnormalities. It is important to know the major milestones of an illness: when the patient last considered himself to be well, when he had to stop work, when he began to use an assistive device, when he was forced to take to his bed. It is often useful to ascertain exactly how and how severely the patient considers himself disabled, as well as what crystallized the decision to seek medical care.

A careful history may uncover previous events, which the patient may have forgotten or may not attach significance to. A history consistent with past vascular events, trauma, or episodes of demyelination may shed entirely new light on the current symptoms. In the patient with symptoms of myelopathy, the episode of visual loss that occurred 5 years previously suddenly takes on a different meaning.

It is useful at some point to ask the patient what is worrying him. It occasionally turns out that the patient is very concerned over the possibility of some disorder that has not even occurred to the physician to consider. Patients with neurologic complaints are often apprehensive about having some dreadful disease, such as a brain tumor, amyotrophic lateral sclerosis, multiple sclerosis, or muscular dystrophy. All these conditions are well known to the lay public, and patients or family members occasionally jump to outlandish conclusions about the cause of some symptom. Simple reassurance is occasionally all that is necessary.

RETAKING THE HISTORY

The history may need to be taken more than once. A good general working rule is that whenever the diagnosis is in doubt, take the history again. The attending effect is when an attending takes the history from a patient after the history has been taken by one or more trainees. History taking improves with experience because the clinician is able to generate more hypotheses to explain the patient's complaint and has more questions available to verify or exclude candidate conditions. It is not uncommon for a great deal of relevant information to suddenly come out under the attending's questioning, sometimes to the chagrin of students and house staff. Although the attending effect may be due to the more highly evolved history-taking skills of an experienced clinician, there are other potential explanations. Patients sometimes forget important details of their history during the initial encounter. They may also be sick, in pain, or inattentive. Many initial histories are taken by trainees at a very late hour. After some sleep, a little breakfast, and some time to ponder, the history has evolved by the time of attending rounds as the patient recalls information prompted by the earlier questioning. The previous history serves as a "warm-up." When working alone, take advantage of the attending effect by simply repeating and verifying the key portions of the history over again after some time has elapsed.

THE PAST MEDICAL HISTORY

The past history is important because neurologic symptoms may be related to systemic diseases. Relevant information includes a statement about general health; history of current, chronic, and past illnesses; hospitalizations; operations; accidents or injuries, particularly head trauma; infectious diseases; venereal diseases; congenital defects; diet; and sleeping patterns. It is surprising what major past medical and surgical history patients sometimes forget to relate. Inquiry should be made about allergies and other drug reactions. Certain situations and comorbid conditions are of particular concern in the patient with neurologic symptomatology. The vegetarian or person with a history of gastric surgery or inflammatory bowel disease is at risk of developing vitamin B_{12} deficiency, and the neurologic complications of connective tissue disorders, diabetes, thyroid disease, and sarcoidosis are protean. A history of cancer raises concern about metastatic disease as well as paraneoplastic syndromes. A history of valvular heart disease or recent myocardial infarction may be relevant in the patient with cerebrovascular disease. In some instances, even in an adult, a history of the patient's birth and early development is pertinent, including any complications of pregnancy, labor and delivery, birth trauma, birth weight, postnatal illness, health and development during childhood, convulsions with fever, learning ability, and school performance.

A survey of current medications, both prescribed and over the counter, is always important. Many drugs have significant neurologic side effects. For example, confusion may develop in an elderly patient simply from the use of beta-blocker ophthalmic solution; nonsteroidal anti-inflammatory drugs can cause aseptic meningitis; many drugs may cause dizziness, cramps, paresthesias, headache, weakness, and other side effects; and headaches are the most common side effect of proton pump inhibitors. Going over the details of the drug regimen may reveal that the patient is not taking a medication as intended. Pointed questions are often necessary to get at the issue of over-the-counter drugs, as many patients do not consider these as medicines. Occasional patients develop significant neurologic side effects from their well-intended vitamin regimen. Patients will take medicines from alternative health care practitioners or from a health-food store, assuming these agents are safe because they are "natural," which is not always the case. Having the patient bring in all medication bottles, prescribed and over the counter, is occasionally fruitful. One patient was shocked to find she had been taking extract of bovine testicle.

THE FAMILY HISTORY

The family history (FH) is essentially an inquiry into the possibility of heredofamilial disorders and focuses on the patient's lineage; it is occasionally quite important in neurologic patients. Information about the nuclear family is also often relevant to the social history (as noted in this section). In addition to the usual questions about cancer, diabetes, hypertension, and cardiovascular disease, the FH is particularly relevant in patients with migraine, epilepsy, cerebrovascular disease, movement disorders, myopathy, and cerebellar disease, to list a few. In some patients, it is pertinent to inquire about an FH of alcoholism or other types of substance abuse. Family size is important. A negative FH is more reassuring in a patient with several siblings and a large extended family than in a patient with no siblings and few known relatives. It is not uncommon to encounter patients who were adopted and have no knowledge of their biologic family.

There are traps, and a negative FH is not always really negative. Some diseases may be rampant in a kindred without any awareness of it by the affected individuals. With Charcot-Marie-Tooth disease, for example, so many family members may have the condition that the pes cavus and stork leg deformities are not recognized as abnormal. Chronic, disabling neurologic conditions in a family member may be attributed to another cause, such as "arthritis." Sometimes, family members deliberately withhold information about a known familial condition.

It is sometimes necessary to inquire about the relationship between the parents, exploring the possibility of consanguinity. In some situations, it is important to probe the patient's ethnic background, given the tendency of some neurologic disorders to occur in particular ethnic groups or in patients from certain geographic regions.

SOCIAL HISTORY

The social history includes such things as the patient's marital status, educational level, occupation, and personal habits. The marital history should include the number of marriages, duration of present marriage, and health of the partner and children. At times, it may be necessary to delve into marital adjustment and health of the relationship as well as the circumstances leading to any changes in marital status.

A question about the nature of the patient's work is routine. A detailed occupational history, occasionally necessary, should delve into both present and past occupations—with special reference to contact with neurotoxins, use of personal protective equipment, working environment, levels of exertion and repetitive motion activities, and coworker illnesses. A record of frequent job changes or a poor work history may be important. If the patient is no longer working, determine when and why he stopped. In some situations, it is relevant to inquire about hobbies and avocations, particularly when toxin exposure or a repetitive motion injury is a diagnostic consideration. Previous residences, especially in the tropics or in areas where certain diseases are endemic, may be relevant.

A history of personal habits is important, with special reference to the use of alcohol, tobacco, drugs, coffee, tea, soft drinks, and similar substances, or the reasons for abstinence. Patients are often not forthcoming about the use of alcohol and street drugs, especially those with something to hide. Answers may range from mildly disingenuous to bald-faced lies. Drugs and alcohol are sometimes a factor in the most seemingly unlikely circumstances. Patients notoriously underreport the amount of alcohol they consume; a commonly used heuristic is to double the admitted amount. To get a more realistic idea about the impact of alcohol on the patient's life, the CAGE questionnaire is useful (Table 3.1). Even one positive response is suspicious, and four are diagnostic of alcohol abuse. The HALT and BUMP are other similar question sets (Table 3.1). The Alcohol Use Disorders Identification Test (AUDIT) is a similar questionnaire; the abbreviated AUDIT-C, focused on the consumption items, is about equal in accuracy to the full AUDIT. Some patients will not admit to drinking alcohol and will only confess when the examiner hits on their specific beverage of choice, for example, gin. Always ask the patient who denies drinking at all some follow-up question: why he doesn't drink, if he ever drank, or when he quit. This may uncover a past or FH of substance abuse, or the patient may admit he quit only the week before. In the patient suspected of alcohol abuse, take a dietary history.

Patients are even more secretive about drug habits. Tactful opening questions might be to ask whether the patient has ever used drugs for other than medicinal purposes, ever abused prescription drugs, or ever ingested drugs other than by mouth. The vernacular is often necessary. Patients understand smoke crack better than inhale cocaine. It is useful to know the street names of commonly abused drugs, but these change frequently as both slang and drugs go in and out of fashion. In addition to such notorious illicit drugs as cocaine, heroin, PCP, methamphetamine, psychedelic mushrooms, and LSD, newer agents constantly appear, such as bath salts and synthetic marijuana. The drugscape evolves. The marijuana now legal in several U.S. states is much more potent than the marijuana of decades ago, and its toxicity is underappreciated. A less refined type of substance abuse is to inhale common substances, such as spray paint, airplane glue, paint thinner, gasoline, and nitrous oxide. It is astounding what some individuals will do. One patient was fond of smoking marijuana and inhaling gasoline—specifically, leaded gasoline—so that he could hallucinate in color. The abuse of prescription drugs has become a major public health problem and is far more prevalent than the abuse of illicit drugs. As much as 20% of the U.S. population is estimated to have abused prescription drugs, including opiate painkillers, sedatives, tranquilizers, dextromethorphan, ketamine, and stimulants. Abuse of such drugs as hydrocodone, oxycodone, Adderall, alprazolam, and clonazepam is common.

Determining if the patient has ever engaged in risky sexual behavior is sometimes important, but the subject is always difficult to broach. Patients are often less reluctant to discuss the topic than the examiner. Useful opening gambits might include how often and with whom the patient has sex, whether the patient engages in unprotected sex, or whether the patient has ever had a sexually transmitted disease (STD).

TABLE 3.1 Questions to Explore the Possibility of Alcohol Abuse

CAGE Questions
Have you ever felt the need to **C**ut down on your drinking?
Have people **A**nnoyed you by criticizing your drinking?
Have you ever felt **G**uilty about your drinking?
Have you ever had a morning "**E**ye-opener" to steady your nerves or get rid of a hangover?
HALT Questions
Do you usually drink to get **H**igh?
Do you drink **A**lone?
Do you ever find yourself **L**ooking forward to drinking?
Have you noticed that you are becoming **T**olerant to alcohol?
BUMP Questions
Have you ever had **B**lackouts?
Have you ever used alcohol in an **U**nplanned way (drank more than intended or continued to drink after having enough)?
Do you ever drink for **M**edicinal reasons (to control anxiety, depression, or the *shakes*)?
Do you find yourself **P**rotecting your supply of alcohol (hoarding, buying extra)?

REVIEW OF SYSTEMS

In primary care medicine, the review of systems (ROS) is designed in part to detect health problems of which the patient may not complain, but which nevertheless require attention. In specialty practice, the ROS is done more to detect symptoms involving other systems of that the patient may not spontaneously complain but that provide clues to the diagnosis of the presenting complaint. Neurologic disease may cause dysfunction involving many different systems. In patients presenting with neurologic symptoms, a neurologic ROS is useful after exploring the present illness to uncover relevant neurologic complaints. Some question areas worth probing into are summarized in Table 3.2. Symptoms of depression are often particularly relevant and are summarized in Table 3.3. A more general ROS may also reveal important information relevant to the present illness (Table 3.4). Occasionally, patients have a generally positive ROS, with complaints in multiple systems out of proportion to any evidence of organic disease. Patients with Briquet's syndrome have a somatization disorder with multiple somatic complaints, which they often describe in colorful, exaggerated terms.

The ROS is often done by questionnaire in outpatients. Another efficient method is to do the ROS during the physical examination, asking about symptoms related to each organ system as it is examined.

TABLE 3.2 A Neurologic System Review: Symptoms Worth Inquiring About in Patients Presenting with Neurologic Complaints

Any history of seizures or unexplained loss of consciousness
Headache
Vertigo or dizziness
Loss of vision
Diplopia
Difficulty hearing
Tinnitus
Difficulty with speech or swallowing
Weakness, difficulty moving, abnormal movements
Numbness, tingling
Tremor
Problems with gait, balance, or coordination
Difficulty with sphincter control or sexual function
Difficulty with thinking or memory
Problems sleeping or excessive sleepiness
Depressive symptoms (Table 3.3)

Modified from Campbell WW, Pridgeon RP. *Practical Primer of Clinical Neurology*. Philadelphia: Lippincott Williams & Wilkins, 2002.

HISTORY IN SOME COMMON CONDITIONS

Some of the important historical features to explore in patients with some common neurologic complaints are summarized in Tables 3.5 through 3.13. There are too many potential neurologic presenting complaints to cover them all, so these tables should be regarded only as a starting point and an illustration of the process. Space does not permit an explanation of the differential diagnostic relevance of each of these elements of the history. Suffice it to say that each of these elements in the history has significance in ruling in or ruling out some diagnostic possibility. Such a "list" exists for every complaint in every patient. Learning and refining these lists is the challenge of medicine.

For example, Table 3.5 lists some of the specific important historical points helpful in evaluating the chronic headache patient. The following features are general rules and guidelines, not absolutes. Patients with migraine tend to have unilateral hemicranial or orbitofrontal throbbing pain associated with gastrointestinal (GI) upset. Those suffering from migraine with aura (classical migraine) have visual or neurologic accompaniments. Patients usually seek relief by lying quietly in a dark, quiet environment. Patients with cluster headache tend to have unilateral nonpulsatile orbitofrontal pain with no visual, GI, or neurologic accompaniments; they tend to get some relief by moving about. Patients with tension-type headaches tend to have nonpulsatile pain, which is band-like or occipitonuchal in distribution and unaccompanied by visual, neurologic, or GI upset.

Table 3.6 lists some of the important elements in the history in patients with neck and arm pain. The primary differential diagnosis is usually between cervical radiculopathy and musculoskeletal conditions such as bursitis, tendinitis, impingement syndrome, and myofascial pain. Patients with a cervical disc usually have pain primarily in the neck, trapezius ridge, and upper shoulder region. Patients with cervical myofascial pain have pain in the same general distribution. Radiculopathy patients may have pain referred to the pectoral or periscapular regions, which is unusual in myofascial pain. Radiculopathy patients may have pain radiating in a radicular distribution down the arm. Pain radiating below the elbow usually means radiculopathy. Patients with radiculopathy have pain on movement of the neck; those with shoulder pathology have pain on movement of the shoulder. Patients with radiculopathy may have weakness or sensory symptoms in the involved extremity.

Tables 3.7 through 3.13 summarize some important historical particulars to consider in some of the other complaints frequently encountered in an outpatient setting.

TABLE 3.3 Some Symptoms Suggesting Depression

Depressed mood, sadness
Unexplained weight gain or loss
Increased or decreased appetite
Sleep disturbance
Lack of energy, tiredness, fatigue
Loss of interest in activities
Anhedonia
Feelings of guilt or worthlessness
Suicidal ideation
Psychomotor agitation or retardation
Sexual dysfunction
Difficulty concentrating or making decisions
Difficulty with memory

Modified from Campbell WW, Pridgeon RP. *Practical Primer of Clinical Neurology*. Philadelphia: Lippincott Williams & Wilkins, 2002.

Table 3.4 Items in the Review of Systems of Possible Neurologic Relevance, with Examples of Potentially Related Neurologic Conditions in Parentheses

General	**Gastrointestinal**
Weight loss (depression, neoplasia)	Appetite change (hypothalamic lesion)
Decreased energy level (depression)	Excessive thirst (diabetes mellitus or insipidus)
Chills/fever (occult infection)	Dysphagia (myasthenia)
Head	Constipation (dysautonomia, mitochondrial neurogastrointestinal encephalomyopathy [MNGIE])
Headaches (many)	Vomiting (increased intracranial pressure)
Trauma (subdural hematoma)	Hepatitis (vasculitis, cryoglobulinemia)
Eyes	**Genitourinary**
Refractive status; lenses, refractive surgery	Urinary incontinence (neurogenic bladder)
Episodic visual loss (amaurosis fugax)	Urinary retention (neurogenic bladder)
Progressive visual loss (optic neuropathy)	Impotence (dysautonomia)
Diplopia (numerous)	Polyuria (diabetes mellitus or insipidus)
Ptosis (myasthenia gravis)	Spontaneous abortion (anticardiolipin syndrome)
Dry eyes (Sjögren's syndrome)	Sexually transmitted disease (neurosyphilis)
Photosensitivity (migraine)	Pigmenturia (porphyria, rhabdomyolysis)
Eye pain (optic neuritis)	**Menstrual history**
Ears	Last menstrual period and contraception
Hearing loss (acoustic neuroma)	Oral contraceptive use (stroke)
Discharge (cholesteatoma)	Hormone replacement therapy (migraine)
Tinnitus (Ménière's disease)	**Endocrine**
Vertigo (vestibulopathy)	Galactorrhea (pituitary tumor)
Vesicles (*H. zoster*)	Amenorrhea (pituitary insufficiency)
Nose	Enlarging hands/feet (acromegaly)
Anosmia (olfactory groove meningioma)	Thyroid disease (many)
Discharge (CSF rhinorrhea)	**Musculoskeletal**
Mouth	Arthritis (connective tissue disease)
Sore tongue (nutritional deficiency)	Muscle cramps (ALS)
Neck	Myalgias (myopathy)
Pain (radiculopathy)	**Hematopoietic**
Stiffness (meningitis)	Anemia (B_{12} deficiency)
Cardiovascular	Deep venous thrombosis (anticardiolipin syndrome)
Heart disease (many)	**Skin**
Claudication (neurogenic vs. vascular)	Rashes (Lyme disease, drug reactions)
Hypertension (cerebrovascular disease)	Insect bites (Lyme disease, rickettsial infection, tick paralysis)
Cardiac arrhythmia (cerebral embolism)	Birthmarks (phakomatoses)
Respiratory	**Psychiatric**
Dyspnea (neuromuscular disease)	Depression (many)
Asthma (systemic vasculitis)	Psychosis (Creutzfeldt-Jakob disease)
Tuberculosis (meningitis)	Hallucination (Lewy body disease)
	Grandiosity (neurosyphilis)

TABLE 3.5	Important Historical Points in the Chronic Headache Patient

If the patient has more than one kind of headache, obtain the information for each type.
Location of the pain (e.g., hemicranial, holocranial, occipitonuchal, band-like)
Pain intensity
Pain quality (e.g., steady, throbbing, stabbing)
Severity
Timing, duration, and frequency
Average daily caffeine intake
Average daily analgesic intake (including over-the-counter medications)
Precipitating factors (e.g., alcohol, sleep deprivation, oversleeping, foods, bright light)
Relieving factors (e.g., rest/quiet, dark room, activity, medications)
Response to treatment
Neurologic accompaniments (e.g., numbness, paresthesias, weakness, speech disturbance)
Visual accompaniments (e.g., scintillating scotoma, transient blindness)
Gastrointestinal accompaniments (e.g., nausea, vomiting, anorexia)
Associated symptoms (e.g., photophobia, phonophobia/sonophobia, tearing, nasal stuffiness)
Any history of head trauma

Modified from Campbell WW, Pridgeon RP. *Practical Primer of Clinical Neurology*. Philadelphia: Lippincott Williams & Wilkins, 2002.

TABLE 3.6	Important Historical Points in the Patient with Neck and Arm Pain

Note: The differential diagnosis is most often between radiculopathy and musculoskeletal pain.

Onset and duration (acute, subacute, chronic)
Pain intensity
Any history of injury
Any history of preceding viral infection or immunization
Any past history of disc herniation, disc surgery, or previous episodes of neck or arm pain
Location of the worst pain (e.g., neck, arm, shoulder)
Pain radiation pattern, if any (e.g., to shoulder, arm, pectoral region, periscapular region)
Relation of pain to neck movement
Relation of pain to arm and shoulder movement
Relieving factors
Any exacerbation with coughing, sneezing, straining at stool
Any weakness of the arm or hand
Any numbness, paresthesias, or dysesthesias of the arm or hand
Any associated leg weakness or bowel, bladder, or sexual dysfunction suggesting spinal cord compression

Modified from Campbell WW, Pridgeon RP. *Practical Primer of Clinical Neurology*. Philadelphia: Lippincott Williams & Wilkins, 2002.

TABLE 3.7	Important Historical Points in the Patient with Back and Leg Pain

Note: The differential diagnosis is most often, as with neck and arm pain, between radiculopathy and musculoskeletal pain.

Onset and duration (acute, subacute, chronic)
Pain intensity
Any history of injury
Any past history of disc herniation, disc surgery, or previous episodes of back/leg pain
Location of the worst pain (e.g., back, buttock, hip, leg)
Pain radiation pattern, if any (e.g., to buttock, thigh, leg, or foot)
Relation of pain to body position (e.g., standing, sitting, lying down)
Relation of pain to activity and movement (bending, stooping, leg motion)
Any exacerbation with coughing, sneezing, straining at stool
Any weakness of the leg, foot, or toes
Any numbness, paresthesias, or dysesthesias of the leg or foot
Relieving factors
Any associated bowel, bladder, or sexual dysfunction suggesting cauda equina compression
Any associated fever, weight loss, or morning stiffness

Modified from Campbell WW, Pridgeon RP. *Practical Primer of Clinical Neurology*. Philadelphia: Lippincott Williams & Wilkins, 2002.

TABLE 3.8 Important Historical Points in the Dizzy Patient

Patient's precise definition of dizziness
Nature of onset
Severity
Presence or absence of an illusion of motion
Symptoms present persistently or intermittently
If intermittently, frequency, duration, and timing of attacks
Relation of dizziness to body position (e.g., standing, sitting, lying)
Any precipitation of dizziness by head movement
Associated symptoms (e.g., nausea, vomiting, tinnitus, hearing loss, weakness, numbness, diplopia, dysarthria, dysphagia, difficulty with gait or balance, palpitations, shortness of breath, dry mouth,* chest pain)
Medications, especially antihypertensives or ototoxic drugs

*Can be a clue to hyperventilation.
Modified from Campbell WW, Pridgeon RP. *Practical Primer of Clinical Neurology.* Philadelphia: Lippincott Williams & Wilkins, 2002.

TABLE 3.9 Important Historical Points in the Patient with Hand Numbness

Note: The primary considerations in the differential diagnosis are carpal tunnel syndrome and cervical radiculopathy.

Symptoms constant or intermittent
If intermittent, timing, especially any relationship to time of day, especially any tendency for nocturnal symptoms, duration and frequency
Relationship to activities (e.g., driving)
What part of hand most involved
Any involvement of the arm, face, leg
Any problems with speech or vision associated with the hand numbness
Neck pain
Hand/arm pain
Hand/arm weakness
Any history of injury, especially old wrist injury
Any involvement of the opposite hand

Modified from Campbell WW, Pridgeon RP. *Practical Primer of Clinical Neurology.* Philadelphia: Lippincott Williams & Wilkins, 2002.

TABLE 3.10 Important Historical Points in the Patient with a Suspected Transient Ischemic Attack

Note: This arises in patients who have had one or more spells of weakness or numbness involving one side of the body, transient loss of vision, symptoms of vertebrobasilar insufficiency, and similar problems.

Date of first spell and number of attacks
Frequency of attacks
Duration of attacks
Specific body parts and functions involved
Any associated difficulty with speech, vision, swallowing, etc.
Other associated symptoms (chest pain, shortness of breath, nausea and vomiting, headache)
Any history of hypertension, diabetes mellitus, hypercholesterolemia, coronary artery disease, peripheral vascular disease, drug abuse
Any past episodes suggestive of retinal, hemispheric, or vertebrobasilar transient ischemic attack
Current medications especially aspirin, oral contraceptives, antihypertensives

Modified from Campbell WW, Pridgeon RP. *Practical Primer of Clinical Neurology.* Philadelphia: Lippincott Williams & Wilkins, 2002.

TABLE 3.11 Important Historical Points in the Patient with Episodic Loss of Consciousness: The Differential Diagnosis of Syncope versus Seizure

Timing of attack (e.g., frequency, duration)
Patient's recollection of events
Circumstances of attack (e.g., in church, in the shower, after phlebotomy)
Events just prior to attack
Body position just prior to attack (e.g., supine, sitting, standing)
Presence of prodrome or aura
Any tonic or clonic activity
Any suggestion of focal onset
Any incontinence or tongue biting
Symptoms following the spell (e.g., sleeping, focal neurologic deficit)
Time to complete recovery
Witness description of attacks
Drug, alcohol, and medication exposure
Family history (FH)

Modified from Campbell WW, Pridgeon RP. *Practical Primer of Clinical Neurology.* Philadelphia: Lippincott Williams & Wilkins, 2002.

TABLE 3.12 Important Historical Points in the Patient with Numbness of the Feet

Note: The differential diagnosis is usually between peripheral neuropathy and lumbosacral radiculopathy. There is a further extensive differential diagnosis of the causes of peripheral neuropathy.
Whether symptoms are constant or intermittent
If intermittent, any relation to posture, activity, or movement
Any associated pain in the back, legs, or feet
Any weakness of the legs or feet
Any history of back injury, disc herniation, back surgery
Symmetry of symptoms
Any bowel, bladder, or sexual dysfunction
Any history of underlying systemic disease (e.g., diabetes mellitus, thyroid disease, anemia, low vitamin B_{12} level)
Any weight loss
Drinking habits
Smoking history
Any history to suggest toxin exposure, vocational or recreational
Dietary history
Medication history, including vitamins
Family history (FH) of similar symptoms
FH of diabetes, pernicious anemia, or peripheral neuropathy

Modified from Campbell WW, Pridgeon RP. *Practical Primer of Clinical Neurology.* Philadelphia: Lippincott Williams & Wilkins, 2002.

TABLE 3.13 Important Historical Points in the Patient Complaining of Memory Loss

Note: The primary consideration is to distinguish Alzheimer's disease from conditions—especially treatable ones—that may mimic it.
Duration of the problem
Getting worse, better, or staying the same
Examples of what is forgotten (minor things such as dates, anniversaries, etc., as compared to major things)
Does the patient still control the checkbook
Any tendency to get lost
Medication history, including over-the-counter drugs
Drinking habits
Any headache
Any difficulty with the senses of smell or taste
Any difficulty with balance, walking, or bladder control
Any depressive symptoms (see Table 3.3)
Any recent head trauma
Past history of stroke or other vascular disease
Past history of thyroid disease, anemia, low vitamin B_{12}, any STDs
Any risk factors for HIV
FH of dementia or Alzheimer's disease

Modified from Campbell WW, Pridgeon RP. *Practical Primer of Clinical Neurology*. Philadelphia: Lippincott Williams & Wilkins, 2002.

BIBLIOGRAPHY

Caplan LC, Hollander J. *The Effective Clinical Neurologist*. 3rd ed. Shelton: People's Medical Publishing House, 2010.

DeGowin RL, Brown DD. *DeGowin's Diagnostic Examination*. 9th ed. New York: McGraw-Hill, 2009.

Duffy DL, Hamerman D, Cohen MA. Communication skills of house officers. A study in a medical clinic. *Ann Intern Med* 1980;93:354–357.

Griffith CH, Rich EC, Wilson JF. House staff's knowledge of their patients' social histories. *Acad Med* 1995;70:64–66.

Haponik EF, Frye AW, Richards B, et al. Sleep history is neglected diagnostic information. Challenges for primary care physicians. *J Gen Intern Med* 1996;11:759–761.

Marvel K, Major G, Jones K, et al. Dialogues in the exam room: medical interviewing by resident family physicians. *Fam Med* 2000;32:628–632.

Meuleman JR, Caranasos GJ. Evaluating the interview performance of internal medicine interns. *Acad Med* 1989;64:277–279.

Meuleman JR, Harward MP. Assessing medical interview performance. Effect of interns' gender and month of training. *Arch Intern Med* 1992;152:1677–1680.

Platt FW, McMath JC. Clinical hypocompetence: the interview. *Ann Intern Med* 1979;91:898–902.

Rich EC, Crowson TW, Harris IB. The diagnostic value of the medical history. Perceptions of internal medicine physicians. *Arch Intern Med* 1987;147:1957–1960.

Robbins AS, Kauss DR, Heinrich R, et al. Interpersonal skills training: evaluation in an internal medicine residency. *J Med Educ* 1979;54:885–894.

Sapira JD. *The Art and Science of Bedside Diagnosis*. Baltimore: Urban & Schwarzenberg, 1990.

Sideris DA, Tsouna-Hadjis P, Toumanidis S, et al. A self-learning approach to history-taking. *Med Educ* 1990;24:46–51.

Swartz MH. *Textbook of Physical Diagnosis: History and Examination*. 6th ed. Philadelphia: W. B. Saunders, 2010.

Woolliscroft JO, Calhoun JG, Billiu GA, et al. House officer interviewing techniques: impact on data elicitation and patient perceptions. *J Gen Intern Med* 1989;4:108–114.

CHAPTER 4

The General Physical Examination

A general physical examination (PE) usually accompanies a neurologic examination (NE). The extent of the general PE done depends on the circumstances; it may range from minimal to extensive. The general PE in a neurologic patient need not be so detailed or painstaking as in a complicated internal medicine patient, but it must be complete enough to reveal any relevant abnormalities. There are many excellent textbooks on physical diagnosis that provide an extensive discussion of general PE techniques.

Even the most compulsive internist doing a "complete physical" performs an NE that the average neurologist would consider cursory. In contrast, the neurologist performs a more complete NE but only as much general PE as the circumstances dictate. Both are concerned about achieving the proper balance between efficiency and thoroughness. The internist or other primary care practitioner would like to learn how to incorporate the NE into the general PE, whereas the neurologist would like to incorporate as much of the general PE as possible into the NE. In fact, any NE, even a cursory one, provides an opportunity to accomplish much of the general PE simply by observation and a few additional maneuvers.

The general examination begins with observation of the patient during the interview. Even the patient's voice may be relevant because hoarseness, dysphonia, aphasia, dysarthria, confusion, and other things of neurologic significance may be apparent even at that early stage. An exam of head, eyes, ears, nose, and throat is a natural by-product of an evaluation of the cranial nerves. When examining the pupils and extraocular movements, take the opportunity to note any abnormalities of the external eye and ocular adnexa, such as conjunctivitis, exophthalmos, lid retraction, lid lag, xanthelasma, or jaundice. When examining the mouth, as an extension of the general PE, search for any intraoral lesions, leukoplakia, or other abnormalities. When examining the optic disc, also examine the retina for any evidence of diabetic or hypertensive retinopathy. While examining neurologic function in the upper extremities, there is ample opportunity to observe for the presence of clubbing, cyanosis, nail changes, hand deformity, arthropathy, and so forth to complete the upper-extremity examination portion of the general PE. Examining the legs and feet for strength, reflexes, sensation, and plantar responses provides an opportunity to coincidentally look at the skin and nails. Check for pretibial edema, leg length discrepancy, swollen or deformed knee or ankle joints, pes cavus, hammer toes, or any other abnormalities. Note the pattern of hair growth, any dystrophic changes in the nails, and feel the pulses in the feet. Do anything else necessary for the lower extremity portion of the general PE. An evaluation of gait and station provides a great deal of information about the musculoskeletal system. Note whether the patient has any orthopedic limitations, such as a varus deformity of the knee, genu recurvatum, or pelvic tilt. Gait testing also provides a convenient opportunity to examine the lumbosacral spine for tenderness and range of motion. After listening for carotid bruits, it requires little additional effort to palpate the neck for masses and thyromegaly.

The NE can thus serve as a core around which a general PE can be built. At the end of a good NE, one has only to listen to the heart and lungs and palpate the abdomen to have also done a fairly complete general PE. Sometimes, it is not so important to do a skillful general PE as it is to be willing to do one at all. Some findings are obvious if one merely takes the trouble to look.

William Osler said, "There are, in truth, no specialties in medicine, since to know fully many of the most important diseases a man must be familiar with their manifestations in many organs." Although there is virtually no part of the general PE that may not occasionally be noteworthy in a particular circumstance, some parts of the general PE are more often relevant and important in patients presenting with neurologic complaints. The general PE, as it is particularly relevant for neurologic patients, follows.

VITAL SIGNS

Determining the blood pressure (BP) in both arms is useful in patients with suspected cerebrovascular disease. Significant asymmetries may reflect extracranial cardiovascular occlusive disease. Measuring the BP with the patient supine, seated, and upright may be necessary in some circumstances. Orthostatic hypotension is a frequent cause of syncope. It may occur in patients with autonomic insufficiency due to peripheral causes, as in diabetic neuropathy, or due to failure of central regulation, as in multisystem atrophy. The most frequent cause of orthostasis is as a side effect of antihypertensive therapy. Increased BP occurs with increased intracranial pressure (Cushing reflex) and in some patients acutely with stroke or subarachnoid hemorrhage before intracranial pressure has risen. Increased BP due to stroke is often because of peripheral attempts to compensate for cerebral ischemia and usually resolves without treatment; overly aggressive treatment in the acute phase may be deleterious. Severe systemic hypotension is seldom because of a neurologic cause, except as a terminal event, and is much more suggestive of a hemodynamic disturbance.

The pulse rate and character are important, especially if increased intracranial pressure is suspected. When intracranial pressure is increased, the pulse usually slows but may occasionally accelerate. A bounding pulse occurs in aortic regurgitation or hyperthyroidism and a small, slow pulse in aortic stenosis. Either of these may have neurologic complications. Detecting the irregular pulse of atrial fibrillation is important in the evaluation of stroke patients. Both bradyarrhythmias and tachyarrhythmias may produce cerebral hypoperfusion. Abnormalities of respiration may be very important in neurologic patients (see below).

GENERAL APPEARANCE

The general appearance of the patient may reveal evidence of acute or chronic illness; fever, pain, or distress; evidence of weight loss; abnormal posture of the trunk, head, or extremities; the general level of motor activity; unusual mannerisms; abnormal movements, bizarre activities; restlessness; or immobility. Weight loss and evidence of malnutrition may indicate hyperthyroidism, Alzheimer's disease, Whipple's disease, celiac disease, or amyloidosis. The body fat level and distribution, together with the hair distribution and the secondary sexual development are important in the diagnosis of endocrinopathies and disorders of the hypothalamus. Note any outstanding deviations from normal development such as gigantism, dwarfism, gross deformities, amputations, contractures, and disproportion or asymmetries between body parts. Short stature can occur in mitochondrial disorders, Schwartz-Jampel syndrome, Refsum's disease, Andersen-Tawil syndrome, Niemann-Pick disease, Turner and Noonan syndromes, and in CADASIL. Excessive height may suggest Marfan's syndrome, homocystinuria, Klinefelter's syndrome, or Sotos syndrome.

Specific abnormal postures may occur in diseases of the nervous system. Spastic hemiparesis causes flexion of the upper extremity with flexion and adduction at the shoulder, flexion at the elbow and wrist, and flexion and adduction of the fingers; in the lower extremity, there is extension at the hip, knee, and ankle, with an equinus deformity of the foot. In Parkinson's disease and related syndromes, there is flexion of the neck, trunk, elbows, wrists, and knees, with stooping, rigidity, masking, slowness of movement, and tremors. In myopathies, there may be lordosis, protrusion of the abdomen, a waddling gait, and hypertrophy of the calves. Peripheral nerve disease may cause wrist or foot drop or a claw hand or pes cavus. These neurogenic abnormalities may be confused with deformities due to such things as Dupuytren's contracture, congenital pes cavus, changes due to trauma or arthritis, developmental abnormalities, habitual postures, and occupational factors.

Occasionally, the general appearance of the patient is so characteristic of a particular process that "diagnosis in a blink of the eye" (augenblickdiagnose) is possible. Familiarity with many clinical conditions underlies this ability to make spot diagnoses simply based on inspection. Goethe said, "Was man weiss, man sieht" (what man knows, man sees). This is the process of pattern recognition, or gestalt, and occurs on many levels in medicine. Examples include the characteristic appearance of the patient with acromegaly, hypothyroidism, hyperthyroidism, hydrocephalus, craniosynostosis syndromes, Down's syndrome, and Parkinson's disease, to name just a few. Similarly, key fragments of history often permit very rapid diagnosis.

HEAD

The skull houses the brain; abnormalities of the head are common and often very important. Inspect the shape, symmetry, and size of the head; note any apparent abnormalities or irregularities. An abnormal turn or tilt of the head may indicate cervical dystonia, a fourth nerve palsy, or ocular tilt reaction. Premature closure of cranial sutures can produce a wide variety of abnormally shaped skulls (see Chapter 2). Other deformities or developmental anomalies include hydrocephaly, macrocephaly, microcephaly, asymmetries or abnormalities of contour, disproportion between the facial and the cerebral portions, scars, and signs of recent trauma. In children, it is informative to measure the head circumference. Dilated veins, telangiectatic areas, or port-wine angiomas on the scalp or face may overlie a cerebral hemangioma, especially when such nevi are present in the trigeminal nerve distribution. In unconscious patients or those with head trauma, ecchymosis over the mastoid (Battle's sign, Figure 4.1) or around the eyes but not extending beyond the orbital rim ("raccoon eyes") suggests basilar skull fracture.

Palpation of the skull may disclose deformities due to old trauma, burr hole, or craniotomy defects, tenderness, or scars. If there is a postoperative skull defect, note any bulging or tumefaction. The size and patency of the fontanelles is important in infants. Bulging of the fontanelles and suture separation can occur with increased intracranial pressure in children. Meningoceles and encephaloceles may cause palpable skull defects. Tumors may involve the scalp and skull. Palpable masses involving the scalp or skull may be metastatic carcinoma, lymphoma, leukemia, dermoid, or multiple myeloma. A turban tumor is an often disfiguring type of dermal cylindroma that may involve the scalp. Neurofibromas of the scalp occur in von Recklinghausen's disease. Localized swelling of the scalp may occur with osteomyelitis of the skull. Exostoses may indicate an underlying meningioma. Hydrocephalus that develops prior to suture closure often results in an enlarged, sometimes massive, head. Frontal bossing is another sign of hydrocephalus. Giant cell arteritis may cause induration and tenderness of the superficial temporal arteries. Transillumination may be useful in the diagnosis of hydrocephalus and hydranencephaly.

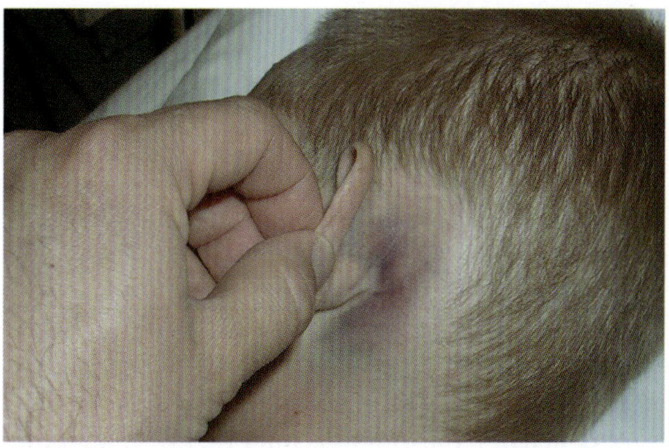

FIGURE 4.1 Battle's sign: superficial ecchymosis over the mastoid process due to basilar skull fracture. (Reproduced from van Dijk GW. The bare essentials: head injury. *Pract Neurol* 2011;11[1]:50–55, with permission from BMJ Publishing Group Ltd.)

Percussion of the skull may disclose dullness on the side of a tumor or subdural hematoma or a tympanitic percussion note in hydrocephalus and increased intracranial pressure in infants and children (Macewen's sign, or "cracked pot" resonance). Auscultatory percussion (percussion over the midfrontal area while listening over various parts of the head with the stethoscope) may reveal relative dullness on the side of a mass lesion or subdural hematoma.

Auscultation of the head is sometimes useful. Bruits may be heard best over the temporal regions of the skull, the eyeballs, and the mastoids. Cephalic bruits may occur with angiomas, aneurysms, arteriovenous malformations, neoplasms that compress large arteries, and in the presence of atherosclerotic plaques that partially occlude cerebral or carotid arteries. They may also occur in the absence of disease. Ocular bruits usually signify occlusive intracranial cerebrovascular disease. A carotid bruit may be transmitted to the mastoid. An ocular bruit in a patient with an arteriovenous aneurysm may disappear on carotid compression. Murmurs may be transmitted from the heart or large vessels; systolic murmurs heard over the entire cranium in children are not always of pathologic significance.

An evaluation of the facies (the facial expression) may aid in neurologic diagnosis. Gross facial abnormalities are found in such conditions as acromegaly (Figure 4.2), myxedema, hyperthyroidism, Down's syndrome, and mucopolysaccharidosis. In

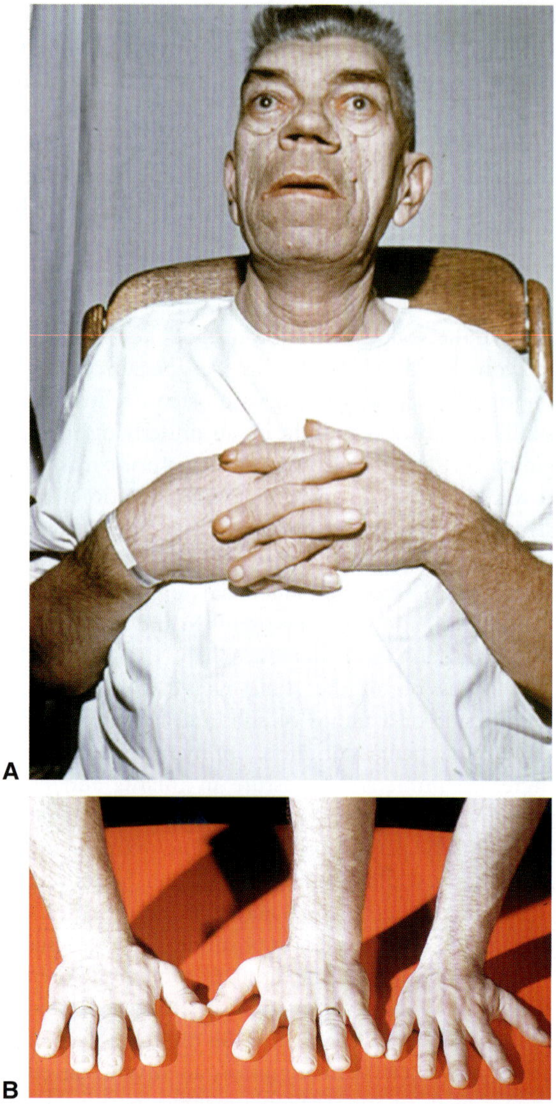

FIGURE 4.2 Acromegaly. **A.** Note coarse facial features. **B.** Patient's large hands at left; single normal hand at right. (Reprinted from McConnell TH, Paulson VA, Valasek MA. *The Nature of Disease: Pathology for the Health Professions.* 2nd ed. Baltimore: Wolters Kluwer Health/Lippincott Williams & Wilkins, 2014, with permission.)

some neurologic disorders, there are characteristic changes in facial expression and mobility such as the fixed ("masked") face of parkinsonism (Figure 30.1), the procerus sign in progressive supranuclear palsy (Chapter 30), the immobile face with precipitate laughter and crying seen in pseudobulbar palsy, the grimacing of athetosis and dystonia, and the ptosis and weakness of the facial muscles seen in some myopathies and myasthenia gravis. The facies of the patient with myotonic dystrophy I are characteristic.

EYES

Ophthalmologic abnormalities can provide clues to the etiology of neurologic disease as well as to the presence of underlying systemic disease causing neurologic symptomatology (see Chapter 13). Examples of findings of possible neurologic relevance include bilateral exophthalmos due to thyroid eye disease in a patient with muscle weakness, unilateral arcus senilis from carotid stenosis, lens dislocation in Marfan's syndrome, or Brushfield spots on the iris due to Down's syndrome. Vesicular lesions on the forehead suggest herpes zoster ophthalmicus (Figure 15.4). Fundoscopic examination is discussed in Chapter 13.

EARS

Examination of the ears is particularly important in patients with hearing loss, vertigo, or a facial nerve palsy. It is important to exclude a perforated tympanic membrane. Examination of the ear canal may reveal a glomus tumor in a patient with jugular foramen syndrome (Figure 21.5), vesicles due to herpes zoster infection (Figure 16.9), or evidence of a posterior fossa cholesteatoma. Cerebrospinal fluid (CSF) otorrhea may cause a clear or bloody ear discharge. Before performing a caloric examination in a comatose patient, it is important to be certain that the ear canals are clear and that the tympanic membranes are intact. Hemorrhage into the middle ear may cause a bulging, blue-red tympanic membrane in patients with basilar skull fracture (Figure 16.10).

NOSE, MOUTH, AND THROAT

Perforation of the nasal septum may be a clue to cocaine abuse. A saddle nose may be a sign of congenital syphilis (Figure 4.3). Evidence of bacterial infection may be a sign of cavernous sinus thrombosis, and watery drainage may be due to CSF rhinorrhea **(Video Link 4.1)**. In pernicious anemia, the tongue is smooth and translucent with atrophy of the fungiform and filiform papillae, along with the associated redness and lack of coating (atrophic glossitis). In thiamine deficiency, the tongue is smooth, shiny, atrophic, and reddened. A trident or triple-furrowed tongue is seen in myasthenia gravis **(Video Link 4.2)**. Lingua plicata occurs in Melkersson-Rosenthal syndrome. Macroglossia occurs in amyloid, myxedema, and

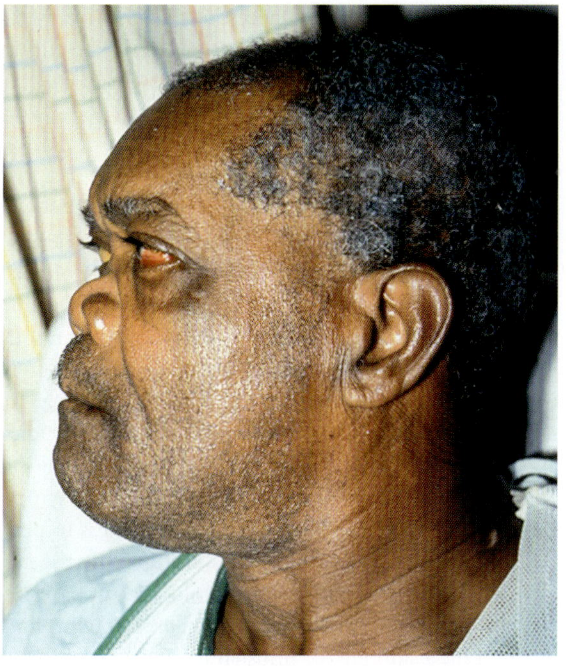

FIGURE 4.3 Saddle nose deformity in a patient with congenital syphilis.

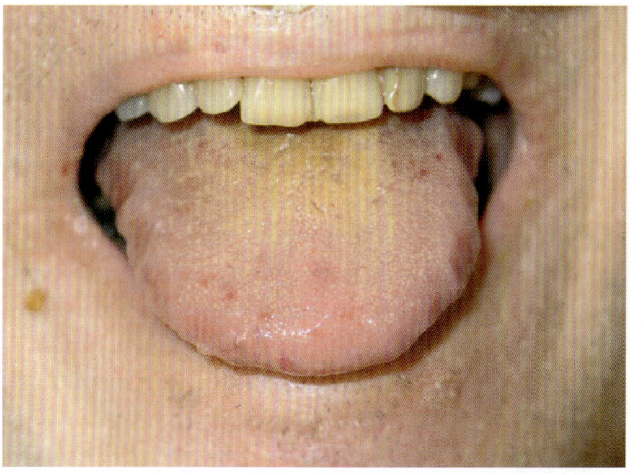

FIGURE 4.4 Massive macroglossia in a patient with systemic AL amyloidosis. (From Sattianayagam P, Gibbs S, Hawkins P, et al. Systemic AL (light-chain) amyloidosis and the gastrointestinal tract. *Scand J Gastroenterol* 2009;44[11]:1384–1385. Reprinted by permission of Taylor & Francis Ltd. http://www.tandfonline.com.)

Down's syndrome (Figure 4.4) and rarely in amyotrophic lateral sclerosis (ALS) (Figure 20.5). Tongue bite marks may indicate a recent seizure and can also occur in neuroacanthocytosis and Lesch-Nyhan syndrome. Other potential findings include xerostomia in Sjögren's syndrome; a lead line along the gums in lead toxicity; trismus in tetanus or polymyositis; and mucosal ulceration in Behçet's disease. Notched teeth are a sign of congenital syphilis (Hutchinson teeth).

NECK

Note any adenopathy, thyroid masses or enlargement, deformities, tenderness, rigidity, tilting or other abnormalities of posture, asymmetries, changes in contour, or pain on movement. Normally, the neck can be flexed so that the chin rests on the chest, and it can be rotated from side to side without difficulty. Meningeal irritation may cause nuchal rigidity, head retraction, and opisthotonos (Figure 52.1). Neck movement may also be restricted with cervical spondylosis, cervical radiculopathy, and dystonias. In meningeal irritation, the primary limitation is in neck flexion; in spondylosis, the limitation is either global or primarily in rotation and lateral bending. In the Klippel-Feil syndrome, syringomyelia, and platybasia, the neck may be short and broad, movement limited, and the hairline low. A short neck may also occur in Chiari malformation, Turner's syndrome, and skull base anomalies. Lhermitte's sign is a sensation of tingling or electric shocks running down the back and legs on flexion of the neck. It is common in multiple sclerosis but can occur with other conditions involving the cervical spinal cord. Two forms of "reverse" Lhermitte's sign have been described. Paresthesias induced by neck extension have been described in extrinsic compression of the cervical spinal cord. Upward moving paresthesias with neck flexion have been described in myelopathy from nitrous oxide inhalation. The carotid arteries should be cautiously and lightly palpated bilaterally, one at a time, and any abnormality or inequality noted, followed by auscultation for carotid bruits.

RESPIRATORY SYSTEM AND THORAX

Neurologic complications of pulmonary disease are common. Note the respiratory rate, rhythm, depth, and character of respirations. Pain on breathing, dyspnea, orthopnea, or shortness of breath on slight activity may be significant. Abnormalities of respiration, such as Cheyne-Stokes, Biot, or Kussmaul breathing may be seen in coma and other neurologic disorders. Either hyperpnea or periods of apnea may occur in increased intracranial pressure and in disturbances of the hypothalamus. In the comatose patient, there are characteristic patterns of respiration that reflect damage at different levels of the nervous system (posthyperventilation apnea, central neurogenic hyperventilation, Cheyne-Stokes, and ataxic breathing). These are discussed further in Chapter 51. Use of accessory muscles of respiration may signal impending ventilatory failure in patients with many neuromuscular disorders, particularly Guillain-Barre syndrome and ALS. Following respiratory function with formal measures of vital capacity and inspiratory and expiratory pressure is often necessary. Evidence of chronic obstructive pulmonary disease (COPD) may be a clue to the etiology of headaches or metabolic encephalopathy or suggest neurologic complications of lung cancer.

CARDIOVASCULAR SYSTEM

The cardiovascular examination is important because of the frequency of neurologic complications of hypertension, atherosclerosis, endocarditis, arrhythmias, and valvular disease. Evidence of atherosclerosis involving the peripheral blood vessels often correlates with cerebrovascular disease.

ABDOMEN

Examination of the abdomen may reveal abnormal masses, enlarged viscera, abnormal pulsations or respiratory movements, or the presence of fluid. Hepatomegaly is common in cirrhosis, hepatitis, carcinoma, and amyloidosis; splenomegaly is common in mononucleosis, amyloidosis, and lymphoma. Ecchymosis of the flank (Grey Turner sign) may be evidence that a lumbosacral plexopathy is due to retroperitoneal hematoma. Ascites may be a clue to hepatic encephalopathy in a patient in coma.

GENITALIA AND RECTUM

Examination of the genitalia, not often called for in neurologic patients, could reveal a chancre or the ulcerations of Behçet's disease. The angiomas in Fabry's disease are often found on the scrotum. A rectal examination to assess sphincter tone and the anal wink reflex is often necessary in patients with evidence of myelopathy or a cauda equina or conus medullaris syndrome.

SPINE

Examination of the spine is often important in neurologic patients. Note any deformity, abnormality of posture or motility, localized tenderness, or muscle spasm. Tuberculosis and neoplasms of the spine may cause a marked kyphosis (gibbus); muscular dystrophy often results in an increased lumbar lordosis (Figure 4.5); and scoliosis is common in syringomyelia and Friedreich's ataxia. Localized rigidity with a slight list or scoliosis and absence of the normal lordosis are frequent symptoms of lumbosacral radiculopathy. Tenderness to percussion over the spinous processes, using either the fist or a reflex hammer, can occur with localized processes such as spinal epidural hematoma or abscess. Dimpling of the skin, a skin tag, or unusual hair growth over the sacrum suggests a spinal dysraphic state such as tethered cord or diastematomyelia (Figure 4.6).

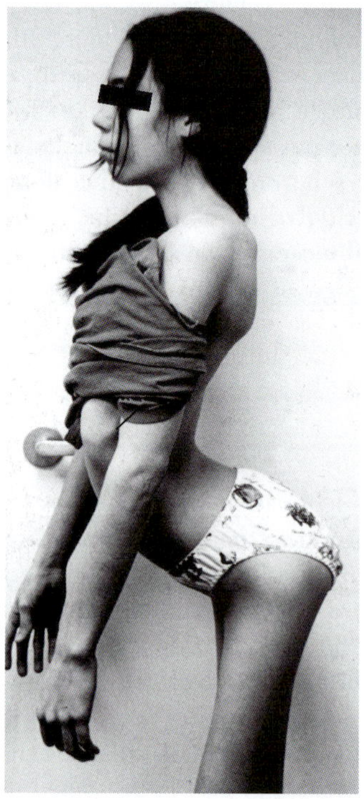

FIGURE 4.5 Marked lumbar lordosis in a 15-year-old girl with FSH dystrophy. (Reprinted from Weinstein SL, Flynn JM, eds. *Lovell and Winter's Pediatric Orthopaedics.* 7th ed. Philadelphia: Wolters Kluwer Health/Lippincott Williams & Wilkins, 2014, with permission.)

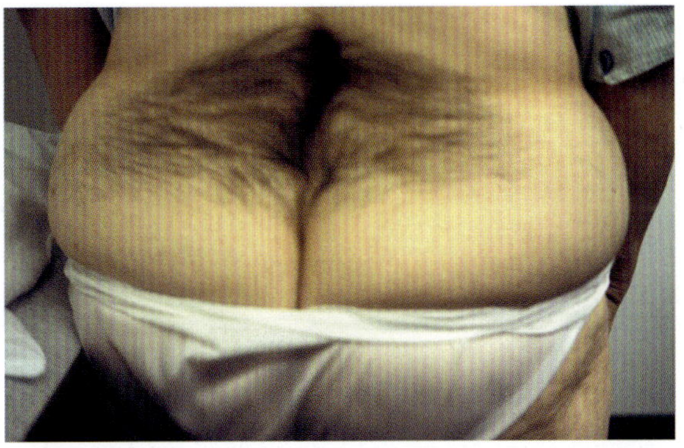

FIGURE 4.6 Giant hairy patch over the lower back in a patient with occult spinal dysraphism. (Reprinted from Campbell WW. *Clinical Signs in Neurology: A Compendium*. Philadelphia: Wolters Kluwer Health, 2016, with permission.)

EXTREMITIES

Note any limb deformities, contractures, edema, or color changes. Any variation from the normal in the size or shape of the hands, feet, or digits, as well as deformities, joint changes, contractures, pain or limitation of movement, localized tenderness, wasting, clubbed fingers, or ulcerations may be significant. Hypermobile joints occur in Marfan's and Ehlers-Danlos syndrome. Edema may be evidence of congestive heart failure or cardiomyopathy. Arthropathy may be a sign of connective tissue disease, sarcoidosis, or Whipple's disease. Painless arthropathy (Charcot joint) occurs when a joint is deafferented; painless enlargement of the shoulder has been reported as the presenting manifestation of syringomyelia. An elbow deformity may signal ulnar neuropathy. Decreased peripheral pulses occur in Takayasu's disease as well as atherosclerosis. Acrocyanosis occurs in ergotism. Palmar erythema may be a clue to alcohol abuse. Diseases of the nervous system are found in association with such skeletal and developmental anomalies as syndactyly, polydactyly, and arachnodactyly.

SKIN

A careful examination of the skin can provide important evidence regarding the nature of a neurologic condition. Findings of possible neurologic relevance include the following: spider angiomas in alcohol abuse; erythema chronicum migrans in Lyme disease; purpura and petechiae in thrombotic thrombocytopenic purpura, meningococcemia, and Rocky Mountain spotted fever (all of which may have prominent neurologic manifestations); livedo reticularis in antiphospholipid syndrome and cryoglobulinemia; hyperpigmentation in Nelson's syndrome, carotenemia, hemochromatosis, pernicious anemia, or Addison's disease; angiokeratomas in Fabry's disease; and the numerous dermatologic manifestations of the neurocutaneous syndromes (see Chapter 53). Other important findings include signs of scleroderma; ichthyosis; xanthelasma, scars, needle marks, or other evidence of intravenous substance abuse; bruises; and trophic change. The degree of moisture or perspiration may be neurologically pertinent, and any localized or generalized increase or decrease in perspiration should be recorded. Skin changes may be of diagnostic significance in the endocrinopathies, diseases of the hypothalamus, and dysautonomia. In parkinsonism, the skin may be greasy and seborrheic. Herpes zoster causes a vesicular eruption in the distribution of the involved root (Figure 4.7). Hemangiomas of the spinal cord may be accompanied by skin nevi in the same metamere. Symmetrically placed, painless,

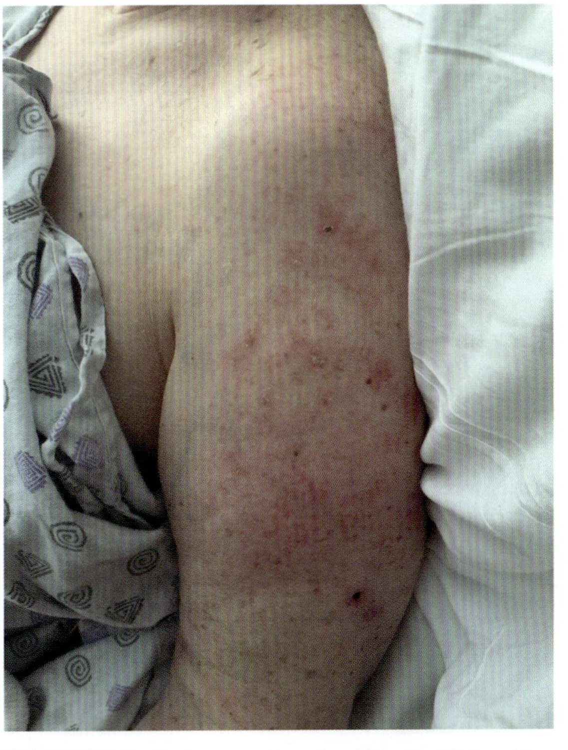

FIGURE 4.7 Healing herpes zoster rash outlining the C5 dermatome in a patient who presented with a severe C5 radiculopathy. (Reprinted from Campbell WW. *Clinical Signs in Neurology: A Compendium*. Philadelphia: Wolters Kluwer Health, 2016, with permission.)

recurring, poorly healing lesions of the extremities may occur in syringomyelia and hereditary sensory neuropathy. Dermatomyositis causes characteristic skin lesions. Peripheral nerve disease, tabes dorsalis, and myelopathy may produce trophic changes in the skin. Skin changes may also be a manifestation of vitamin deficiency. Some of the other conditions of neurologic importance that cause skin abnormalities include pseudoxanthoma elasticum, Refsum's disease, Sweet's syndrome, Degos disease, and xeroderma pigmentosum.

HAIR AND NAILS

Hair texture and distribution are important in the evaluation of endocrinopathies. Premature graying of the hair may be familial and of no clinical significance, but is frequently observed in pernicious anemia, and may occur in hypothalamic and other disorders. Alopecia, or balding, occurs in several disorders with neurologic features or complications, including myotonic dystrophy, hypothyroidism, Leigh's disease, sarcoidosis, secondary syphilis, and SLE. Hypertrichosis can occur in POEMS syndrome, porphyria, and other conditions.

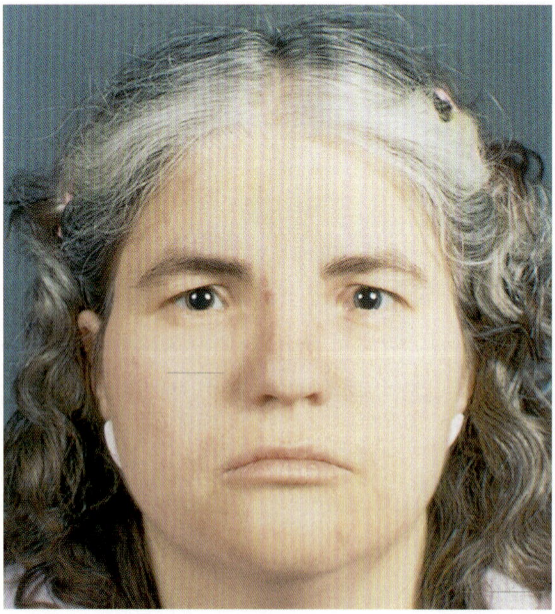

FIGURE 4.8 Poliosis in a patient with Waardenburg syndrome. (Reprinted from Gold DH, Weingeist TA. *Color Atlas of the Eye in Systemic Disease*. Baltimore: Lippincott Williams & Wilkins, 2001, with permission.)

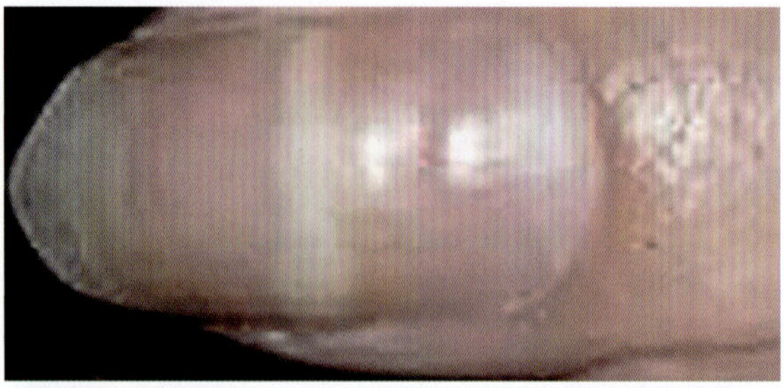

FIGURE 4.9 Mees' lines. These are transverse lines, usually one per nail, with curves similar to the lunula, not the cuticle. The line often disappears if pressure is placed over the line. They emerge from under the proximal nail folds and grow out with the nails. Mees' lines occur with arsenic poisoning, thallium poisoning, and to a lesser extent other heavy metal poisoning. They may also follow any acute or severe illness. (Reprinted from Campbell WW. *Clinical Signs in Neurology: A Compendium*. Philadelphia: Wolters Kluwer, 2016, with permission.)

Poliosis occurs with Vogt-Koyanagi-Harada disease (Figure 4.8). Kinky hair occurs in Menkes disease and giant axonal neuropathy. Transverse discoloration of the nails (Mees' lines) may occur with arsenic poisoning and debilitated states (Figure 4.9). Clubbing of the nails occurs with bronchogenic carcinoma or heart disease. Abnormal nail bed capillary loops may be a sign of dermatomyositis.

NODES

Lymphadenopathy may occur in lymphoma, mononucleosis, HIV, Lyme disease, Niemann-Pick disease, Gaucher's disease, phenytoin pseudolymphoma, sarcoidosis, Whipple's disease, and in many other conditions that may also have neurologic manifestations.

Video Links

Video Link 4.1. CSF rhinorrhea. http://www.nejm.org/doi/full/10.1056/NEJMicm0708178#t=article

Video Link 4.2. Triple-furrowed tongue in myasthenia gravis. http://neurosigns.org/wiki/Triple_furrow_tongue_in_myasthenia_gravis

BIBLIOGRAPHY

Boulet JR, McKinley DW, Whelan GP, et al. Clinical skills deficiencies among first-year residents: utility of the ECFMG clinical skills assessment. *Acad Med* 2002;77:S33–S35.

Campbell WW. Augenblickdiagnose. *Semin Neurol* 1998;18:169–176.

Drago F, Ciccarese G, Agnoletti AF, et al. Neuro sweet syndrome: a systematic review. A rare complication of Sweet syndrome. *Acta Neurol Belg* 2017;117:33–42.

Dyken PR, Miller M. *Facial Features of Neurologic Syndromes.* St. Louis: Mosby, 1980.

Edelstein DR, Ruder HJ. Assessment of clinical skills using videotapes of the complete medical interview and physical examination. *Med Teach* 1990;12:155–162.

Fagan MJ, Griffith RA, Obbard L, et al. Improving the physical diagnosis skills of third-year medical students: a controlled trial of a literature-based curriculum. *J Gen Intern Med* 2003;18:652–655.

Goldstein LB, Matchar DB. The rational clinical examination. Clinical assessment of stroke. *JAMA* 1994;271:1114–1120.

Haring CM, van der Meer JW, Postma CT. A core physical examination in internal medicine: what should students do and how about their supervisors? *Med Teach* 2013;35:e1472–e1477.

Hatala R, Smieja M, Kane SL, et al. An evidence-based approach to the clinical examination. *J Gen Intern Med* 1997;12:182–187.

Kempster PA, Rollinson RD. The Lhermitte phenomenon: variant forms and their significance. *J Clin Neurosci* 2008;15: 379–381.

LeBlond RF, DeGowin RL, Brown DD. *DeGowin's Diagnostic Examination.* 9th ed. New York: McGraw-Hill, 2009.

Mangione S, Peitzman SJ. Revisiting physical diagnosis during the medical residency: it is time for a logbook—and more. *Acad Med* 1999;74:467–469.

Reeves AG, Swenson RS. *Disorders of the Nervous System: A Primer. Online Version.* Hanover: Dartmouth, 2008. http://www.dartmouth.edu/~dons/index.html

Tham WY, Oh CC, Koh HY. Pernicious anaemia presenting as hyperpigmentation. *Clin Exp Dermatol* 2015;40: 626–628.

Wiener S, Nathanson M. Physical examination. Frequently observed errors. *JAMA* 1976;236:852–855.

Wray NP, Friedland JA. Detection and correction of house staff error in physical diagnosis. *JAMA* 1983;249:1035–1037.

CHAPTER 5

General Outline of the Neurologic Examination

The neurologic examination, as commonly done, includes the major categories listed in Table 5.1. The examination does not have to be performed in any particular sequence, and every physician develops his own routine for the examination. It is customary to record the neurologic examination in the general format outlined in Table 5.1 or with minor modifications.

The complete neurologic examination can be a complex and arduous undertaking. In fact, few neurologists do a truly complete exam on every patient. As with the general physical examination, the history focuses the neurologic examination so that certain aspects are emphasized in a given clinical situation. The exam done on a typical patient with headache is not the same as that done on a patient with low back pain, or dementia, or cerebrovascular disease. The examination should also be adapted for the circumstances. If the patient is in pain or feels apprehensive, it may initially focus on the area of complaint, followed later by a more thorough assessment. Only a brief examination may be possible for unstable or severely ill persons until their condition stabilizes. With comatose, combative, or uncooperative patients, a compulsively complete examination is an impossibility. However, in each of these situations, at least some maneuvers are employed to screen for neurologic dysfunction that is not necessarily suggested by the history. A rapid screening or mini neurologic examination may initially be adequate for persons with minor or intermittent symptoms. Every patient does not require every conceivable test, but all require a screening examination. The findings on such a screening examination determine the emphasis of a more searching subsequent examination. There are a number of ways to perform a screening examination. Table 5.2 details such an abbreviated examination from previous editions of this book.

There are two basic ways to do a traditional neurologic examination—regional and systemic. A system approach evaluates the motor system, then the sensory system, and so on. A regional approach evaluates all the systems in a given region, such as the upper extremities and then the lower extremities. The screening exam outlined in Table 5.3 is an amalgam of the regional and system approaches geared for speed and efficiency. The concept is an examination that requires the nervous system to perform at a high level, relying heavily on sensitive signs, especially the flawless execution of complex functions. If the nervous system can perform a complex task perfectly, it is very unlikely there is significant pathology present, and going through a more extensive evaluation is not likely to prove productive. A neurologic examination that assesses complex functions and seeks signs that are sensitive indicators of pathology is efficient and not overly time consuming.

Educators have proposed a third type of exam, especially for teaching: the hypothesis-driven examination. This approach evolves naturally with experience but has not been used previously in teaching the exam. Teaching a hypothesis-driven neurologic exam evolved from a similar approach to the general physical exam. Examination maneuvers were focused by the history. Using the hypothesis-driven approach produced greater sensitivity but lower specificity and was performed in less time. Learning to develop a hypothesis from the history and how to test it is of course a paramount challenge in neurology.

The examination begins with taking the medical history, which serves as a fair barometer of the mental status. Patients who can relate a logical, coherent,

TABLE 5.1 Major Sections of the Neurologic Examination

Mental status
Cranial nerves
Motor
Sensory
Reflexes
Cerebellar function, coordination
Gait and station
Other signs

pertinent, and sensible narrative of their problem will seldom have abnormalities on more formal bedside mental status testing. On the other hand, a rambling, disjointed, incomplete history may be a clue to the presence of some cognitive impairment, even though there is no direct complaint of thinking or memory problems from the patient or the family. Similarly, psychiatric disease is sometimes betrayed by the patient's demeanor and style of history giving. If there is any suggestion of abnormality from the interaction with the patient during the history-taking phase of the encounter, then a more detailed mental status examination should be carried out. Other reasons to do a formal mental status examination are discussed in Chapter 8. Simple observation is often useful. The patient's gait, voice, mannerisms, ability to dress and undress, and even handshake (grip myotonia) may suggest the diagnosis.

Functions requiring the use of the penlight having been completed, observe the nasolabial folds for depth and symmetry and compare the forehead wrinkles on both sides. Then have the patient grimace, vigorously baring the teeth, while closing the eyes tightly. Note the symmetry of the grimace, how many teeth are seen on each side, and the relative amplitude and velocity of the lower facial contraction, as well as the symmetry of the upper facial contraction (see Chapter 16). How completely the patient buries the eyelashes on the two sides is a sensitive indicator of orbicularis oculi strength.

If the patient has no complaints of hearing loss, tinnitus, vertigo, facial numbness, or weakness and there is no specific reason suggested by the history to do so, routine examination of hearing is seldom productive. Examination of hearing is discussed further in Chapter 17. Complete the cranial nerve examination by checking the visual fields and fundi (see Chapter 13).

The screening examination detailed in Table 5.3 continues by doing everything that requires use of a penlight. Begin by noting the position of the eyelids and the width of the palpebral fissures bilaterally. Check the pupils for light reaction with the patient fixing at distance. If the pupillary light reaction is normal and equal in both eyes, checking the pupillary near reaction is not necessary. Continue by assessing extraocular movements in the six cardinal positions of gaze, having the patient follow the penlight. Be sure that the patient has no diplopia or limitation of movement and that ocular pursuit movements are smooth and fluid. With the eyes in primary and eccentric positions, look for any nystagmus. The eye examination is discussed in more detail in Chapter 14. With the light still in hand, prepare to examine the pharynx and oral cavity. Examination of the trigeminal motor function is accomplished merely by watching the patient's jaw drop open prior to examining the mouth and throat. When the pterygoids are unilaterally weak, the jaw invariably deviates toward the weak side on opening. This deviation, while subtle, is a sensitive indicator of trigeminal motor root pathology (see Chapter 15). Observe the tongue for atrophy or fasciculations (see Chapter 20). Have the patient phonate, and be sure the median raphe of the palate elevates in the midline (see Chapter 18). There is little to be gained by checking the gag reflex if the

TABLE 5.2 Components of a Screening Initial Neurologic Examination (Abnormalities or Specific Symptoms Should Lead to More Complete Evaluations)

1. Mentation and communication during conversation with examiner
2. Cranial nerves II, III, IV, VI: visual acuity, gross fields, funduscopic, pupillary reactions, extraocular movements
3. Cranial nerves VII, VIII, IX, X, XII: facial musculature and expression, gross hearing, voice, inspection of the tongue
4. Muscle tone, strength, and bulk proximally and distally in all extremities; abnormal movements
5. Sensory: pain or temperature medially and laterally in all extremities; vibration at ankles
6. Coordination: rapid alternating movements of hands, finger-nose test, gait, station
7. Reflexes: biceps, triceps, brachioradialis, quadriceps, Achilles, plantar, clonus

TABLE 5.3 Steps in a Screening Neurologic Examination

Mental status examination (during history taking or dispersed during the rest of the examination)
Using a penlight
Pupils (at distance)
Extraocular movements
Pharynx and tongue (watch the jaw on mouth opening to be sure it drops vertically to screen for trigeminal motor dysfunction)
Facial motor functions (grimace, close eyes tightly)
Visual fields
Fundi
Upper extremity formal strength examination—deltoid, triceps, wrist extensors, and hand intrinsics
Examination for pronator drift, eyes closed
Examination of upper extremity stereognosis and upper and lower extremity double simultaneous stimulation, while waiting for drift, eyes closed (evaluate fine motor control during the patient's manipulation of the stereognosis test objects)
Examination of finger-to-nose coordination, eyes closed
Examination of arm and finger roll
Examination of lower extremity strength
Completion of the sensory assessment
Examination of deep tendon reflexes, upper and lower extremities
Elicitation of plantar responses
Examination of station and gait, heel and toe walking, hopping on each foot, tandem gait, Romberg or eyes closed tandem

Modified from Campbell WW, Pridgeon RP. *Practical Primer of Clinical Neurology.* Philadelphia: Lippincott Williams & Wilkins, 2002.

patient has no complaints of dysphagia or dysarthria and if there is no reason from the history to suspect a brainstem or cranial nerve lesion. Routine elicitation of the gag reflex is rarely informative and is unpleasant for the patient. Have the patient protrude the tongue and move it from side to side.

Screening examination of motor function, sensory function, and coordination in the upper extremities can be completed as one compound, multifaceted maneuver. In most clinical situations in which a screening examination is appropriate, the primary concern is to detect a lesion involving the corticospinal tract (CST). The CST preferentially innervates certain muscle groups, and these are the groups most likely to be weak because of an upper motor neuron lesion. In the upper extremity, the CST-innervated muscles are the finger extensors, wrist extensors, forearm supinators, external rotators of the shoulder, triceps, and deltoid. The cardinal CST muscles in the lower extremity are the hip flexors, the hamstrings, and the dorsiflexors of the foot and toes. In addition, one of the most important functions of the CST is to provide fine motor control to distal muscles. Fine motor control, including rapid alternating movements, would furthermore be impossible without normal cerebellar function. The screening examination focuses on detecting weakness in the CST distribution and impaired distal fine motor control. In the upper extremity, the best muscles for strength testing are the deltoid, triceps, wrist and finger extensors, and intrinsic hand muscles, especially the interossei. Although commonly done, it is very poor technique to use grip power to assess strength. The finger and wrist flexors are not corticospinal innervated, and they are not likely to be weak with a mild CST lesion. In addition, grip is a complex function with many different muscles involved, so it is insensitive to peripheral pathology as well. Although strength is the primary focus of the motor examination, it is important to note any changes in muscle bulk, for example, atrophy, hypertrophy, or pseudohypertrophy; or muscle tone, for example, rigidity, spasticity, or hypotonia; and to note any abnormal involuntary movements, for example, tremor, fasciculations, or chorea.

When patients with mild CST lesions retain normal strength, ancillary maneuvers may detect the deficit. The most important of these is the examination for pronator drift (see Chapter 27). With the patient's upper extremities outstretched to the front, palms up, and with the eyes closed, observe the position of each extremity. Normally, the palms will remain flat, the elbows straight, and the limbs horizontal. With a CST lesion, the strong muscles are the pronators, the biceps, and the internal rotators of the shoulder. As these overcome the weakened CST-innervated muscles, the hand pronates, the elbow flexes, and the arm drifts downward.

A screening sensory examination assesses sensory function by tasking the nervous system with performing a complex and difficult function. If this function is executed flawlessly, the likelihood of finding clinically significant sensory loss through a more detailed examination is low. Testing for stereognosis and performing double simultaneous stimulation are efficient and sensitive screening tools. The period of time waiting for pronator drift to occur is a convenient time to begin examining upper extremity sensory functions. While the patient is still in "drift position"—arms outstretched in front, palms up, and eyes closed—ask him to indicate which side is touched. Then lightly touch first one hand, then the other, and then both, using minimal finger pressure, a cotton wisp, or a tissue. A set of stimuli to the lower extremities is also convenient at this point. Continue by testing for stereognosis. Place an object, such as a coin, a key, a safety pin, or a paper clip, into one of the patient's still upturned palms, and ask him to feel and identify it. Stereognosis is the ability to recognize and identify an object by feel; the inability to do so is astereognosis. Stereognosis can only be normal when all the peripheral sensory pathways and the parietal lobe association areas are intact; only when the primary sensory modalities are normal does astereognosis indicate a parietal lobe lesion. A patient with severe carpal tunnel syndrome and numb fingers may not be able to identify a small object by feel; this finding is NOT astereognosis. As a screening test, stereognosis is an excellent modality because it tests the entire sensory pathway, from the fingertips to the parietal lobe. If stereognosis is rapid and accurate, then all the sensory pathways must be functioning normally, and detailed examination is not likely to be productive. If a deficit is found on this preliminary assessment, a detailed examination of sensory function is necessary to localize the site of the abnormality. Additional useful information can be gained by dropping the small stereognosis object more or less in the center of the palm. A patient with normal fine motor control will adroitly manipulate the object, move it to the fingertips, rub it between the thumb and opposed fingers, and announce the result. A patient with a mild corticospinal lesion, producing relatively subtle clinical signs without major weakness, may be clumsy in manipulating the object and will occasionally drop it. The sensory examination is discussed further in Chapters 31 to 36.

After testing double simultaneous stimulation and stereognosis, with the patient's eyes still closed, the hand and arm position is examined to determine if any drift has occurred. Then, eyes still closed, the patient is instructed to spread the fingers and touch first one index finger and then the other to the tip of the nose. This is the finger-to-nose (FTN) test, which is used to look for intention tremor, incoordination, and past-pointing. Ordinarily, the FTN test is carried out with the patient's eyes open. For purposes of the screening exam, the more difficult maneuver of eyes closed FTN is performed first. If it is done perfectly, then neither cerebellar nor vestibular disease is likely. Complete the upper extremity examination by examining forearm roll, finger roll, and rapid alternating movements (see Chapter 27).

After completing examination of motor, sensory, and cerebellar function in the upper extremities, attention is turned to strength assessment of the lower extremities. The important muscles to examine are the CST-innervated groups: hip flexors, knee flexors, and the dorsiflexors of the foot. Further sensory testing is convenient at this point, comparing primary modality sensibility on the two sides; comparing proximal to distal in the lower extremities if peripheral neuropathy is a diagnostic consideration; and examining vibratory sensation over the great toes.

Continue by eliciting the biceps, triceps, brachioradialis, knee, and ankle reflexes; then assess the plantar responses. Conclude the examination by checking station and gait. Excellent tests for gait and balance functions are tandem walking with eyes closed and hopping on either foot (see Chapter 44).

The rest of this book is devoted to the detailed assessment of the functions touched on in the screening examination.

BIBLIOGRAPHY

Campbell WW. *Clinical Signs in Neurology: A Compendium.* Philadelphia: Wolters Kluwer Health, 2016.

Campbell WW, Pridgeon RP. *Practical Primer of Clinical Neurology.* Philadelphia: Lippincott Williams & Wilkins, 2002.

Caplan LC, Hollander J. *The Effective Clinical Neurologist.* 3rd ed. Shelton: People's Medical Publishing House-USA, 2011.

Dhand A, Engstrom J, Dhaliwal G. How experienced community neurologists make diagnoses during clinical encounters. *Neurology* 2013;81:1460–1466.

Fuller G. *Neurological Examination Made Easy*. 5th ed. Edinburgh: Churchill Livingstone, 2013.

Gilman S. *Clinical Examination of the Nervous System*. New York: McGraw-Hill, 2000.

Glick TH. Toward a more efficient and effective neurologic examination for the 21st century. *Eur J Neurol* 2005;12:994–997.

Kamel H, Dhaliwal G, Navi BB, et al. A randomized trial of hypothesis-driven vs screening neurologic examination. *Neurology* 2011;77:1395–1400.

Louis ED, Pascuzzi RM, Roos KL, eds. The neurological examination (with an emphasis on its historical underpinnings). *Semin Neurol* 2002;22:329–418.

Massey EW, Pleet AB, Scherokman BJ. *Diagnostic Tests in Neurology: A Photographic Guide to Bedside Techniques*. Chicago: Year Book Medical Publishers, Inc., 1985.

Moore FG, Chalk C. The essential neurologic examination: what should medical students be taught? *Neurology* 2009; 72:2020–2023.

Nishigori H, Masuda K, Kikukawa M, et al. A model teaching session for the hypothesis-driven physical examination. *Med Teach* 2011;33:410–417.

Ross RT. *How to Examine the Nervous System*. 4th ed. Totowa: Humana Press, 2006.

Strub RL, Black FW. *The Mental Status Examination in Neurology*. 4th ed. Philadelphia: F.A. Davis, 2000.

Wartenberg R. *The Examination of Reflexes: A Simplification*. Chicago: Year Book Medical Publishers, 1945.

Wartenberg R. *Diagnostic Tests in Neurology: A Selection for Office Use*. Chicago: Year Book Medical Publishers, 1953.

Weibers DO, Dale AJD, Kokmen E, et al., eds. *Mayo Clinic Examinations in Neurology*. 7th ed. St. Louis: The C.V. Mosby Co., 1998.

Yudkowsky R, Otaki J, Lowenstein T, et al. A hypothesis-driven physical examination learning and assessment procedure for medical students: initial validity evidence. *Med Educ* 2009; 43:729–740.

SECTION C Mental Status Examination and Higher Cortical Functions

CHAPTER 6

Gross and Microscopic Anatomy of the Cerebral Hemispheres

The major fissures and sulci of the cerebral hemispheres are shown in Figures 6.1 and 6.2. Cytoarchitectonic maps are based on regional differences in the microscopic anatomy of the cortical layers (Figure 6.3). The frontal lobe extends from the frontal pole to the central sulcus above the sylvian fissure. It makes up about the anterior one-half of each hemisphere. The frontal lobe is made up of four principal gyri: precentral, superior frontal, middle frontal, and inferior frontal. The precentral gyrus (motor strip) lies just anterior to the central sulcus (Figure 6.4). A homunculus is a distorted figure with the size of an anatomical part proportional to the amount of the cortex to which it is related. The motor homunculus depicts the organization of the motor strip according to body part innervated (Figure 6.5). On the medial surface, the frontal lobe extends down to the cingulate sulcus (Figure 6.2). The paracentral lobule consists of the extensions of the precentral and postcentral gyri onto the medial hemispheric surface above the cingulate sulcus; it is important in bladder control. The supplementary motor and premotor regions lie in area 6, anterior to the precentral gyrus. The supplementary motor area is a portion of the superior frontal gyrus that lies on the medial surface; the premotor area lies on the lateral surface. The frontal eye fields lie in the middle frontal gyrus, in part of area 8. The inferior frontal gyrus is divided into the pars orbitalis, pars triangularis, and the pars opercularis. The pars opercularis and triangularis of the inferior frontal gyrus of the dominant hemisphere contain the motor (Broca's) speech area (areas 44 and 45). On the inferior surface of the frontal lobe, medial to the inferior frontal gyrus, are the orbital gyri. They are separated by the olfactory sulcus from the gyrus rectus, which is the most medial structure on the orbital surface (Figure 6.6). The olfactory bulbs and tracts overlie the olfactory sulcus.

The parietal lobe lies posterior to the central sulcus, anterior to the occipital lobe, and superior to the temporal lobe. An imaginary line drawn between the parietooccipital sulcus and the preoccipital notch separates the parietal and occipital lobes. An imaginary line extending from the sylvian fissure to the midpoint of the preceding line separates the parietal lobe above from the temporal lobe below. The parietal lobe consists of the following five principal parts: the postcentral gyrus, the superior parietal lobule, the inferior parietal lobule, the precuneus, and the posterior portion of the paracentral lobule. The postcentral gyrus (areas 1, 2, and 3) is the primary sensory cortex; it lies between the central sulcus and the postcentral sulcus. The sensory homunculus depicts the representation of body parts in the primary sensory cortex; it is similar but not identical to the motor homunculus (Figure 6.7). The secondary somatosensory cortex lies in the inferior portion of the postcentral gyrus,

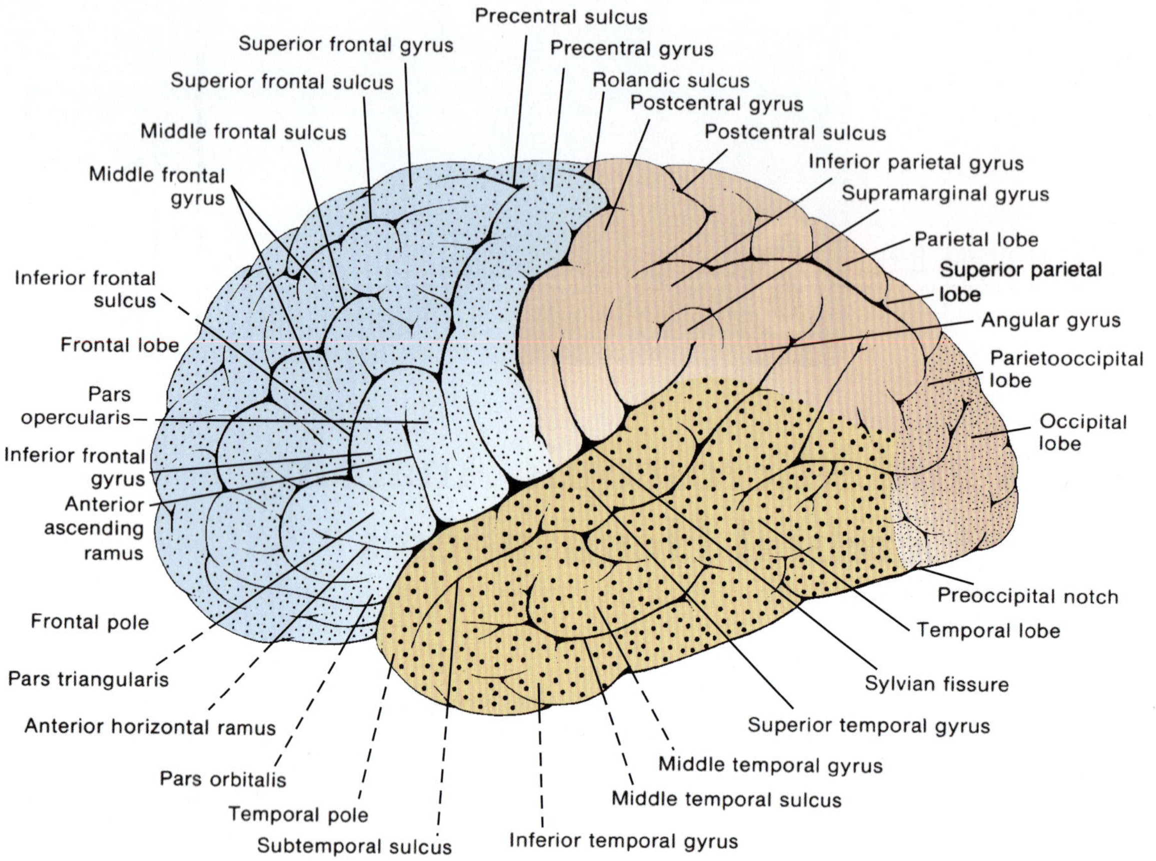

FIGURE 6.1 Lobes, sulci, and gyri of the lateral aspect of the cerebral hemisphere. The frontal and occipital lobes are *finely stippled*, the temporal lobe *coarsely stippled*, and the parietal lobe *unstippled*.

abutting the sylvian fissure. The superior parietal lobule is a somatosensory association area that lies posterior to the trunk and upper extremity segments of the postcentral gyrus. The inferior parietal lobule lies posterior to the face and tongue segments of the postcentral gyrus, and it has the following two major components: the supramarginal gyrus, which caps the upturned end of the sylvian fissure, and the angular gyrus, which is at the end of the parallel superior temporal sulcus (Figure 6.1). The inferior parietal lobule is association cortex for somatosensory, visual, and auditory functions. The precuneus is an area of the cortex just anterior to the occipital lobe on the medial hemispheric surface.

The temporal lobe is a tongue-shaped anterior projection that originates as an evagination of the developing cerebral hemisphere; it carries along its central cavity, forming the temporal horn of the lateral ventricle. The temporal lobe lies below the sylvian fissure, extending from the temporal pole to the arbitrary limits of the parietal and occipital lobes. The ventral surface lies on the floor of the middle cranial fossa. The lateral surface has three gyri: the superior, middle, and inferior, which are separated by the superior, middle, and inferior temporal sulci (Figure 6.1). Buried in the sylvian fissure at the posterior end of the superior temporal gyrus on its dorsal surface—running at right angles to the gyrus and stretching toward the medial geniculate body—are the transverse temporal gyri (of Heschl). The transverse temporal gyri are the primary auditory cortex (areas 41 and 42). Immediately adjacent to the primary auditory cortex is the auditory association cortex (area 22); in the dominant hemisphere, part of this is the Wernicke's speech area. The planum temporale lies just behind the Heschl gyri and is part of Wernicke's area. The planum temporale is larger in the left hemisphere in most individuals and is probably related to cerebral dominance for language. On the base of the temporal lobe, the inferior temporal

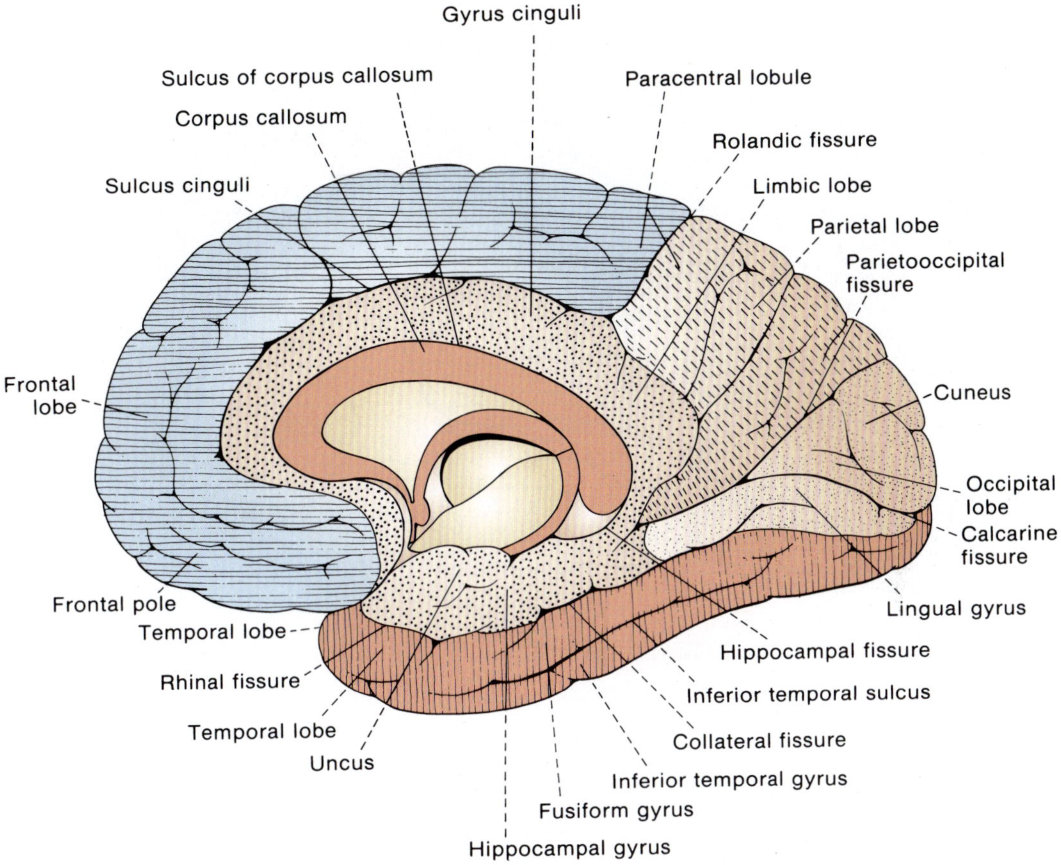

FIGURE 6.2 Lobes, sulci, and gyri of the medial aspect of the cerebral hemisphere. The frontal lobe is *lined horizontally* and the temporal *vertically*, the parietal lobe is *dashed*, the limbic lobe is *stippled*, and the occipital lobe *plain*.

gyrus is continuous medially with the lateral occipitotemporal gyrus. The occipitotemporal sulcus separates the lateral occipitotemporal (inferior temporal) gyrus from the medial occipitotemporal (fusiform) gyrus. Medial to the fusiform gyrus, separated by the collateral sulcus, is the parahippocampal (hippocampal) gyrus, part of the limbic lobe. Posterior to the isthmus of the cingulate, the parahippocampal gyrus stretches toward the occipital pole and becomes the lingual gyrus.

The occipital lobe is only a small part of the dorsolateral surface of the hemisphere, but it occupies a large triangular field on the medial aspect of the brain between the parietal and temporal lobes. The calcarine fissure separates the medial surface of the occipital lobe into the cuneus above and the lingual (medial occipitotemporal) gyrus below. The occipital lobe is the visual cortex (areas 17, 18, and 19). The cuneus forms the upper bank, and the lingual gyrus the lower bank, of the calcarine cortex.

The limbic lobe is sometimes considered a separate lobe of the brain, more because of its function than its anatomy. Components of the limbic lobe include the following: the hippocampus, which lies deep in the medial temporal lobe and becomes continuous with the fornix; the mammillary bodies (part of the hypothalamus); the anterior nucleus of the thalamus; the cingulate gyrus; and the parahippocampal gyrus. As with several other central nervous system (CNS) structures, the limbic lobe morphologically is a C-shaped structure. It begins anteriorly and superiorly in the paraterminal gyrus and subcallosal area beneath the rostrum of the corpus callosum. The body of the C is formed by the cingulate gyrus, which merges at the isthmus of the cingulate into the parahippocampal (hippocampal) gyrus. The end of the C is the hippocampal formation. The cingulate gyrus lies just above the corpus callosum. The parahippocampal gyrus begins at the isthmus of the cingulate and runs to the temporal tip, lying between

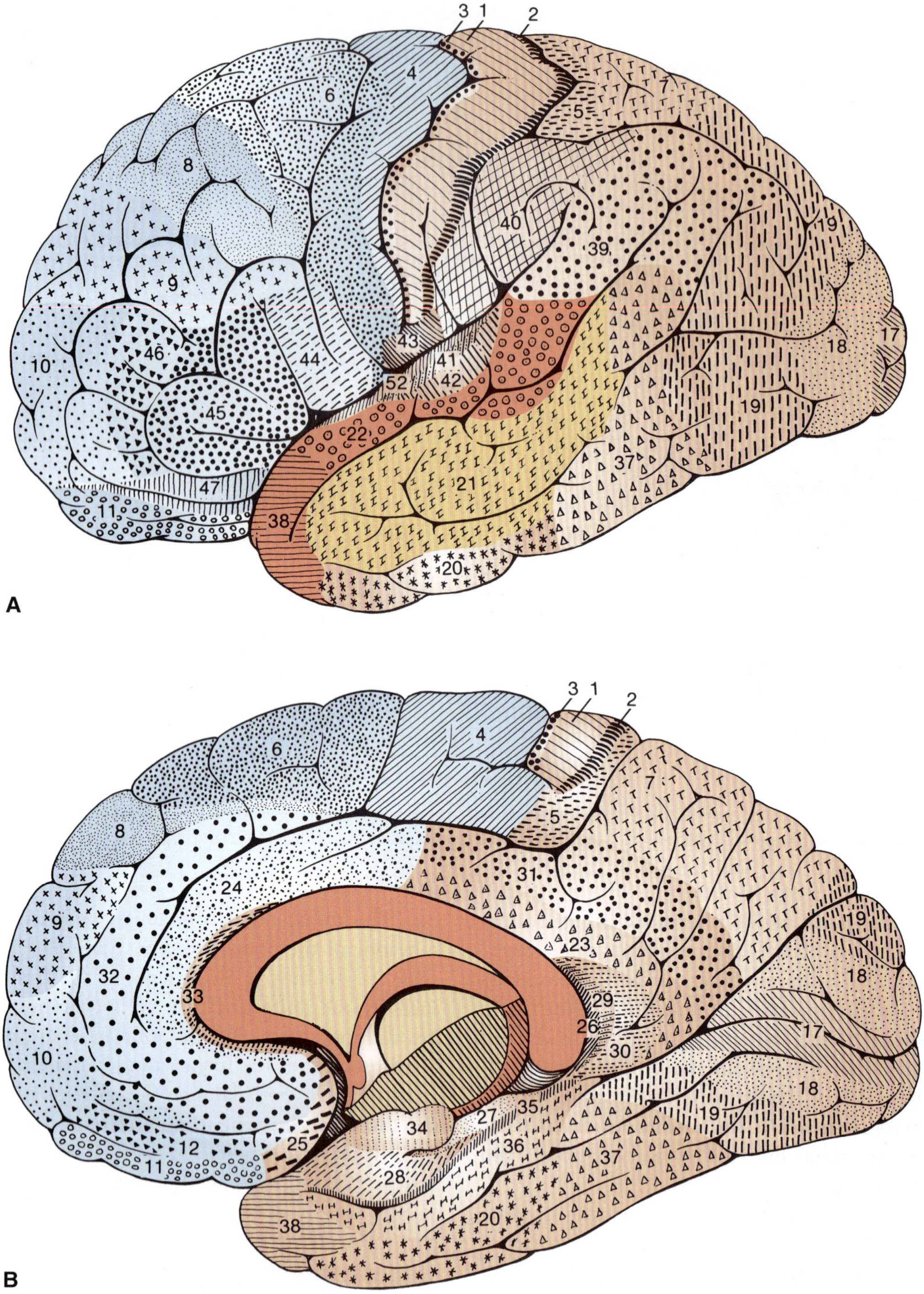

FIGURE 6.3 Areas of the cerebral cortex, each of which possesses a distinctive structure. **A.** Lateral surface. **B.** Medial surface. (Modified from Brodmann K. *Vergleichende Lokalisationslehre der Grosshirnrinde in ihren Prinzipien dargestellt auf Grund des Zellenbaues*. Leipzig: Johann Ambrosius Barth, 1909.)

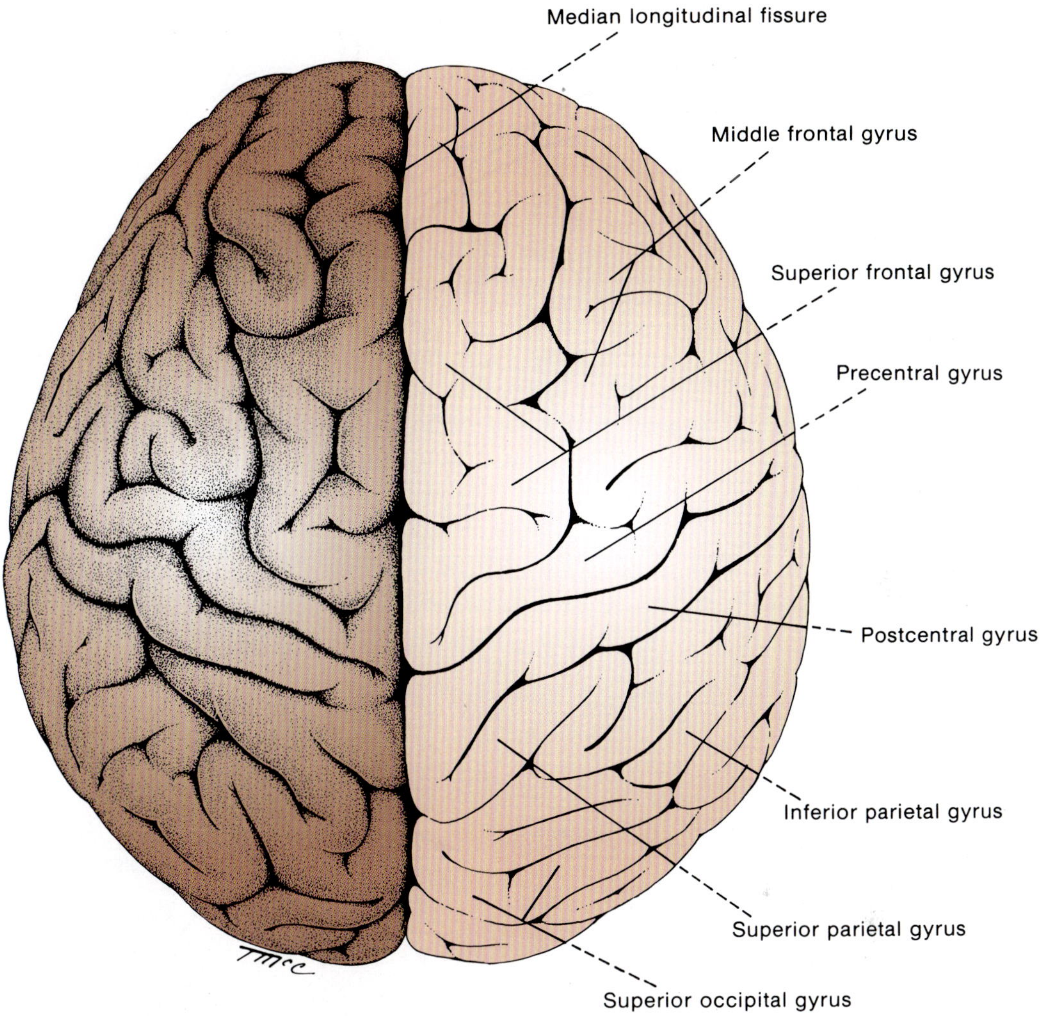

FIGURE 6.4 Gross structure of the cerebral hemispheres as seen from above.

the collateral sulcus and the hippocampus; it curls around the hippocampal fissure to form the uncus. The hippocampal formation is composed of the hippocampus proper (Ammon's horn), the dentate gyrus, and the subiculum. When not regarded as part of the limbic lobe, the anterior and posterior parts of the cingulate gyrus are considered parts of the frontal and parietal lobes, respectively. The parahippocampal gyrus and hippocampal formation are considered part of the temporal lobe. The structures of the limbic lobe are connected in Papez circuit (cingulate gyrus → parahippocampal gyrus → hippocampus → fornix → mammillary body → anterior nucleus of the thalamus → cingulate gyrus).

The rhinencephalon (nose brain) is a primitive, basal forebrain region involved with olfaction and emotion that is closely related to the limbic lobe. It consists of the olfactory bulbs and tracts, the olfactory stria, olfactory trigone (olfactory tubercle, anterior perforated substance, and diagonal band of Broca), the piriform lobe (uncus, entorhinal area, and limen insulae), and part of the amygdala. The hippocampal formation is sometimes included as part of the rhinencephalon.

CORTICAL LAYERS

The cerebral cortex begins as an outpouching of the rostral end of the neural tube, and it culminates as a complex cellular layer that covers the surface of the brain. After formation of the marginal and mantle

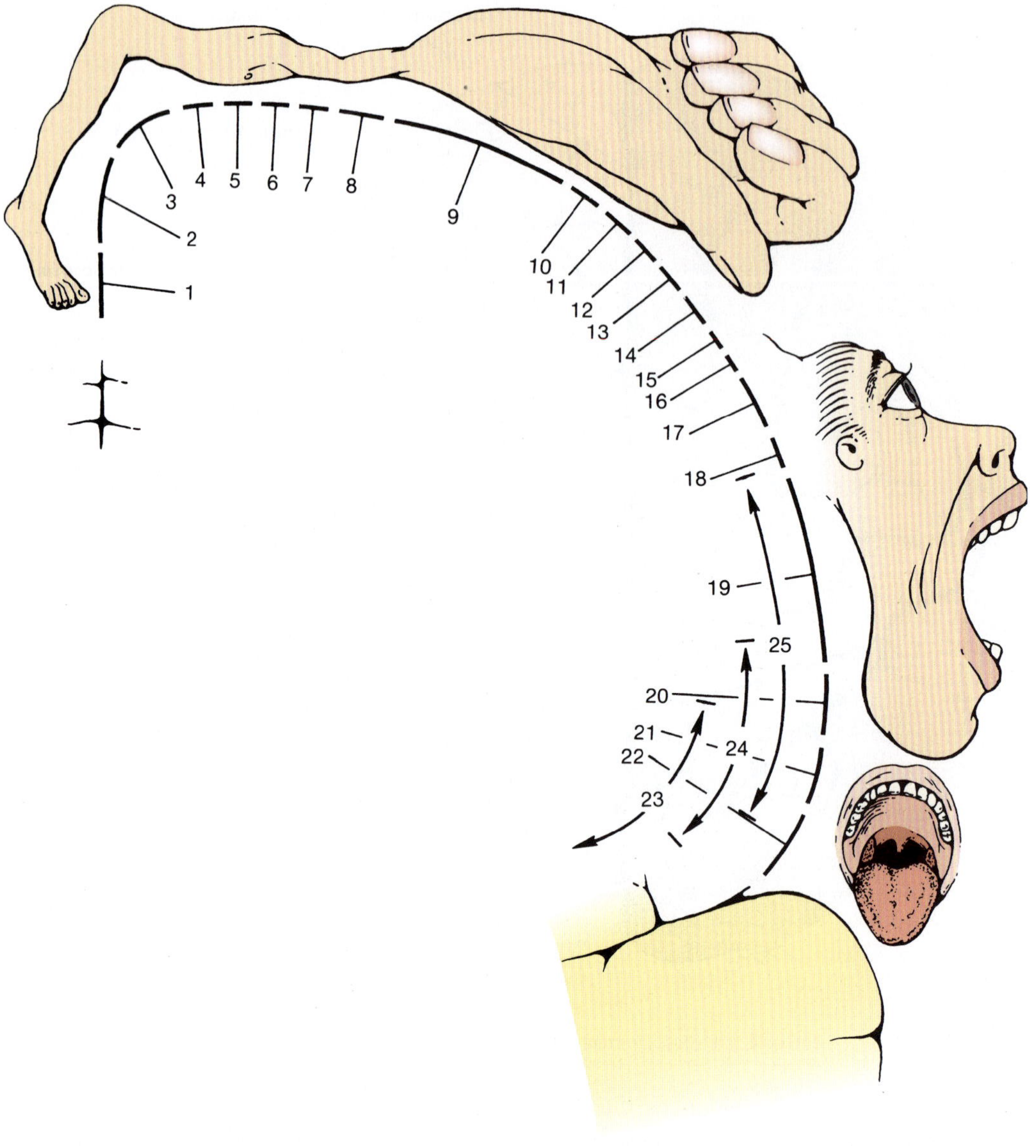

FIGURE 6.5 Motor homunculus, showing the relationship of the motor centers to cortical representation. *1*, toes; *2*, ankle; *3*, knee; *4*, hip; *5*, trunk; *6*, shoulder; *7*, elbow; *8*, wrist; *9*, hand; *10*, little finger; *11*, ring finger; *12*, middle finger; *13*, index finger; *14*, thumb; *15*, neck; *16*, brow; *17*, eyelid and eyeball; *18*, face; *19*, lips; *20*, jaw; *21*, tongue; *22*, swallowing; *23*, mastication; *24*, salivation; *25*, vocalization. (Modified from Penfield W, Rasmussen T. *The Cerebral Cortex of Man*. New York: Macmillan, 1950.)

layers, cells migrate from the marginal layer to form the cerebral cortex. Migrational defects are a common cause of congenital brain malformations, such as gray matter heterotopias. Between the 6th and 8th month of fetal life, the migrating cells reach the cortex and become organized into strata, which eventually become the cortical layers. The cortex covers the gyri and convolutions and dips into the fissures and sulci. About one-third is on the exposed surface, and the rest is buried in the fissures and sulci. There are about 15 to 30 billion nerve cells in the cortex. Its thickness varies from 4.5 mm in the precentral gyrus to 1.3 mm near the occipital pole.

Most of the cortical mantle has six identifiable layers; some areas of the brain have less (Figure 6.8). Six-layered cortex is referred to as neocortex, isocortex, or heterogenetic cortex. The six layers, from superficial to deep, are as follows: (I) molecular

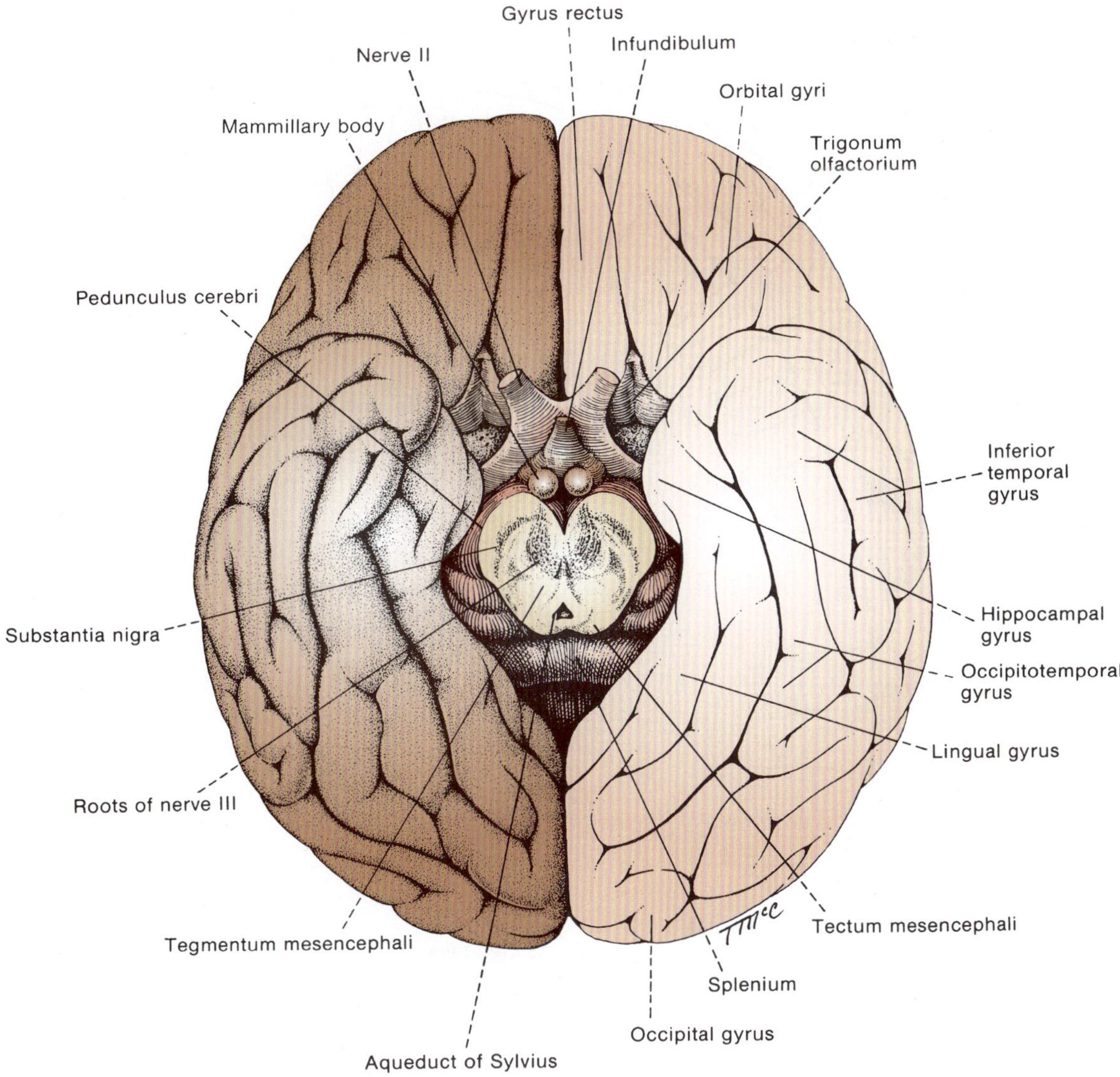

FIGURE 6.6 Base of the human brain.

(plexiform), (II) external granular, (III) external pyramidal, (IV) internal granular, (V) internal pyramidal (ganglion), and (VI) multiform. The molecular layer is most superficial, covered by pia. It consists of a dense tangle of fibers composed of dendrites of deeper lying cells. Pyramidal cells are sparse and small. Layer 2, the external granular layer, is made up of small, densely packed neurons. Layer 3, the external pyramidal layer, consists of medium to large pyramidal-shaped neurons. It is sometimes subdivided into a superficial layer of medium pyramidal cells and a deep layer of large pyramidal cells. Layer 4, the internal granular layer, consists of many small, multipolar granule cells with short axons and scattered small pyramidal cells. Granule cells are most numerous in this layer. Layer 5, the internal pyramidal (ganglion cell) layer, consists of medium and large pyramidal cells, among which are the largest neurons found in the cortex. In the precentral gyrus, this layer contains the giant pyramidal cells of Betz, the neurons whose axons form the corticospinal and corticobulbar tracts. The deepest cortical layer is the multiform layer, which consists of polymorphic cells whose short axons enter the subjacent white matter.

Isocortex is found in the neopallium, which makes up about 90% of the cortical surface. Severe compromise of brain energy supplies, such as in hypoxia, ischemia, or hypoglycemia, may lead to

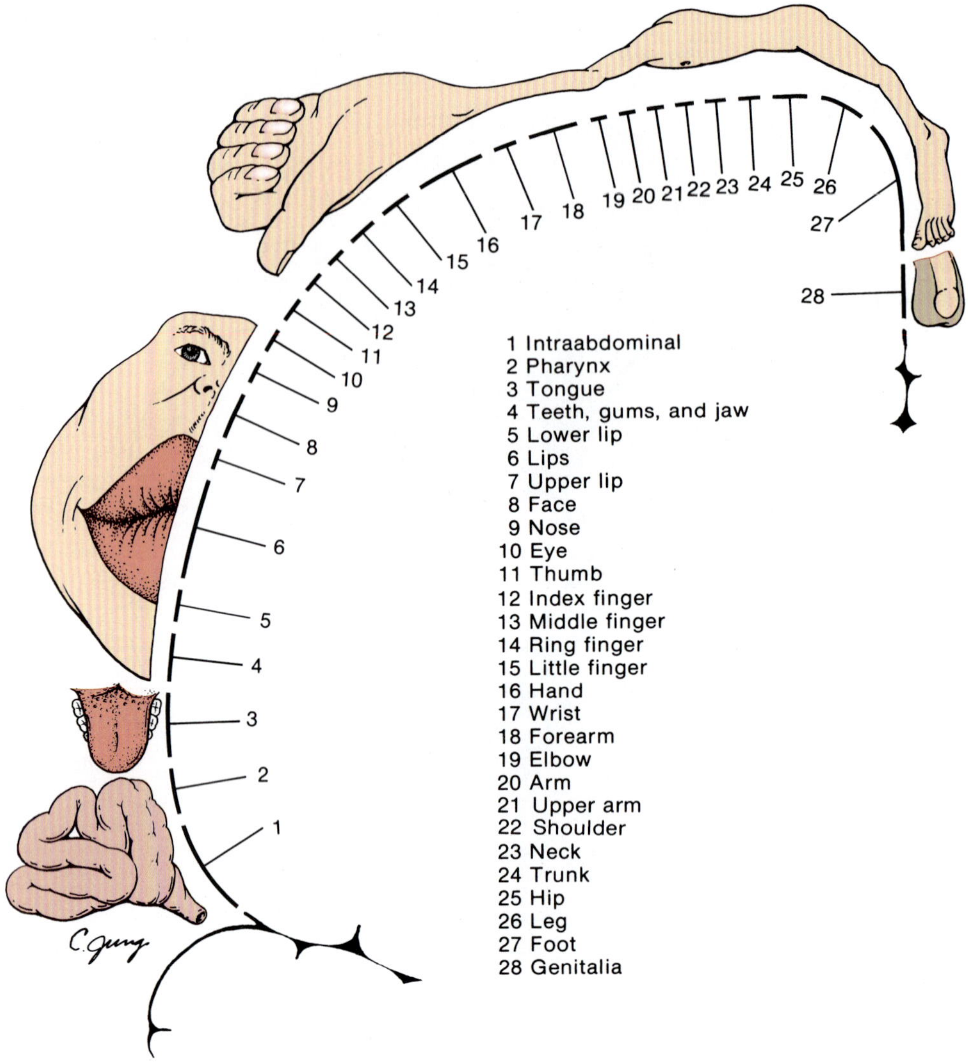

FIGURE 6.7 Homunculus showing cortical sensory representation. (Modified from Penfield W, Rasmussen T. *The Cerebral Cortex of Man*. New York: Macmillan, 1950.)

selective destruction of certain cortical layers, mainly the third—a condition termed cortical laminar necrosis. The archipallium and paleopallium both have three-layered cortex, referred to as allocortex.

Different areas of the cortex have characteristic appearances, with differences in the overall thickness of the cortical layer, the thickness and arrangement of specific cellular layers, the cell structure, the number of afferent and efferent myelinated fibers, and the number and position of white stria. How regional differences in the cytoarchitecture correlate with differences in function remains a matter of conjecture. Maps based on differences in cellular structure are referred to as cytoarchitectonic and on differences in fiber structure as myelotectonic. The best known cytoarchitectonic map is that of Brodmann (Figure 6.3). Modern imaging and the use of other cortical markers may lead to a newer generation of more accurate maps.

The cortex sends and receives fibers to and from other areas of the brain. Layer 4 contains a dense horizontal band of fibers—the external band of Baillarger. This band contains the terminal ramifications of the thalamocortical projections from the specific thalamic relay nuclei. The external band of Baillarger is particularly prominent in the calcarine cortex, forming a grossly visible white stripe—the line or band of Gennari—that gives the striate cortex its name.

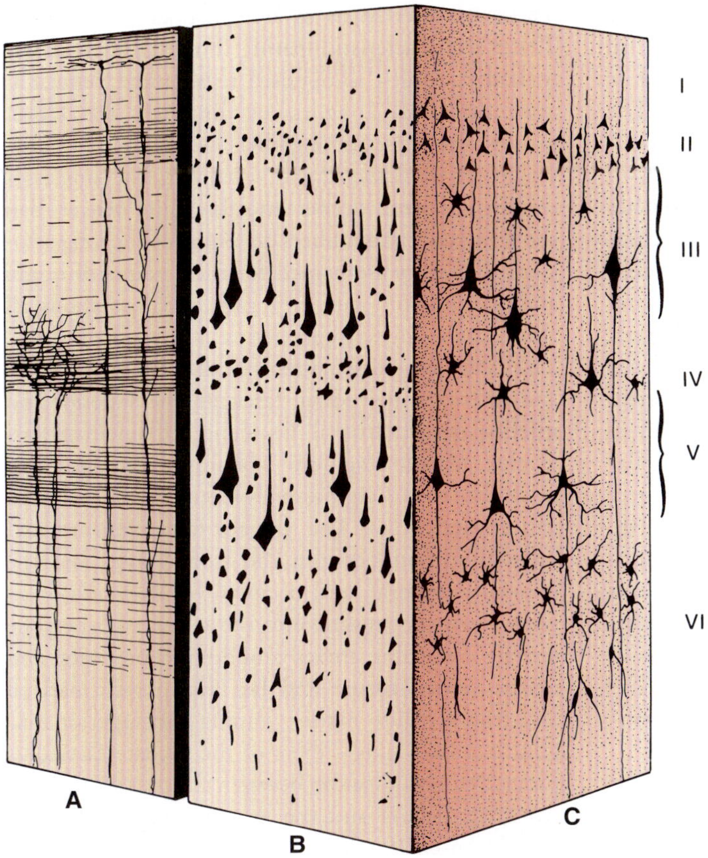

FIGURE 6.8 Cell layers and fiber arrangement of the cerebral cortex. **A.** Weigert stain. **B.** Nissl stain. **C.** Golgi stain. Layers: *I*, molecular layer; *II*, external granular layer; *III*, external pyramidal layer; *IV*, internal granular layer; *V*, internal pyramidal layer; *VI*, multiforme layer.

The specific thalamic sensory nuclei synapse in layer 4. The external band of Baillarger is made up of the terminal ramifications of thalamic nuclei that subserve specific sensory modalities, such as vision and exteroceptive sensation. In contrast, the nonspecific thalamic nuclei (reticular, intralaminar) project diffusely to all layers of the cortex.

Isocortex can also be simply divided into supragranular and infragranular layers. Layers above layer 4 (the dense internal granular layer) are supragranular; those below layer 4 are infragranular. The supragranular cortex (primarily layer 2 and layer 3) is highly differentiated and phylogenetically recent. Supragranular afferents and efferents are primarily associative; they are concerned with higher-level integrative functions and corticocortical connections. The infragranular cortex is more primitive. It is well developed in lower forms, and it primarily sends descending projection fibers to lower centers. Six-layered isocortex is formed essentially by the presence of supragranular cortex atop three-layered allocortex. The supragranular layers are not present in the archipallium and paleopallium.

Isocortex may be either homotypical, in which six layers can be easily discerned, or heterotypical, in which lamination is less obvious. The cortex can also be divided into granular and agranular types. In agranular cortex, the granule cell layers are poorly developed, whereas the pyramidal cell layers are prominent. Agranular cortex is characteristic of the precentral gyrus. Granular cortex (koniocortex) is thin and contains dense granule cell layers; the pyramidal cell layers are less conspicuous. Granular cortex is characteristic of areas that receive heavy afferent input, such as the calcarine cortex. There is a striking paucity of granule cells in the agranular cortex, for example, the motor strip, and a paucity of pyramidal cells in the granular cortex, for example, the primary sensory areas. Koniocortex is seen only in areas that receive projections from the specific thalamic relay nuclei. Cortical areas that receive thalamocortical projections from the specific thalamic relay nuclei therefore have the following two morphologic characteristics: granular type cortex and a prominent external band of Baillarger.

In addition to its horizontal, laminated organization, the cortex is also organized vertically into columns. Neurons subserving the same modality and with similar receptive fields are organized into vertical rows that extend from the cortical surface to the white matter, which is referred to as cortical columns. The vertical column organization is particularly prominent in the occipital, parietal, and temporal lobes.

Beneath the cortical mantle of gray matter lies the white matter, which consists of association, commissural, and projection axons—as well as glial cells and blood vessels. The association and commissural fibers connect one area of the cortex with another. Association fibers connect cortical areas within the same hemisphere; commissural fibers connect to areas in the opposite hemisphere. Association and commissural fibers come primarily from the supragranular cortex (layer 1 to layer 3). Projection fibers connect the cortex with lower centers (Figures 6.9 and 6.10). Projection fibers arise primarily from the infragranular cortex (layer 5 and layer 6) and go to lower centers of the nervous system. The corticospinal tract is composed of projection fibers that arise from neurons in the deeper layers of the precentral gyrus. The number of projection fibers is surprisingly small in comparison to the total number of neurons in the cortex.

Corticocortical association fibers may be short or long. Some association fibers are very short, synapsing near their origin and remaining within the cortex. Other short association fibers loop from one gyrus to an adjacent gyrus, running in the depths of a sulcus in the most superficial layer of the cortical white matter. These are referred to as arcuate fibers or U-fibers. There is characteristic sparing of the U-fibers in the leukodystrophies, as opposed to acquired demyelinating disorders. Long association fibers travel over greater distances. Some gather into discrete bundles, which can be dissected and visualized. The long association fibers run deeper into the white matter than the short association fibers do. Some of the long association bundles are named for their points of origin and termination, but they gain and lose axons all along their course, connecting intermediate areas. The major long association bundles are the superior and inferior longitudinal fasciculi, the superior and inferior occipitofrontal fasciculi, the uncinate fasciculus, and the cingulum. The superior longitudinal fasciculus runs longitudinally between the occipital and frontal poles. The arcuate fasciculus provides communication between the frontal lobe and the parietal, temporal, and occipital lobes. Many of its fibers curve downward into the temporal lobe. The arcuate fasciculus arches around the posterior end of the sylvian fissure and lies deep in the parietal and frontal white matter, joining the superior longitudinal fasciculus. Fibers of the arcuate fasciculus provide communication between the posterior, receptive (Wernicke's) and the anterior, motor (Broca's) speech centers (Figure 9.1). The inferior longitudinal (occipitotemporal) fasciculus is a thin layer of fibers that runs inferiorly, near the geniculocalcarine tract, connecting the occipital and temporal lobes. The

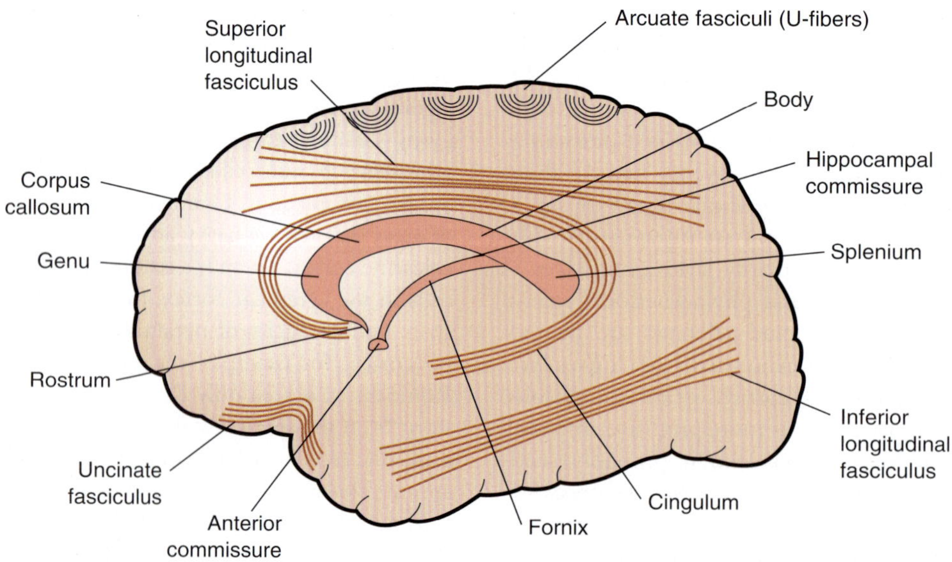

FIGURE 6.9 Sagittal view demonstrating short association fibers (arcuate or U-fibers), long association bundles, and major commissures.

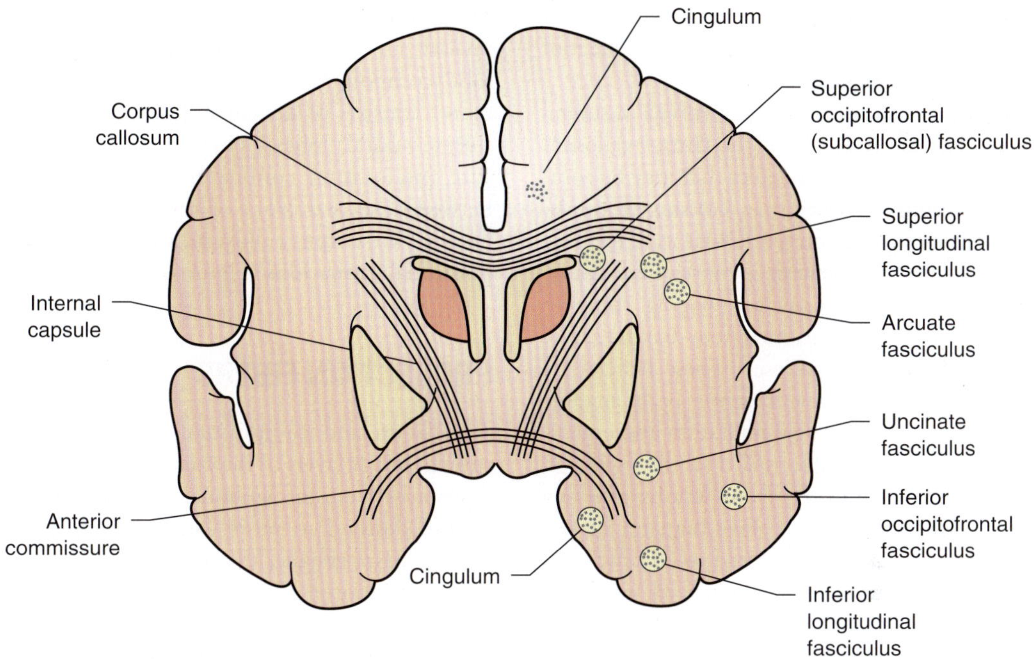

FIGURE 6.10 Coronal view demonstrating major association, commissural, and projection fiber systems.

superior occipitofrontal (subcallosal) fasciculus is a compact bundle that lies deep in the hemisphere just below the corpus callosum; it connects the posterior portions of the hemisphere with the frontal lobe. The inferior occipitofrontal fasciculus runs near the temporal lobe. The uncinate fasciculus arches through the stem of the sylvian fissure to connect the inferior temporal lobe to the orbital surface of the frontal lobe. The cingulum is a white matter tract that runs deep to the cortex of the cingulate gyrus. It is part of the limbic system and interconnects the cingulate gyrus, parahippocampal gyrus, and the septal area. Lesions involving these long association bundles are responsible for cortical disconnection syndromes—disorders in which a clinical deficit occurs because of the inability of one portion of the hemisphere to communicate normally with another portion.

COMMISSURAL FIBERS

Commissural fibers connect an area of one hemisphere with the corresponding, mirror-image area of the other hemisphere. The primary brain commissures are the corpus callosum, the anterior commissure, and the hippocampal commissure (Figures 6.9 and 6.10). There are many smaller commissures.

The corpus callosum is the largest of the commissural systems. It consists of a broad band of fibers located at the bottom of the interhemispheric fissure that connects the neocortical areas of the two hemispheres. It is composed of the body, the major portion; the anterior genu, which tapers into the rostrum; and a thickened posterior termination, the splenium. Fibers connecting the anterior portions of the frontal lobes, including the speech areas, course through the anterior third; the body carries fibers from the posterior portions of the frontal lobes and the parietal lobes; the splenium contains fibers from the temporal and occipital lobes. Fibers that sweep around the anterior portion of the interhemispheric fissure, forming the genu, are referred to as the forceps minor (forceps frontalis); fibers that sweep around posteriorly, forming the splenium, are referred to as the forceps major (forceps occipitalis). The corpus callosum does not contain crossing fibers from the striate cortex or the hand area of the motor or sensory cortices. These areas communicate by the transcallosal connections of their respective association cortex. The rostrum lies just below the frontal horn of the lateral ventricle. It is continuous with the lamina terminalis, which forms the anterior wall of the third ventricle. The subcallosal and paraterminal gyri, part of the limbic system, lie just beneath the rostrum.

The tapetum is a thin sheet of radiating callosal fibers that forms the roof of the temporal horn and the roof and lateral wall of the occipital horn.

The corpus callosum may be involved in several clinical syndromes. Agenesis of the corpus callosum is a common developmental defect that may be complete or incomplete. Rather than crossing, commissural fibers cluster along the ventricular wall, forming the bundle of Probst. Agenesis is most often discovered incidentally by autopsy or imaging study in patients with no symptoms, but there may be severe clinical deficits in some patients. These deficits are likely related to other, accompanying brain malformations or defects of neuronal migration and organization. There may be intellectual disability, seizures, and motor deficits resulting from lesions affecting contiguous structures. Marchiafava-Bignami disease is a rare condition, probably related to chronic alcoholism and undernutrition, characterized by necrosis and degeneration of the middle two-thirds of the corpus callosum. Clinical manifestations range from dementia, apraxia, gait abnormalities, spasticity, seizures, incontinence, and psychiatric disturbances to stupor and coma. Tumors, particularly gliomas, may involve the corpus callosum (butterfly glioma). Anterior cerebral artery thrombosis may cause softening of a large portion of the corpus callosum. Neurocognitive symptoms are prominent and include the following: apathy, drowsiness, loss of memory, difficulty in concentration, personality changes, and other manifestations typical of a frontal lobe lesion.

Commissurotomy is division of the corpus callosum, now rarely used, to treat intractable epilepsy. Commissurotomy disrupts the major corticocortical connections between the two hemispheres. Patients with split-brain syndrome—with agenesis of the corpus callosum or postcommissurotomy—have been used to investigate hemispheric lateralization and interhemispheric communication, because stimuli can be presented selectively to one hemisphere and the functions of the two hemispheres studied separately.

The anterior commissure arose phylogenetically as part of the rhinencephalon; it connects the olfactory bulbs, amygdala, and basal forebrain regions of the two sides. It lies in the lamina terminalis, forming part of the anterior wall of the third ventricle, above the optic chiasm, behind and below the rostrum of the corpus callosum (Figure 6.9). The fornix splits around the anterior commissure into pre- and postcommissural parts. The anterior commissure connects the olfactory bulbs and temporal lobes of the two hemispheres. It has several subsystems connecting different temporal lobe components; the major component in primates consists of neocortical connections between the temporal lobes. The hippocampal commissure (psalterium, commissure of the fornix) runs between the two crura of the fornix, beneath the body of the corpus callosum, and connects the hippocampal formations (Figure 6.9).

PROJECTION FIBERS

Association and commissural fibers arise from the supragranular layers of the cortex. Efferent projection fibers arise from infragranular cortex, primarily layer 5, and descend to more caudal structures, including the basal ganglia, thalamus, reticular formation, brainstem motor nuclei, and spinal cord. Afferent projection fibers ascend from deeper structures, such as the thalamus and striatum, and project to the cortex. Afferent projection fibers terminate in the supragranular cortex.

THE INTERNAL CAPSULE

The various fibers coming to and proceeding from the cortex make up the fan-shaped corona radiata. Fibers of the corona radiata converge into a broad band, which is the internal capsule. Early CNS dissectors saw the profusion of fibers going in all directions as a "radiating crown" perched atop the internal capsule. The internal capsule contains most of the fibers, both efferent and afferent, that communicate with the cerebral cortex. A large part of the internal capsule is composed of the thalamic radiations; the rest consists of efferent fibers to lower structures. Below the level of the thalamus, the internal capsule becomes the cerebral peduncle of the midbrain. In horizontal section, the internal capsule, from anterior to posterior, has three parts: anterior limb, genu, and posterior limb. The shorter anterior limb (lenticulocaudate division) lies between the lenticular nucleus laterally and the caudate nucleus anteromedially. Early in development, the caudate and putamen are fused. They separate but remain attached by strands of gray matter. The fibers of the anterior limb of the capsule weave between the gray matter bridges, giving the anterior limb a striated appearance in some sections. The marbling created by the internal capsule fibers led to the name corpus striatum for the caudate and putamen (see Chapter 26). The junction between the anterior and posterior limbs is the genu, the apex of the obtuse angle formed by the two limbs. The apex of the globus pallidus fits into the angle of the genu. A line drawn between the genua of the two internal capsules lies just posterior to the foramen of Monro. The longer posterior limb of the internal capsule (lenticulothalamic division) lies between the lenticular nucleus laterally and the thalamus posteromedially. The posterior limb has a retrolenticular portion, which projects behind the lenticular nucleus to reach the occipital cortex, and a sublenticular portion, which passes below the posterior part of the nucleus to reach the temporal lobe.

The anterior limb of the internal capsule is composed of the frontopontine tract and the anterior thalamic radiations. Fibers of the frontopontine tract arise in the motor and premotor regions of the frontal cortex. They descend in the medial part of the cerebral peduncle to the ipsilateral pontine nuclei. After a synapse, an impulse is transmitted through the middle cerebellar peduncle to the opposite cerebellar hemisphere. Related fibers from other cortical areas, the parietotemporopontine and occipitopontine tracts, travel in the retrolentiform part of the capsule and descend in the lateral portion of the cerebral peduncle. The anterior limb also contains the corticostriatal projections.

In general, any area of the cortex that receives thalamic afferents sends efferents back to the same thalamic nucleus, and these also run in the thalamic radiations. The anterior thalamic radiations (anterior thalamic peduncle) primarily consist of fibers connecting the dorsomedial (DM) thalamic nucleus and the prefrontal cortex. There are also connections between the frontal lobe and the anterior thalamic nuclei, the hypothalamus, and limbic structures.

The genu of the internal capsule contains the corticobulbar tracts, which carry impulses from the lower portion of the precentral (and premotor) cortex to the motor nuclei of the cranial nerves. The corticobulbar fibers pass largely, but not entirely, to contralateral nuclei.

The posterior limb of the internal capsule has many important components, most notably the corticospinal tract. Since observations by Charcot, Dejerine, and Dejerine-Klumpke, the corticospinal fibers were thought to lie in the anterior two-thirds of the posterior limb. It now appears that the fibers of the corticospinal tract lie in scattered bundles more posteriorly. The tract lies more anteriorly in its course through the rostral capsule and shifts posteriorly as it descends. Fibers destined for the upper limb are more anterior. The somatotopic organization in the rostral internal capsule, from anterior to posterior, is face/arm/leg. In its descent, the frontopontine tract gradually moves from the anterior limb to the anterior part of the posterior limb as the corticospinal tract transitions to a more posterior position. Other descending fibers in the posterior limb include corticostriatal, corticorubral, corticoreticular, and cortico-olivary. Ascending fibers in the posterior limb include the middle thalamic radiations (middle thalamic peduncle), which carry fibers from the ventral posterior thalamic nuclei to the sensory cortex, and fibers from the ventral anterior (VA) and ventral lateral (VL) thalamic nuclei to the motor, premotor, and supplementary motor areas.

The posterior thalamic radiations (posterior thalamic peduncle), composed mainly of the optic radiations (geniculocalcarine tract), make up most of the retrolenticular part of the internal capsule. The optic radiations are separated from the temporal horn of the lateral ventricle by the tapetum of the corpus callosum. Other retrolenticular fibers include the parietopontine, occipitopontine, occipitocollicular, occipitotectal, and connections between the occipital lobes and the pulvinar. The sublenticular part of the capsule is made up primarily of the auditory radiations (inferior thalamic peduncle), carrying fibers from the medial geniculate body below and behind the lenticular nucleus to the auditory cortex in the temporal lobe. Other sublenticular fibers include temporopontine, thalamopallidal, and pallidothalamic.

The internal capsule is frequently involved in cerebrovascular disease, especially small vessel lacunar infarcts related to hypertension. Because all of the descending motor fibers are grouped compactly together, a single small lesion may impair the function in all of them and produce a hemiparesis with equal involvement of face, arm, and leg without sensory abnormalities: the syndrome of capsular pure motor hemiparesis.

Lateral to the lenticular nuclei lie, in order, the external capsule, claustrum, and extreme capsule. The external and extreme capsules are part of the subcortical white matter of the insula. Their function is largely unknown. The external capsule contains some corticostriatal and corticoreticular fibers.

THALAMUS

The thalamus serves primarily as a relay station that modulates and coordinates the function of various systems. It is a locus for integration, modulation, and intercommunication between various systems and has important motor, sensory, arousal, memory, behavioral, limbic, and cognitive functions. The largest source of afferent fibers to the thalamus is the cerebral cortex, and the cortex is the primary destination for thalamic projections. Many systems and fibers converge on the thalamus (Gr. "meeting place" or "inner chamber"). Except for olfaction, all of the ascending sensory tracts end in the thalamus, from which projections are sent to the cortex. The thalamus allows crude appreciation of most sensory modalities; only very fine discriminative sensory functions such as stereognosis, two-point discrimination, graphesthesia, and precise tactile localization require the cortex (see Chapter 32). Similarly, the thalamus synchronizes the motor system, integrating the activity of the motor cortex, basal ganglia, and cerebellum. The motor cortex in turn sends fibers to the thalamus. The thalamus also integrates function between the limbic, emotional brain, and the cortex; it is important in arousal mechanisms, subserves important memory circuits, and has specialized relay nuclei for visual and auditory function.

The thalamus lies medially in the cerebrum (Figures 6.11 and 6.12). It is the largest constituent of the diencephalon. Its dorsal aspect forms the floor of the lateral ventricle, and it is bounded medially by the third ventricle and laterally by the internal capsule and basal ganglia; ventrally, it is continuous with the subthalamus. The lateral dorsal wall, at the point of attachment of the roof of the third ventricle, is demarcated by the stria medullaris thalami. The stria medullaris thalami carry projections from the septal area to the habenular nuclei. Neuroanatomists often divide the thalamus into the dorsal thalamus, the thalamus proper, and the ventral thalamus, which consists of the subthalamic region, including the zona incerta, the fields of Forel, and other structures. The epithalamus is made up of the paraventricular nuclei, the habenular nuclei, the stria medullaris thalami, the posterior commissure, and the pineal body.

The superior surface of the thalamus is covered by a thin layer of white matter, the stratum zonale. The upper, lateral border is separated from the body of the caudate nucleus by the stria terminalis and thalamostriate vein. Laterally, the posterior limb of the internal capsule separates the thalamus and the lenticular nucleus. The lateral wall of the third ventricle makes up the medial surface of the thalamus, which is usually connected to the opposite thalamus by the interthalamic adhesion (massa intermedia). The hypothalamic sulcus separates the thalamus above from the hypothalamus below. Inferiorly, the thalamus merges with the rostral midbrain tegmentum. Laterally, the thalamus is covered by a thin layer of myelinated axons, the external medullary lamina. Scattered within it are the cells of the reticular nucleus of the thalamus.

The thalamus is divided by internal medullary lamina into large nuclear groups—medial, lateral, and anterior—which are in turn divided into component nuclei (Figure 6.12). The intralaminar nuclei lie scattered along the internal medullary laminae; they essentially comprise a rostral extension of the brainstem reticular formation. The intralaminar nuclei receive input from the reticular formation and

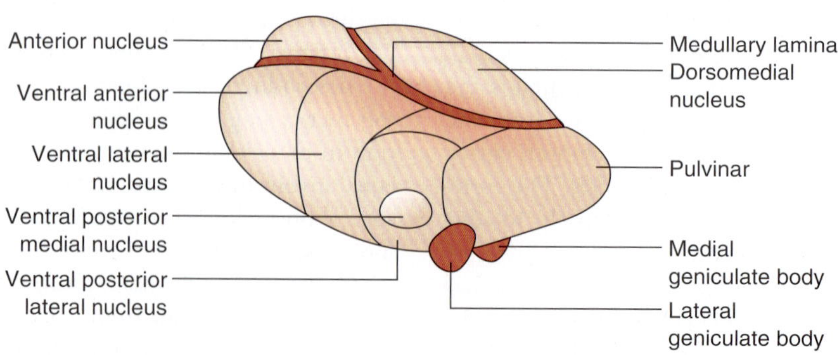

FIGURE 6.11 The thalamus showing major nuclei. The internal medullary lamina fork anteriorly to enclose the anterior nucleus. (Reprinted from Campbell WW, Pridgeon RP. *Practical Primer of Clinical Neurology*. Philadelphia: Lippincott Williams & Wilkins, 2002, with permission.)

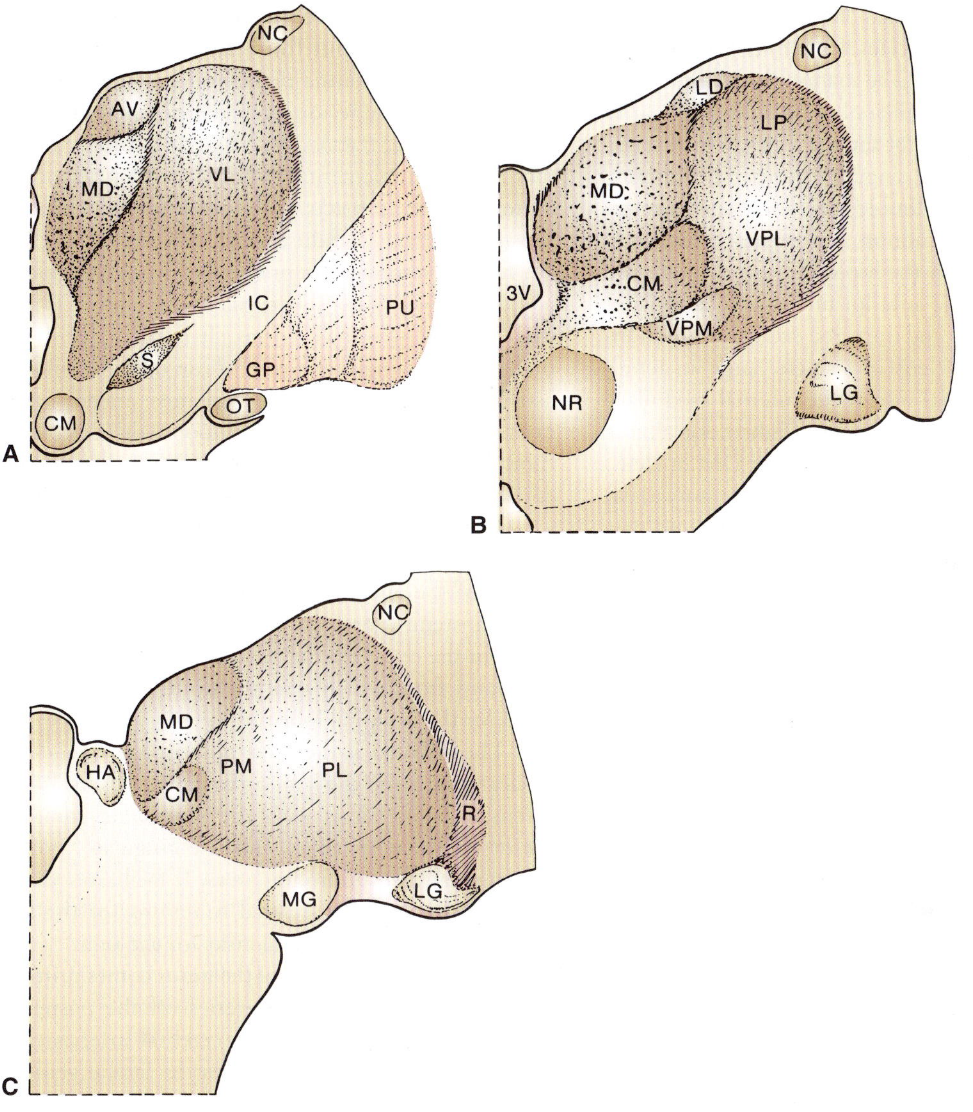

FIGURE 6.12 Cross section of the human thalamus showing the principal nuclear masses at three levels. **A.** Anterior thalamus. **B.** Midthalamus. **C.** Posterior thalamus. 3V, third ventricle; AV, nucleus anteroventralis; CM, nucleus centrum medianum; GP, globus pallidus; HA, habenula; IC, internal capsule; LD, nucleus lateralis dorsalis; LG, lateral geniculate body; LP, nucleus lateralis posterior; MD, nucleus medialis dorsalis; MG, medial geniculate body; NC, caudate nucleus; NR, red nucleus; OT, optic tract; PL, lateral nuclear group of pulvinar; PM, medial nuclear group of pulvinar; PU, putamen; R, nucleus reticularis; S, subthalamic nucleus; VL, nucleus ventralis lateralis; VPL, nucleus ventralis posterolateralis; VPM, nucleus ventralis posteromedialis.

the ascending reticular activating system and project widely to the neocortex. These nuclei are primarily concerned with arousal. The reticular and intralaminar nuclei are classified as nonspecific nuclei, as their projections are diffuse. The specific nuclei receive afferents from specific systems and project to dedicated cortical areas, for example, somatic sensation, the ventral posterior nuclei, and the somatosensory cortex. The largest and most easily identified of the intralaminar nuclei is the centromedian nucleus. It has connections with the motor cortex, globus pallidus, and striatum, and it has extensive projections to the cortex. Lesions involving the intralaminar nuclei, especially the centromedian-parafascicular complex, may cause thalamic neglect, with neglect of the contralateral body and extrapersonal space. Bilateral lesions involving the posterior intralaminar nuclei may produce akinetic mutism.

The internal medullary lamina diverges anteriorly, and the anterior nucleus lies between the arms of this Y-shaped structure. The mammillothalamic tract ascends from the mammillary bodies bound primarily for the anterior nucleus of the thalamus, which sends its major output to the cingulate gyrus. The anterior nucleus is part of the limbic lobe and Papez circuit, and it is related to emotion and memory function. It receives input from the hippocampus through the fornix. Lesions of the anterior nucleus are associated with loss of memory and impaired executive function.

The medial nucleus is a single, large structure that lies on the medial side of the internal medullary lamina. Because its position is also slightly dorsal, it is usually referred to as the mediodorsal or DM nucleus. It sends or receives projections from the amygdala, olfactory and limbic systems, hypothalamus, and prefrontal cortex. There are extensive connections with the intralaminar nuclei. The DM has functions related to cognition, judgment, affect, olfaction, emotions, sleep and waking, executive function, and memory.

In contrast to the straightforward anterior and medial nuclear groups, the lateral nuclear group is subdivided into several component nuclei. The major division is into the dorsal tier and the ventral tier. In general, the lateral nuclei serve as specific relay stations between motor and sensory systems and the related cortex. The dorsal tier nuclei consist of the lateral dorsal and lateral posterior nuclei and the pulvinar. The pulvinar is a large mass that forms the caudal extremity of the thalamus; it is the largest nucleus in the thalamus. Fibers project to it from other thalamic nuclei, from the geniculate bodies, and from the superior colliculus; and it has connections with the peristriate area and the posterior parts of the parietal lobes. The lateral posterior nucleus and the pulvinar have reciprocal connections with the occipital and parietal association cortex; they may play a role in extrageniculocalcarine vision.

The ventral tier subnuclei of the lateral nucleus are true relay nuclei, connecting lower centers with the cortex and vice versa. The ventral posterior lateral (VPL) nucleus and ventral posterior medial (VPM) nucleus are the major sensory relay nuclei. The VPL receives the termination of the lemniscal and spinothalamic sensory pathways for the body; it projects in turn to the somesthetic cortex (Brodmann areas 1, 2, and 3). VPM serves the same function for the head, receiving the trigeminothalamic tracts as well as taste fibers from the solitary nucleus; it projects to the somesthetic cortex.

The VL nucleus coordinates the motor system. The VL receives input from the basal ganglia (globus pallidus), substantia nigra, and cerebellum (dentate nucleus via superior cerebellar peduncle and the dentatothalamic tract). The VL then projects to the motor and supplementary motor areas. The motor cortex, in turn, projects to the striatum, which projects to the globus pallidus, which projects to VL. The VA nucleus also receives projections from the globus pallidus, as well as the substantia nigra; it projects primarily to the premotor cortex. It is via VL and VA that the basal ganglia and cerebellum influence motor activity (Chapter 26). The thalamus anchors two extensive sensorimotor control loops: the cerebello-rubro-thalamo-cortico-pontocerebellar loop and the cortico-striato-pallido-thalamo-cortical loop.

The geniculate bodies are also part of the ventral tier. The medical geniculate body receives the termination of the auditory pathways ascending through the brainstem; it projects to the auditory cortex. The axons in the optic tract synapse in the lateral geniculate body, from which arise the optic radiations destined for the occipital lobe.

The pulvinar is the most posterior of the lateral nuclear group and the largest thalamic nucleus. It has extensive connections with the visual and somatosensory association areas, and the cingulate, posterior parietal, and prefrontal areas. It facilitates visual attention for language-related functions for the left hemisphere and visuospatial tasks for the right.

The blood supply to the thalamus comes primarily via thalamoperforating arteries off the posterior communicating and posterior cerebral arteries; the anterior choroidal artery supplies the lateral geniculate body.

BIBLIOGRAPHY

Bogousslavsky J. Frontal stroke syndromes. *Eur Neurol* 1994;34:306–315.

Brazis PW, Masdeu JC, Biller J. *Localization in Clinical Neurology*. 7th ed. Philadelphia: Wolters Kluwer/Lippincott Williams & Wilkins, 2017.

Carpenter MB. *Core Text of Neuroanatomy*. 4th ed. Baltimore: Lippincott Williams & Wilkins, 1991:115–223.

Corballis MC, McLean A. Interhemispheric comparisons in a man with complete forebrain commissurotomy. *Neuropsychology* 2000;14:519–525.

Ferracci F, Conte F, Gentile M, et al. Marchiafava-Bignami disease: computed tomographic scan, 99mTc HMPAO-SPECT, and FlAIR MRI findings in a patient with subcortical aphasia, alexia, bilateral agraphia, and left-handed deficit of constructional ability. *Arch Neurol* 1999;56:107–110.

FitzGerald MJT, Folan-Curran J. *Clinical Neuroanatomy and Related Neuroscience*. 4th ed. Edinburgh: W. B. Saunders, 2002.

Gilman S, Newman SW. *Manter and Gatz's Essentials of Clinical Neuroanatomy and Neurophysiology*. 10th ed. Philadelphia: FA Davis, 2003.

Gould DJ, Fix JD. *Neuroanatomy*. 5th ed. Philadelphia: Wolters Kluwer Health/Lippincott Williams & Wilkins, 2014.

Hanaway J, Young RR. Localization of the pyramidal tract in the internal capsule of man. *J Neurol Sci* 1977;34:63–70.

Kiernan JA, Rajakumar N. *Barr's The Human Nervous System: An Anatomical Viewpoint*. 10th ed. Philadelphia: Wolters Kluwer Health/Lippincott Williams & Wilkins, 2014.

Macchi G, Jones EG. Toward an agreement on terminology of nuclear and subnuclear divisions of the motor thalamus. *J Neurosurg* 1997;86:670–685.

Parent A. *Carpenter's Human Neuroanatomy*. 9th ed. Baltimore: Lippincott Williams & Wilkins, 1996.

Ross ED. Localization of the pyramidal tract in the internal capsule by whole brain dissection. *Neurology* 1980;30:59–64.

Sakakibara R, Hattori T, Yasuda K, et al. Micturitional disturbance after acute hemispheric stroke: analysis of the lesion site by CT and MRI. *J Neurol Sci* 1996;137:47–56.

Serrano Ponz M, Ara Callizo JR, Fayed Miquel N, et al. Hypoxic encephalopathy and cortical laminar necrosis. *Rev Neurol* 2001;32:843–847.

Standring S, ed. *Gray's Anatomy: The Anatomical Basis of Clinical Practice*. 41st ed. New York: Elsevier Limited, 2016.

Tham WW, Stevenson RJ, Miller LA. The role of the mediodorsal thalamic nucleus in human olfaction. *Neurocase* 2011; 17:148–159.

Turk DJ, Heatherton TF, Kelley WM, et al. Mike or me? Self-recognition in a split-brain patient. *Nat Neurosci* 2002;5: 841–842.

Van der Werf YD, Scheltens P, Lindeboom J, et al. Deficits of memory, executive functioning and attention following infarction in the thalamus; a study of 22 cases with localised lesions. *Neuropsychologia* 2003;41:1330–1344.

Van der Werf YD, Witter MP, Groenewegen HJ. The intralaminar and midline nuclei of the thalamus. Anatomical and functional evidence for participation in processes of arousal and awareness. *Brain Res Brain Res Rev* 2002;39(2–3):107–140.

Ward R, Arend I. An object-based frame of reference within the human pulvinar. *Brain* 2007;130(Pt 9):2462–2469.

Ward R, Calder AJ, Parker M, et al. Emotion recognition following human pulvinar damage. *Neuropsychologia* 2007;45: 1973–1978.

Zilles K, Amunts K. Centenary of Brodmann's map—conception and fate. *Nat Rev Neurosci* 2010;11:139–145.

Zimmerman RS, Sirven JI. An overview of surgery for chronic seizures. *Mayo Clin Proc* 2003;78:109–117.

CHAPTER 7

Functions of the Cerebral Cortex and Regional Cerebral Diagnosis

It has not always been accepted that parts of the brain have specific functions. Flourens (1823) thought that all cerebral tissue was equipotential, and his influential views held sway for the better part of a century. Broca's seminal aphasic patient (1861) demonstrated that speech functions were localized to the left inferior frontal gyrus. Based on his studies of epilepsy, Hughlings Jackson was the first to point out that there is a motor cortex. Many subsequent experiments have amply demonstrated that certain areas of the cerebral cortex have specific functions. Brodmann created maps based on regional histologic differences (Figure 6.3). The correlation between histology and function is imprecise. Many areas with identical histology have differing functions. Disease involving specific areas can cause widely differing clinical manifestations. Destruction of an inhibitory area can cause the same clinical manifestations as overactivity of the area inhibited. Because of the plasticity of the nervous system, other structures or areas may assume the function of a diseased or injured part.

In addition to being localized in a specific brain region, a function can also be lateralized to one or the other hemisphere. The hemisphere to which a function is lateralized is said to be dominant for that function. In lower animals, both hemispheres seem to have equal influence. A particular attribute of the human brain, however, is the dominance of one hemisphere over the other for certain functions. This is especially true for language, gnosis (the interpretation of sensory stimuli), and praxis (the performance of complex motor acts).

Modern functional imaging techniques such as positron emission tomography (PET), functional magnetic resonance imaging (fMRI), and other methods of studying the metabolic activity of the brain have provided another dimension to the traditional notions of cerebral localization. For even simple tasks, such studies have shown a pattern of involvement of multiple brain regions overlapping the anatomical divisions into discrete lobes. The fact that a lesion produces defects in a particular function does not necessarily imply that under normal circumstances, that function is strictly localized to a particular region. Despite these limitations, it remains clinically useful to retain the traditional concepts of localization of functions in the various lobes of the dominant and nondominant hemispheres.

THE FRONTAL LOBES

Chapter 6 discusses the gross anatomy of the frontal lobe. Clinically, important areas include the motor strip, the premotor and supplementary motor areas (SMAs), the prefrontal region, the frontal eye fields, and the motor speech areas. The frontal lobe anterior to the premotor area is referred to as the prefrontal cortex. The anterior portion of the cingulate gyrus is sometimes considered part of the frontal lobe, although its connections are primarily with limbic lobe structures. Frontal lobe areas related to motor function are discussed in Chapter 25. The frontal eye fields are discussed in Chapter 14, and the motor speech area is covered in Chapter 9. Figure 7.1 shows some of these areas.

THE PREFRONTAL AREA

The portions of the frontal lobe anterior to area 6, area 8, and the motor speech centers are areas referred to as the prefrontal cortex. It includes areas 9 to 12,

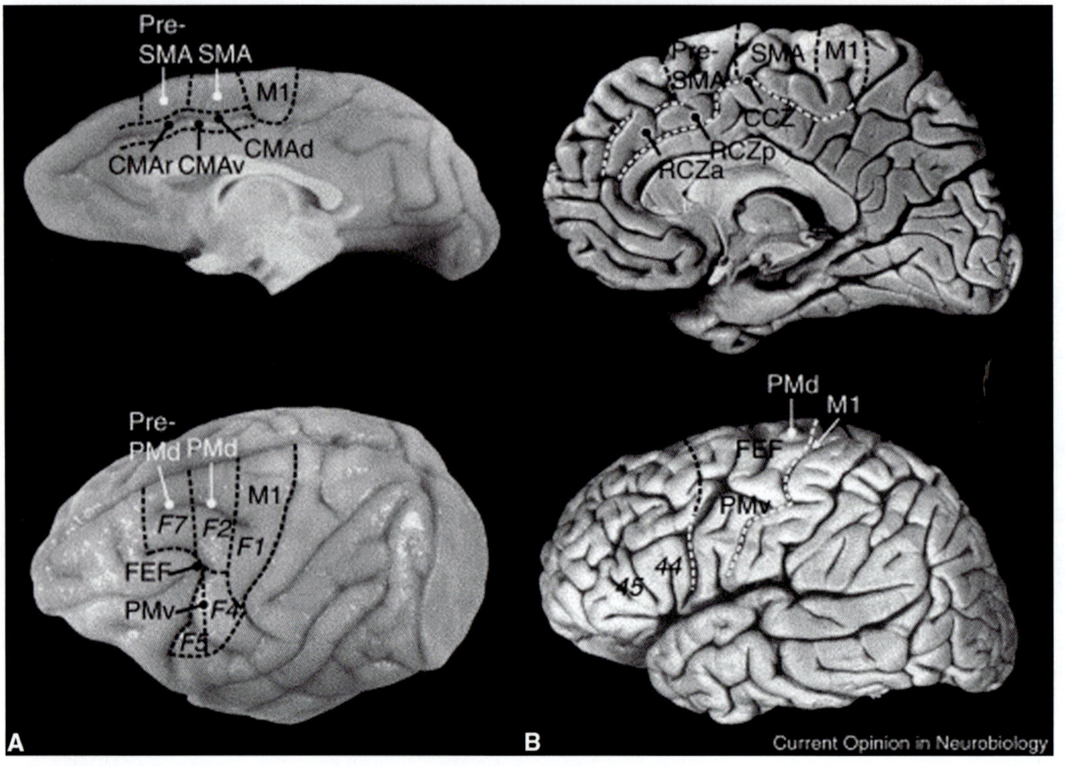

FIGURE 7.1 Motor areas of the frontal lobe in monkeys **(A)** and homologous areas in the human **(B)**. In humans, the border between areas 6 and 4 on the lateral surface is located in the anterior bank of the central sulcus. FEF, frontal eye field; M1, primary motor cortex; PMd, dorsal premotor cortex; PMv, ventral premotor cortex; RCZa, anterior rostral cingulate zone; RCZp, posterior rostral cingulate zone; SMA, supplementary motor area. (Reprinted from Picard N, Strick PL. Imaging the premotor areas. *Curr Opin Neurobiol* 2001;11[6]:663–672. Copyright © 2001 Elsevier. With permission.)

32, 45, 47, and others. These areas are connected with the somesthetic, visual, auditory, and other cortical areas by long association bundles and with the thalamus and the hypothalamus by projection fibers. The prefrontal cortex is the main projection site for the dorsomedial nucleus of the thalamus. The prefrontal cortex projects to the basal ganglia and substantia nigra; it receives dopaminergic fibers that are part of the mesocortical projection from the midbrain. The dopaminergic neurons are associated with reward, attention, short-term memory tasks, planning, and drive.

Clinically, the prefrontal region can be divided into the dorsolateral prefrontal cortex (DLPFC), the medial prefrontal cortex (MPC), and the orbitofrontal cortex (OFC). The cellular structure of the prefrontal region is strikingly different from areas 4 and 6 (the motor and premotor areas). The cortex is thin and granular; the pyramidal cells in layer 5 are reduced in both size and number. These brain areas are highly developed in humans, and they have long been considered the seat of higher intellectual functions. Much of the information about the functions of the frontal association areas has come from clinical observation of patients with degeneration, injuries, or tumors of the frontal lobes and from examination of patients who have had these regions surgically destroyed. Beginning with Phineas Gage, many examples of patients with dramatic changes in personality or behavior after frontal lobe damage have been reported (Figure 7.2; Box 7.1). Mataro et al. reported a modern case similar to Phineas Gage with a 60-year follow-up.

There is a paucity of information regarding the functions of the different regions of the prefrontal cortex. The DLPFC is important in the organization of self-ordered tasks. It plays a critical role in the neural network subserving working memory (Chapter 8). The responsibility for executive function largely resides with the DLPFC and its connections. Frontal lobe executive function is the ability to plan, carry out, and monitor a series of actions intended to accomplish a goal. It is concerned with planning and organizational skills, the ability to benefit from

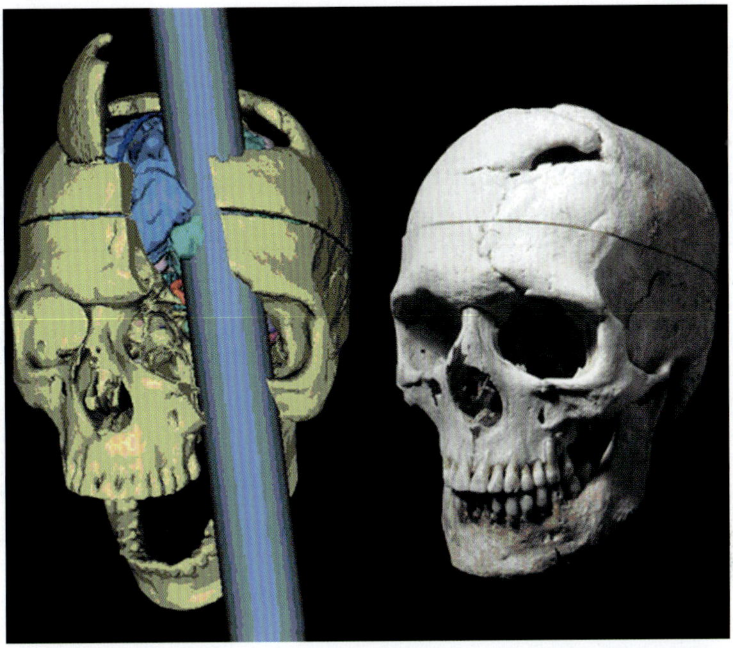

FIGURE 7.2 Phineas Gage, a three-dimensional computer reconstruction of the original skull from a thin-slice computed tomographic image and of the tamping iron. (Reprinted from Ratiu P, Talos IF. Images in clinical medicine. The tale of Phineas Gage, digitally remastered. *N Engl J Med* 2004;351:e21. Copyright © 2004 Massachusetts Medical Society. Reprinted with permission from Massachusetts Medical Society.)

BOX 7.1

Frontal Lobotomy

In a famous incident in 1848, Mr. Phineas Gage, a 25-year-old railroad worker, sustained severe damage to his frontal lobes when a metal tamping rod was blasted through his head after a freak accident (the "case of the crowbar skull"). The rod entered through the left cheek and exited in the midline near the intersection of the sagittal and coronal sutures. Surprisingly, he survived and has become a celebrated patient in the annals of medicine. Following the accident, there was a dramatic change in his character and personality. He died 13 years later after having traveled extensively and having been, for a period of time, exhibited in a circus. He reportedly became irreverent, profane, impatient, and unable to hold a job. He was "a child in his intellectual capacities, with the general passions of a strong man." Reports of the case strengthened prevailing ideas about cerebral localization, particularly about the importance of the frontal lobes in personality. Gage's accidental frontal lobotomy laid some of the groundwork for the surgical procedure of frontal (prefrontal) lobotomy or leukotomy, which was thought to decrease emotional and affective responses and relieve anxiety, apprehension, and "nervous tension." The operation consisted of cutting the white matter coronally in each frontal lobe, dividing the association fibers that connect the prefrontal areas with other brain regions. This operation became popular in the mid-20th century; it was done extensively over a period of years as a treatment not only for psychosis but also for neurosis and depression. It was even used to control the behavior of criminals and recommended for "difficult" children. A popular procedure was the "ice-pick" lobotomy in which an ice pick was inserted above the eye and pounded through the orbital roof with a mallet, then swept to and fro to sever the connections of the prefrontal region from the rest of the brain. The primary proponent of this technique used a gold-plated ice pick and kept speed records for the procedure. A lobotomy was once done on an eccentric actress who had no mental illness. The abuse of frontal lobotomy was dramatized in the motion picture One Flew Over the Cuckoo's Nest. The procedure has been abandoned. See Ginat for an illustration of the neuroradiologic sequelae.

experience, abstraction, motivation, cognitive flexibility, and problem solving. Disturbed executive function is common with frontal lobe lesions. Defects in executive function occur with frontal lobe lesions, but may occur with lesions elsewhere because of the extensive connections of the frontal lobes with all other parts of the brain. The DLPFC is also important in oculomotor control, which is responsible for decision-making regarding voluntary eye movements and inhibiting unwanted reflex saccades. It may also play a role in pain perception. There is evidence of DLPFC dysfunction in schizophrenia. The prefrontal region likely plays a role as well in the ability to predict the consequences of actions, emotional expression (affect), "go/no-go" decision-making, personality, and the sense of time. Widespread changes in prefrontal activation are associated with calculating and thinking.

The MPC has connections with the several thalamic nuclei, particularly the dorsomedian, and with the superior temporal cortex. There are connections with other portions of the frontal lobe, including the OFC, the DLPFC, and the medial motor areas. The MPC is important in auditory and visual associations. The ventrolateral prefrontal cortex is concerned with mnemonic processing of objects. The OFC has important connections with the limbic system, including the amygdala. Disinhibition syndromes, ranging from mildly inappropriate social behavior to full-blown mania, may occur with dysfunction of the OFC, particularly of the right hemisphere. Patients with OFC dysfunction are also prone to display emotional lability, poor judgment and insight, and distractibility.

Frontal association areas may be involved in various degenerative processes, especially those such as frontotemporal dementia, which are likely to affect frontal lobe function. The earliest change is often a loss of memory, especially of recent memory or of retention and immediate recall. This may be followed by impaired judgment, especially in social and ethical situations. Absence of the inhibitions acquired through socialization may lead to inappropriate behavior and carelessness in dress and personal hygiene. Sexual promiscuity may develop. Loss of ability to carry out business affairs and attend to personal finance is common. The ability to perceive abstract relationships is impaired early. The patient may carry out simple well-organized actions, but he may be incapable of dealing with new problems within the scope and range expected for a person of similar age and education. Tasks requiring a deviation from established routine and adaptation to unfamiliar situations are the most difficult. There is loss of attentiveness, and distractibility may be marked. There are problems with comprehension and loss of ability to make associations. Acquisition and synthesis of new material is difficult. The time needed for solving intellectual problems is prolonged, and the patient fatigues rapidly.

Emotional lability may be prominent, with vacillating moods and outbursts of crying, rage, or laughter, despite a previously even temperament. There may be marked irritability. The mood is often euphoric, with an increased sense of well-being. Facetiousness, levity, and senseless joking and punning (witzelsucht) or moria (Gr. "silliness"), or apathy, indifference, emotional blunting, and lack of initiative and spontaneity may be present. Abulia refers to difficulty in initiating and sustaining spontaneous movements and reduction in emotional responsiveness, spontaneous speech, and social interaction. It is characteristic of frontal lobe and basal ganglia lesions. The patient may fail to link immediate impressions with past experience, leading to confusion and disorientation. There is usually progressive deterioration and increasing difficulty with intellectual functions. Extensive bilateral prefrontal lesions may culminate in akinetic mutism or a state of persistent unresponsiveness (see Chapter 51).

Similar symptoms may occur with frontal lobe neoplasms. Either witzelsucht and euphoria or indifference and apathy are early manifestations, and they may be evident before memory loss and difficulties with judgment become apparent. There are often other signs of intracranial disease, such as weakness, focal or generalized seizures, frontal ataxia, forced grasping, anosmia, or visual field defects. Evidence of increased intracranial pressure usually occurs late. Although severe impairment of function may occur with lesions of the anterior frontal lobes, further localization may not be possible from the examination alone. There is no definite focus for which removal leads to dementia, and massive lesions of the frontal lobe, especially if unilateral, may cause few symptoms, particularly if the lesion is in the nondominant hemisphere.

The severe disability that may result from a frontal lobe lesion is strikingly illustrated by Eslinger and Damasio's patient "EVR" (Box 7.2). Following frontal lobotomy, patients often developed indifference, lack of insight, euphoria, emotional outbursts,

BOX 7.2

Frontal Lobe Dysfunction

At the age of 35, a previously healthy patient, "EVR," underwent removal of a large orbitofrontal meningioma. Surgical recovery was uneventful, and there was never any evidence of tumor recurrence. Although he seemed superficially normal, with a verbal IQ of 120 and normal neuropsychological testing, the patient's behavior, judgment, and social interactions were forever impaired. He invested and lost his life's savings in an ill-advised business venture. He was fired from a succession of jobs because of tardiness and disorganization. His wife divorced him, and, unemployed, he moved back in with his parents. He required 2 hours to prepare for work each morning. He took job 100 miles from his home but was fired for lack of punctuality. He spent entire days shaving and washing his hair. Minor decisions were scrutinized ad infinitum, including simple purchases and deciding where to eat. He collected outdated and useless items (see also Volle et al.), including dead houseplants, old phone books, 6 broken fans, 5 broken television sets, 3 bags of empty orange juice cans, 15 cigarette lighters, and countless stacks of old newspapers. The New York Times provided a poignant and very personalized description of the personality changes and other effects of frontal lobe dysfunction in *When Illness Makes a Spouse a Stranger* (D. Grady, May 5, 2012), an article on frontotemporal dementia.

tactlessness, and social ineptitude, but without demonstrable memory or cognitive deficits.

FRONTAL MOTOR AREAS

The motor areas of the frontal lobe include the primary motor cortex (area 4) as well as the premotor and SMAs. The motor cortex contains the large motor neurons (Betz cells) that give rise to the corticospinal and corticobulbar tracts. The premotor cortex lies just anterior to the primary cortex, squeezed between the precentral gyrus and the posterior border of the prefrontal area (area 6); it is involved in the planning and execution of movements, particularly sequences of movements (the basis for Luria's hand sequence or fist-edge-palm test, Chapter 8). It receives afferents from other areas of the cortex, including the sensory cortex and elsewhere in the frontal cortex, and projects to the motor cortex and the motor thalamus. Some fibers descend and make up part of the extrapyramidal system.

The SMA consists of areas of cortex lying on the medial aspect of the hemisphere just anterior to the primary motor cortex at the posterior medial aspect of the frontal lobe (area 6). The SMA functions in planning motor movements, such as a sequence of actions provided from memory. The SMA areas are crucial for the temporal organization of multiple movements. In animals, lesions of the SMA impair memory-based sequencing of movements. The SMA also coordinates movements between the hands, and lesions in this area may cause the alien hand syndrome (see Chapter 10). Lesions of the more anterior and medial parts of the motor cortex cause less paralysis and more spasticity and may allow the emergence of primitive reflexes, such as grasping and groping responses.

The syndrome of the SMA is not well recognized and can easily be confused with corticospinal weakness. Patients have reduced spontaneous movements and difficulty in performing volitional motor acts to command in the contralateral limbs, although the limbs function normally in automatic motor activities, for example, dressing. Hemineglect and apraxia may also be present, but the deficit results from a frontal lobe rather than a parietal lobe lesion. Unilateral prefrontal lesions may cause imitation and utilization behavior (Chapter 8).

Seizures may arise from the frontal lobe and may either be simple partial or complex partial. Seizures arising from the motor cortex typically produce focal Jacksonian epilepsy of the contralateral limbs. Partial complex seizures arising from the frontal lobe resemble those arising from the temporal lobe but are more bizarre and likely to be confused with pseudoseizures. Seizures arising from the SMA often involve tonic posturing that is either unilateral or asymmetric and often accompanied by facial grimacing and automatisms, as well as vocal symptoms such as laughing or speech arrest. Seizures arising from the orbitofrontal or frontopolar area often involve pedaling, thrashing movements easily confused with pseudoseizures. Seizures arising from the DLPFC are often adversive, with turning of the head and eyes to the contralateral, less commonly ipsilateral, side.

The frontal eye fields lie in the middle frontal gyrus and control movement of the eyes to the contralateral side. Destructive lesions in this area cause gaze deviation ipsilaterally, whereas epileptiform activity causes gaze deviation contralaterally. Gaze palsies and gaze deviations are discussed more fully in Chapter 14. The motor speech areas (Broca's area) lie in the inferior frontal gyrus anterior to the motor strip. Lesions in this area cause aphasia (Chapter 9). Lesions of the frontal lobe may also cause incontinence, particularly with involvement of the paracentral lobule, or a gait disorder (Chapter 44).

THE PARIETAL LOBES

Chapter 6 discusses the gross anatomy of the parietal lobe. The primary sensory (somesthetic) cortex (S1; areas 3, 1, and 2) occupies all but the lowest part of the postcentral gyrus, continuing onto the medial surface into the adjoining part of the paracentral lobule. Recent work suggests that the designation primary sensory cortex should be restricted to area 3. The secondary somatosensory cortex (S2) lies in the parietal operculum adjacent to the lower portion of S1 near the sylvian fissure. In the depth of the central sulcus, area 3 abuts area 4. The postcentral cortex is homotypical (granular) cortex with six well-developed layers. The interparietal sulcus extends posteriorly from the midpoint of the postcentral gyrus and divides the remainder of the parietal lobe into the superior parietal lobule above and the inferior parietal lobule below. Area 5a—the preparietal area, in the upper part of the parietal lobe just posterior to area 2—contains large, deep pyramidal cells, some as large as the smaller Betz cells in area 4. Area 5b, the superior parietal area, occupies a large part of the superior parietal lobule, extending over the medial surface of the hemisphere to include the precuneus. Area 7, the inferior parietal area, constitutes the major portion of the parietal lobule; it includes the supramarginal and angular gyri and receives many afferents from the occipital lobe. S1 receives enormous projections from the ventral posterolateral and ventral posteromedial nuclei of the thalamus. These relay impulses from the spinothalamic tracts, medial lemnisci, and trigeminothalamic tracts, which send fibers through the posterior limb of the internal capsule to the postcentral gyrus. Body regions are represented in specific parts of the postcentral gyrus; the pattern roughly parallels the motor homunculus localization of the precentral gyrus but is not as well defined (Figure 6.7). Cortical sensory functions are discussed further in Chapter 35. The superior and inferior parietal lobules are sensory association areas. They connect with the postcentral gyrus by means of the association pathways, and they receive fibers from the nuclei lateralis dorsalis and posterior.

The functions of the parietal lobe are essentially those of reception, correlation, analysis, synthesis, integration, interpretation, and elaboration of the primary sensory impulses received from the thalamus. S1 is the initial reception center for afferent impulses, especially for tactile, pressure, and position sensations. It is necessary for discriminating finer, more critical grades of sensation and for recognizing intensity. Stimulation produces paresthesias on the opposite side of the body, with tactile and pressure sensations, numbness, tingling, sensations of constriction and movement, and occasional thermal sensations, but rarely pain. Such sensations may precede or accompany Jacksonian convulsions as part of a seizure; the spread of the sensory disturbance follows the same general pattern as in the motor area.

The sensory association areas are essential for the synthesis and interpretation of impulses, appreciation of similarities and differences, interpretation of spatial relationships and two-dimensional qualities, evaluations of variations in form and weight, and localization of sensation. Overactivity of these areas causes minimal symptoms, for example, vague paresthesias or hyperesthesias on the opposite side of the body. Destructive lesions affect mainly the gnostic (knowing, recognition) aspects of sensation. Simple appreciation of primary sensations remains, but associative functions are impaired. These deficits are discussed further in Chapters 10 and 35. Parietal lobe lesions produce abnormalities of higher-level sensory functions, which require association cortex: stereognosis, graphesthesia, two-point discrimination, and tactile localization. Patients with nondominant parietal lobe lesions may display various forms of apraxia, hemi-inattention, hemineglect, and denial of disability, culminating in the striking syndrome of anosognosia, in which patients may deny owning their contralateral limbs (see Chapter 10). The parietal lobes, through connections with the temporal and occipital lobes, integrate somatosensory with visual and auditory information.

The inferior parietal lobule—especially the angular and supramarginal gyri and the areas in close proximity to the occipital and temporal lobes—is functionally associated with the visual and auditory systems. The angular and supramarginal gyri of the dominant hemisphere are important in relation to language and related functions. Lesions in these areas may cause aphasia, agnosia, and apraxia; these are discussed in Chapter 10. The optic radiations course through the deep parietal lobe to reach the visual cortex. A deeply placed parietal lesion may cause either an inferior quadrantic or hemianopic visual field defect. Parietal lesions have been reported to cause contralateral muscular atrophy and trophic skin changes. Deafferentation may produce hypotonia, slowness of movement—especially of the proximal muscles—ataxia, updrift (Figure 27.59), and pseudoathetoid movements (sensory wandering) of the opposite side of the body (Figure 30.6). Incoordination of movement because of sensory loss from a parietal lobe lesion may mimic cerebellar ataxia (pseudocerebellar syndrome). Dystonia has also been described. Focal motor seizures and partial paralysis involving the contralateral parts of the body can occur with parietal lesions. These may be due to impaired communication with areas 6 and 4, or they may indicate that the parietal lobes also possess some motor function.

THE OCCIPITAL LOBES

Chapter 6 discusses the gross anatomy of the occipital lobe, which is more nearly a structural and functional entity than the other cerebral lobes; all of its functions are concerned either directly or indirectly with vision. It is composed of Brodmann's areas 17, 18, and 19. The primary visual cortex (area 17) is located on the lips of the calcarine fissure and adjacent portions of the cuneus above and the lingual gyrus below. The cortex is granular in type and extremely thin. Layer 4 is relatively thick with a prominent outer band of Baillarger (line or band of Gennari), which is visible grossly and gives the area its designation of striate cortex. Area 17 receives the geniculocalcarine projection, which is retinotopically organized (see Chapter 13). The striate area receives primary visual impressions: color, size, form, motion, and illumination. Ictal activity or electrical stimulation of the calcarine cortex produces unformed visual hallucinations, such as scotomas and flashes of light. Destructive lesions cause defects in the visual field supplied by the affected areas. The most familiar and classical deficit is a congruous, contralateral, macular-sparing hemianopia with a preserved optokinetic nystagmus response.

The parastriate region (area 18) and the peristriate region (area 19) receive and interpret impulses from area 17. Areas 18 and 19 are visual association cortex, essential for the recognition and identification of objects. The visual association cortex projects to the angular gyrus, lateral and medial temporal gyri, the frontal lobe, the limbic system, and to corresponding areas in the opposite hemisphere through the splenium of the corpus callosum. Interruption of these pathways leads to disconnection syndromes (see Chapter 10). There are other extrastriate visual areas beyond areas 18 and 19. Some cortical areas mediate special visual functions. The posterior parts of the lingual and fusiform gyri are important for color vision, the posterior portion of the middle temporal gyrus is involved in recognition of movement (motor vision), and the fusiform gyrus is important in facial recognition.

Visual memories are stored in the association cortex. It functions in more complex visual recognition and perception, revisualization, visual association, and spatial orientation. The association cortex is thicker than the striate cortex, with an increase in the size and number of cells in layer 3, but almost complete absence of large cells in layer 5; no line of Gennari is present. Stimulation of these regions causes formed visual hallucinations. Destruction causes difficulty with ocular fixation and with maintaining visual attention, loss of stereoscopic vision, impairment of visual memory, difficulty with accurate localization and discernment of objects, and disturbances in the spatial orientation of the visual image, especially for distance. There is loss of ability to discriminate size, shape, and color. The patient may lose the ability to localize either himself or objects in space, and he may have impaired perception of visual spatial relationships. There may be distortion of objects (metamorphopsia).

Lesions involving the occipital lobes bilaterally result in various degrees of visual loss, often accompanied by other deficits (cortical blindness, biposterior syndrome). Adjacent parietal and temporal cortical areas are often involved as well. There may be bilateral hemianopia with or without macular sparing, bilateral superior or bilateral inferior altitudinal hemianopia, or bilateral homonymous scotomas. Pupillary light reflexes are preserved. Patients with bilateral occipital or occipitoparietal lesions may have other defects of higher cortical function, such as color agnosia, prosopagnosia, and simultanagnosia (see Chapter 10). In addition, patients may lack awareness of their deficit, or they may have awareness but deny that the deficit exists (Anton's or denial visual hallucination syndrome; cortical blindness; anosognosia for blindness). The patient may behave as if he can see—try to walk, bump into objects, and fall over things. There is the belief that the patient confabulates or "hallucinates his environment." Cortical blindness may occur after stroke, cardiorespiratory arrest, head trauma, bacterial meningitis, progressive multifocal encephalopathy, and even as a postictal phenomenon. The occipital lobe is also important in ocular motility. The central control of eye movements is discussed in the chapter on the ocular motor nerves (see Chapter 14). Balint's (Balint-Holmes) syndrome consists of higher-order impairment of visual fixation and alterations in visual attention. The patient has an inability to reach for objects using visual guidance despite normal visual acuity and intact visual fields (optic ataxia) and an inability to voluntarily direct gaze (optic apraxia). The patient can see only one object and cannot move his eyes from it, but he cannot reach out and take it. Balint's syndrome is typically seen in patients with bilateral parietooccipital lesions. Recovery from cortical blindness typically evolves through a stage of visual agnosia (see Chapter 10).

THE TEMPORAL LOBES

The temporal lobe includes the superior, middle and inferior temporal, lateral occipitotemporal, fusiform, lingual, parahippocampal, and hippocampal gyri. Heschl's gyri and the planum temporale lie on the superior surface. The superior temporal gyrus subserves auditory and language functions. The middle and inferior gyri receive abundant projections from the occipital lobe and serve to integrate vision with temporal lobe auditory and language functions. The hippocampal formation is a center for learning and memory. There are abundant connections between the temporal lobe and the limbic system.

The auditory radiations run from the medial geniculate body to the auditory cortex (areas 41 and 42) in the superior temporal gyrus. Area 41 is composed of granular cortex similar to that in the parietal and occipital regions; area 42 has large pyramidal cells in layer 3. Hearing is bilaterally represented in the temporal lobes, although there is a contralateral predominance. Nearby areas in the superior temporal gyrus allow for the differentiation and the interpretation of sounds. The superior temporal gyrus may also receive vestibular impulses. Electrical stimulation of the auditory area causes vague auditory hallucinations (tinnitus, sensations of roaring and buzzing), and stimulation of adjacent areas causes vertigo and a sensation of unsteadiness. Because hearing is bilaterally represented, unilateral destruction of the auditory cortex does not cause deafness, although there may be difficulty with sound localization and a bilateral dulling of auditory acuity. Sophisticated audiometric testing may reveal mild hearing defects in the contralateral ear in a patient with a unilateral temporal lobe lesion. Bilateral temporal lobe destruction may cause deafness. Patients with cortical deafness may seem unaware of their deficit similar to the way in which patients with Anton's syndrome are unaware of their blindness. Temporal lobe lesions that do not disturb hearing may cause auditory distortions and illusions. Auditory hallucinations may also occur, especially in temporal lobe epilepsy, sometimes with accompanying visual, olfactory, and gustatory hallucinations. Involvement of the temporal lobe vestibular areas may cause difficulty with equilibrium and balance. A destructive lesion in the posterior superior temporal area of the dominant hemisphere causes Wernicke's aphasia (see Chapter 9).

Lesions involving the temporal lobe geniculocalcarine pathways (Meyer's loop) may have contralateral upper visual field defects. Bilateral ablation of the temporal lobes, particularly the anterior regions, in experimental animals causes a characteristic constellation of abnormalities referred to as the Kluver-Bucy syndrome. Affected animals have psychic blindness or visual agnosia. They can see objects but do not recognize them until they are explored and identified nonvisually, particularly orally. There is loss of fear and rage reactions, hypersexuality, bulimia, and severe memory loss. There is an excessive tendency to attend and react to every visual stimulus. Partial forms of Kluver-Bucy syndrome occur in patients with temporal lobe lesions, but the complete syndrome occurs only rarely.

Patients with temporal lobe lesions may have visual hallucinations and perversions. These occur most often during complex partial (partial complex, temporal lobe, psychomotor) seizures (CPS). The visual hallucinations in temporal lobe CPS are complex and often include the patient (autoscopy). Autoscopy has been invoked as an explanation for some of the phenomenology of near death experiences. Visual perceptions may be distorted with objects appearing too large (macropsia) or too small (micropsia), or too near or too far away. The complex hallucinations may have an auditory component; the hallucinated figure may speak. Electrical stimulation of the temporal lobe may cause hallucinations, illusions, automatisms, and emotional responses, and call forth memories. Hughlings Jackson described seizures characterized by olfactory and visual hallucinations, dreamy states and reminiscences, automatisms, and gastric and autonomic symptoms. He observed that these occurred with lesions involving the medial temporal lobe in the region of the uncus and referred to them as uncinate fits. Currently, the term uncinate fits is generally used only for those CPS that include olfactory hallucinations. CPS may include some or all of the following: automatisms; illusions and hallucinations (visual, auditory, olfactory, or gustatory); and pilomotor erection (gooseflesh). Automatisms are common and consist of brief or prolonged inappropriate but seemingly purposeful automatic movements such as chewing, swallowing, and lip smacking. There is alteration of consciousness, usually with amnesia for the period of the event. Disorders of recognition and recall are common. Déjà vu (Fr. "already seen") refers to the delusion or misperception that something new and novel has been seen or experienced before. There are many variations on the theme of déjà, of something new seeming strangely familiar (déjà pensée, déjà vacu, and others), but déjà vu is typically used to include all of them. The converse, jamais vu, is the misperception or illusion that something familiar is strange or new. Tornado epilepsy refers to vertigo due to involvement of the vestibular cortex in a seizure discharge.

CPS may include psychic manifestations, such as anxiety, fear, rage, obsessive thoughts, compulsive speech or actions, or feelings of unreality. These phenomena are associated with abnormal electrical discharges or lesions involving the anterior and medial portions of the temporal lobes, including the hippocampal gyrus, uncus, amygdaloid complex, parahippocampal gyrus, or the connections of these structures. Impulses from these structures may be relayed to the thalamus, hypothalamus, or mesencephalic reticular formation. Some instances of CPS may also involve the insula, posterior orbital surface of the frontal lobe, basal ganglia, frontal association areas, or contiguous structures. Surgical extirpation of abnormal foci may be curative. A syndrome similar to that described by Kluver and Bucy in animals has been seen in humans when temporal lobe surgery was attempted bilaterally. A variety of tools are currently used to localize and characterize abnormal seizure foci, including imaging—MRI, PET, and single photon emission computed tomography—and electroencephalographic recordings, both from the scalp and intracranially.

Neoplasms of the temporal lobe are second only to those of the frontal lobes in the frequency with which they cause mental symptoms. These may include the following: psychic manifestations varying from vague personality changes to frank behavioral disturbances; emotional abnormalities such as anxiety, depression, fear, and anger; paranoia; memory defects; learning and cognitive disabilities; and apathy.

BIBLIOGRAPHY

Alexander MP, Stuss DT. Disorders of frontal lobe functioning. *Semin Neurol* 2000;20:427–437.

Bannur U, Rajshekhar V. Post operative supplementary motor area syndrome: clinical features and outcome. *Br J Neurosurg* 2000;14:204–210.

Bell B, Lin JJ, Seidenberg M, et al. The neurobiology of cognitive disorders in temporal lobe epilepsy. *Nat Rev Neurol* 2011;7:154–164.

Benson DF, Stuss DT, Naeser MA, et al. The long-term effects of prefrontal leukotomy. *Arch Neurol* 1981;38:165–169.

Berthoz S, Armony JL, Blair RJ, et al. An fMRI study of intentional and unintentional (embarrassing) violations of social norms. *Brain* 2002;125(Pt 8):1696–1708.

Bisley JW, Goldberg ME. Attention, intention, and priority in the parietal lobe. *Annu Rev Neurosci* 2010;33:1–21.

Brazis PW, Masdeu JC, Biller J. *Localization in Clinical Neurology*. 7th ed. Philadelphia: Wolters Kluwer/Lippincott Williams & Wilkins, 2017.

Carr VA, Rissman J, Wagner AD. Imaging the human medial temporal lobe with high-resolution fMRI. *Neuron* 2010; 65:298–308.

Chatterjee A, Southwood MH. Cortical blindness and visual imagery. *Neurology* 1995;45(12):2189–2195.

Damasio H, Grabowski T, Frank R, et al. The return of Phineas Gage: clues about the brain from the skull of a famous patient. *Science* 1994;264:1102–1105.

Dolan RJ, Bench CJ, Liddle PF, et al. Dorsolateral prefrontal cortex dysfunction in the major psychoses; symptom or disease specificity? *J Neurol Neurosurg Psychiatry* 1993;56:1290–1294.

El-Hai J. *The Lobotomist: A Maverick Medical Genius and His Tragic Quest to Rid the World of Mental Illness*. Hoboken: John Wiley, 2005.

Eslinger PJ, Damasio AR. Severe disturbance of higher cognition after bilateral frontal lobe ablation: patient EVR. *Neurology* 1985;35:1731–1741.

Filley CM. Clinical neurology and executive dysfunction. *Semin Speech Lang* 2000;21:95–108.

Fogassi L, Luppino G. Motor functions of the parietal lobe. *Curr Opin Neurobiol* 2005;15:626–631.

Fraser JA, Newman NJ, Biousse V. Disorders of the optic tract, radiation, and occipital lobe. *Handb Clin Neurol* 2011;102:205–221.

Freund HJ. Somatosensory and motor disturbances in patients with parietal lobe lesions. *Adv Neurol* 2003;93:179–193.

Gaber TA. Rehabilitation of cortical blindness secondary to stroke. *NeuroRehabilitation* 2010;27:321–325.

Ginat DT. Frontal lobotomy. *Neurology* 2012;79:1830.

Godefroy O. Frontal syndrome and disorders of executive functions. *J Neurol* 2003;250:1–6.

Godefroy O, Brigitte A, Philippe A, et al. Frontal dysexecutive syndromes. *Rev Neurol (Paris)* 2004;160:899–909.

Goldberg E, Bougakov D. Neuropsychologic assessment of frontal lobe dysfunction. *Psychiatr Clin North Am* 2005;28:567–569.

Goldenberg G, Oder W, Spatt J, et al. Cerebral correlates of disturbed executive function and memory in survivors of severe closed head injury: a SPECT study. *J Neurol Neurosurg Psychiatry* 1992;55:362–368.

Haas LF. Phineas Gage and the science of brain localisation. *J Neurol Neurosurg Psychiatry* 2001;71:761.

Joseph JM, Louis S. Transient ictal cortical blindness during middle age. A case report and review of the literature. *J Neuroophthalmol* 1995;15:39–42.

Kaga K, Nakamura M, Takayama Y, et al. A case of cortical deafness and anarthria. *Acta Otolaryngol* 2004;124:202–205.

Kaufman LD, Pratt J, Levine B, et al. Antisaccades: a probe into the dorsolateral prefrontal cortex in Alzheimer's disease. A critical review. *J Alzheimers Dis* 2010;19:781–793.

Kroger JK, Sabb FW, Fales CL, et al. Recruitment of anterior dorsolateral prefrontal cortex in human reasoning: a parametric study of relational complexity. *Cereb Cortex* 2002;12:477–485.

Leiguarda RC. Apraxias and the lateralization of motor functions in the human parietal lobe. *Adv Neurol* 2003;93:235–248.

Manes F, Sahakian B, Clark L, et al. Decision-making processes following damage to the prefrontal cortex. *Brain* 2002;125 (Pt 3):624–639.

Mataro M, Jurado MA, Garcia-Sanchez C, et al. Long-term effects of bilateral frontal brain lesion: 60 years after injury with an iron bar. *Arch Neurol* 2001;58:1139–1142.

McGeoch PD, Brang D, Song T, et al. Xenomelia: a new right parietal lobe syndrome. *J Neurol Neurosurg Psychiatry* 2011;82:1314–1319.

Mega MS, Cummings JL. Frontal-subcortical circuits and neuropsychiatric disorders. *J Neuropsychiatry Clin Neurosci* 1994;6:358–370.

Mirsky JB, Heuer HW, Jafari A, et al. Anti-saccade performance predicts executive function and brain structure in normal elders. *Cogn Behav Neurol* 2011;24:50–58.

Nielsen JM. Tornado epilepsy simulating Meniere's syndrome: report of 4 cases. *Neurology* 1959;9:794–796.

Olson IR, Berryhill M. Some surprising findings on the involvement of the parietal lobe in human memory. *Neurobiol Learn Mem* 2009;91:155–165.

Paradiso S, Chemerinski E, Yazici KM, et al. Frontal lobe syndrome reassessed: comparison of patients with lateral or medial frontal brain damage. *J Neurol Neurosurg Psychiatry* 1999;67:664–667.

Picard N, Strick PL. Imaging the premotor areas. *Curr Opin Neurobiol* 2001;11:663–672.

Pochon JB, Levy R, Poline JB, et al. The role of dorsolateral prefrontal cortex in the preparation of forthcoming actions: an MRI study. *Cereb Cortex* 2001;11:260–266.

Pryse-Phillips W. *Companion to Clinical Neurology*. 3rd ed. Oxford: Oxford University Press, 2009.

Rafal RD. Oculomotor functions of the parietal lobe: effects of chronic lesions in humans. *Cortex* 2006;42(5):730–739.

Ratiu P, Talos IF. Images in clinical medicine. The tale of Phineas Gage, digitally remastered. *N Engl J Med* 2004;351:e21.

Ropper AH, Samuels MA, Klein J. *Adams and Victor's Principles of Neurology*. 10th ed. New York: McGraw-Hill Education Medical, 2014.

Shima K, Tanji J. Both supplementary and presupplementary motor areas are crucial for the temporal organization of multiple movements. *J Neurophysiol* 1998;80:3247–3260.

Spierer L, Meuli R, Clarke S. Extinction of auditory stimuli in hemineglect: space versus ear. *Neuropsychologia* 2007;45: 540–551.

Standring S, ed. *Gray's Anatomy: The Anatomical Basis of Clinical Practice*. 41st ed. New York: Elsevier Limited, 2016.

Stuss DT. Traumatic brain injury: relation to executive dysfunction and the frontal lobes. *Curr Opin Neurol* 2011;24:584–589.

Stuss DT, Alexander MP. Is there a dysexecutive syndrome? *Philos Trans R Soc Lond B Biol Sci* 2007;362(1481):901–915.

Sveinbjornsdottir S, Duncan JS. Parietal and occipital lobe epilepsy: a review. *Epilepsia* 1993;34:493–521.

Tanji J. Sequential organization of multiple movements: involvement of cortical motor areas. *Annu Rev Neurosci* 2001;24: 631–651.

Tanji J, Shima K. Supplementary motor cortex in organization of movement. *Eur Neurol* 1996;36(Suppl 1):13–19.

Thiebaut de Schotten M, Dell'Acqua F, Ratiu P, et al. From Phineas Gage and Monsieur Leborgne to H.M.: revisiting disconnection syndromes. *Cereb Cortex* 2015;25:4812–4827.

Thimble MR. Psychopathology of frontal lobe syndromes. *Semin Neurol* 1990;10:287–294.

Vijayaraghavan L, Krishnamoorthy ES, Brown RG, et al. Abulia: a delphi survey of British neurologists and psychiatrists. *Mov Disord* 2002;17:1052–1057.

Volle E, Beato R, Levy R, et al. Forced collectionism after orbitofrontal damage. *Neurology* 2002;58:488–490.

Wunderlich G, Suchan B, Volkmann J, et al. Visual hallucinations in recovery from cortical blindness: imaging correlates. *Arch Neurol* 2000;57:561–565.

CHAPTER 8

The Mental Status Examination

The mental status examination (MSE) is used to help determine if a patient has neurologic disease as opposed to psychiatric disease, to identify psychiatric disease possibly related to underlying neurologic disease, and to distinguish focal neurologic deficits from diffuse processes. Abnormalities of mental status could be caused by a focal lesion such as a stroke or a tumor; diffuse disease, such as metabolic encephalopathy; or a degenerative process, such as Alzheimer's disease (AD). The extent of the MSE should be appropriate for the patient and the presenting problem. The psychiatric MSE is longer and more involved than the neurologic MSE; it explores elements of psychiatric function that are not usually included in a neurologic mental evaluation. One possible organization of the psychiatric interview and the elements of the structured MSE is shown in Table 8.1. The additional elements of the psychiatric mental status are listed in Table 8.2.

MENTAL STATUS EXAMINATION

The MSE begins with careful observation of the patient during the history, which may aid in evaluating emotional status, memory, intelligence, powers of observation, character, and personality. Observe the general appearance, attitude, and behavior. Note the patient's manner, speech, and posture, and look for abnormalities of facial expression. There may be odd or unusual dress, gait, and mannerisms; prominent tattoos; excessive jewelry; or other evidence of eccentricity. Unkempt, disheveled patients may have dementia, frontal lobe dysfunction, a confusional state, or schizophrenia. Depression and substance abuse may lead to evidence of self-neglect. Flamboyant dress may suggest mania. Patients with visuospatial disturbances or dressing apraxia due to a nondominant parietal lesion may not be able to get into their clothes properly.

The patient may show interest in the interview, understand the situation, and be in touch with the surroundings or may appear anxious, distracted, confused, absorbed, preoccupied, or inattentive. The patient may be engaged, cooperative, and pleasant or indifferent, hostile or belligerent. She may be alert, even hypervigilant, or dull, somnolent, or stuporous. Patients who are disinhibited, aggressive, or overly familiar may have frontal lobe lesions. Silliness and incessant joking and punning (witzelsucht) may occur with frontal lobe lesions, as may apathy and emotional blunting. Abnormal motor activity may include restlessness; repetitive, stereotypical movements; bizarre mannerisms; catatonia; and posturing. Inertia and psychomotor slowing suggest depression, dementia, or parkinsonism. Restlessness, agitation, and hyperactivity may occur with mania or drug ingestion. Patients who are jumpy and hyperalert with autonomic hyperactivity may be in drug withdrawal. Note any tendency to emotional lability (pseudobulbar affect) or apparent unconcern (la belle indifference).

If there is any suggestion of abnormality from the interaction with the patient during the history-taking phase of the encounter, then a more formal MSE should be carried out. The formal MSE is a more structured process that expands on the information from the history. A detailed MSE should also be carried out if there is any complaint from the patient or family of memory difficulties, cognitive slippage, or a change in character, behavior, or personality. For instance, formerly personable and affable patients who have become irascible and contentious may have early dementia. Other reasons to proceed further include symptoms that are vague and circumstantial, known or suspected psychiatric disease or substance abuse, or when other aspects of the neurologic investigation indicate subtle or covert cognitive impairment could be present, such as anosmia, suggesting a frontal lobe tumor.

TABLE 8.1 Sample Organization of the Psychiatric Interview and the Mental Status Examination (MSE)

Interview	MSE
Appearance	Attention and concentration
Motoric behavior	Language
Mood and affect	Memory
Verbal output	Constructions
Thought	Calculation skills
Perception	Abstraction
	Insight and judgment
	Praxis

A number of short screening mental status evaluation instruments have been developed for bedside use. The most widely used of these is the Folstein Mini–Mental State Examination (MMSE, Table 8.3), but there are many others, such as the Cognistat and the Montreal Cognitive Assessment (MoCA) battery. The MoCa includes executive function testing. The Blessed Short Orientation Memory Concentration (SOMC) test is simple, efficient and useful (Table 8.4). The SOMC is easier to incorporate into the other elements of the neurologic exam than the MMSE **(Video 8.1)**. The MMSE takes about 10 minutes to administer, and the maximum score is 30. Minimum normal performance depends on age and educational level, but it has been variously stated as between 24 and 27 (Table 8.5). One heuristic is an MMSE score of ≥27 for high school graduates and ≥29 for college graduates. A "one-minute" MSE comparing verbal fluency for semantic (category) naming compared with letter (phonemic) naming has been proposed to identify patients with probable AD. In one study, there were fewer scoring errors with the SOMC than with the MMSE.

The MMSE has limitations in both sensitivity and specificity and should not be used as more than a screening instrument for diagnosis. It is affected not only by age and education but also by gender and cultural background. A cutoff score of 23 has a sensitivity of 86% and a specificity of 91% for detecting dementia in a community sample. But this score is insensitive and will not detect mild cognitive impairment (MCI), especially in well-educated or high-functioning patients (ceiling effect). An average or above average MMSE score does not reliably exclude dementia. There is also a relatively high false-positive rate. The MMSE is not sensitive to nondominant hemisphere or frontal lobe pathology. Weaknesses of the MMSE are an overemphasis on language functions and an underemphasis on memory, constructions, and abstract reasoning. A 15-item extension, the modified MMSE, addresses some of the limitations of the traditional MMSE.

A comparison of the MMSE, Abbreviated Mental Test, and Short Portable Mental Status Questionnaire showed sensitivities of 80%, 77%, and 70% and specificities of 98%, 90%, and 89%, respectively. The Dementia Rating Scale, a 36-item measure of cognition with five subsets, takes longer to administer but assesses more cognitive domains and is less likely to miss impairments. In patients in whom there is a question of cognitive impairment or a change in behavior and the MMSE or a similar instrument is normal, formal neuropsychological testing may provide more detail regarding the mental status. Formal neuropsychological testing may be useful in other situations as well (Box 8.1). The MMSE score in typical presenting adults is reasonably stable over time; in patients with AD, it declines at an average rate of three points per year.

Before making judgments about the patient's mental status, especially memory, the examiner should ensure that the patient is alert, cooperative, and attentive

TABLE 8.2 Elements of the Psychiatric Mental Status Interview

Attitude	Cooperative, hostile, evasive, threatening, obsequious, belligerent
Affect	Range (expansive, flat); appropriateness; stability (labile, shallow); quality (silly, anxious)
Mood	Stated mood in response to questions such as "How are your spirits?" and "How's your mood been?"
Behavior	Psychomotor agitation or retardation
Speech	Rate (rapid, slow, pressured); volume (loud, soft, monotonous, histrionic); quality (fluent, neologisms, word salad)
Thought process	Disorganized, illogical, loose associations, tangential, circumstantial, flight of ideas, perseveration, incoherent
Thought content	Preoccupations, obsessions, ideas of reference, delusions, thought broadcasting, suicidal or homicidal ideation
Perception	Delusions, illusions, hallucinations (auditory, visual, other); spontaneously reported or in response to direct question, patient attending or responding to hallucination

TABLE 8.3 Mini-Mental State Exam

Maximum Score	Procedure
	Orientation
5	What are the day, date, month, season, and year?
5	Where are we? Country, state, city, hospital, floor?
	Registration
3	Name 3 objects: 1 s to say each. Then ask the patient to repeat all three. Give 1 point for each correct answer. Then repeat until all three are registered.
	Attention and calculation
5	Serial 7s. One point for each correct. Stop after 5 answers. Alternatively, spell *world* backward.
	Recall
3	Ask for the 3 objects repeated above. Give 1 point for each correct.
	Language
9	Name a pencil and a watch. (2 points.) Repeat the following: "No its, ands, or buts." (1 point.) Follow a three-stage command: "Take a piece of paper in your right hand, fold it in half, and put it on the floor." (3 points.) Read and obey the following: "Close your eyes." (1 point.) Write a sentence. (1 point.) Copy design. (1 point.)

Reprinted from Folstein MF, Folstein S, McHugh P. "Mini-mental state": a practical method for grading the cognitive state of patients for the clinician. *J Psychiatr Res* 1975;12(3):189–198. Copyright © 1975 Elsevier. With permission.

TABLE 8.4 Short Orientation-Memory-Concentration Test for Cognitive Impairment

Ask the patient to:

1. Name the month
2. Name the year
3. State the time of day
4. Remember the following memory phrase: "John Brown, 42 Market Street, Chicago"
5. Count backward from 20 to 1
6. Name the months of the year in reverse
7. Recall the memory phrase

See Katzman R, Brown T, Fuld P, et al. Validation of a short orientation-memory-concentration test of cognitive impairment. *Am J Psychiatry* 1983;140:734, for expected scores in various age groups.

TABLE 8.5 Mean (Standard Deviation) Mini-Mental State Examination Scores

	55–59	60–64	65–69	70–74	75–79	80–84	>85
9–12 y or high school diploma	28 (2.2)	28 (2.2)	28 (2.2)	27 (1.6)	27 (1.5)	25 (2.3)	26 (2.0)
College experience or higher degree	29 (1.5)	29 (1.3)	29 (1.0)	28 (1.6)	28 (1.6)	27 (0.9)	27 (1.3)

Adapted from Crum RM, Anthony JC, Bassett SS, et al. Population-based norms for the mini-mental state examination by age and educational level. *JAMA* 1993;269:2386–2391.

BOX 8.1

Neuropsychological Testing

Formal neuropsychological testing is a long and complex undertaking that requires many hours of patient and neuropsychologist time. Testing is often done as a battery of individual tests that provide a structured assessment of mental status. The two batteries in widespread use are the Halstead-Reitan battery (HRB) and the Luria-Nebraska neuropsychological battery (LNNB). The HRB is the most commonly used. It consists of 13 subtests (intelligence, abstract reasoning, tactile performance, tactile/visuospatial memory, rhythm perception and memory, speech-sound perception, psychomotor speed, sequencing abilities, language function, sensory function, primary motor speed, grip strength, and personality functioning). The HRB is not sensitive for MCI, and localization is imprecise. The LNNB grew out of the pioneering work of Aleksander Luria, a Russian neurologist. There are 14 scales that measure various functions. The LNNB requires less time to administer and score than does the HRB, but reference values and reliability are not as well accepted.

The Wechsler Adult Intelligence Scale (WAIS) is the most commonly performed intelligence test in adults; it provides summary measures of verbal IQ, performance IQ, and full-scale IQ. For each, the mean score is 100, and the standard deviation is 15. Patients with an IQ score of more than two standard deviations below the mean are generally considered to have cognitive impairment. The verbal IQ score has been thought to reflect dominant hemisphere and the performance IQ nondominant hemisphere integrity, but this is an oversimplification. The performance pattern on the WAIS subtests may also have diagnostic significance.

and has no language impairment. Mental status cannot be adequately evaluated in a patient who is not alert or is aphasic. Evaluation of patients with altered consciousness is discussed in Chapter 51. To avoid upsetting the patient, it is desirable, when possible, to examine the mental functions unobtrusively by asking questions that gently probe memory, intelligence, and other important functions without obvious inquisition.

ORIENTATION AND ATTENTION

The formal MSE usually begins with an assessment of orientation. Normally, patients are said to be "oriented times three" if they know who they are, their location, and the date. Some examiners assess insight or the awareness of the situation as a fourth dimension of orientation. The details of orientation are sometimes telling. The patient may know the day of the week but not the year. Orientation can be explored further when necessary by increasing or decreasing the difficulty level of the questions. Patients may know the season of the year if not the exact month; conversely, they may be oriented well enough to know their exact location down to the street address. Most patients can estimate the time within 1 hour. Orientation questions can be used as a memory test for patients who are disoriented. If the patient is disoriented, she may be told the day, the month, the year, the city, etc., and implored to try to remember the information. Failure to remember this information by a patient who is attentive and has registered it suggests a severe memory deficit. Occasionally, patients cannot remember very basic information, such as the year or the city, despite being repeatedly told, for more than a few seconds. In the presence of disease, orientation to time is impaired first and then orientation to place; only rarely is there disorientation to person.

Poor performance on complex tests of higher intellectual function cannot be attributed to cortical dysfunction if the patient is not attentive to the tasks. Defective attention taints all subsequent testing. Patients may appear grossly alert but are actually inattentive, distractible, and unable to concentrate. An early manifestation of toxic or metabolic encephalopathy is often a lack of attention and concentration in an apparently alert patient, which may progress to delirium or to a confused state. Confusion, inattention, and poor concentration may also be seen with frontal lobe dysfunction, posterior nondominant hemisphere lesions, and increased intracranial pressure. Lesions causing apathy or abulia also impair attention. Patients with dementing illnesses are not typically inattentive until the cognitive deficits are severe. Consider the possibility of a central nervous system toxic or metabolic disturbance when the patient is inattentive.

Having the patient signal whenever the letter A is heard from a string of random letters dictated by the examiner or having the patient cross out all of the A's on a written sheet may reveal a lack of attention or task impersistence. In the line cancellation, or line bisection, test, the patient is requested to bisect several lines randomly placed on a page. Inattentive, distractible patients may fail to complete the task. Patients with hemineglect may fail to see the left half of the line and bisect all of the lines off center, or they may ignore the lines on one side of the page. The proportion and placement of lines left uncrossed relates to the severity of the neglect and localization of the lesion.

Digit span forward is a good test of attention, concentration, and immediate memory. The examiner dictates a series of random numbers of increasing length, beginning with 3 or 4, at a rate of about one per second; the patient is asked to repeat them. Backward digit span is a more complex mental process that involves working memory; it requires the ability to retain and manipulate the string of numbers. Expected performance is 7 ± 2 forward and 5 ± 1 backward. Reverse digit span should not be more than two digits less than the forward span. Forward digit span is also a test of repetition and may be impaired in aphasic patients. Another test of attention and concentration is a three-step task. For instance, tear a piece of paper in half, then tear half of it in half, and then tear one half in half again, so that there are three different sizes. Give the patient an instruction such as "Give the large piece of paper to me, put the small piece on the bed, and keep the other piece" (Marie's paper test, see Chapter 9). Other multistep tasks might be "Stand up, face the door, and hold out your arms" or "Touch your right ear with your left thumb and put out your tongue."

Attention has an important spatial component, and patients may fail to attend to one side of space (hemi-inattention or hemineglect). The nondominant hemisphere has special responsibilities regarding attention. It seems to maintain attention in both right and left hemispace. The dominant hemisphere in contrast only attends to contralateral hemispace. Patients with right parietal lesions often have hemineglect for the left side of space. They may also ignore even a profound neurologic deficit involving the left side of the body (anosognosia). With dominant lesions, the nondominant hemisphere can attend well enough to both sides of space that hemineglect does not occur as a prominent feature. Bilateral lesions may be required to cause neglect of right hemispace. Thalamic lesions, especially those involving the medial thalamus, may produce similar findings, often accompanied by a tendency not to use the involved limbs without any weakness (thalamic neglect).

Mental control or concentration is a higher-level function that requires the patient not only to attend to a complex task but also to marshal other intellectual resources, such as the ability to mentally manipulate items. Tests of mental control and working memory include serial 7s or 3s, spelling world backward (part of MMSE), and saying the days of the week or months of the year in reverse. The average adult can recite the months of the year backward in less than 30 seconds. When underlying functions, for example, calculation ability, are intact, defective mental control may indicate dorsolateral frontal lobe (executive) dysfunction, usually on the left.

LANGUAGE

Evaluation of language includes assessment of fluency, comprehension, naming, repetition, reading, and writing. Language function is discussed further in Chapter 9.

MEMORY

Structures important in memory function include the hippocampus, the parahippocampal gyrus, the fornix, the septal nucleus, the mammillary bodies, the mammillothalamic tract, the cingulate gyrus, and the anterior and medial dorsal nuclei of thalamus (Chapter 6). Memory has many facets and may be tested in different ways. Memory terminology is not used consistently, with different terms in use in general neurology and in behavioral neurology. A precise description of the task attempted is often more useful than describing the patient's "recent memory." The generally used classification includes immediate, short-term or recent, and long-term or remote memory. These correspond approximately to the terms working, episodic, and semantic memory used by behavioral neurologists and cognitive neuropsychologists. These designations attempt to reflect the neurophysiology of memory. Remote memory is typically much better than recent memory in patients with memory disturbances.

Memory terminology is not used consistently, and a precise description of the task attempted is often more useful than describing the patient's "recent memory." A commonly used memory classification includes immediate (working) memory, recent (short-term) memory, and remote (long-term) memory. Episodic memory refers to the system involved in remembering particular episodes or experiences, such as the movie you saw last weekend or the meeting you attended yesterday.

The first stage of memory—immediate or working memory—involves the circuits used to register, recall, and mentally manipulate transitory information. The prefrontal cortex mediates much of this function. This is a short-lived operation in which material is not actually committed to memory. People can typically retain seven digits, a telephone number, in immediate memory. Retaining longer numbers, or *supraspan numbers*, and tasks such as reverse digit span require more active memory processing. Working memory tends to decline with advancing age. Working memory also depends on executive function, the ability to remain focused on the task despite distractions. The second stage of memory—short-term, recent, episodic, or declarative memory—involves retaining and recalling information or events for minutes to hours. The medial temporal lobe mediates much of this second stage of memory. The familiar test of the ability to recall three items after 5 minutes assesses episodic or short-term memory. The term episodic memory is also used to refer to the system involved in remembering particular episodes or experiences, such as the movie seen last weekend; episodic memory involves specific personal experiences. In the third stage, memories are consolidated and stored more permanently. The lateral temporal region and other cortical areas subserve this storage function. The fund of information stored in remote, long-term memory includes basic school facts, such as state capitals, past presidents, and important dates; current events; and personal information, such as address, phone number, and the names of relatives. This long-term stage of memory is commonly referred to as semantic memory, a confusing term at best. Semantic memory includes generalized knowledge and factual information not related to memory of a specific thing or event, such as what a movie is. Semantic memory is distinct from personal long-term memory.

Digit span is a test of attention and immediate, working memory. Episodic (recent, short-term) memory is tested by giving the patient items to recall. The recall items may be simple objects, such as orange, umbrella, and automobile, or more complex, such as "John Brown, 42 Market St., Chicago" (part of Blessed SOMC). Apple, table, penny is a favorite three-item list. The items should be in different categories. Maurice Victor preferred a simple "one"-item list, an appointment: Dr. Victor, Saturday, 8 o'clock. After ensuring the patient has registered the items, proceed with other testing. After approximately 5 minutes, ask the patient to recall the items. Investigators have found considerable variability when using such three-word lists; some typical presenting subjects may recall zero or one word. Better tests for the bedside evaluation of memory are supraspan list learning tasks with delayed recall and recognition conditions. Asking the patient to recall that morning's breakfast is another test of short-term memory. Assessing memory is frequently difficult in patients who work in very specialized fields and who have few outside interests. Patients with major cognitive impairment may still recall some deeply ingrained, overlearned memories, for example, days of the week, months of the year, nursery rhymes, and jingles.

Patients with severe memory deficits may not only fail to recall the items but also fail to recall being asked to recall. Some patients may fail to remember the items, but they can improve performance with hints or pick the items from a list. Patients who are able to remember items with cuing or by picking from a list are able to retain the information but not retrieve it. When cuing or picking do not improve performance, the defect is in retention. Patients with early dementing processes may have only a failure of retrieval. Another memory test is to ask the patient to remember the Babcock sentence ("One thing a nation must have to be rich and great is a large, secure supply of wood") after 5 minutes. Typical patients can do this in three attempts. Tests of nonverbal memory include hiding objects in the patient's room as she watches and then having her remember where the objects are hidden, or asking her to remember shapes, colors, or figures.

In confabulation, a patient with memory loss, most classically Wernicke-Korsakoff syndrome, "fills in the gaps" in memory by saying whatever comes to mind, having no idea whether it is actually true or not. There is memory impairment out of proportion to other cognitive functions. Unable to recall things, the patient makes up wild tales without an intent to deceive and without any awareness whether the information is or is not true. The confabulation may range from minor deviations from actual events to blatant falsehoods. Two forms are recognized: spontaneous and provoked. The provoked type typically emerges during memory testing.

CONSTRUCTIONAL TASKS

Brain disease commonly causes impaired visuospatial abilities, and constructional ability can be tested by drawing shapes, the clock drawing test (CDT), or copying the Rey-Osterrieth figure (see Chapter 10). Drawing a cube or interlocking pentagons (part of the MMSE) are commonly used constructional tasks. The CDT is a test of visuospatial capability and mental status. Originally developed as a test of constructional and visuospatial function, the CDT has evolved into a simple and quick test of general cognitive abilities. Given a circle, the patient is asked to insert the numbers and draw the hands indicating a specific time. Points are assessed for each element of the task. An abnormal CDT increases the probability of dementia. Errors on the CDT develop early in AD and worsen progressively. Studies have shown a sensitivity of 36% to 75%, a specificity of 72% to 98%, and a positive likelihood ratio of 5.3. Testing of constructional ability is discussed more fully in Chapter 10.

CALCULATIONS

Ability to count and calculate may be evaluated by asking the patient to count forward or backward, to count coins, or to make change. Patients may be asked to select a certain amount from a handful of change. More formal testing might include having the patient perform simple arithmetic, either mentally or on paper. The ability to calculate depends on native intelligence, innate number sense or mathematical ability, and educational level. Basic calculations, such as 2 + 2, are often rote, overlearned items from early schooling; these test remote memory more than calculating ability. The average patient can perform mental calculations that involve two-digit operations and require simple carrying and borrowing. A patient who succeeds with simple calculations should be pressed to at least a moderate level of difficulty, for example, 12 + 3, 13 + 7, 17 + 11, and 26 + 14. Another test is to sequentially double a number until failure. Adding or subtracting a column of two- or three-digit numbers on paper further requires the ability to correctly align and manipulate a column of numbers. It gives insight not only into calculating skill but also into visuospatial ability, which may be particularly impaired with nondominant parietal lesions. Simple math problems may be presented; for example, if apples are a quarter apiece, how many can you buy for a dollar? How many quarters are in $1.50? If a loaf of bread costs 89 cents and you paid with a dollar, what change would you get back? A commonly used calculation task is subtracting serial 7s from 100 (failing that, serial 3s). This function also requires attention and concentration. Counting to 20 is more of a remote memory test and counting backward from 20 more of an attentional task. There is little difference in calculating ability across age groups and little impairment in early AD. However, advancing disease dramatically alters calculation ability.

Aphasic patients may have difficulty with calculations because they make paraphasic errors involving the numbers. Impaired calculating ability may occur with posterior dominant hemisphere lesions, either as an isolated defect or as part of Gerstmann's syndrome (see Chapter 10). These patients have a true anarithmetria, a primary disturbance of calculating ability.

ABSTRACT THINKING

The ability to think abstractly is typically tested by asking the patient to describe similarities and differences, to find analogies, and to interpret proverbs and aphorisms. The patient may be asked how an apple and a banana, a car and an airplane, a watch and a ruler, or a poem and a statue are alike, or to tell the difference between a lie and a mistake. To test for the ability to find analogies, the patient might be asked: "Table is to leg as car is to what?" The patient may be unable to interpret a proverb or may interpret it concretely or literally. When interpreting "Don't cry over spilt milk," the patient thinking concretely will talk about accidents, milk, spillage, cleanup, and other things that miss the point. Some commonly used proverbs include the following: a rolling stone gathers no moss, a stitch in time saves nine, and people who live in glass houses shouldn't throw stones. The usefulness of proverb interpretation has been questioned. It seems many examiners are not precisely sure themselves what some of the proverbs mean. Only late in life did either of the authors learn what Thoreau meant by "Some circumstantial evidence is very strong, as when you find a trout in the milk" (meaning the milk has been watered down). Bizarre, peculiar proverb interpretations may be given by patients with psychiatric disease, or by people who are simply not familiar with the idiomatic usage. It may be useful to throw in a concatenated, mixed, and confused proverb or saying such as "The hand that rocks the cradle shouldn't throw stones" to test both the patient's abstraction ability and sense of humor. Impaired abstraction occurs in many conditions but is particularly common with frontal lobe disorders.

INSIGHT AND JUDGMENT

Common insight and judgment questions—such as asking what the patient would do if she found a sealed, addressed, stamped letter on the sidewalk, or smelled smoke in a crowded theater—may be less useful than determining if the patient has insight into her illness and the implications of any functional impairment. Historical information from family members about the patient's actual judgment in real-life situations may be more enlightening than these artificial constructs. Patients with no concern about their illness have impaired judgment. Patients with poor judgment may behave impulsively or inappropriately during the examination. Many neurologic conditions may impair judgment, particularly processes that affect the orbitofrontal regions. Lack of insight into the illness, to the point of denial of any disability, may occur with nondominant parietal lesions.

FRONTAL LOBE (EXECUTIVE) FUNCTION

Executive function refers to "supervisory" cognitive processes that involve high-level organization and execution of complex thoughts and behavior, including such processes as planning, problem solving, multitasking, and monitoring of actions. These functions primarily reflect frontal lobe function, although other systems are involved. Concepts of the executive system have arisen largely by observations of patients such as Phineas Gage, who display disorganized actions and strategies for everyday tasks (dysexecutive syndrome), without deficits on formal tests of cognition.

Frontal lobe dysfunction may be subtle. The usual methods of bedside testing, including formal neuropsychological assessment, may fail to detect even significant frontal lobe dysfunction (see Box 7.2). Comparison with the patient's premorbid personality and behavior is often more telling than assessment based on population-derived reference information. In addition to the standard tests of abstract thinking and proverb interpretation, special techniques designed to evaluate frontal lobe function may be useful. Tests helpful for evaluating frontal lobe function include verbal fluency by word list generation, assessment of the ability to alternate tasks or switch between tests, abstraction ability, motor sequencing, and tests for perseveration, apathy, and impulsivity. The Frontal Assessment Battery is a test battery that can be administered in a few minutes that covers five executive tests plus the grasp reflex.

Some commonly used executive function measures include the Wisconsin Card Sorting Test, verbal fluency by word list generation, and response inhibition tests. Patients with frontal lobe dysfunction who do not have anomia when tested by other methods may not be able to generate word lists (see Chapter 9). Patients may be asked to name items as quickly as possible from a particular category, such as animals or furniture (semantic or category fluency), or think of as many words as possible beginning with a particular letter, for example, F, A, or S (letter or phonemic fluency). Semantic category fluency has been found to rely on lateral and inferior temporal lobe regions known to be involved in object perception, recognition, imagery, and naming. In contrast, first-letter verbal fluency tests the ability to use phonemic and/or graphemic cues to guide retrieval. This requires greater effort and a more active strategic search than does semantic category fluency. Consistent with its prominent executive demands, letter fluency has been found to correlate more with prefrontal lobe functioning than semantic fluency. Category fluency (naming animals) was found to be a very useful one-minute MSE and identified dementia better than did phonemic fluency. Typical patients should be able to name a minimum of 12 items in a category; some adjustment may be necessary for poorly educated and older patients (Chapter 9). In a relatively well-educated study group, a cutoff score of 15 on the category fluency test had a sensitivity of 0.87 and a specificity of 0.96. In the MoCA, letter fluency of $\geq$11 is considered normal.

The Wisconsin Card Sort Test is used by neuropsychologists to determine if the patient can shift between tasks (shift sets). The formal test requires the patient to discover through trial and error the expected sorting of cards by color, shape, or number and then to recognize and adapt to a change in the scheme. A bedside variation is to ask the patient to detect a pattern when the examiner switches a coin between hands behind her back—for example, twice in the right hand, once in the left—and then to change the pattern and see if the patient detects the new scheme. Perseveration is the abnormal, inappropriate repetition of words or actions. Patients with frontal lesions, especially those involving the dominant dorsolateral prefrontal cortex, have difficulty abandoning the initial pattern of responses and tend to perseverate.

In trail-making tests, the patient is required to connect in sequence either letters or numbers scattered around a page (Trails A) or to alternate connecting letters and numbers, for example, A-1-B-2-C-3 (Trails B). In another test of alternating ability, the patient writes a string of Ms and Ns, all connected. In Luria's fist-edge-palm test, the patient is asked to repetitively place the hand down in a series of motions: fist, edge of hand palm, over and over. There is a tendency to perseveration and difficulty accurately executing the sequences of hand positions, particularly with frontal lobe lesions. In copying tasks involving drawing simple figures with multiple loops, patients with perseveration may insert extra loops.

A common manifestation of frontal lobe dysfunction is lack of response inhibition. Automatic responses are a type of defective response inhibition. The ability to inhibit automatic responses can be measured in several ways. The Stroop color word interference test assesses the patient's ability to inhibit automatic responses. In the "little-big" test, the words little and big are printed on separate cards in both upper- and lowercase letters. The patient is required to answer "big" aloud if the print is upper case, even in response to the word "little," or vice versa. A variation is to write several color names in nonmatching colors, for example, write the word "blue" with a red marker and then ask the patient to read the cards by stating the color of the print, not the written name of the color. Patients with frontal lobe dysfunction have trouble inhibiting the tendency to read the color name. Another response inhibition task is to have the patient respond oppositely to the examiner, for example, asking the patient to tap once if the examiner taps twice and vice versa, or telling the patient to point to her chin as the examiner points to her nose.

The Go/No-Go test is another test for detect defective response inhibition. The patient is asked to perform an action in response to a stimulus (Go) and do nothing in response to a different stimulus (No Go). If Go stimuli exceed No-Go stimuli, the patient with frontal lobe disease has difficulty inhibiting the response on the No-Go stimuli. Then the rules are changed, and the patient is challenged to adapt. Any number of stimulus-responses paradigms are possible. The antisaccade task is another measure of the ability to inhibit automatic responses (see Chapter 14).

The applause sign is an inability to stop clapping after being asked to clap three times and was initially touted as a way to distinguish progressive supranuclear palsy (PSP) from Parkinson's disease (PD) and frontotemporal dementia (FTD) **(Video Link 8.1)**. Later studies found the applause sign was a nonspecific sign of frontal lobe dysfunction. Lhermitte first described utilization behavior and imitation behavior in patients with frontal lobe damage. Patients with utilization behavior will reach out and use objects in the environment in an automatic manner and are not able to inhibit this response. Similarly, patients with imitation behavior will imitate the examiner's gestures, even if specifically told to refrain from doing so.

OTHER MENTAL STATUS TESTS

Other procedures used to evaluate cognitive function include assessment of visuospatial and constructional ability, praxis, language disturbances, recognition (visual, tactile, and auditory), right-left orientation, and finger identification. These are discussed in subsequent chapters.

ABNORMAL MENTAL STATUS EXAMINATION

The MSE may be abnormal for a number of reasons, including metabolic disorders, drug intoxication or withdrawal, psychiatric conditions, neurologic disorders, especially degenerative conditions, or following traumatic brain injury. Dementia refers to the loss of cognitive abilities in a previously average functioning individual. The term implies a progressive disorder, in contrast to the cognitive impairment that may follow brain trauma or a hypoxic insult, although in vascular dementia, the onset may be sudden and the progression stepwise.

Many disorders may cause dementia (see Chapter 53). AD, dementia with Lewy bodies (DLB, diffuse Lewy body disease) and vascular dementia account for the majority of cases. The distribution of etiologies is somewhat age dependent. Overall, AD accounts for about 60% to 80%, DLB for about 10%, cerebrovascular disease for about 10%, "treatable" dementias (e.g., normal pressure hydrocephalus, drug effects, metabolic disorders) for about 2%, FTD for about 1%, and Creutzfeldt-Jakob disease for less than 1%. These diseases, especially AD and vascular dementia, may coexist. MCI refers to patients with demonstrable cognitive abnormalities, especially difficulty with memory, that do not appreciably interfere with daily functioning. The current construct of MCI is that it is an intermediate stage between the cognitive changes of aging and the very earliest features of AD.

Dementia is sometimes divided into cortical and subcortical types, although recent research questioned the clinical, neuropsychological, neuroimaging, and neuroanatomical basis of the distinction. AD is the prototype cortical dementia; aphasia, apraxia, and agnosia are commonly present. Subcortical dementia lacks these features and is characterized by slowness of mental processing, forgetfulness, impaired cognition, apathy, and depression; vascular dementia and the intellectual impairment in PD are the most common examples.

ALZHEIMER'S DISEASE

AD typically manifests as an insidiously progressive deterioration of higher intellectual function, with memory loss and alterations in mood and behavior, evolving over 5 to 10 years to a state of severe, diffuse cortical dysfunction. Other cognitive deficits may appear with or after the development of memory impairment. Language function and visuospatial skills tend to be affected relatively early, whereas deficits in executive function and behavioral symptoms often manifest later in the disease course. These deficits appear and progress insidiously. Clinical assessment and modern imaging allow for accurate diagnosis in 80% to 90% of cases.

Although diffuse cognitive changes are typical, especially in the mid and later stages, AD causes two particularly distinct findings on MSE: rapid forgetting on tests of episodic memory and impaired category fluency compared with letter fluency. Difficulty consolidating new memories causes rapid forgetting. Patients may have relatively intact immediate recall, but much of the information is lost after delays of a little as a few minutes. Decreased category fluency with relatively preserved letter fluency is another prominent feature of AD; the reverse pattern occurs in FTD and vascular dementia.

DEMENTIA WITH LEWY BODIES

DLB typically causes recurrent visual hallucinations, fluctuations in attention and alertness, episodes of confusion, parkinsonian features, visuospatial impairments, and a particular sensitivity to neuroleptic medications (Chapter 30). The pathology resembles that of PD dementia, and DLB is classified as an alpha-synucleinopathy. Symptoms characteristically fluctuate ("good days and bad days"). In one study, daytime drowsiness and lethargy, naps of 2 or more hours, staring into space for long periods, and episodes of disorganized speech occurred in 63% of DLB patients compared with 12% of AD patients and 0.5% of normal elderly persons. Findings on MSE are similar to AD, but patients with DLB have relatively greater deficits in attention, executive function, visuospatial and constructional skills, psychomotor speed, and verbal fluency. Impaired visual perception may be involved in the visual hallucinations as well as the impaired visuospatial capability. Cognitive impairment occurs in half or more of patients with advanced idiopathic PD. Hallucinations can also occur in PD, particularly in relation to medications. The relationship between DLB and PD with dementia remains unsettled.

FRONTOTEMPORAL DEMENTIA

FTD is a group of disorders with prominent involvement of the frontal and temporal lobes. Onset is typically in the late 50s or early 60s; in patients under age 65, FTD is as common as AD. Two subtypes are currently recognized: the behavioral variant of FTD (FTDbv), and primary progressive aphasia (PPA). Pick's disease is the same as FTDbv. The term FTD is variably used to refer to FTDbv or the entire frontotemporal lobar degeneration (FTLD) complex. Patients with PPA may have a nonfluent aphasia similar to Broca's or a fluent aphasia termed semantic dementia.

FTDbv is characterized by deterioration in personal and social conduct, lack of insight, hyperorality, and apathy or irritability and disinhibition. Patients with FTDbv have more impairment of executive functioning compared to patients with AD. They perform worse on letter fluency compared to category fluency. They are prone to repetition errors and tend to deviate from test instructions. They perform relatively better on tests of spatial ability, episodic memory, and semantic tasks. Semantic dementia, or the temporal variant of FTLD, causes progressive difficulty with recalling the meaning of words. Verbal output is fluent and grammatically correct, but with an empty quality because of severe word-finding difficulty. On mental status testing, they demonstrate severe naming deficits and loss of word knowledge, but visual memory and visuospatial abilities are relatively preserved. Category fluency is particularly impaired. FTLD is classified into a group with tau inclusions and a group with ubiquitin inclusions. FTD signs can be seen in patients with amyotrophic lateral sclerosis (ALS), implying clinical overlap between these disorders. Both FTD and ALS are heterogeneous and there is increasing evidence that they share some clinical, neuropathologic, and genetic features.

Video Links

Video Link 8.1. The applause sign. https://www.youtube.com/watch?v=Qn4VrJRiBOk

BIBLIOGRAPHY

Alvarez JA, Emory E. Executive function and the frontal lobes: a meta-analytic review. *Neuropsychol Rev* 2006;16:17–42.

Anthony JC, LeResche L, Niaz U, et al. Limits of the 'Mini-Mental State' as a screening test for dementia and delirium among hospital patients. *Psychol Med* 1982;12:397–408.

Ballard C, Gauthier S, Corbett A, et al. Alzheimer's disease. *Lancet* 2011;377(9770):1019–1031.

Blessed G, Black SE, Butler T, et al. The diagnosis of dementia in the elderly. A comparison of CAMCOG (the cognitive section of CAMDEX), the AGECAT program, DSM-III, the mini-mental state examination and some short rating scales. *Br J Psychiatry* 1991;159:193–198.

Campbell WW. *Clinical Signs in Neurology: A Compendium.* Philadelphia: Wolters Kluwer Health, 2016.

Canning SJ, Leach L, Stuss D, et al. Diagnostic utility of abbreviated fluency measures in Alzheimer disease and vascular dementia. *Neurology* 2004;62:556–562.

Chauvire V, Even C, Thuile J, et al. Frontotemporal dementia: a review. *Encéphale* 2007;33:933–940.

Cullen B, Fahy S, Cunningham CJ, et al. Screening for dementia in an Irish community sample using MMSE: a comparison of norm-adjusted versus fixed cut-points. *Int J Geriatr Psychiatry* 2005;20:371–376.

Crum RM, Anthony JC, Sassett SS, et al. Population-based norms for the mini-mental state examination by age and educational level. *JAMA* 1993;269:2386–2391.

Cummings JL. The one-minute mental status examination. *Neurology* 2004;62:534–535.

Cummings JL, Benson DF. Subcortical dementia. Review of an emerging concept. *Arch Neurol* 1984;41:874–879.

Daffner KR, Gale SA, Barrett AM, et al. Improving clinical cognitive testing: report of the AAN Behavioral Neurology Section Workgroup. *Neurology* 2015;85:910–918.

Delbeuck X, Debachy B, Pasquier F, et al. Action and noun fluency testing to distinguish between Alzheimer's disease and dementia with Lewy bodies. *J Clin Exp Neuropsychol* 2013;35:259–268.

Dubois B, Slachevsky A, Litvan I, et al. The FAB: a frontal assessment battery at bedside. *Neurology* 2000;55:1621–1626.

Dubois B, Slachevsky A, Pillon B, et al. "Applause sign" helps to discriminate PSP from FTD and PD. *Neurology* 2005;64:2132–2133.

Ferman TJ, Smith GE, Boeve BF, et al. DLB fluctuations: specific features that reliably differentiate DLB from AD and normal aging. *Neurology* 2004;62:181–187.

Ferrari R, Kapogiannis D, Huey ED, et al. FTD and ALS: a tale of two diseases. *Curr Alzheimer Res* 2011;8(3):273–294.

Fillenbaum GG, Heyman A, Wilkinson WE, et al. Comparison of two screening tests in Alzheimer's disease. The correlation and reliability of the mini-mental state examination and the modified Blessed test. *Arch Neurol* 1987;44:924–927.

Fillenbaum GG, Landerman LR, Simonsick EM. Equivalence of two screens of cognitive functioning: the Short Portable Mental Status Questionnaire and the Orientation-Memory-Concentration test. *J Am Geriatr Soc* 1998;46:1512–1518.

Hanson JC, Lippa CF. Lewy body dementia. *Int Rev Neurobiol* 2009;84:215–228.

Hodges JR. Frontotemporal dementia (Pick's disease): clinical features and assessment. *Neurology* 2001;56(11 Suppl 4):S6–S10.

Holl AK, Ille R, Wilkinson L, et al. Impaired ideomotor limb apraxia in cortical and subcortical dementia: a comparison of Alzheimer's and Huntington's disease. *Neurodegener Dis* 2011;8:208–215.

Jurado MB, Rosselli M. The elusive nature of executive functions: a review of our current understanding. *Neuropsychol Rev* 2007;17:213–233.

Katzman R, Brown T, Fuld P, et al. Validation of a short Orientation-Memory-Concentration Test of cognitive impairment. *Am J Psychiatry* 1983;140:734–739.

Kilada S, Gamaldo A, Grant EA, et al. Brief screening tests for the diagnosis of dementia: comparison with the mini-mental state exam. *Alzheimer Dis Assoc Disord* 2005;19:8–16.

Kokmen E, Smith GE, Petersen RC, et al. The short test of mental status. Correlations with standardized psychometric testing. *Arch Neurol* 1991;48:725–728.

Krueger CE, Kramer JH. Mental status examination. In: Miller BL, Boeve BF, eds. *The Behavioral Neurology of Dementia.* New York: Cambridge University Press, 2011.

Lashley T, Rohrer JD, Mead S, et al. Review: an update on clinical, genetic and pathological aspects of frontotemporal lobar degenerations. *Neuropathol Appl Neurobiol* 2015;41:858–881.

Laureno R. *Foundations for Clinical Neurology.* New York: Oxford University Press, 2017.

McGee, S. *Evidence Based Physical Diagnosis.* 3rd ed. Philadelphia: Elsevier/Saunders, 2012.

Mesulam MM. Frontal cortex and behavior. *Ann Neurol* 1986;19:320–325.

Nyhus E, Barcelo F. The Wisconsin Card Sorting Test and the cognitive assessment of prefrontal executive functions: a critical update. *Brain Cogn* 2009;71:437–451.

Petersen RC. Clinical practice. Mild cognitive impairment. *N Engl J Med* 2011;364:2227–2234.

Prasad K, Yadav R, Spillane J, eds. *Bickerstaff's Neurological Examination in Clinical Practice.* 7th ed. New Delhi: Wiley India, 2013.

Queally VR, Evans JJ, McMillan TM. Accuracy in scoring vignettes using the mini mental state examination and the short orientation memory concentration test. *J Geriatr Psychiatry Neurol* 2010;23:160–164.

Reverberi C, Cherubini P, Baldinelli S, et al. Semantic fluency: cognitive basis and diagnostic performance in focal dementias and Alzheimer's disease. *Cortex* 2014;54:150–164.

Rossetti HC, Lacritz LH, Cullum CM, et al. Normative data for the Montreal Cognitive Assessment (MoCA) in a population-based sample. *Neurology* 2011;77:1272–1275.

Shibasaki H. *Hallett Mark. The Neurological Examination: Scientific Basis for Clinical Diagnosis.* New York: Oxford University Press, 2016.

Strub RL, Black FW. *The Mental Status Examination in Neurology.* 4th ed. Philadelphia: F.A. Davis, 2000.

Swain DG, O'Brien AG, Nightingale PG. Cognitive assessment in elderly patients admitted to hospital: the relationship between the Abbreviated Mental Test and the Mini-Mental State Examination. *Clin Rehabil* 1999;13:503–508.

Tschanz JT, Welsh-Bohmer KA, Plassman BL, et al. Cache County Study Group. An adaptation of the modified mini-mental state examination: analysis of demographic influences and normative data: the cache county study. *Neuropsychiatry Neuropsychol Behav Neurol* 2002;15:28–38.

Turner MA, Moran NF, Kopelman MD. Subcortical dementia. *Br J Psychiatry* 2002;180:148–151.

Umetsu A, Okuda J, Fujii T, et al. Brain activation during the fist-edge-palm test: a functional MRI study. *Neuroimage* 2002;17:385–392.

Vendrell P, Junque C, Pujol J, et al. The role of prefrontal regions in the Stroop task. *Neuropsychologia* 1995;33:341–352.

Wade DT, Vergis E. The Short Orientation-Memory-Concentration Test: a study of its reliability and validity. *Clin Rehabil* 1999;13:164–170.

Watson RT, Valenstein E, Heilman KM. Thalamic neglect. Possible role of the medial thalamus and nucleus reticularis in behavior. *Arch Neurol* 1981;38:501–506.

Weisman D, McKeith I. Dementia with Lewy bodies. *Semin Neurol* 2007;27:42–47.

CHAPTER 9

Disorders of Speech and Language

Phonation, strictly defined, is the production of vocal sounds without word formation; it is entirely a function of the larynx. Howls of rage, the squeals of little girls, and singing a note with the mouth open are phonation. A vocalization is the sound made by the vibration of the vocal folds, modified by workings of the vocal tract. Speech consists of words, which are articulated vocal sounds that symbolize and communicate ideas. Articulation is the enunciation of words and phrases; it is a function of organs and muscles innervated by the brainstem. Language is a mechanism for expressing thoughts and ideas as follows: by speech (auditory symbols), by writing (graphic symbols), or by gestures and pantomime (motor symbols). Language may be regarded as any means of expressing or communicating feeling or thought using a system of symbols. Grammar (or syntax) is the set of rules for organizing the symbols to enhance their meaning.

Language is a function of the cerebral cortex. Linguistic communication requires not only the motor acts necessary for execution; it also requires the reception and interpretation of these acts when they are carried out by others—along with the retention, recall, and visualization of the symbols. Speech is as dependent upon the interpretation of the auditory and visual images—and the association of these images with the motor centers that control expression—as it is upon the motor elements of expression.

In neurologic patients, the speech abnormalities most often encountered are dysarthria and aphasia. The essential difference is that aphasia is a disorder of language and dysarthria is a disorder of the motor production or articulation of speech. The common vernacular phrase "slurred speech" could be due to either. Aphasia usually affects other language functions such as reading and writing. Dysarthria is defective articulation of sounds or words of neurologic origin. In dysarthria, language functions are normal and the patient speaks with proper syntax, but pronunciation is faulty because of a breakdown in performing the coordinated muscular movements necessary for speech production. A good general rule is that no matter how garbled the speech, if the patient is speaking in correct sentences—using grammar and vocabulary commensurate with his dialect and education—he has dysarthria and not aphasia. In dysarthria, there are often other accompanying bulbar abnormalities—such as dysphagia—and a brainstem lesion is usually a prominent clinical consideration. Dysarthria is a problem with articulation of speech; aphasia is a problem with language function. The implications of these two conditions are quite different. Disturbed language function is always due to brain disease, but dysfunction limited to the speech mechanisms may occur with many conditions, neurologic and nonneurologic.

Difficulty talking is a common neurologic symptom, and many conditions could be responsible. The following sections discuss the anatomy, physiology, clinical examination, and disorders of articulation. They also include a review of the following: the anatomy of the cerebral language centers, the examination of the aphasic patient, and the different types of aphasia. Other disturbances of higher cortical function include apraxias, agnosias, and various disconnection syndromes, which are discussed in Chapter 10.

ANATOMY AND PHYSIOLOGY OF ARTICULATION

Sounds are produced by expired air passing through the vocal cords. Properly articulated speech requires coordination between the respiratory muscles and the muscles of the larynx, pharynx, soft palate, tongue, and lips. All of these components are referred to as the vocal (oral) tract. Respiratory movements determine the strength and rhythm of the voice. Variations in pitch are accomplished by alterations in the tension and length of the vocal cords and the rate and character of the vibrations transmitted to the column of air that passes between them. Modifications in sound are produced by changes in the size and shape of the glottis, pharynx, and mouth and by changes in the position of the tongue, soft palate, and lips. The oropharynx, nasopharynx, and mouth act as resonating chambers and further influence the timbre and character of the voice.

Speech may be possible in the absence of vocal cords, and whispered speech may be possible in inspiration as well as expiration. Esophageal speech is used by patients who cannot move air over the vocal cords, such as after tracheostomy or laryngectomy. The patient swallows a bolus of air and then allows it to escape in a controlled fashion. The escaping air causes vibrations in the walls of the esophagus and pharynx, particularly the cricopharyngeal sphincter, producing a sound that can be articulated by the mouth and lips to produce speech.

Articulation is one of the vital bulbar functions. Several cranial nerves (CNs) are involved in speech production, and an adequate appraisal of speech requires evaluating the function of each. The trigeminal nerves control the muscles of mastication and open and close the mouth. The facial nerves control the muscles of facial expression, especially the branches to the orbicularis oris and other smaller muscles about the mouth that control lip movement. The vagus nerves and glossopharyngeal nerves control the soft palate, pharynx, and larynx, and the hypoglossal nerves control tongue movements. Other factors include the following: the upper cervical nerves, which communicate with the lower CNs and, in part, supply the infrahyoid and suprahyoid muscles; the cervical sympathetic nerves that contribute to the pharyngeal plexus; and the phrenic and intercostal nerves, which also contribute to normal speech.

TYPES OF SPEECH SOUNDS

Voiced sounds are produced by narrowing the glottis so that the vocal cords are approximated. Voiceless sounds are made with the glottis open. Either type of sound may be modulated by adjusting the size and shape of the vocal cavities. Vowels are largely of laryngeal origin but are modified by the resonance of the vocal cavities. Certain vowel sounds such as i, a, and y are modified by the soft palate. Consonants may be either voiced or voiceless; they are enunciated by constriction or closure at one or more points along the vocal tract.

Speech sounds may be placed in different categories related to the place of articulation (e.g., labiodental, interdental, alveolar, palatal, alveopalatal, velar, and uvular). From an anatomic and neurologic viewpoint, it is more important to recognize how various sounds are produced. Articulated labials (b, p, m, and w) are formed principally by the lips. Modified labials (o and u, and to a lesser extent i, e, and a) are altered by lip contraction. Labiodentals (f and v) are formed by placing the teeth against the lower lip. Linguals are sounds formed with tongue action. T, d, l, r, and n are tongue-point, or alveolar, sounds, formed by touching the tip of the tongue to the upper alveolar ridge. S, z, sh, zh, ch, and j are dentals, or tongue-blade sounds. To hear distorted linguals, place the tip of your tongue against the back of your bottom teeth, hold it there and say "top dog," "go jump," and "train." To hear distorted labials, hold your upper lip between the thumb and forefinger of one hand and your bottom lip similarly with the other and say "my baby." Gutturals (velars, or tongue-back sounds, such as k, g, and ng) are articulated between the back of the tongue and the soft palate. Palatals (German ch and g, and the French gn) are formed when the dorsum of the tongue approximates the hard palate.

EXAMINATION OF ARTICULATION

Examination of articulation begins with noting the patient's spontaneous speech in normal conversation, usually during taking of the history. The accuracy of pronunciation, rate of speech, resonance, and prosody (variations in pitch, rhythm, and stress of pronunciation) are noted. Abnormalities of articulation include tremulousness, stuttering, slurring, or sliding of letters or words, scanning, explosiveness, and difficulties with specific sound formations. Some difficult-to-enunciate phrases have been traditionally used. These require the pronunciation of labials, linguals, and, to a lesser extent, velars. The nonsense phrase "puhtuhkuh" or "pataka" tests all the three: labials (puh/pa), linguals (tuh/ta), and velars (kuh/ka).

Traditional phrases have been selected to test primarily the labials and linguals, such letters as l, r, b, p, t, and d. As the patient repeats these phrases, various aspects of the dysarthria may become more evident. These phrases are time-honored, perhaps above their actual value, and are to a certain extent colloquial. Nonetheless, they are often useful. Pronouncing r's requires a facile tongue, and many of the test phrases are loaded with this letter. The best test words and phrases have the significant consonants and vowels placed in the initial, middle, and final positions. Commonly used words and phrases include *third riding artillery brigade, Methodist Episcopal, West Register Street, liquid electricity, truly rural, voluntary retribution, baby hippopotamus*, and *irretrievable ball.* Phrases such as "my baby ate a cupcake on the train" contain all of the pertinent elements.

Have the patient repeat a syllable such as "puh" over and over as rapidly as possible. Normally, the syllable can be pronounced accurately at a rate of 5 to 7 Hz. Then try for "tuh" and "kuh." Listen for abnormally slow or rapid repetition, regularity and evenness, uniform loudness, or tremulousness. Speech pathologists count how long it takes for the patient to pronounce a syllable such as "puh" 20 times to determine the diadochokinetic syllable rate.

Weakness and fatigueability of articulation, such as might occur in myasthenia gravis (MG), may be brought out by having the patient count to 100 at about one number per second, enunciating each number clearly. Listen for the voice to become hoarse, hypernasal, slurred, or breathy. Disturbances of laryngeal function and of speech rhythm may be elicited by having the patient attempt prolonged phonation, such as by singing and holding a high "a" or "e" or "ah" sound. Assess loudness, pitch, quality (hoarseness, breathiness), steadiness, nasality, and duration. The voice may break, waver, or flutter excessively, particularly when there is cerebellar dysfunction. Note whether the pitch of the voice is appropriate for the patient's age and sex. Ability to hold a high note indicates the vocal cords are adducting normally.

Normal coughing requires normal vocal cord movement. A normal cough indicates that vocal cord innervation is intact. Dysphonia with a normal cough suggests laryngeal disease or a nonorganic speech disturbance. The glottal coup (glottic click, coup de glotte) is the sharp sound at the beginning of a cough. The intensity of the glottic click reflects the power of vocal cord adduction. The glottic click may also be elicited by asking the patient to say "oh-oh" or to make a sharp, forceful grunting sound. A cough without a glottal coup (bovine cough) suggests vocal cord palsy.

Resonance is an important voice quality. Normal resonance depends on an adequate seal between the oropharynx and nasopharynx (velopharyngeal competence). When palatal weakness causes an inadequate seal on pronouncing sounds that require high oral pressure, the voice has a nasal quality. An audible nasal emission is nasal air escape that causes a snorting sound. Hypernasality is more noticeable when the head is tipped forward; it is less evident when the patient lies with his head back because the weakened soft palate falls back by its own weight and closes off the nasopharynx. To check for nasal air leakage, hold a smooth glass or metal surface, such as one lens of a pair of spectacles, under the patient's nostrils. Pronouncing sounds with a nasal component (m, n, ng) as in the phrase "ming, ping, ring, sing," will normally produce slight condensation and fogging of the surface. Have the patient say a phrase with no sounds having a nasal component ("we see three geese"). Clouding of the surface suggests an abnormal nasal component of the voice. Velopharyngeal incompetence is common in patients with cleft palate.

DISORDERS OF ARTICULATION

Lesions of the nervous system may cause various abnormalities of sound production and word formulation (Table 9.1). Laryngeal disorders may alter the volume, quality, or pitch of the voice (dysphonia). Laryngitis causes dysphonia. Aphonia is complete voice loss. A central or peripheral disturbance of the innervation of the articulatory muscles may cause dysarthria. Lesions may involve the peripheral nerves, brainstem nuclei, or the central corticobulbar, extrapyramidal, or cerebellar pathways. Anarthria is a total inability to articulate because of a defect in the control of the peripheral speech musculature. Videostroboscopy has become a standard technique for evaluating articulatory disturbances.

Lesions of the cerebral centers and connections that subserve language function may cause aphasia, an abnormality of language, even though the articulation mechanisms may be intact. Mutism is a total inability to speak; usually the patient appears to make no attempt to speak or make sounds. Mutism is usually of psychogenic origin if present in an apparently otherwise normal patient, but it may occur with lesions of the cerebrum, brainstem, and cerebellum (especially in children). In akinetic mutism, the patient is mute and unmoving (akinetic). The patient

TABLE 9.1 Differential Diagnosis of Abnormal Speech in the Absence of Obvious Oral Abnormality

- Speech abnormal
  - Language functions (syntax, naming, comprehension, etc.) abnormal → aphasia
  - Language functions normal
    - Voice volume, pitch, timbre abnormal
      - Dysphonia
        - High-pitched, strained, choking → adductor spasmodic dysphonia
        - Hoarse, whispery, mute
          - Cough abnormal → vocal cord palsy
          - Cough normal
            - Abductor spasmodic dysphonia
            - Local laryngeal disease
            - Nonorganic dysphonia
    - Voice volume and pitch normal
      - Speech rhythm, prosody abnormal
        - Speech slurred, drunken sounding → cerebellar dysfunction vs. intoxication
        - Speech flat, monotonous, without normal inflection or emotionality → Extrapyramidal dysfunction vs. right frontal lobe lesion
      - Speech rhythm, prosody normal
        - Speech hypernasal
          - Palatal weakness
        - Abnormal labials (puh, papa, mama, baby hippopotamus)
          - Facial weakness
        - Abnormal linguals (tuh, daddy, darn it)
          - Anterior tongue weakness
        - Abnormal velars (kuh, cupcake, coke)
          - Palatal or posterior tongue weakness

appears awake but is mute, immobile, and unresponsive. Akinetic mutism most often occurs with damage to the frontal lobes. Selective (elective) mutism is a disorder of childhood characterized by a total lack of speech limited to certain situations—such as school—despite normal speech in other settings. The present discussion is limited to disorders limited to the motor components of speech; disorders of language are discussed subsequently.

Abnormalities of articulation may be caused by many different pathologic conditions. Disturbances in the respiratory rhythm interfere with speech, and respiratory muscle weakness causes a feeble voice with abnormalities in regularity and rhythm. Laryngeal disease may cause severe speech impairment, but whispered speech may still be possible. In children, articulation disturbances may be developmental and are often temporary. Structural abnormalities of the vocal tract, such as congenital craniofacial defects (cleft palate, cleft lip), ankyloglossia (abnormal shortness of the frenulum of the tongue; "tongue-tie"), adenoidal hypertrophy, vocal cord edema or nodules, nasal obstruction, or perforated nasal septum may cause abnormalities in sound production. The importance of the teeth in articulation is apparent in the speech of edentulous patients.

Neurologic disturbances of articulation may be caused by the following: primary muscle diseases affecting the tongue, larynx, and pharynx; neuromuscular junction disorders; lower motor neuron disease involving either the CN nuclei or the peripheral nerves that supply the muscles of articulation; cerebellar dysfunction; basal ganglia disease; or disturbances of the upper motor neuron control of vocalization. A commonly used classification separates dysarthria into flaccid, spastic, ataxic, hypokinetic, hyperkinetic, and mixed types.

Lesions of the hypoglossal nerve or nucleus—or local disorders of the tongue such as ankyloglossia—may cause impairment of all enunciation, but with special difficulty in pronouncing lingual sounds. The speech is lisping in character and is clumsy and indistinct. Paralysis of the laryngeal musculature causes hoarseness, and the patient may not be able to speak above a whisper; there is particular difficulty pronouncing vowels. Similar changes occur in laryngitis and in tumors of the larynx. With unilateral laryngeal muscle weakness, such as in recurrent laryngeal nerve lesions, the voice is usually low-pitched and hoarse. However, occasionally severe unilateral vocal cord weakness may be present without much effect on speech because the normal vocal cord is able to adduct across the midline and approximate the abnormal cord. Hoarseness because of slight vocal cord weakness may be brought out by having the patient talk with his head turned to one side. With paralysis of the cricothyroid, the voice is hoarse and deep and fatigues quickly. Diplophonia is one sound being produced at two different frequencies because of differences in vibration when one vocal cord is weak and the other normal. In bilateral abductor paresis, speech is moderately affected, but in bilateral total paralysis it is lost.

Paralysis limited to the pharynx causes little detectable impairment of articulation. Weakness of the soft palate results in nasal speech (rhinolalia, Gr. lalia "speech"), caused by inability to seal off the nasal from the oral cavity. Voice sounds have an added abnormal resonance. There is special difficulty with the velar sounds, but labials and linguals are also affected because much of the air necessary for their production escapes through the nose. The speech resembles that of a patient with a cleft palate.

Characteristically, b becomes m, d becomes n, and k becomes ng. Amyotrophic lateral sclerosis and MG are common causes of this type of speech difficulty.

Seventh nerve paralysis causes difficulty in pronouncing labials and labiodentals. Dysarthria is noticeable only in peripheral facial palsy; the facial weakness in the central type of facial palsy is usually too mild to interfere with articulation. Bell's palsy occasionally causes marked dysarthria because of inability to close the mouth, purse the lips, and distend the cheeks. Similar articulatory defects are found in myopathies involving the labial muscles (e.g., facioscapulohumeral or oculopharyngeal dystrophy), in cleft lip and with wounds of the lips. There is little impairment of articulation in trigeminal nerve lesions unless the involvement is bilateral; in such cases, there are usually other characteristics of bulbar speech. Trismus may affect speech because the patient is unable to open the mouth normally.

Lower motor neuron disorders causing difficulty in articulation may occur in cranial neuropathies. Lesions of the ninth and eleventh nerves usually do not affect articulation. A unilateral lesion of CN X causes hypernasality. Lesions involving the vagus bilaterally distal to the origin of the superior laryngeal nerve may leave the vocal cords paralyzed in adduction, resulting in a weak voice with stridor. With more proximal lesions, there is no stridor, but the voice and cough are weak.

Neuromuscular disorders, particularly neuromuscular junction disorders, often interfere with speech. In MG, prolonged speaking, such as counting, may cause progressive weakness of the voice with a decrease in volume and at times the development of a bulbar or nasal quality, which may even proceed to anarthria. As the voice fatigues, the speech of a patient with bulbar myasthenia may be reduced to an incoherent whisper. Thomas Willis, who provided one of the first descriptions of MG in 1672, wrote of a woman who, when she tried to talk for a prolonged period, "temporarily lost her power of speech and became mute as a fish." An occasional myasthenic patient must hold his jaw closed with his hand in order to enunciate.

Motor neuron disease commonly causes dysarthria. The type varies from a primarily flaccid dysarthria in bulbar palsy to a primarily spastic dysarthria in primary lateral sclerosis; most patients have classical amyotrophic lateral sclerosis, and the dysarthria is of mixed type with both flaccid and spastic components; that is, there are both bulbar palsy and pseudobulbar palsy (see below). In bulbar palsy, dysarthria results from weakness of the tongue, pharynx, larynx, soft palate, and, to a lesser extent, the facial muscles, lips, and muscles of mastication. Both articulation and phonation may be affected; speech is slow and hesitant with failure of correct enunciation, and all sounds and syllables may be indistinct. The patient talks as though his mouth were full of mashed potatoes. Speech is thick and slurred, often with a nasal quality and a halting, drawling, monotonous character. The tongue lies in the mouth, more or less immobile, shriveled, and fasciculating; the palate rises very little. The dysarthria may progress to a stage where there is phonation but no articulation. Speech is reduced to unmodified, unintelligible laryngeal noises. Often at this stage, the jaw hangs open and the patient drools. The condition may eventually reach the stage of anarthria. Dysphagia is typically present as well. For a video of flaccid dysarthria, see **Video Link 9.1**.

Supranuclear lesions involving the corticobulbar pathways may also cause dysarthria. Unilateral cortical lesions do not usually affect speech unless they are in the dominant hemisphere and cause aphasia. Occasionally, some dysarthria accompanies aphasia. Rarely, lesions in the cortical motor areas for articulation may cause severe dysarthria without aphasia. Both dysarthria and dysprosody, a defect in rhythm, melody, and pitch, have been described with localized frontal lobe lesions; these may be due to an apraxia of speech (AOS). In acute hemiplegia, there may be transient slurring or thickness of speech depending on the degree of face and tongue weakness.

Bilateral supranuclear lesions involving the cortex, corona radiata, internal capsule, cerebral peduncles, pons, or upper medulla may cause pseudobulbar palsy with spastic dysarthria. The muscles that govern articulation are both weak and spastic. Phonation is typically strained-strangled, and articulation and diadochokinesis are slow. There is a thick bulbar type of speech, similar to that in progressive bulbar palsy, but more explosive; it rarely progresses to complete anarthria. The tongue is protruded and moved from side to side with difficulty. There may also be spasticity of the muscles of mastication; mouth opening is restricted and speech seems to come from the back of the mouth. The jaw jerk, gag reflex, and facial reflexes often become exaggerated and emotional incontinence commonly occurs (pseudobulbar affect). For a video of spastic dysarthria, see **Video Link 9.2**.

The Foix-Chavany-Marie (bilateral anterior opercular) syndrome is the loss of voluntary bulbar movements, with preservation of involuntary movements and reflexes, due to a lesion involving the frontal opercular regions bilaterally. Unilateral lesions of the dominant frontal operculum may cause "cortical dysarthria" or AOS (see below).

Lesions of the basal ganglia may affect speech. Athetotic grimaces of the face and tongue may interfere with speech. Irregular spasmodic contractions of the diaphragm and other respiratory muscles, together with spasms of the tongue and pharynx, may give the speech a curious jerky and groaning character. In addition, there may be a pseudobulbar element with slurred, indistinct, spastic speech. When chorea is present, the violent movements of the face, tongue, and respiratory muscles may make the speech jerky, irregular, and hesitant. The patient may be unable to maintain phonation, and occasionally, there is loss of the ability to speak. Dysarthria is one of the most common neurologic manifestations of Wilson's disease, and frequently the presenting complaint. It is typically mixed with spastic, ataxic, hypokinetic, and dystonic elements. The type of dysarthria often corresponds with other manifestations, with spasmodic dysphonia in those with dystonic features, hypokinetic in those with parkinsonism, and ataxic in those with tremor as the primary manifestation. Pantothenate kinase-associated neurodegeneration (Hallervorden-Spatz syndrome) may cause a similar mixed spastic-extrapyramidal dysarthria.

Speech in parkinsonism is often mumbled, hesitant, rapid, and soft (hypophonic). Parkinsonian patients tend to be soft, fast, mumbly talkers. There may sometimes be bradylalia, with feeble, slow, slurred speech because of muscular rigidity and immobility of the lips and tongue. There is dysprosody, and the speech lacks inflections, accents, and modulation. The patient speaks in a monotone, and the words are slurred and run into one another. The voice becomes increasingly weak as the patient talks, and he may become unable to speak above a whisper; as the speech becomes more indistinct it may become inaudible or practically disappear. Words may be chopped off. There may be sudden blocks and hesitations, or speech may stop abruptly. There may be pathologic repetition of syllables, words, or phrases (palilalia). Like the parkinsonian gait, the speech may show festination, with a tendency to hurry toward the end of sentences or long words.

Voice tremor produces rhythmic alterations in loudness and pitch. There may be associated tremor of the extremities or head, or other signs of neurologic dysfunction. Voice tremor may further complicate the other speech disturbances of parkinsonism. Voice tremor occurs commonly in essential tremor, a frequently familial syndrome that most often affects the hands. Fine voice tremors are characteristic of essential tremor; coarse tremors are more commensurate with cerebellar disease. Essential voice tremor is probably more common than generally suspected, and many cases appear to go unrecognized or misdiagnosed, most often as spasmodic dysphonia. Voice tremor is a common manifestation of anxiety. Lip and chin tremors, when severe, may interfere with speech. In habit spasms, Tourette's syndrome, and obsessive-compulsive states, there may be articulatory tics causing grunts, groans, or barking sounds. In Tourette's syndrome, palilalia may also occur.

Cerebellar dysfunction causes a defect of articulatory coordination (scanning speech, ataxic dysarthria, or speech asynergy). Many studies have attempted to localize speech functions in the cerebellum. The superior regions bilaterally appear to mediate speech motor control and the right cerebellar hemisphere has a putative role in speech planning and processing. Lesion mapping studies have shown that dysarthria occurs with pathology affecting the upper paravermal areas, or lobules V and VI. Subtypes of ataxic dysarthria are recognized, common to all is an impairment of articulation and prosody.

Ataxic dysarthria causes a lack of smooth coordination of the tongue, lips, pharynx, and diaphragm. Ataxic speech is slow, slurred, irregular, labored, and jerky. Words are pronounced with irregular force and speed, with involuntary variations in loudness and pitch lending an explosive quality. There are unintentional pauses, which cause words and syllables to be erratically broken. Excessive separation of syllables and skipped sounds in words produce a disconnected, disjointed, faltering, staccato articulation (scanning speech). The speech pattern is reminiscent of a person who is sobbing or breathing hard from exertion. The unusual spacing of sounds with perceptible pauses between words and irregular accenting of syllables may cause a jerky, singsong cadence that resembles the reading of poetry. Ataxic speech is particularly characteristic of multiple sclerosis. It may be accompanied by grimaces and irregular respirations. Ataxia of the voice and scanning speech may be more apparent when the patient repeats a fairly long sentence.

Specific speech abnormalities may occur in various neurologic conditions. The disturbance varies in individual cases and depends upon the site of the predominant pathologic change. In multiple sclerosis, the speech is characteristically ataxic; there are explosive and staccato elements, with slowness, stumbling, halting, slurring, and a cerebellar type of speech ataxia. Spastic-ataxic and mixed dysarthrias are also common. In Friedreich's ataxia, the ataxic, staccato, and explosive elements predominate. Speech is clumsy, often scanning, and the pitch may suddenly change in the middle of a sentence. In alcohol intoxication, the speech is slurred and indistinct. There is difficulty with labials and linguals, and there may be tremulousness of the voice. Conversation is often characterized by a tendency to garrulousness. The patient may repeatedly use words he can pronounce correctly, avoiding the use of other words. This results from loss of cerebral cortical control over thought and word formulation and speech, rather than from a primary articulatory disturbance. In delirium tremens, the speech is tremulous and slurred. Other types of intoxication also produce speech that is thick and slurred. Rarely, the inability to relax muscles in myotonia causes slight speech impairment. Myxedema may cause a low-pitched, harsh, husky, slow, and monotonous voice. General paresis may cause a tremulous, slurring type of dysarthria, with special difficulties with the linguals and labials. Letters, syllables, and phrases are omitted or run together. The speech is slovenly, with ataxia, stumbling, and alliteration, often accompanied by tremors of the lips, tongue, and face.

Patients with some forms of aphasia, dysarthria, dysprosodia, and speech apraxia may begin to sound as if they have developed an unusual accent. The foreign accent syndrome during recovering facial diplegia made one patient from Virginia sound for several months as if she were a Bavarian countess. The foreign accent syndrome has been reported as the only manifestation of a cortical lesion and as the presenting manifestation of primary progressive aphasia (PPA).

Spasmodic dysphonia is a focal dystonia characterized by a striking abnormality of voice production. In adductor dysphonia, irregular involuntary spasms of the vocal muscles cause erratic adduction of the cords. As the patient strains to speak through the narrowed vocal tract, his voice takes on a high-pitched, choked quality that varies markedly during the course of a sentence. It is most marked in stressed vowels. The dysphonia may lessen or disappear when the patient sighs or whispers. For a video of spasmodic dysphonia, see **Video Link 9.3**.

The much rarer abductor spasmodic dysphonia causes excessive abduction of the involved cord, and the voice is hoarse and breathy. In both types, there is often a dramatic improvement in the voice during shouting, whispering, or singing. The difference in adductor and abductor spasmodic dysphonia is nicely demonstrated in the audio/video posted by Reich and Meyer. Both types may respond dramatically to the injection of botulinum toxin into the involved muscle.

Secondary speech disturbances may also occur without abnormalities or specific dysfunction of the articulatory apparatus, as seen in individuals with hearing defects, delayed physical development, intellectual disability, and psychogenic disturbances. Severe hearing loss, especially when it occurs early in life before speech patterns are ingrained, can result in abnormalities of speech. The nature and severity of the speech abnormality depend largely upon the degree of hearing loss, the time at which it occurred, and the individual's ability to compensate. The speech disorder may range from a mild abnormality of articulation to the indistinct and often unintelligible speech of deaf-mutism. A child with slow physical development or psychological problems may retain childish speech until later years. Childish speech may persist in mild intellectual disability. With moderate disability, speech develops late, and the vocabulary is limited. It may be slow, labored, indistinct, and difficult to understand. With severe disability, speech is babbling and grunting in character, with a tendency toward echolalia. In delayed puberty and in eunuchism, the male voice retains juvenile or feminine characteristics, whereas in the virilized woman, it may be low-pitched and coarse.

Stuttering refers to faulty, spasmodic, interrupted speech characterized by involuntary hesitations in which the speaker is unable to produce the next expected sound. The flow of speech is broken by pauses during which articulation is entirely arrested. Stammering may happen to anyone in certain circumstances, as with embarrassment. Stuttering implies a more severe disturbance of speech, with faltering or interrupted speech characterized by difficulty in enunciating syllables and joining them together. Interference with communication may be profound and the social consequences severe. Stuttering speech is stumbling and hesitant in character, with habitual and spasmodic repetitions of consonants or syllables, alternating with pauses. There may be localized cramps, spasms, and tic-like contractions of the muscles essential to articulation, which may be accompanied by grimaces, spasms and contractions of the muscles of the head and extremities, and spasm and incoordination of the respiratory muscles. The individual may be unable to pronounce certain consonants, with particular difficulty in using dentals and labials. Often the first syllable or consonant of a word is repeated many times. The individual may remain with his mouth open until the articulatory spasm relaxes, then the words explode out until the breath is gone. He then takes another breath, and the process is repeated. Stuttering is markedly influenced by emotional excitement and by the presence of strangers. In spite of difficulty in speaking, the individual may be able to sing without hesitation. There have been accomplished professional singers who stuttered severely in ordinary speech. Britain's King George VI stuttered severely, as memorably depicted in the motion picture *The King's Speech*. Many theories have been offered regarding the etiology of stuttering.

In lalling (lallation, "baby talk"), the speech is childish, babbling, and characterized by a lack of precision in pronouncing certain consonants, especially the letters r and l. A uvular is substituted for a lingual-palatal r, so that "broken reed" is pronounced "bwoken weed." The diphthong ow or other sounds may be substituted for the l sound, or sometimes l may be substituted for r. T and d may be substituted for s, g, and the k sound. Lalling may occur because of hearing defects, intellectual or physical disability, or from psychogenic disorders. In lisping, the sibilants are imperfectly pronounced, and th is substituted for s; a similar defect in articulation may be associated with partial edentulism. Lalling and lisping are usually because of imperfect action of the articulatory apparatus (as in children), persistent faulty habits of articulation, imitation of faulty patterns of articulation, poor speech training, habit, or affectation.

NONORGANIC (FUNCTIONAL) SPEECH DISORDERS

Emotional and psychogenic factors influence articulation. Speech, but not language, disorders may occur on a nonorganic basis. Nonorganic voice disorders can take many different forms and can be caused by a variety of factors. The most common functional voice disorders are dysphonia and aphonia. Dysarthria, lalling, stuttering, mutism, or anarthria occurs rarely. Psychogenic foreign accent syndrome has been reported. There may be infantile language wherein the objective pronoun is used as the subject (e.g., "Me want to go home"). Onset is often abrupt, perhaps in association with emotional trauma; there may be periods of remission, and the condition may suddenly disappear. The speech defect may vary in type from time to time. It is often bizarre, and does not correspond to any organic pattern. The patient may fail to articulate and speak only by whispering. Speech may be lost but the patient is able to sing, whistle, and cough. There may be associated dysphagia and globus hystericus.

In anxiety and agitation the speech may be broken, tremulous, high-pitched, uneven, and breathless. Stuttering and stammering are common. The speech may be rapid and jumbled (tachyphemia or tachylalia), or there may be lalling or mutism. In psychogenic aphonia, there is profound speech difficulty but no disturbance of coughing or respiration. Manic patients may have a rapid flow of words (pressured speech), often with an abrupt change of subject. In depression speech may be slow, sometimes with mutism. True organic aphasia is occasionally confused with psychogenic or simulated mutism. The aphasic patient, no matter how speechless, at least occasionally tries to speak; in psychogenic mutism there may be the appearance of great effort without the production of so much as a tone; in simulated mutism, the patient does not even make an effort. Mutism may also occur in catatonia. In schizophrenia there may be hesitancy with blocking, or negativism with resulting mutism (alalia). Two common nonorganic dysphonias seen in children and adolescents are the whispering syndrome, seen primarily in girls, and mutational falsetto (high-pitched voice), seen primarily in boys.

Palilalia, echolalia, and perseveration are often manifestations of psychosis, but they can occur with organic lesions, especially of the frontal lobes. Palilalia is the repetition of one's own speech. Echolalia is the meaningless repetition of heard words. Perseveration is the persistence of one reply or one idea in response to various questions. Neologisms are new words, usually meaningless, coined by the patient, and usually heard in psychotic states or in aphasic patients. Idioglossia is imperfect articulation with utterance of meaningless sounds; the individual may speak with a vocabulary all his own. Idioglossia may be observed in patients with partial deafness, aphasia, and congenital word deafness. Alliterative sentences, repetition, and confusion are found in delirium and in psychosis. Dyslogia refers to abnormal speech because of psychiatric disease, and it is most often used to refer to abnormal speech in dementia.

APHASIA

When focal brain disease affects primary cortex, the resulting deficit reflects the area involved (e.g., hemiparesis with conditions affecting the posterior frontal lobe, or visual field defects with conditions affecting the occipital lobe). When disease affects association cortex or areas of the brain that subserve high-level integrative function, a variety of abnormalities of higher cortical function may result. Aphasia (dysphasia) refers to a disorder of language, including various combinations of impairment in the ability to spontaneously produce, understand, and repeat speech, as well as defects in the ability to read and write. A deficit affecting only speech is usually dysarthria, because of cerebellar disease or weakness or spasticity of the speech-producing musculature.

In the late 18th century, Russian clinicians began to report aphasia. Broca (1861) noted loss of speech associated with a lesion of the left inferior frontal convolution, and Trousseau (1862) first used the term aphasia. Wernicke's seminal ideas laid the groundwork for many of the current concepts of aphasia. In 1874, he described loss of speech comprehension (word deafness) from a lesion of the left superior temporal gyrus, and he later reported that a lesion posterior to the superior temporal gyrus, in the region of the angular gyrus, was followed by inability to comprehend written words (alexia, or word blindness). Wernicke also provided the first description of what is now known as conduction aphasia. Lichtheim proposed a model of the cortical speech areas based on Wernicke's ideas (the Wernicke-Lichtheim model). This model was further described and popularized by Benson, Geschwind, and others at the Boston Aphasia Research Center to create what is now referred to as the Wernicke-Geschwind model, or the Boston classification.

Overall, functional neuroimaging has shown that the 19th-century model of language is remarkably insightful, confirming the importance of the left posterior inferior frontal (PIF) and posterior superior temporal (PST) cortices as predicted by Broca, Wernicke, and Lichtheim. However, the Wernicke-Geschwind model has a number of limitations, for example, it does not account for language disturbances caused by subcortical lesions other than conduction aphasia; it does not account for the often significant recovery after stroke, possibly because of plasticity with speech functions taken over by other areas of the cortex; and it does not account for the diverse nature of most aphasias, for example, comprehension deficits in Broca's aphasia.

A simple definition of aphasia is a disorder of previously intact language abilities because of brain damage. A more comprehensive definition considers it a defect in or loss of the power of expression by speech, writing, or gestures or a defect in or loss of the ability to comprehend spoken or written language or to interpret gestures, because of brain damage. Aphasia implies that the language disorder is not due to paralysis or disability of the organs of speech or of muscles governing other forms of expression. The term dysphasia is not helpful and is easily confused with dysphagia; therefore, it has fallen into disuse.

There are three cortical levels involved in language comprehension. The first is the level of arrival, a function of the primary cortical reception areas; at this level, language symbols are perceived, seen, or heard, without further differentiation of the impulses. The second level is that of knowing, or gnostic function, concerned with the recognition of impulses, formulation of engrams for recall of stimuli, and revisualization. The third level, the one of greatest importance in aphasia, has to do with recognition of symbols in the form of words, or the higher elaboration and association of learned symbols as a function of language.

There are also three levels of motor speech function. In aphasia, the most elementary of these is least frequently affected, and the most complex most often involved. Most primitive is the emotional level; the patient may respond to a painful stimulus with an "ouch," even though other language functions are entirely absent. Emotional language may be preserved when all other language functions are lost. Next is the automatic level, which is concerned with casual, automatic speech; the patient may be able to answer questions with words such as "yes" and "no," and be able to count or recite the days of the week, even though other elements of speech are severely impaired. The highest level is propositional, volitional, symbolic, or intellectualized language, which is most easily disrupted and most difficult to repair. Language requires the use of symbols (sounds, marks, gestures) for communication. Propositional language is the communication of thoughts, ideas, feelings, and judgments using words, syntax, semantics, and rules of conversation. A normal individual is able to understand complex sentences and make statements that require thought and concentration.

ANATOMY OF THE LANGUAGE CENTERS

The classical language centers are located in the perisylvian areas of the language-dominant hemisphere (Figure 9.1). Although these anatomical constructs are useful, current evidence is that language functions involve widespread neural networks in many parts of both hemispheres. This may help explain the many clinical nuances found in language disorders. The language areas form a C-shaped mass of tissue around the lips of the Sylvian fissure extending from Broca's area to Wernicke's area. The central sulcus intersects the Sylvian fissure near its posterior ramus. The PIF language areas lie in front of the central sulcus in the frontal lobe and are referred to as anterior or prerolandic. The PST areas lie posterior to the central sulcus and are referred to as posterior or postrolandic. The anterior speech areas subserve the motor—or expressive—aspects, and the posterior areas subserve the sensory—or perceptive—aspects of language. Broca's speech area lies in the inferior frontal gyrus. It is essentially the motor association cortex, the executive area for language function that lies just anterior to the primary motor areas for the lips, tongue, and face. The region of the left precentral gyrus of the

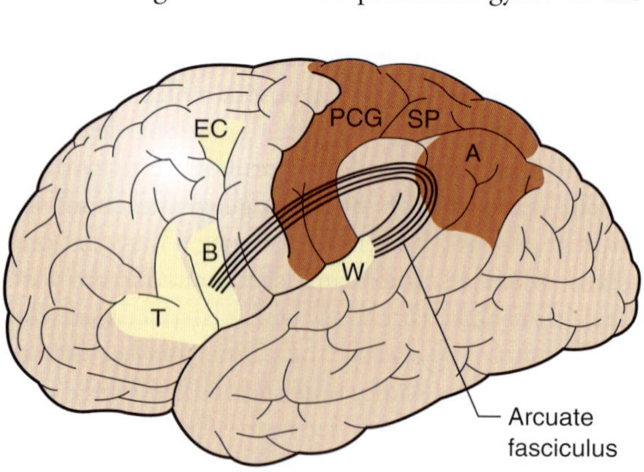

FIGURE 9.1 Centers important in language. A, angular gyrus; B, Broca's area; EC, Exner's writing center; SP, superior parietal lobule, which with the PCG (postcentral gyrus) is important in tactile recognition; T, pars triangularis; W, Wernicke's area.

insula, a cortical area beneath the frontal and temporal lobes, seems to be important in the motor planning of speech.

Wernicke's speech area lies in the superior temporal gyrus. It is essentially the sensory association cortex that lies just posterior to the primary auditory cortex. The arcuate fasciculus (AF) is a deep white matter tract that arches from Wernicke's area around the posterior end of the Sylvian fissure and through the subcortical white matter of the insula to Broca's area. Other tracts in the subcortical white matter of the insula provide additional connections between the PIF and PST areas. The angular gyrus is part of the inferior parietal lobule; it caps the posterior ramus of the Sylvian fissure and lies between Wernicke's area and the visual cortex. The angular gyrus is important for reading and similar nonverbal language functions. The supramarginal gyrus also lies between the visual cortex and the posterior perisylvian language areas and is involved with visual language functions. Exner's center is a purported cortical area concerned with writing that lies in the middle frontal gyrus of the language-dominant frontal lobe very near the frontal eye field, just anterior to the primary motor cortex for the hand. There may be white matter tracts connecting Wernicke's and Exner's areas analogous to the AF.

Although the cortical areas and connections described above are important language centers, the clinicopathologic correlations are not so exact as to permit precise localization in all instances. The degree of deficit seems to correlate with the size of the lesion as well as its location. Language functions are not as discretely localized in the brain as are things such as vision and elemental sensation, but they are more localized than such faculties as intelligence, judgment, and creativity. There is evidence that propositional speech depends on left hemisphere regions remote from the classic perisylvian language areas. The 2012 meta-analysis of more than 100 functional imaging studies done by Dewitt and Rauschecker implicates a much broader portion of the superior temporal gyrus in speech comprehension than has been previously appreciated, challenging the classical scheme that word recognition occurs in the PST gyrus.

The perisylvian language areas are perfused by the middle cerebral artery (MCA); the anterior language areas are supplied by the superior division and the posterior areas by the inferior division. Most cases of aphasia are due to ischemia in the MCA distribution. Aphasia occurs in as many as 40% of stroke patients but can also occur in other disorders, such as neoplasms, degenerative disorders, and demyelinating disease. Aphasia due to a tumor is generally less severe than aphasia due to a stroke in the same region. Dysphagia is common in patients with nonfluent aphasia, and strokes causing aphasia have twice the mortality as nonaphasic strokes.

EXAMINATION OF THE PATIENT WITH APHASIA

Initial appraisal of language function takes place during the taking of the history. Obvious deficits require exploration, but there may be language deficits that are not readily apparent during history taking. For example, the inability to repeat, which is the essential characteristic of conduction aphasia, may not be apparent during history taking. Some degree of formal assessment is usually prudent. In evaluating aphasia, it is important to know about the patient's handedness, cultural background, languages spoken, vocabulary, and intellectual capacity. It is difficult to evaluate language status in a person who has altered mental status, inattention, agitation, or severe depression. Patients with emotional problems may have language disturbances on a nonorganic basis. Any apparent speech or language difficulty must of course be correlated with the findings on other parts of the neurologic examination. The evaluation of hearing is discussed in Chapter 17. Aphasia is sometimes mistaken for dementia and vice versa.

About 90% to 95% of the population is right-handed. The left cerebral hemisphere is dominant for language in 99% of right-handers, and 60% to 70% of left-handers. Of the remaining left-handers, about half are right-hemisphere dominant and about half have mixed dominance. Shifted sinistrals (anomalous dextrals) are naturally left-handed individuals forced by parents or teachers early in life to function right-handed, primarily for writing. This approach to dealing with left-handedness has largely died out, but shifted sinistrals are still encountered, primarily in the older population. One can therefore encounter right-handed patients (dextrals) who are left-hemisphere dominant for language, left-handed patients (sinistrals) who are still left-hemisphere dominant, "right-handed" patients who are right-hemisphere dominant (anomalous dextrals), and left-handed patients who are right-hemisphere dominant (true sinistrals). Because clinical abnormalities of higher cortical function, especially language, are heavily influenced by dominance, determination of the patient's handedness and dominance status is paramount. Only about 2% of cases of aphasia are due to unilateral right hemisphere lesions.

Cerebral dominance and handedness are at least in part hereditary. Failure to develop clear hemispheric dominance has been offered as an explanation for such things as dyslexia, stuttering, mirror writing, learning disability, and general clumsiness. Many patients are at least to some degree ambidextrous, and it may be difficult, short of a Wada test, to be certain which hemisphere is language dominant. Various "foolproof" markers of true handedness have been proposed, but all are suspect. In right-handed patients, aphasia will be due to a left hemisphere lesion in 99% of the cases; the other 1% are crossed aphasics. In left-handers, the situation is much more variable. In one series of left-handed aphasics, 60% had lesions of the left hemisphere. There may be a degree of mixed dominance for language in non–right-handed individuals. Aphasia may tend to be less severe in left-handers and recover better; just a family history of left-handedness in a right-handed aphasic may predict better recovery. Basso has challenged the concept of better recovery in non–right-handed patients.

Multilingual aphasics require examination in all of their languages. Polyglots may have several centers for speech in somewhat discrete but overlapping cortical areas. Neurophysiologic and neuroimaging studies are gradually adding to our knowledge of the regions of the brain involved in the various speech-related processes. In bilinguals, the cerebral representation of some functions is similar for both languages, but the areas concerned with other functions may be different depending on when the languages were acquired. Which language recovers best in multilingual aphasics is variable. Pitres' law states that recovery from aphasia will be best for the language most used, but Ribot's rule holds that recovery will be best for the native language. In fact, most patients show parallel recovery in both languages.

There are six separate components of language function that are typically tested in the clinical arena: spontaneous (conversational) speech, auditory comprehension, naming, reading, writing, and the ability to repeat. It is often useful to assess these components individually before trying to synthesize the findings into a diagnostic entity. There are several instruments available for more detailed examination of the aphasic patient, such as the Boston Diagnostic Aphasia Examination, Western Aphasia Battery, and others. The Western Aphasia Battery produces a summary score reflecting overall severity (aphasia quotient). For clinical purposes, it is not clear these add a great deal to the bedside examination.

SPONTANEOUS SPEECH

In addition to high-level propositional speech, spontaneous utterances may include the lower-level functions of emotional and automatic speech. Emotional speech is spontaneous speech prompted by a high emotional charge. It is present in animals, especially higher primates, and in humans before they acquire propositional language. Some patients with aphasia, primarily nonfluent aphasia, even when severe, may swear and curse eloquently when angry, often to the shock and surprise of friends and family. Automatic speech refers to the recitation of simple overlearned items from early childhood or to a specific retained speech fragment that an aphasic patient is still capable of saying even in the presence of severe nonfluency. Even when unable to produce propositional speech, an aphasic patient may be able to automatically count, say the days of the week or months of the year, repeat the alphabet, say his name, or recite nursery rhymes. Some aphasic patients are able to sing simple overlearned songs, such as Happy Birthday, even when they are unable to speak.

A retained fragment that an aphasic patient repeats over and over has been referred to as a monophasia (recurring utterance, verbal stereotypy, verbal automatism, verbigeration). In monophasia, the individual's vocabulary is limited to a single word, phrase, or sentence, such as "do-do-do" or "Oh, God." Verbal automatisms occur most often in global aphasia. The recurrent utterance may be a real word or a neologism. Sometimes the monophasia is an outrageous expletive that bursts from an otherwise dignified and respectable patient under socially awkward circumstances. Some verbal automatisms are unusual and difficult to understand. One aphasic patient would say "Pontius Pilate" in response to any and all questions. Other examples include "no pasta," "television," and "gotta go." Broca's original aphasic patient, M. Leborgne, was nicknamed "Tan" because that was the only word he could say. According to Critchley, Hughlings Jackson first became interested in aphasia when his family vacationed in a house where the aphasic landlady could utter only the neologistic stereotypy "watty." A patient may have several stereotypies in their repertoire, and preservation of stereotypic social responses ("hello," "fine") may trick the careless or rushed clinician into believing the patient is linguistically intact. Speech automatisms can also occur as an ictal phenomenon.

A paraphasia is a speech error in which the patient substitutes a wrong word or sound for the intended word or sound. Paraphasic errors are common in aphasic patients. In a phonemic (phonologic, literal) paraphasia, there is the addition, deletion, or substitution of a phoneme; however, the word is recognizable and may be clearly pronounced. Substitution of the wrong phoneme would cause the patient to say "blotch" instead of watch, or "thumbness" instead of numbness. Technically, a literal paraphasia is a single-letter substitution. Phonemic paraphasia is the preferable term because a single-letter substitution also changes the phoneme, and the brain thinks in phonemes, not letters. Illiterate patients commit phonemic paraphasias despite their ignorance of letters. In a semantic (verbal) paraphasia, the patient substitutes the wrong word. A semantic paraphasia would cause the patient to say "ring" instead of watch. Paraphasias are similar to the malapropisms, spoonerisms, and sniglets everyone occasionally utters, but aphasic patients make them more often and may not recognize them as wrong. A neologism is a novel utterance, a nonword made up on the spot. The patient might call a watch a woshap. Phonemic paraphasias are more typical of anterior, and semantic paraphasias more typical of posterior, perisylvian lesions.

In evaluating propositional speech, note pronunciation, word and sentence formation, fluency, cadence, rhythm, prosody, omission or transposition of syllables or words, misuse of words, circumlocutions, repetition, perseveration, paraphasias, jargon, and the use of neologisms. Aphasic patients may use unusual synonyms or circumlocutions in order to avoid the use of a word that cannot be recalled. There may be omissions of words; hesitations and inappropriate pauses; perseveration; difficulty understanding the implication of words; verbal automatisms; agrammatism; jargon; or gibberish. When the patient is having difficulty with fluency, it is difficult to evaluate propositional spontaneous speech. Fluency refers to the volume of speech output. Normal speech is 100 to 115 words per minute. Speech output is often as low as 10 to 15 words per minute, sometimes less, in patients with nonfluent aphasia. If the maximum sentence length is fewer than seven words, then the patient is nonfluent. Patients are usually aware of nonfluency and frustrated by it. Their speech may tend toward the laconic, answering questions but trying to speak no more than necessary. Patience and open-ended questions are the best approaches in persuading the patient to converse. Patients unable to express themselves through speech may use pantomime or gesture, shaking, or nodding the head, shrugging the shoulders, or demonstrating visible emotional reactions. In severe aphasia, the patient may be unable to utter a single word.

COMPREHENSION

The patient's responses to verbal requests and commands and to everyday questions and comments give information about his ability to understand speech. Comprehension may be tested by having the patient follow verbal commands ("show me your teeth," "stick out your tongue," "close your eyes," or "point to the ceiling"). Comprehension can be judged to be reasonably intact if the patient follows a complicated, multistep command. However, failure to follow a command, even a simple one, does not necessarily prove that comprehension is impaired. A patient may not comply because of apraxia. Patients with a left hemisphere lesion may even have apraxia for functions of their nonparetic left hand. They may be unable to salute, wave goodbye, or perform other simple functions on command using the left hand because of involvement of fibers that transmit information from the language areas on the left to the motor areas on the right (sympathetic apraxia). When the patient does not follow simple commands, establish whether he can say or shake his head yes and no. Then ask ridiculously simple questions, such as—"Are you from the planet Jupiter?," "Did you have nails for breakfast?," "Are you riding in a taxicab?," or "Are you a man (or a woman)?" Include obvious "no" questions, as some aphasic patients will agree with almost anything. The responses may be nonverbal. An elderly woman who laughs when asked "Are you pregnant?" has understood the question. More complex yes-no questions might include the following: "Is a mother older than her daughter?," "Do you have dinner before breakfast?," "Can you fly in a car?," "Did the sun come up this morning?," or "Do you have feet on the ends of your legs?" Because the chance of a correct response is 50%, it is important to ask enough questions to exclude lucky answers.

Impaired comprehension may result from difficulty understanding grammar and syntax, words in relation to other words, difficulty with semantics or understanding individual words. The patient may have more difficulty with polysyllabic words and long sentences than with simple words and short sentences. Compound sentences and double or complex commands may be used to see if comprehension is more than superficial. The aphasia examination begins to overlap with the mental status examination with commands such as "place one coin on the table, give me the second, and keep the third in your hand" or "here is a piece of paper; tear it in four parts and place one on the table, give one to me, and keep two for yourself" (Marie's paper test). Both comprehension and retention are evaluated by telling a short story and then asking questions about it. Patients with impaired comprehension have particular difficulty with passive constructions (e.g., "The lion was killed by the tiger; which animal is dead?" or "The boy was slapped by the girl; who got hit?") and possessives (e.g., "Is my wife's brother a man or a woman?"). Patients who are unable to comprehend spoken or written language may understand pantomime, gestures, and symbols. They may imitate the examiner in placing a finger to the nose or sticking out the tongue. Imitation, however, is a more lower-level function than comprehension.

Many aphasic patients have difficulty with right-left orientation, especially with posterior lesions. Right-left confusion is part of Gerstmann's syndrome. Testing right-left orientation might include such commands as "show me your right thumb" or "touch your right ear with your left thumb." It is important to determine baseline function before concluding a patient has right-left confusion.

NAMING

Testing naming ability is an important part of the aphasia examination. Naming is a delicate function, and most aphasic patients have some difficulty with it. However, naming defects are nonspecific. In anomic aphasia, an inability to name is an isolated defect, but more often misnaming occurs as part of some other aphasic, or even nonaphasic, syndrome. In confrontation naming, the patient is asked to name simple objects such as a key, pencil, coin, watch, parts of the body (nose, ear, chin, fingernail, knuckle), or to name colors. When lost for the name of an object, the patient may describe it or tell its use. The patient may be able to name an object, such as a watch, but be unable to identify the component parts, such as the band or buckle. Some caution is necessary, as there are age, cultural, and even gender influences at work. For whatever reason, many normal women are unable to identify a watch crystal. Many normal men (with intact color vision) are unable to name more than primary and very simple secondary colors. Before including something as a naming test item, the examiner should ensure that nonaphasic people of all ages and both sexes are normally able to identify it. Some normal patients use unusual names for various parts of the body, especially the fingers. Some of this is related to educational level and region of origin. Individuals may refer to the index finger or pointer as "the finger next to the thumb," or call it the "dog finger," "poison finger," or "statue of liberty finger." These patients are not aphasic. Many normal individuals cannot name the index, middle, and ring fingers. When unable to retrieve a name, an aphasic patient may be able to select the correct name from a list. Another naming test is to have the patient point to something named by the examiner (e.g., the telephone, the window).

A sensitive method of testing spontaneous naming ability is word list generation. The patient is asked to name as many items as possible in a certain category in 1 minute. Animals are a common category for testing spontaneous naming. The patient may name any types of animals (e.g., farm, zoo), but groups should not be suggested ahead of time because there may be an inability to shift groups. It is wise to check more than one item category; other useful categories include tools, foods, countries, and modes of transportation. Spontaneous naming ability also depends on age and educational level. Normal patients should name a minimum of 12 items in a category; some adjustment may be necessary for poorly educated and older patients. Another measure of spontaneous naming is to ask the patient to list all of the words he can think of that begin with a certain letter. The FAS test is popular. The patient thinks of words beginning with one of these letters, excluding proper nouns or morphologic variants. For FAS, a person of average education should produce 12 or more words per letter in 1 minute, or 36 words with all three letters in 3 minutes. Standardization and reference values for testing naming are imperfect. Language competence depends on education, dialect, experience, and other factors. Often the reference population does not include less well-educated people nor every dialect. Poor word list generation may also occur with dementia, depression, parkinsonism, and prefrontal lesions. Responsive naming is also useful, and it uses audition rather than vision. The patient may be asked for nouns (e.g., "Where do teachers work?"), verbs (e.g., "What do you do with a cup?"), or adjectives (e.g., "How does sugar taste?").

REPETITION

The ability to repeat may be selectively involved or paradoxically preserved in certain aphasic syndromes. Most often the inability to repeat is proportional to the defect in comprehension or fluency, and repetition is a good screening test for aphasia. The patient is asked to repeat words or phrases back to the examiner. A patient's repetition span (i.e., the number of words he can repeat) is usually two more than his digit span. Simple repetition tasks might include counting, avoiding numbers that might be repeated by automatic speech, or repeating single words. More complex tasks include polysyllabic words (e.g., catastrophe), phrases (e.g., "If he were here, I would go away"), or tongue twisters (e.g., Popocatepetl [po-pó-cah-té-petl], a volcano in Mexico). The stock phrases used to test for dysarthria work for this purpose as well. A popular phrase for testing repetition in aphasia is "no ifs, ands, or buts." Omitting the s in each of these words may not be an error in some dialects of English. A better repetition test is "they heard him speak on the radio last night" (modified from the Boston diagnostic aphasia examination). Patients with impaired repetition may omit words, change the word order, or commit paraphasic errors. Repetition is preserved in anomic, transcortical, and some cases of subcortical aphasia.

WRITING

The patient's ability to use written language should also be assessed. Accompanying impairment of fine motor control of the dominant hand often hampers the ability to evaluate writing. Writing may be disturbed in conjunction with abnormalities of spoken language, or separately. Patients who are aphasic in speech are also aphasic in writing, but writing may be preserved in patients with dysarthria or verbal apraxia. In all aphasias, reading and writing are typically worse than understanding and speaking, probably because they are secondarily acquired skills. The patient may be asked to write spontaneously or to dictation. A spontaneous writing sample might include a few words, a sentence, or a paragraph. The writing sample usually reveals the same sorts of naming difficulties and paraphasias evident in the patient's speech. Patients may be able to write elementary, overlearned things such as name, address, days of the week, and months of the year but be unable to write more complex material. There may be a difference in the patient's ability to print and to write in cursive. The ability to write to dictation is analogous to the ability to repeat verbal material. Copying written material also assesses the ability to transfer information from the visual system to the language areas. Having the patient copy written material may also test the connections between the receptive language areas and Exner's writing center. However, copying does not require much processing; one can copy material in another language despite not speaking the language, as long as the alphabet is the same. An inability to copy may be due to apraxia. Naming can also be tested by having the patient write down the names of things in a manner similar to that for speech.

Modern electronic communications have brought to light new aphasic disturbances: difficulty writing mobile phone texts, an entity called dystextia, and difficulty typing on a computer, dystypia. These have been reported in both stroke and complex migraine. Aphasia can also affect sign language.

READING

The patient's ability to comprehend written language symbols can be tested by having him read. Written language is perceived by the visual system and the information conveyed to the perisylvian language centers. Dysfunction of the language centers or interruption of the connections with the visual system may cause an inability to read (alexia). Reading difficulty because of acquired alexia is unrelated to the developmental (congenital) dyslexia seen most often in school-age boys that may cause severe reading disability. Patients may have alexia without any accompanying inability to comprehend speech—the syndrome of pure word blindness. Alexia may occur with or without a hemianopia. Alexia may occur with or without accompanying agraphia. Most patients with alexia also have difficulty with writing (alexia with agraphia). Some patients have alexia without agraphia (see Chapter 10). Judging reading ability by having the patient follow a written command such as close your eyes involves a praxis element and should be interpreted with caution. For patients unable to read aloud, use questions that can be answered by "yes" or "no," or by gestures. It is also important to determine whether the patient is able to read his own writing.

Reading aloud is a different task from reading comprehension. Oral reading (visual input-oral output) is comparable to copying (visual input-manual output), repetition (auditory input-oral output), and transcribing dictation (auditory input-manual output) and may be preserved despite impaired reading comprehension.

CLASSIFICATION OF THE APHASIAS

Classification of the aphasias is problematic. These disorders vary in severity, even with a lesion in the same location, and are frequently mixed in type. There have been many attempts at classification from anatomic, physiologic, and psychological points of view. None is entirely satisfactory. A strictly anatomic classification does not apply in all instances, for a small lesion may cause severe impairment of both fluency and comprehension, whereas an extensive lesion sometimes causes an isolated defect. Lesions similar in size and location on imaging studies may be associated with different aphasic syndromes even in persons with identical cerebral dominance for speech. Lesions in different locations and of variable size may produce similar aphasic syndromes. Nevertheless, some general relationships exist between anatomic sites and the type of aphasia.

One common classification divides aphasias into expressive and receptive types. In expressive aphasia, the patient has difficulty with speech output and struggles to talk (nonfluent); in receptive aphasia, the primary difficulty is with understanding language, whereas speech output is unaffected (fluent). A major problem with the expressive-receptive classification of aphasia is that all aphasic patients have difficulty expressing themselves. This causes difficulty, particularly for trainees and nonneurologists. There is a tendency to classify almost all aphasias as expressive, even when they are flagrantly receptive. It requires some clinical experience to recognize that a patient may be having difficulty expressing himself linguistically because of a defect in the reception (comprehension) of spoken language. Other simple dichotomous classifications proposed include fluent/nonfluent, motor/sensory, and anterior/posterior. Although each of these is useful, none adequately describes most aphasic patients, who have some evidence of both types. Pure forms of aphasia are uncommon; most patients with sensory aphasia have some motor deficit, posterior lesions can cause nonfluency, anterior lesions can cause comprehension deficits, and aphasic disorders can occur with pathology that does not directly affect the classical perisylvian language centers, such as subcortical and even nondominant hemisphere lesions. In the mid-19th century, John Hughlings Jackson expressed a preference for the fluent and nonfluent subtypes. Most aphasia experts discourage the expressive-receptive scheme.

The Wernicke-Geschwind model (Boston classification) recognizes eight aphasia syndromes: Broca's, Wernicke's, conduction, global, transcortical motor, transcortical sensory, transcortical mixed (isolation of the speech area), and anomic. It divides aphasias into fluent and nonfluent varieties (Tables 9.2 and 9.3). If speech output is high and articulation facile, the aphasia is referred to as fluent; if speech output is sparse and effortful, the aphasia is classified as nonfluent. Nonfluency occurs when a lesion involves the anterior speech areas in the region of Broca's area in the frontal lobe. When these areas are relatively spared, fluency is preserved. Broca's is a type of nonfluent aphasia. Many aphasic patients fail to fulfill the criteria for a specific subtype other than fluent/nonfluent.

When the posterior speech areas in the region of Wernicke's area in the temporal lobe are involved, auditory comprehension is impaired. When this area is spared, comprehension is relatively preserved. The most common fluent aphasia is Wernicke's. In global or total aphasia, there is both nonfluency and impaired comprehension; the lesion may involve both

TABLE 9.3 Organization of Common Aphasia Syndromes

Nonfluent	
Good comprehension	
Good repetition	Transcortical motor
Poor repetition	
Aphasic writing	Broca's
Writing intact	Verbal apraxia
Poor comprehension	
Good repetition	Mixed transcortical
Poor repetition	Global
Fluent	
Good comprehension	
Good repetition	Anomic
Poor repetition	Conduction
Poor comprehension	
Good repetition	Transcortical sensory
Poor repetition	
Poor reading comprehension	Wernicke's
Intact reading comprehension	Pure word deafness

According to whether spontaneous speech is fluent or nonfluent and whether auditory comprehension and repetition are good or poor.

TABLE 9.2 The Major Aphasia Syndromes

	Aphasia Classification					
	Relative Severities					
	Fluency	Auditory Comprehension	Repetition	Naming	Reading	Writing
Broca's	–	+	–	–	–	–
Global	–	–	–	–	–	–
Wernicke's	+	–	–	–	–	–
Conduction	+	+	–	±	+	+
Anomic	+	+	+	–	+	–
Transcortical, mixed	–	–	+	–	–	–
Transcortical, motor	–	+	+	–	–	–
Transcortical, sensory	+	–	+	–	–	–
Verbal apraxia	–	+	–	–	–	+

+, function is relatively intact; –, function is abnormal; ±, involvement is mild or impairment equivocal.
Modified from Campbell WW, Pridgeon RP. *Practical Primer of Clinical Neurology*. Philadelphia: Lippincott Williams & Wilkins, 2002.

anterior and posterior speech areas. Difficulty arises because not all patients can be satisfactorily placed into one of these categories. The clinical features of aphasia evolve over time. For example, global aphasia can occur with a purely anterior lesion, but it usually evolves into a Broca's aphasia. If seen acutely, about 60% to 80% of aphasic patients fit into the anterior-nonfluent/posterior-fluent classification.

This aphasia classification can also be divided into central, or perisylvian, and paracentral, or extrasylvian, types. The central aphasias (Broca's, Wernicke's, and conduction) have in common loss of repetition. The paracentral aphasias (transcortical syndromes and anomic aphasia) have in common preserved repetition. The central aphasias are due to lesions involving the perisylvian cortical structures, and the paracentral aphasias by lesions surrounding the perisylvian areas, for example, border zone (watershed) infarction (BZI). The central and paracentral aphasias are distinguished by testing repetition. Without testing repetition, difficulty will arise in distinguishing Broca's from transcortical motor, Wernicke's from transcortical sensory, anomic from conduction, and global from isolation.

Critchley described the normal changes in linguistic ability that accompany advancing age. Aphasia may be a feature of degenerative and other diffuse neurologic disorders. Aphasia is common in Alzheimer's disease. The language disorder in Alzheimer's disease most resembles transcortical sensory aphasia, and it grows progressively worse as the disease advances. The presence of aphasia has been suggested as a diagnostic criterion for the disorder. Prominent aphasia may be associated with an earlier date of onset and more rapid progression. Patients typically display a paucity of information content in their spontaneous speech and anomia, particularly for spontaneous naming tasks. When dementia complicates Parkinson's disease, aphasia may also develop. In addition, parkinsonian patients have superimposed motor speech abnormalities related to the extrapyramidal dysfunction.

Aphasia most often results from stroke but can be caused by any pathologic process involving the language areas. PPA is a condition in which patients present with a progressive loss of specific language functions with relative sparing of other cognitive domains, eventually resulting in severe aphasia, even mutism, or evolving into dementia. Three variants of PPA are recognized: semantic variant (semantic dementia), logopenic variant, and a nonfluent-agrammatic variant. In contrast to the aphasia of Alzheimer's disease, the nonfluent variant of PPA tends to affect the anterior speech areas initially, resulting in impaired and anomia but relative preservation of comprehension. In the early stages, nonverbal cognitive abilities are preserved. Patients who present with PPA may eventually develop evidence of other degenerative neurologic disorders, most often frontotemporal lobar degeneration, occasionally corticobasal degeneration or progressive supranuclear palsy.

Broca's Aphasia (Nonfluent, Expressive, Motor, Anterior, Prerolandic, Executive)

Broca's aphasia is a nonfluent type of aphasia due to a lesion involving the anterior perisylvian speech areas in the PIF region (Figure 9.2). Patients have labored, uninflected, nonfluent spontaneous speech with a decreased amount of linguistic output: few words, short sentences, and poor grammar **(Video 9.1)**. In severe Broca's aphasia, the speech consists of nouns and substantive verbs produced with great effort. Patients are aware of and frustrated by their difficulty speaking. There is a tendency to leave out nonessential words such as adjectives, adverbs, and functor words (i.e., articles, pronouns, conjunctions, and prepositions that serve primarily to provide sentence structure rather than to convey meaning). Such parsimonious, agrammatical language is sometimes referred to as telegraphic speech. It has been likened to the speech of someone learning a new language, or of Tarzan. The patient knows what he wishes to say but is unable to say it or to say it correctly. There is an inability to use proper

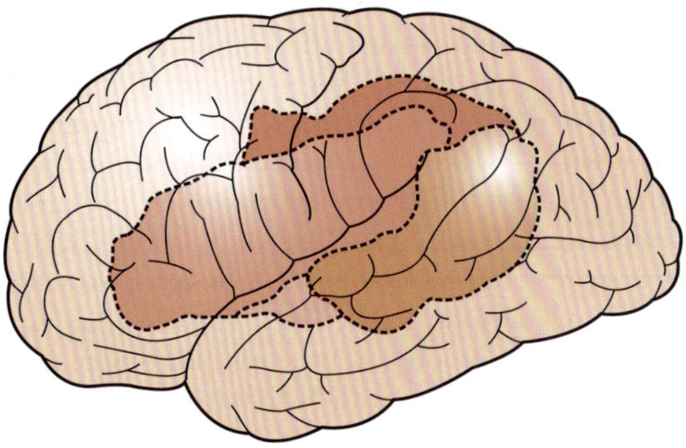

FIGURE 9.2 The extent of the lesion classically causing global aphasia is indicated by the *dashed outer line;* the lesion causing Broca's aphasia by the *light red area;* and the lesion causing Wernicke's aphasia by the *dark brown area.*

syntax, so that sentence structure is defective (paragrammatism). The resultant misuse of words and defective syntax is termed agrammatism. The ability to comprehend speech is relatively unimpaired. When challenged with difficult material, some comprehension defects usually emerge. The comprehension defect is greater for grammar than semantics. For a video of a patient with Broca's aphasia, see **Video Link 9.4**.

Because of the severe nonfluency, patients are unable to repeat what they hear and unable to read aloud. The patient can identify objects but not name them. Although the patient is nonfluent for propositional speech, there may be preservation of emotional and automatic speech, and the patient may be able to sing. Occasionally, speech is reduced to monophasia or recurrent utterances. The patient is aphasic in writing as in speech, even when using the nonparetic (usually left) hand. Preservation of writing suggests verbal apraxia.

In mild cases, there may be only slight errors in word formation, occasional circumlocutions, or word-finding difficulty, often brought out only by stressing the patient by requesting specific information in a rapid-fire manner. Patients with Broca's aphasia classically have a contralateral hemiparesis or faciobrachial paresis but no visual field deficit. Dysarthria is sometimes present in aphasic patients—either because of coincidental lesions affecting the articulatory apparatus at a lower level or as the result of apraxia of the muscles of articulation. There may be an accompanying buccofacial apraxia causing the patient to have difficulty executing mouth and lip movements on command. Sympathetic apraxia involving the nonparalyzed hand is common. Some patients with Broca's aphasia have an accompanying alexia (third alexia of Dejerine).

Occasionally, lesions affect areas of the brain that control speech but not language. The patient may have difficulty with speech, but comprehension is perfect and writing is not affected. Emotional and automatic speech functions are preserved. The problem is essentially an isolated apraxia for speech, which may or may not be accompanied by other evidence of buccofacial apraxia. The lesion in these cases may be confined to Broca's area, whereas in the more typical case of Broca's aphasia, the lesion is usually more extensive. This condition has been called apraxia of speech (AOS; verbal apraxia, cortical dysarthria, acquired AOS, Broca's area aphasia, mini-Broca, or baby-Broca). Lesions limited to Broca's area may cause the Broca's area infarction syndrome with initial mutism rapidly evolving into apractic and effortful speech without a persistent language impairment.

Patients with AOS appear to have forgotten how to make the sounds of speech. There is speech sound distortion as their articulatory muscles grope for the right position. There is defective control but no weakness of the vocal tract. Prosody may be impaired, and speech may have a stuttering quality. The speech pattern may change so that the patient sounds as though he has developed a foreign accent. There is greater difficulty with polysyllabic words and complex phrases than with simple words. The patient with AOS may be able to repeat short, common words but will fail longer, polysyllabic words. Syllable transposition is common ("pasghetti"). With puhtuhkuh, the patient may interpose a syllable or perseverate on one syllable. The speech resembles the hesitant nonfluency seen in Broca's aphasia, but the patient speaks in correct English sentences, using proper grammar and syntax. Indeed, some of the speech difficulty in Broca's aphasia may be due to an element of AOS. Closely related to AOS is the syndrome of pure word mutism (aphemia, pure motor aphasia of Dejerine). The patient is totally unable to speak, but auditory comprehension, reading, and writing are normal. The usual cause is a small lesion of the PIF area.

Modern imaging and clinicopathologic studies have shown that lesions restricted to Broca's area more likely cause predominantly AOS or Broca's area infarction syndrome rather than aphasia. The development of Broca's aphasia seems to require a large perisylvian lesion that involves Broca's area and the subjacent white matter, as was present in his original patient. With large, acute lesions, mutism may occur initially. Persistence of aphasia after stroke is usually associated with larger lesions.

Wernicke's Aphasia (Fluent, Receptive, Sensory, Posterior, Postrolandic)

Wernicke's aphasia is due to a lesion in the PST region that involves the auditory association cortex and the angular and supramarginal gyri (Figure 9.2). Patients are unable to understand speech (word deafness) or unable to read (word blindness). They are relatively fluent, with a normal or even increased word output (logorrhea, hyperlalia), but there is loss of the ability to comprehend the significance of spoken words or recall their meaning. Speech production is effortless; phrase and sentence length and prosody are normal. Although speech is abundant, it is devoid of meaningful content. The patient can still hear and can recognize voices but not the words they utter. Paraphasic errors are frequent, resulting in incorrect or unintelligible words, unconventional and gibberish sounds, and senseless combinations. The speech abounds in neologisms. There may be circumlocution and an excess of small filler words. In its mildest form, there are mild paraphasias and minimal difficulty understanding grammatically complex material (mini-Wernicke's).

Speech may be fluent, but the patient cannot understand his own speech; he is not aware of, and does not correct, his errors in speaking. The frequent paraphasias and neologisms, combined with agrammatism, along with the high word output, may lead to completely unintelligible gibberish, termed jargon aphasia, or word salad. Hughlings Jackson described this type of aphasia as "plentiful words wrongly used." This is an example of speech from a patient with Wernicke's, "We stayed with the water over here at the moment and talked with the people with the them over there, they're giivving for them at the moment." Naming and repetition deficits arise from poor comprehension. There is usually an accompanying proportional alexia. Rarely, there is dissociation between the comprehension defects for spoken and written language. Often the patient lacks awareness of the deficit and may actually appear euphoric. Patients with Wernicke's aphasia often have a visual field deficit but no hemiparesis. When due to vascular disease, the ischemia is usually in the distribution of the inferior division of the MCA. With large, acute lesions, Wernicke's aphasia may evolve from a state of mutism. As with Broca's aphasia, lesions causing Wernicke's aphasia usually extend beyond the superior temporal gyrus. Patients with acute Wernicke's aphasia may become agitated because of their comprehension difficulty. The agitated patient, speaking gibberish and with no gross neurologic deficit, is frequently thought to be psychotic. Psychotic speech is distinguished by bizarre content, few paraphasic errors, and minimal comprehension difficulties. For a video of Wernicke's aphasia, see **Video Link 9.5**.

Global (Total, Expressive-Receptive, Complete) Aphasia

In global aphasia, most commonly a large lesion has destroyed the entire perisylvian language center, or separate lesions have destroyed both the PIF and PST regions (Figure 9.2). Grossly nonfluent speech is combined with a severe comprehension deficit and inability to name or repeat. Speech is often reduced to expletives or monophasia. Typically, there is both a hemiplegia and a field cut. Global aphasia is usually due to internal carotid or proximal MCA occlusion. In some patients, comprehension improves, leaving a deficit resembling Broca's aphasia.

Conduction (Associative, Commissural, Central, Deep) Aphasia

Conduction aphasia was described by Carl Wernicke, who called it leitungsaphasie. It is due to a lesion that interrupts the conduction of impulses between Wernicke's and Broca's areas. The characteristic deficit is poor repetition with relative preservation of other language functions. Comprehension is often impaired but not to the degree seen in Wernicke's. The patient is relatively fluent, but the speech is contaminated by paraphasic errors (primarily literal, with incorrect phonemes); comprehension is unaffected, and naming is variable. Repetition is worst for multisyllabic words and sentences, and it is during repetition that paraphasic errors are most apt to appear. Patients are aware of and try to correct the pronunciation errors. Patients have difficulty reading aloud and writing to dictation. The remainder of the neurologic examination is often normal or shows mild hemiparesis. The lesion most often lies in the deep white matter in the region of the supramarginal gyrus and involves the AF and other fiber tracts that run from the posterior to the anterior language areas (Figure 9.3). In addition, conduction aphasia can occur with cortical injury and no subcortical extension. The etiology is

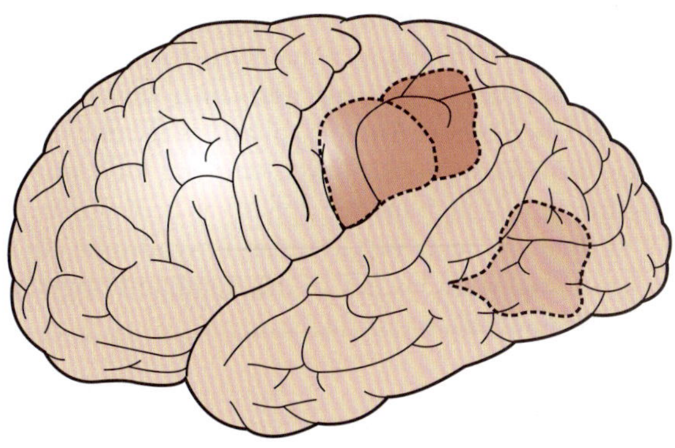

FIGURE 9.3 The lesion classically causing conduction aphasia is indicated by the lightly shaded area; the lesion causing anomic aphasia by lightly shaded area at right; and the lesion causing the angular gyrus syndrome by the darkly shaded area.

usually an embolic occlusion of a terminal branch of the MCA. Because it disconnects the anterior from the posterior perisylvian language areas, conduction aphasia represents one of the disconnection syndromes (see Chapter 10).

Conduction aphasia may evolve from Wernicke's aphasia. Although conduction aphasia results primarily from lesions that disrupt communication between Wernicke's and Broca's areas, the most severe and persistent repetition disturbance follows damage to Wernicke's area itself.

Anomic (Amnesic, Amnestic, Nominal) Aphasia

In anomic aphasia, there is a deficit in naming ability with preservation of other language functions. The patients are fluent, have good comprehension, and are able to repeat. Speech may be relatively empty and circumlocutory because of the word-finding deficit. Anomic aphasia is the most common but least specific type of aphasia. Anomia occurs with every type of aphasia. Patients with any aphasia type, as it develops or recovers, may pass through a stage in which anomia is the primary finding, and it may be the most persistent deficit. In anomic aphasia, the patient usually is simply at a loss for a name; anomia associated with other aphasia types often provokes a paraphasia. Only when anomia occurs as an isolated deficit throughout the course of the illness is the designation anomic aphasia appropriate. Dysnomia is sometimes used to refer to mild difficulty with naming. Associated neurologic findings vary widely; many patients have none. Anomic aphasia is regarded as nonlocalizing syndrome; the lesion cannot be readily localized to any particular cortical area. Patients may have naming difficulty as a manifestation of lesions that are outside the language areas or of generalized cerebral dysfunction. Anomic aphasia as the only language disorder suggests a lower temporal lobe lesion (Figure 9.3). When anomic aphasia is accompanied by all four elements of Gerstmann's syndrome, the lesion virtually always lies in the dominant angular gyrus (Figure 9.3).

Transcortical (Extrasylvian) Aphasia

The transcortical aphasias (TCAs) are syndromes in which the perisylvian language area is preserved but disconnected from the rest of the brain (Figure 9.4). The usual etiology is a BZI. Because the PIF and PST

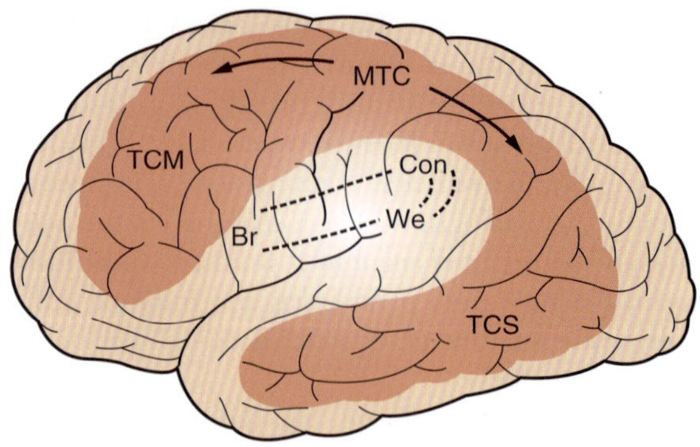

FIGURE 9.4 Areas typically involved in transcortical aphasias; these correspond to the watershed zones between major arterial distributions. Br, Broca's; Con, conduction; MTC, mixed transcortical; TCM, transcortical motor; TCS, transcortical sensory; We, Wernicke's. (From Benson DF, Geschwind N. The aphasias and related disturbances. In: Joynt RJ, ed. *Clinical Neurology*. Philadelphia: J.B. Lippincott, 1990:1–34.)

areas and the connecting AF are intact, the patients are aphasic but have a paradoxical preservation of the ability to repeat. Repetition can be so well preserved that the patients display echolalia, repeating everything they hear. When the condition is severe and the entire perisylvian language complex is separated from the rest of the brain, the patients are not fluent in spontaneous speech and are unable to comprehend. This syndrome has been termed isolation of the speech area, or mixed TCA. When the lesion is primarily anterior, the syndrome resembles Broca's aphasia with nonfluency in spontaneous speech but intact comprehension. Repetition is better than spontaneous speech. This is the syndrome of transcortical motor aphasia (anterior isolation syndrome). The supplementary motor area and dorsolateral prefrontal cortex, which are responsible for the planning and initiation of speech, are isolated from the PIF region. In transcortical sensory aphasia (posterior isolation syndrome), there is greater involvement of the posterior language areas. The PST region is isolated from the surrounding parietal, occipital, and temporal cortex that store word associations. The patients are fluent but have difficulty with comprehension; repetition is better than spontaneous speech. Associated neurologic findings are much like those in Broca's aphasia. The TCAs are more common than is often appreciated. There are reports of a fairly specific pattern of aphasia in BZI, with patients having mixed TCA initially, then evolving to motor TCA or sensory TCA depending on the individual anatomy. Exceptions to the pattern have been reported, for example, transcortical sensory aphasia due to a frontal lobe lesion. These may be because of anomalous location of language centers and variability in the anatomy of the AF.

Subcortical Aphasia

Subcortical (extrasylvian) aphasia refers to language disorders that arise not from damage to the perisylvian language areas, but from lesions—usually vascular—involving the thalamus, caudate, putamen, periventricular white matter, or internal capsule of the language-dominant hemisphere. Subcortical aphasia is not a new concept; it was recognized by Lichtheim in the 19th century. The speech disorder is difficult to categorize in the Wernicke-Geschwind scheme and may most resemble a TCA. Two types have been described: an anterior and a posterior syndrome. The anterior syndrome (caudate or striatocapsular aphasia) is characterized by slow dysarthric speech with preserved phrase length, that is, not telegraphic, preserved comprehension, and poor naming. In the posterior syndrome (thalamic aphasia), there is fluent speech without dysarthria, poor comprehension, and poor naming. In both forms, repetition is relatively preserved, and the patients usually have an accompanying hemiplegia. The anterior syndrome resembles a transcortical motor aphasia, and the posterior syndrome resembles Wernicke's or transcortical sensory aphasia but accompanied by a hemiplegia. It is the relative preservation of repetition that indicates a link between the subcortical and transcortical syndromes. The anterior syndrome shows more clinical variability than the posterior. The mechanism by which subcortical lesions cause aphasia remains conjectural, but it may involve secondary dysfunction of the perisylvian language areas because of interruption of fibers that communicate between cortical and subcortical structures. Modern imaging has shown that cortical hypoperfusion is common in subcortical aphasia. In a single-photon emission computed tomography study, left cerebral cortical hypoperfusion was observed in all patients with striatocapsular infarction.

NONDOMINANT HEMISPHERE LANGUAGE DISTURBANCES

How much language function resides in the nondominant hemisphere remains a matter of debate. Non–right-handers, particularly, are thought to have some speech function in the nondominant hemisphere. Some of the recovery from aphasia and the persistence of emotional and automatic speech suggest some language function may be present in the minor hemisphere. Lesions of the nondominant hemisphere cause speech disturbances that affect the nonlinguistic elements of language. There is loss or impairment of the rhythm and emotional elements of language. Prosody refers to the melodic aspects of speech—the modulation of pitch, volume, intonation, and inflection that convey nuances of meaning and emotional content. Hyperprosody is exaggeration, hypoprosody a decrease, and aprosody an absence of the prosodic component of speech. Dysprosody, typically hypoprosody or aprosody, may occur with right hemisphere lesions. Patients lose the ability to convey emotion in speech or to detect the emotion expressed by others. They are unable to say the same neutral phrase (e.g., "I am going to the store") in an angry or happy way. Dysprosodic speech is flat and monotonous, without inflection or emotion. The speech in parkinsonism is typically hypoprosodic. Patients with nondominant lesions may also have difficulty in understanding figurative meanings and in distinguishing the implicit and implied meaning of a phrase such as "Can you tell me the time?" There is often difficulty processing nonliteral, context bound, complex aspects of language, such as understanding figurative language, stories, and jokes.

ALEXIA AND AGRAPHIA

A lesion of the primary visual cortex causes loss of visual perception. With a lesion involving the visual association cortex, visual perception is intact, but there may be impairment of the ability to recognize and interpret visual stimuli. The region of the angular gyrus and the adjacent cortex in the dominant hemisphere (Figure 9.1) is important for the recognition and interpretation of symbols in the form of letters and words. Connections between the visual cortex and the dominant angular gyrus are vital for visual recognition of language symbols. Geschwind said that the angular gyrus, "turns written language into spoken language and vice versa." Loss of the ability to read in the absence of actual loss of vision is alexia (word blindness, visual receptive aphasia, visual sensory aphasia). There are other disorders of visual recognition in addition to alexia; these are discussed in Chapter 10.

A lesion of the angular or supramarginal gyrus, or its connections to the visual cortex, causes alexia. There is loss of the ability to recognize, interpret, and recall the meaning of visual language symbols. Printed words have no meaning, although the patient may talk without difficulty and understand what is said to him. In verbal alexia, the patient can read individual letters but not words. In some patients, the recognition of letters and syllables as well as of words may be impaired; in some, number reading may be less affected than letter identification and word reading. Reading sometimes improves when the patient traces over a letter with his finger (kinesthetic facilitation), and occasionally a patient with alexia can read by touch, recognizing embossed letters by feel even though he cannot identify them visually. Syntactic alexia is the inability to comprehend meaning that depends on syntax. The left supramarginal gyrus is particularly important for comprehension of language where the syntax conveys much of the meaning. In hemialexia, the patient ignores half of the word. Types of alexia commonly recognized include alexia with agraphia, alexia without agraphia, frontal alexia, deep alexia, and pure alexia. Patients with pure alexia may suffer from a specific word form–processing deficit; they see "wrods with trasnpsoed letters." Alexia with agraphia is classically associated with a dominant angular gyrus lesion, and alexia without agraphia with an occipitotemporal lesion with disconnection between the visual cortex and the angular gyrus.

Loss of the ability to write not because of weakness, incoordination, or other neurologic dysfunction of the arm or hand is called agraphia. Milder involvement may be referred to as dysgraphia. There are three types of agraphia: aphasic, constructional (because of visuospatial compromise), and apractic. Agraphia is seen in all types of aphasia except pure word blindness and pure word mutism. Although agraphia typically accompanies aphasia, it may occur as an isolated finding (pure agraphia) and as part of other syndromes in which the patient is not aphasic. Agraphia without alexia is a feature of Gerstmann's syndrome. A lesion involving the writing center or its connections may cause agraphia. In aphasia, writing is often even more impaired than speech. Patients may lose the ability to write even though speech is retained. The defect is essentially an apraxia of the writing hand.

Aphasic agraphia causes spelling and grammatical errors, with contraction of words, omission of letters or syllables, transposition of words, or mirror writing. Having the patient write spontaneously will usually bring out all the errors present in speech as well as spelling and letter formation errors. In dissociated agraphia, there may be difficulty in writing spontaneously or to dictation, with retention of the ability to copy written or printed material. Patients with constructional apraxia may also have difficulty writing. Constructional agraphia interferes with the proper alignment and orientation of the text. Apractic agraphia is due to inability to properly use the writing hand in the absence of other deficits. The Japanese language has two separate but parallel writing systems: kana (phonograms, syllabograms), which is similar to alphabet-based languages; and kanji (morphograms, logograms, ideograms), which consists of 1,945 symbols or characters. Patients may have alexia or agraphia to different degrees for the two systems.

AMUSIA

Loss of musical ability, either production or comprehension, may occur in patients with aphasia or agnosia, or acquired amusia may develop independently. One classification of amusia includes vocal amusia, instrumental amnesia, musical agraphia, musical amnesia, disorders of rhythm, and receptive amusia. Melody and rhythm may be affected independently. There has been speculation as to the site of the lesion producing amusia. The centers that control musical ability are largely undefined compared to the centers that control verbal language. Evaluation is hindered by the fact that the patient must not have any significant other type of aphasia, and must have had premorbid musical ability. The examiner must have some degree of appreciation of music to assess the patient. Wertheim described a comprehensive test for the evaluation of amusia. Different features of musical ability appear to be distributed between the two hemispheres; thus, elements of amusia may develop from lesions of either. Maurice Ravel, the French composer, developed amusia, probably because of a degenerative neurologic disease primarily affecting his left hemisphere. His final compositions may demonstrate the influence of the disease on his creative process. The mesmerizing *Boléro,* his most famous composition, features a predominance of changes in pitch and rhythm (more right hemisphere), with few changes in melody (more left hemisphere).

Video Links

Video Link 9.1. Flaccid dysarthria. http://neurosigns.org/wiki/Flaccid_dysarthria
Video Link 9.2. Spastic dysarthria. http://neurosigns.org/wiki/Spastic_dysarthria
Video Link 9.3. Spasmodic dysphonia. http://neurosigns.org/wiki/Spasmodic_dysphonia
Video Link 9.4. Broca'saphasia.http://neurosigns.org/wiki/Broca%27s_aphasia
Video Link 9.5. Wernicke's aphasia. http://neurosigns.org/wiki/Wernicke%27s_aphasia

BIBLIOGRAPHY

Al Hadidi S, Towfiq B, Bachuwa G. Dystextia as a presentation of stroke. *BMJ Case Rep* 2014;2014. pii: bcr2014206987.

Aladdin Y, Snyder TJ, Ahmed SN. Pearls & Oy-sters: selective postictal aphasia: cerebral language organization in bilingual patients. *Neurology* 2008;71:e14–e17.

Alexander MP, Naeser MA, Palumbo CL. Correlations of subcortical CT lesion sites and aphasia profiles. *Brain* 1987;110(Pt 4):961–991.

Amaducci L, Grassi E, Boller F. Maurice Ravel and right-hemisphere musical creativity: influence of disease on his last musical works? *Eur J Neurol* 2002;9:75–82.

Ardila A. A review of conduction aphasia. *Curr Neurol Neurosci Rep* 2010;10:499–503.

Ayotte J, Peretz I, Rousseau I, et al. Patterns of music agnosia associated with middle cerebral artery infarcts. *Brain* 2000;123(Pt 9):1926–1938.

Bakar M, Kirshner HS, Wertz RT. Crossed aphasia. Functional brain imaging with PET or SPECT. *Arch Neurol* 1996;53:1026–1032.

Bang OY, Heo KG, Kwak Y, et al. Global aphasia without hemiparesis: lesion analysis and its mechanism in 11 Korean patients. *J Neurol Sci* 2004;217:101–106.

Barr A, Brandt J. Word-list generation deficits in dementia. *J Clin Exp Neuropsychol* 1996;18:810–822.

Basso A, Farabola M, Grassi MP, et al. Aphasia in left-handers. Comparison of aphasia profiles and language recovery in non-right-handed and matched right-handed patients. *Brain Lang* 1990;38:233–252.

Becker A, Hardmeier M, Steck AJ, et al. Primary lateral sclerosis presenting with isolated progressive pseudobulbar syndrome. *Eur J Neurol* 2007;14:e3.

Benson DF. *Aphasia, Alexia, and Agraphia*. New York: Churchill Livingstone, 1980.

Bernal B, Ardila A. The role of the arcuate fasciculus in conduction aphasia. *Brain* 2009;132(Pt 9):2309–2316.

Berthier ML, Lambon Ralph MA, Pujol J, et al. Arcuate fasciculus variability and repetition: the left sometimes can be right. *Cortex* 2011;48:133–143.

Blank SC, Scott SK, Murphy K, et al. Speech production: Wernicke, Broca and beyond. *Brain* 2002;125:1829–1838.

Blanken G, Wallesch CW, Papagno C. Dissociations of language functions in aphasics with speech automatisms (recurring utterances). *Cortex* 1990;26:41–63.

Bonner MF, Ash S, Grossman M. The new classification of primary progressive aphasia into semantic, logopenic, or nonfluent/agrammatic variants. *Curr Neurol Neurosci Rep* 2010;10:484–490.

Brazis PW, Masdeu JC, Biller J. *Localization in Clinical Neurology*. 7th ed. Philadelphia: Wolters Kluwer/Lippincott Williams & Wilkins, 2017.

Buckingham HW. The mechanisms of phonemic paraphasia. *Clin Linguist Phon* 1992;6:41–63.

Burns MS, Fahy J. Broca's area: rethinking classical concepts from a neuroscience perspective. *Top Stroke Rehabil* 2010;17:401–410.

Cauquil-Michon C, Flamand-Roze C, Denier C. Borderzone strokes and transcortical aphasia. *Curr Neurol Neurosci Rep* 2011;11:570–577.

Choi JY, Lee KH, Na DL, et al. Subcortical aphasia after striatocapsular infarction: quantitative analysis of brain perfusion SPECT using statistical parametric mapping and a statistical probabilistic anatomic map. *J Nucl Med* 2007;48:194–200.

Confavreux C, Croisile B, Garassus P, et al. Progressive amusia and aprosody. *Arch Neurol* 1992;49:971–976.

Critchley M. And all the daughters of Musick shall be brought low: language function in the elderly. *Arch Neurol* 1984;41:1135–1139.

Croquelois A, Bogousslavsky J. Stroke aphasia: 1,500 consecutive cases. *Cerebrovasc Dis* 2011;31:392–399.

Damasio AR. Aphasia. *N Engl J Med* 1992;326:531–539.

Dewitt I, Rauschecker JP. Phoneme and word recognition in the auditory ventral stream. *Proc Natl Acad Sci U S A* 2012;109:E505–E514.

Dronkers NF. A new brain region for coordinating speech articulation. *Nature* 1996;384:159–161.

Dronkers NF, Plaisant O, Iba-Zizen MT, et al. Paul Broca's historic cases: high resolution MR imaging of the brains of Leborgne and Lelong. *Brain* 2007;130(Pt 5):1432–1441.

Duffy JR. Language and motor speech. In: Weibers DO, Dale AJD, Kokmen E, Swanson JW, eds. *Mayo Clinic Examinations in Neurology*. 7th ed. St. Louis: Mosby, 1998:53–85.

Dyukova GM, Glozman ZM, Titova EY, et al. Speech disorders in right-hemisphere stroke. *Neurosci Behav Physiol* 2010;40:593–602.

Espay AJ, Aybek S, Carson A, et al. Current concepts in diagnosis and treatment of functional neurological disorders. *JAMA Neurol* 2018;75(9):1132–1141.

Fabbro F. The bilingual brain: bilingual aphasia. *Brain Lang* 2001;79:201–210.

Flamand-Roze C, Cauquil-Michon C, Roze E, et al. Aphasia in border-zone infarcts has a specific initial pattern and good long-term prognosis. *Eur J Neurol* 2011;18:1397–1401.

Foundas AL, Bollich AM, Corey DM, et al. Anomalous anatomy of speech-language areas in adults with persistent developmental stuttering. *Neurology* 2001;57:207–215.

Fridriksson J, Bonilha L, Rorden C. Severe Broca's aphasia without Broca's area damage. *Behav Neurol* 2007;18:237–238.

Geschwind N. Current concepts: aphasia. *N Engl J Med* 1971;284:654–656.

Glozman JM. A.R. Luria and the history of Russian neuropsychology. *J Hist Neurosci* 2007;16:168–180.

Goodglass H, Kaplan E, Barresi B, et al. *The Assessment of Aphasia and Related Disorders*. Philadelphia: Lippincott Williams & Wilkins, 2001.

Grossman M. Primary progressive aphasia: clinicopathological correlations. *Nat Rev Neurol* 2010;6:88–97.

Henderson VW. Jules Dejerine and the third alexia. *Arch Neurol* 1984;41(4):430–432.

Hillis AE, Barker PB, Wityk RJ, et al. Variability in subcortical aphasia is due to variable sites of cortical hypoperfusion. *Brain Lang* 2004;89:524–530.

Hoffmann M, Chen R. The spectrum of aphasia subtypes and etiology in subacute stroke. *J Stroke Cerebrovasc Dis* 2013;22: 1385–1392.

Jonkers R, Bastiaanse R. Action naming in anomic aphasic speakers: effects of instrumentality and name relation. *Brain Lang* 2007;102:262–272.

Jordan LC, Hillis AE. Aphasia and right hemisphere syndromes in stroke. *Curr Neurol Neurosci Rep* 2005;5:458–464.

Jordan LC, Hillis AE. Disorders of speech and language: aphasia, apraxia and dysarthria. *Curr Opin Neurol* 2006;19: 580–585.

Joseph PR. Selective mutism—the child who doesn't speak at school. *Pediatrics* 1999;104(2 Pt 1):308–309.

Kent RD, Kent JF, Duffy JR, et al. Ataxic dysarthria. *J Speech Lang Hear Res* 2000;43:1275–1289.

Kertesz A, Poole E. The aphasia quotient: the taxonomic approach to measurement of aphasic disability. 1974. *Can J Neurol Sci* 2004;31:175–184.

Keulen S, Verhoeven J, De Page L, et al. Psychogenic foreign accent syndrome: a new case. *Front Hum Neurosci* 2016;10:143.

Kim EJ, Suh MK, Lee BH, et al. Transcortical sensory aphasia following a left frontal lobe infarction probably due to anomalously represented language areas. *J Clin Neurosci* 2009;16: 1482–1485.

Kluin KJ, Foster NL, Berent S, et al. Perceptual analysis of speech disorders in progressive supranuclear palsy. *Neurology* 1993;43(3 Pt 1):563–566.

Kluin KJ, Gilman S, Lohman M, et al. Characteristics of the dysarthria of multiple system atrophy. *Arch Neurol* 1996;53:545–548.

Konstantopoulos K, Vikelis M, Seikel JA, et al. The existence of phonatory instability in multiple sclerosis: an acoustic and electroglottographic study. *Neurol Sci* 2010;31:259–268.

Kreisler A, Godefroy O, Delmaire C, et al. The anatomy of aphasia revisited. *Neurology* 2000;54:1117–1123.

Krishnan G, Rao SN, Rajashekar B. Apraxic agraphia: an insight into the writing disturbances of posterior aphasias. *Ann Indian Acad Neurol* 2009;12:120–123.

Kuljic-Obradovic DC. Subcortical aphasia: three different language disorder syndromes? *Eur J Neurol* 2003;10:445–448.

Kumral E, Ozdemirkiran T, Alper Y. Strokes in the subinsular territory: clinical, topographical, and etiological patterns. *Neurology* 2004;63:2429–2432.

Lazar RM, Marshall RS, Prell GD, et al. The experience of Wernicke's aphasia. *Neurology* 2000;55:1222–1224.

Li EC, Williams SE. Repetition deficits in three aphasic syndromes. *J Commun Disord* 1990;23:77–88.

Liotti M, Ramig LO, Vogel D, et al. Hypophonia in Parkinson's disease: neural correlates of voice treatment revealed by PET. *Neurology* 2003;60:432–440.

Ludlow CL. Spasmodic dysphonia: a laryngeal control disorder specific to speech. *J Neurosci* 2011;31:793–797.

Mark VW. Perisylvian aphasias. In: Roos RP, ed. *MedLink Neurology*. San Diego: MedLink Corporation, 2016. Available at: www.medlink.com. Last updated: August 13, 2016.

Martnez-Sanchez F. Speech and voice disorders in Parkinson's disease. *Rev Neurol* 2010;51:542–550.

Matas M. Psychogenic voice disorders: literature review and case report. *Can J Psychiatry* 1991;36:363–365.

Matsuo K, Kato C, Sumiyoshi C, et al. Discrimination of Exner's area and the frontal eye field in humans—functional magnetic resonance imaging during language and saccade tasks. *Neurosci Lett* 2003;340:13–16.

Mesulam MM. Primary progressive aphasia. *Ann Neurol* 2001;49:425–432.

Mohr JP, Pessin MS, Finkelstein S, et al. Broca aphasia: pathologic and clinical. *Neurology* 1978;28:311–324.

Mulroy E, Murphy S, Lynch T. Alexia without agraphia. *Ir Med J* 2011;104:124.

Murdoch BE. *Acquired Speech and Language Disorders: A Neuroanatomical and Functional Neurological Approach*. 2nd ed. Chichester, West Sussex; Hoboken: Wiley-Blackwell, 2010.

Ochfeld E, Newhart M, Molitoris J, et al. Ischemia in broca area is associated with broca aphasia more reliably in acute than in chronic stroke. *Stroke* 2010;41:325–330.

Ogawa K, Yoshihashi H, Suzuki Y, et al. Clinical study of the responsible lesion for dysarthria in the cerebellum. *Intern Med* 2010;49:861–864.

Ohyama M, Senda M, Kitamura S, et al. Role of the nondominant hemisphere and undamaged area during word repetition in poststroke aphasics. A PET activation study. *Stroke* 1996;27:897–903.

Pearce JM. Selected observations on amusia. *Eur Neurol* 2005;54:145–148.

Peters AS, Remi J, Vollmar C, et al. Dysprosody during epileptic seizures lateralizes to the nondominant hemisphere. *Neurology* 2011;77:1482–1486.

Pflugshaupt T, Suchan J, Mandler MA, et al. Do patients with pure alexia suffer from a specific word form processing deficit? Evidence from 'wrods with trasnpsoed letetrs'. *Neuropsychologia* 2011;49:1294–1301.

Pool KD, Freeman FJ, Finitzo T, et al. Heterogeneity in spasmodic dysphonia. Neurologic and voice findings. *Arch Neurol* 1991;48:305–309.

Price CJ. Functional-imaging studies of the 19th century neurological model of language. *Rev Neurol (Paris)* 2001;157(8–9 Pt 1): 833–836.

Pryse-Phillips W. *Companion to Clinical Neurology*. 3rd ed. Oxford: Oxford University Press, 2009.

Ravi A, Rao VR, Klein JP. Dystextia: acute stroke in the modern age. *JAMA Neurol* 2013;70:404–405.

Reich SG, Meyer T. Teaching video NeuroImage: spasmodic dysphonia: adductor and abductor. *Neurology* 2008;70:e78.

Rodriguez-Fornells A, Rotte M, Heinze HJ, et al. Brain potential and functional MRI evidence for how to handle two languages with one brain. *Nature* 2002;415:1026–1029.

Rohrer JD, Knight WD, Warren JE, et al. Word-finding difficulty: a clinical analysis of the progressive aphasias. *Brain* 2008;131(Pt 1):8–38.

Sakurai Y, Ichikawa Y, Mannen T. Pure alexia from a posterior occipital lesion. *Neurology* 2001;56:778–781.

Sakurai Y, Asami M, Mannen T. Alexia and agraphia with lesions of the angular and supramarginal gyri: evidence for the disruption of sequential processing. *J Neurol Sci* 2010;288:25–33.

Schiff HB, Alexander MP, Naeser MA, et al. Aphemia. Clinical-anatomic correlations. *Arch Neurol* 1983;40:720–727.

Selnes OA, Hillis A. Patient Tan revisited: a case of atypical global aphasia? *J Hist Neurosci* 2000;9:233–237.

Sheldon CA, Malcolm GL, Barton JJ. Alexia with and without agraphia: an assessment of two classical syndromes. *Can J Neurol Sci* 2008;35:616–624.

Shinoura N, Onodera T, Kurokawa K, et al. Damage to the upper portion of area 19 and the deep white matter in the left inferior parietal lobe, including the superior longitudinal fasciculus, results in alexia with agraphia. *Eur Neurol* 2010;64:224–229.

Shipley KG, McAfee JG. *Assessment in Speech-Language Pathology*. 4th ed. Clifton Park: Delmar Cengage Learning, 2009.

Sommer M, Koch MA, Paulus W, et al. Disconnection of speech-relevant brain areas in persistent developmental stuttering. *Lancet* 2002;360:380–383.

Song X, Dornbos D III, Lai Z, et al. Diffusion tensor imaging and diffusion tensor imaging-fibre tractography depict the mechanisms of Broca-like and Wernicke-like conduction aphasia. *Neurol Res* 2011;33:529–535.

Spencer KA, Slocomb DL. The neural basis of ataxic dysarthria. *Cerebellum* 2007;6:58–65.

Starrfelt R, Behrmann M. Number reading in pure alexia—a review. *Neuropsychologia* 2011;49:2283–2298.

Sugishita M, Otomo K, Kabe S, et al. A critical appraisal of neuropsychological correlates of Japanese ideogram (kanji) and phonogram (kana) reading. *Brain* 1992;115(Pt 5):1563–1585.

Sulica L, Louis ED. Clinical characteristics of essential voice tremor: a study of 34 cases. *Laryngoscope* 2010;120:516–528.

Takayama Y, Sugishita M, Kido T, et al. A case of foreign accent syndrome without aphasia caused by a lesion of the left precentral gyrus. *Neurology* 1993;43:1361–1363.

Thomas NWD, Mestre TA. Impact of new technologies in a stroke presentation: a case of dystextia and dystypia. *Can J Neurol Sci* 2017;44:458–460.

Timmann D, Konczak J, Ilg W, et al. Current advances in lesion-symptom mapping of the human cerebellum. *Neuroscience* 2009;162:836–851.

Tomik B, Guiloff RJ. Dysarthria in amyotrophic lateral sclerosis: a review. *Amyotroph Lateral Scler* 2010;11:4–15.

Tudor L, Sikiric P, Tudor KI, et al. Amusia and aphasia of Bolero's creator–influence of the right hemisphere on music. *Acta Med Croatica* 2008;62:309–316.

Urban PP, Hopf HC, Zorowka PG, et al. Dysarthria and lacunar stroke: pathophysiologic aspects. *Neurology* 1996;47:1135–1141.

von Keyserlingk AG, Naujokat C, Niemann K, et al. Global aphasia-with and without hemiparesis. A linguistic and CT scan study. *Eur Neurol* 1997;38:259–267.

Wise RJ, Greene J, Buchel C, et al. Brain regions involved in articulation. *Lancet* 1999;353:1057–1061.

Yamada K, Nagakane Y, Mizuno T, et al. MR tractography depicting damage to the arcuate fasciculus in a patient with conduction aphasia. *Neurology* 2007;68:789.

Yang ZH, Zhao XQ, Wang CX, et al. Neuroanatomic correlation of the post-stroke aphasias studied with imaging. *Neurol Res* 2008;30:356–360.

Zhang Y, Wang Y, Wang C, et al. Study on the pathogenic mechanism of Broca's and Wernicke's aphasia. *Neurol Res* 2006;28:59–65.

Zhang Y, Wang C, Zhao X, et al. Diffusion tensor imaging depicting damage to the arcuate fasciculus in patients with conduction aphasia: a study of the Wernicke-Geschwind model. *Neurol Res* 2010;32:775–778.

CHAPTER 10

Agnosia, Apraxia, and Related Disorders of Higher Cortical Function

Gnosia (Gr. gnosis, "knowledge") refers to the higher synthesis of sensory impulses, with the resulting perception, appreciation, and recognition of stimuli. Agnosia refers to the loss or impairment of the ability to know or recognize the meaning or import of a sensory stimulus, even though it has been perceived. Agnosia occurs in the absence of any impairment of cognition, attention, or alertness. The patients are not aphasic and do not have word-finding or a generalized naming impairment. Hughlings Jackson saw agnosia as a nonlanguage form of aphasia. Agnosias are usually specific for a given sensory modality and can occur with any type of sensory stimulus. Agnosias that involve the primary sensory modalities may represent disconnection syndromes that disrupt communication between a specific cortical sensory area and the language areas, which causes a restricted anomia. Agnosias are frequently due to bilateral or diffuse processes such as multiple stroke, hypoxic ischemic encephalopathy, and degenerative disorders.

Tactile agnosia refers to the inability to recognize stimuli by feel; visual agnosia is the inability to recognize visually; and auditory (acoustic) agnosia is the inability to know or recognize by audition. Body-image agnosia (autotopagnosia) is loss or impairment of the ability to name and recognize body parts. Finger agnosia is a type of autotopagnosia involving the fingers. Auditory agnosia is the loss of recognition of sounds. A patient with auditory agnosia may not be able to distinguish between the sound of a baby crying and the noise of traffic. Phonagnosia is the loss of recognition of familiar voices. Amusia is a form of auditory agnosia (Chapter 9). Time agnosia refers to loss of time sense without disorientation in other spheres. Visuospatial agnosia is loss or impairment in the ability to judge direction, distance, and motion and the inability to understand three-dimensional spatial relationships. Because of the impaired spatial judgment and visual disorientation, the patient cannot find her way in familiar surroundings. Multimodal agnosias may occur with dysfunction of the association areas in the parietal and temporal lobes that assimilate sensory information from more than one domain.

Astereognosis (stereoanesthesia) is loss of the ability to recognize and identify an object by touch despite intact primary sensory modalities. There is no loss of perceptual ability. The patient can feel the object, sensing its dimensions, texture, and other relevant information. However, she is unable to synthesize this information and correlate it with past experience and stored information about similar objects in order to recognize and identify it. Stereognosis is tested by asking the patient to identify, with eyes closed, common objects placed into the hand (e.g., coin, key, button, safety pin, paper clip). The most convincing deficit is when the patient is able to identify with the other hand an object that she was unable to identify with the tested hand. When primary sensory modalities in the hand are impaired, as by radiculopathy or neuropathy, failure to identify an object by touch is not astereognosis. Astereognosis usually indicates a lesion involving the contralateral parietal lobe. Rarely, a lesion of either parietal lobe can produce astereognosis bilaterally. It has also been reported to occur with lesions involving the anterior corpus callosum and the thalamic radiations. If there is hand weakness, the examiner may hold and move the object between the patient's fingers. It is striking to see a patient with a paralyzed hand from a pure motor capsular stroke demonstrate exquisitely intact stereognosis when tested in this fashion. In tactile agnosia, the patient is unable to identify the object with either hand but can identify it visually. Graphesthesia is a similar function. It is tested by writing numbers on the patient's palm or fingertips. The inability to recognize the numbers is referred to as agraphesthesia; in the presence of intact primary sensory modalities, it usually indicates a lesion involving the contralateral parietal lobe. Cortical sensory functions and abnormalities are discussed further in Chapter 35.

Finger agnosia refers to the loss or impairment of the ability to recognize, name, or select individual fingers of the patient's own hands or the hands of the examiner. The patient loses the ability to name individual fingers, point to fingers named by the examiner, or move named fingers on request, in the absence of any other naming deficit. Testing for finger agnosia may be conveniently combined with assessment of right-left orientation. The simplest test of right-left orientation is to ask the patient to raise a specific hand. A more challenging test is to have the patient touch a body part on one side (e.g., the right ear) with a specific digit of the other side (e.g., the left thumb). Even more strenuous is when the examiner faces the patient, crosses her forearms with hands and fingers extended, and requests the patient to touch one of the examiner's fingers on a specific side (e.g., the left index finger). A very challenging test is to ask the patient to touch a specific finger as the examiner faces away from the patient with forearms crossed behind the back. Using a confusing syntax, the examiner might say, "with your left hand, touch my right index finger."

Finger agnosia and right-left confusion, along with agraphia and acalculia, make up Gerstmann's syndrome. Finger agnosia alone is not highly localizing, but when all components of the syndrome are present, the lesion is likely to lie in the dominant inferior parietal lobule, particularly in the region of the angular gyrus and subjacent white matter. Current thinking is that pure Gerstmann's syndrome likely results from a lesion of the subcortical parietal white matter causing disconnection of separate but colocalized fiber tracts disrupting intraparietal cortical networks, rather than a focal cortical lesion.

In the visual agnosias, there is loss or impairment of the ability to recognize things visually, despite intact vision (psychogenic blindness or mind blindness). Area 18 and area 19 are particularly important for visual gnostic functions. Visual agnosia is not a sensory defect but a problem in recognition. There is impairment in the higher visual association processes necessary for recognition and naming, not explicable by any deficit in visual perception or in naming ability. Patients can see but cannot make sense of the visual world. Teuber said visual agnosia was a "percept stripped of its meaning." Oliver Sacks provided an entertaining and informative description of the clinical picture of visual agnosia in *The Man Who Mistook His Wife for a Hat.*

The specifics of which visual functions are preserved or involved vary from patient to patient. Lissauer divided the visual agnosias into apperceptive and associative types. Apperceptive visual agnosia occurs when there is some perceptual defect distorting the visual image so that the object is unrecognizable. It most often follows lesions involving the parietooccipital regions bilaterally and may evolve during recovery from cortical blindness. In apperceptive agnosia, there is lack of recognition because of a visual perceptual impairment above the level of a basic visual function such as acuity, color perception, and visual fields. There is impairment of the more complex perceptions that allow for the synthesis of visual elements. The patient may be able to see parts but not the whole. She may not be able to distinguish a circle from a square or match an object with its picture.

Associative visual agnosia refers to a global inability to identify objects in the absence of visual impairment, aphasia, or anomia. It is a defect in the association of the object with past experience and memory. Patients can readily identify the same objects using other sensory modalities. Associative visual agnosia occurs with bilateral occipitotemporal junction lesions, often involving fusiform gyri. It may also occur when the visual cortex is disconnected from the language centers by a lesion involving the splenium of the corpus callosum and the left occipital lobe, similar to the lesion causing alexia without agraphia. Patients often have related recognition deficits, such as color agnosia and prosopagnosia. The apperceptive-associative scheme has been applied to other types of agnosia as well.

Visual object agnosia (optic aphasia) is an associative visual agnosia causing an inability to recognize things seen that is not because of visual impairment, cognitive deficit, inattention, aphasic misnaming, or unfamiliarity. The patient is unable to identify familiar objects presented visually and cannot correctly identify a seen object from a pick list. She may be able to see the object, even describe it, but have no idea what it is or what it is called. But she recognizes it immediately if allowed to handle it or hear any sound it might make. Visual object agnosia must be distinguished from anomia. The patient with anomia cannot recognize the object when presented by another modality (e.g., touch), and she will have other defects in naming, such as impairment in spontaneous naming with inability to generate word lists (e.g., naming animals). The anomic patient may also be able to demonstrate what the object is by gesture (e.g., appropriately apply a comb to her hair), yet not be able to call it a comb. The patient with agnosia doesn't recognize the comb as a comb and has no idea what to do with it. Visual object agnosia is often accompanied by right homonymous hemianopia and alexia without agraphia.

Some occipital lobe lesions, particularly of the primary visual cortex, cause color blindness (central achromatopsia). Lesions of the association areas may cause color agnosia. In color agnosia, the patient cannot name or identify colors, although she is not color blind and can discern the numbers on color plates. In prosopagnosia (face or facial agnosia), there is an inability to recognize familiar faces. The patient may not be able to identify people, even close family members, by looking at their faces. However, she may immediately identify the person by the sound of the voice. The patient may recognize a face as a face but cannot associate it with a particular individual. She learns to identify people using other cues. In extreme examples, the patient is unable to recognize herself in a mirror or a photograph. Patients with prosopagnosia, and other visual agnosias, usually have bilateral lesions of the occipitotemporal area involving the lingual, fusiform, and parahippocampal gyri. Prosopagnosia can occur with unilateral right posterior hemispheric lesions. Recent literature suggests that a hereditary form may affect about 2.5% of the population, and perhaps up to 10% in a very mild form. A common complaint is the inability to keep track of characters in movies. Transient prosopagnosia has been reported after focal electrical stimulation of the right inferior occipital gyrus.

Simultagnosia is the ability to perceive only one object at a time or specific details but not a picture in its entirety. The patient may perceive parts but not the whole of a pattern. They may be able to read letter-by-letter but not recognize an entire word. Area 19 is thought to be important in revisualization, and lesions in this region cause a visual agnosia characterized by inability to revisualize, or a loss of visual memory. An object may be identified when seen, but the patient cannot describe it afterward. In the Charcot-Wilbrand syndrome, there is loss of revisualization; the patient cannot draw or construct from memory. Patients may not be able to remember the color of common things (e.g., the sky).

Apraxia (Gr. praxis "action") is defined in several ways. Common to all definitions is the inability to carry out on request a motor act in the absence of any weakness, sensory loss, or other deficit involving the affected part. The patient must have intact comprehension and be cooperative and attentive to the task. One definition requires the task be high level, learned, familiar, and purposeful, such as saluting or using an implement. But the term is also used to refer to loss of the ability to execute some very elemental functions, such as opening or closing the eyes (eyelid apraxia), glancing to the side (ocular motor or gaze apraxia), walking (gait apraxia), or a behavior as basic as smacking the lips (buccofacial apraxia). Another definition of apraxia is the inability to perform an act on command that the patient is able to perform spontaneously. But the patient with gait apraxia cannot walk spontaneously any better than to command. So, all the definitions and applications of the term suffer in one respect or another. There are many varieties of apraxia. The ones seen most often are ideomotor, buccofacial, constructional, and dressing apraxia. Apraxia of speech is discussed in Chapter 9.

The major limb apraxias are limb kinetic, ideomotor, and ideational. The simplest form is limb kinetic apraxia. This category probably should not exist. These patients have difficulty with fine motor control. They typically have very mild lesions involving the corticospinal tract that are not severe enough to cause detectable weakness, but they are severe enough to impair coordination and dexterity. Limb kinetic apraxia is due to dysfunction of the primary motor pathways. In other forms of apraxia, the primary motor and sensory functions are intact. Pryse-Phillips referred to limb kinetic apraxia as, "an entity of doubtful validity, the clumsiness… probably being due to paresis."

In ideomotor apraxia, the patient is unable to perform a complex command (e.g., salute, wave goodbye, comb hair, use scissors, flip a coin, show how to hitchhike) with the involved extremity, sometimes with either extremity. The patient may be unable to pantomime how to use common implements (e.g., hammer, toothbrush, comb) or how to kick or throw a ball. She may substitute a hand or finger for the imagined object, thus using a body part as the tool (e.g., raking her fingers through her hair instead of showing how to use a comb or snapping her fingers together as the blades when asked to show how to use scissors). The patient may be unable to carry out the act on command but be able to imitate it. Rarely, the patient may be unable to carry out an act on command or imitation—such as showing how to use a comb—but be able to use the actual object, referred to as dissociation or disconnection apraxia.

In ideomotor apraxia, there may be a disconnection between the language or visual centers that understand the command and the motor areas tasked with carrying it out. Patients may have apraxia for whole body movements. They are unable to, on command, do such things as stand up, take a bow, or stand like a boxer. Lack of apraxia for whole body movements in the presence of apraxia for limb movements has been attributed to sparing of the bundle of Turck, a tract from the posterior superior temporal area to the pontine nuclei (temporopontine tract). As many as 40% of aphasic patients have ideomotor ataxia if correctly tested, but it frequently goes undetected. Depending on the anatomy of the lesion, ideomotor apraxia may affect only contralateral or all four limbs plus midline functions. Some authorities distinguish between parietal and disconnection variants of ideomotor apraxia.

Sympathetic apraxia is the inability of a patient to perform a complex motor act with the nonparetic limb in the presence of a unilateral dominant hemisphere lesion. For instance, a patient with a left hemisphere lesion causing Broca's aphasia may be unable to show how to wave goodbye using the left hand. This is because the fibers connecting the language areas of the left hemisphere with the motor areas of the right hemisphere are disrupted. The patient understands the request, has no weakness of the left hand, but is unable to execute because the right hemisphere never receives the command.

In ideational apraxia, the patient is able to carry out individual components of a complex motor act, but she cannot perform the entire sequence properly. The patient may perform each step correctly, but in attempting the sequence, she omits steps or gets the steps out of order. There is an inability to correctly sequence a series of acts leading to a goal. Ideational apraxia seems to be an impairment in conceptualizing the overall goal of the activity sequence or an inability to plan the series of steps. For instance, in showing how to drive a car, the patient might try to put the car in drive before starting the engine. When asked to demonstrate how to mail a letter, the patient may seal the envelope before inserting the letter, or mail the letter before affixing the stamp. Ideational apraxia may occur with damage to the left posterior temporoparietal junction or in patients with generalized cognitive impairment. In daily life, patients with ideational apraxia may choose the wrong tool for a task, for example, eat soup with fork, or perform tasks out of sequence, for example, brush teeth before applying toothpaste. In one reported case, a woman trying to light a gas stove first struck the match, then blew it out, then lit the burner. On another occasion, she turned on the gas, filled the kettle, then struck the match, causing a minor explosion.

In buccofacial (oral) apraxia, patients are unable to execute on request complex acts involving the lips, mouth, and face; this may include such activities as whistling, coughing, pursing the lips, sticking out the tongue, blowing a kiss, pretending to blow out a match, or sniffing a flower. There is no weakness of the mouth, lips, or face, but the patients are unable to make the requested movement. The patient may spontaneously lick her lips or stick out her tongue, but she is unable to do so on command. Apraxia of such midline functions is common in patients with lesions involving either hemisphere. Failure to execute such acts should not necessarily be construed as evidence of impaired comprehension in aphasic patients.

Other common types of apraxia include dressing and constructional. Constructional or dressing apraxia usually occurs with parietal lobe lesions, occasionally with frontal lesions that interfere with the patient's ability to comprehend spatial relationships. In constructional apraxia, the patient is unable to copy geometric forms of any complexity because of impaired visuospatial skills. She may be able to draw a square but not a three-dimensional cube. She may be able to draw individual shapes, but she cannot synthesize them into a more complex geometric figure (e.g., a square with a triangle perched on its upper-right corner and a circle attached to the lower-right corner, all touching). The patient may also be asked to draw actual things, such as a three-dimensional house with a roof and chimney, a clock, or a daisy.

Patients with hemineglect may fail to put petals on one side of the daisy. A test for both praxis and cognition is to have the patient draw a clock face, insert the numbers, and draw the hands at a specific time (e.g., 3:10, or "10 minutes past 3"). Patients with hemineglect may fail to put the numbers on one side of the clock. Patients with frontal lobe dysfunction or a confusional state may have a disorganized and confused approach to the task, making multiple errors. A patient with cognitive impairment may forget the proper arrangement of numbers or how to indicate a specific time. Some patients cannot interpret 3:10 and will put one hand on the 10 and the other on the 3, indicating 2:50 or 10:15. The clock drawing test is discussed further in Chapter 8. The Rey-Osterrieth figure is very complex and can bring out subtle constructional apraxia (Figure 10.1). Constructional tasks are particularly useful for differentiating psychiatric from neurologic disease. Impaired constructional ability is a sensitive indicator of lesions involving various parts of the brain, but in patients with psychiatric disease, constructional ability is preserved.

In dressing apraxia, the patient loses the ability to don clothing correctly. Dressing requires bimanual cooperation to solve a complex spatial problem. There is loss of the ability to manipulate the clothing in space and to understand its three-dimensional relationships. Patients with hemineglect may fail to dress one side of the body. A useful test for dressing apraxia is to turn one sleeve of the hospital gown or robe inside out and then ask the patient to put it on. Patients with dressing apraxia are often baffled. Dressing apraxia can be particularly disabling, as the patient struggles for a long period of time each morning simply to get dressed. Constructional apraxia would be very disabling for a patient who was an artist or craftsman. Dressing apraxia often occurs in conjunction with constructional apraxia.

DISCONNECTION SYNDROMES

Disconnection syndromes are disorders in which the fiber tracts that interconnect primary cortical areas are disrupted, with preservation of the cortical areas of origin. Neurologic dysfunction occurs not because of destruction of cortex but because of defects in intrahemispheric or interhemispheric communication. In 1874, Wernicke was the first to suggest that such a pathoanatomic mechanism might exist when he described conduction aphasia in his MD thesis, written at the age of 26. Dejerine added alexia without agraphia in 1892. In his 1965 paper, *Disconnection syndromes in animals and man*, which became the manifesto of behavioral neurology, Geschwind expanded and popularized the concept, describing several new examples. Other disconnection syndromes include ideomotor apraxia, sympathetic apraxia, pure word deafness, and the transcortical aphasias. The modality-specific agnosias may be disconnection syndromes in which the primary sensory area for a given modality is disconnected from the language and memory areas of the brain that are responsible for recognition and naming. Disconnection syndromes may result from any process that disrupts subcortical white matter, including infarction, hemorrhage, neoplasm, and trauma. There have been reports of patients with double disconnection syndromes.

In alexia without agraphia, a left occipital lobe lesion, usually an infarction, extends anteriorly to involve the splenium of the corpus callosum or the adjacent white matter. Patients usually have a right

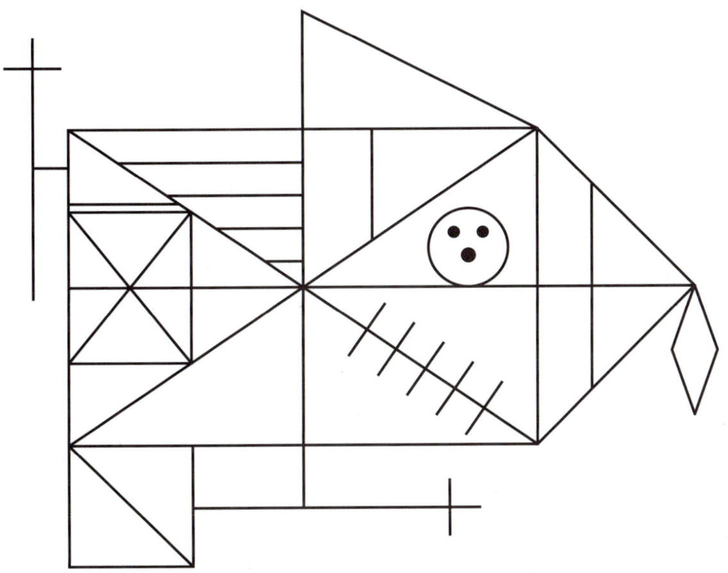

FIGURE 10.1 The Rey-Osterrieth complex figure for evaluating constructional ability.

homonymous hemianopia because of the occipital lobe lesion. Although the right occipital lobe and left visual field are intact, fibers from the right occipital lobe are disconnected from the language centers in the left parietal lobe because of disruption of commissural fibers in the splenium. The patients are unable to read because the visual information from the right occipital lobe cannot be transferred to the region of the opposite angular gyrus. They are typically better able to read letters than words, and individual letters better than letter strings. Preservation of number reading may occur. Because the angular gyrus is itself intact, patients are able to write without difficulty but are unable to read what they may have just written. Rarely, alexia without agraphia occurs without an accompanying hemianopia.

In pure word deafness (auditory verbal agnosia), patients are unable to understand speech, but other language modalities are unimpaired. Spontaneous speech, reading, and writing are preserved in the face of a severe auditory comprehension deficit. Hearing is intact, and nonlanguage auditory processing (e.g., for music) is undisturbed. Responsible pathology is typically bitemporal or dominant temporal, causing disconnection of Wernicke's area from the primary auditory cortex. In pure word blindness, the patient cannot read, but other language functions are intact. The lesion disconnects the visual cortex from the language centers. There is conjecture that the dysphagia in Wallenberg's lateral medullary syndrome may be due to a disconnection between premotor neurons related to swallowing and the bulbar nuclei responsible for execution.

In callosal disconnection syndromes, there is evidence of interhemispheric disconnection causing deficits in corpus callosum function that resemble those seen in split-brain patients. Patients with anterior callosal lesions may have unilateral tactile anomia, unilateral agraphia, unilateral apraxia, difficulty in copying drawings, dyscalculia, abnormalities of somesthetic transfer, and the alien hand phenomenon. Posterior callosal lesions may cause left tactile anomia, left visual anomia, and agraphia of the left hand. A patient with infarction of the total length of the corpus callosum had unilateral verbal anosmia, hemialexia, unilateral ideomotor apraxia, unilateral agraphia, unilateral tactile anomia, unilateral constructional apraxia, lack of somesthetic transfer, and dissociative phenomena. Callosal apraxia refers to impaired ability to pantomime to command, imitate, or use actual objects with the left hand, with spared ability to perform these tasks with the right hand, because of a callosal lesion. Evidence of callosal disconnection has been reported in infarction, hemorrhage, Marchiafava-Bignami disease, multiple sclerosis, and Alzheimer's disease.

Attentional Deficits

In addition to the generalized defects in attention seen in patients with altered mental status and other diffuse cerebral disturbances, there may be selective defects of attention in patients with focal cerebral lesions. These are seen primarily in right-handed patients with right (nondominant) hemisphere lesions, especially those that involve the inferior parietal lobule. A variety of terms has been used to describe the phenomenon, including extinction, neglect, hemineglect, hemi-inattention, denial, and spatial inattention. Hemiattention may be modality specific. The mildest manifestation of a right parietal lesion is extinction of the contralateral stimulus with double simultaneous stimulation on visual field or somatosensory testing. Although primary sensory modalities are intact, when touched simultaneously on both sides, the patient fails to appreciate the stimulus on the involved side or fails to see the stimulus in the involved visual hemifield.

Patients with multimodal hemineglect may extinguish all types of contralesional stimuli, and they may completely ignore the left side of space. On the line bisection test, they fail to see the left half of the line (Chapter 8). They bisect the right half, drawing their vertical tick about one-quarter of the way down the line from the right. If lines are drawn all over the page, patients may fail to bisect any of the lines on the left. When presented with a complex drawing, such as the cookie theft picture, they may describe what is taking place on the right side of the picture, but they may fail to notice the cookie theft happening on the left. It appears that the right parietal lobe is dominant for spatial attention; subtle ipsilateral deficits may also occur. In addition, the left hemisphere plays a role in attention to contralateral stimuli only. With a right-sided lesion, the left hemisphere still adequately attends to the right side of space, and the deficit appears in contralateral hemispace left unguarded by the right hemisphere. In motor neglect (hemiakinesia), all of the patient's motor activities are directed to one side of space.

Babinski introduced the cumbersome term anosognosia to refer to a patient's lack of awareness of a neurologic deficit. It occurs particularly in patients with nondominant parietal lesions. It has been estimated at seven times more common with nondominant than dominant lesions, a difference not wholly explicable by associated aphasia with dominant lesions. It is not uncommon to see patients with a right parietal infarction on imaging studies but no clinical history of the event, in part because of this lack of recognition of deficits involving the left side of the body. Occasionally, a patient with severe left hemiplegia may deny there is anything wrong with the involved limbs. Even when the examiner dangles the patient's paralyzed left hand before her face and asks if there is anything wrong with this hand, the patient may deny it. The most severe form of anosognosia is when the patient denies owning the hand (asomatognosia). Occasionally, patients become belligerent in denying that the hand dangling before them is theirs. They commonly say the hand belongs to the examiner. One patient stated it was, "Queen Elizabeth's hand." When asked where Queen Elizabeth was, the patient replied, "behind the curtain." Patients with anosognosia may refuse to remain in the bed with this "other person." One patient thought her left arm was her grandbaby lying beside her. One patient, convinced her left arm was not her own, threw it over the side rail of the bed, fracturing the humerus (see section on "Alien Hand Syndrome"). In misoplegia, also seen with right hemisphere lesions, patients hate and may reject their paralyzed limbs. A possibly related disorder, also attributed to a right parietal lesion, is apotemnophilia, in which otherwise apparently rational individuals seek amputation of healthy limbs.

Patients with persistent anosognosia typically have large right hemisphere strokes causing severe left hemisensory loss and left spatial neglect. Anosognosia for the hemiplegia may result from impaired proprioceptive mechanisms that leave the patient unaware of the position and movement of the affected limbs. Anosognosia for hemiplegia has also been reported with pontine lesions. Using special techniques to compensate for aphasia, it may be detected more often in dominant hemisphere lesions than previously suspected. Patients may deny or neglect other neurologic deficits as well, particularly loss of vision due to bilateral occipital lobe lesions (cortical blindness, Anton's syndrome).

Alien Hand Syndrome

In alien hand syndrome, there is complex but involuntary activity in one hand; the hand moves as if it had a mind of its own. There is debate about whether the activity need appear purposeful and goal directed. Alien hand syndrome is usually due to interruption of the cortical connections that control smooth bimanual operations. The hands no longer work as a team. The affected hand begins to function autonomously and loses the ability to cooperate with its fellow. The patient feels a loss of ownership of the extremity. There may be outright intermanual conflict. The affected hand acts as if possessed by a poltergeist. If the patient tries to eat with the good hand, the alien hand may grasp the good hand and force it away from the mouth. If the good hand tries to write, the alien hand may snatch the pen.

There are at least two forms of alien hand syndrome. In the callosal form, there is a lesion in the anterior corpus callosum. Intermanual conflict is typical of the callosal form, and it nearly always affects the left hand (anarchic hand). In the frontal form, there is a lesion of the medial frontal lobe, near or involving the supplementary motor area. The alien hand is uncooperative but not contentious. It may display reflex grasping and other autonomous behavior, but there is little or no intermanual conflict. Patients may complain of the hand's behavior and may criticize it or even slap the alien hand with the good hand. Other patients regard the hand's behavior as amusing.

A sensory or posterior alien hand syndrome has also been described following parietal lobe lesions. There are typically parietal sensory deficits and hemineglect involving the left side of the body, which resemble anosognosia. The left arm may then involuntarily attack the right side of the body. There have been reports of patients with a callosal lesion feeling as though they had a second left hand.

Other neurologic examination abnormalities help indicate the alien hand subtype. Nonfluent aphasia and a prominent grasp reflex suggest the frontal lobe variant. Ideomotor apraxia of the nondominant hand suggests the callosal form. A hemisensory deficit and other parietal lobe findings suggest the sensory alien hand variant. Potential etiologies include stroke, corpus callosotomy, hypoglycemic encephalopathy, diabetic hypermolar syndrome, Marchiafava-Bignami disease, MS, migraine, and posterior reversible encephalopathy syndrome. Alien hand syndrome occurs in degenerative cerebral disorders, including corticobasal syndrome, Alzheimer's disease, and Creutzfeldt-Jakob disease. The incidence of alien hand in corticobasal syndrome has been reported as high as 40% to 50%, making corticobasal syndrome potentially the commonest etiology for alien hand syndrome.

The alien hand syndrome has appeared many times in pop culture. In Dr. Strangelove, Peter Sellers constantly has to restrain his alien hand from giving the Nazi party salute and alien hand syndrome has been referred to as Dr. Strangelove syndrome.

BIBLIOGRAPHY

Absher JR, Benson DF. Disconnection syndromes: an overview of Geschwind's contributions. *Neurology* 1993;43:862–867.

Adair JC, Na DL, Schwartz RL, et al. Anosognosia for hemiplegia: test of the personal neglect hypothesis. *Neurology* 1995;45:2195–2199.

Anonymous. Alien hand syndrome. http://en.wikipedia.org/wiki/Alien_hand_syndrome

Ardila A. A proposed reinterpretation of Gerstmann's syndrome. *Arch Clin Neuropsychol* 2014;29:828–833.

Aydogdu I, Ertekin C, Tarlaci S, et al. Dysphagia in lateral medullary infarction (Wallenberg's syndrome): an acute disconnection syndrome in premotor neurons related to swallowing activity? *Stroke* 2001;32:2081–2087.

Brang D, McGeoch PD, Ramachandran VS. Apotemnophilia: a neurological disorder. *Neuroreport* 2008;19:1305–1306.

Buxbaum LJ. Ideomotor apraxia: a call to action. *Neurocase* 2001;7:445–458.

Catani M, Ffytche DH. The rises and falls of disconnection syndromes. *Brain* 2005;128(Pt 10):2224–2239.

Catani M, Mesulam M. The arcuate fasciculus and the disconnection theme in language and aphasia: history and current state. *Cortex* 2008a;44:953–961.

Catani M, Mesulam M. What is a disconnection syndrome? *Cortex* 2008b;44:911–913.

Chan JL, Liu AB. Anatomical correlates of alien hand syndromes. *Neuropsychiatry Neuropsychol Behav Neurol* 1999;12(3):149–155.

Cherrier MM, Mendez MF, Dave M, et al. Performance on the Rey-Osterrieth complex figure test in Alzheimer disease and vascular dementia. *Neuropsychiatry Neuropsychol Behav Neurol* 1999;12:95–101.

Cocchini G, Beschin N, Cameron A, et al. Anosognosia for motor impairment following left brain damage. *Neuropsychology* 2009;23:223–230.

Critchley M. Misoplegia, or hatred of hemiplegia. *Mt Sinai J Med* 1974;41:82–87.

Degos JD, Gray F, Louarn F, et al. Posterior callosal infarction. Clinicopathological correlations. *Brain* 1987;110:1155–1171.

Delrieu J, Payoux P, Toulza O, et al. Sensory alien hand syndrome in corticobasal degeneration: a cerebral blood flow study. *Mov Disord* 2010;25:1288–1291.

Epelbaum S, Pinel P, Gaillard R, et al. Pure alexia as a disconnection syndrome: new diffusion imaging evidence for an old concept. *Cortex* 2008;44:962–974.

Estañol B, Baizabal-Carvallo JF, Sentíes-Madrid H. A case of tactile agnosia with a lesion restricted to the post-central gyrus. *Neurol India* 2008;56:471–473.

Evyapan D, Kumral E. Pontine anosognosia for hemiplegia. *Neurology* 1999;53:647–649.

Fitzgerald LK, McKelvey JR, Szeligo F. Mechanisms of dressing apraxia: a case study. *Neuropsychiatry Neuropsychol Behav Neurol* 2002;15:148–155.

Gasquoine PG. Blissfully unaware: anosognosia and anosodiaphoria after acquired brain injury. *Neuropsychol Rehabil* 2016;26:261–285.

Geschwind N. Disconnection syndromes in animals and man, parts I and II. *Brain* 1965;88:237–294, 585–644.

Geschwind N. The organization of language and the brain. *Science* 1970;170:940–944.

Geschwind N. The Apraxias: neural mechanisms of disorders of learned movement: the anatomical organization of the language areas and motor systems of the human brain clarifies apraxic disorders and throws new light on cerebral dominance. *Am Sci* 1975;63:188–195.

Geschwind N, Kaplan E. A human cerebral deconnection syndrome. *Neurology* 1962;12:675–685.

Goldenberg G, Mullbacher W, Nowak A. Imagery without perception—a case study of anosognosia for cortical blindness. *Neuropsychologia* 1995;33:1373–1382.

Gruter T, Gruter M, Carbon CC. Neural and genetic foundations of face recognition and prosopagnosia. *J Neuropsychol* 2008;2(Pt 1):79–97.

Hartmann JA, Wolz WA, Roeltgen DP, et al. Denial of visual perception. *Brain Cogn* 1991;16:29–40.

Heilman KM. Apraxia. *Continuum (Minneap Minn)* 2010;16(4 Behavioral Neurology):86–98.

Jonas J, Descoins M, Koessler L, et al. Focal electrical intracerebral stimulation of a face-sensitive area causes transient prosopagnosia. *Neuroscience* 2012;222:281–288.

Kararizou E, Lykomanos D, Kosma A, et al. Stereoanesthesia or astereognosia? *Neurol Sci* 2009;30:409–411.

Kim YD, Lee ES, Lee KS, et al. Callosal alien hand sign following a right parietal lobe infarction. *J Clin Neurosci* 2010;17:796–797.

Kirshner HS. Agnosias. In: Daroff RB, Jankovic J, et al., eds. *Bradley's Neurology in Clinical Practice*. 7th ed. Philadelphia: Elsevier, 2016.

Kleinschmidt A, Rusconi E. Gerstmann meets Geschwind: a crossing (or kissing) variant of a subcortical disconnection syndrome? *Neuroscientist* 2011;17:633–644.

Kloesel B, Czarnecki K, Muir JJ, et al. Sequelae of a left-sided parietal stroke: posterior alien hand syndrome. *Neurocase* 2010;16:488–493.

Lausberg H, Gottert R, Munssinger U, et al. Callosal disconnection syndrome in a left-handed patient due to infarction of the total length of the corpus callosum. *Neuropsychologia* 1999;37:253–265.

Lavados M, Carrasco X, Pena M, et al. A new sign of callosal disconnection syndrome: agonistic dyspraxia. A case study. *Neurocase* 2002;8:480–483.

Leiguarda R, Starkstein S, Berthier M. Anterior callosal hemorrhage: a partial interhemispheric disconnection syndrome. *Brain* 1989;112:1019–1037.

Levine DN, Calvanio R, Rinn WE. The pathogenesis of anosognosia for hemiplegia. *Neurology* 1991;41:1770–1781.

Luzzi S, Piccirilli M, Pesallaccia M, et al. Dissociation apraxia secondary to right premotor stroke. *Neuropsychologia* 2010;48:68–76.

Marangolo P, De Renzi E, Di Pace E, et al. Let not thy left hand know what thy right hand knoweth. The case of a patient with an infarct involving the callosal pathways. *Brain* 1998;121:1459–1467.

Mark VW. Alien hand syndrome. In: Gilman S, ed. *MedLink Neurology*. San Diego: MedLink Corporation. Available at www.medlink.com. Last updated: May 2, 2017.

Meador KJ, Loring DW, Feinberg TE, et al. Anosognosia and asomatognosia during intracarotid amobarbital inactivation. *Neurology* 2000;55:816–820.

Mendez MF, Deutsch MB. Limb apraxias and relates disorders. In: Daroff RB, Jankovic J, et al., eds. *Bradley's Neurology in Clinical Practice*. 7th ed. Philadelphia: Elsevier, 2016.

Motomura N, Yamadori A. A case of ideational apraxia with impairment of object use and preservation of object pantomime. *Cortex* 1994;30:167–170.

Mulroy E, Murphy S, Lynch T. Alexia without agraphia. *Ir Med J* 2011;104:124.

Murdoch BE. *Acquired Speech and Language Disorders: A Neuroanatomical and Functional Neurological Approach*. 2nd ed. Chichester, West Sussex/Hoboken: Wiley-Blackwell, 2010.

Nocentini U, Borghese NA, Caltagirone C, et al. A callosal disconnection syndrome of vascular origin. *J Neurosurg Sci* 1997;41:107–111.

Ochipa C, Rothi LJ, Heilman KM. Ideational apraxia: a deficit in tool selection and use. *Ann Neurol* 1989;25:190–193.

Pryse-Phillips W. *Companion to Clinical Neurology*. 3rd ed. Oxford: Oxford University Press, 2009.

Rizzo M, Hurtig R. Looking but not seeing: attention, perception, and eye movements in simultanagnosia. *Neurology* 1987;37: 1642–1648.

Ropper AH, Samuels MA, Klein J. *Adams and Victor's Principles of Neurology*. 10th ed. New York: McGraw-Hill Education Medical, 2014.

Rusconi E, Pinel P, Dehaene S, et al. The enigma of Gerstmann's syndrome revisited: a telling tale of the vicissitudes of neuropsychology. *Brain* 2010;133(Pt 2):320–332.

Sacks O. The man who mistook his wife for a hat. *Br J Psychiatry* 1995;166:130–131.

Schmahmann JD, Nitsch RM, Pandya DN. The mysterious relocation of the bundle of Turck. *Brain* 1992;115: 1911–1924.

Schnider A, Benson F, Rosner LJ. Callosal disconnection in multiple sclerosis. *Neurology* 1993;43:1243–1245.

Takahashi N, Kawamura M, Shinotou H, et al. Pure word deafness due to left hemisphere damage. *Cortex* 1992;28: 295–303.

Thiebaut de Schotten M, Dell'Acqua F, Ratiu P, et al. From Phineas Gage and Monsieur Leborgne to H.M.: revisiting disconnection syndromes. *Cereb Cortex* 2015;25: 4812–4827.

Vincent FM, Sadowsky CH, Saunders RL, et al. Alexia without agraphia, hemianopia, or color-naming defect: a disconnection syndrome. *Neurology* 1977;27:689–691.

Zhang Y, Wang C, Zhao X, et al. Diffusion tensor imaging depicting damage to the arcuate fasciculus in patients with conduction aphasia: a study of the Wernicke-Geschwind model. *Neurol Res* 2010;32:775–778.

An Overview of Brainstem and Cranial Nerve Anatomy

Except for cranial nerve (CN) I (olfactory) and CN II (optic), the anatomy of the CNs is inextricably linked to that of the brainstem. This chapter provides an overview of the organization and general features of the brainstem. Detailed discussion about each of the CNs follows in subsequent chapters. Gates offered a mnemonic, the rule of 4 of the brainstem, to remember the basic anatomy and the vascular syndromes (Box 11.1).

EMBRYOLOGY OF THE BRAINSTEM

A brief review of the pertinent embryology helps in understanding the structure and organization of the brainstem. A longitudinal groove, the sulcus limitans, appears in the lateral wall of the neural tube in the 4th week. As it deepens, it divides the tube into a dorsal and a ventral half throughout its length. Thickening of the mantle layer dorsal to the sulcus limitans forms the alar plate, and a thickening ventrally forms the basal plate (Figure 11.1). Development of the spinal cord is a simplified example of the ontogeny of the brainstem. The alar plate contains sensory neuroblasts and becomes the posterior gray horns of the spinal cord; the basal plate contains motor neuroblasts and becomes the anterior gray horns of the spinal cord. The sulcus limitans is not present in the adult spinal cord, but it is present in the brainstem where it continues to demarcate the zones of motor and sensory neurons.

As the brainstem develops, the expansion of the cavity of the fourth ventricle pushes the alar plate outward and downward. This causes the alar plate to retroflex so that it comes to lie lateral to, rather than dorsal to, the basal plate. The two plates are separated by the sulcus limitans (Figure 11.2). In the mature brainstem, the motor neurons derived from the basal plate lie medially, and the sensory neurons derived from the alar plate lie laterally. The neurons form cell columns, which are divided by anatomists into functional categories. The formal anatomical classification is somewhat arcane, seldom used by clinicians, but its conceptual framework is useful. The cell columns are divided into motor (efferent) and sensory (afferent) and into general and special, somatic and visceral cell types.

Referring to Figure 11.2 and moving from medial to lateral, the first cell column is general somatic efferent (GSE), which contains somatic motor cells. The GSE cells innervate skeletal muscles, which are derived from myotomes. For the head and neck, these are the extraocular muscles and the tongue. The next cell column laterally is general visceral efferent (GVE). This contains visceral motor or autonomic (parasympathetic) neurons supplying smooth muscles and glands of the head and neck, and the thoracic and abdominal viscera as far as the

BOX 11.1

The Rule of 4 of the Brainstem

In brief, the rule of 4 states that there are 4 midline or medial structures beginning with M, 4 structures to the side beginning with S, 4 cranial nerves (CNs) in the medulla, 4 in the pons, and 4 above the pons. The 4 medial structures are the motor pathway (corticospinal tract), medial lemniscus (ML), medial longitudinal fasciculus (MLF), and motor nuclei and nerves. The 4 lateral (side) structures are the spinocerebellar tracts, spinothalamic tract, sensory nucleus of CN V, and sympathetics. The 4 CNs in the medulla are IX, X, XI, and XII; the 4 in the pons are V, VI, VII, and VIII; and the remainder are above the pons. See Gates P at http://www.boutlis.com/files/UnderstandingTheBrainstem.pdf for details.

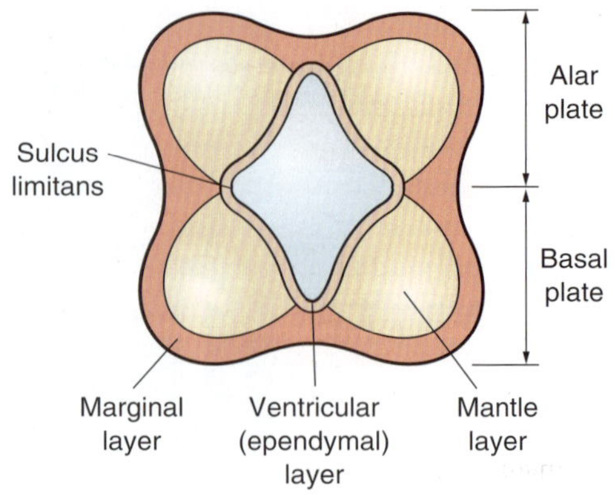

FIGURE 11.1 The sulcus limitans divides the neural tube into the dorsal alar plate, which contains sensory neuroblasts, and the ventral basal plate, which contains motor neuroblasts. In the brainstem, the sulcus limitans separates the motor nuclei from the sensory nuclei.

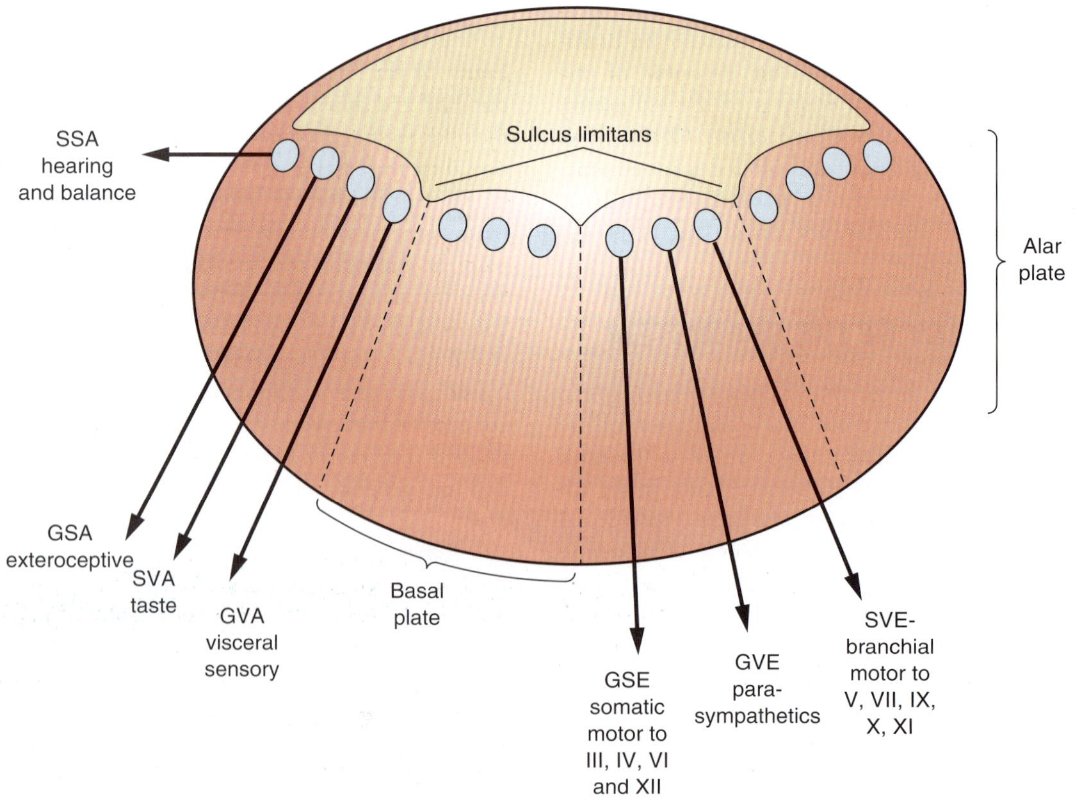

FIGURE 11.2 The cell columns of the brainstem with motor nuclei medial and sensory nuclei lateral. GSA, general somatic afferent; GSE, general somatic efferent; GVA, general visceral afferent; GVE, general visceral efferent; SSA, special somatic afferent; SVA, special visceral afferent; SVE, special visceral efferent.

splenic flexure of the colon. The GVE nuclei are the cranial portion of the craniosacral autonomic system, and they include the superior and inferior salivatory nuclei and the dorsal motor nucleus of the vagus.

Lateral to the GVE column is the special visceral efferent (SVE) column. Nuclei-innervating muscles of branchial (pharyngeal) arch origin were designated visceral because the gills in fish are derived from the embryonic branchial arches (Gr. branchia "gills"). Gills are viscera, primordial lungs, so branchial arch–derived muscles in humans were considered visceral, and branchiomeric neurons were designated as SVE. In the course of ontogeny and phylogeny, the branchiomotor cell column drifted ventrally from a location just under the ventricular floor to a position in the tegmentum. The motor nuclei of CNs V and VII and the nucleus ambiguus lie about midway between the somatic motor nuclear column and the point of exit of their respective nerves. The nucleus ambiguus is obscured by the fibers of the reticular formation (RF), making it inconspicuous and difficult to identify. Because of the displacement of their nuclear columns, branchiomotor axons have a tendency to form internal loops, for example, the encirclement of the CN VI nucleus (GSE) by the axons leaving the CN VII nucleus (SVE). Somatic motor fibers exit the brainstem anteriorly; branchiomotor fibers exit laterally.

The sulcus limitans separates the most lateral motor cell column from the most medial sensory cell column. Most medial are the general visceral afferent—or visceral sensory—cell columns, which receive sensory input from the viscera. The special visceral afferent—or special sensory—cell column receives fibers subserving taste. The general somatic afferent column receives exteroceptive input (i.e., touch, pressure, pain, temperature, vibration, and proprioception) from the head and neck. The most lateral sensory column is for special somatic afferent functions subserving the special sensations (i.e., hearing and vestibular function).

External Anatomy

Selected major features of the external anatomy of the brainstem are shown in Figures 11.3 and 11.4. On

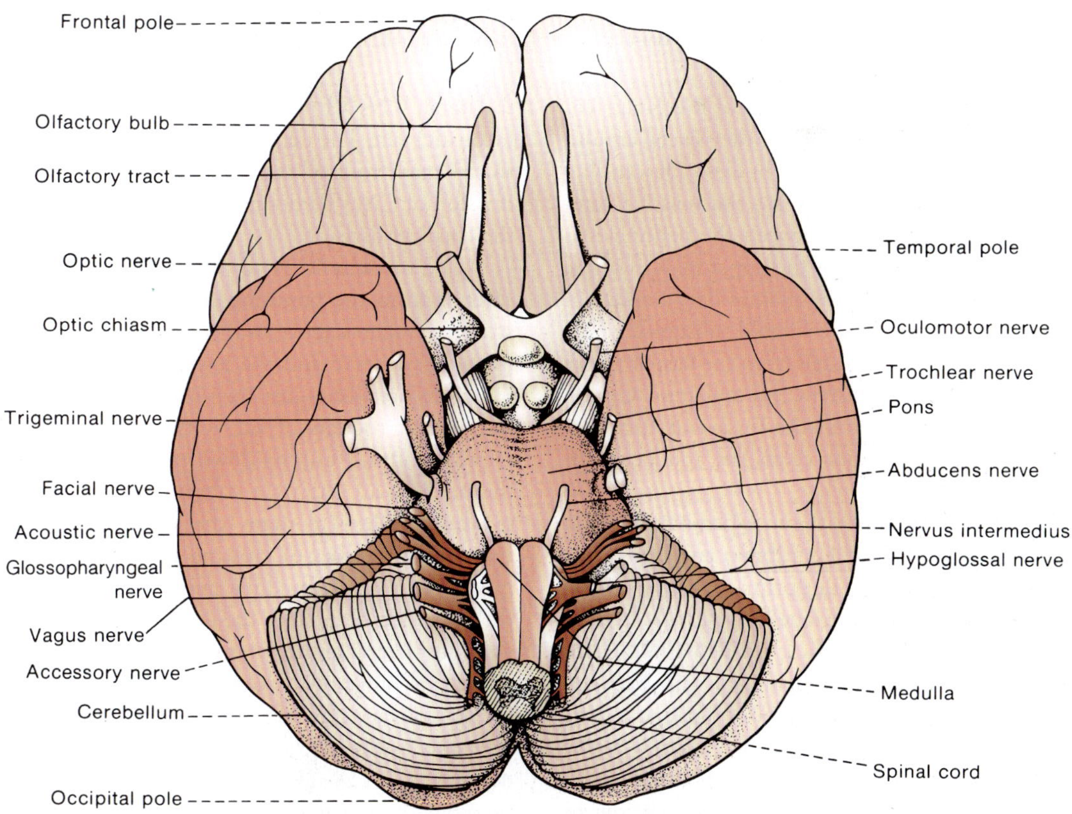

FIGURE 11.3 The base of the brain showing the sites of emergence of the cranial nerves.

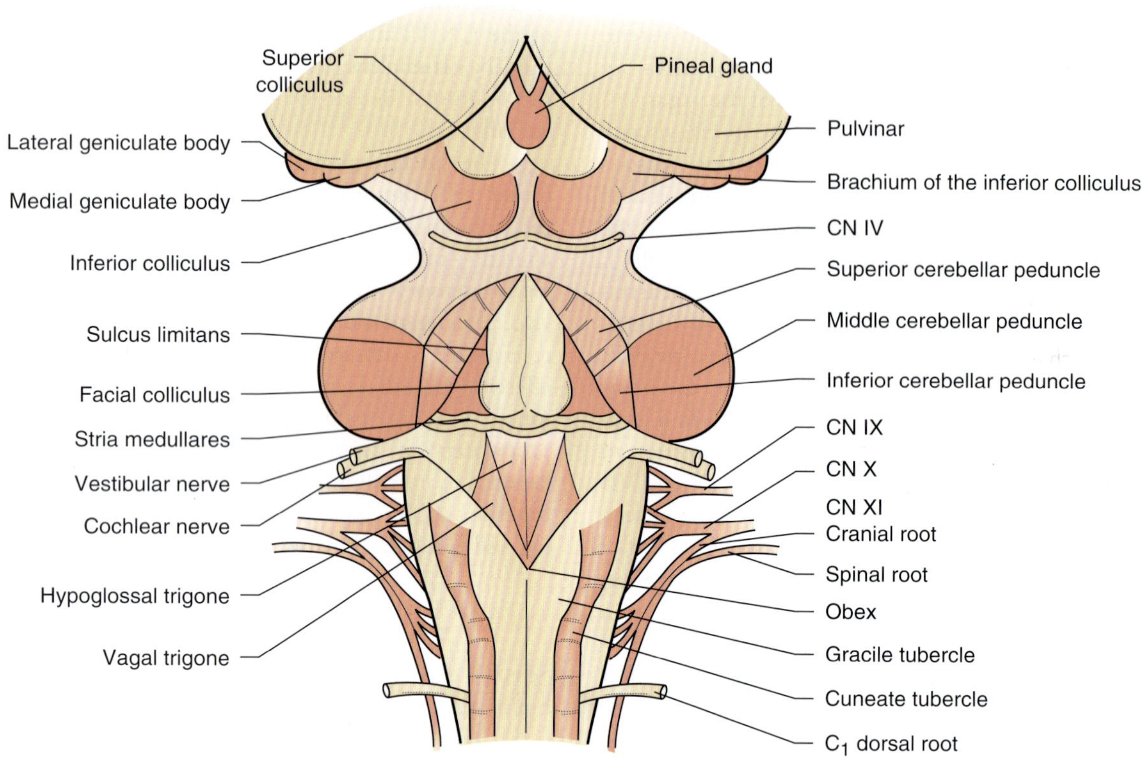

FIGURE 11.4 Dorsal view of the brainstem and rhomboid fossa.

the ventral surface, the rostral limit of the brainstem is demarcated by the optic tracts as they sweep around to reach the lateral geniculate bodies. Descending from beneath the optic tracts are the massive cerebral peduncles. The space between the peduncles is the interpeduncular fossa. At the upper margin of the interpeduncular fossa are the mammillary bodies. In its depths is the posterior perforated substance where paramedian perforating vessels from the basilar artery penetrate the upper brainstem and thalamus. CN III (oculomotor) emerges from the fossa and runs forward between the superior cerebellar and posterior cerebral arteries.

At the caudal limit of the interpeduncular fossa is the junction between the midbrain and pons. The bulge of the anterior pons, due primarily to the underlying fibers of the middle cerebellar peduncle (MCP) (brachium pontis), bridges the space between the two cerebellar hemispheres and spans the gap between the midbrain and medulla (L. pons "bridge"). The root of CN V (trigeminal) is attached laterally at the level of the midpons. The furrow of the basilar artery, the basilar sulcus, grooves the pons from below to above. At the pontomedullary junction, from medial to lateral, CNs VI (abducens), VII (facial), and VIII (acoustic) exit. The nervus intermedius lies just lateral to the main root of the facial nerve. The vestibular division of CN VIII lies medial and slightly rostral to the cochlear division.

The medulla is 24 to 30 mm in length, and it extends from the pontomedullary junction and the striae medullares above to the lowermost roots of the hypoglossal nerve and the lowest plane of the pyramidal decussation—just rostral to the emergence of the highest rootlets of C1 at the level of the foramen magnum. Running down the anterior aspect of the medulla are the twin columns of the medullary pyramids, which contain the corticospinal tracts. Interlacing bundles of crossing fibers at the caudalmost extent of the medulla mark the decussation of the pyramids. Caudal to the decussation is the spinal cord. Just lateral to the pyramids in the upper medulla is the oval bulge of the olive, beneath which lies the inferior olivary nucleus. The CN XII (hypoglossal) filaments exit in the gutter between the pyramid and the olive. CNs IX (glossopharyngeal), X (vagus), and the cranial root of XI (accessory) exit in the retro-olivary sulcus, in sequence from rostral to caudal.

Figure 11.4 shows the brainstem with the cerebellum removed and the fourth ventricle opened. The most rostral extent of the brainstem is marked by its junction with the pulvinar of the thalamus. The prominent mounds of the superior and inferior colliculi form the quadrigeminal plate. The pineal body extends caudally between the superior colliculi. The superior colliculus is connected to the lateral geniculate body by the brachium of the superior colliculus, and the inferior colliculus to the medial geniculate by its brachium. Just caudal to the inferior colliculus CN IV (trochlear) exits.

The fourth ventricular floor is rhomboid or diamond shaped and is called the rhomboid fossa. The superior cerebellar peduncle (SCP) forms the upper, lateral walls of the fourth ventricular cavity, and the inferior cerebellar peduncle (ICP) forms the walls elsewhere. At the lateral recesses of the ventricle, near the foramina of Luschka, the vestibular and cochlear nerves enter. In the ventricular floor, there are longitudinal fissures or sulci separating ridges and protuberances. The medial longitudinal fissure lies in the midline and separates the two sides. The paired grooves of the sulcus limitans, separating basal plate (motor) structures from alar plate (sensory) structures, lie laterally.

The striae medullares of the fourth ventricle (stria medullares medullares) is a band of myelinated fibers running across the ventricular floor. The fibers arise from the external arcuate nucleus, which lies anterior to the medullary pyramids, and are bound for the ICP. Paired midline humps in the ventricular floor rostral to the stria medullares are the facial colliculi, beneath which are the nuclei of CN VI and the internal genu of CN VII. Along the same meridians caudal to the striae are the hypoglossal trigones, beneath which lie the nuclei of CN XII. Lateral to the hypoglossal trigones are the vagal trigones (ala cinerea), beneath which are the dorsal motor nuclei of the vagus nerves. The area postrema (chemoreceptor trigger zone) is a narrow strip along the caudal aspect of the vagal trigone. Far laterally, near the entry zones of CN VIII, are the vestibular areas. At the caudal tip of the fourth ventricle is the obex, the point at which the fourth ventricle communicates with the central canal of the spinal cord. The shape of the rhomboid fossa at the caudal end of the ventricle resembles a writing pen; it is referred to as the calamus scriptorius. On the dorsal surface caudal to the ventricle are the gracile tubercles in the midline and the cuneate tubercles just laterally; these merge into the gracile and cuneate fasciculi inferiorly. Lateral to the gracile and cuneate tubercles are the ICPs.

Brainstem Organization

The brainstem, throughout its length, is composed of three parts: tectum (roof), tegmentum (midportion), and base (Figure 11.5). In the midbrain, the tectum consists of the quadrigeminal plate. In the pons and medulla, the tectum devolves into nonfunctional tissue forming the roof plate of the fourth ventricle, the anterior (superior) medullary velum in the pons, and the posterior (inferior) medullary velum in the medulla. The contents of the tegmentum are variable from level to level and include the CN motor and sensory nuclei. Running throughout the length of the tegmentum is the RF. The reticular activating system is part of this loose network and is responsible for controlling arousal. Coursing through the tegmentum are the long ascending and descending tracts (e.g., ML, spinothalamic tract, rubrospinal tract, and others). The base consists of descending corticospinal and corticobulbar fibers in different configurations.

Reticular Formation

The core of the brainstem is the RF, a loose network of cells and fibers that has extensive interconnections with other brainstem structures as well as complex, polysynaptic projections rostrally and caudally.

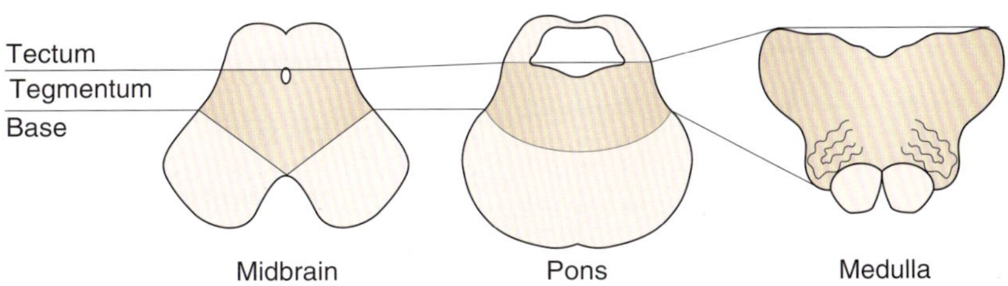

FIGURE 11.5 Three levels of the brainstem showing what constitutes the tectum, tegmentum, and base at each level. (Reprinted from Campbell WW, Pridgeon RM. *Practical Primer of Clinical Neurology*. Philadelphia: Lippincott Williams & Wilkins, 2002, with permission.)

The RF terminates as the intralaminar nuclei of the thalamus. There are three cell populations in the RF: the raphe nuclei, the medial reticular nucleus, and the lateral reticular nucleus. The raphe nuclei are a detached series of individual nuclear groups that lie in the midline (Gr. raphe "seam") from the rostral midbrain to the caudal medulla. All the raphe nuclei send serotonergic projections widely throughout the nervous system. As a generalization, the midbrain raphe nuclei project to the hemispheres, those in the pons to the brainstem and cerebellum, and those in the medulla to the spinal cord.

The lateral reticular nucleus contains small neurons and is primarily afferent; it receives collateral projections from ascending and descending long tracts. These parvocellular neurons are essentially a continuation of the system of interneurons in the spinal cord. The lateral reticular nucleus projects primarily to the medial reticular nucleus. The cells of the medial reticular nucleus are larger, and these magnocellular neurons send projections up and down the neuraxis. An expansion of the nucleus in the upper medulla forms the medullary gigantocellular nucleus, and in the pons the pontine gigantocellular nucleus. The medial reticular nucleus gives rise to two major descending tracts. The medial reticulospinal (bulbospinal) tract arises from the medullary nucleus and the lateral reticulospinal (pontospinal) tract from the pontine nucleus.

Brainstem Nuclei

The major brainstem nuclei are depicted in Figure 11.6. Some exist as focal collections, others as cell columns

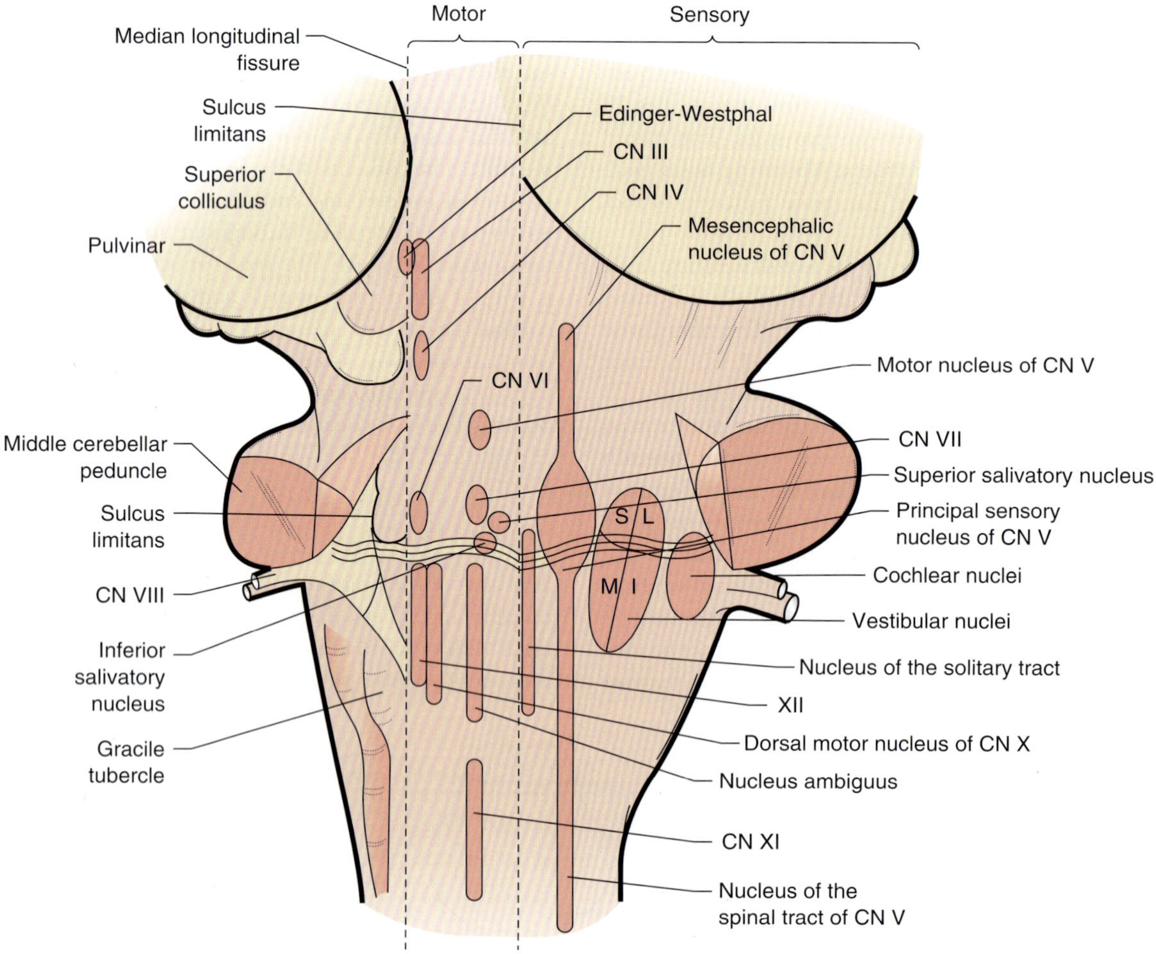

FIGURE 11.6 Gross representational brainstem view on the left demonstrates the relationships of the external structures. On the right, the expanded diagrammatic view shows the location of the various cell columns that lie interiorly, motor nuclei medially, and sensory nuclei laterally, separated by the sulcus limitans.

TABLE 11.1 The Motor Nuclei of the Brainstem

Nucleus	Type	Location	Efferents
Oculomotor	Somatic motor (GSE)	Midbrain; level of superior colliculus	CN III
Trochlear	Somatic motor (GSE)	Midbrain; level of inferior colliculus	CN IV
Abducens	Somatic motor (GSE)	Pons	CN VI
Hypoglossal	Somatic motor (GSE)	Medulla	CN XII
Edinger-Westphal	Parasympathetic (GVE)	Midbrain; level of superior colliculus	CN III
Superior salivatory	Parasympathetic (GVE)	Pons	CN VII
Inferior salivatory	Parasympathetic (GVE)	Pons	CN IX
Dorsal motor nucleus of the vagus	Parasympathetic (GVE)	Medulla	CN X
Trigeminal motor	Branchiomotor (SVE)	Pons	CN V
Facial	Branchiomotor (SVE)	Pons	CN VII
Ambiguus	Branchiomotor (SVE)	Medulla	CN IX, X, cranial root of XI

GSE, general somatic efferent; GVE, general visceral efferent; SVE, special visceral efferent.

that range longitudinally over an extensive span. The location, composition, and function of these nuclei are summarized in Tables 11.1 and 11.2.

Long Tracts

The long tracts are fiber systems that run through the brainstem over several segments. Some are ascending sensory pathways coming from the spinal cord, such as the ML and spinothalamic tracts. Others are descending pathways going to the spinal cord, such as the corticospinal tract. Some fiber tracts are more complex, carrying both ascending and descending fibers, such as the MLF. The major long tracts of the brainstem are summarized in Table 11.3 and illustrated in Figure 11.7.

Cross-Sectional Anatomy

The internal details of the brainstem are best appreciated as a series of cross sections at different levels (Figure 11.8). The following paragraphs review the

TABLE 11.2 The Sensory Nuclei of the Brainstem

Nucleus	Type	Location	Afferents	Efferents
Mesencephalic root of V	Somatic afferent (GSA)	Midbrain	Proprioceptive fibers from all cranial nerves	Trigeminothalamic tract; reflex connections
Principal sensory nucleus of V	Somatic afferent (GSA)	Pons	Touch and pressure sensation from the head, via CNs V, VII, IX, and X	Trigeminothalamic tract
Nucleus of the spinal tract of V	Somatic afferent (GSA)	Pons, extending through medulla to upper cervical cord	Pain and temperature sensation from the head, via CNs V, VII, IX, and X	Trigeminothalamic tract
Nucleus of the solitary tract, rostral portion (gustatory nucleus)	Taste (SVA)	Pons	Taste sensation via CNs VII, IX, and X	Central tegmental tract
Nucleus of the solitary tract, caudal portion	Visceral afferent (GVA)	Medulla	General visceral sensation via CNs IX, X	Local reflex connections
Cochlear nuclei	Hearing (SSA)	Pontomedullary junction	Auditory fibers from spiral ganglion of the cochlea via CN VIII	Central auditory pathways, primarily the lateral lemniscus
Vestibular nuclei	Balance and equilibrium (SSA)	Pontomedullary junction	Vestibular fibers from Scarpa's ganglion via CN VIII	Vestibulospinal and vestibulocerebellar tracts

GSA, general somatic afferent; SVA, special visceral afferent; GVA, general visceral afferent; SSA, special somatic afferent.

TABLE 11.3 The Major Ascending and Descending Long Tracts of the Brainstem

	Origin	Destination	Description
Ascending Tracts			
Medial lemniscus	Nucleus gracilis and cuneatus	VPL nucleus of the thalamus	GSA; begins as internal arcuate fibers in caudal medulla, is vertical and midline in medulla, becomes horizontal and lateral in the midbrain, somatotopically organized with homunculus erect in medulla, in sitting position in pons, horizontal then Trendelenburg in midbrain
Lateral spinothalamic tract	Posterior horn of the spinal cord (laminae I, II, V)	VPL nucleus of the thalamus	GSA; cells of origin in posterior horn; decussates in anterior white commissure; ascends contralaterally; anterolateral in medulla, moves more laterally at rostral levels; somatotopically organized, sacral fibers most lateral and dorsal
Lateral lemniscus	Cochlear nuclei	Inferior colliculus	SSA; courses laterally, becoming more dorsal approaching the midbrain
Medial longitudinal fasciculus	PPRF and VI nucleus, vestibular nuclei	III nucleus	Crosses just above VI nucleus, ascends in midline in dorsal tegmentum
Descending Tracts			
Corticobulbar tract	Motor cortex	Cranial nerve nuclei	Lies medially in central three-fifths of cerebral peduncle, decussates at local level; many nuclei also have uncrossed innervation
Corticospinal tract	Motor cortex	Spinal cord	In cerebral peduncles in midbrain, basis in pons, pyramids in medulla
Rubrospinal tract	Red nucleus	Spinal cord	Near center of tegmentum initially, moves laterally as it descends, lies near lateral corticospinal tract in the spinal cord
Medical longitudinal fasciculus	Reticular formation (RF) and vestibular nuclei	RF and spinal cord	Descending MLF contains vestibulospinal and reticulospinal fibers, mediates reflex head and neck movements in response to visual and vestibular stimuli
Central tegmental tract	Red nucleus	Inferior olivary nucleus	Prominent fasciculus in the anterior tegmentum

GSA, general somatic afferent; MLF, medial longitudinal fasciculus; PPRF, pontine paramedian reticular formation; SSA, special somatic afferent; VPL, ventral posterolateral.

cross-sectional anatomy at the level of the superior colliculus, inferior colliculus, midpons, and midmedulla.

Midbrain

The midbrain is composed of tectum, tegmentum, and base. The tectum is the quadrigeminal plate and the base the crus cerebri. There are two segmental levels with different characteristics.

Superior Colliculus Level

A cross section at the level of the superior colliculi is shown in Figure 11.8. The functions of the superior colliculi are closely related to those of the pretectum. In addition, they subserve visual reflexes, tracking, and orienting behavior. The medial geniculate bodies are located just lateral to the colliculi. They are part of the thalamus and are important relay nuclei in the auditory system. In the tegmentum at this level, the most prominent structure is the red nucleus, which gives rise to a major descending motor pathway, the rubrospinal tract (Figure 11.7). After decussating, the rubrospinal tract descends in the brainstem and then in the lateral funiculus of the spinal cord, lying just beside the pyramidal tract; it functions to facilitate flexor tone.

The third nerve nuclei lie in the midline anterior to the aqueduct; they send axons that stream through and around the red nucleus to exit anteriorly in the interpeduncular fossa. The extraocular motor nuclei (CNs III, IV, and VI) are GSE fibers. At this level, the long ascending sensory tracts lie far laterally. The ML, so named because it was in the midline in the medulla, has by now in its ascent drifted laterally, and been joined by ascending fibers of the anterolateral (spinothalamic) system and trigeminothalamic tract. The MLF courses posteriorly in the midline, bound for the medial rectus subnucleus of the oculomotor complex. Lying in the area adjacent to the aqueduct is

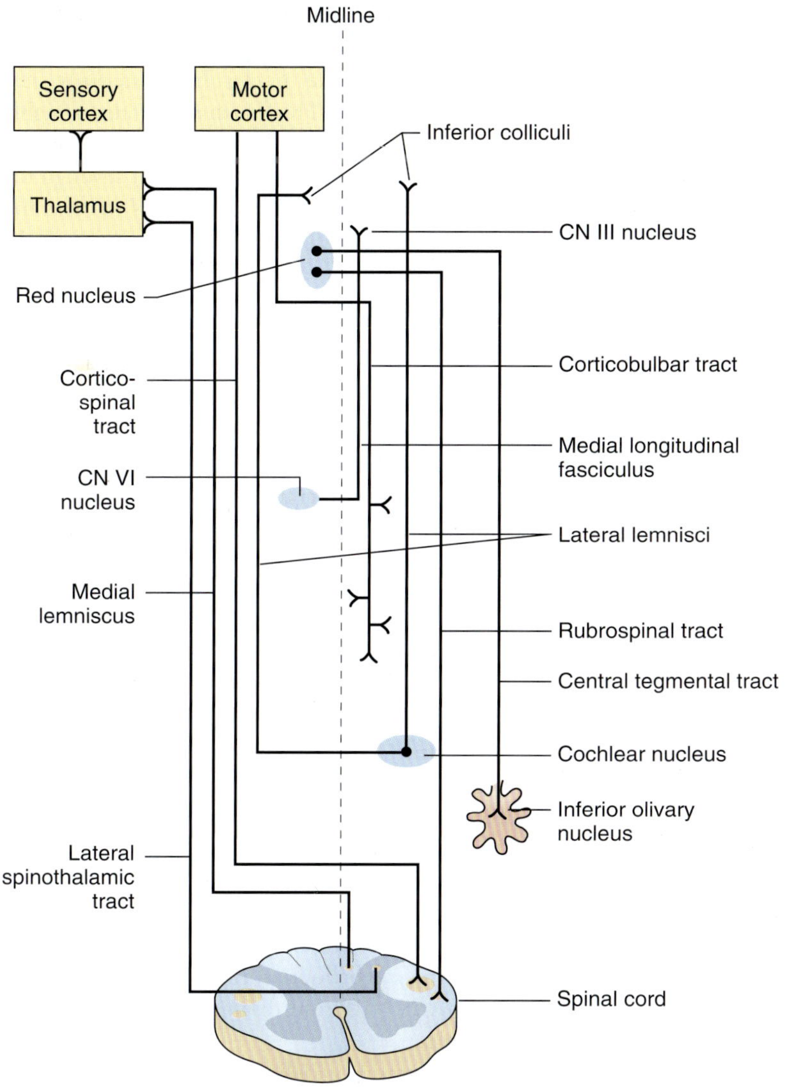

FIGURE 11.7 Some of the major long tracts that ascend and descend through the brainstem.

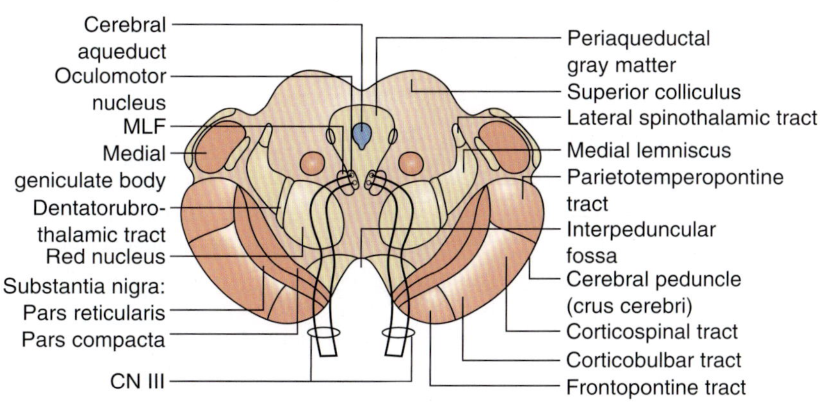

FIGURE 11.8 The midbrain at the superior collicular level, showing the oculomotor nucleus, the red nucleus, and the fibers of the third nerve as they exit through the interpeduncular fossa. (Modified from Fix JD. *Neuroanatomy*. Baltimore: Williams & Wilkins, 1992, with permission.)

the SCP, the major efferent pathway from the cerebellum. The gray matter immediately surrounding the aqueduct is one of the characteristic sites for lesions in Wernicke's encephalopathy.

Anteriorly, at this level, the base of the midbrain is composed of the cerebral peduncle, which consists of the substantia nigra and crus cerebri. The crus cerebri is a direct continuation of the internal capsule and conveys mostly descending corticospinal and corticobulbar fibers. It can be approximately divided into fifths. The lateral fifth contains the parietotemperopontine tract; the corticospinal and corticobulbar tracts occupy the middle three-fifths; and the medial fifth consists of the frontopontine tract. The middle three-fifths is somatotopically organized. The homunculus lies in Trendelenburg position with the head medial (corticobulbar fibers) and the feet above and lateral (corticospinal fibers). In the space between the peduncles—the interpeduncular fossa—the third nerve emerges.

Inferior Colliculus Level

The inferior colliculus is a relay station in the auditory pathway; it receives fibers from the lateral lemniscus and sends fibers to the medial geniculate body through the brachium of the inferior colliculus. The medial geniculate body in turn sends fibers to the auditory cortex. In the tegmentum at this level, the most prominent morphologic feature is the decussation of the SCP (Figure 11.9). The major component of the SCP is the dentatothalamic (dentatorubrothalamic) tract, which is crossing in the midline, coming from the cerebellum, primarily the dentate nucleus, en route to the contralateral ventral lateral nucleus of the thalamus, with collaterals to the red nucleus. The decussating fibers of the SCP surround the caudal red nucleus, completely obscuring it.

The fourth nerve nuclei lie posteriorly just beneath the aqueduct. The fourth nerve takes a highly aberrant course out of the brainstem, curving posteriorly to decussate in the tectum and exit through the dorsal surface. The fourth is the only CN to cross and the only one to exit dorsally. The remainder of the tegmentum and base are essentially the same as at the superior collicular level.

Pons

At the level of the pons, the tectum consists of the nonfunctional anterior medullary velum. The base is rounded and protuberant (the "belly" of the pons) and consists of descending corticospinal and corticobulbar fibers admixed with crossing pontocerebellar fibers entering the MCP (Figure 11.10). The tegmentum of the pons contains numerous important structures. The major long tracts include the medial and lateral lemnisci, the spinothalamic tracts, and the MLF. Near the midline in the gray matter lies the nucleus of CN VI, encircled by the fibers of CN VII. Just within or adjacent to the CN VI nucleus in the pontine paramedian RF lies the pontine lateral gaze center. Fibers of CN VI exit anteriorly, in the same manner as fibers of CN III exit the midbrain into the interpeduncular fossa. After looping around the CN VI nucleus, CN VII fibers exit the pons laterally, cross the cerebellopontine angle (CPA) in company with CN VIII, and disappear into the internal auditory meatus.

The trigeminal ganglion lies just beside the pons in a depression in the petrous ridge, called Meckel's

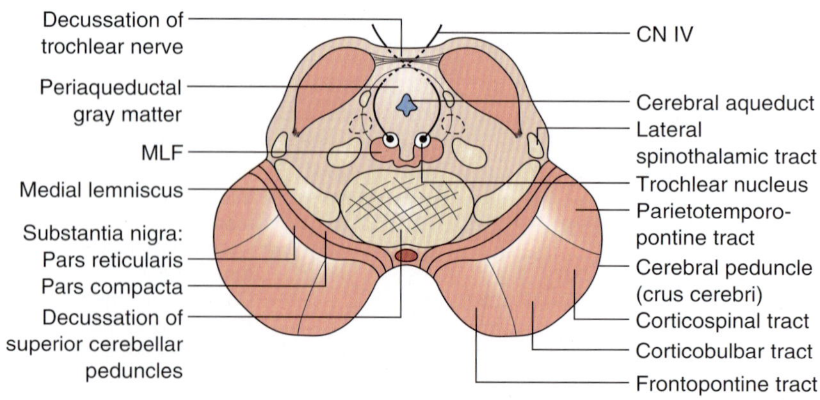

FIGURE 11.9 The midbrain at the inferior collicular level, showing the decussation of the superior cerebellar peduncle, the medial longitudinal fasciculus, and the fibers of the fourth nerve as they exit through the tectum. (Modified from Fix JD. *Neuroanatomy*. Baltimore: Williams & Wilkins, 1992, with permission.)

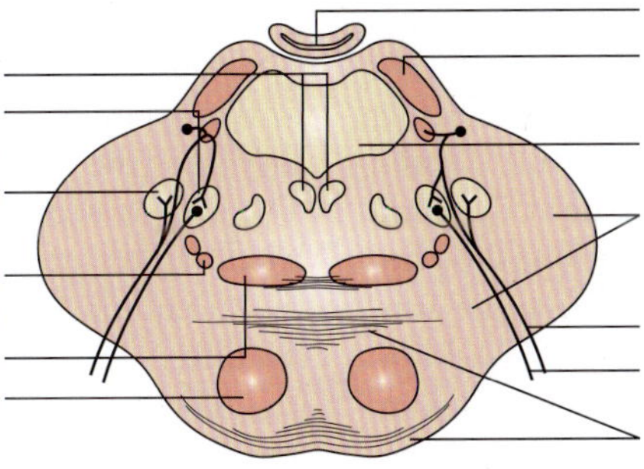

FIGURE 11.10 The midpons, showing the cavity of the fourth ventricle, trigeminal nucleus, medial longitudinal fasciculus, transverse pontine fibers, and cerebellar peduncles. (Modified from Fix JD. *Neuroanatomy.* Baltimore: Williams & Wilkins, 1992, with permission.)

cave. A large sensory and a smaller motor root join the ganglion to the pons. The motor fibers are derived from the trigeminal motor nucleus in the lateral pontine tegmentum and are destined for the nerve's mandibular division. Afferent fibers conveying light touch and pressure enter the principal sensory nucleus, which lies beside the trigeminal motor nucleus, there to synapse and give rise to second order neurons that cross the midline en route to the ventral posterior medial (VPM) thalamic nucleus. Fibers conveying pain and temperature enter the spinal tract of the trigeminal, where they descend to various levels, depending on their somatotopic origin, and synapse in the adjacent nucleus of the spinal tract. The axons of second order neurons cross the midline, aggregate as the trigeminothalamic tract, and ascend to VPM running in proximity to the ML and spinothalamic tracts.

At the junction of pons and medulla, CN VIII enters far laterally after crossing the CPA. The cochlear component consists of fibers from the organ of Corti and the spiral ganglion of the cochlea, which synapse in the cochlear nuclei. From the cochlear nuclei a complex, crossed and uncrossed, ascending pathway with multiple nuclear relays arises. Most auditory fibers eventually ascend in the lateral lemniscus en route to the inferior colliculus, then to the medial geniculate, and on to the auditory cortex in the temporal lobe. The vestibular component consists of fibers from the vestibular ganglion, which synapse in one of the four vestibular nuclei. Fibers from these nuclei ascend and descend the brainstem and spinal cord as vestibulospinal tracts and as part of the MLF.

Medulla

In the medulla, the tectum consists of the posterior medullary velum. The velum is continuous inferiorly with the tela choroidea, to which the choroid plexus is attached, which makes up the caudal part of the ventricular roof. The base consists of the medullary pyramids, which are made up of fibers of the corticospinal tract (Figure 11.11). About 90% of the corticospinal

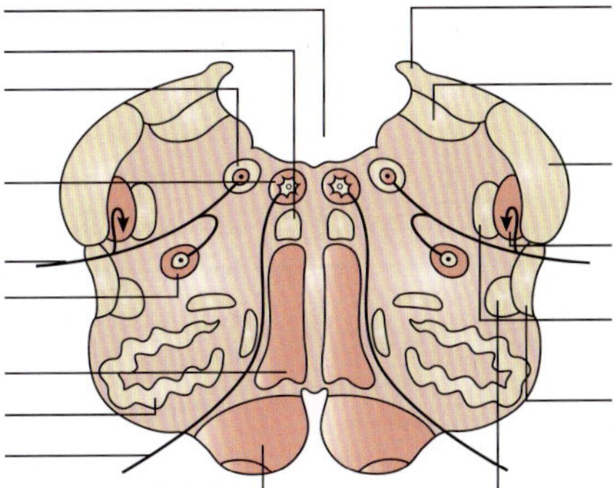

FIGURE 11.11 The medulla at midolivary level, showing the pyramids, olives, hypoglossal and ambiguus nuclei, medial lemniscus, medial longitudinal fasciculus, and spinal tract of the trigeminal. (Modified from Fix JD. *Neuroanatomy.* Baltimore: Williams & Wilkins, 1992, with permission.)

tract crosses to the other side at this level, forming the decussation of the pyramids, and continues as the lateral corticospinal tract. The remainder of the corticospinal fibers descend ipsilaterally in the anterior corticospinal tract and then decussate at the local spinal level. At the level of the decussation, the arm fibers lie medial and rostral to the leg fibers; the arm fibers decussate first and then assume a position medially in the lateral corticospinal tract in the spinal cord (Figure 11.12). Because of the complexity of the decussation, unusual clinical deficits can occur with lesions in this region.

The tegmentum of the medulla is conveniently divided into medial and lateral portions, especially because of differences in their blood supply. The medial medulla contains the ML in a vertical midline position (homunculus erect) with the MLF capping it posteriorly. The hypoglossal nerve nucleus lies in the midline and projects axons that exit anteriorly in the groove between the pyramid and the olive. The olive is a prominent, wrinkled structure lying just posterior to the pyramids. Neurons in the olive project axons that cross the midline to enter the contralateral ICP. The ICP is a prominent structure arising from the lateral aspect of the medulla; it receives fibers from the ascending spinocerebellar tracts as well as from the olive.

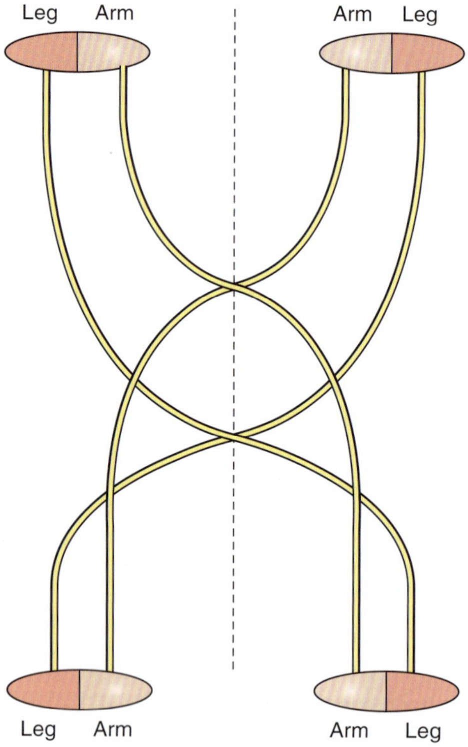

FIGURE 11.12 At the decussation of the pyramids in the lower medulla, the arm fibers lie medial to the leg fibers. Arm fibers decussate first and come to lie in the medial portion of the lateral corticospinal tract in the upper cervical spinal cord. Leg fibers decussate more caudally and come to lie in the lateral portion of the lateral corticospinal tract. The syndrome of the pyramidal decussation (cruciate or crossed paralysis) is spastic weakness of one arm and the contralateral leg because of a lesion at the decussation.

The lateral medulla contains the spinal tract and nucleus of CN V; nearby run ascending spinothalamic (anterolateral system) fibers. The nucleus ambiguus, because of its branchial arch origin, lies deep in the tegmentum anterolaterally, in a position analogous to that of the CN VII nucleus in the pons. It extends from the level of entry of CN VIII at the upper border of the medulla to the level of the decussation of the ML or even to the beginning of the corticospinal decussation. From the nucleus ambiguus, motor fibers exit laterally to enter both the ninth and tenth nerves. The dorsal motor nucleus of the vagus, the autonomic component of CN X, sends fibers laterally to join the exiting ambiguus fibers. The solitary tract lies lateral to the dorsal motor nucleus of the vagus, and it receives entering taste fibers from CNs VII and IX. Descending in the reticular core are sympathetic fibers destined for the intermediolateral gray column of the thoracic and lumbar cord.

OVERVIEW OF CRANIAL NERVES III–XII

This section provides a brief overview of the CNs that arise or terminate in the brainstem. The nerves are covered in more detail in succeeding chapters.

Oculomotor (CN III)

CN III arises from the oculomotor complex in the midbrain and conveys motor fibers to extraocular muscles, plus parasympathetic fibers to the pupil and ciliary body. It exits the midbrain in the interpeduncular fossa, travels between the posterior cerebral and superior cerebellar artery, and runs alongside the posterior communicating artery. The nerve travels through the cavernous sinus where it has important relationships with the carotid artery, ascending pericarotid sympathetics, and CNs IV, V, and VI. After exiting the cavernous sinus and passing through the superior orbital fissure, the third nerve innervates the medial rectus, inferior oblique and superior and inferior recti, and the levator palpebrae. Long ciliary nerves swerve off to the ciliary ganglion, from which short ciliary nerves arise to innervate the iris and ciliary body.

Trochlear (CN IV)

CN IV arises from the trochlear nucleus at the level of the inferior colliculus and travels backward and around to decussate and exit through the tectum. The nerve winds around the brainstem, then runs forward, passes through the cavernous sinus in proximity to CN III, traverses the superior orbital fissure, and enters the orbit to supply the superior oblique.

Trigeminal (CN V)

Motor fibers of CN V arise from the motor nucleus in the midpons, exit laterally, pass through the gasserian ganglion, and travel with the mandibular sensory branch to exit the skull through the foramen ovale. Trigeminal motor fibers innervate the masseter, temporalis, and pterygoids.

Sensory trigeminal fibers arise from the ophthalmic, maxillary, and mandibular divisions supplying the face. Ophthalmic division fibers enter the skull via the superior orbital fissure, and maxillary fibers enter through the foramen rotundum; both pass through the cavernous sinus before joining the ganglion. The mandibular fibers enter through the foramen ovale. Sensory fibers terminate in the principal sensory nucleus in the pons and in the nucleus of the spinal tract, which extends from the pons to the upper cervical spinal cord.

Abducens (CN VI)

The cells of origin of the CN VI lie in the pons near the pontine lateral gaze center. Axons pass forward through the substance of the pons, weaving among descending corticospinal fibers, and exit anteriorly. CN VI ascends the clivus, traverses the cavernous sinus in company with the CNs III, IV, and V, and then passes through the superior orbital fissure and enters the orbit to innervate the lateral rectus.

Facial (CN VII)

Axons of CN VII arise from the facial nucleus in the pontine tegmentum, travel backward, up and around the nucleus of CN VI, and then cross the pons to exit laterally. In the company of CN VIII, CN VII crosses the CPA, enters the internal auditory meatus, and travels along the internal auditory canal. It curves down and away from CN VIII at the external genu in the vicinity of the geniculate ganglion. After traversing the remainder of the petrous bone, CN VII exits through the stylomastoid foramen, turns forward, passes under the parotid gland, and ramifies into upper and lower divisions to supply the muscles of facial expression. Running in company with the facial nerve is the nervus intermedius; its primary component is the chorda tympani, which provides taste sensation to the anterior two-thirds of the tongue.

Vestibulocochlear (CN VIII)

Auditory stimuli activate hair cells in the organ of Corti. Nerve fibers supplying the hair cells are the peripheral processes of the bipolar neurons that make up the spiral ganglion lying in the center of the cochlea. The central processes of these neurons form the auditory nerve, which follows a direct course through the internal auditory canal and across the CPA, enters the brainstem at the pontomedullary junction, and synapses in the cochlear nuclei.

The vestibular nerve arises from the vestibular (Scarpa's) ganglion. The peripheral processes of its bipolar neurons receive impulses from the utricle, saccule, and three semicircular canals; the central processes convey these impulses through the vestibular portion of CN VIII.

Glossopharyngeal (CN IX)

The nucleus ambiguus sends axons via CN IX to innervate the pharyngeal plexus. The functions of CNs IX and X are virtually inseparable in this regard. The only muscle innervated solely by CN IX is the stylopharyngeus. In company with CNs X and XI, the nerve exits the skull through the jugular foramen. CN IX also conveys taste fibers from the posterior third of the tongue and supplies parasympathetics to the parotid gland.

Vagus (CN X)

CN X carries motor fibers from the nucleus ambiguus to the palate, pharynx, and larynx. In addition, a heavy input arises from the dorsal motor nucleus of the vagus, which conveys parasympathetic fibers to innervate viscera of the thorax and abdomen. The vagus also carries visceral afferents and taste fibers.

Accessory (CN XI)

The accessory nerve has two parts. The spinal portion arises from lower motor neurons in the upper cervical cord. Because of its branchial arch origin, it exits laterally, runs upward to enter the skull through the foramen magnum, and ascends to the jugular foramen. These fibers ultimately innervate the sternomastoid and trapezius muscles. The cranial portion of CN XI arises from the nucleus ambiguus, exits laterally, joins the spinal root briefly, and then quickly turns off to join IX and X. Its functions are not separable from those of the vagus.

Hypoglossal (CN XII)

CN XII arises from motor neurons in the hypoglossal nucleus, exits the medulla anteriorly in the groove between the pyramid and the olive, leaves the skull through the hypoglossal foramen, and runs forward to innervate the tongue.

BIBLIOGRAPHY

Carpenter MB. *Core Text of Neuroanatomy*. 4th ed. Baltimore: Williams & Wilkins, 1991:115–223.

Dickman CA, Hadley MN, Pappas CTE, et al. Cruciate paralysis: a clinical and radiographic analysis of injuries to the cervicomedullary junction. *J Neurosurg* 1990;73:850–858.

FitzGerald MJT, Folan-Curran J. *Clinical Neuroanatomy and Related Neuroscience*. 4th ed. Edinburgh: W. B. Saunders, 2002.

Gates P. The rule of 4 of the brainstem: a simplified method for understanding brainstem anatomy and brainstem vascular syndromes for the non-neurologist. *Intern Med J* 2005;35:263–266.

Gilman S, Winans S. *Manter and Gatz's Essentials of Clinical Neuroanatomy and Neurophysiology*. 10th ed. Philadelphia: F. A. Davis Publishers, 2003:77–118.

Gould DJ, Fix JD. *Neuroanatomy*. 5th ed. Philadelphia: Wolters Kluwer Health/Lippincott Williams & Wilkins, 2014.

Kiernan JA, Rajakumar N. *Barr's The Human Nervous System: An Anatomical Viewpoint*. 10th ed. Philadelphia: Wolters Kluwer Health/Lippincott Williams & Wilkins, 2014.

Parent A. *Carpenter's Human Neuroanatomy*. 9th ed. Baltimore: Williams & Wilkins, 1996.

Standring S, ed. *Gray's Anatomy: The Anatomical Basis of Clinical Practice*. 41st ed. New York: Elsevier Limited, 2016.

CHAPTER 12

The Olfactory Nerve

ANATOMY AND PHYSIOLOGY

The first-order neurons of the olfactory system are bipolar sensory cells that lie in the olfactory epithelium, which occupies a small area on the superior nasal concha, upper nasal septum, and roof of the nose. Their peripheral ramifications are ciliated processes that penetrate the mucous membrane of the upper nasal cavity. Tiny knobs on the cilia are the sites of chemosensory signal transduction. Odorant binding to receptors causes ion fluxes, excitation, and the activation of messenger systems. Specific odorants stimulate specific receptor cells, and specific cells respond to particular odorants.

Most nasally inspired air fails to reach the olfactory epithelium because of its location in the nasal attic. Sniffing creates a better airflow pattern for reaching the olfactory endings. The central processes of the olfactory neurons are unmyelinated axons that form approximately 20 branches on each side. These are the olfactory nerves. They penetrate the cribriform plate of the ethmoid bone, acquire a sheath of meninges, and synapse in the olfactory bulbs (Figure 12.1). Basal cells in the olfactory epithelium can regenerate, an unusual neuronal property. Olfactory receptor cells are continuously replaced by newly formed cells. The olfactory apparatus is sensitive to processes such as chemotherapy that affect rapidly replicating cell systems. Receptor regeneration with recovery of olfactory function can occur after some insults.

Within the olfactory bulbs, axons of incoming fibers synapse on dendrites of mitral and tufted cells in the olfactory glomeruli. The mitral and tufted cells are the output cells of the olfactory bulb. The axons of the second-order neurons, mainly the mitral cells, course posteriorly through the olfactory tracts, which lie in the olfactory grooves, or sulci, beneath the frontal lobes in the floor of the anterior cranial fossa.

The olfactory bulbs and tracts are sometimes mistakenly called the olfactory nerves. The olfactory nerves are the unmyelinated filaments, wrapped by a special type of glia called olfactory ensheathing glia, that pass through the cribriform plate. The olfactory tracts are mainly formed by axons myelinated by oligodendrocytes and are thus part of the central nervous system (CNS). The bulbs and tracts are part of the rhinencephalon. The proximity of the olfactory tracts to the inferior surface of the frontal lobes is an important anatomic relationship (see Figure 11.3).

Olfactory information is processed in primitive areas of the brain. Olfaction is the only sensation not directly processed in the thalamus. The olfactory tracts divide into medial and lateral olfactory striae that run on either side of the anterior perforated substance. The triangular area thus formed is called the olfactory trigone. Some olfactory stria fibers decussate in the anterior commissure to join the fibers from the opposite side; some go to the olfactory trigone and tuberculum olfactorium within the anterior perforated substance. Fibers of the medial olfactory stria terminate on the medial surface of the cerebral hemisphere in the parolfactory area, subcallosal gyrus, and inferior part of the cingulate gyrus. The lateral olfactory stria courses obliquely along the anterior perforated space and beneath the temporal lobe to terminate in the uncus, anterior hippocampal gyrus, piriform cortex, entorhinal cortex, and amygdaloid nucleus (Figures 12.2 and 12.3). Structures collectively referred to as the primary olfactory cortex include the anterior olfactory nucleus, the piriform cortex, the anterior cortical nucleus of the amygdala, the periamygdaloid complex, and the rostral entorhinal cortex.

The parahippocampal gyrus sends impulses to the hippocampus. The hippocampi and amygdaloid nuclei on the two sides are intimately related through the anterior commissure. These nuclei send

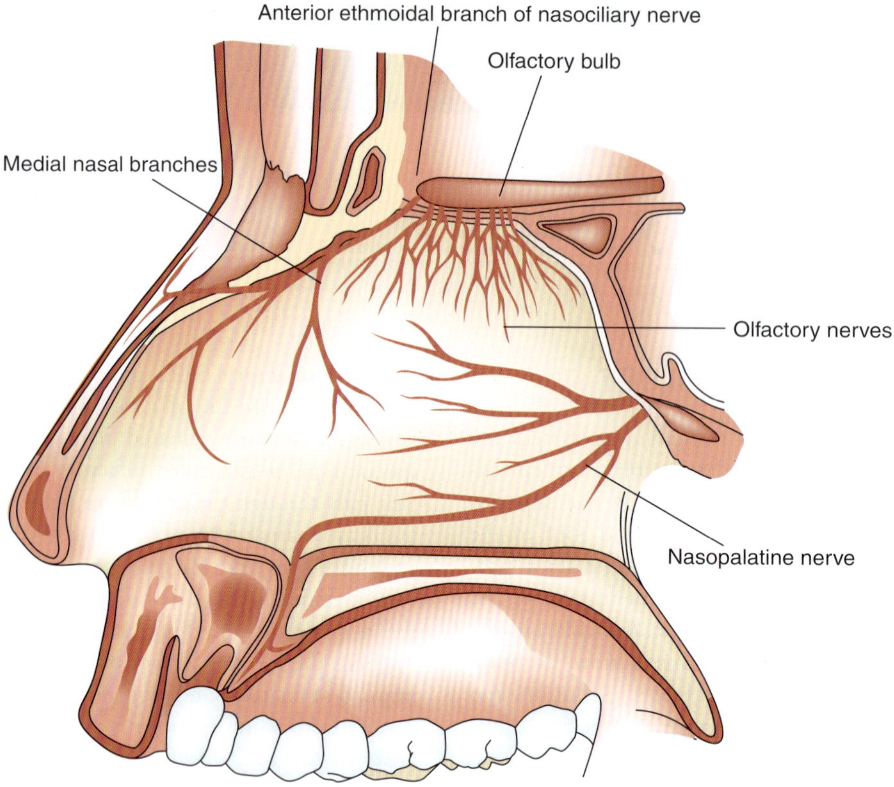

FIGURE 12.1 The distribution of the olfactory nerves within the nose.

projection fibers to the anterior hypothalamic nuclei, mammillary bodies, tuber cinereum, and habenular nucleus. These in turn project to the anterior nuclear group of the thalamus, interpeduncular nucleus, dorsal tegmental nucleus, striatum, cingulate gyrus, and mesencephalic reticular formation. Functional magnetic resonance imaging has shown that chemosensory signals cause activation of cortical areas not previously known to have olfactory functions. Communications with the superior and inferior salivatory nuclei are important in reflex salivation. Pheromones are also detected by neurons in the vomeronasal organ. These project via the olfactory tract to the accessory olfactory bulb, then to the piriform cortex and amygdala.

Olfaction is a phylogenetically ancient sensation. In lower mammals in whom olfaction is extremely important, the olfactory cortex constitutes a large part of the cerebral hemispheres. The connections between the olfactory system, hypothalamus, certain brainstem nuclei, and autonomic centers are pertinent to the understanding of many visceral functions.

The olfactory nerve is a sensory nerve with but one function—smell. The ability to perceive and identify various odors differs from person to person. Only volatile substances soluble in lipids or water are perceived as odors. In true anosmia, there is loss of ability to perceive or recognize not only scents but also flavors, for much of what is interpreted as taste involves smell. Flavor is a synthesis of sensations derived from the olfactory nerves, taste buds, and other sensory end organs. A patient with olfactory impairment may complain of loss of taste rather than of smell. Patients with unilateral anosmia may be unaware of any impairment.

CLINICAL EXAMINATION

Impairments because of anosmia are not trivial. The problem is not merely that patients with disturbances of smell sensation miss out on some of life's pleasures; they may also miss olfactory danger signals, such as spoiled food, smoke, and leaking gas. As with hearing, olfactory deficits are sometimes divided into (a)

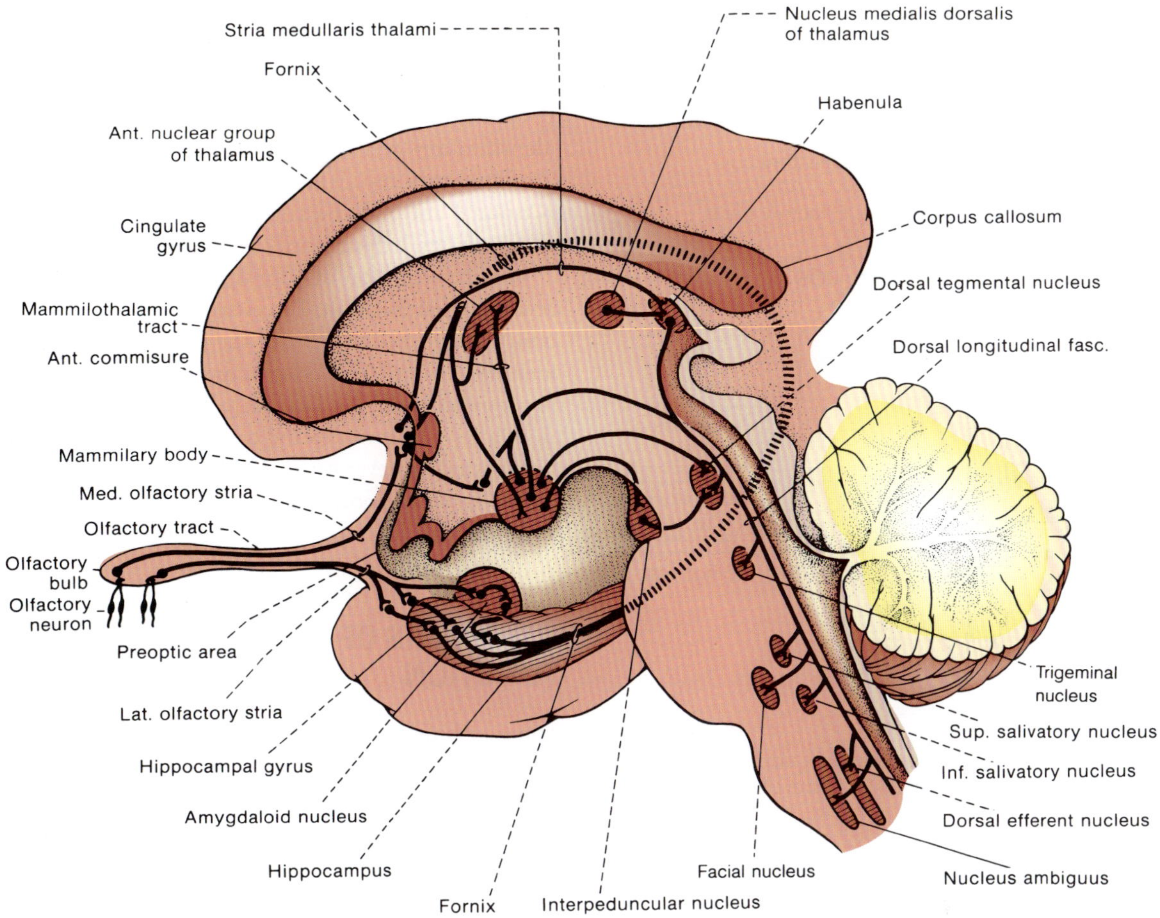

FIGURE 12.2 The olfactory pathway and its central connections.

conductive deficits, because of processes interfering with the ability of odorants to contact the olfactory epithelium, such as nasal polyps; and (b) sensorineural or neurogenic deficits, because of dysfunction of the receptors or their central connections.

Important historical points to address in a patient with a smell or taste disturbance include past head injury; smoking; recent upper respiratory tract infection (URI); systemic illness; nutrition; and exposure to toxins, medications, or illicit drugs. Feldman contends that changes in the flavor of coffee may be particularly informative. Unilateral loss of smell is more significant than bilateral, which may be caused by many conditions, primarily conductive (Table 12.1).

Before evaluating smell, ensure that the nasal passages are open. Most cases of impaired smell are due to intranasal obstructions. Acute or chronic rhinitis and chronic sinusitis may seriously interfere with olfaction.

Smell is tested using nonirritating stimuli. Avoid substances such as ammonia that may stimulate the trigeminal nerve instead of the olfactory nerve, causing a response that can be confused with olfaction. The nasal passages are richly innervated by free nerve endings from the trigeminal system, which respond to many substances. Some patients with impaired taste and smell enjoy spicy food because of its stimulation of the trigeminal system.

Examine each nostril separately while occluding the other. With the patient's eyes closed and one nostril occluded, bring the test substance near the open one. Ask the patient to sniff and indicate whether she smells something and, if so, to identify it. Repeat for the other nostril and compare the two sides. The side that might be abnormal should be examined first. Many substances can be used to test smell (e.g., wintergreen, cloves, coffee, and cinnamon). At the bedside or in the clinic, one can use mouthwash,

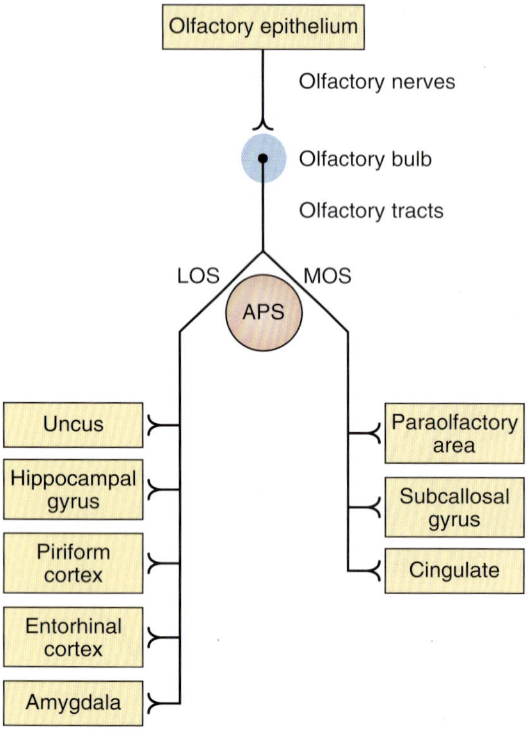

FIGURE 12.3 The olfactory pathways. APS, anterior perforated substance; LOS, lateral olfactory stria; MOS, Medial olfactory stria.

toothpaste, alcohol, soap, and similar substances. Commercial scratch-and-sniff strips are available. Commercially available quantitative smell and taste tests include the University of Pennsylvania smell identification test (UPSIT) and the Connecticut chemosensory test. The UPSIT requires no trained personnel and may be self-administered. Its forced-choice design helps identify malingering.

The perception of odor is more important than accurate identification. Perceiving the presence of an odor indicates continuity of the olfactory pathways; identification of the odor indicates intact cortical function as well. Because there is bilateral innervation, a lesion central to the decussation of the olfactory pathways never causes loss of smell, and a lesion of the olfactory cortex does not produce anosmia. The appreciation of the presence of a smell, even without recognition, excludes anosmia.

DISORDERS OF OLFACTORY FUNCTION

Some definitions regarding disorders of smell are reviewed in Table 12.2. Loss of smell may occur in a variety of conditions (Table 12.1). Common causes of impaired smell are URI, trauma, nasal and sinus disease, and normal aging. Persistent olfactory

TABLE 12.1 Some Causes of Persistent Loss of Smell

Olfactory groove meningioma	Smoking
Frontal lobe tumor, especially glioma	Chronic rhinitis
Sellar/parasellar tumor	Deviated nasal septum
Neuro-olfactory tumor (esthesioneuroblastoma)	Nasal polyps
Korsakoff's syndrome	Intranasal tumors (e.g., epidermoid carcinoma)
Vitamin deficiency (B_6, B_{12}, A)	Postviral
Zinc or copper deficiency	General anesthesia
Craniocerebral trauma, including surgery	Dental trauma
Alzheimer's disease	Chemical burns of the olfactory epithelium
Parkinson's disease	Normal aging
Multiple sclerosis	Pregnancy
Congenital anosmia	Meningitis
Arhinencephaly	Chemotherapeutic agents
Olfactory dysgenesis	Cadmium toxicity
Kallmann's syndrome (hereditary hypogonadism with anosmia)	Antihistamines
Familial dysautonomia	Propylthiouracil
Refsum's syndrome	Antibiotics
Psychiatric conditions (depression, conversion disorder, schizophrenia)	Levodopa
Chronic sinus disease	Cocaine
	Amphetamines
	Radiation therapy

TABLE 12.2 Terms and Definitions Related to Olfactory Abnormalities

Anosmia	No sense of smell
Hyposmia	A decrease in the sense of smell
Hyperosmia	An overly acute sense of smell
Dysosmia	Impairment or defect in the sense of smell
Parosmia	Perversion or distortion of smell
Phantosmia	Perception of an odor that is not real
Presbyosmia	Decrease in the sense of smell because of aging
Cacosmia	Inappropriately disagreeable odors
Coprosmia	Cacosmia with a fecal scent
Olfactory agnosia	Inability to identify or interpret detected odors

loss following a URI is the most common etiology, accounting for 15% to 25% of cases.

Age is the strongest correlate of olfactory decline, and decreased smell function occurs in the otherwise healthy elderly. Such decline often goes noticed and unreported. In those under the age of 65, about 2% of the population has impaired olfaction; the prevalence rises to about 50% between 65 and 80 and to nearly 75% in those over 80. This impaired olfaction may be related to ossification of the foramina in the cribriform plate, early neurodegenerative disease (see below), and degradation of receptor function related to repeated viral infections and other insults over the span of time.

Chronic intranasal cocaine use may cause anosmia. Toxins such as cadmium, chromium, or toluene may cause anosmia, usually accompanied by other neurologic abnormalities. Exposure, especially when chronic, to herbicides, pesticides, and solvents may lead to impaired smell. Disturbances of taste and smell may result from deficiency of vitamin B_{12}, B_6, or A and from the effects of some drugs. Decreased sense of smell has been often attributed to abnormalities in zinc metabolism.

Craniocerebral trauma may cause damage to the olfactory nerves at the cribriform plate because of coup or contrecoup forces. The incidence of trauma-related olfactory dysfunction in the general population is 4% to 15%. The likelihood of smell impairment after head trauma is directly related to the severity. The incidence of anosmia may be as high as 80% in patients with cerebrospinal fluid (CSF) rhinorrhea. Head trauma accounted for about 20% of all chemosensory disorders in one referral center.

Neurologic causes of impaired smell are rare but important. Lesions involving the orbital surface of the brain may cause unilateral anosmia. Meningiomas of the sphenoidal ridge or olfactory groove and gliomas of the frontal lobe may damage the olfactory bulbs or tracts. A typical clinical picture with sphenoidal ridge meningioma consists of unilateral optic atrophy or papilledema and exophthalmos, and ipsilateral anosmia. In meningiomas of the olfactory groove or cribriform plate area, unilateral anosmia occurs early, progressing to bilateral anosmia, often accompanied by optic neuropathy. Anosmia may also occur with other frontal lobe tumors, with parasellar and pituitary lesions and with other mass lesions, such as giant anterior cerebral aneurysm.

The Foster Kennedy syndrome consists of anosmia accompanied by unilateral ipsilateral optic atrophy and contralateral papilledema, classically because of a large tumor involving the orbitofrontal region, such as an olfactory groove meningioma. It was first described by Sir William Gowers; later and more thoroughly by R. Foster Kennedy. The anosmia and optic atrophy are due to direct compression; the contralateral papilledema occurs late when intracranial pressure increases. The atrophic optic disk cannot swell and the unusual picture of optic atrophy in one eye and papilledema in the fellow eye develops. This ophthalmologic picture, without the anosmia, is more often due to anterior ischemic optic neuropathy, arteritic or nonarteritic, involving first one eye, leading to atrophy, then the other, leading to disk edema (the pseudo–Foster Kennedy syndrome). A mass causing asymmetric compression of both optic nerves may cause a similar picture.

Anosmia may accompany some degenerative dementias, especially Alzheimer's disease (AD). Dopamine is one of the neurotransmitters in the olfactory bulbs and Lewy bodies appear in the olfactory bulb early in Parkinson's disease (PD). Olfactory dysfunction has been recognized as a common finding in patients with PD and may help distinguish PD from atypical Parkinson syndromes. Deficits may involve odor detection, identification, and discrimination. In AD and PD, the deficit is present in 85% to 90% of patients even in the early stages of the disease. The sensitivity of olfactory testing in detecting PD has been estimated as high as 0.91. In fact, Hawkes suggested that impaired smell identification is so common in PD that its absence should prompt reconsideration of the diagnosis. The prevalence of anosmia may be even higher in Lewy body dementia than in AD. Anosmia and visual hallucinations are both strong independent predictors of Lewy body pathology. Impaired smell may occur in other neurologic disorders (Box 12.1).

BOX 12.1

Other Neurologic Causes of Impaired Smell

Impaired smell has been found to occur in many other neurologic conditions, including Huntington's disease, Korsakoff's syndrome, hydrocephalus, disease of the anterior cerebral artery near its origin, basilar meningitis, frontal lobe abscess, Refsum's disease, Wilson's disease, corticobasal degeneration, spinocerebellar ataxias, narcolepsy, MS, pure autonomic failure, and following temporal lobectomy. Creutzfeldt-Jakob disease may cause anosmia, and prion protein immunoreactivity has been detected by olfactory biopsy to confirm the diagnosis. Kallmann's syndrome is a hereditary disorder that causes hypogonadism, anosmia, and mirror movements associated with developmental anomalies of the corticospinal tracts.

Anosmia sometimes occurs in conversion disorder; taste is usually not affected. In psychogenic anosmia, irritating substances, such as ammonia, that stimulate the trigeminal endings are detected no better than subtle aromas.

Disorders of smell other than hyposmia or anosmia occasionally occur. Hyperosmia is usually functional, but it can occur with certain types of substance abuse and in migraine. Parosmia and cacosmia are often due to psychiatric disease but occasionally follow head trauma and may accompany conductive dysosmia. Olfactory hallucinations are most often due to psychosis, but they can result from a lesion of the central olfactory system, usually neoplastic or vascular, or as a manifestation of seizure. So-called uncinate fits are complex partial or temporal lobe seizures preceded by an olfactory or gustatory aura, usually disagreeable, and often accompanied, as the patient loses awareness, by smacking of the lips or chewing movements. Such attacks are typically because of a seizure focus involving medial temporal lobe structures. There is never objective loss of smell interictally.

BIBLIOGRAPHY

Anholt RRH. Molecular physiology of olfaction. *Am J Physiol* 1989;257:1043.

Boesveldt S, Postma EM, Boak D, et al. Anosmia-A clinical review. *Chem Senses* 2017;42:513–523.

Brazis PW, Masdeu JC, Biller J. *Localization in Clinical Neurology*. 7th ed. Philadelphia: Wolters Kluwer/Lippincott Williams & Wilkins, 2017.

Campbell WW. *Clinical Signs in Neurology: A Compendium*. Philadelphia: Wolters Kluwer Health, 2016.

Deems DA, Doty RL, Settle RG, et al. Smell and taste disorders: a study of 750 patients from the University of Pennsylvania Smell and Taste Center. *Arch Otolaryngol Head Neck Surg* 1991;117:519–528.

Demarquay G, Ryvlin P, Royet JP. Olfaction and neurological diseases: a review of the literature. *Rev Neurol (Paris)* 2007;163:155–167.

Devanand DP, Lee S, Manly J, et al. Olfactory deficits predict cognitive decline and Alzheimer dementia in an urban community. *Neurology* 2015;84:182–189.

Doty RL. The olfactory system and its disorders. *Semin Neurol* 2009;29:74–81.

Doty RL. Olfactory dysfunction in neurodegenerative diseases: is there a common pathological substrate? *Lancet Neurol* 2017;16:478–488.

Doty RL, Shaman P, Dann M. Development of the University of Pennsylvania Smell Identification Test: a standardized microencapsulated test of olfactory function. *Physiol Behav* 1984;32:489–502.

Doty RL, Golbe LI, McKeown DA, et al. Olfactory testing differentiates between progressive supranuclear palsy and idiopathic Parkinson's disease. *Neurology* 1993;43:962.

Feldman JI, Wright HN, Leopold DA. The initial evaluation of dysosmia. *Am J Otolaryngol* 1986;7:431.

Fullard ME, Morley JF, Duda JE. Olfactory dysfunction as an early biomarker in Parkinson's disease. *Neurosci Bull* 2017;33:515–525.

Garcia-Gonzalez D, Murcia-Belmonte V, Clemente D, et al. Olfactory system and demyelination. *Anat Rec* 2013;296:1424–1434.

Hawkes C. Olfaction in neurodegenerative disorder. *Mov Disord* 2003;18:364–372.

Hussey HH. Taste and smell deviations: importance of zinc. *JAMA* 1974;226:1669.

Lafaille-Magnan ME, Poirier J, Etienne P, et al. Odor identification as a biomarker of preclinical AD in older adults at risk. *Neurology* 2017;89:327–335.

Levy M, Henkin RI, Hutter A, et al. Functional MRI of human olfaction. *J Comput Assist Tomogr* 1997;21:849–856.

Lucassen EB, Turel A, Knehans A, et al. Olfactory dysfunction in multiple sclerosis: a scoping review of the literature. *Mult Scler Relat Disord* 2016;6:1–9.

Manconi M, Paolino E, Casetta I, et al. Anosmia in a giant anterior communicating artery aneurysm. *Arch Neurol* 2001;58:1474–1475.

Marine N, Boriana A. Olfactory markers of depression and Alzheimer's disease. *Neurosci Biobehav Rev* 2014;45:262–270.

Mesholam RI, Moberg PJ, Mahr RN, et al. Olfaction in neurodegenerative disease: a meta-analysis of olfactory functioning in Alzheimer's and Parkinson's diseases. *Arch Neurol* 1998;55:84–90.

Olichney JM, Murphy C, Hofstetter CR, et al. Anosmia is very common in the Lewy body variant of Alzheimer's disease. *J Neurol Neurosurg Psychiatry* 2005;76:1342–1347.

Pardini M, Huey ED, Cavanagh AL, et al. Olfactory function in corticobasal syndrome and frontotemporal dementia. *Arch Neurol* 2009;66:92–96.

Roberts RO, Christianson TJ, Kremers WK, et al. Association between olfactory dysfunction and amnestic mild cognitive impairment and Alzheimer disease dementia. *JAMA Neurol* 2016;73:93–101.

Ross GW, Petrovitch H, Abbott RD, et al. Association of olfactory dysfunction with risk for future Parkinson's disease. *Ann Neurol* 2008;63:167–173.

Ruggiero GF, Wick JY. Olfaction: new understandings, diagnostic applications, *Consult Pharm* 2016;31:624–632.

Scangas GA, Bleier BS. Anosmia: differential diagnosis, evaluation, and management. *Am J Rhinol Allergy* 2017;31:3–7.

Schiffman SS. Taste and smell losses in normal aging and disease. *JAMA* 1997;278:1357–1362.

Schon F. Involvement of smell and taste in giant cell arteritis. *J Neurol Neurosurg Psychiatry* 1988;51:1594.

Shibasaki H, Hallett M. *The Neurological Examination: Scientific Basis for Clinical Diagnosis.* Oxford; New York: Oxford University Press, 2016.

Silveira-Moriyama L, Mathias C, Mason L, et al. Hyposmia in pure autonomic failure. *Neurology* 2009;72:1677–1681.

Stiasny-Kolster K, Doerr Y, Moller JC, et al. Combination of 'idiopathic' REM sleep behaviour disorder and olfactory dysfunction as possible indicator for alpha-synucleinopathy demonstrated by dopamine transporter FP-CIT-SPECT. *Brain* 2005;128(Pt 1):126–137.

Stiasny-Kolster K, Clever SC, Moller JC, et al. Olfactory dysfunction in patients with narcolepsy with and without REM sleep behaviour disorder. *Brain* 2007;130(Pt 2):442–449.

Tabaton M, Monaco S, Cordone MP, et al. Prion deposition in olfactory biopsy of sporadic Creutzfeldt-Jakob disease. *Ann Neurol* 2004;55:294–296.

Vale TC, Pedroso JL, Rivero RLM, et al. Lack of decussation of pyramids in Kallmann syndrome presenting with mirror movements. *J Neurol Sci* 2017;372:220–222.

Velayudhan L. Smell identification function and Alzheimer's disease: a selective review. *Curr Opin Psychiatry* 2015;28:173–179.

Zanusso G, Ferrari S, Cardone F, et al. Detection of pathologic prion protein in the olfactory epithelium in sporadic Creutzfeldt-Jakob disease. *N Engl J Med* 2003;348:711–719.

Zatorre RJ, Jones-Gotman M, Evans AC, et al. Functional localization and lateralization of human olfactory cortex. *Nature* 1992;360:339–340.

CHAPTER 13

The Optic Nerve

ANATOMY AND PHYSIOLOGY

The optic nerve is a central nervous system (CNS) fiber pathway connecting the retina and the brain. The peripheral receptors, retinal rods and cones, are stimulated by light rays that pass through the cornea, lens, and vitreous. They send impulses to the inner nuclear or bipolar layer; cells there send axons to the ganglion cell layer (Figure 13.1). There are nearly 1.2 million ganglion cells and their axons that make up the optic nerve. The photoreceptor layer is the deepest layer of the retina; it lies adjacent to the choroid, and light must pass through the more superficial layers to reach it. The rods, more numerous than the cones, are scattered diffusely throughout the retina but are absent in the macula. They respond to low-intensity stimulation and mediate night vision, peripheral vision, and perception of movement. They cannot perceive color. Cones are also present throughout the retina but are concentrated in the macula lutea. The macula consists entirely of cones; it is the point of central fixation and the site of greatest visual acuity and color perception. The macular cones have a 2:1 ratio with ganglion cells, the highest in the eye. The macula (L. "spot") is a small shallow depression in the retina that lies temporal to the disk (Figure 13.2). It has a slightly different color than the surrounding retina that can be seen with the ophthalmoscope. The fovea (L. "pit") centralis is a tiny depression that lies in the center of the macula. The foveola is an even tinier depression in the center of the fovea. It is the point of most acute vision because the overlying retinal layers are pushed aside and light falls directly on the receptors; the foveola is the optical center of the eye. The macula is responsible for the central 15 degrees of vision and the discrimination of colors and fine visual details; its cones are stimulated by light of relatively high intensity and colors. The optic disk, or papilla, is the ophthalmoscopically visible tip of the intraocular portion of the optic nerve. The nerve head is a 1.5 × 1.8 mm vertical ellipse, and it appears as a pink to yellowish-white disk. The disk normally inserts into the retina perpendicularly. When the angle is less than 90 degrees, a rim or crescent of choroid or sclera appears on the temporal side and the nasal side may appear elevated (tilted disk). It contains no receptor cells, does not respond to visual stimuli, and is responsible for the physiologic blind spot. The macula, not the disk, forms the center of the retina, and the macular fixation point is the center of the clinical visual field (VF).

The retinal ganglion cell axons form the retinal nerve fiber layer (NFL) as they stream toward the disk to exit through the lamina cribrosa (L. "sieve"), the collagenous support of the optic disk. Loss of axons and other abnormalities involving the NFL can sometimes be appreciated ophthalmoscopically. Using the red-free light of the ophthalmoscope helps visualize the NFL. Myelin in the optic nerve is CNS myelin, formed by oligodendroglia. The axons are unmyelinated in the retina and on the papillary surface but become myelinated at the posterior end of the optic nerve head as they pass through one of 200 to 300 holes in the lamina cribrosa. In about 1% of individuals, myelin extends into the peripapillary retinal NFL (myelinated nerve fibers). Optic nerve axons primarily carry visual impulses, but they also transmit the impulses that mediate accommodation and reflex responses to light and other stimuli. Optic nerve signals are coded spatially because of the location of cells in the retina, and they are also coded temporally because the frequency and pattern of firing relays information.

Macular vision is a critical function, and the projection of the macula to the optic nerve is massive. There are approximately 1.2 million fibers in each optic nerve; about 90% arise from the macula. Because

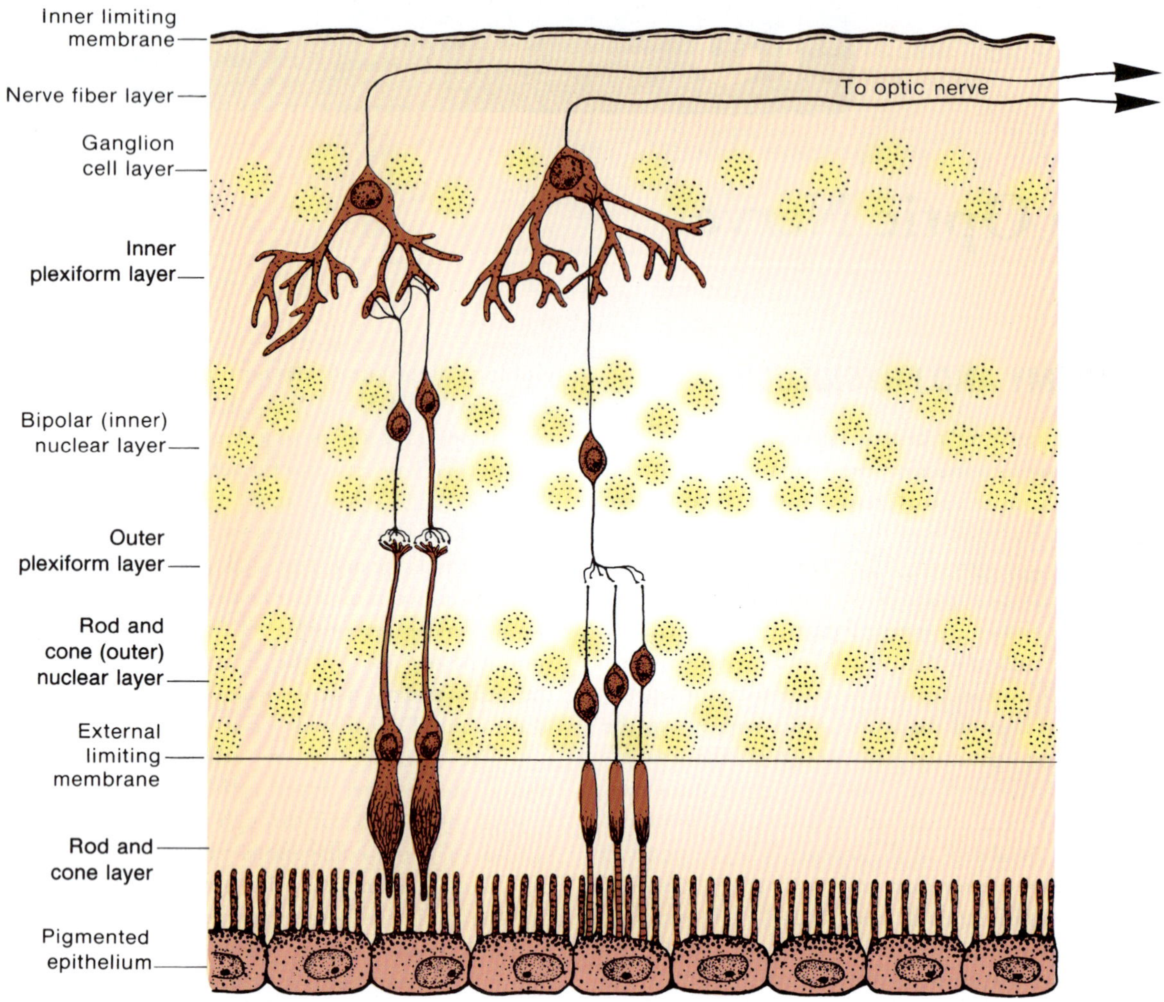

FIGURE 13.1 The layers of the retina and their relationship to the optic nerve. The inner limiting membrane is the most superficial structure; light must pass through the other layers to reach the rod and cone layer. (Modified from Ramon y Cajal S. *Histologie du Système Nerveux de l'Homme et Des Vertebres, vol 2.* Paris: A. Maloine, 1909, 1911.)

of this preponderance of macular fibers, early signs of optic nerve disease reflect macular function: impaired color vision, impaired acuity, and central scotoma. A dense collection of axons, the papillomacular bundle (PMB), travels from the nasal hemimacula to enter the temporal aspect of the disk (Figure 13.3). Fibers from the temporal hemiretina and hemimacula arch around the macula and enter the disk as the superior and inferior retinal arcades. Lesions involving these arcades may create arcuate VF defects that have an arching shape. The horizontal temporal raphe demarcates superiorly from inferiorly sweeping axons traveling from the temporal hemimacula to the disk. All of the axons from the macula gather into the PMB as it enters the optic nerve. The fibers of the PMB are very vulnerable to toxins, ischemia, and pressure.

The organization of the visual afferent system is not random. Tight retinotopic correlation prevails throughout the system; each point on the retina has a specific representation in the optic nerve, the chiasm, the tract, the radiations, and the cortex. The PMB, which forms the bulk of optic nerve axons, runs as a discrete bundle inside the optic nerve. The VF maintains its basic shape and structure throughout the system, although its orientation within the visual pathways changes (Figure 13.4). Fibers from the temporal hemiretina are located in the temporal half of the optic nerve, whereas fibers from the nasal hemiretina

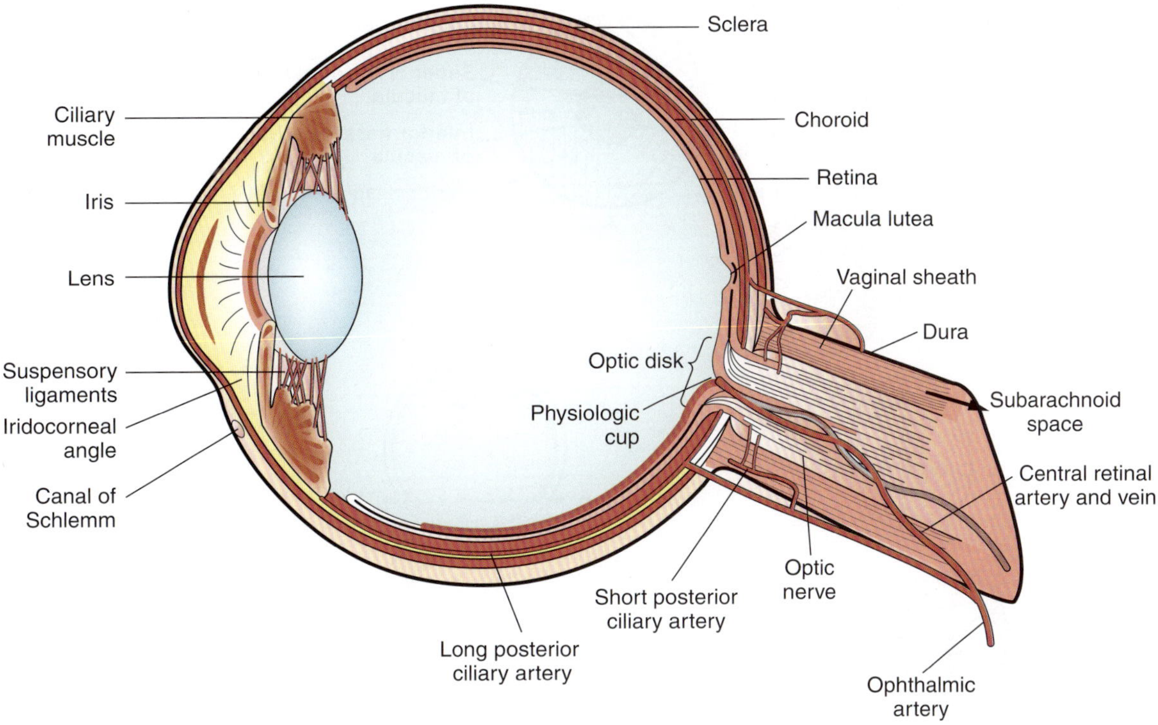

FIGURE 13.2 Structure of the eyeball.

are located medially. Upper retinal fibers are located superiorly and lower retinal fibers inferiorly in the optic nerve; this relationship is retained except in the optic tract and lateral geniculate body (LGB).

The optic nerve extends from the retina to the optic chiasm; it is approximately 5 cm long. It is conventionally divided into four portions: intraocular (1 mm; the disk), intraorbital (about 25 mm), intracanalicular (about 9 mm), and intracranial (12 to 16 mm). The nerve is organized into 400 to 600 fascicles separated by connective tissue septa. The intraorbital portion is surrounded by fat (Figure 13.5).

The intracranial dura is continuous with the investments of the optic nerve; at the posterior globe, the dura fuses with Tenon's capsule, and at the optic foramen, it is adherent to the periosteum. The pia and arachnoid also continue from the brain and envelop the optic nerve. They fuse with the sclera where the nerve terminates. The intracranial meninges extend forward along the optic nerves for a variable distance,

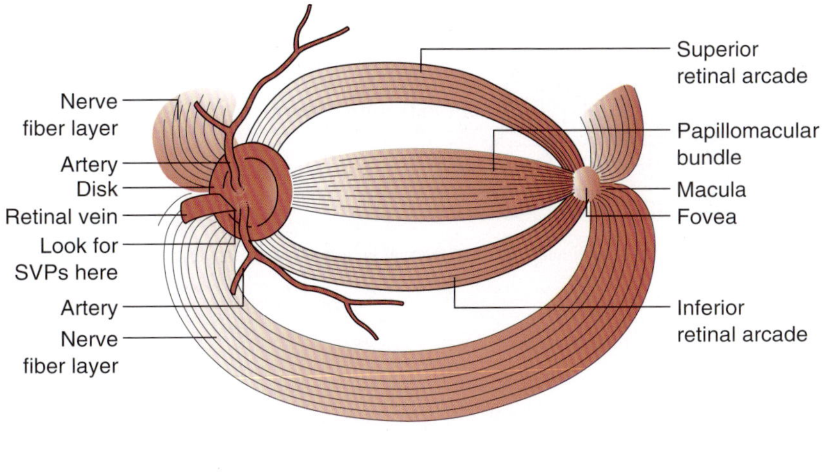

FIGURE 13.3 The optic disk and associated structures. Axons destined to form the bulk of the fibers in the optic nerve arise from the macula, those from the nasal side form the papillomacular bundle, and those from the temporal hemimacula enter the disk as superior and inferior arcades. Spontaneous venous pulsations are best seen by looking at the tip of the column of one of the large veins on the disk surface.

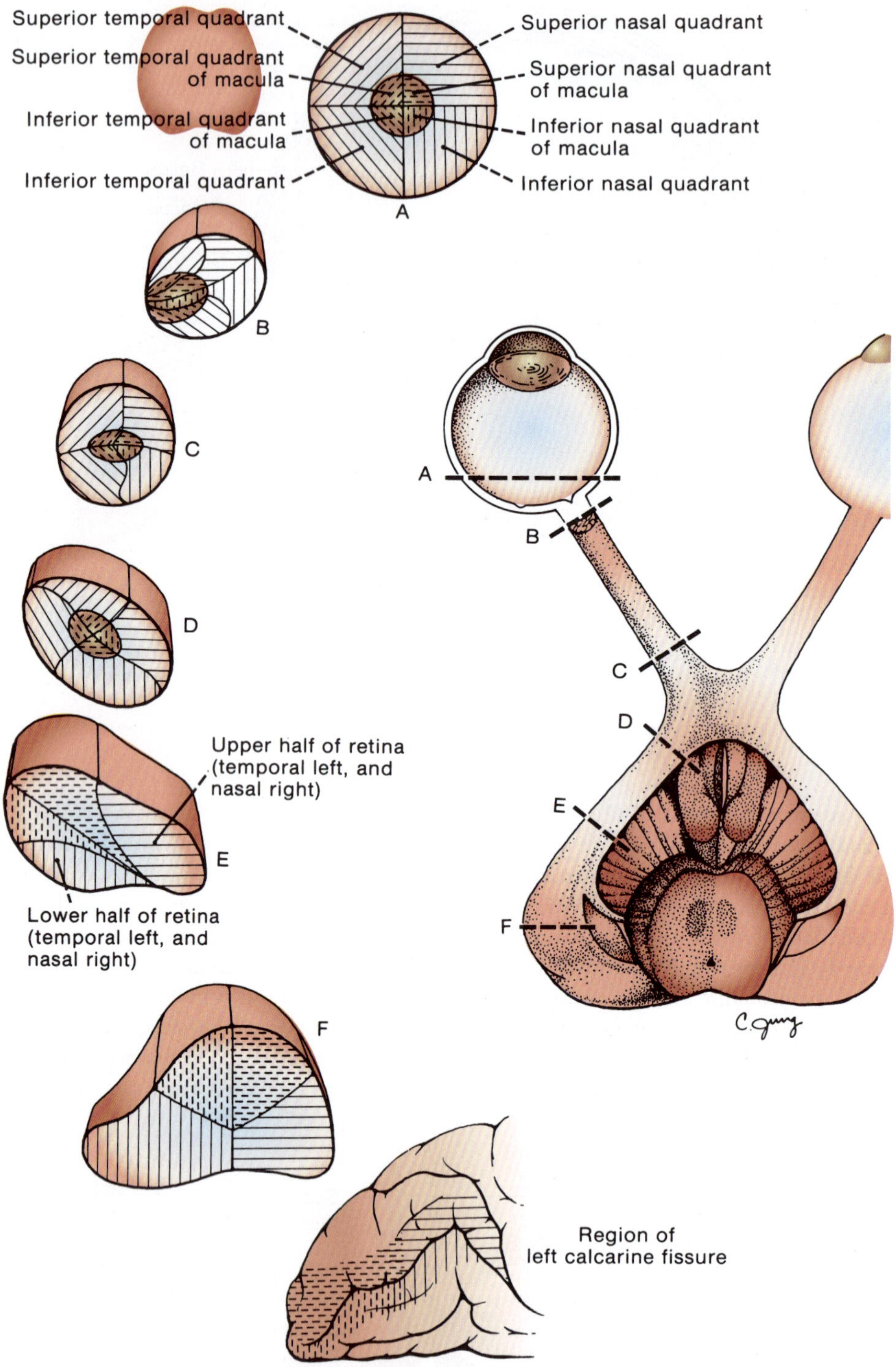

FIGURE 13.4 The grouping of visual fibers from the retinal quadrants and macular area in the optic nerve, optic tract, lateral geniculate body (LGB), and occipital cortex.

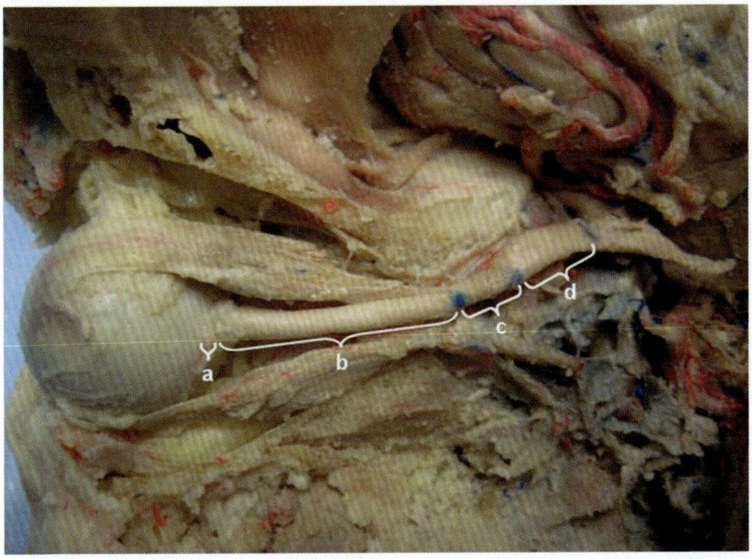

FIGURE 13.5 Optic nerve exposed from above with fat and the roof and lateral wall removed. The intraocular segment (*a*) is within the globe. The intraorbital segment (*b*) runs through the orbit to the entrance of the optic canal depicted by the left-most *blue dot*. The short intracanalicular segment (*c*) courses between the *two blue dots*. The intracranial segment (*d*) continues to its junction with the optic chiasm (*blue bar*). (Courtesy Dr. John B. Selhorst.)

forming the vaginal sheaths (Figure 13.2). Through these sheaths, the intracranial subarachnoid space continues along the nerves and may transmit increased intracranial pressure, causing papilledema. Variations in vaginal sheath anatomy may explain the occasional asymmetry of papilledema. Decompression of the optic nerves by opening the sheaths is sometimes done to treat papilledema that threatens vision. The intervaginal space lies between the dura and the pia, divided by the arachnoid into a small subdural and a larger subarachnoid space. The ophthalmic artery, the ciliary ganglion and nerves, and the nerves to the extraocular muscles lie close to the optic nerve in the orbital apex. The intraorbital optic nerve is sinuous, with about 8 mm of redundant length to accommodate eye movement. This excess of length allows about 9 mm of proptosis before the nerve begins to tether.

In the peripheral portion of the nerve, near the eye, the PMB is positioned laterally and slightly inferiorly; this separates the temporal fibers into dorsal and ventral quadrants. These in turn crowd and somewhat displace the nasal quadrants (Figure 13.4). As the nerve approaches the chiasm, the PMB moves toward its center.

The intracanalicular portion of the optic nerve begins as it traverses the optic foramen at the orbital apex. The orbital opening of the canal is a vertical ellipse; the intracranial end is a horizontal ellipse. The intracanalicular portion is fixed tightly inside the optic canal with little room to move; intracanalicular lesions can compress the optic nerve while they are still small and difficult to visualize on imaging studies (the "impossible meningioma"). The ophthalmic artery and some filaments of the sympathetic carotid plexus accompany the nerve through the canal.

After traversing the orbit and optic canal, the two optic nerves exit from the optic canals and rise at an angle of about 45 degrees to unite at the optic chiasm, so named because of its resemblance to the Greek letter chi (χ) (Figure 13.6). The orbital surface of the frontal lobes lies just above the intracranial

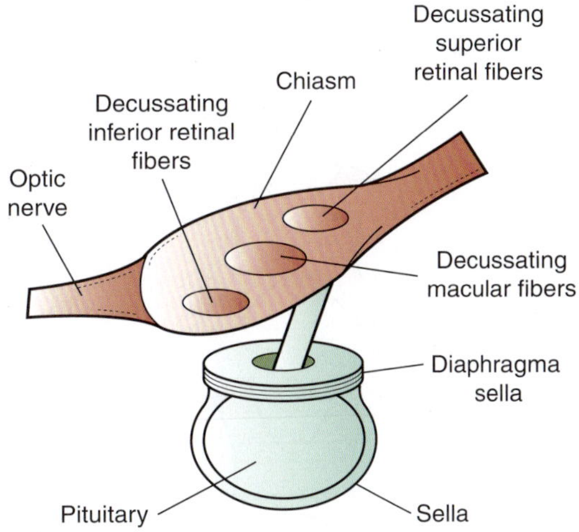

FIGURE 13.6 The macular fibers decussate as a separate compact bundle, inferior retinal (superior visual field [VF]) fibers cross inferiorly, and superior retinal (inferior VF) fibers cross superiorly. Masses impinging from below (e.g., pituitary adenoma) tend to cause early defects in the superior temporal fields; masses impinging from above (e.g., craniopharyngioma) tend to cause early defects in the inferior temporal fields.

optic nerves. The chiasm typically lies about 10 mm above the pituitary gland, separated by the suprasellar cistern. Fibers from the temporal retina continue directly back to enter the ipsilateral optic tract. Fibers from the nasal retina decussate to enter the opposite optic tract.

In 80% of the population, the chiasm rests directly above the sella. In 10%, the chiasm sits forward over the tuberculum sellae with short optic nerves and long optic tracts (prefixed); in the other 10%, the chiasm sits posteriorly over the dorsum sellae with long optic nerves and short optic tracts (postfixed) (Figure 13.7). The position of the chiasm in relation to the sella and the neoplasia-prone pituitary gland influences the clinical presentation of masses in the region.

The basic scheme of the chiasm with temporal hemiretinal fibers continuing ipsilaterally and nasal hemiretinal fibers decussating is straightforward (Figure 13.8). But there are intricacies in the chiasmal crossing. In the process of decussating, fibers from the inferior nasal quadrant loop forward into the opposite optic nerve for a short distance before turning back again, forming Wilbrand's knee (Figure 13.9, see junctional scotoma in "Scotomas" section). In addition, some of the upper nasal fibers loop back briefly into the ipsilateral optic tract before decussation.

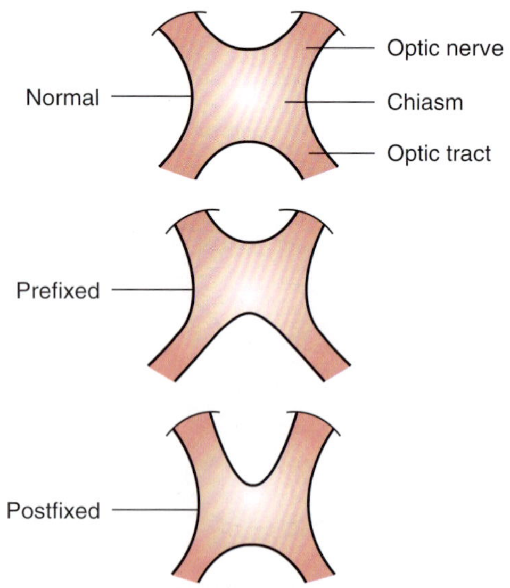

FIGURE 13.7 The normal position of the chiasm is shown in the top drawing. When the chiasm is prefixed, the optic nerves are short, the chiasm sits forward over the sella, and the optic tracts are long. When the chiasm is postfixed, the optic nerves are long, the chiasm sits posteriorly over the sella, and the optic tracts are short.

In the chiasm, the fibers from the upper retinal quadrants lie superior and those from the lower quadrants inferior (Figure 13.6). Inferior nasal fibers decussate anteriorly and inferiorly in the chiasm, whereas superior nasal fibers cross posteriorly and superiorly, accounting for the difference in the pattern of evolution of the field defect in infrachiasmatic versus suprachiasmatic lesions (Figure 13.9). Macular fibers more or less decussate as a group, forming a miniature chiasm within the chiasm, primarily in the posterior superior portion.

The cavernous sinuses and carotid siphons lie just lateral to the chiasm on either side. The anterior cerebral and anterior communicating arteries are in front and above, and the third ventricle and hypothalamus are behind and above. The sella turcica and sphenoid sinus lie below. The circle of Willis lies above, sending numerous small perforators to supply the chiasm. The ophthalmic artery runs alongside the optic nerve within the same dural sheath through the canal and orbit. About 8 to 12 mm posterior to the globe, the artery enters the nerve and runs along its center to the optic disk, where it becomes the central retinal artery, which pierces the nerve and runs forward onto the disk. The central retinal artery divides at the disk head into superior and inferior branches, which supply the retina. Other terminal branches of the ophthalmic, the short posterior ciliary arteries and choroidal vessels, form an arterial network, the circle of Zinn-Haller, which supplies the disk; the central retinal artery makes only a minimal contribution to the vascular supply of the optic disk.

Posterior to the optic chiasm, the uncrossed fibers from the ipsilateral temporal hemiretina and the crossed fibers from the contralateral nasal hemiretina form the optic tract. About 55% of the axons of the optic tract arise from the contralateral nasal retina and 45% from the ipsilateral temporal retina, which roughly corresponds to the ratio of the area of the temporal field to the nasal field. The tracts contain approximately 80% visual afferents and 20% pupillary afferents. The tracts extend from the chiasm to the LGB, where the majority of fibers terminate. Retinotopic organization is maintained in the optic tract, but the orientation changes. There is a gradual inward rotation, so fibers from the upper retina assume a medial position, whereas those from the inferior retina lie lateral. Fibers of the PMB gradually assume a dorsal and lateral position, wedged between the upper and lower retinal fibers (Figure 13.4). The retinotopic organization in optic tracts is not

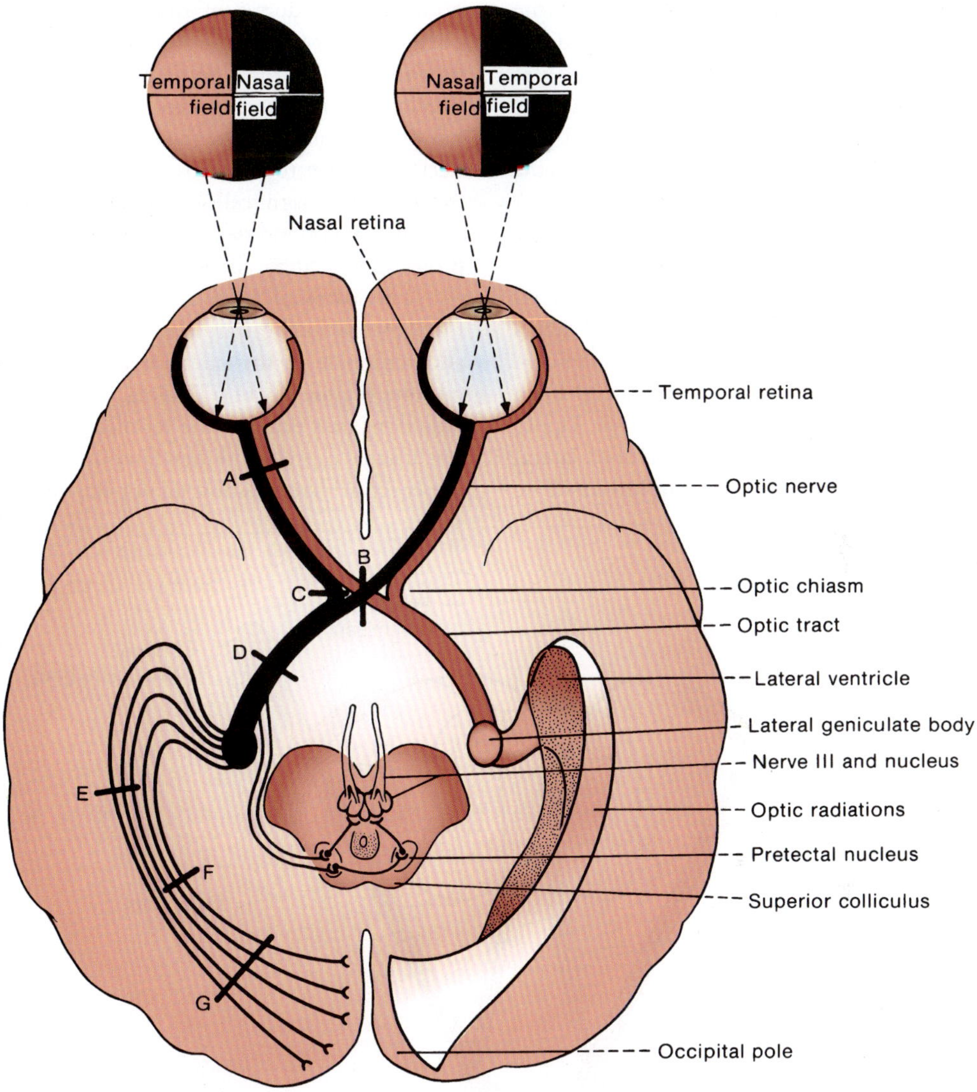

FIGURE 13.8 The course of the visual fibers from the retina to the occipital cortex. *A* to *G* show the sites of various lesions that may affect the fields of vision.

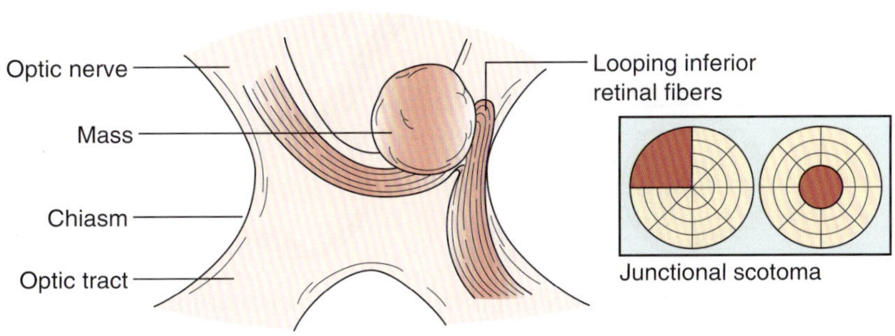

FIGURE 13.9 A mass impinging on the optic nerve at its junction with the chiasm, producing a junctional scotoma.

as precise as elsewhere, which may contribute to the incongruity of VF defects that are characteristic of optic tract lesions.

Afferent fibers from the pupil leave the tract just anterior to the geniculate to enter the pretectal area of the midbrain (Figure 13.10). The visual afferents synapse in the geniculate on second-order neurons, which give rise to the geniculocalcarine pathway (optic radiations).

There are six neuronal layers in the LGB, separated by myelinated nerve fibers. Uncrossed fibers from the ipsilateral temporal hemiretina synapse in layers 2, 3, and 5; those from the contralateral nasal hemiretina synapse in layers 1, 4, and 6. Upper retinal fibers remain medial and lower ones lateral (Figure 13.4). Macular fibers occupy an intermediate position in the dorsal, middle, and somewhat caudal portion. The LGB has large magnocellular and small parvocellular neurons. Some of the visual fibers pass over or through the LGB to terminate in the pulvinar of the thalamus, but the significance of this connection has yet to be determined for vision or visual reflexes. The magnocellular projections seem to process movement and depth, whereas the parvocellular projections mediate shape, pattern, and color.

The axons of LGB neurons pass posteriorly to form the geniculocalcarine tract, or optic radiations, and terminate in the calcarine cortex of the occipital lobe (Figure 13.11). Leaving the LGB, the optic radiations pass through the retrolenticular portion of the internal capsule and then fan out. Retinotopically, upper retinal fibers resume an upper, and lower retinal

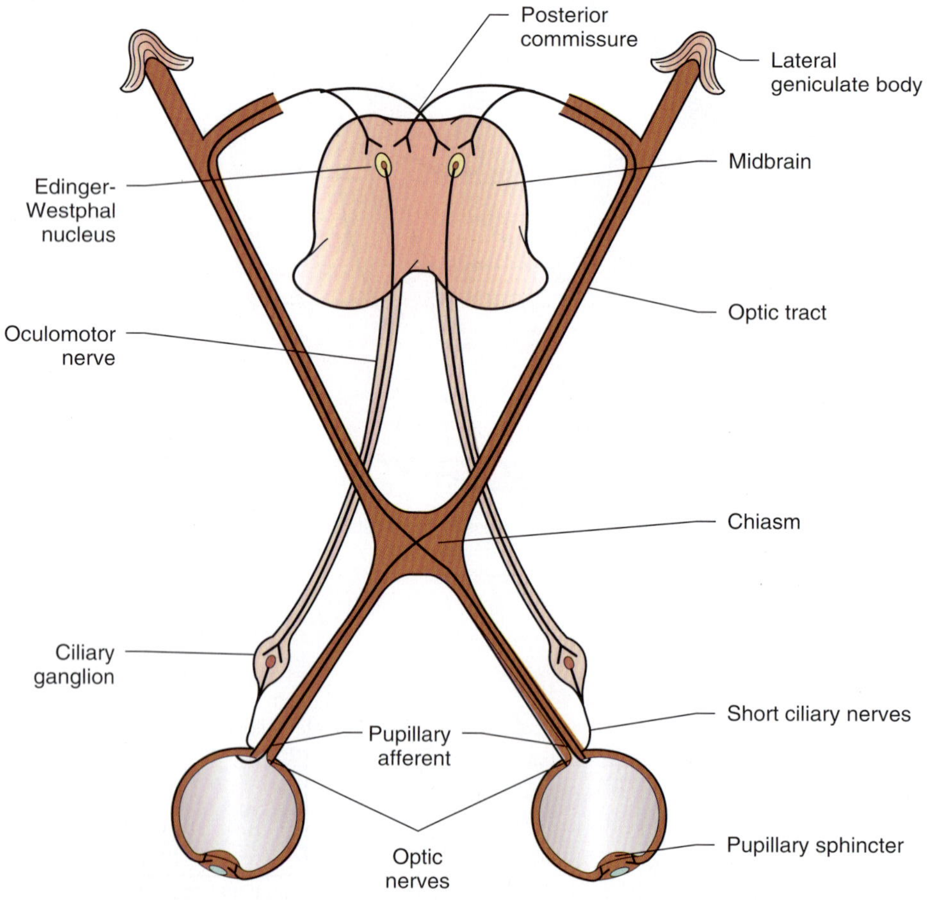

FIGURE 13.10 Pupillary afferent fibers from the right eye are crossed and uncrossed and run in both optic tracts. They leave the tract before the LGB and send projections to the pretectal region bilaterally. The Edinger-Westphal nucleus sends pupillomotor fibers through the third cranial nerve to the ciliary ganglion, and postganglionic fibers innervate the pupil sphincter. Because of the bilaterality of the pathways, a light stimulus in the right eye causes pupillary constriction in both eyes.

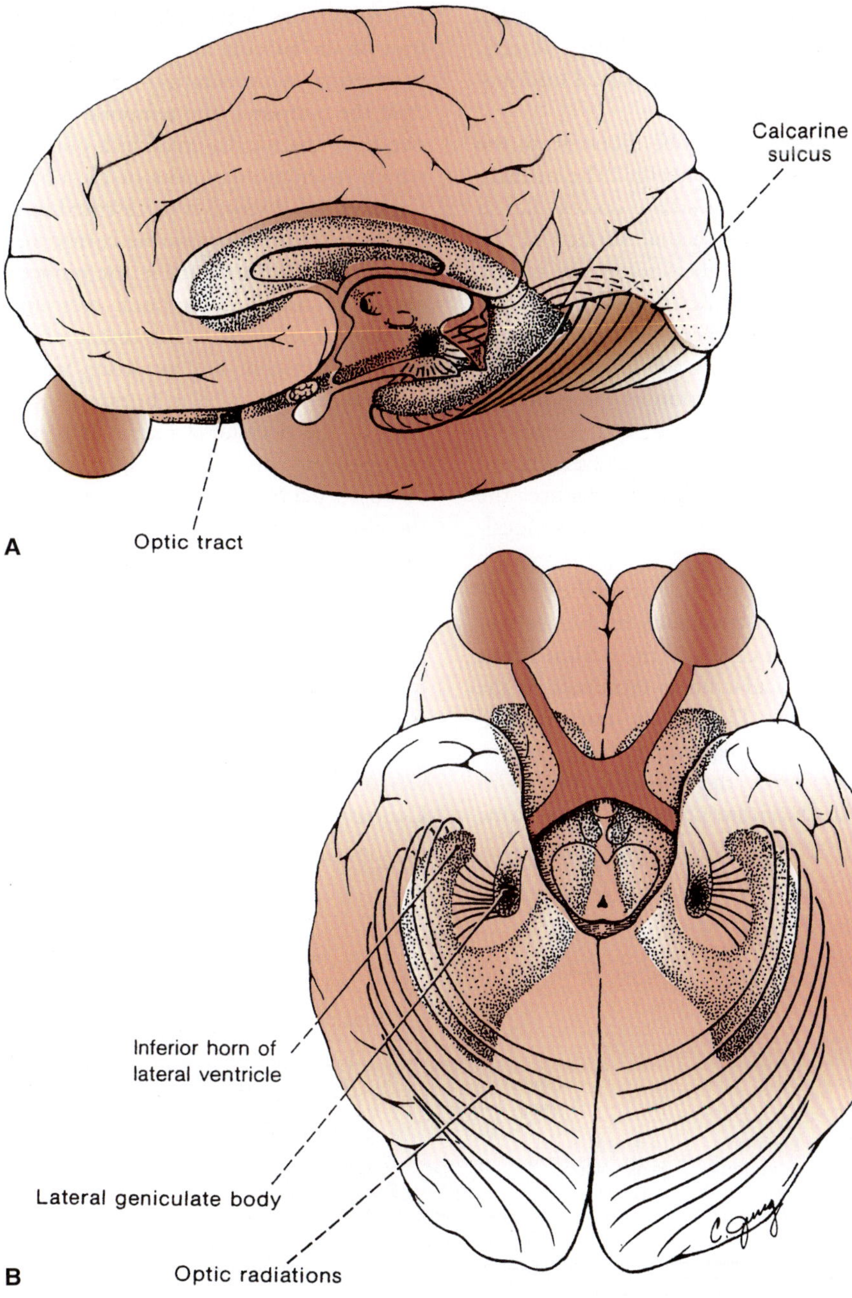

FIGURE 13.11 The course of the geniculocalcarine fibers. **A.** Medial view. **B.** Inferior view.

fibers a lower, position in the radiations, with fibers subserving central vision intermediate between the two other bundles. Inferior retinal fibers arch anteriorly into the temporal lobe, sweeping forward and laterally above the inferior horn of the ventricle to run within 5 to 7 cm of the temporal tip, then laterally, down, and backward around the inferior horn. This creates a great arching shape referred to as Meyer's loop (loop of Meyer and Archambault). The inferior retinal fibers then course through the temporal and occipital lobes. Peripheral retinal fibers loop further forward than macular fibers. Fibers from the superior retina run directly back in the deep parietal lobe in the external sagittal stratum, lateral to the posterior horn of the lateral ventricle. The inferior, or ventral, radiations may mediate recognition of visual objects, whereas the dorsal pathway processes spatial information and recognition of movement.

Approaching the occipital lobe, fibers from the upper and lower retina again converge. The primary visual cortex (calcarine area or striate cortex) lies in Brodmann's area 17 on the medial surface of the occipital lobe. Lower retinal fibers terminate on the lower lip of the calcarine fissure (lingual gyrus) and upper retinal fibers on the upper lip of the calcarine fissure (cuneus). Macular fibers are first lateral and then form the intermediate portion of the geniculocalcarine pathway, continuing to the posterior pole of the occipital lobe. The divergence and convergence of fibers throughout the visual pathway influences the shape and congruity of VF defects, which have localizing value.

Fibers that carry visual impulses from the peripheral portions of the retina terminate on the anterior third or half of the visual cortex of the occipital lobe in concentric zones; macular fibers terminate in the posterior portion (Figure 13.12). The most peripheral parts of the retina are represented most anteriorly in the calcarine cortex; the closer a retinal point lies to the macula, the more posterior its calcarine representation. This culminates in the representation of the macula at the occipital pole. The nasal hemiretina representation extends farther forward than the temporal (the temporal field is more extensive than the nasal), creating a portion of retina for which no homology exits in the opposite eye. This unpaired nasal retina is represented in the most anterior portion of the calcarine cortex, near the area of the tentorium, just outside the binocular VF, which creates an isolated temporal crescent in each VF. Sparing or selective involvement of this monocular temporal crescent has localizing value. The macula has a wider cortical distribution in the striate cortex than in the peripheral retina. It is represented in a wedge-shaped area with its apex anterior. The central 10 to 15 degrees of the VF occupy 50% to 60% of the visual cortex.

To summarize the retinotopic organization of the visual system, upper retinal fibers remain upper and lower fibers lower throughout except in the tract and LGB where upper becomes medial and lower becomes lateral. The corresponding VF abnormalities can be deduced.

The striate cortex is the sensory visual cortex. It receives afferents via the myelinated stripe or line of Gennari, because of the abundant myelinated fibers

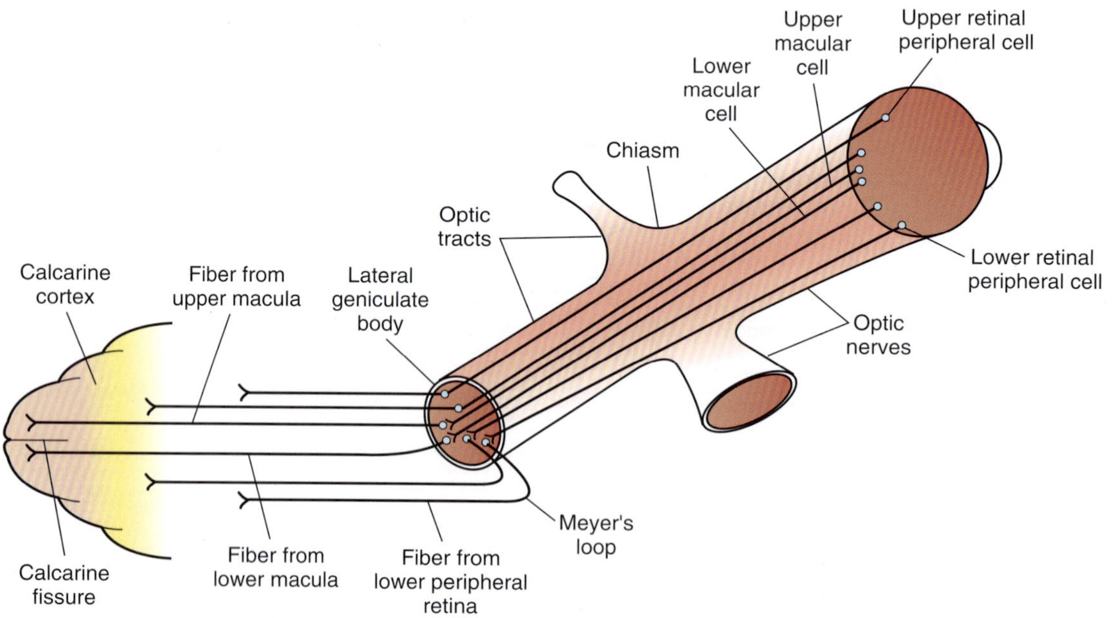

FIGURE 13.12 Fibers from the macula synapse in the geniculate and then project to the occipital tip. The most peripherally located retinal ganglion cells synapse in the geniculate and then loop far forward in Meyer's loop before terminating in the most anterior portion of the calcarine cortex. The most anterior and medial portions of the cortex receive projections from the monocular temporal crescent, which represents the nasal portion of the retina that extends far forward and is the most peripheral part of the retina.

in the fourth layer of the calcarine cortex, which gives this area its distinctive appearance and name. Its physiology is complex. Neurons are arranged in parallel, vertically oriented, ocular dominance columns and complex units called hypercolumns. One hypercolumn can process information from a focal region of the VF. There may be interhemispheric connections through the corpus callosum to synchronize information generated from the two sides. Surrounding the striate cortex are the visual association areas. Area 18, the parastriate or parareceptive cortex, receives and interprets impulses from area 17. Area 19, the peristriate or perireceptive cortex, has connections with areas 17 and 18 and with other portions of the cortex. It functions in more complex visual recognition, perception, revisualization, visual association, size and shape discrimination, color vision, and spatial orientation.

The anterior choroidal artery from the internal carotid and thalamoperforators from the posterior cerebral supply the optic tract. The geniculate is perfused by the anterior choroidal and thalamogeniculate branches from the posterior cerebral. Perhaps because of this redundant blood supply, vascular disease only rarely affects the optic tract or lateral geniculate. Meyer's loop receives blood supply primarily from the inferior division of the middle cerebral artery, whereas the optic radiations in the parietal lobe are perfused via the superior division. The occipital lobe is supplied primarily by the posterior cerebral artery. Collaterals from the anterior and middle cerebral may provide additional perfusion to the macular areas at the occipital tip. The parietal smooth pursuit optomotor center and its projections are supplied by the middle cerebral.

Optic Reflexes

Fibers subserving the pupillary light reflex and other optic reflexes pass through the pregeniculate pathways in the same fashion as fibers subserving vision. They leave the optic tract just before it reaches the LGB. Pupillary light reflex fibers travel to the pretectal nuclei, just rostral to the superior colliculus; from the pretectum, axons are sent to synapse on the Edinger-Westphal nuclei. Some light reflex fibers project to the ipsilateral pretectal nucleus to mediate the direct light reflex; others decussate through the posterior commissure to mediate the consensual light reflex (Figures 13.8 and 13.10). Parasympathetic fibers from the Edinger-Westphal nuclei are carried by the oculomotor nerve to the pupillary sphincter.

Fibers controlling somatic visual reflexes, such as turning of the head and eyes toward a visual stimulus, synapse in the superior colliculus. From there tectospinal tract fibers descend to more caudal brainstem nuclei to execute the reflex response. The internal corticotectal tract is made up of fibers that run from areas 18 and 19 of the occipital cortex to the superior colliculus to subserve reflex reactions through connections with the eye muscle nuclei and other structures. Fibers that carry impulses having to do with visual-palpebral reflexes (such as blinking in response to light) go to the facial nuclei.

CLINICAL EXAMINATION AND DISORDERS OF FUNCTION

Optic nerve function is tested by examining the various modalities of vision: the visual acuity, the VFs, and special components of vision, such as color vision and day and night vision. The optic nerve is the one cranial nerve that can be visualized directly, and no neurologic, or indeed general, physical examination is complete without an ophthalmoscopic inspection of the optic disk and the retina.

Before performing the optic nerve examination, look for local ocular abnormalities such as conjunctival irritation, corneal scarring or opacity, foreign bodies, photophobia, or an ocular prosthesis. The presence of a unilateral arcus senilis with ipsilateral carotid disease has been reported. In Wilson's disease (hepatolenticular degeneration), a yellowish-orange brown coloration 1 to 3 mm wide (Kayser-Fleischer ring) may be seen around the rim of the cornea, more easily in light-eyed individuals (Chapter 30). It is due to copper deposition in the posterior stroma and in Descemet's membrane and best seen with a slit lamp. Cataracts may be present in patients with myotonic dystrophy, certain rare hereditary conditions with disturbed lipid or amino acid metabolism, and in many other conditions. Lisch nodules are pigmented iris hamartomas that are highly suggestive of NF1 (Figure 13.13). Proptosis, chemosis, and tortuous ("corkscrew") blood vessels in the conjunctiva occur with carotid cavernous fistula (Chapter 21). Other causes of unilateral proptosis include thyroid eye disease, meningocele, encephalocele, and histiocytosis X. Other potentially relevant findings might include jaundice, evidence of iritis, dysmorphic changes (e.g., epicanthal folds), xanthelasma due to hypercholesterolemia, corneal clouding from

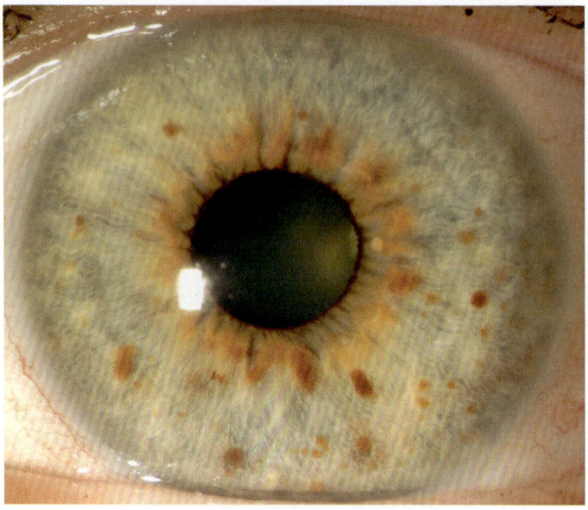

FIGURE 13.13 Lisch nodules are elevated, pale brown lesions that vary in appearance depending on the underlying color of the iris. The prevalence in patients with NF1 increases from birth to about 50% of 5-year-olds, 75% of 15-year-olds, and 95% to 100% of adults over the age of 30. (Reprinted from Gerstenblith AT, Rabinowitz MP. *The Wills Eye Manual: Office and Emergency Room Diagnosis and Treatment of Eye Disease*. 6th ed. Philadelphia: Wolters Kluwer Health/Lippincott Williams & Wilkins, 2012, with permission.)

mucopolysaccharidosis, keratoconjunctivitis sicca due to Sjögren's syndrome or other collagen vascular diseases, ocular complications of upper facial paralysis, depositions of amyloid in the conjunctiva, pigmented pingueculae due to Gaucher's disease, tortuous conjunctival vessels in ataxia telangiectasia, scleritis in Wegener's granulomatosis, lens dislocation in Marfan's syndrome, homocystinuria or Ehlers-Danlos syndrome, and nonsyphilitic interstitial keratitis in Cogan's syndrome. Hypertelorism can be seen in a number of neurologic conditions. Blue sclera can occur in Ehlers-Danlos syndrome, osteogenesis imperfecta, and occasionally in Marfan's syndrome. Basal skull fractures often cause bilateral periorbital ecchymosis (raccoon eyes).

Visual Acuity

Ideally, the eyes are examined individually. When testing acuity and color vision, it is important to occlude the eye not being tested. Visual acuity is a measure of the eye's ability to resolve details; it depends on several functions. The intensity threshold reflects the sensitivity of the retina to light; the minimum visibility is the smallest area that can be perceived, and the minimum separability is the ability to recognize the separateness of two close points or lines. Visual acuity charts, such as the Snellen chart for distance and the near card for near, consist of letters, numbers, or figures that get progressively smaller and can be read at distances from 10 to 200 ft by normal individuals (Figure 13.14). Snellen charts have certain limitations, the most critical is the nonlinear variation in the sizes of the letters from line to line, and the Early Treatment in Diabetic Retinopathy Study (ETDRS) charts have become increasingly popular.

The difference between near and distance vision and between vision with and without correction are points of primarily ophthalmologic interest. For

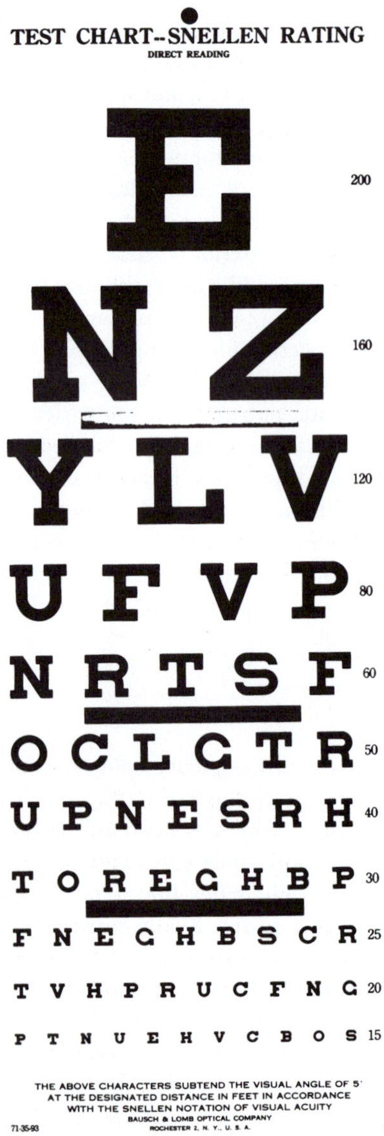

FIGURE 13.14 Snellen test chart.

neurologic purposes, only the patient's best-corrected visual acuity is pertinent. Near acuity is not as accurate as distant, especially if the card is not held at the required 14 in. Refractive errors, media opacities, and similar optometric problems are irrelevant. Acuity is always measured using the patient's accustomed correction. Ophthalmologists and neuro-ophthalmologists often employ more detailed methods (e.g., full refraction) to clarify the refractive component of a patient's visual impairment. In infants and children, acuity can be estimated by blink to threat or bright light, following movements, and the pupillary reactions. At the age of 4 months, acuity may be 20/400; it gradually increases, reaching normal levels at about age 5.

For distance vision measurement in the United States, a Snellen chart or similar is placed 20 ft from the patient; at that distance, there is relaxation of accommodation, and the light rays are nearly parallel. The eyes are tested separately, and by convention, the right eye is tested first. In countries using the metric system, the distance is usually given as 6 m. The ability to resolve test characters (optotypes) approximately 1-in high at 20 ft is normal (20/20 or 6/6) visual acuity. These characters subtend 5 minutes of visual arc at the eye; the components of the characters (e.g., the crossbar on the A) subtend 1 minute of arc. The acuity is the line where more than half of the characters are accurately read. If the patient can read the 20/30 line and two characters on the 20/25 line, the notation is 20/30 + 2. Two mistakes or two extra letters are allowed per line. By conventional notation, the distance from the test chart, 20 or 6, is the numerator, and the distance at which the smallest type read by the patient should be seen by a person with normal acuity is the denominator. An acuity of 20/40 (6/12) means the individual must move in to 20 ft to read letters a normal person can read at 40 ft. This does not mean the patient's acuity is one-half of normal. In fact, an individual with a distance acuity of 20/40 has only a 16.4% loss of vision.

Because few neurology clinics, offices, or hospital rooms have 20-ft eye lanes, testing is commonly done at a closer distance. Neurologists frequently assess vision with a near card. Though examination of distance vision is preferable, the requisite devices are generally not at hand. There are pocket cards designed for testing at 6 ft, a convenient distance that usually eliminates the need for presbyopic correction. Near vision is tested with a near card, such as the Rosenbaum pocket vision screening card, held at the near point (14 in or 35.5 cm). Jaeger reading cards are still used occasionally (Box 13.1). Good lighting is essential. A penlight shone directly on the line being read is useful for bedside testing.

BOX 13.1

Jaeger Notation

Jaeger's test types are ordinary printer's types, graded from fine (Jaeger 0) to coarse, also used for near testing. The physical optics of the Jaeger system are crude. The numbers refer to the boxes in the Austrian print shop from which Jaeger selected the type in 1854. Jaeger 0 corresponds approximately to an acuity of 20/20. As a rough approximation of near vision, the examiner may use different sizes of ordinary print. Newspaper want-ad text is approximately J-0, regular newsprint J-6, and newspaper headlines J-17.

If the patient cannot read the 20/200 line at 20 ft, the distance may be shortened and the fraction adjusted. Ability to read the line at 5 ft is vision of 5/200, equivalent to 20/800. Vision worse than the measurable 20/800 is described as count fingers (CFs), hand motion (HM), light perception (LP), or no light perception (NLP). The average finger is approximately the same size as the 20/200 character, so ability to count fingers at 5 ft is equivalent to an acuity of 20/800.

When a patient has impaired vision, an attempt should be made to exclude refractive error by any available means. If the patient has corrective lenses, they should be worn. In the absence of correction, improvement of vision by looking through a pinhole suggests impairment related to a refractive error. Commercial multi-pinhole devices are available. A substitute can be made by making three or four holes with a pin in a 3 × 5 card in a circle about the size of a quarter. The multiple pinholes help the patient locate one. The patient should then attempt to read further down the acuity card through the pinhole. The pinhole permits only central light rays to enter the eye. These are less likely to be disrupted by refractive errors such as presbyopia and astigmatism. If a pinhole was used, make some notation, such as 20/20 (ph). If the visual impairment is due to a neurologic process, such as optic neuritis (ON), vision will not improve with a pinhole. Under some circumstances, such as with opacities in the media (e.g., cataract), vision may get worse with pinhole.

Other ocular causes of reduced visual acuity include a macular lesion, media opacity such as cataract or vitreous hemorrhage, and corneal opacities or irregularities. Neurologic processes that affect the optic nerve or chiasm may cause impaired acuity. Retrochiasmal lesions affect visual acuity only if they are bilateral. Suspected functional visual loss because of conversion disorder or malingering is best evaluated by an ophthalmologist, who has the proper tools to answer the question. Clever and determined patients with functional visual loss present a major challenge. There may be certain clues (Box 13.2).

The term amblyopia refers to impaired vision because of an organic process in the absence of a demonstrable lesion. The mechanism is poorly understood. Suppression amblyopia is the visual impairment in one eye because of preferential use of the opposite eye in a patient with congenital strabismus. Suppression amblyopia is also referred to as amblyopia ex anopsia (amblyopia from disuse). Many other varieties of amblyopia have been described, including alcoholic, toxic, traumatic, and uremic amblyopia. Amaurosis means blindness of any type, but in general usage, it means blindness without primary eye disease or loss of vision secondary to disease of the optic nerve or brain.

Color Vision; Day and Night Vision

Color blindness (achromatopsia) is an X-linked condition present in about 3% to 4% of males. The most common hereditary dyschromatopsia is an X-linked red-green defect. Disturbances of color vision may also occur in neurologic conditions. Loss of color vision may precede other visual deficits. Color deficits may be partial or total. Color plates or pseudoisochromatic plates (Ishihara, Hardy-Ritter-Rand [HRR], or similar) formally and quantitatively assess color vision. Pseudoisochromatic plates were originally designed to screen for congenital dyschromatopsias. The HRR plates, which contain blue and purple figures that screen for tritan defects, may be more helpful in detecting acquired dyschromatopsia because of some optic neuropathies. Having the patient identify the colors in a fabric, such as a tie or a dress, can provide a crude estimate of color vision.

Acquired dyschromatopsia may result from macular, retinal, optic nerve, chiasmal, or retrochiasmal lesions. Monocular loss of acuity, deficits in color vision, and an afferent pupillary defect (APD) are highly characteristic of an ipsilateral optic neuropathy. Acquired optic nerve diseases usually cause a red/green color deficiency, but there are several exceptions, such as glaucoma and dominant optic atrophy. Impaired color vision with only mildly reduced acuity is suggestive of optic neuropathy; color deficits associated with more severe acuity loss suggest maculopathy.

Fading or bleaching of colors is a real but uncommon complaint in optic nerve disease. Red perception is usually lost first. Desaturation to red, or red washout, describes a graying down or loss of

BOX 13.2

Nonorganic (Functional) Visual Loss

A truly blind person can sign his name without difficulty. A functionally blind patient often cannot. A truly blind person asked to look at his hand will look wherever proprioception tells him his hand should be; a functionally blind person may gaze in any direction and perhaps never where the hand actually is (Schmidt-Rimpler test). A truly blind person can touch his forefingers together without difficulty; a functionally blind person may make half-hearted inaccurate thrusts. The presence of normal visual, menace, fixation, and emergency light reflexes (see Chapter 16) excludes organic blindness. A functionally blind person ignorant of the laws of reflection may have much improved vision reading the image of an acuity chart held to his chest in a mirror 10 ft away compared to reading the actual chart at 20 ft; the acuity in fact should be the same. Some patients with functional blindness can suppress optokinetic nystagmus (OKN) responses and the visual evoked response (VER). An excellent test is to have the patient look into a large mirror that can be held and moved. Tilting and moving the mirror will elicit OKN responses because the entire visual environment is moving. The patient cannot suppress or "blur out" by willfully failing to fixate on a single target, as he may be able to do with OKN or VER.

intensity of red. The bright red cap on a bottle of mydriatic drops is a common test object. The patient compares the brightness or redness in right versus left hemifields, temporal versus nasal hemifields, or central versus peripheral fields. No right/left or temporal/nasal desaturation to red occurs normally. Red does normally look brighter in the center of the VF than off center; reversal of this pattern suggests impairment of central vision. The normal red appears washed out, or changes to pink to orange to yellow to colorless as color perception is lost. Because optic neuropathies affect macular fibers, patients lose the ability to read pseudoisochromatic plates. The flight of colors phenomenon is the series of color perceptions that follows shining a bright light into the eye. With impaired color vision, the flight of colors may be reduced or absent. Patients may also compare the brightness or intensity of an examining light in one eye versus the other. A diminution of brightness on one side suggests optic nerve dysfunction; it is sometimes referred to as a subjective APD, relative APD, or Marcus-Gunn pupil. Its significance is the same as for red desaturation. The APD is discussed in more detail in Chapter 14.

Day blindness (hemeralopia) is a condition in which vision is better in dim lighting than in bright. It occurs in various conditions causing a central scotoma, in early cataracts; it is a rare side effect of trimethadione. Night blindness (nyctalopia) is much poorer vision in feeble illumination than occurs normally. It is common in retinitis pigmentosa and can occur in chronic alcoholism, Leber's hereditary optic neuropathy (LHON), and xerophthalmia due to vitamin A deficiency.

The Visual Fields

The VF examination is a very important and, unfortunately, often omitted part of the neurologic examination. The VF is the limit of peripheral vision, the area in which an object can be seen while the eye remains fixed. Macular vision is sharp. Peripheral images are not as distinct, and objects are more visible if they are moving. The normal VF extends to 90 to 100 degrees temporally, about 60 degrees nasally, 50 to 60 degrees superiorly, and 60 to 75 degrees inferiorly. The field is wider in the inferior and temporal quadrants than in the superior and nasal quadrants (Figure 13.15). There are individual variations in the field of vision, dependent to some extent on the facial configuration, the shape of the orbit, the position of the eye in the orbit, the width of the palpebral fissure, and the amount of brow projection or the size of the nose. However, these changes are seldom clinically relevant. With binocular vision, the VFs of the two eyes overlap except for the unpaired temporal crescent extending from 60 to 90 degrees on the horizontal meridian, which is seen by one eye only. The monocular temporal crescent exists because of the anatomy of the retina. The nasal retina extends

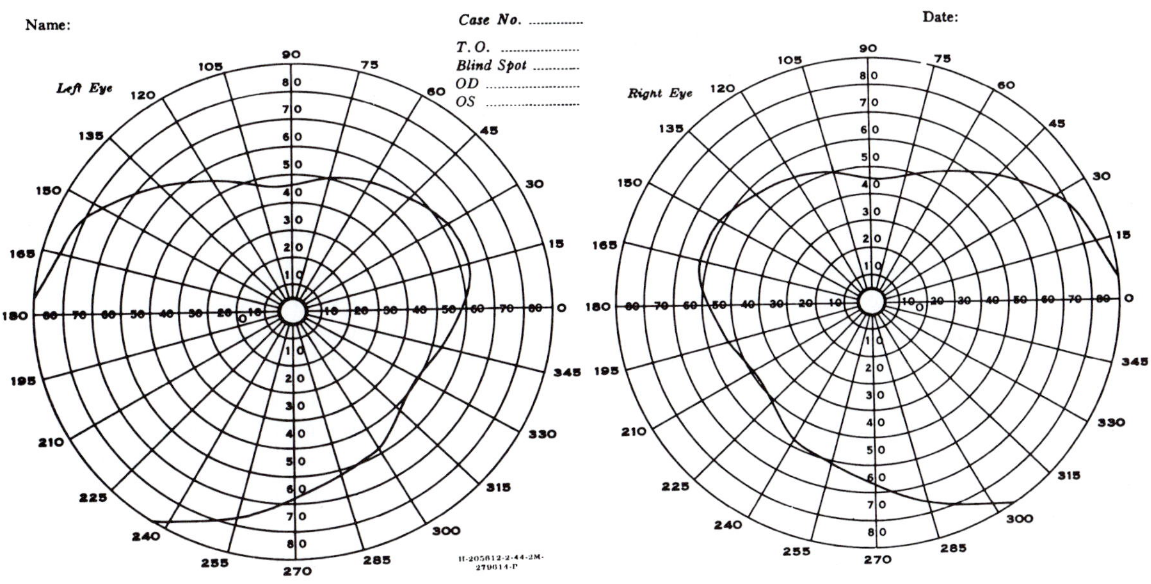

FIGURE 13.15 The normal VFs.

farther forward, more peripherally, than the temporal. This is the true reason that the temporal VF is more expansive, not because the nose is blocking the nasal field.

VF examination results are most accurate in an individual who is alert and cooperative and will maintain fixation. Wandering of the eye impairs the evaluation. Crude assessment is possible even in uncooperative patients if the target is interesting enough (e.g., food or paper money). Fatigue and weakness may lengthen the latency between perception of the test object and the response to it, giving a false impression of VF deficit. Close cooperation, good fixation, and adequate illumination are essential for mapping of the blind spot and delineation of scotomas.

Clinicians use several different methods for VF evaluation. The time and energy expended on bedside confrontation testing depends on the patient's history and on the facilities available for formal field testing with tangent (Bjerrum) screen (central 30 degrees) or perimetry (entire field). Even sophisticated confrontation testing cannot approach the accuracy of formal fields.

The confrontation VF exam can be tailored to the circumstances and done as superficially or as thoroughly as the situation requires. Sophisticated bedside techniques can explore the VFs in detail if circumstances warrant. If the patient has no specific visual complaint, and if other aspects of the history and examination do not suggest a field defect is likely, then a screening exam is appropriate. This can be accomplished rapidly and with great sensitivity using small amplitude finger movements in the far periphery of the VF. Recall that the VFs extend temporally to 90+ degrees. Extending elbows and index fingers, the examiner should position the fingers nearly directly lateral to the lateral canthus at a distance of about 24 in. Superficially, this appears to be a binocular examination, but, properly placed, the finger targets are actually in the unpaired monocular temporal crescent part of the VF. With the targets positioned, make a small amplitude flexion movement with the tip of one index finger, perhaps 2 cm in amplitude. Have the patient "point to the finger that moves." This language is more efficient than attempting a right-left verbal description where the patient's and examiner's rights and lefts are reversed. Stimuli should be delivered in each upper quadrant individually, then both together, and then similarly for the lower quadrants. Including bilateral simultaneous stimuli is necessary to detect subtle defects, which may be manifested only by extinction of one stimulus on double simultaneous stimulation. This technique of small finger movements in the far periphery in both upper and lower quadrants is an excellent screen; when properly done, even binocularly, this technique misses few VF defects. Large amplitude finger wiggles near the center are insensitive. Always bear in mind that primary ophthalmologic disorders such as glaucoma, diabetic retinopathy, and retinal detachment can also alter the VFs.

With any hint of abnormality, or if the patient has or could be expected to have a visual problem, higher-level testing is in order. Examining monocularly, techniques include having the patient assess the brightness and clarity of the examiner's hands as they are held in the right and left hemifields, in both upper and lower quadrants, or having the patient count fingers fleetingly presented in various parts of the field. Because of the over-representation of central vision in the CNS, assessing each quadrant within the central 10 to 20 degrees is important.

More exacting techniques compare the patient's field dimensions with the examiner's, using various targets—still or moving fingers, the head of a cotton swab, colored pinheads, or similar objects. Impairment of color perception also occurs with lesions of the posterior visual pathways. Loss of VF to testing with a red object may be apparent even when the fields are intact to a white object. Positioning the patient and examiner at the same eye level, and gazing eyeball to eyeball over an 18- to 24-in span, targets introduced midway between and brought into the VF along various meridians should appear to both people simultaneously in all parts of the field except temporally, where the examiner must simply develop a feel for the extent of a normal field (Figure 13.16). Even in expert hands, confrontation fields are relatively gross and more precision required perimetry.

For obtunded, uncooperative, or aphasic patients, paper money (the larger the denomination the better) makes a compelling target. Even if the examiner has only a $1 bill, suggest to the patient that it might be $100. The patient who can see will glance at or reach for the object. Children may respond to keys (no jingling), candy, or other visually interesting objects. Infants may turn the head and eyes toward a diffuse light within a few days after birth. Moving a penlight into the VF and noting when the patient blinks is sometimes useful. Checking for blink to threat—the menace reflex—provides a crude last resort method. The examiner's hand or fingers are brought in rapidly from the side, as if to strike the patient or poke

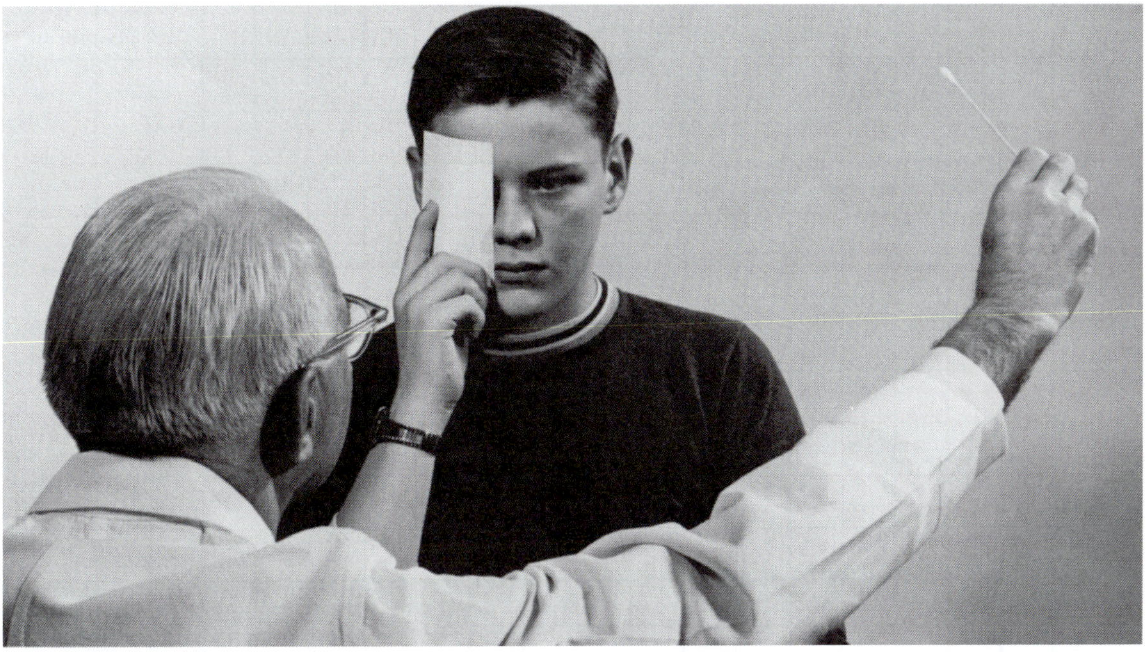

FIGURE 13.16 Confrontation method of testing the VFs.

him in the eye. The patient may wince, drawback, or blink. The threatening movement should be deliberate enough to avoid stimulating the cornea with an induced air current.

Testing central fields can include having the patient gaze at the examiner's face and report any defects, such as a missing or blurred nose. Having the patient survey a grid work (Amsler grid, graph paper, or a quickly sketched homemade version) while fixing on a central point is a sensitive method to detect scotomas (Figure 13.17). Probing the central field with a small white or red object may detect moderate or large scotomas. With a cooperative patient, one can estimate the size of the blind spot. Amsler grid testing is helpful in detecting central and paracentral scotomas. Small deficits suggest macular disease and may be missed on perimetry.

Pandit et al. compared the sensitivity of seven confrontation VF examining methods in patients whose formal fields showed small or shallow defects. The most sensitive method was examining the central VF with a 5-mm red target; the next most sensitive was comparing red color intensity. These together had a sensitivity of 76%. Description of the examiner's face and quadrant finger counting were the least sensitive. All of the confrontation methods had high specificity. In a similar study, Kerr et al. compared seven common confrontation VF tests to Humphrey VF in 301 eyes in patients recruited from a neuro-ophthalmology clinic, and therefore at high risk for having a VF defect. Anterior visual pathway lesions accounted for 78% of the defects, and of these, glaucoma was the underlying cause in 81%; how applicable the findings are to a general neurologic practice is debatable. Most confrontation tests were relatively insensitive. All tests were more sensitive for posterior than anterior lesions. Although very commonly done, finger counting had a sensitivity of only 35%, but a specificity of 100%. The most sensitive single test was red comparison. Testing with a kinetic red target had the highest combined sensitivity and specificity of any individual test. The combination of kinetic testing with a red target combined with static finger wiggle was the best combination, with a sensitivity of 78% while retaining a specificity of 90%. The combination was significantly better than any single test. Description of the examiner's face and finger counting, while simple tests, had low sensitivity and negative predictive values; it was recommended these tests not be used in isolation to exclude VF loss.

By convention, VFs are depicted as seen by the patient (i.e., right eye drawn on the right). This convention is backward from most things in clinical medicine, and violations of the rule occur sufficiently often that labeling notations are prudent. When confrontation fields are not adequate for the

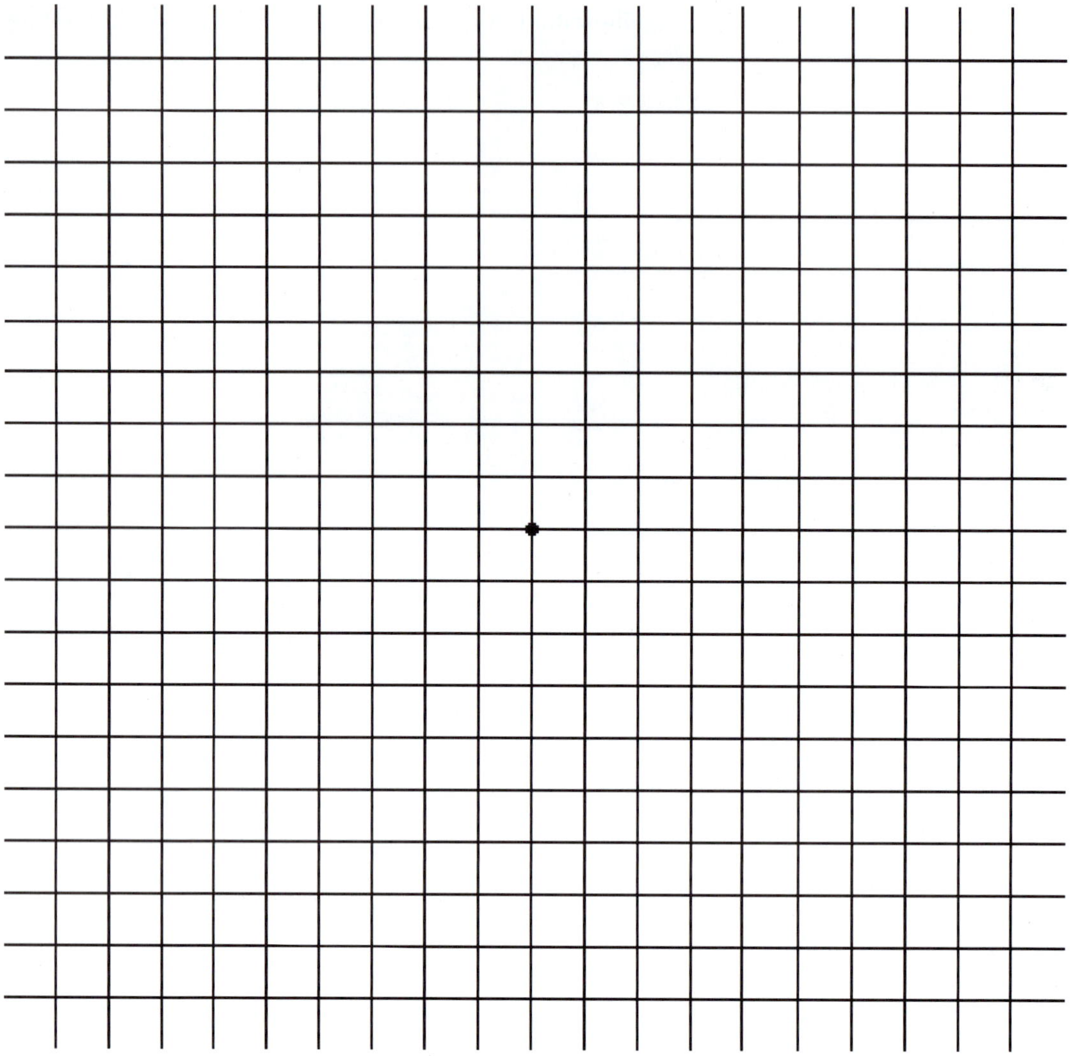

FIGURE 13.17 The Amsler grid for testing the central VFs. (1) Test vision with one eye at a time, and use normal glasses for reading. (2) Hold chart at normal reading distance. (3) Stare at *central dot* and look for distortion or blind spots in the grid.

clinical circumstances, formal fields are done. These might include tangent screen examination, kinetic perimetry, or computerized automated static perimetry (Box 13.3).

Visual Field Abnormalities

For neurologic purposes, VF abnormalities can be divided into scotomas, hemianopias, altitudinal defects, and concentric constriction or contraction of the fields. Figure 13.19 depicts some examples of different types of field defects. Because of the anatomy and organization of the visual system, neurologic disorders tend to produce straight-edged defects that respect either the horizontal or vertical meridian or have a characteristic shape because of the arrangement of the NFL. Respect of the horizontal meridian may occur because of the horizontal temporal raphe and the arching sweep of NFL axons above and below the macula. This pattern is characteristic of optic nerve, optic disk, and NFL lesions. The vascular supply of the retina consists of superior and inferior branches of the central retinal artery, which supply the upper and lower retina, respectively. Vascular disease characteristically causes altitudinal field defects that are sharply demarcated horizontally. The calcarine cortex is organized into a superior and an inferior bank, and lesions involving only one bank may produce

BOX 13.3

Formal Visual Field Testing

Perimetry is the measurement of the visual field (VF) on a curved surface. Campimetry is the measurement of the VF on a flat surface. The tangent screen is the standard method for performing campimetry. For tangent screen examination, a black screen, blackboard, or other flat surface is used to examine the central 30 degrees of vision. The central fields can be evaluated more accurately with the tangent screen, the peripheral fields more accurately with perimetry. The patient is seated 1 to 2 m from the tangent screen; objects of various sizes and colors are brought into view using a black wand that blends into the background. Testing is now often done with a laser pointer. The test object is the only thing of visual interest against the black background. As with perimetry, the notation numerator is the test object size and the denominator the distance from the screen, often followed by a letter to indicate the target color. A field notation of 2/1,000 r indicates the field was done with a 2-mm red test object, and the patient was seated 1 m away from the screen. The tangent screen is especially valuable for measuring the size of the physiologic blind spot and for demonstrating central defects. Defects may be easier to detect when the VF is done at 2 m, because the dimensions of the field and the dimensions of the defect are doubled. The Amsler grid is another sensitive method for testing the central 10 degrees of the VF (Figure 13.17).

A perimeter is useful for testing the peripheral VFs, which cannot be done by tangent screen. Many different types of perimeters and perimetric techniques have been described. Perimetry may be kinetic or static. Kinetic perimetry entails moving a test object along various meridians and noting when it is detected. For standard kinetic perimetry (e.g., Goldmann), the patient gazes at a fixation point and various test objects are brought into the field of vision through multiple meridians in a hemispheric dome. White and colored test objects varying in size from 1 to 5 mm are used. The points at which a target of given size and color is first seen are recorded, and a line is drawn joining these points to outline the VF. The line representing the limits of the field for a given size and color test object is called an isopter. The smaller the test object, the smaller the VF. Mapping isopters for test objects of varying sizes and colors creates an image resembling a topographic map. Perimetric readings are expressed in fractions; the numerator indicates the target size and the denominator the distance away from the patient in millimeters. If the size of a VF defect is the same with all test objects, it is said to have steep, or abrupt, margins. If the defect is larger with smaller test objects, its margins are said to be gradual, or sloping, in character.

Limits of the VF vary according to the size, color, and brightness of the test object, the intensity of illumination, the state of adaptation of the eye, and the cooperation of the patient. The VF for a colored test object is smaller than the VF for a white object of the same size. The size of the VF is different for different colors. Changes in color fields precede gross field changes (color desaturation). Altered responses to color may help differentiate between retinal lesions and neurologic conditions. Formal fields provide permanent objective documentation of the VFs. They may be repeated periodically to look for progression or improvement.

The Goldmann perimeter uses a kinetic paradigm. Modern quantitative automated perimetry uses static perimeters, and automated perimetry has largely replaced manual perimetry. Static perimetry measures the threshold for perception of various targets at various locations in the VF with the aid of a computer and statistical analysis. The Humphrey Visual Field Analyzer is in widespread use in the United States. Statistical analysis of the VF data allows determination of the probability that a VF is normal. Automated perimetry is very sensitive for detecting VF defects. However, normal patients may appear to have an abnormal VF because of the large number of erroneous responses that can occur during automated testing. The instruments include reliability indices determined by the false-positive and false-negative responses (Figure 13.18).

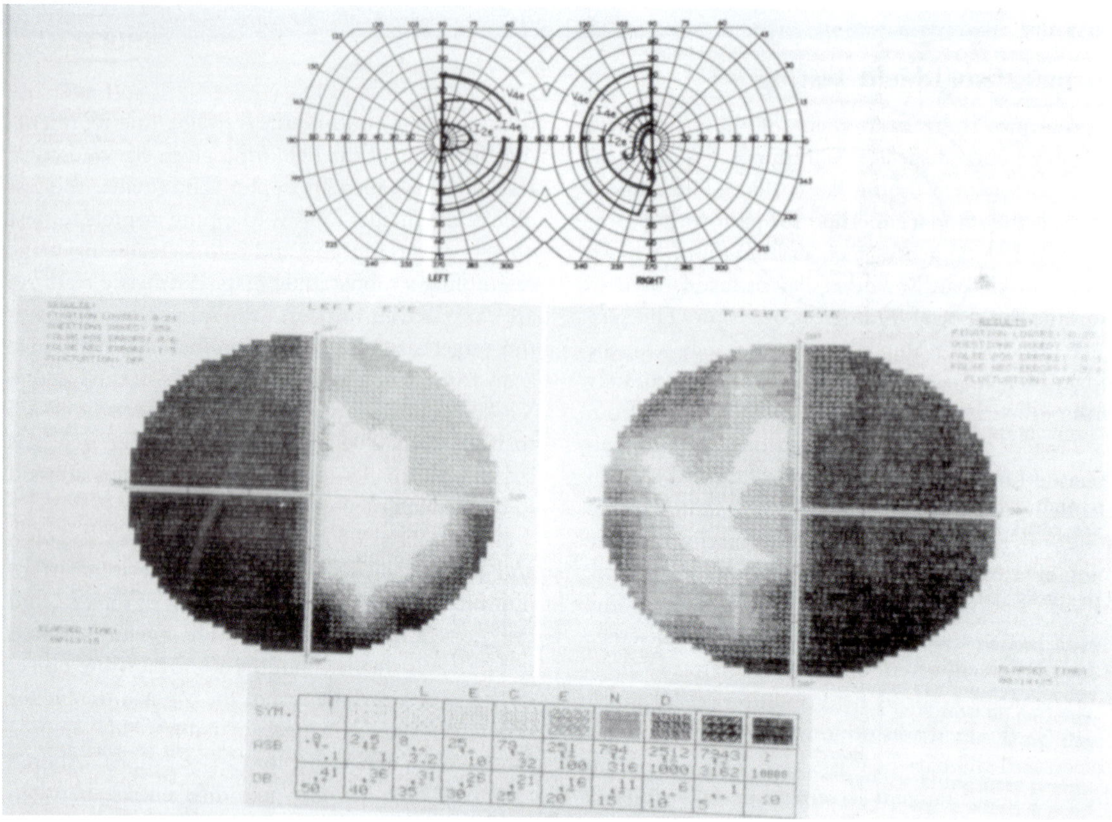

FIGURE 13.18 **Top.** VF performed on a Goldmann perimeter in a patient with a chiasmal lesion. **Bottom.** Humphrey perimeter field in the same patient. (Reprinted from Beck RW, Bergstrom TJ, Lichter PR. A clinical comparison of visual field testing with a new automated perimeter, the Humphrey Field Analyzer, and the Goldmann perimeter. *Ophthalmology* 1985;92[1]:77–82. Copyright © 1985 American Academy of Ophthalmology, Inc. With permission.)

VF defects that respect the horizontal meridian. The vertical meridian is respected because of the division into nasal and temporal hemiretinas that occurs at the chiasmal decussation and is maintained through the retrochiasmal visual pathways.

Scotomas

A scotoma (Gr. "darkness") is an area of impaired vision in the field, with normal surrounding vision. With an absolute scotoma, there is no visual function within the scotoma to testing with all sizes and colors of objects. With a relative scotoma, visual function is depressed but not absent; smaller objects and colored objects are more likely to detect the abnormality. A positive scotoma causes blackness or a sense of blockage of vision, as though an object were interposed; it suggests disease of the retina, especially the macula or choroid. Positive scotomas are often due to exudate or hemorrhage involving the retina or opacity in the media. A negative scotoma is an absence of vision, a blank spot as if part of the field had been erased; it suggests optic nerve disease but can occur with lesions more posteriorly. With a negative scotoma, the defect may not be perceived until a VF examination is done.

A scotoma can often be demonstrated on confrontation VF testing using small objects and carefully exploring the central fields, but they are best demonstrated by the use of the tangent screen. The physiologic blind spot (Mariotte's spot) is a scotoma corresponding to the optic nerve head, which contains no rods or cones and is blind to all visual impressions. The physiologic blind spot is situated 15 degrees lateral to and just below the center of fixation because the disk lies nasal to the macula and the blind spot is projected into the temporal field. Elliptical in shape, it averages 7 to 7½ degrees vertically and 5 to 5½ degrees horizontally and extends 2 degrees above and 5 degrees below the horizontal meridian. On a tangent screen with the patient 1 m away using a 1-mm white object, the average measurements for the blind spot are from 9 to 12 cm horizontally and 15 to 18 cm vertically. The blind spot is enlarged in papilledema and ON.

Scotomas are described by their location or their shape. A central scotoma involves the fixation point and is seen in macular or optic nerve disease. It is typical for ON but can occur in vascular and compressive lesions (Figure 13.19A). A paracentral scotoma involves the areas adjacent to the fixation point, and it has the same implications as for a central scotoma. A cecocentral scotoma extends from the blind spot to fixation. It is usually accompanied by loss of all central vision with preservation of a small amount of peripheral vision, and it strongly suggests optic nerve disease (Figures 13.19B and 13.20). Central, paracentral, and cecocentral scotomas are all suggestive of a process involving the PMB. Any scotoma involving the blind spot implies optic neuropathy.

An arcuate scotoma is a crescent defect arching out of the blind spot, usually because of optic neuropathy with the brunt of damage falling on the fibers forming the superior and inferior NFL arcades. A nasal step defect is a scotoma that involves the nasal part of the VF away from fixation, usually respecting the horizontal meridian, which is due to optic neuropathy and often progresses to become a broad arcuate scotoma. Nasal step defects are common, especially in optic neuropathy because of glaucoma. A junctional scotoma is an optic nerve defect in one eye (central, paracentral, or cecocentral scotoma) and a superior temporal defect in the opposite eye (syndrome of Traquair). This is due to a lesion (usually a mass) that involves one optic nerve close to the chiasm, which damages the inferior nasal fibers from the opposite eye (Wilbrand's knee) as they loop forward into the proximal optic nerve on the side of the lesion (Figures 13.9 and 13.19C). The temporal VF defect in the contralateral eye may be subtle and easily missed. The anatomic evidence supporting the existence of Wilbrand's knee has been questioned, but clinical cases continue to suggest it exists. No junctional scotoma could be detected in three patients whose optic nerves were surgically divided at the optic nerve-chiasm junction.

Although scotomas most often result from disease of the retina or optic nerve, they may also be caused by cerebral lesions. Occipital pole lesions primarily affecting the macular area can produce contralateral homonymous hemianopic scotomas (Figure 13.19D). Because the bulk of fibers in the chiasm come from the macula, early compression may preferentially affect central vision producing bitemporal heteronymous paracentral scotomas (Figure 13.19E); with progression of the lesion, a full blown bitemporal hemianopia will appear (Figure 13.19G). Optic nerve lesions such as glioma and drusen (hyaline excrescences that may be buried in or on the surface of the nerve) may cause scotomas, contraction of the VFs, or sector defects. Enlargement of the physiologic blind spot is referred to as a peripapillary scotoma.

Other types of scotomas occur from primary ocular disease, such as retinitis, chorioretinitis, and glaucoma, which are not related directly to disease of the nervous system (Box 13.4).

Subjective scotomas cannot be delineated in the field examination. Subjective scotomas include the scintillating scotomas, or teichopsias, of migraine, and the annoying but harmless vitreous floaters that many normal individuals experience.

Hemianopia

Hemianopia is impaired vision in half the VF of each eye; hemianopic defects do not cross the vertical meridian. Hemianopias may be homonymous or heteronymous. A homonymous hemianopia causes impaired vision in corresponding halves of each eye (e.g., a right homonymous hemianopia is a defect in the right half of each eye). Homonymous hemianopias are caused by lesions posterior to the optic chiasm, with interruption of the fibers from the temporal half of the ipsilateral retina and the nasal half of the contralateral retina. Vision is lost in the ipsilateral nasal field and the contralateral temporal field (Figure 13.21). A heteronymous hemianopia is impaired vision in opposite halves of each eye (e.g., the right half in one eye and the left half in the other). Unilateral homonymous hemianopias, even those with macular splitting, do not affect visual acuity. Patients can read normally with the preserved half of the macula, but those with left-sided hemianopias may have trouble finding the line to be read. Occasionally, patients with homonymous hemianopia will read only half of the line on the acuity chart.

A homonymous hemianopia may be complete or incomplete. If incomplete, it may be congruous or incongruous. A congruous hemianopia shows similar-shaped defects in each eye (Figure 13.19H). The closer the optic radiations get to the occipital lobe, the closer lie corresponding visual fibers from the two eyes. The more congruous the field defect, the more posterior the lesion is likely to be. An incongruous hemianopia is differently shaped defects in the two eyes

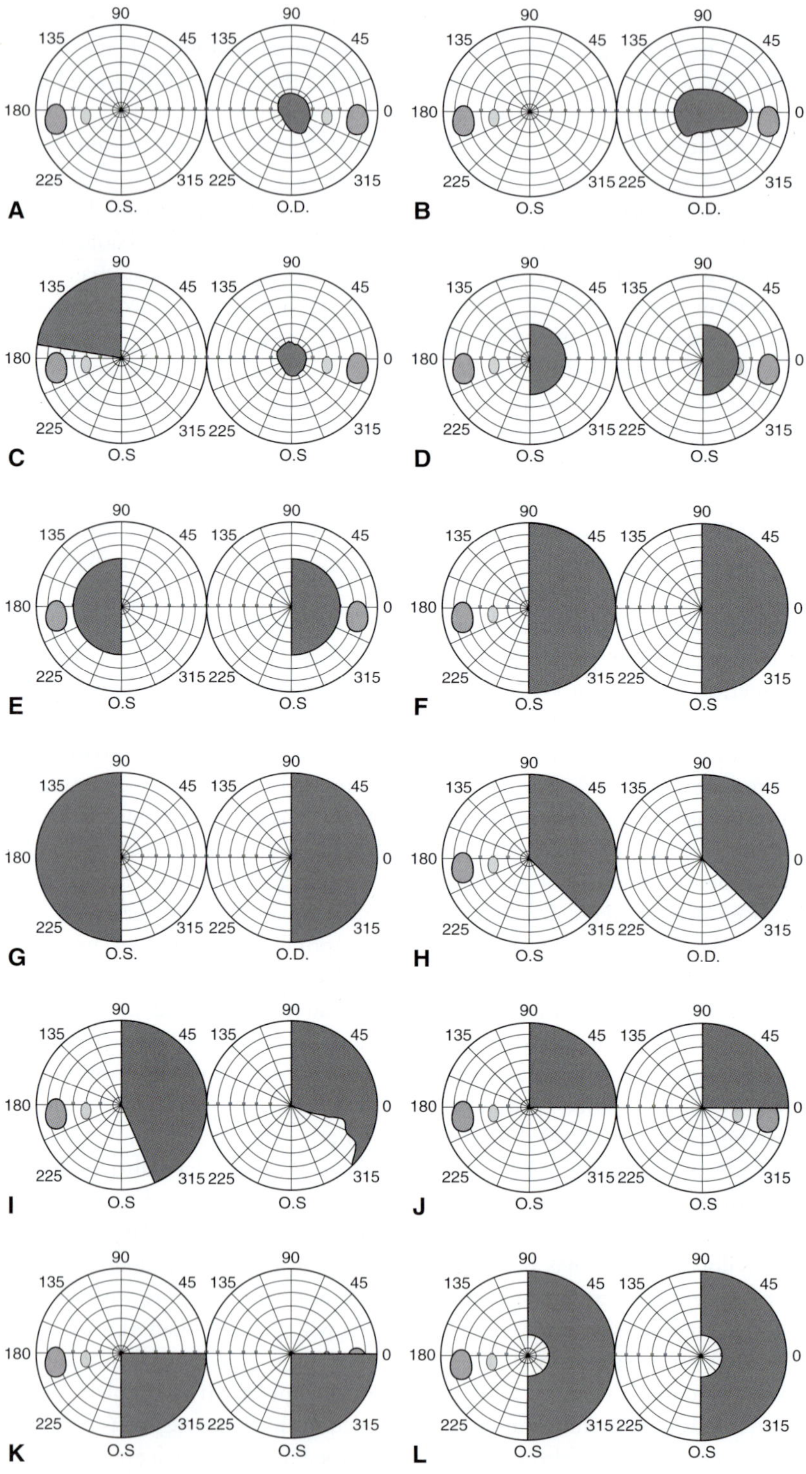

FIGURE 13.19 Types of VF defects. **A.** Central scotoma. **B.** Cecocentral scotoma. **C.** Junctional scotoma. **D.** Homonymous scotomas. **E.** Heteronymous scotomas. **F.** Right homonymous hemianopia. **G.** Bitemporal hemianopia. **H.** Congruous right homonymous hemianopia. **I.** Incongruous right homonymous hemianopia. **J.** Right superior quadrantanopia ("pie in the sky"). **K.** Right inferior quadrantanopia. **L.** Macular-sparing right homonymous hemianopia.

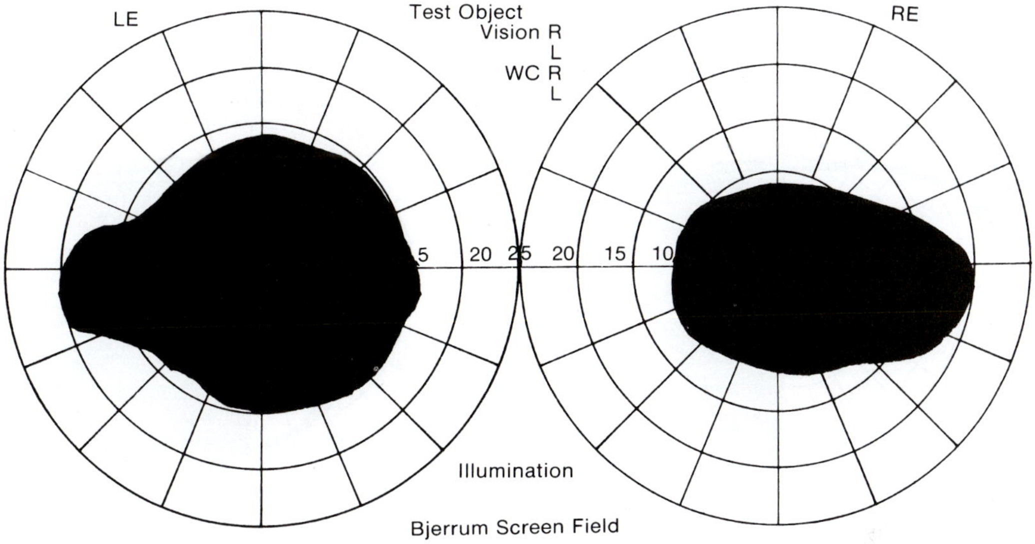

FIGURE 13.20 Bilateral cecocentral scotomas in a patient with bilateral optic neuritis.

(Figure 13.19I). The more incongruous the defect, the more anterior the lesion. The most incongruous hemianopias occur with optic tract and lateral geniculate lesions. With a complete hemianopia, congruity cannot be assessed; the only localization possible is to identify the lesion as contralateral and retrochiasmal. A superior quadrantanopia implies a lesion in the temporal lobe affecting Meyer's loop (inferior retinal fibers): "pie in the sky" (Figure 13.19J). Such a defect may occur after temporal lobe epilepsy surgery because of damage to the anteriorly looping fibers. An inferior quadrantanopia ("pie on the floor") implies a parietal lobe lesion affecting superior retinal fibers (Figure 13.19K). A macular-sparing hemianopia is one that spares the area immediately around fixation; it implies an occipital lobe lesion (Figure 13.19L). The explanation for macular sparing remains unclear. There has been conjecture about dual representation of the macula in each occipital pole, but this has never been confirmed anatomically. More likely it is collateral blood supply from the anterior or middle cerebral artery, which protects the macular region from ischemia. Or it could simply be that the extensive cortical representation of the macula both at the occipital pole and anteriorly in the depths of the calcarine fissure makes it difficult for a single lesion to affect all macular function. A small amount of macular sparing may be due to fixation shifts during testing.

BOX 13.4

Other Types of Scotomas

Glaucoma may cause arcuate, cuneate, comma-shaped, or other partially ring-shaped scotomas. A Seidel scotoma arises from the blind spot and has a thin and well-demarcated arcuate tail, the shape resembling a comma. A Bjerrum scotoma is shaped like a bow, extending from the blind spot to near fixation. Both are common in glaucoma. Peripheral scotomas may be present anywhere in the field of vision. In annular, or ring, scotomas, there is a loss of vision in a doughnut shape with relative sparing of fixation and of the far periphery. These types of scotomas are typically due to retinitis pigmentosa, a condition primarily affecting the rods that are concentrated in the midzone of the retina. Ring scotomas also occur in optic neuropathy, macular lesions, cancer-associated retinopathy, choroiditis, and myopia. Many ophthalmologic conditions produce a global depression of retinal function and concentric constriction of the VF, rather than a discrete defect. Ophthalmoscopic examination generally reveals the nature of such conditions.

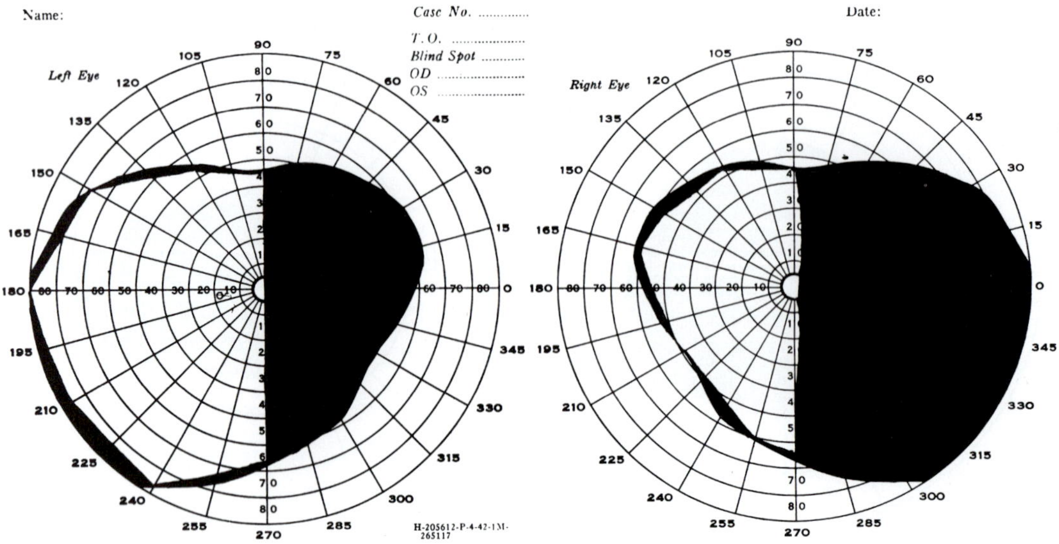

FIGURE 13.21 Macular-splitting right homonymous hemianopia in a patient with a neoplasm of the left occipital lobe.

Incomplete homonymous VF defects are common. These include partial or irregular defects in one or both of the hemifields, relative rather than absolute loss of vision, an inability to localize the visual stimulus, and hemianopia only for objects of a certain color (hemiachromatopsia). Extinction (visual inattention) is hemianopic suppression of the visual stimulus in the involved hemifield when bilateral simultaneous stimuli are delivered. Visual extinction is most characteristic of lesions involving the nondominant parietooccipital region. Riddoch's phenomenon is a dissociation between the perception of static and kinetic stimuli. The patient may not perceive a stationary object but detect it instantly when it moves.

Heteronymous hemianopias are usually bitemporal; only rarely are they binasal. A bitemporal hemianopia is usually due to chiasmatic disease, such as a pituitary tumor growing up out of the sella turcica and pressing on the underside of the chiasm (Figure 13.18). Bitemporal field defects can usually be detected earliest by demonstrating bitemporal desaturation to red. Because of the anterior inferior position of decussating inferior nasal fibers, lesions impinging from below produce upper temporal field defects, which evolve into a bitemporal hemianopia (Figure 13.6). Lesions encroaching from above tend to cause inferior temporal defects initially. The defect will be first and worst in the upper quadrants with infrachiasmatic masses (e.g., pituitary adenoma), and it will be first and worst in the lower quadrants with suprachiasmatic masses (e.g., craniopharyngioma). Patients with postfixed chiasms and pituitary tumors may present with optic nerve defects, and those with prefixed chiasms may have optic tract defects.

The most common cause of bitemporal hemianopia is a pituitary adenoma; occasionally, it results from other parasellar or suprasellar lesions such as meningioma and craniopharyngioma, as well as glioma of the optic chiasm, aneurysms, trauma, and hydrocephalus. Other VF defects that may simulate bitemporal hemianopia include tilted optic disks, bilateral cecocentral scotomas, and bilaterally enlarged blind spots. Binasal hemianopias may occur from disease impinging on the lateral aspect of the chiasm bilaterally (e.g., bilateral intracavernous carotid aneurysms), but they are more likely to be due to bilateral optic neuropathy.

An altitudinal VF defect is one involving the upper or lower half of vision, usually in one eye, and usually due to retinal vascular disease (central retinal artery or branch occlusion or anterior ischemic optic neuropathy [AION]). A partial altitudinal defect may approximate a quadrantanopia. Altitudinal defects do not cross the horizontal meridian.

Constriction of the VFs is characterized by a narrowing of the range of vision, which may affect one or all parts of the periphery. Constriction may be regular or irregular, concentric or eccentric, temporal or nasal, and upper or lower. Symmetric concentric contraction is most frequent and is characterized by a more or less even, progressive reduction in field diameter through all meridians. Such constriction is referred to as funnel vision, as opposed to tunnel vision (see below). Concentric constriction of the VFs may occur with optic atrophy, especially secondary to papilledema or late glaucoma, or with retinal disease, especially retinitis pigmentosa. Narrowing of the fields because of fatigue, poor attention, or inadequate illumination must be excluded, as must spurious contraction because of decreased visual acuity or delayed reaction time. Slight constriction of the VF may occur when there is a significant refractive error. Diffuse depression is the static perimeter equivalent of constriction on kinetic perimetry.

Concentric constriction of the fields is sometimes seen in conversion disorder. A suspicious finding is when the fields fail to enlarge as expected with testing at increasing distance (tubular or tunnel fields). Normally, the field of vision widens progressively as the test objects are held farther away from the eye. However, in nonorganicity, this normal widening is not seen, and the entire width of the field is as great at 1 ft from the eye as it is at 2, 5, 10, or 15 ft. The normal VF is a funnel; the nonorganic VF is a tunnel. The tubular field can be demonstrated either by testing the extent of the VF at varying distances from the patient, or it can be shown by using test objects of different sizes at a constant distance. Spiral contraction is a progressive narrowing of the VF during the process of testing. It may be a sign of nonorganicity, but it is probably more suggestive of fatigue. A similar pattern field is the star-shaped VF, where there is an irregularity of outline. This may be seen in nonorganicity, fatigue, or poor attention.

The Ophthalmoscopic Examination

The physician using a direct ophthalmoscope is like a one-eyed person peering into a dark room from the entryway with a flashlight. Only a narrow sector of the posterior pole is visible, and there is no stereopsis. Pupil dilation significantly increases the field of view. Indirect ophthalmoscopy, used by ophthalmologists, can stereoscopically view almost the entire vista of the fundus. PanOptic direct ophthalmoscopes (Welch-Allyn) give the advantage of a broader view but still reveal only the posterior pole. See Box 13.5 for a brief discussion of the techniques of direct ophthalmoscopy. It is important to become facile by practicing direct ophthalmoscopy on all patients, as the examination is inevitably most technically difficult in situations where fundus examination is most critical.

BOX 13.5

Direct Ophthalmoscopy

The standard direct ophthalmoscope has dials that adjust the light apertures and filters and allow the examiner to focus. The small aperture is for examining an undilated pupil, the large aperture for examining a dilated pupil. Using the small aperture may help minimize reflections from the cornea. The red-free filter is useful for examining blood vessels, looking for hemorrhages, and examining the nerve fiber layer (NFL). The red reflex can be assessed from a distance of 12 to 15 in. Opacities in the media (e.g., cataract) appear as black dots against the red background. The ocular fundus is the only place in the body where blood vessels can be visualized directly. Changes in the retinal vasculature in conditions such as diabetes and hypertension mirror the status of the systemic circulation. The fundus may also reveal important findings in systemic diseases such as endocarditis and AIDS.

In the neurologic examination, the areas of primary concern are the disk, the macula, and the arteries. The disk is normally round or a vertically oriented slight oval. The nasal margin is normally slightly blurred compared to the temporal. The disk consists of a peripheral neuroretinal rim and a central cup. The neuroretinal rim consists of axons streaming from the retina to enter the optic nerve. The physiologic cup is a slight depression in the center of the disk that is less pinkish than the rim and shows a faint latticework because of the underlying lamina cribrosa. The rim is elevated slightly above the cup. The cup normally occupies about a third of the temporal aspect of the disk. To locate the disk, a helpful technique is to find a retinal blood vessel, focus on it, and then follow it to the disk. In severe myopia, the disk may appear larger and paler than normal. In the aphakic eye, the disk looks small and far away.

The myelinated axons making up its substance render the normal optic disk yellowish-white. It is paler temporally where the papillomacular bundle (PMB) enters. The normal disk lies flat and well

(continued)

BOX 13.5

Direct Ophthalmoscopy *(Continued)*

demarcated against the surrounding retina, with arteries and veins crossing the margins and capillaries staining the surface a faint pink. The size of the scleral opening varies from individual to individual. When the opening is small, the disk consists entirely of neuroretinal tissue, and the cup is inconspicuous or nonexistent. Such a small cupless disk is more vulnerable to anterior ischemic optic neuropathy and is termed a disk at risk. The normal cup-to-disk ratio is about 0.1 to 0.5. In patients with glaucoma, the cup-to-disk ratio is increased and the cup is more prominent and often nasally displaced.

The central retinal artery enters the eye through the physiologic cup and divides into superior and inferior branches, which in turn divide into nasal and temporal branches, yielding four prominent arterial trunks emanating from the disk. Beyond the second branch, the retinal vessels are arterioles, visible because of the 14× magnification provided by the patient's lens and cornea. Cilioretinal arteries are present in many normal individuals. These vessels arise from posterior ciliary arteries, enter the eye along the disk margin, and perfuse the peripapillary retina. They may become prominent as shunt vessels when there is optic nerve compression. Varying amounts of pigmentation are present in the retina near the temporal border of the disk, especially in dark-skinned persons. At times a pigment ring may completely surround the disk. White scleral and dark choroidal rings may sometimes be seen.

The macula is a dark area that lies about two disk diameters temporal to and slightly below the disk. The macula appears darker than the surrounding retina because the depression of the macula and fovea means the retina is thinner in that area, allowing more of the deeply colored choroid to show through. The area of the macula is devoid of large blood vessels. The fovea centralis appears as a pinpoint of light reflected from the center of the macula. The macula may be seen more easily with a red-free filter. It is sometimes easier to visualize the macula if the patient looks directly into the light.

The routine fundus examination in neurologic patients is generally done through the undilated pupil. The fundus examination is more challenging when the patient has a small pupil, myopia, or opacities in the media such as cataract. One or more of these are commonly present in older individuals. In some circumstances, the benefits of an adequate fundus exam outweigh the minimal risk of precipitating an attack of acute narrow angle glaucoma by using mydriatic drops. A crude estimate of the narrowness of the iridocorneal angle can be made by shining a light from the temporal side to see if a shadow is cast on the nasal side of the iris and sclera. The risk of an attack of acute narrow-angle glaucoma because of the use of mydriatic drops has been estimated at 0.1%. Mydriatic drops are best avoided in situations where assessment of pupillary function is critical, such as patients with head injury or other causes of depressed consciousness. Their use in such situations must be obtrusively documented, even to the point of writing "eye drops in" on the patient's forehead.

LOCALIZATION AND DISORDERS OF VISUAL FUNCTION

Disorders of the afferent visual system can be divided into prechiasmal, chiasmal, and retrochiasmal. Disease in each of these locations has characteristic features that usually permit its localization. The etiologic processes affecting these different segments of the afferent visual system are quite different. As a generalization, prechiasmal lesions cause monocular visual loss; impaired color perception; a central, paracentral, or cecocentral VF defect; and an APD. The disk may or may not appear abnormal depending on the exact location of the lesion. Chiasmal lesions cause heteronymous VF defects, most often bitemporal hemianopia, with preservation of visual acuity and color perception and a normal appearing optic disk. Retrochiasmal lesions cause a contralateral homonymous hemianopia and have no effect on acuity or disk appearance. There is usually no effect on color vision, but some central lesions may cause achromatopsia. A summary of the features of disease involving the macula, optic nerve, chiasm, optic tract, LGB, optic radiations, and calcarine cortex can be found in Table 13.1.

TABLE 13.1 Clinical Characteristics of Acute Lesions Involving Different Parts of the Afferent Visual Pathway

	Visual Acuity	Color Vision	Visual Field Defect	Pupillary Function	Disk Appearance	Comment
Macula	Decr	Decr	Ipsilateral central scotoma	Possible mild APD	Normal	May have metamorphopsia; macula may be abnormal on ophthalmoscopy; common etiologies: age-related macular degeneration, central serous retinopathy, macular hole, cystoid macular edema, trauma, toxic retinopathy
Optic Nerve						
Papillopathy	Decr	Decr	Ipsilateral central, paracentral, or cecocentral scotoma	APD	Edema	With ON may have pain on eye movement; common etiologies: idiopathic ON, MS, AION, postviral, sarcoid, LHON, collagen vascular disease, neurosyphilis, diabetes, papillophlebitis
Retrobulbar neuropathy	Decr	Decr	Same as papillopathy	APD	Normal	May have proptosis; common etiologies: ON, MS, optic nerve compression, glioma, infiltrative lesions, trauma, sarcoid, toxins, collagen vascular disease, infection, posterior ischemic optic neuropathy
Distal optic nerve, near chiasm	Decr	Decr	Junctional scotoma	APD	Normal	May have evidence of a sellar/parasellar mass; common etiology: mass lesion
Chiasm	Normal	Normal	Bitemporal hemianopia	Normal	Normal	May develop bow-tie atrophy; APD can occur in eye with greatest VF loss; common etiologies: tumor (e.g., pituitary adenoma, suprasellar meningioma), demyelination, trauma, radionecrosis, aneurysm, ischemia, chiasmal glioma, sarcoid, optochiasmatic arachnoiditis
Optic tract	Normal	Normal	Contralateral incongruous homonymous hemianopia	Mild APD in contralateral eye	Normal	May be involved with disease involving the posterior chiasm; common etiologies: demyelinating disease, trauma, mass lesion, stroke
Lateral geniculate body	Normal	Normal	Contralateral incongruous homonymous hemianopia	Normal	Normal	Common etiologies: ischemia, trauma, mass lesion
Optic Radiations						
Temporal lobe	Normal	Normal	Contralateral superior quadrantanopia	Normal	Normal	May have visual hallucinations in the affected hemifield; common etiologies: tumor, stroke, hematoma, trauma, mass lesion
Parietal lobe	Normal	Normal	Contralateral inferior quadrantanopia	Normal	Normal	May have asymmetric OKN; patient may be unaware of the deficit, especially with nondominant hemisphere lesions; common etiologies: tumor, stroke, trauma, hematoma
Calcarine cortex	Normal	Normal	Contralateral congruous homonymous hemianopia	Normal	Normal	Macula sparing frequent; common etiologies: stroke, trauma, tumor, demyelinating disease

AION, anterior ischemic optic neuropathy; APD, afferent, papillary defect; decr, decreased; LHON, Leber hereditary optic neuropathy; MS, multiple sclerosis; OKN, optokinetic nystagmus; ON, optic neuritis.

Prechiasmal Lesions

Prechiasmal disorders affect the optic nerve. Disorders can be divided into those that affect the disk (papillopathy) and those that affect the retrobulbar segment between the globe and the chiasm. The macula gives rise to the majority of the fibers in the optic nerve, and disease of the macula itself can cause a clinical picture that is at times difficult to distinguish from optic neuropathy. Common causes of maculopathy include age-related macular degeneration and central serous retinopathy (Table 13.1). Macular disease causes marked impairment of central acuity and impaired color vision. There may be a central scotoma. A distinct central scotoma with normal field between the central defect and the blind spot is more common in macular than in optic nerve disease. Macular disease often causes metamorphopsia, a distortion of visual images. When severe, maculopathy can cause an APD. Prolongation of the time to recover vision after direct, intense light stimulation (photostress test) can sometimes help to distinguish macular from optic nerve disease (Box 13.6). Other retinal lesions severe enough to cause monocular VF defects are almost all visible ophthalmoscopically.

A macular star is a radial pattern of exudates in the perimacular retina. They are common in hypertension, papilledema, and in other conditions. Neuroretinitis refers to the association of ON with a macular star and is commonly of viral origin. Chorioretinitis is inflammation involving choroid and retina, which is most often due to infections such as tuberculosis, syphilis, toxoplasmosis, cytomegalovirus, and HIV. Chorioretinitis often leaves whitish scars surrounded by clumps of pigment. Cytomegalovirus chorioretinitis is common in AIDS.

Monocular altitudinal defects are characteristic of disease in the distribution of the central retinal artery. Central vision may be spared because the macula is often perfused by the cilioretinal arteries. AION (see below) is another cause of an altitudinal defect. Bilateral altitudinal defects may occur with bilateral lesions in certain parts of the visual pathway, for example, bilateral occipital infarction or a large prechiasmal lesion compressing both optic nerves. A checkerboard pattern is a superior altitudinal defect in one eye and an inferior altitudinal defect in the other eye.

BOX 13.6

The Photostress Test

In macular disease, the photoreceptors require longer to recover from bleaching of the retinal pigments after exposure to a bright light. The photostress test is done by determining a baseline visual acuity, then shining a bright light (e.g., a fresh penlight) into the eye for 10 seconds, and then determining the time required for the visual acuity to return to baseline. Reliable reference values are not available; the test is mainly useful with unilateral disease when the unaffected eye can be used for comparison. In optic nerve disease, the photostress test is normal. Recovery times may reach several minutes in macular disorders such as macular edema, central serous retinopathy, and macular degeneration.

Disorders of the Optic Disk

The color and appearance of the disk may change in a variety of circumstances. The disk may change color—to abnormally pale in optic atrophy or to abnormally red with disk edema. The margins may become obscured because of disk edema or the presence of anomalies. Edema of the disk is nonspecific. It may reflect increased intracranial pressure, or it may occur because of optic nerve inflammation, ischemia, or other local processes. By convention, disk swelling because of increased intracranial pressure is referred to as papilledema; under all other circumstances, the noncommittal terms disk edema or disk swelling are preferred. Visual function provides a critical clue to the nature of disk abnormalities. Patients with acute papilledema and those with disk anomalies have normal visual acuity, VFs, and color perception. Impairment of these functions is the rule in patients suffering from optic neuropathies of any etiology. The first step in evaluating a questionably abnormal disk is therefore a careful assessment of vision.

Papilledema

Increased intracranial pressure exerts pressure on the optic nerves, which impairs axoplasmic flow and produces axonal edema and an increased volume of axoplasm at the disk. The swollen axons impair venous return from the retina, engorging first the capillaries on the disk surface, then the retinal veins, and ultimately causing splinter- and flame-shaped hemorrhages as well as cotton wool exudates in the retinal NFL. Further axonal swelling eventually leads to elevation of the disk above the retinal surface. Transient visual obscurations, momentary graying out or blacking out of vision, often precipitated by postural changes, are classical symptoms of papilledema, especially in pseudotumor cerebri (idiopathic intracranial hypertension [IIH]). Obscurations may be due to microvascular compromise at the nerve head.

The four stages of papilledema are early, fully developed, chronic, and atrophic. Fully developed papilledema is obvious, with elevation of the disk surface, humping of vessels crossing the disk margin, obliteration of disk margins, peripapillary hemorrhages, cotton wool exudates, engorged and tortuous retinal veins, and marked disk hyperemia. The recognition of early papilledema is much more problematic (Figure 13.22). Occasionally, the only way to resolve the question of early papilledema is by serial observation. The earliest change is loss of previously observed spontaneous venous pulsations (SVPs). Venous pulsations are best seen where the large veins dive into the disk centrally. The movement is a back-and-forth rhythmic oscillation of the tip of the blood column, which resembles a slowly darting snake's tongue. Side-to-side expansion of a vein is much more difficult to see. The presence of SVPs indicates an intracranial pressure less than approximately 200 mm H_2O. However, because they are absent in 10% to 20% of normals, only the disappearance of previously observed SVPs is clearly pathologic.

As papilledema develops, increased venous back pressure dilates the capillaries on the disk surface, transforming its normal yellowish-pink color to fiery red. Blurring of the superior and inferior margins evolves soon after. However, because these margins are normally the least distinct areas of the disk, blurry margins alone are not enough to diagnose papilledema. There is no alteration of the physiologic cup with early papilledema. With further evolution, the patient with early papilledema will develop diffuse disk edema, cup obscuration, hemorrhages, exudates, and venous engorgement. Frank disk elevation then ensues as the fundus ripens into fully developed papilledema (Figure 13.23). In chronic papilledema, hemorrhages and exudates resolve and leave a markedly swollen "champagne cork" disk bulging up from the plane of the retina. If unrelieved, impaired axoplasmic flow eventually leads to death of axons and visual impairment, which evolves into the stage of atrophic papilledema, or secondary optic atrophy. Papilledema ordinarily develops over days to weeks. With acutely increased intracranial pressure because of subarachnoid or intracranial hemorrhage, it may develop within hours. Measuring diopters of disk elevation ophthalmoscopically has little utility.

The changes in the optic nerve head in papilledema are both mechanical and vascular in nature. The mechanical signs of disk edema include blurring of the disk margins, filling in of the physiologic cup, protrusion of the nerve head, edema of the NFL and retinal or choroidal folds, or both. The vascular signs include venous congestion, hyperemia of the nerve head, papillary and peripapillary hemorrhages, NFL infarcts (cotton-wool spots), and hard exudates of the optic disk.

Acute papilledema causes no impairment of visual acuity or color vision. The typical patient has

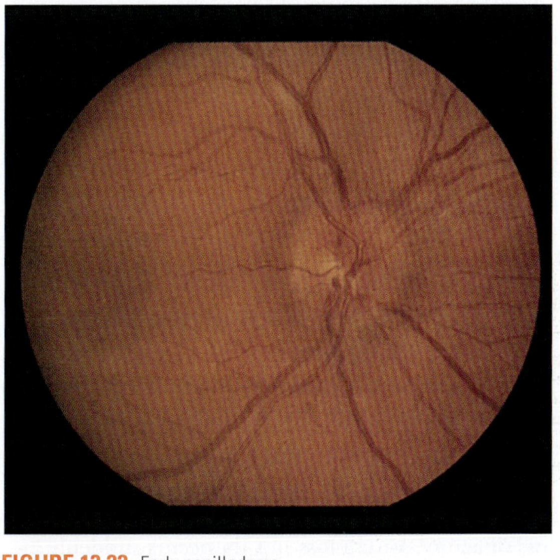

FIGURE 13.22 Early papilledema.

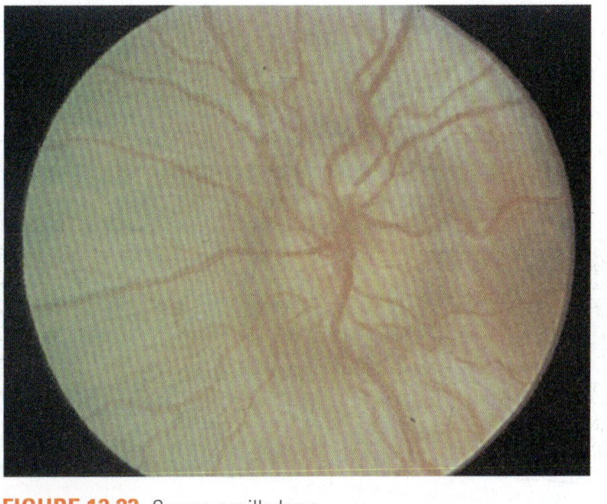

FIGURE 13.23 Severe papilledema.

no symptoms related to its presence except for obscurations. The blind spot may be enlarged, but VF testing is otherwise normal. In patients who develop optic atrophy following papilledema, the visual morbidity can be severe and may include blindness.

With current technology, imaging has usually detected intracranial mass lesions before the development of increased intracranial pressure. As a result, IIH is the most common cause of papilledema in the developed world. IIH can occur without papilledema, or with asymmetric papilledema, rarely with unilateral papilledema. The typical patient with IIH is an obese, young female with headaches, no focal findings on neurologic examination, normal imaging except for small ventricles, and normal CSF except for elevated opening pressure. Without adequate treatment, visual loss is a common sequel.

Other Causes of Disk Edema

Changes ophthalmoscopically indistinguishable from papilledema occur when conditions primarily affecting the optic nerve papilla cause disk edema. Papilledema is usually bilateral; other causes of disk edema are often unilateral (Table 13.2). Optic neuropathies generally cause marked visual impairment, including loss of acuity, central or cecocentral scotoma, loss of color perception, and an APD. Disease of the optic nerve head is usually due to demyelination, ischemia, inflammation, or compression. ON and AION are two common conditions that cause impaired vision and disk edema. Both are usually unilateral. Compressive lesions of the optic nerve in the orbit may cause disk edema, but intracanalicular and intracranial compression usually does not. ON with disk edema is sometimes called papillitis. Papillitis may occur as an isolated abnormality, as a manifestation of multiple sclerosis (MS), or as a complication of some systemic illness. Demyelinating optic neuropathies causing papillopathy are common as a feature of MS, but they also can occur as an independent disease process or complicate other disorders such as acute disseminated encephalomyelitis and neuromyelitis optica (NMO), which includes Devic's disease. There are many other causes of optic neuropathy; some of the more common conditions are listed in Table 13.3.

TABLE 13.2 Some Causes of Unilateral Disk Edema

Optic neuritis
Anterior ischemic optic neuropathy
Compression of the optic nerve in the orbit
Central retinal vein occlusion
Optic nerve infiltration
Diabetic papillopathy
Syphilis
Leber's hereditary optic neuropathy (LHON)

TABLE 13.3 Some Causes of Optic Neuropathy

Optic neuritis
Ischemic optic neuropathy
Optic nerve compression
Papillophlebitis
Optic nerve infiltration (carcinomatous, lymphomatous)
Sarcoidosis
Diabetic papillopathy
Tobacco-alcohol amblyopia
Nutritional deficiency, especially vitamin B_{12}
Drugs
Toxins
Hereditary optic neuropathy (Leber, Kjer)
Glaucoma

Optic Neuritis

Inflammation or demyelination of the optic nerve can occur in a variety of conditions, including MS, postviral syndromes, sarcoidosis, collagen vascular disease, neurosyphilis, and others. Many cases are idiopathic. The majority of patients are women in the 20 to 50 age range. ON occurs sometime during the course of MS in 70% of patients and is the presenting feature in 25%. Some 50% to 70% of patients presenting with ON eventually develop other evidence of MS. Factors that increase the likelihood of underlying MS in patients with ON include the presence of Uhthoff's phenomenon (increased symptoms with elevation of body temperature or after exercise), HLA-DR2 positivity, and a recurrent episode. Decreased acuity, impaired color perception, central or cecocentral scotoma, disk edema, and an APD are the typical findings. For a video of an APD, see **Video Link 13.1** (from Kathleen B. Digre, MD at the University of Utah Neuro-Ophthalmology Virtual Education Library: NOVEL). Color vision loss usually parallels acuity loss, but in ON, the loss of color vision may be more severe than expected for the loss of acuity. Visual loss in ON occurs suddenly and tends to progress over 1 to 2 weeks, with substantial recovery over 2 to 12 weeks. Severe visual loss acutely does not necessarily portend poor recovery. Eye pain is present in 90% of patients, and many have positive visual phenomena with colors or flashing lights (photopsias, phosphenes). The eye pain is usually mild but can become severe and more debilitating than the visual loss. The pain may precede or begin concomitantly with the visual loss and is usually worsened with eye movement, particularly upgaze. The absence of pain suggests a noninflammatory type of optic neuropathy. In about 65% of cases of ON, the disk appears normal; in the remainder, there is mild disk edema and occasional NFL hemorrhages. Pain can occur whether or not there is disk edema. Optic atrophy ensues over the next several weeks in 50% of patients. Improvement to normal or near normal acuity occurs in 90% of patients. ON may rarely involve the chiasm (chiasmal neuritis).

In NMO, there are lesions of the optic nerves and the spinal cord. It is a distinct entity from MS, but separating the two clinically may be difficult. The spinal cord lesion extends over three or more vertebral segments (longitudinally extensive transverse myelitis [LETM]). The spinal cord syndrome is usually sudden and severe and may be permanent. In one series of 60 patients, ON was the initial feature in 53.3%.

NMO is increasingly being seen as a spectrum of neurologic conditions defined by serologic tests. The term NMO spectrum disorder (NMOSD) emphasizes that patients with ON or LETM alone are often antibody positive and that some patients have brain lesions. The brain MRI abnormalities differ from those typical of MS. Autoantibodies against aquaporin-4 and myelin-oligodendrocyte glycoprotein have been identified so far.

Anterior Ischemic Optic Neuropathy

AION is the most common syndrome of optic nerve ischemia, and the most common optic neuropathy in adults over 50 after glaucoma. In AION, microangiopathy produces occlusion of the short posterior ciliary arteries and infarction of all or part of the disk. Visual loss is sudden, painless, nonprogressive, and generally does not improve. Decreased acuity, impaired color perception, an altitudinal field defect, usually inferior, and pallid disk edema are the typical findings acutely; evolving subsequently into optic atrophy. In the acute phase, a pale disk with hemorrhage will virtually always be due to AION. Other useful findings suggesting AION are altitudinal swelling and arterial attenuation.

AION is due to disease involving the posterior ciliary arteries, not the central retinal artery, and is divided into two forms: arteritic and nonarteritic. Arteritic AION most commonly complicates giant cell arteritis (GCA), accounting for about 10% to 15% of patients. Usually, these patients are over 65 and have more severe visual loss than patients with nonarteritic AION. A history of headache, jaw claudication, and scalp tenderness is very suspicious. Evidence of polymyalgia rheumatica, such as malaise, weight loss, myalgias, and an elevated ESR, increases the likelihood that AION is due to GCA. In a meta-analysis of 21 studies, jaw claudication and diplopia were the only historical features that substantially increased the likelihood of GCA. Predictive physical findings included temporal artery beading, prominence, and tenderness; the absence of any temporal artery abnormality was the only clinical factor that modestly reduced the likelihood of disease. There is evidence that varicella-zoster virus infection may trigger the inflammatory cascade that characterizes GCA.

Premonitory amaurosis fugax is more common in the arteritic form. They do not have a small disk in the fellow eye (disk at risk, see below). Involvement of the opposite eye occurs in approximately 15% of patients within 5 years. Although no treatment affects the outcome in the involved eye, recognition and management of underlying vasculitis may prevent a future attack in the opposite eye.

Nonarteritic AION is most often caused by a microvasculopathy related to hypertension, diabetes, tobacco use, arteriosclerosis, or atherosclerosis. Some cases are due to impaired microvascular perfusion related to systemic hypotension or increased intraocular pressure. There is a syndrome of posterior ischemic optic neuropathy, lacking disk edema, but it is rare and much less well defined than the anterior ischemic syndromes. It may be difficult to distinguish ON from ischemic optic neuropathy. In contrast to ON, the visual loss in AION is usually permanent, although one-third of patients may improve somewhat.

Other Optic Neuropathies

Numerous other conditions may affect the optic nerve head, causing visual loss and disk abnormalities (e.g., glaucoma; LHON and other hereditary optic atrophies; toxins and drugs; primary and metastatic tumors; malnutrition and deficiency states; neurodegenerative disorders; leukodystrophies; sarcoid; optic perineuritis; and congenital anomalies). Dysthyroid

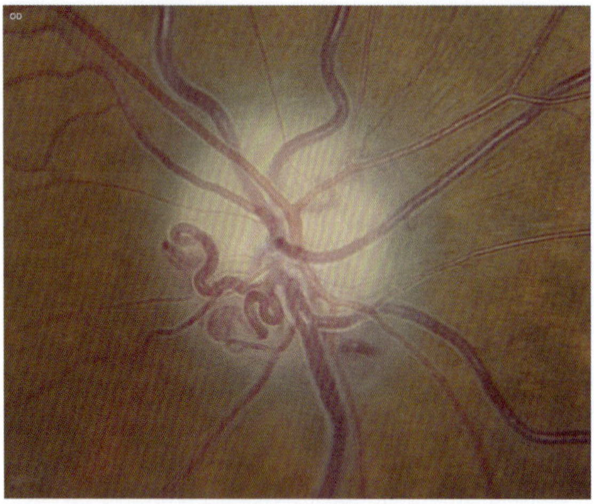

FIGURE 13.24 Pale, elevated optic disk with optociliary shunt vessels in a blind eye; the typical findings of an optic nerve meningioma. (Reprinted from Savino PJ, Danesh-Meyer HV; Wills Eye Hospital [Philadelphia, PA]. *Neuro-Ophthalmology*. 2nd ed. Philadelphia: Wolters Kluwer Health/Lippincott Williams & Wilkins, 2012, with permission.)

optic neuropathy occurs as a late complication of thyroid orbitopathy when enlarged ocular muscles compress the nerve at the orbital apex. See Table 13.3. It is important to distinguish ON from compressive lesions of the optic nerve. One characteristic feature of compressive optic neuropathy is that the condition continues to progress, often insidiously. Large, abnormal-appearing veins on the disk surface because of collateral venous drainage between the retinal and ciliary venous systems (optociliary shunt vessels) may provide a telltale clue to a compressive lesion (Figure 13.24). The triad of progressive visual loss, optic atrophy, and optociliary shunt vessels is highly suggestive.

Pseudopapilledema

Some conditions affecting the nerve head cause striking disk changes of little or no clinical import. This circumstance arises frequently when routine ophthalmoscopy unexpectedly reveals an abnormal-appearing disk in a patient with migraine or some seemingly benign neurologic complaint. Such patients generally have normal vision and no visual complaints. Common causes of pseudopapilledema include optic nerve drusen and myelinated nerve fibers.

Optic nerve drusen, or hyaloid bodies, are acellular, calcified hyaline deposits within the optic nerve that may elevate and distort the disk (Figure 13.25). Drusen occur in about 2% of the population and are bilateral in 70% of cases. They are familial, inherited as an irregular dominant with incomplete penetrance,

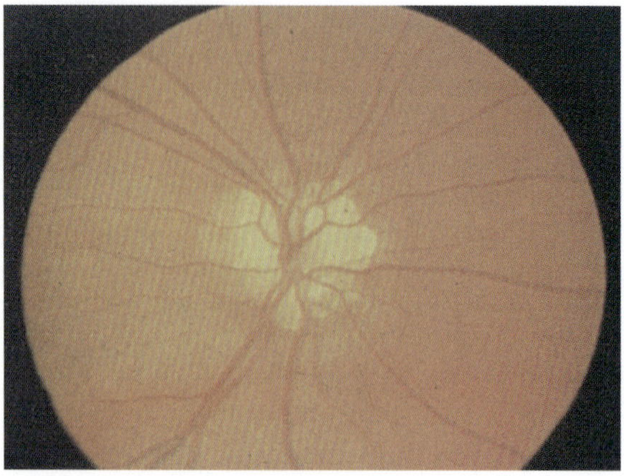

FIGURE 13.25 Drusen of the optic nerve head simulating papilledema.

and occur almost exclusively in Caucasians. On the disk surface, drusen have a highly refractile, rock-candy appearance. But when buried beneath the surface, drusen may produce only disk elevation and blurred margins, causing confusion with papilledema. Optic nerve drusen are not to be confused with retinal drusen, which are an age-related abnormality consisting of yellowish-white, round spots of variable size concentrated at the posterior pole. Myelinated nerve fibers occasionally extend beyond the disk margin into the retina, which causes a very striking disk picture but signifies nothing (Figure 13.26). Other causes of pseudopapilledema include remnants of the

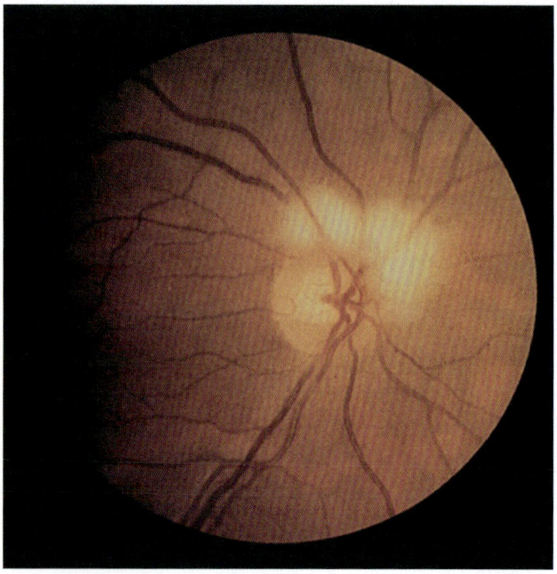

FIGURE 13.26 Myelinated nerve fibers.

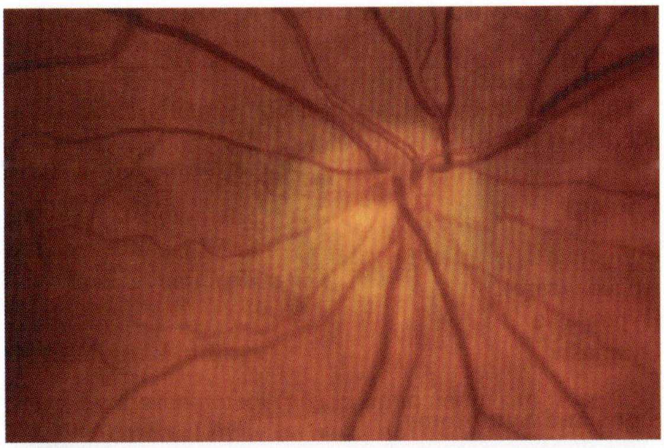

FIGURE 13.27 The congenital tilted optic disk is apparent as the oval of nerve tissue superiorly. There is no apparent optic cup. (Reprinted from Chern KC, Saidel MA. *Ophthalmology Review Manual.* 2nd ed. Philadelphia: Wolters Kluwer Health/Lippincott Williams & Wilkins, 2012, with permission.)

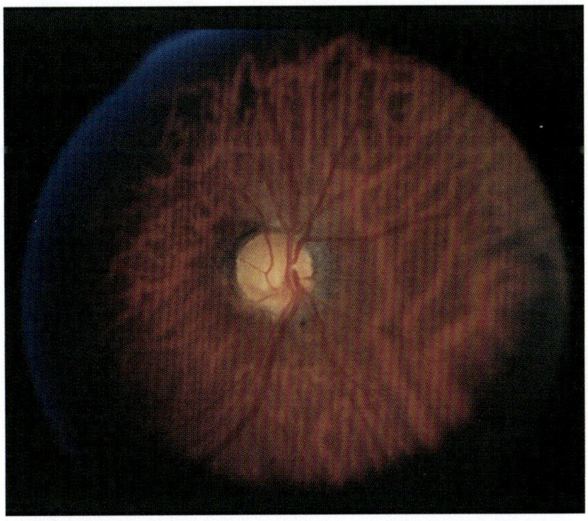

FIGURE 13.28 Primary optic atrophy.

primitive hyaloid artery (Bergmeister's papilla), tilted disks (Figure 13.27), and extreme hyperopia.

Distinguishing pseudopapilledema from acquired disk edema can be difficult. Features that may be helpful include the following: in papilledema, the disk is usually hyperemic; the disk margin blurriness is at the superior and inferior poles early in the process; blood vessels look normal except for fullness of the veins; SVPs are absent; and the NFL is dull with the retinal blood vessels obscured because of retinal edema. In pseudopapilledema, the disk color remains normal; blurriness of the disk margin may be irregular, and the disk may have a lumpy appearance; SVPs are usually present; the blood vessels on the disk frequently look anomalous; and the NFL is clear. Hemorrhages are common in papilledema and extremely rare in pseudopapilledema. If in doubt, consult an ophthalmologist.

Optic Atrophy

In optic atrophy, the disk is paler than normal and more sharply demarcated from the surrounding retina, sometimes having a punched-out appearance (Figure 13.28). The disk margins stand out distinctly; the physiologic cup may be abnormally prominent and extend to the margin of the disk. Loss of myelinated axons and their supporting capillaries with replacement by gliotic scar produce the lack of color, which may vary from a dirty gray to a blue-white color to stark white. Loss of axons causes involution of the capillary bed of the disk and allows the sclera to show through, contributing to the pallor. Dark choroidal pigment deposits may be present about the margin of the disk. The depth of color of the choroid will influence the perception of the degree of contrast between the disk and retina. An atrophic disk may appear perceptibly smaller. Pallor of the temporal portion of the disk—a classical finding in MS—may precede definite atrophy, but normal physiologic temporal pallor makes this finding often equivocal.

Optic atrophy may follow some other condition (ON, AION, or papilledema) and is then referred to as secondary or consecutive optic atrophy. Primary optic atrophy, appearing de novo, occurs as a heredofamilial condition (e.g., LHON) or after toxic, metabolic, nutritional, compressive, or glaucomatous insult to the nerve. Some causes of optic atrophy are listed in Table 13.4. The term cavernous, or pseudoglaucomatous, optic atrophy is used if there is marked recession of the disk. Glaucoma is a common cause of optic atrophy; it produces both an increase

TABLE 13.4 Some Causes of Optic Atrophy

Optic neuritis
Glaucoma
Trauma
Chronic papilledema
Ischemic optic neuropathy
LHON
Drugs
Toxins
Optic nerve compression
Deficiency states
Central nervous system syphilis

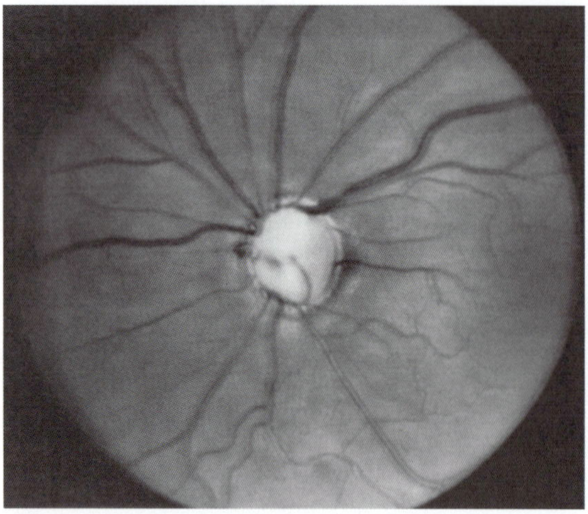

FIGURE 13.29 Glaucomatous optic atrophy. (Courtesy Richard A. Lewis.)

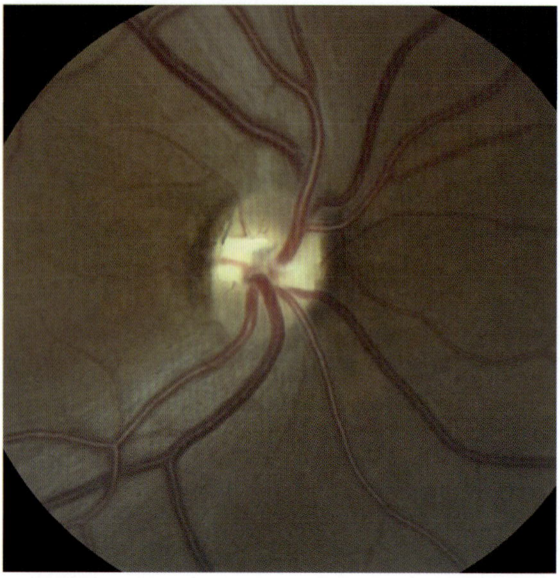

FIGURE 13.30 "Band" or "bow-tie" atrophy of the right optic disk in a patient with a temporal hemianopia caused by a pituitary adenoma. Note horizontal band of atrophy across the right disk, with preservation of the superior and inferior portions of the disk. (Reprinted from Miller NR, Biousse V, Newman NJ, et al. *Walsh and Hoyt's Clinical Neuro-Ophthalmology: The Essentials*. 2nd ed. Philadelphia: Wolters Kluwer Health/Lippincott Williams & Wilkins, 2008, with permission.)

in the depth of the physiologic cup and atrophy of the nerve (Figure 13.29). LHON is an uncommon mitochondriopathy that affects only males; it may cause the appearance of disk edema acutely but evolves into optic atrophy. It typically affects young men and causes sudden unilateral visual loss with involvement of the fellow eye within days to months. Characteristic peripapillary telangiectasias are frequently present, even in the uninvolved eye. Bow-tie or band optic atrophy refers to pallor of the disk that may develop in an eye with temporal VF loss following a lesion of the optic chiasm or tract (Box 13.7, Figure 13.30).

BOX 13.7

Bow-Tie (Band) Optic Atrophy

The macula lies temporal to the disk, and fibers from the nasal hemimacula enter the temporal aspect of the disk. These papillomacular fibers are responsible for the normal pallor of the temporal aspect of the disk, and the pallor is accentuated with NFL axon loss. There is also atrophy of the nasal hemiretinal NFL. Fibers from the peripheral nasal hemiretina enter the nasal aspect of the disk, and axon loss causes nasal disk pallor. With axon loss involving both nasal hemimacula and nasal hemiretina, the result is a transverse band of atrophy across the disk. The appearance is reminiscent of a white bow tie.

A patient may have disk edema in one eye and optic atrophy in the other eye. Foster Kennedy syndrome is due to an olfactory groove meningioma, causing anosmia (see Chapter 12), with optic atrophy because of direct compression ipsilateral to the neoplasm, and late contralateral papilledema because of increased intracranial pressure. Optic atrophy in one eye with disk edema in the other eye is now much more commonly seen with AION or ON (pseudo–Foster Kennedy syndrome), when the disease strikes the opposite eye weeks to months after an initial episode renders the originally affected disk atrophic.

Retrobulbar Optic Neuropathy

The retrobulbar portion of the nerve may be affected by most of the diseases that affect the optic disk. The clinical picture is similar except that there is no disk edema acutely, but optic atrophy may follow later. When ON strikes the retrobulbar portion of the nerve, marked visual impairment occurs, but the disk appearance remains normal, because the pathology is posterior to the papilla. Optic papillopathy thus causes impaired vision and an abnormal disk; retrobulbar optic neuropathy causes impaired vision and a normal disk; and papilledema causes an abnormal disk but does not affect vision acutely. An old saw describes these differences aptly: when the patient sees (has normal vision) and the doctor sees (observes disk abnormalities), it is papilledema; when the patient doesn't see (has impaired vision) and the doctor sees (observes disk abnormalities), it is papillitis; when the patient doesn't see (has impaired vision) and the doctor doesn't see (observes no disk abnormality), it is retrobulbar neuritis.

A major difference between retrobulbar neuropathy and papillopathy is the increased incidence of compression as an etiology in the former. Mass lesions of many types, particularly neoplasms, can affect the retrobulbar optic nerve. Common causes include meningiomas of the optic nerve sheath or sphenoid wing, pituitary tumors, and distal carotid aneurysms. The possibility of compression always figures prominently in the differential diagnosis of patients with optic neuropathy. Insidious visual loss producing decreased acuity; impaired color perception; and central, cecocentral, or arcuate scotoma is typical. Compressive neuropathies may evolve more acutely in patients with metastatic lesions, particularly lymphoma. The optic neuropathy in low-pressure glaucoma may simulate the picture of compression.

Distal (Prechiasmal) Optic Neuropathy

Disorders that affect the distal portion of the optic nerve near its junction with the chiasm are similar to other retrobulbar optic neuropathies except that involvement of the Wilbrand's knee fibers may produce a junctional scotoma, which is highly localizing when present (Figure 13.19C). For this reason, it is important to pay particular attention to the temporal field of the opposite eye when examining a patient with optic neuropathy. The most common cause is pituitary tumor.

Chiasmal Lesions

Pituitary tumors, craniopharyngiomas, meningiomas, gliomas, and carotid aneurysms are the lesions that commonly involve the chiasm. Uncommon causes include demyelination, ischemia, radionecrosis, and a host of other conditions. Because the chiasm lies about a centimeter above the diaphragma sella, visual system involvement indicates suprasellar extension; chiasmatic mass effect is a late, not an early, manifestation of a pituitary tumor (Figure 13.6). Involvement of macular fibers may produce bitemporal scotomas. Chiasmal lesions rarely produce textbook bitemporal hemianopias. There is often a combination of chiasm and optic nerve or optic tract defects depending on whether the chiasm is prefixed, postfixed, or in normal position and the particular attributes of the mass and its force vectors (Figure 13.7). Generally, the defects are binocular and usually heteronymous. The deficit may develop so slowly as to pass unnoticed by the patient. Acuity, color vision, and pupillary function are not affected unless there is optic nerve involvement. Although binasal hemianopias can occur from chiasmal disease, optic neuropathy, glaucoma, and congenital anomalies are more common causes.

Retrochiasmal Lesions

Retrochiasmal lesions produce contralateral homonymous VF defects that respect the vertical meridian. Except for optic tract lesions, they do not cause any deficit of visual acuity, color perception, pupillary reactions, or disk appearance.

Optic tract and LGB lesions occur rarely, perhaps because of generous collateral blood supply; they are characterized by incongruous homonymous hemianopias that split the macula. Optic tract lesions may be accompanied by a mild APD in the contralateral eye because of a greater percentage of crossed pupillomotor fibers (see Chapter 14). Tract lesions may also result in bow-tie pattern disk pallor in the contralateral eye (Box 13.7) and more generalized pallor in the ipsilateral eye. Visual acuity remains normal. Etiologies of optic tract lesions include masses (e.g., meningioma, glioma, craniopharyngioma), aneurysms, AVMs, demyelinating disease, and trauma. Rarely, an APD can be seen with lesions elsewhere in the retrochiasmal pathways and even in the midbrain. Behr's pupil refers to a slightly dilated pupil because of an optic tract lesion, usually associated with a contralateral hemiparesis.

LGB lesions are rare and usually because of vascular disease. They cause a contralateral homonymous hemianopia that is somewhat incongruous, occasionally with a wedge-shaped or hour-glass pattern along the horizontal meridian pointing to fixation (sectoranopia or keyhole defect) and splits the macula. The unusual pattern is due to the organization of the LGB and to its dual blood supply. Etiologies of an LGB lesion include ischemia, neoplasm, AVM, demyelinating disease, and trauma.

In geniculocalcarine pathway (optic radiation) lesions, temporal lobe pathology typically produces contralateral superior quadrantanopias, or homonymous hemianopia, worse in the upper quadrants; and parietal lobe processes contralateral inferior quadrantanopias, or homonymous hemianopia, worse in the lower quadrants (Figure 13.19). The more posterior the lesion, the more congruous the defect. Parietal lesions are associated with asymmetric OKN responses. Parietal lobe lesions may be accompanied by other evidence of parietal lobe dysfunction, such as cortical sensory loss, aphasia, apraxia, agnosia, anosognosia, and hemispatial neglect (Chapters 9, 10, and 35).

In the occipital lobe, the upper retinal fibers (lower VF) synapse on the upper bank, and the lower retinal fibers synapse on the lower bank of the calcarine cortex, which is separated by the calcarine fissure (Figure 13.12). The macular representation is massive, taking up the occipital pole and about 40% to 50% of the contiguous cortex. Occipital lobe lesions cause contralateral homonymous hemianopias that are highly congruous, tend to spare the macula, and do not affect OKN responses. Macular sparing is thought to be due in part to middle cerebral artery collaterals that help to preserve macular function despite a posterior cerebral artery territory infarct. Conversely, the occipital pole is an area of border zone perfusion between the middle and posterior cerebral arteries, and hypotensive watershed infarctions may cause contralateral homonymous paracentral scotomas because of ischemia limited to the macular cortex (Figure 13.19D). Bilateral occipital lobe lesions causing bilateral hemianopias may cause decreased visual acuity. Bilateral occipital infarcts with macular sparing may leave only constricted tunnels of central vision, as though looking through pipes. Although acuity may be normal, the functional visual impairment is extreme because of the constricted peripheral vision, analogous to end-stage retinitis pigmentosa. Occipital lobe lesions may spare the monocular temporal crescent if the damage does not involve the anterior part of the cortex. Conversely, small far anteriorly placed lesions may involve only the temporal crescent in the contralateral eye (half [quarter might be more appropriate] moon or temporal crescent syndrome). Preservation of the temporal crescent results in strikingly incongruous fields. Preservation of the temporal crescent has been called an "endangered" finding because it requires the now seldom used kinetic (Goldmann) perimetry; the currently used static perimetric techniques that concentrate on the central 30 degrees of the VF tend to miss this phenomenon (Figure 13.31).

Bilateral occipital lesions may also cause some dramatic defects of cortical function in addition to the visual loss. Anton's syndrome is cortical blindness because of bilateral homonymous hemianopias, with extreme visual impairment in which the patient is unaware of, and denies the existence of, the deficit. Anton's syndrome and related disorders are discussed in Chapter 10.

Most occipital lesions are vascular. Many anterior temporal lobe lesions are neoplastic. Parietal lesions may be either. The greater likelihood of tumor in the parietal lobe gives rise to Cogan's rule regarding OKNs (see Chapter 14). Trauma, vascular malformations, abscesses, demyelinating disease, metastases, and other pathologic processes can occur in any location.

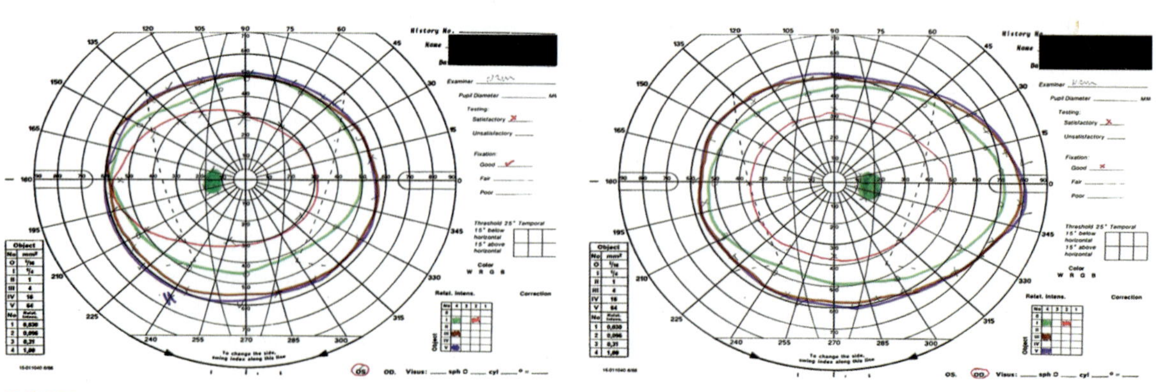

FIGURE 13.31 Loss of the temporal crescent in a patient with an infarct in the right anterior occipital lobe. Kinetic perimetry demonstrates a full peripheral field in the right eye **(right)**, but there is loss of the far temporal field (the temporal crescent) in the left eye **(left)**. (Reprinted from Miller NR, Biousse V, Newman NJ, et al. *Walsh and Hoyt's Clinical Neuro-Ophthalmology: The Essentials.* 3rd ed. Philadelphia: Wolters Kluwer, 2016, with permission.)

Other Abnormalities of the Ocular Fundus

Other abnormalities of the fundus are also important to detect in neurologic patients. The fundus may reveal evidence of hypertensive retinopathy in the patient with stroke, especially in the lacunar syndromes. In the patient with hypertensive encephalopathy, there may be spasm of retinal arterioles. Retinal emboli may be seen in the patient with possible cerebrovascular disease. In the patient with acute severe headache, the finding of subhyaloid (preretinal) hemorrhage is pathognomonic for subarachnoid hemorrhage (Figure 13.32). The presence of a cherry red spot indicates a condition such as gangliosidosis, lipid storage disease or mucopolysaccharidosis in the younger patient (e.g., Tay-Sachs disease), or a central retinal artery occlusion in the older patient (Figure 13.33). In storage diseases, the cherry red spot is seen because of the accumulation of abnormal material within the cell layers of the retina. Because of the relative transparency of the macula, the underlying choroid is visible. In central retinal artery occlusion, the preservation of blood supply to the macula from the choroidal circulation makes it stand out against the retina made pale by ischemia. Pigmentary retinopathy is seen in such conditions as Kearns-Sayre syndrome and other mitochondriopathies.

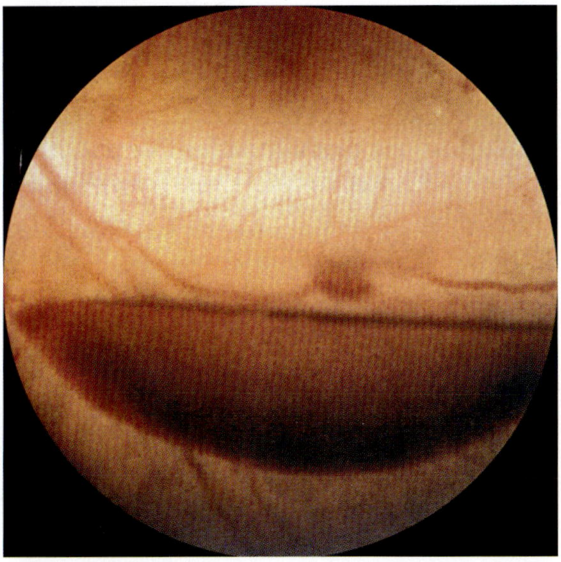

FIGURE 13.32 Subhyaloid hemorrhage in a patient with subarachnoid hemorrhage (Terson's syndrome). The hemorrhage occurs between the posterior layer of the vitreous and the retina, is globular, and often forms a meniscus.

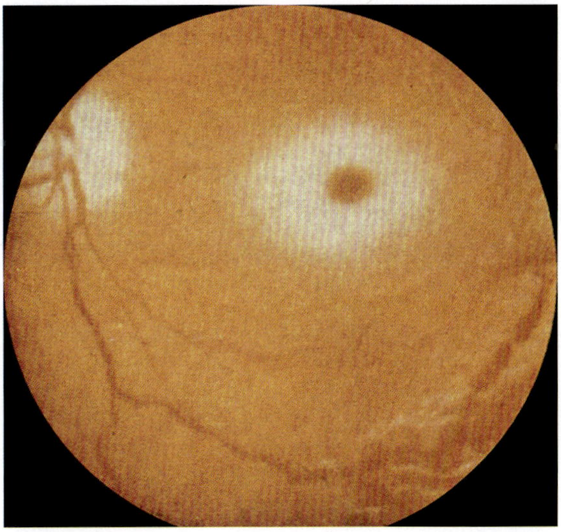

FIGURE 13.33 Cherry red spot in a patient with a lipid storage retinopathy.

Video Links

Video Link 13.1. Afferent pupillary defect. https://collections.lib.utah.edu/details?id=180307&q=sort_type_t%3A%2AMovingImage%2A+AND+afferent+pupillary+defect&fd=type_t%2Ctitle_t%2Cdescription_t%2Csubject_t%2Ccollection_t&rows=50&sort=sort_title_t+asc&facet_setname_s=ehsl_novel_%2A

BIBLIOGRAPHY

Anonymous. The clinical profile of optic neuritis. Experience of the Optic Neuritis Treatment Trial. Optic Neuritis Study Group. *Arch Ophthalmol* 1991;109:1673–1678.

Bell RA, Thompson HS. Relative afferent pupillary defect in optic tract hemianopias. *Am J Ophthalmol* 1978;85:538–540.

Benton S, Levy I, Swash M. Vision in the temporal crescent in occipital infarction. *Brain* 1980;103:83–97.

Brazis PW, Masdeu JC, Biller J. *Localization in Clinical Neurology*. 7th ed. Philadelphia: Wolters Kluwer/Lippincott Williams & Wilkins, 2017.

Brody J, Hellmann MA, Marignier R, et al. Neuromyelitis optica spectrum disorder: disease course and long-term visual outcome. *J Neuroophthalmol* 2016;36:356–362.

Burde RM. Optic disk risk factors for nonarteritic anterior ischemic optic neuropathy. *Am J Ophthalmol* 1993;116:759–764.

Campbell WW. *Clinical Signs in Neurology: A Compendium*. Philadelphia: Wolters Kluwer Health, 2016.

Chavis PS, al-Hazmi A, Clunie D, et al. Temporal crescent syndrome with magnetic resonance correlation. *J Neuroophthalmol* 1997;17:151–155.

Chen CJ, Scheufele M, Sheth M, et al. Isolated relative afferent pupillary defect secondary to contralateral midbrain compression. *Arch Neurol* 2004;61:1451–1453.

Clearkin LG, Watts MT. Ocular involvement in giant cell arteritis. *Br J Hosp Med* 1990;43:373–376.

Downer JJ, Leite MI, Carter R, et al. Diagnosis of neuromyelitis optica (NMO) spectrum disorders: is MRI obsolete? *Neuroradiology* 2012;54:279–285.

Egan RA, Lessell S. A contribution to the natural history of optic nerve sheath meningiomas. *Arch Ophthalmol* 2002;120:1505–1508.

Feldman M, Todman L, Bender MB. 'Flight of colours' in lesions of the visual system. *J Neurol Neurosurg Psychiatry* 1974;37:1265–1272.

Frisen L, Hoyt WF. Insidious atrophy of retinal nerve fibers in multiple sclerosis. Funduscopic identification in patients with and without visual complaints. *Arch Ophthalmol* 1974;92:91–97.

Fujino T, Kigazawa KI, Yamada R. Homonymous hemianopia: a retrospective study of 140 cases. *Neuroophthalmology* 1986;6:17–21.

Gilden D, White T, Khmeleva N, et al. Prevalence and distribution of VZV in temporal arteries of patients with giant cell arteritis. *Neurology* 2015;84:1948–1955.

Giuseppe G. The spectrum of the visual field defects in the tilted disc syndrome: clinical study and review. *Neuroophthalmology* 1986;10:239–246.

Glaser JS, Savino PJ, Sumers KD, et al. The photostress recovery test in the clinical assessment of visual function. *Am J Ophthalmol* 1977;83:255–260.

Hackelbusch R, Nover A, Scherer U. Bitemporal visual field defects in the tilted disk syndrome. *Neuroophthalmology* 1986;6:125–127.

Hayreh SS. Anterior ischemic optic neuropathy. *Arch Neurol* 1981;38:675–678.

Horton JC, Hoyt WF. The representation of the visual field in human striate cortex. A revision of the classic Holmes map. *Arch Ophthalmol* 1991;109:816–824.

Hoyt WF, Schlicke B, Eckelhoff RJ. Fundoscopic appearance of a nerve-fibre-bundle defect. *Br J Ophthalmol* 1972;56:577–583.

Ichhpujani P, Rome JE, Jindal A, et al. Comparative study of 3 techniques to detect a relative afferent pupillary defect. *J Glaucoma* 2011;20:535–539.

Karanjia N, Jacobson DM. Compression of the prechiasmatic optic nerve produces a junctional scotoma. *Am J Ophthalmol* 1999;128:256–258.

Katz J, Tielsch JM, Quigley HA, et al. Automated perimetry detects visual field loss before manual Goldmann perimetry. *Ophthalmology* 1995;102:21–26.

Keane JR. Patterns of hysterical hemianopia. *Neurology* 1998;51:1230–1231.

Keltner JL, Johnson CA. Automated and manual perimetry—a six-year overview. Special emphasis on neuro-ophthalmic problems. *Ophthalmology* 1984;91:68–85.

Kerr NM, Chew SS, Eady EK, et al. Diagnostic accuracy of confrontation visual field tests. *Neurology* 2010;74:1184–1190.

Kim HJ, Paul F, Lana-Peixoto MA, et al. MRI characteristics of neuromyelitis optica spectrum disorder: an international update. *Neurology* 2015;84:1165–1173.

Lakhanpal A, Selhorst JB. Bilateral altitudinal visual fields. *Ann Ophthalmol* 1990;22:112–117.

Landau K, Wichmann W, Valavanis A. The missing temporal crescent. *Am J Ophthalmol* 1995;119:345–349.

Lee JH, Tobias S, Kwon JT, et al. Wilbrand's knee: does it exist? *Surg Neurol* 2006;66:11–17.

Lee MS, Balcer LJ, Volpe NJ, et al. Laser pointer visual field screening. *J Neuroophthalmol* 2003;23:260–263.

Liu GT, Volpe NJ, Galetta S. *Neuro-Ophthalmology: Diagnosis and Management*. 2nd ed. Philadelphia: Saunders Elsevier, 2010.

Lepore FE. The origin of pain in optic neuritis. Determinants of pain in 101 eyes with optic neuritis. *Arch Neurol* 1991;48:748–749.

Lepore FE. The preserved temporal crescent: the clinical implications of an "endangered" finding. *Neurology* 2001;57:1918–1921.

Lessell S. Optic neuropathies. *N Engl J Med* 1978;299:533–536.

Levin BE. The clinical significance of spontaneous pulsations of the retinal vein. *Arch Neurol* 1978;35:37–40.

Masuyama Y, Kodama Y, Matsuura Y, et al. Clinical studies on the occurrence and the pathogenesis of optociliary veins. *J Clin Neuroophthalmol* 1990;10:1–8.

Miller NR, Biousse V, Newman NJ, et al. *Walsh and Hoyt's Clinical Neuro-Ophthalmology: The Essentials*. 2nd ed. Philadelphia: Lippincott Williams & Wilkins, 2008.

Muci-Mendoza R, Arevalo JF, Ramella M, et al. Optociliary veins in optic nerve sheath meningioma. Indocyanine green videoangiography findings. *Ophthalmology* 1999;106:311–318.

Nakashima I, Fukazawa T, Ota K, et al. Two subtypes of optic-spinal form of multiple sclerosis in Japan: clinical and laboratory features. *J Neurol* 2007;254:488–492.

Neville RG, Greenblatt SH, Kollartis CR. Foster Kennedy syndrome and an optociliary vein in a patient with a falx meningioma. *J Clin Neuroophthalmol* 1984;4:97–101.

Newman NJ. Neuro-ophthalmology: the afferent visual system. *Curr Opin Neurol* 1993;6:738–746.

Newman NJ. Leber's hereditary optic neuropathy. New genetic considerations. *Arch Neurol* 1993;50:540–548.

Newman SA, Miller NR. Optic tract syndrome. Neuro-ophthalmologic considerations. *Arch Ophthalmol* 1983;101:1241–1250.

Newman NJ, Lessell S, Winterkorn JM. Optic chiasmal neuritis. *Neurology* 1991;41:1203–1210.

Osaguona VB. Differential diagnoses of the pale/white/atrophic disc. *Community Eye Health* 2016;29:71–74.

Pandit RJ, Gales K, Griffiths PG. Effectiveness of testing visual fields by confrontation. *Lancet* 2001;358:1339–1340.

Papais-Alvarenga RM, Carellos SC, Alvarenga MP, et al. Clinical course of optic neuritis in patients with relapsing neuromyelitis optica. *Arch Ophthalmol* 2008;126:12–16.

Rizzo JF III, Lessell S. Optic neuritis and ischemic optic neuropathy. Overlapping clinical profiles. *Arch Ophthalmol* 1991;109:1668–1672.

Rosenberg MA, Savino PJ, Glaser JS. A clinical analysis of pseudopapilledema. I. Population, laterality, acuity, refractive error, ophthalmoscopic characteristics, and coincident disease. *Arch Ophthalmol* 1979;97:65–70.

Sadun AA, Currie JN, Lessell S. Transient visual obscurations with elevated optic discs. *Ann Neurol* 1984;16:489–494.

Salinas-Garcia RF, Smith JL. Binasal hemianopia. *Surg Neurol* 1978;10:187–194.

Sato DK, Lana-Peixoto MA, Fujihara K, et al. Clinical spectrum and treatment of neuromyelitis optica spectrum disorders: evolution and current status. *Brain Pathol* 2013;23:647–660.

Savino PJ, Glaser JS, Rosenberg MA. A clinical analysis of pseudopapilledema. II. Visual field defects. *Arch Ophthalmol* 1979;97:71–75.

Savino PJ, Paris M, Schatz NJ, et al. Optic tract syndrome. A review of 21 patients. *Arch Ophthalmol* 1978;96:656–663.

Selhorst JB, Chen Y. The optic nerve. *Semin Neurol* 2009;29: 29–35.

Shamir RR, Friedman Y, Joskowicz L, et al. Comparison of Snellen and Early Treatment Diabetic Retinopathy Study charts using a computer simulation. *Int J Ophthalmol* 2016;9:119–123.

Smetana GW, Shmerling RH. Does this patient have temporal arteritis? *JAMA* 2002;287:92–101.

Susac JO, Smith JL, Walsh FB. The impossible meningioma. *Arch Neurol* 1977;34:36–38.

Thompson HS, Corbett JJ, Cox TA. How to measure the relative afferent pupillary defect. *Surv Ophthalmol* 1981;26:39–42.

Trobe JD, Acosta PC, Krischer JP, et al. Confrontation visual field techniques in the detection of anterior visual pathway lesions. *Ann Neurol* 1981;10:28–34.

Vongphanit J, Mitchell P, Wang JJ. Population prevalence of tilted optic disks and the relationship of this sign to refractive error. *Am J Ophthalmol* 2002;133:679–685.

Warner JE, Lessell S, Rizzo JF III, et al. Does optic disc appearance distinguish ischemic optic neuropathy from optic neuritis? *Arch Ophthalmol* 1997;115:1408–1410.

Watnick RL, Trobe JD. Bilateral optic nerve compression as a mechanism for the Foster Kennedy syndrome. *Ophthalmology* 1989;96:1793–1798.

Wilhelm H, Peters T, Ludtke H, et al. The prevalence of relative afferent pupillary defects in normal subjects. *J Neuroophthalmol* 2007;27:263–267.

Wingerchuk DM, Lennon VA, Pittock SJ, et al. Revised diagnostic criteria for neuromyelitis optica. *Neurology* 2006;66:1485–1489.

Whiting AS, Johnson LN. Papilledema: clinical clues and differential diagnosis. *Am Fam Physician* 1992;45:1125–1134.

Yan Y, Li Y, Fu Y, et al. Autoantibody to MOG suggests two distinct clinical subtypes of NMOSD. *Sci China Life Sci* 2016;59: 1270–1281.

Zhang X, Kedar S, Lynn MJ, et al. Homonymous hemianopias: clinical-anatomic correlations in 904 cases. *Neurology* 2006;66:906–910.

CHAPTER 14

The Ocular Motor Nerves

ANATOMY AND PHYSIOLOGY

By convention, the phrase ocular motor nerves refers to cranial nerves (CNs) III, IV, and VI, and the term oculomotor nerve refers specifically to CN III. The orbits and the globes lie in the skull divergently, making the anatomic axes of the eyes diverge slightly from the visual axes, which lie straight ahead for distance vision and convergently for near vision. In sleep and coma, the eyes rest in the divergent position of anatomic neutrality. In wakefulness, cerebral cortical activity influencing the extraocular muscles lines the eyes up for efficient, binocular vision. Phorias and tropias are manifestations of the latent or manifest tendency, respectively, of the eyes to drift away from the visual axis (see Box 14.4).

The four rectus muscles arise from a common structure in the orbital apex, the annulus of Zinn. The annulus is a thickening of the periosteum that forms a circular tendon, its center pierced by the optic nerve, central retinal artery and CNs III and VI, and the recti arising from its body. The rectus muscles insert on the sclera 5 to 7 mm posterior to the limbus.

The nervous system attempts to maintain visual fusion of images by controlling precisely the movements of the two eyes. The extraocular muscles work in pairs that are yoked together and work in concert to perform a certain action. The superior and inferior recti lie in the orbit, and insert into the globe, along the anatomic axis, exerting their maximally efficient pull when the eye is slightly abducted (Figure 14.1). The superior and inferior obliques insert into the globe at an angle of about 30 degrees from medial to lateral; they exert maximal pull with the eye slightly adducted. The obliques insert posteriorly into the globe: the superior oblique pulls the back of the eye up, producing downgaze; the inferior oblique pulls the back of the eye down, producing upgaze. The superior oblique therefore works as a depressor of the adducted eye, the inferior oblique as an elevator; they move the globe in the direction opposite their names (Figure 14.2).

To achieve conjugate downgaze to one side, the superior oblique of the adducting eye is yoked to the inferior rectus of the abducting eye (Figure 14.3). In fact, even in adduction, most of ocular elevation and depression is accomplished by the superior and inferior rectus, and the major action of both obliques is torsional (cyclotorsional, rotational). The primary action—some contend the only action—of the superior oblique is to intort (incyclotort) and of the inferior oblique to extort (excyclotort). Because of its angle of insertion along the anatomic axis, when the eye is in primary gaze, the inferior rectus acts not only to depress the eye but also to extort it. The yoked superior oblique, through its intorsion action, counteracts the extorsion effect of the inferior rectus so that downgaze is smooth and linear. Likewise, the superior rectus and the inferior oblique.

Because of the anatomical arrangement of the obliques and vertically acting recti, examination of extraocular movement should include gaze to the right and left plus upgaze and downgaze in eccentric position to both sides: the six cardinal directions of gaze (Figure 14.3). The levator palpebrae superioris supplies the striated muscles of the eyelid and elevates the lid.

THE OCULOMOTOR NERVE

The oculomotor, or third cranial nerve (CN III), arises from the oculomotor nuclear complex in the midbrain and conveys motor fibers to extraocular muscles, plus parasympathetic fibers to the pupil and ciliary body. These nuclear centers are situated in the periaqueductal gray matter just anterior to the aqueduct of Sylvius, at the level of the superior colliculi

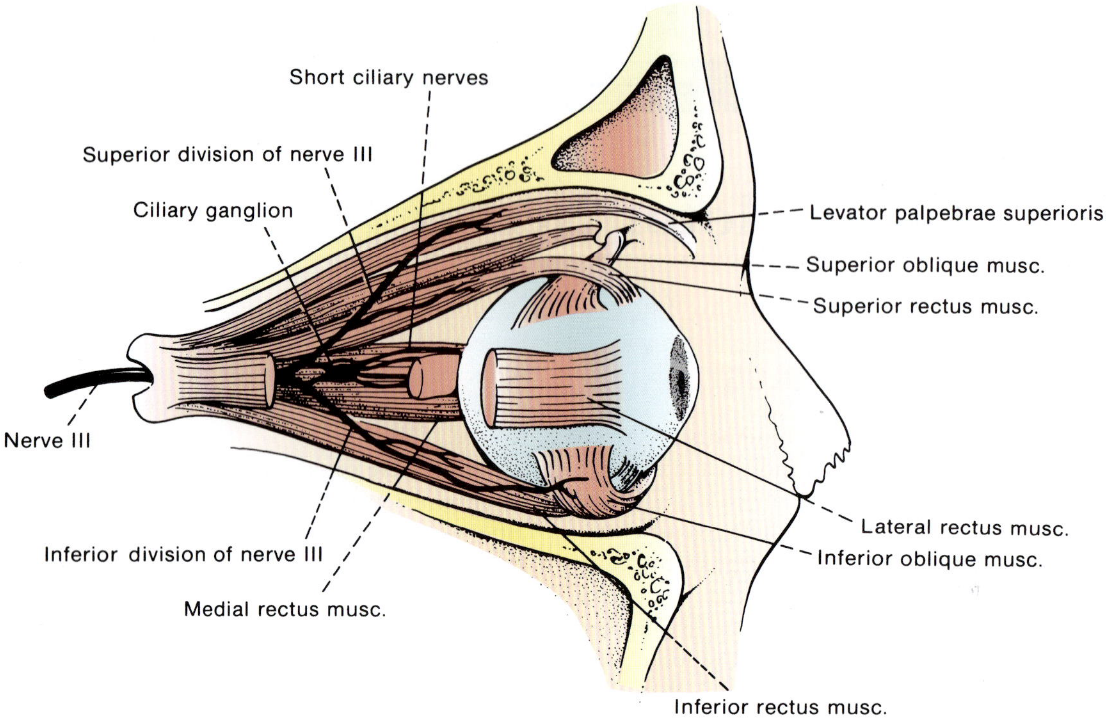

FIGURE 14.1 The extraocular muscles and the third nerve in the orbit.

(anterior quadrigeminal bodies). The median longitudinal fasciculus (MLF) abuts the nucleus laterally and ventrally (Figure 14.4). Each oculomotor nucleus consists of multiple adjacent subnuclei that innervate specific ocular muscles. The neurons are somatic motor (general somatic efferent). The paired lateral nuclei are the largest and are situated anterior and lateral to the others; their medial portions are fused into an unpaired mass. CN III has a superior and an inferior division. The superior division supplies the levator palpebrae superioris and superior rectus muscles. The inferior division supplies the medial and inferior recti, the inferior oblique, and the pupil. The lateral subnucleus innervates the ipsilateral inferior oblique and medial and inferior recti; its axons make up the inferior division of CN III. The superior rectus muscle is innervated by the contralateral medial subnucleus. Because of its crossed innervation, a major clue to the presence of a nuclear third nerve palsy is superior rectus weakness in the opposite eye.

A single midline structure, the central caudal nucleus, supplies the levator palpebrae muscles on

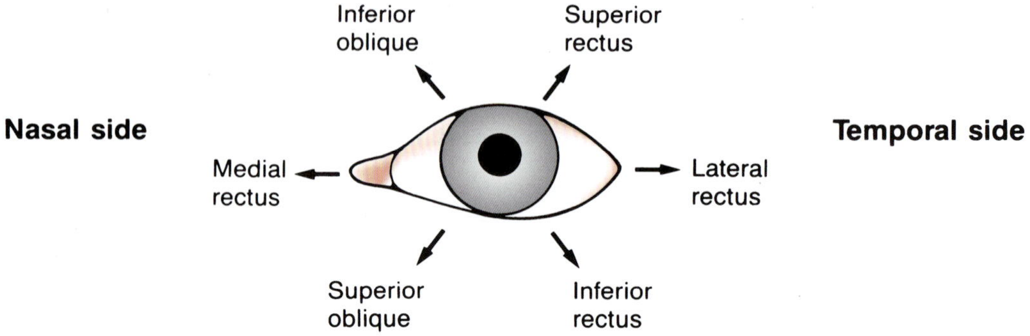

FIGURE 14.2 Actions of the extraocular muscles on the left eye. *Arrows* denote the main directions of action for each muscle, resulting from a combination of movements of the globe in the three dimensions.

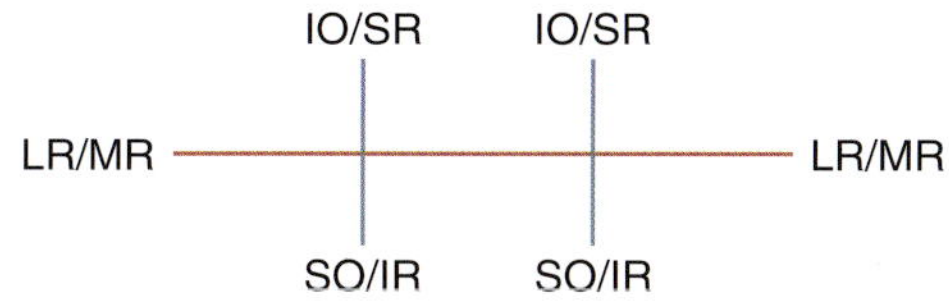

FIGURE 14.3 The yoke muscles control extraocular movement in the six cardinal directions of gaze.

both sides. The periaqueductal gray matter is also involved with eyelid function; destructive lesions there may cause ptosis. A supraoculomotor area in the ventral periaqueductal gray matter controlling levator function has been proposed. The Edinger-Westphal (EW) nuclei are part of the craniosacral, or parasympathetic, division of the autonomic nervous system. The EW subnucleus is a single structure that provides parasympathetic innervation to both sides. It is spread throughout the length of the oculomotor complex with a paired rostral portion and an unpaired medial and caudal portion. Preganglionic fibers from the EW nuclei go to the ciliary ganglion (Figure 13.9). Postganglionic fibers derived from cells in the rostral part of the subnucleus supply the pupillary sphincter; those derived from the anteromedial nucleus supply the ciliary muscle and function in accommodation. Fibers from the medial, EW, and central caudal subnuclei form the superior division of CN III.

Fibers from the ipsilateral lateral subnucleus, from the contralateral medial subnucleus (superior rectus), and from both central caudal (levator palpebrae) and EW (parasympathetics) nuclei join to form the filaments of CN III, which course anteriorly through the mesencephalon, traversing the medial portion of the red nucleus and the substantia nigra. The nerve exits from the interpeduncular fossa on the anterior surface of the midbrain just above the pons (Figure 11.3). It travels anteriorly and passes between the superior cerebellar and posterior cerebral arteries (Figure 14.5). It runs forward parallel to the posterior communicating artery. Third nerve palsy is a classic and important sign of posterior communicating aneurysm. In its course toward the cavernous sinus, it lies on the free edge of the tentorium cerebelli, medial to the temporal lobe. Here, it is at risk of compression because of uncal herniation. Through the nerve's subarachnoid course, the parasympathetic fibers lie superficially on the dorsomedial surface. The location of these fibers influences whether a third nerve palsy will or will not involve the pupil, an important differential diagnostic point. CN III penetrates the dura just lateral and anterior to the posterior clinoid processes and enters the cavernous sinus, where it lies in the upper aspect, close to the lateral wall (Figure 14.6). In the cavernous sinus, CN III has important relationships with the carotid artery, ascending pericarotid sympathetics, and CNs IV, V,

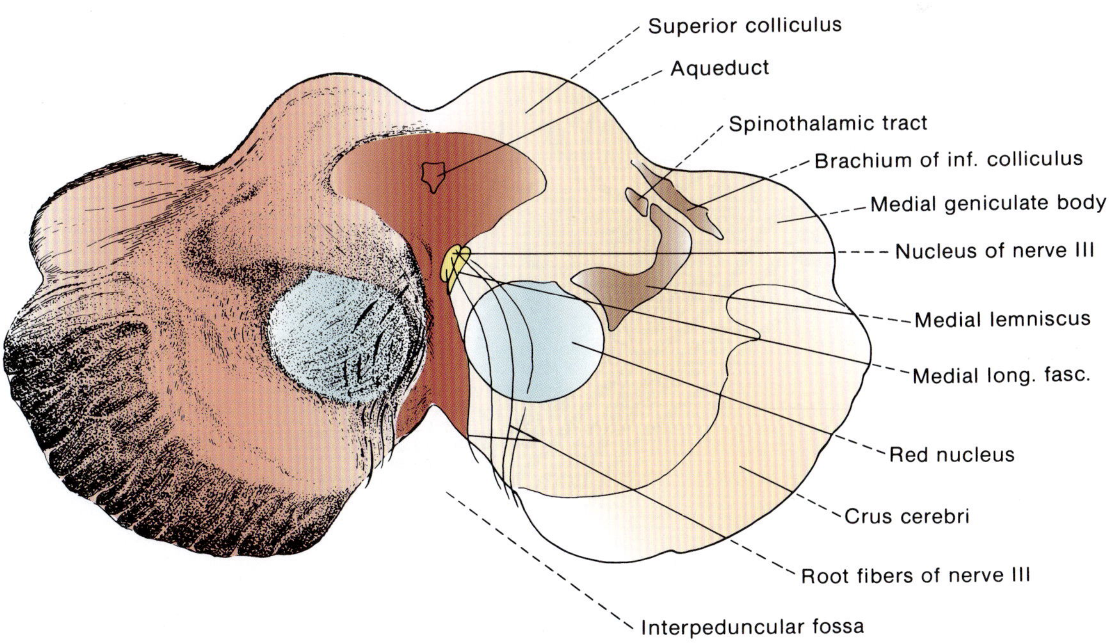

FIGURE 14.4 Section through the mesencephalon at the level of the superior colliculus and oculomotor nucleus.

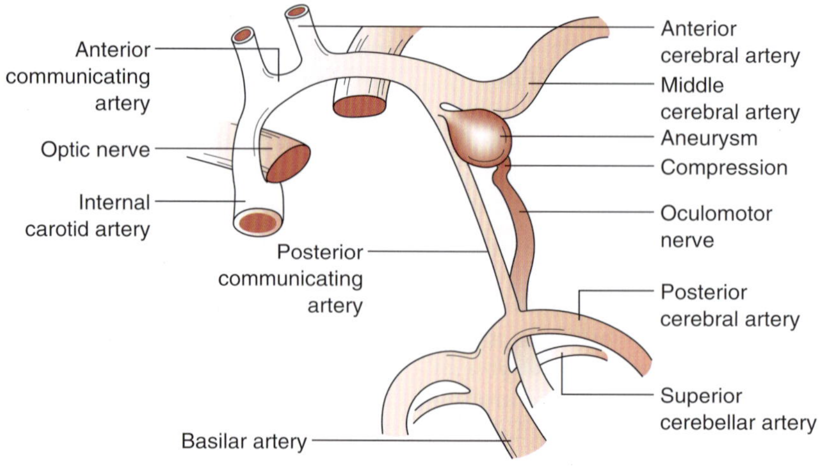

FIGURE 14.5 Anatomy of the oculomotor nerve in relation to the major arteries at the base of the brain. An aneurysm arising from the posterior communicating artery is compressing and distorting the nerve.

and VI. CN III separates into its superior and inferior divisions in the anterior cavernous sinus, then enters the orbit through the superior orbital fissure, and passes through the annulus of Zinn. It sends a short root to the ciliary ganglion, from which postganglionic fibers go as the short ciliary nerves to supply the ciliary muscle and the sphincter pupillae (Figure 14.1). The sphincter pupillae causes constriction of the pupil. Contraction of the ciliary muscle causes relaxation of the ciliary zonule, decreasing the tension on the lens

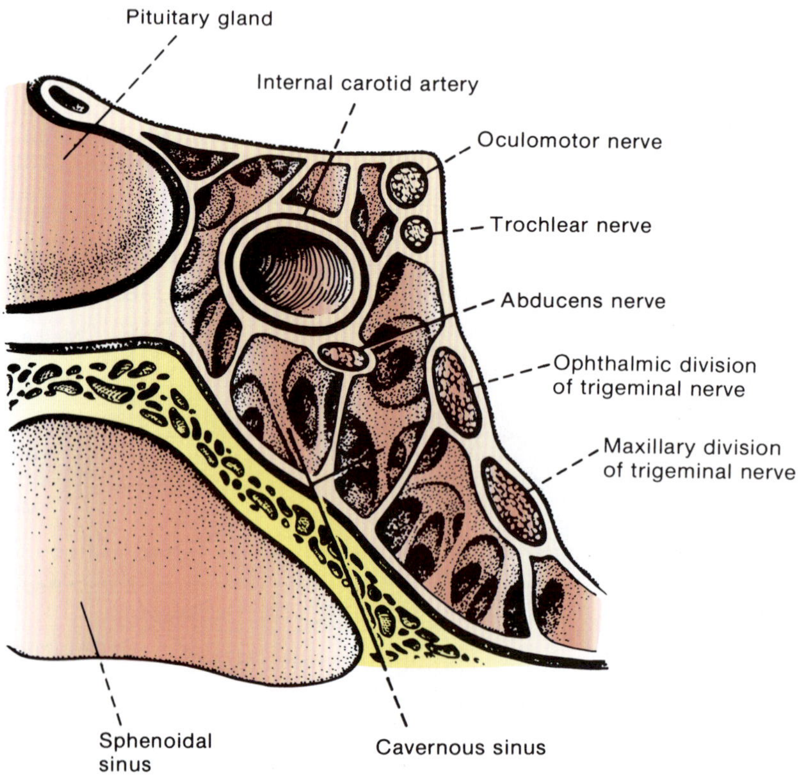

FIGURE 14.6 Oblique section through the cavernous sinus.

capsule and allowing it to become more convex to accommodate for near vision. Pupillary constriction, convergence, and accommodation are all part of the near reflex.

THE TROCHLEAR NERVE

The trochlear, or fourth cranial nerve (CN IV), is the smallest CN. It arises from the trochlear nucleus located just anterior to the aqueduct in the gray matter of the lower mesencephalon at the level of the inferior colliculus, immediately above the pons (Figure 14.7) and caudal to the lateral nucleus of CN III but separated by a short distance. The nucleus contains somatic motor neurons. The nerve filaments curve posteriorly around the aqueduct, decussate in the anterior medullary velum, and exit through the tectum. It is the only CN to exit from the brainstem posteriorly, and because of this extra distance, CN IV has the longest intracranial course of any of the CNs. The nerve circles the brainstem, then turns and runs forward, passing between the posterior cerebral and superior cerebellar arteries, and then courses along the tentorium. It penetrates the dura just behind and lateral to the posterior clinoid processes and enters the cavernous sinus in proximity to CN III. In the sinus, it is located superolaterally, below CN III but above the trigeminal branches. Leaving the cavernous sinus, it traverses the superior orbital fissure, enters the orbit, and crosses over CN III to supply the superior oblique. It does not pass through the annulus of Zinn.

CN IV terminates on the superior oblique muscle on the side opposite the nucleus of origin. In a nuclear lesion of the fourth nerve, the contralateral superior oblique muscle is weakened; in an extramedullary lesion along the course of the nerve, the ipsilateral muscle is involved.

THE ABDUCENS NERVE

The nucleus of the abducens, or sixth cranial nerve (CN VI), lies in the mid to lower pons, in the gray matter of the dorsal pontine tegmentum in the floor of the fourth ventricle, encircled by the looping fibers of the facial nerve (Figure 14.8). The nucleus is made up of somatic motor neurons. The nerve exits

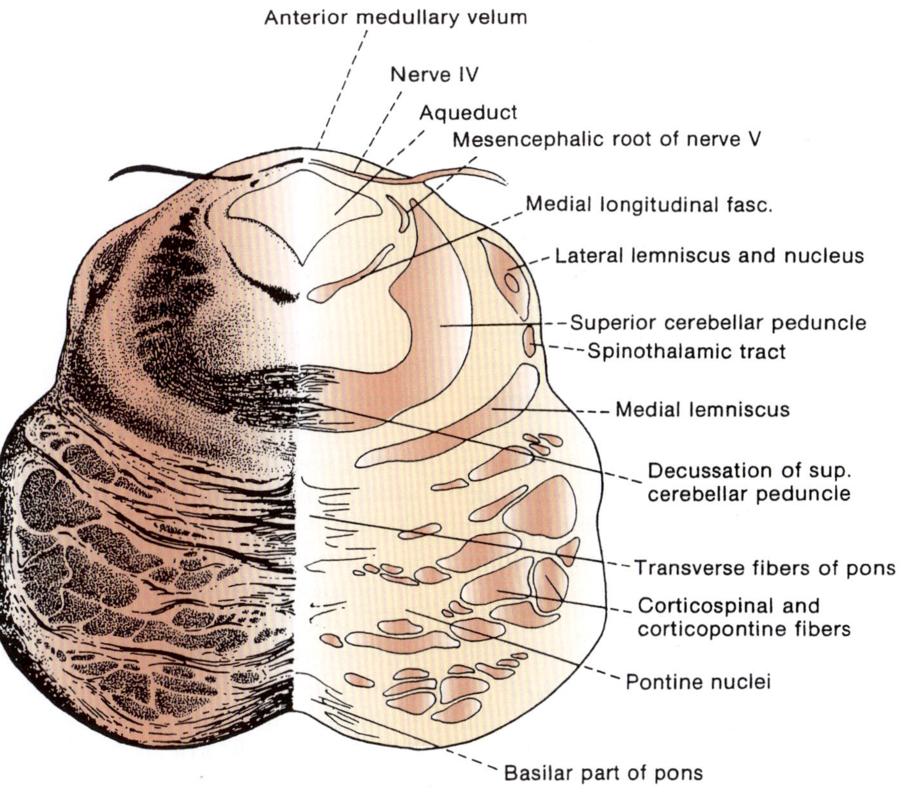

FIGURE 14.7 Section through the mesencephalon at the border of the pons, showing the trochlear nerve.

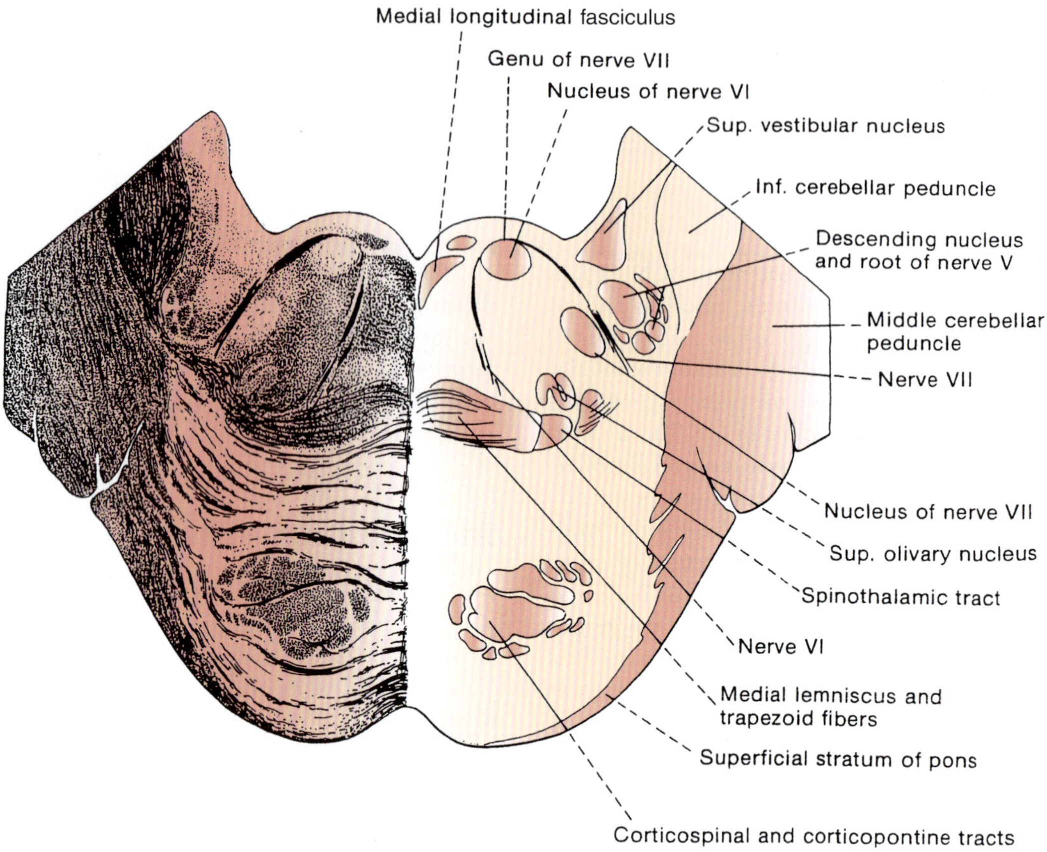

FIGURE 14.8 Section through the pons showing fibers of the abducens and facial nerves.

anteriorly at the pontomedullary junction, crosses the internal auditory artery, and then ascends the clivus in the prepontine cistern. It passes near the gasserian ganglion, makes a sharp turn over the petrous apex, pierces the dura at the dorsum sellae, and traverses the Dorello's canal between the posterior clinoid process and the petrous apex. The petroclinoid ligament forms the roof of the canal. The nerve enters the cavernous sinus in company with CNs III and IV, where it lies below and medial to CN III and just lateral to the internal carotid artery. CN VI is the only nerve that lies free in the lumen of the sinus; the others are in the wall (Figure 14.6). It enters the orbit through the superior orbital fissure and the annulus of Zinn to innervate the lateral rectus.

SUPRANUCLEAR CONTROL OF GAZE

The supranuclear mechanisms that control gaze are designed to ensure that the fovea maintains fixation on the object of interest despite movements of the object, the eyes, or the head. A saccade (Fr. "jerk") is a quick, small-amplitude eye movement used to acquire a target. Smooth pursuit mechanisms use slower eye movements to track a target once acquired. Saccades are designed to rapidly shift gaze to the target; pursuit movements are designed to maintain foveation of a moving target. The CN VI nucleus is the final common pathway controlling horizontal eye movements. The vertical gaze centers lie in the midbrain. There are six currently recognized eye movement control systems: saccadic, smooth pursuit, vergence, fixation, optokinetic, and vestibuloocular reflex (VOR).

Four interconnected cortical areas are involved in the generation of saccades: the frontal eye field (FEF), which lies anterior to the motor strip in the premotor cortex in the second frontal gyrus; the supplementary eye field, which lies in the supplementary motor area; the dorsolateral prefrontal cortex, which lies anterior to the FEF in the second frontal gyrus; and the posterior eye field, which lies in the parietal lobe.

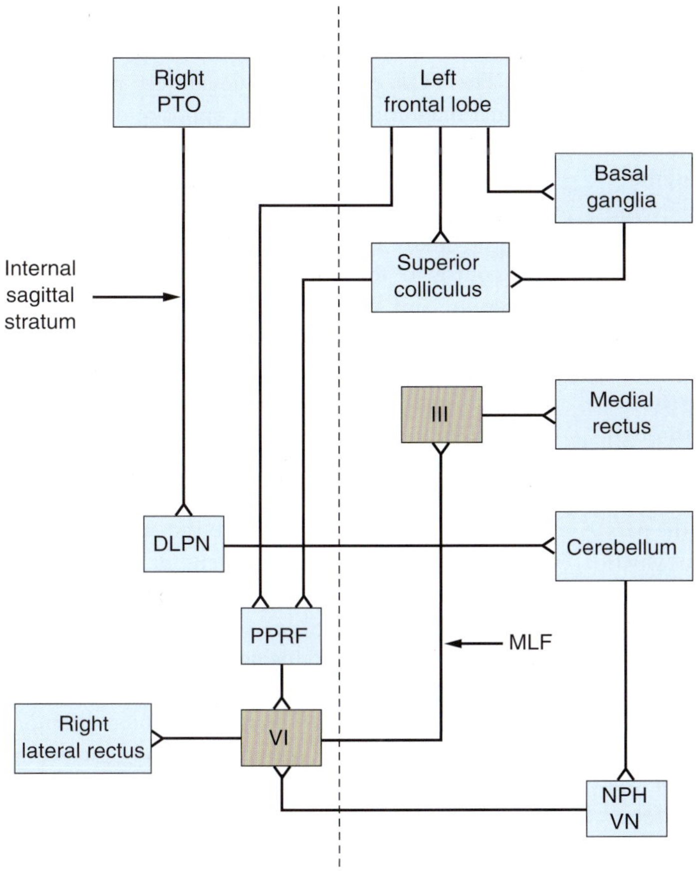

FIGURE 14.9 Diagram of the major supranuclear gaze pathways. The saccadic pathway arises in the frontal lobe and descends to the contralateral pons. The pursuit pathway arises in the region of the parietotemporal-occipital junction (PTOJ) and descends to the ipsilateral pons. Vertical dashed line represents the midline. III, nucleus of CN III; VI, nucleus of cranial nerve (CN) VI; DLPN, dorsolateral pontine nuclei; MLF, medial longitudinal fasciculus; NPH, nucleus prepositus hypoglossi; PPRF, pontine paramedian reticular formation; VN, vestibular nuclei.

The FEF controls horizontal conjugate saccades to the opposite side. Fibers descend and decussate en route to the pontine paramedian reticular formation (PPRF) (Figure 14.9). Other fibers descend to the superior colliculus and are then relayed to the contralateral PPRF. The FEF to the superior colliculus pathway and the posterior eye fields are likely involved in reflex saccades. The PPRF (horizontal gaze center, lateral gaze center, pontine gaze center) is a premotor area that consists of cells lying ventrolateral to the MLF from the level of the abducens nucleus extending rostrally to near the trochlear nucleus. Signals from the PPRF activate both motor neurons and interneurons in the adjacent CN VI nucleus. The CN VI motor neurons activate the ipsilateral lateral rectus, whereas the interneurons simultaneously send impulses up the MLF, which decussates just rostral to the PPRF and runs to the medial rectus subnucleus of the contralateral oculomotor nuclear complex in the midbrain to activate the medial rectus. The ipsilateral lateral rectus and contralateral medial rectus then contract synchronously to produce conjugate horizontal gaze. A left FEF-initiated command to look right is thus transmitted down to the right PPRF, which simultaneously influences the right sixth nerve to contract the lateral rectus and the left third nerve to contract the yoked medial rectus—both contract, according to Hering's law, exactly the same amount.

The PPRF contains burst and pause neurons. The burst neurons fire a high-frequency pulse of discharges to initiate an ipsilateral saccade. The burst neurons determine saccadic velocity. The pause neurons lie in the nucleus raphe interpositus. Their tonic discharges prevent the burst cells from initiating extraneous saccades, and the tonic firing pauses just before and during saccades. Smooth pursuit signals to the PPRF come from the vestibular nuclei and the nucleus prepositus hypoglossi, which lies in the perihypoglossal nuclear complex. Step cells in the perihypoglossal nuclei control the impulses that maintain the eyes in an eccentric position following a saccade. To acquire and maintain an eccentric stationary target, the CN VI motor neurons would have a pulse of activity generated by the burst cells to create the saccade, followed by a step-up of firing generated by the step cells to maintain the new position. All movements would be conjugate and synchronous because of coordination with the fellow eye by the MLF.

The dorsolateral prefrontal cortical area may be involved in mechanisms responsible for inhibiting unwanted saccades. Antisaccades are voluntary saccades away from a target. Patients with frontal lobe disease, progressive supranuclear palsy (PSP), Parkinson's disease, Alzheimer's disease, and schizophrenia, when asked to look away from a visual stimulus, may be unable to inhibit a saccade toward the target (prosaccade) and are therefore unable to make an antisaccade or make it only after a prosaccade. Another system involved in saccades works through the basal ganglia. Collaterals from the FEF go to the head of the caudate and putamen, which send fibers to the ipsilateral substantia nigra. Neurons in the pars reticulata project to the superior colliculus, which then projects to the PPRF. Disturbances in this system may explain some of the abnormalities of ocular motor control that occur in basal ganglia disorders, particularly Parkinson's disease.

The FEF to the contralateral PPRF system controls saccadic eye movements. The smooth pursuit system originates ipsilaterally in the region of the parietotemporal-occipital junction (PTOJ) and functions to maintain foveation of a moving target. The visual cortex sends information about the target to the extrastriate cortex at the PTOJ. From there, fibers descend in the internal sagittal stratum adjacent to the atrium of the lateral ventricle down to the ipsilateral dorsolateral pontine nuclei. The system then double decussates. The dorsolateral pontine nuclei project to the contralateral cerebellum. Signals from the cerebellum then activate the medial vestibular nucleus and the nucleus propositus hypoglossi, which in turn project to the contralateral PPRF. The PPRF then coordinates conjugate horizontal pursuit movements. The PTOJ also sends corticocortical fibers to the ipsilateral frontal lobe. Smooth pursuit to the right is controlled by the right occipital region. Quick refixation saccades back to the left are mediated by the right FEF, so the process of following a series of moving objects (as in optokinetic nystagmus [OKN], or railroad nystagmus) is all accomplished in the same cerebral hemisphere.

The vergence system controls the degree of convergence or divergence of the eyes, maintaining macular fixation no matter what the distance to the target. The vestibular system has a large input into the oculomotor system in order to maintain proper eye orientation in relation to head and body position. The VOR produces conjugate eye movements of equal magnitude but in the opposite direction to compensate for head movements in order to maintain foveation during motion of the head. The VOR is discussed in more detail in Chapter 17.

The pathways controlling upgaze and downgaze course in the region of the rostral midbrain, pretectum, and posterior commissure. The vertical gaze equivalent of the PPRF is the rostral interstitial nucleus of the MLF (riMLF), which lies in the midbrain near the red nucleus. The lateral portion of the riMLF is concerned with upgaze, the medial portion with downgaze. The riMLF send impulses to the nuclei of CNs III and IV. Connections via the posterior commissure coordinate the activity on the two sides. The interstitial nucleus of Cajal (INC) lies caudal to the riMLF. Its neurons connect to the riMLF and are involved in vertical pursuit and gaze holding. Upgaze and downgaze pathways occupy different positions, and abnormalities may affect one without the other. The upgaze centers lie more dorsally. Lesions in the region of the posterior commissure may disturb vertical gaze, especially upgaze (Parinaud's syndrome). The downgaze centers lie more ventrally, and lesions there may primarily affect downgaze.

Bhidayasiri et al. developed a hypothetical scheme to account for clinical disorders of vertical gaze based on recent insights gained from experimental studies. Vertical saccades are generated by burst neurons in the riMLF, with unilateral innervation of depressor muscles but bilateral innervation of elevator muscles. The riMLF is also a torsional saccade generator. Torsional deviation during an attempted vertical saccade, together with a vertical gaze palsy, occurs with lesions involving the riMLF. The INC acts similar to the step neurons in the PPRF, holding the eye in the new position after a vertical saccade. The INC projects to ocular motoneurons via the posterior commissure. Bilateral INC or posterior commissure lesions cause defects of vertical gaze.

Reflex upgaze occurs with forceful eyelid closure (Bell's phenomenon), and in some conditions, reflex upgaze may be preserved when upgaze is otherwise paralyzed. Levator palpebrae and superior rectus muscle tone are normally matched. In extreme downgaze, both are maximally inhibited, but in reflex upgaze, the normal parallel innervation becomes reversed.

THE MEDIAL LONGITUDINAL FASCICULUS

The oculomotor, trochlear, and abducens nuclei make up one more or less continuous cell column. They are united for coordinated and conjugate action by the MLF, an extensive and prominent fiber tract that runs in the midline in the dorsal tegmentum of the brainstem. The MLF extends from the midbrain down to the upper thoracic spinal cord. It has many connections. Its primary function is to coordinate lateral gaze by connecting the sixth nerve nucleus on one side with the third and fourth nerve nuclei on the opposite side in order to allow the two eyes to move synchronously. Signals from the PPRF activate interneurons in the adjacent sixth nerve nucleus, which send axons up the MLF. The MLF crosses in the pons, soon after beginning its ascent to the contralateral third nerve complex. Lesions of the MLF disrupt communication between the two nuclei, causing internuclear ophthalmoplegia (INO). The MLF also has extensive connections with CNs V, VII, VIII, XI, and XII, and with the motor nuclei of the upper cervical nerves. Nuclear groups in the rostral midbrain are involved in MLF function, including the nucleus of the posterior commissure (nucleus of Darkshevich), INC (the nucleus of the MLF), and the riMLF. These connections coordinate movement of the two eyes, as well as head and eye, and even body movements. The MLF mediates reflex head and eye movements in response to various stimuli and is important in auditory-ocular, vestibular-ocular, and righting reflexes.

SYMPATHETIC INNERVATION

The sympathetic pathway to the eye begins in the hypothalamus. Fibers of the first-order neuron descend through the brainstem and upper cervical spinal cord. The second-order neuron lies in the intermediolateral gray column at C8-T2 of the upper thoracic spinal cord (ciliospinal center of Budge). Axons exit through the anterior roots and transverse the gray rami communicantes, and then arch over the apex of the lung and beneath the subclavian artery to enter the cervical sympathetic chain, where they ascend to synapse on the third-order neuron in the superior cervical ganglion at the level of the carotid bifurcation.

Postganglionic fibers of the third-order neuron lie on the wall of the common carotid artery, forming the pericarotid sympathetic plexus. Sympathetic fibers innervating facial structures follow the external carotid at the bifurcation. Sympathetic fibers destined for the eye follow the internal carotid artery. A lesion proximal to the carotid bifurcation causes Horner's syndrome (ptosis, miosis, and anhidrosis), and a lesion distal to the bifurcation causes oculosympathetic paresis (Horner's syndrome minus facial anhidrosis). The effects on the eye of oculosympathetic paresis and Horner's syndrome are the same, and the terms are often used interchangeably; subsequent discussion refers to Horner's syndrome. The pericarotid sympathetic plexus continues along the internal carotid artery in its course through the cavernous sinus. Sympathetic fibers migrate to CN VI for a short distance, then join the nasociliary branch of CN V_1, and enter the orbit through the superior orbital fissure. They continue as long ciliary nerves to the pupillodilator muscle (Figure 14.10).

Sympathetically innervated smooth muscle is present in both the upper and lower lids to serve as accessory retractors. The upper lid muscle is better organized and identified, and it is referred to as the accessory levator palpebrae superioris, superior tarsal muscle, or Müller's muscle. The inferior tarsal muscle in the lower lid is less distinct.

CLINICAL EXAMINATION AND DISORDERS OF FUNCTION OF THE OCULAR MOTOR NERVES AND THE CERVICAL SYMPATHETIC SYSTEM

Examination of the eyes begins with inspection—looking for any obvious ocular malalignment, abnormal lid position, or abnormalities of the position of the globe within the orbit. Abnormalities of the external eye may occasionally be of diagnostic significance in neurologic patients (see Chapter 13).

EXOPHTHALMOS AND ENOPHTHALMOS

The globe may be abnormally positioned within the orbit so that it protrudes (exophthalmos, proptosis) or recedes (enophthalmos). Subtle proptosis can often be better appreciated by looking down at

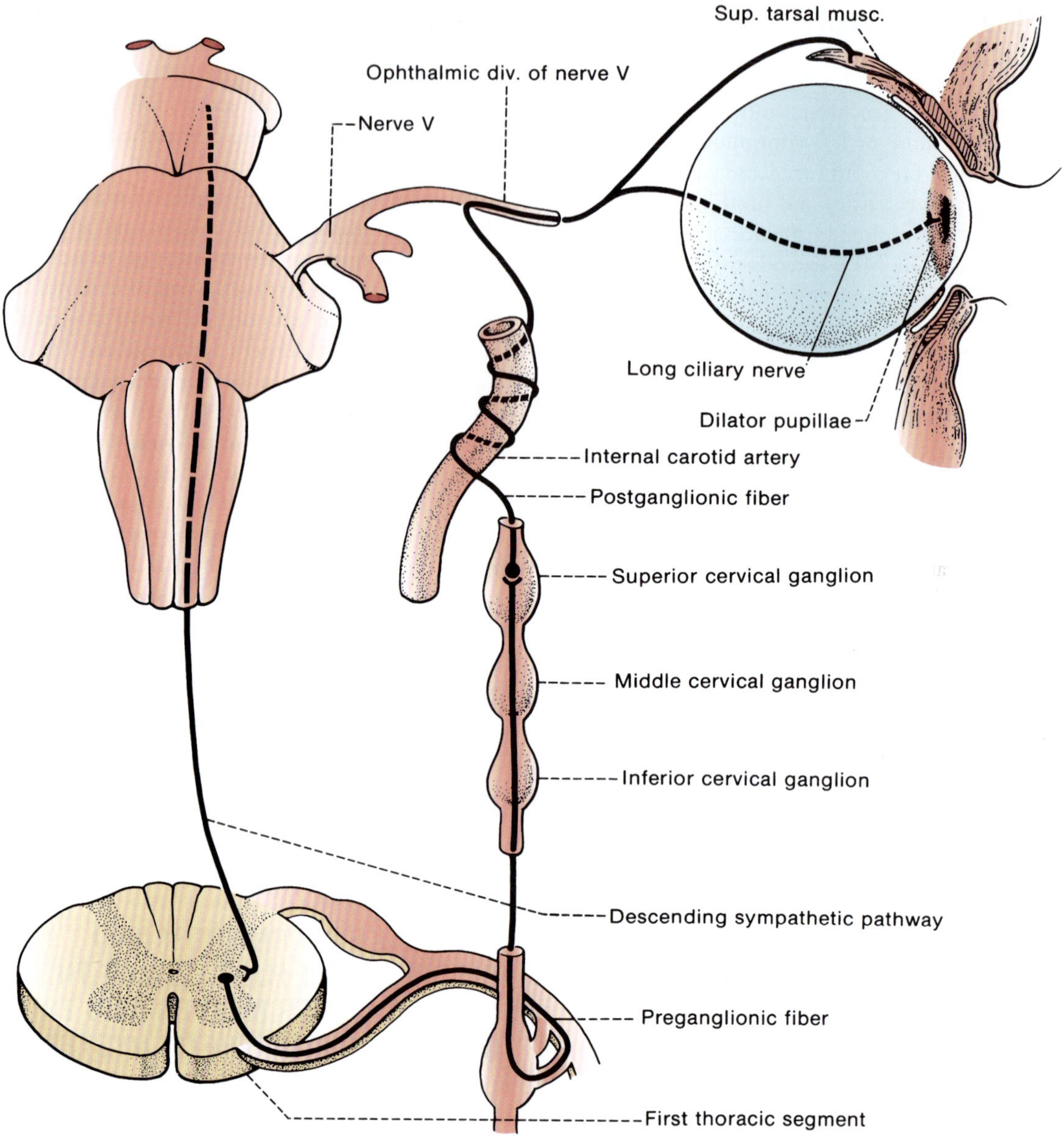

FIGURE 14.10 The cervical portion of the sympathetic division of the autonomic nervous system.

both eyes from above the vertex of the head or by comparing side views. Exophthalmos is usually bilateral and most commonly due to thyroid eye disease (TED, Graves' ophthalmopathy, Graves' orbitopathy). Other conditions associated with neurologic complications and exophthalmos include the craniosynostosis syndromes and Hand-Schüller-Christian disease. Although TED can occasionally cause unilateral exophthalmos, the likelihood of other conditions increases in this situation. Orbital pseudotumor is an idiopathic inflammatory condition that affects the tissues of the orbit. It is common, and second only to TED as a cause of unilateral proptosis. Some of the neurologically significant causes of unilateral proptosis include orbital mass lesion, carotid cavernous fistula (Figure 14.11), cavernous sinus thrombosis, sphenoid wing meningioma, meningocele, and mucormycosis.

Other causes of exophthalmos include orbital neoplasm and vascular malformation of the orbit.

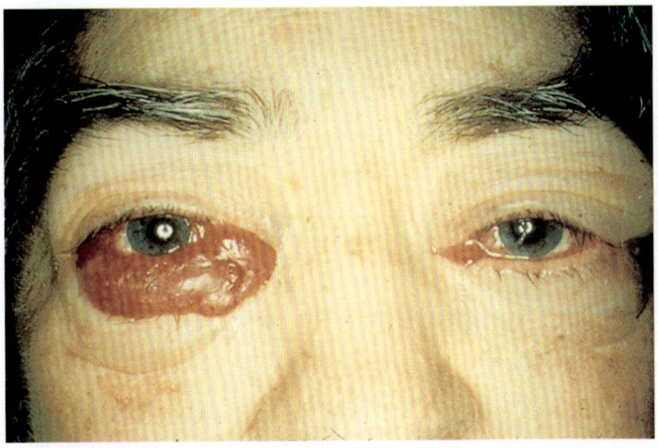

FIGURE 14.11 Proptosis and chemosis in a direct, high-flow, right carotid cavernous fistula following trauma. (Courtesy N. Schatz. Reprinted from Gold DH, MD, and Weingeist TA, MD, PhD. *Color Atlas of the Eye in Systemic Disease.* Baltimore: Lippincott Williams & Wilkins, 2001, with permission.)

Intraorbital varicosities may cause intermittent, positional exophthalmos because of decreased venous return in certain head postures. Pulsatile proptosis may occur with an orbital vascular malformation or when there is a defect in the orbital roof that transmits cerebral pulsations, which can occur in neurofibromatosis. Diplopia can occur in conditions where the movement of the eyeball is restricted. Pseudoproptosis is the appearance of proptosis in the absence of any orbital disease; it may occur with lid retraction or high myopia.

Few conditions of neurologic interest cause enophthalmos. Horner's syndrome causes apparent enophthalmos because the upper lid is ptotic and the lower lid elevated because of hypotonicity of the accessory eyelid retractors. This may cause the eye to appear sunken in the orbit, but it is an optical illusion and the actual globe position is normal.

THE EYELIDS

Patients may couch the complaint of ptosis (blepharoptosis) in ways other than droopy eyelid (e.g., eye has shrunk). Fluctuating ptosis may suggest myasthenia gravis (MG), although many varieties of ptosis, as in Horner's syndrome, may get worse when the patient is fatigued. Ptosis may have been present for a very long time before coming to the patient's attention. Looking at old photographs is often helpful. The eyes on a driver's license photo can be seen quite well by using the ophthalmoscope on magnification.

The position of the eyelids is important and can reveal significant information. Note the position of the eyelids and the width of the palpebral fissures bilaterally. The width of the palpebral fissures should be equal on both sides, although a slight difference occurs in many normal individuals. Any asymmetry of lid position should be noted, such as ptosis or lid retraction. Note the amount of iris or pupil covered by the lid. Patients may compensate for ptosis by contracting the frontalis muscle. If the examiner fixes the frontalis muscle with her finger, the patient may be unable to raise the eyelid. Ptosis may cause an artefactual superior altitudinal visual field defect that disappears when the eyelid is raised.

The normal upper eyelid in primary position crosses the iris between the limbus (junction of the iris and sclera) and the pupil, usually 1 to 2 mm below the limbus; the lower lid touches or crosses slightly above the limbus. Normally, there is no sclera showing above the iris. The palpebral fissures are normally 9 to 12 mm from upper to lower lid margin at the midpoint. Measurement can also be made from the lid margin to the corneal light reflex. The upper lid margin is normally 3 to 4 mm above the light reflex. Levator function can be assessed by measuring the upper lid excursion from full downgaze to full upgaze just to the point where the frontalis begins to contract. This excursion is typically 10 to 12 mm. Upper lid excursion of 4 mm or less indicates poor levator function; 8 mm or more indicates good function.

With ptosis, the lid droops down and may cross at the upper margin of the pupil or cover the pupil partially or totally. With complete ptosis, the eyelid is down and the eye appears closed (Figure 14.12). Patients with ptosis often display telltale wrinkling of the ipsilateral forehead as they attempt to hold the eye open using the frontalis muscle. Ptosis may be unilateral or bilateral, partial or complete, and occurs in many neurologic conditions (Figure 14.13). With eyelid retraction, the upper lid pulls back and frequently exposes a thin crescent of sclera between the upper limbus and the lower lid margin. Lid retraction is a classic sign of thyroid disease but occurs in neurologic disorders as well.

The width of the palpebral fissures is normally equal on the two sides. Sometimes, inequality results from subtle lid retraction or a widened palpebral fissure on one side, not to be confused with ptosis on the other side. When in doubt, measure the width of the palpebral fissures with a ruler, in both primary position and in upgaze. In addition to observing the

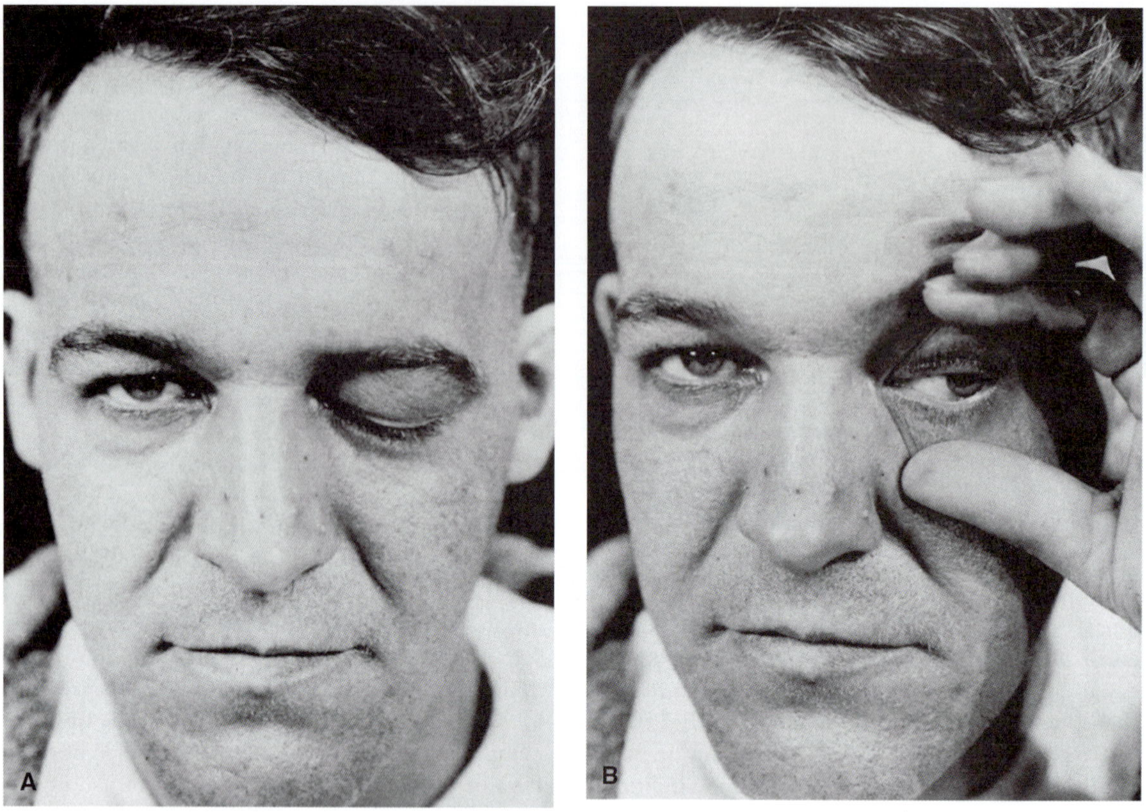

FIGURE 14.12 Paralysis of the left oculomotor nerve in a patient with an aneurysm of the left internal carotid artery. **A.** Only ptosis can be seen. **B.** On elevating the eyelid, it is seen that the pupil is dilated and the eyeball is deviated laterally.

lid position at rest, notice the relationships of the lid to the globe during eye movement. CN VII, via contraction of the orbicularis oculi, closes the eye. Facial weakness never causes ptosis. In fact, the palpebral fissure on the weak side is often wider than normal, and unilateral widening of one palpebral fissure may be an early sign of facial palsy.

Total unilateral ptosis only occurs with complete third nerve palsy. Mild to moderate unilateral ptosis occurs as part of Horner's syndrome, or with partial third nerve palsy. Ptosis may rarely be the only manifestation of an oculomotor nerve palsy. Mild to moderate bilateral ptosis occurs in some neuromuscular disorders, such as MG, muscular dystrophy, or ocular myopathy. The ptosis in MG is frequently asymmetric and may be unilateral, though it will tend to shift from side to side (Figure 14.14). It characteristically fluctuates from moment to moment and is worsened by prolonged upgaze (fatigable ptosis). Cogan's lid twitch sign, characteristic of myasthenia, consists of a brief overshoot twitch of lid retraction following sudden return of the eyes to primary position after a period of downgaze (see **Video Link 14.1**). In a series of 117 patients, the specificity of the lid twitch sign was 99%, the sensitivity was 75%, and the false-positive rate was 1%. A similar upward twitch may occur on glancing quickly to the side from primary position (eyelid hopping). When the ptosis is asymmetric, the driving discharges attempting to keep the more ptotic eyelid open are also transmitted, per Hering's law, to the less ptotic eyelid. Manually raising the more ptotic lid causes relaxation, and the eye with less ptosis, sometimes even no ptosis, may suddenly crash (curtain sign, seesaw ptosis, enhanced ptosis, see **Video Link 14.2**). Because of the law of equal innervation, compensation for mild ptosis on one side may cause the involved eye to appear normal and the other eye to have lid retraction. Ptosis in MG may respond dramatically to edrophonium (Figure 14.15, also see *Bilateral Ptosis* from Dr. Shirley Wray,

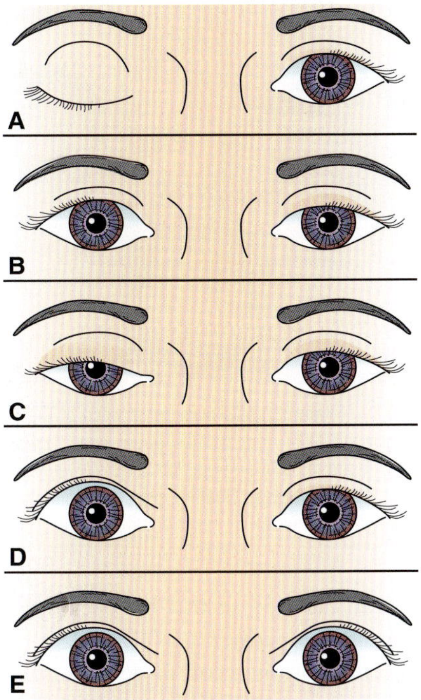

FIGURE 14.13 Characteristics of different causes of abnormal lid position. **A.** Right third CN palsy with complete ptosis. **B.** Left Horner's syndrome with drooping of upper lid and slight elevation of lower lid. **C.** Bilateral, asymmetric ptosis in myasthenia gravis (MG). **D.** Right lid retraction in thyroid eye disease. **E.** Bilateral lid retraction with a lesion in the region of the posterior commissure (Collier's sign).

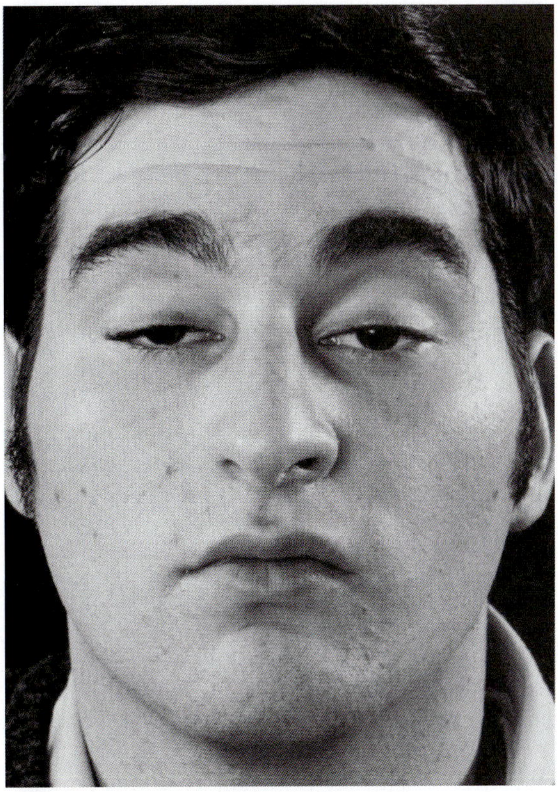

FIGURE 14.14 Bilateral ptosis in a patient with MG.

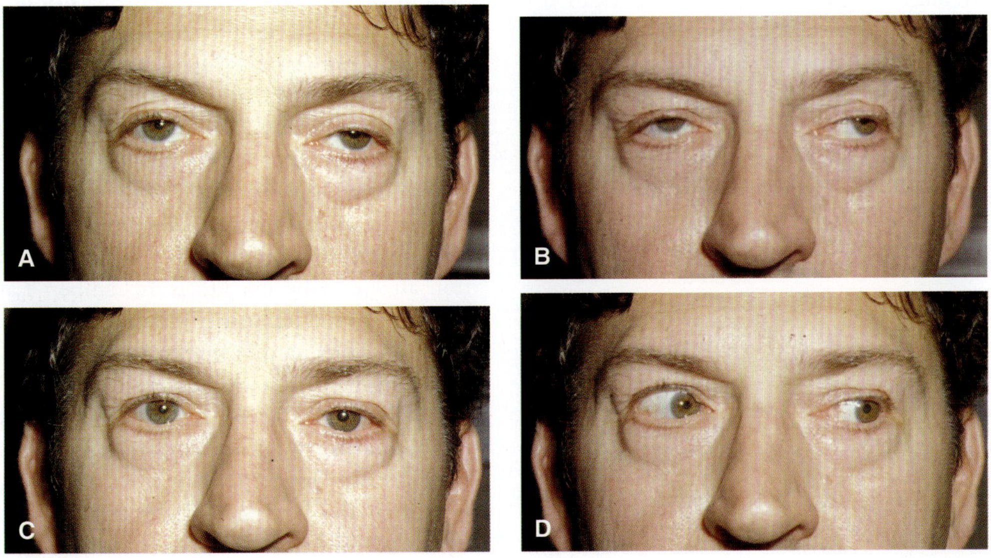

FIGURE 14.15 Results of a Tensilon (edrophonium chloride) test in a 34-year-old man with recent onset of ptosis and diplopia. **A.** The patient has bilateral ptosis, left more than right. Note also bilateral inferior scleral show from laxity of the lower eyelids. **B.** The patient can adduct the right eye only to the midline when attempting to look to the left (pseudointernuclear ophthalmoplegia). **C.** One minute after intravenous injection of 2 mg of Tensilon, the patient's ptosis has markedly improved and the inferior scleral show has resolved. **D.** At the same time, the patient's right eye adduction has become full. (Reprinted from Miller NR, Subramanian PS, Patel VR. *Walsh and Hoyt's Clinical Neuro-ophthalmology: The Essentials.* 3rd ed. Philadelphia: Wolters Kluwer, 2016, with permission).

Neuro-ophthalmology Virtual Education Library [NOVEL], University of Utah, **Video Link 14.3**).

Cerebral ptosis is due to supranuclear lesions. Unilateral cerebral ptosis occurs with lesions, usually ischemic, of the opposite hemisphere, and is more common with right hemisphere lesions. Bilateral supranuclear ptosis may occur with unilateral or bilateral hemispheric lesions. Ptosis has been reported in as many as 37.5% of patients with hemispheric strokes. Because of the anatomy of the central caudal nucleus, bilateral ptosis can occur as the only ocular motility abnormality with some midbrain lesions.

Senile or involutional ptosis is very common. Asymmetric lids and redundant lid tissue are more the rule than the exception in the elderly. The levator aponeurosis attaches the levator muscle to the tarsal plate, which forms the eyelid. The lid crease, or upper lid fold, is the skin fold at the upper part of the lid at the site of levator insertion. Aging may cause levator dehiscence-disinsertion (LDD)—with stretching, thinning, or detachment of the aponeurosis. Normally, with the eyelids gently closed, the upper lid margin lies 5 to 7 mm below the lid crease. An increase in this distance suggests LDD (Figures 14.16 and 14.17). The lid excursion is normal, usually 9 mm or more. Trauma to the eyelid, as from contact lenses, may cause LDD in younger patients. Blepharochalasis (dermatochalasis) refers to age-related lax, baggy skin around the eyelids; it can also simulate ptosis but levator function is normal. Other nonneurologic conditions that may be confused with ptosis include blepharitis, lid edema, lid infiltration, and eyelid tumor. Patients with neurofibromatosis may have diffuse neurofibroma in the eyelid, causing a characteristic S-shaped lid. Chronic use of steroid

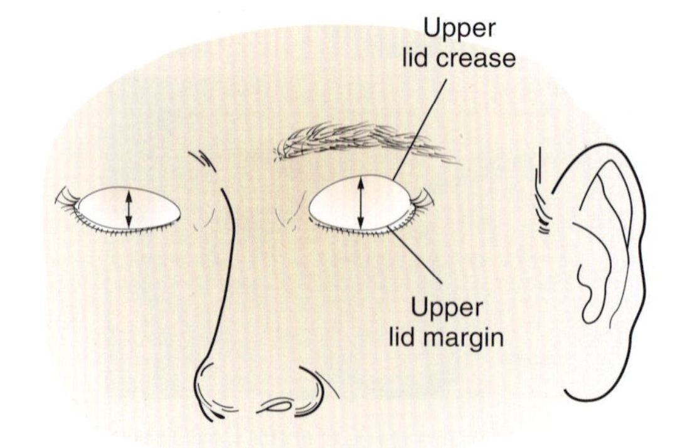

FIGURE 14.16 Levator dehiscence disinsertion on the left. The distance between the upper lid margin and the upper lid crease is increased compared to the normal right side.

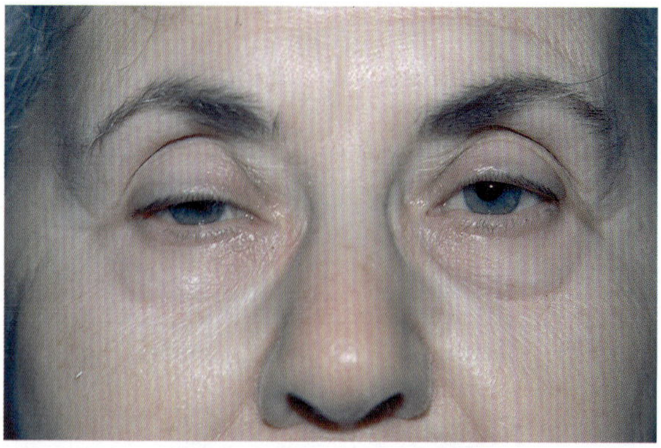

FIGURE 14.17 Bilateral ptosis from dehiscence of the levator aponeurosis. Note the high, very defined upper eyelid crease. Levator function was 18 mm. (Reprinted from Penne RB. *Oculoplastics*. 2nd ed. Philadelphia: Wolters Kluwer Health/Lippincott Williams & Wilkins Health, 2012, with permission.)

eye drops can cause ptosis that has been attributed to a focal steroid myopathy.

Congenital ptosis is common; because of levator fibrosis, it may be associated with lid lag in downgaze that is unusual in acquired ptosis. Jaw winking (Marcus Gunn phenomenon, for R. Marcus Gunn, Scottish ophthalmologist) occurs when there is congenital ptosis with abnormal communication between CN V and the levator palpebrae. The ptotic lid opens with jaw movement (see Chapter 15). Synkinesia between CN V and the levator more rarely causes ptosis on mouth opening (inverse Marcus Gunn phenomenon). Marin Amat syndrome is a facial nerve aberrant innervation syndrome with levator inhibition with mouth opening (see Chapter 16). Orbicularis oculi contraction causing eye closure on smiling is another common synkinesia. Eyelid myotonia may cause transient difficulty opening the eyes after a forceful contraction or transient lid retraction after looking up. Ptosis in Lambert-Eaton syndrome may temporarily improve after a brief period of upgaze. Blepharospasm is a focal dystonia causing involuntary eye closure; levator function is normal. In apraxia of lid opening, the patient has difficulty in voluntarily initiating lid elevation although there is no levator impairment or blepharospasm. A fine tremor of the lid (Rosenbach's sign) may occur in hyperthyroidism.

Pseudoptosis is the appearance of ptosis in the absence of levator abnormality. A narrow palpebral fissure can occur because of mechanical limitation of levator excursion or enophthalmos. In vertical strabismus with the hypertropic eye fixing, the lid of the hypotropic eye may seem to be ptotic, but is not. In Duane's syndrome (Box 14.9), the palpebral fissure narrows on ocular adduction because of globe retraction causing dynamic enophthalmos (see *Type I Duane's syndrome* from Dr. Kathleen B. Digre, John A. Moran Eye Center, Neuro-ophthalmology Virtual Education Library [NOVEL], University of Utah, **Video Link 14.4**). The eyelids may also be intrinsically abnormal because of inflammation, trauma, or other factors, and these lid disorders may be mistaken for ptosis. Nonorganic ptosis is rare; it can occur because of voluntary unilateral blepharospasm. A telltale clue is that there is contraction of the orbicularis oculi or relaxation of the eyebrow elevators causing brow ptosis in addition to the appearance of lid ptosis.

Lid Retraction

Lid position is abnormal if there is a rim of sclera showing above the limbus, indicating either lid retraction or lid lag. TED is a common cause of lid abnormalities, including lid retraction in primary gaze (Dalrymple's sign), infrequent blinking (Stellwag's sign), and lid lag in downgaze (von Graefe's sign). Lid retraction in primary gaze also occurs with lesions involving the posterior commissure (Collier's sign, posterior fossa stare; see discussion of Parinaud's syndrome). Lid retraction with posterior commissure lesions is bilateral but may be asymmetric. With Collier's sign, the levators relax appropriately and the lids usually descend normally on downgaze without lagging behind as they do in TED. In addition, the lid retraction may worsen with attempted upgaze (Figure 14.18). Circumscribed midbrain lesions may cause eyelid retraction with minimal impairment of vertical gaze.

In Parkinson's disease, there is infrequent blinking and there may be some lid retraction. Topical instillation of sympathomimetic agents may cause lid retraction. Very weak sympathomimetics (e.g., tetrahydrozoline) may cause the lid with denervation supersensitivity, as in Horner's syndrome, to elevate. Apraclonidine may also improve the ptosis (see below). In vertical strabismus, the lid of the hypertropic eye may appear to be retracted when the hypotropic eye is fixing. Aberrant regeneration of CN III may cause lid retraction on adduction (the opposite of Duane's syndrome) or on downgaze. Lid retraction may also be mechanical, because of trauma or surgery. The plus minus lid syndrome is ptosis on one side and lid retraction on the other because of a unilateral lesion of the third nerve nucleus extending rostrally to involve the region of the posterior commissure. Lid retraction may be confused with ipsilateral proptosis or contralateral ptosis.

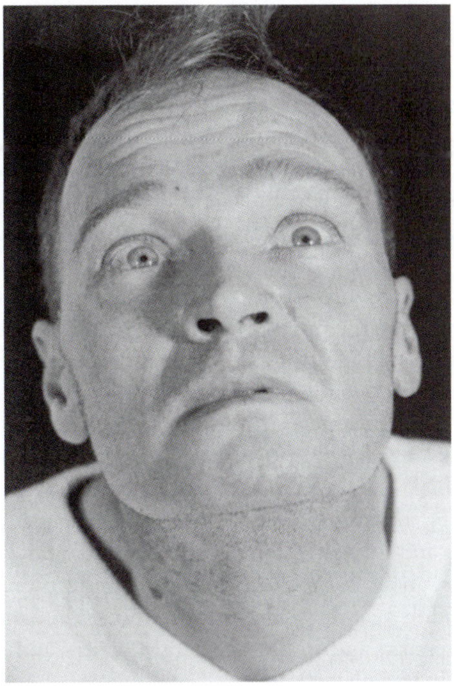

FIGURE 14.18 Paresis of upward gaze and lid retraction in a patient with a neoplasm of the posterior third ventricle.

The Pupils

The function of the pupil is to control the amount of light entering the eye, ensuring optimal vision for the lighting conditions. The pupils should be equal in size, round, regular, centered in the iris, and should exhibit specific reflex responses. Large, small, and abnormally reactive pupils are discussed in this section. Normal pupils may display constant, small amplitude fluctuations in size under constant illumination (hippus, pupillary play). Hippus is of no clinical significance, even when pronounced, but can cause confusion in the evaluation of an afferent pupillary defect (APD) (see discussion of afferent pupillary defect).

Pupil examination should first assess pupillary size and equality. If they are unequal, determine whether the difference is greater in light or darkness. Compare the pupillary reactions to light and to near. Assess whether the pupils constrict and redilate with the same velocity. Finally, determine whether an APD is present.

Size

Pupillary size depends primarily on the balance between sympathetic and parasympathetic innervation and the level of ambient illumination. The most important determinants are the level of illumination and the point at which the eyes are focused. Accurate measurements are important. Measurements should be made with a pupil gauge or a millimeter ruler; estimates are surprisingly inaccurate. Special cameras can measure the pupil to within 0.1 mm. The size of the pupils should be determined at distance in ambient and dim light and at near. The normal pupil is 2 to 6 mm in diameter. In ordinary ambient light, the pupils are usually 3 to 4 mm in diameter. The pupils are small and poorly reactive at birth and in early infancy, becoming normal size around ages 7 to 8. They are normally larger in adolescents and young adults, about 4 mm in diameter and perfectly round. In middle age, they are typically 3.5 mm in diameter and regular, and in old age 3 mm or less and often slightly irregular.

Pupils less than 2 mm in diameter are miotic. Common causes of acquired miosis include old age, hyperopia, alcohol abuse, and drug effects. Neurologically significant causes of miosis include neurosyphilis, diabetes, levodopa therapy, and Horner's syndrome. Acute, severe brainstem lesions, such as pontine hematoma, may cause bilaterally tiny, "pinpoint" pupils that still react. Primary ophthalmologic conditions commonly cause miosis when there is external eye disease. Spastic or irritative miosis is due to spasm of the pupillary sphincter, often in association with corneal or intraocular foreign bodies or eye trauma. Other ophthalmologic disorders causing miosis include iridocyclitis, miotic drops, spasm of the near reflex, chronic anterior segment ischemia, and an old Adie's pupil. Synechia are adhesions that may develop in the eye, usually after inflammation such as iritis. The scarring may bind the pupil down to the cornea (anterior synechia) or lens (posterior synechia) and cause miosis and pupillary irregularity. Paralytic miosis is due to paralysis of the pupillary dilator muscle (oculosympathetic paresis).

Pupils more than 6 mm in diameter are dilated. Common causes of bilateral mydriasis include anxiety, fear, pain, myopia, and drug effects—especially anticholinergics. Large pupils were once considered a sign of youth and beauty, and the anticholinergic belladonna (Ital. "fair lady") alkaloids were named for their ability to produce this effect. Persons with light irises have larger pupils than those with dark irises. Only severe, bilateral lesions of the retina or anterior visual pathways, enough to cause near blindness, will affect the resting pupil size. Neurologically significant bilateral mydriasis occurs in midbrain lesions, in comatose patients following cardiac arrest, in cerebral anoxia, and as a terminal condition.

Shape

The normal pupil is round, with a smooth, regular outline. Gross abnormalities in shape are usually the result of ocular disease such as iritis or eye surgery. Synechia, a congenital coloboma (a gap in the iris), prior trauma, or iridectomy may all cause pupil irregularity. A slight change in shape, however, such as an oval pupil, slight irregularity in outline, serration of the border, or slight notching, may be significant in the diagnosis of neurologic disease.

Equality

The pupils are generally of equal size. A difference of 0.25 mm in pupil size is noticeable, and a difference of 2 mm is considered significant. Physiologic anisocoria (aniso, "unequal"; cor, "pupil"), mild degrees of inequality with less than 1 mm of difference between the two sides, occurs in 15% to 20% of normal individuals. With such physiologic anisocoria, the degree of inequality remains about the same in light and dark, and the pupils react normally to all stimuli and to instilled drugs (Figures 14.19 and 14.20). Slightly greater asymmetry in the dark sometimes occurs with physiologic anisocoria. Unequal pupils may be caused by primary eye disorders, such as iritis. Unilateral mydriasis is never due to isolated, unilateral visual loss. The reactivity of the normal eye and the consensual light reflex will ensure that pupil size remains equal. Anisocoria may result from damage to the iris sphincter or pupillodilator muscles or to their nerve supply. Unilateral mydriasis can occur with local ocular trauma (traumatic iridoplegia).

Position

The pupil is normally situated in the center of the iris. An eccentric pupil (corectopia) usually signifies local eye disease, but it can occur with neurologic disease, especially disorders of the midbrain.

Etiologic Factor	Ambient Light		Strong Light		Dark		Conclusion
Physiologic anisocoria	•	●	•	●	●	⬤	Same relative asymmetry under all conditions
Right Horner syndrome	•	●	•	•	•	●	More asymmetry in the dark; abnormal pupil can not dilate
Left third cranial nerve palsy	•	●	•	●	⬤	⬤	More asymmetry in the light; abnormal pupil cannot constrict

FIGURE 14.19 Behavior of unequal pupils in light and dark conditions.

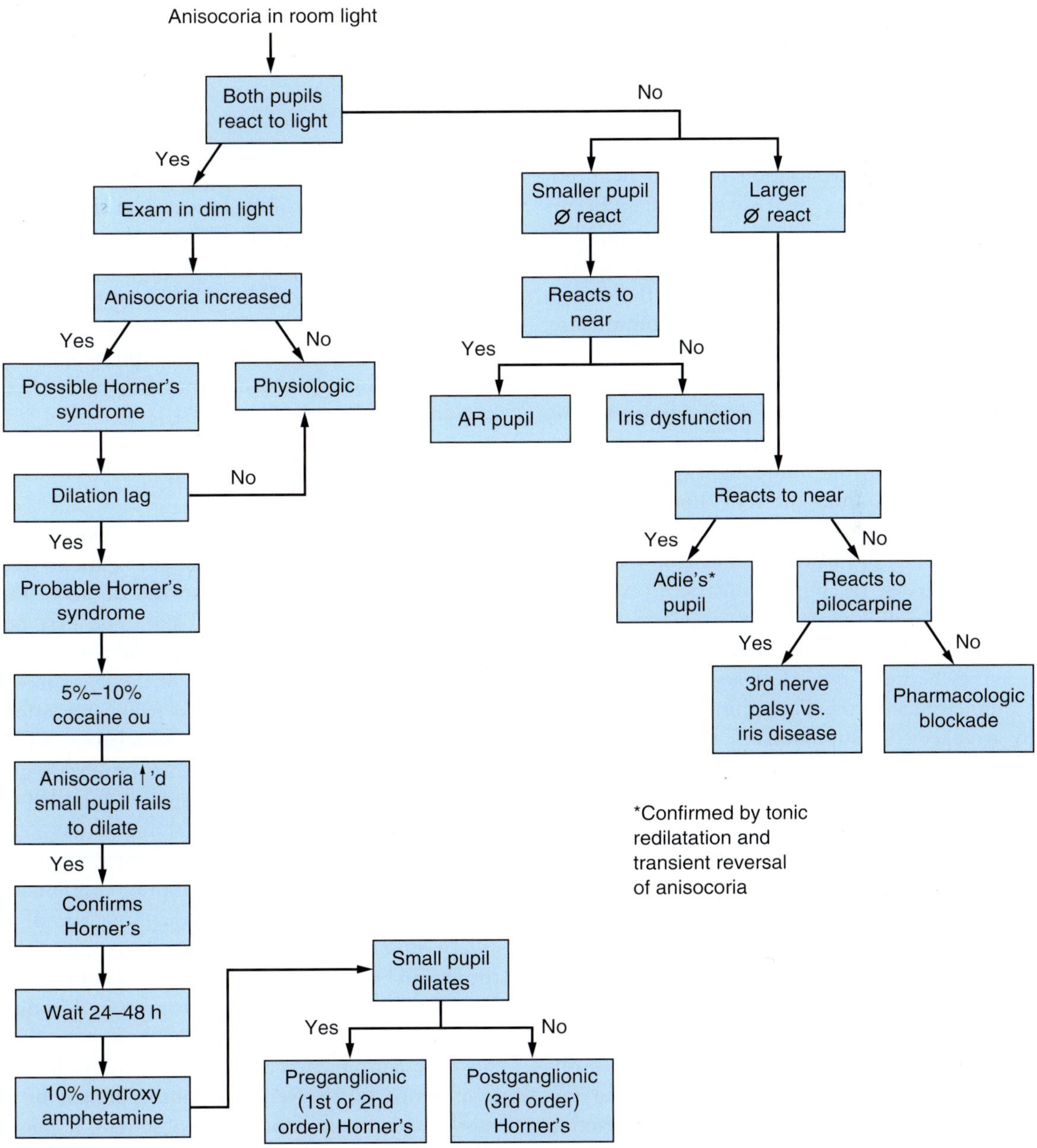

FIGURE 14.20 Flow diagram for the evaluation of anisocoria.

The Pupillary Reflexes

The principal pupillary reflex responses assessed on examination are the light response and the near response ("accommodation"). The normal pupil constricts promptly in response to light. Pupillary constriction also occurs as part of the near response, along with convergence and rounding up of the lens for efficient near vision. Normally, the light and near responses are of the same magnitude.

The Light Reflex

The pupillary light reaction is mediated by the macula, optic nerve, chiasm, and optic tract. Before reaching the lateral geniculate body, pupil afferents leave the optic tract to synapse in the pretectum. In addition to the decussation of nasal hemiretinal pupillary afferents, extensive crossing occurs through the posterior commissure with pupillary afferents synapsing both ipsilaterally and contralaterally. Because of the decussation in the chiasm and the decussation in the posterior commissure, pupillary fibers are extensively commingled and the reflex is bilateral, both direct and consensual (crossed) (Figure 13.9). Fibers project from the pretectum to the EW subnucleus of the oculomotor nuclear complex in the midbrain. Parasympathetic pupillary efferents from the EW subnucleus enter the third nerve and travel through the cavernous sinus and along the inferior branch of III in the orbit to innervate the pupilloconstrictor muscle of the iris. The pupillomotor fibers travel to the ciliary ganglion, then through the short posterior ciliary nerves between the sclera and the choroid to the pupillary sphincter. The sphincter is concentrically arranged; the pupillodilator muscle is radially arranged. Balancing parasympathetic input from the EW subnucleus is sympathetic input ascending from the superior cervical ganglion.

The light reflex should be tested in each eye individually. The examining light should be shone into the eye obliquely with the patient fixing at distance to avoid eliciting a confounding near response. A common error in pupil examination is to have the patient fixing at near, as by instructing her to look at the examiner's nose. This technique provides both a light stimulus and a near stimulus simultaneously, and the pupils may well constrict to the near target of the examiner's nose even when the reaction to light is impaired or absent. Using this technique, the examiner would invariably miss light-near dissociation. Always have the patient fix at a distance when checking the pupillary light reaction. Having the patient look up while directing the light forward to move the corneal light reflex away from the axis of the pupil may help to visualize the pupils in very dark irides. Another technique is to use ambient light by covering the eyes, then withdrawing the cover alternately, and looking for pupil constriction. The normal pupillary light reflex is brisk constriction followed by slight dilatation back to an intermediate state (pupillary escape). Escape may occur because of adaptation of the visual system to the level of illumination. The responses may be noted as prompt, sluggish, or absent, graded from 0 to 4+, or measured and recorded numerically (e.g., 4 mm → 2 mm). In comatose patients, it is often important, but difficult, to see if the pupillary light reaction is preserved, especially if there is a question of brain death. A useful technique is to use the ophthalmoscope: focus on the pupil with high positive magnification, dim the ophthalmoscope, and then rapidly reilluminate. Even a small residual reaction may be seen. Obliquely illuminating the pupil by holding a dim light source to the side may help evaluate the consensual light reflex.

The Accommodation Reflex

The accommodation reflex (near response, near reflex) is elicited by having the patient relax accommodation by gazing into the distance, then shifting gaze to some near object. The best near object is the patient's own finger or thumb. The response consists of thickening of the lens (accommodation), convergence of the eyes, and miosis. The primary stimulus for accommodation is blurring. Without the near response, attempting to focus on a close object would result in blurred vision or frank diplopia. With special techniques, each component of the response can be tested separately. Routine bedside testing elicits all three components. Accommodation occurs because contraction of the ciliary muscle relaxes the zonular fibers, permitting the lens to become more convex because of its inherent elasticity. Accommodation is measured in diopters (Box 14.1).

The convergence movement of the near reflex is mediated by the vergence subcomponent of the supranuclear ocular motor control system. It consists of a long latency, slow dysconjugate eye movement

BOX 14.1

Myopia and Hyperopia

The near point of accommodation (NPA) is the closest point at which an object can be seen clearly. The NPA lengthens distressingly with advancing presbyopia. The far point of accommodation (FPA) is the distance at which a distant image is focused on the retina with no accommodative effort. An emmetrope (person with a perfectly normal eye) has an FPA of infinity, and distant objects are properly focused on the fovea. In hyperopia (farsightedness, hypermetropia), the eyeball is too short, the FPA is behind the eye, accommodation can bring far objects into focus but may fail with near objects, and the correction is with positive lenses to add refractive power. In myopia (nearsightedness), the eyeball is too long or refractive power is excessive, the FPA falls in front of the fovea, relaxation of accommodation can bring near objects into focus but fails for distant objects, and the correction is with negative lenses to reduce refractive power. To quickly tell if a patient who uses correction has hyperopia or myopia, use the patient's glasses to look at some object about an arm's length away. Hyperopic glasses magnify, myopic lenses minify.

to foveate the near object by contracting both medial rectus muscles. Convergence spasm causes excessive convergence for the distance of the object, and the patient cannot focus at distance. Convergence insufficiency causes inadequate convergence, and the patient cannot focus at near.

The pupils constrict at near to increase the depth of focus. The pathways are less certain than for the pupillary light reflex, but they involve the visual cortex with impulses probably descending through the corticotectal tract to near response cells in the pretectum. The midbrain mechanisms for pupillary constriction to near are separate from those for the light reflex; one response may be abnormal, whereas the other is preserved.

Other Pupillary Reflexes

The ciliospinal reflex consists of dilation of the pupil on painful stimulation of the skin of the ipsilateral neck. Local cutaneous stimulation (e.g., scratching the neck) activates sympathetics through connections with the ciliospinal center at C8-T2 that cause the ipsilateral pupil to dilate. An intact ciliospinal reflex is evidence of brainstem integrity when evaluating a comatose patient. The response is minimal and may be difficult to see even when normal. The oculosensory or oculopupillary reflex is pupil constriction in response to painful stimulation of the eye or its adnexa. The pupils normally constrict on attempted lid closure. Pupil dilation may occur in response to a loud noise (cochleopupillary reflex) or labyrinthine stimulation (vestibulopupillary reflex). The pupils may dilate in response to fear, anxiety, mental concentration, and sexual arousal because of sympathetic activity.

Effects of Drugs on the Pupil

Many systemically acting as well as locally acting drugs may influence pupil size and reactivity. An abnormal pupil may fail to respond appropriately or respond excessively because of denervation supersensitivity. Pupil pharmacology is complex. In brief, sympathomimetics and anticholinergics cause pupillary dilation, and parasympathomimetics or sympathetic blockers cause pupillary constriction. Agents that cause mydriasis include the anticholinergics atropine, homatropine, and scopolamine and the sympathomimetics epinephrine, norepinephrine, phenylephrine, hydroxyamphetamine, and cocaine. Agents that cause miosis include the cholinomimetics pilocarpine, methacholine, muscarine, and opiates, and the cholinesterase inhibitors physostigmine and neostigmine. Ergot derivatives block postganglionic adrenergic nerves and can cause pupil constriction. Pupillary pharmacology can be applied in the neurologic examination, primarily in the evaluation of Horner's syndrome and Adie's pupil (see Table 14.1).

TABLE 14.1 Summary of Pharmacologic Pupillary Testing for Horner's Syndrome

	First Order	Second Order	Third Order
Cocaine	No response	No response	No response
Hydroxyamphetamine	Dilates	Dilates	No response

DISORDERS OF THE PUPIL

Pupils can be abnormal for numerous reasons. Common problems include pupils that are too large or too small, unilaterally or bilaterally, or pupils that fail to demonstrate normal reflex responses.

Large Pupils

The two conditions most commonly causing a unilaterally large pupil are third CN palsy and Adie's pupil. In CN III palsy, the large pupil has impaired reactions to light and to near; abnormalities of extraocular movement and eyelid position generally betray the origin of the abnormal pupil. With total CN III palsy, there is complete ptosis; lifting the eyelid reveals the eye resting in a down and out position (Figure 14.12). Although CN III palsies often affect the pupil more than other functions, some ptosis and ophthalmoparesis is usually present. Because the pupillary parasympathetics occupy a position on the dorsomedial periphery of the nerve as it exits the brainstem, compressive lesions such as aneurysms generally affect the pupil prominently. Ischemic lesions tend to affect the interior of the nerve and spare the pupil, as in diabetic third nerve palsies, because the periphery of the nerve has a better vascular supply. This rule is not absolute: pupil-sparing third nerve palsies have been reported with aneurysms (in up to 10% of cases), as have diabetic palsies involving the pupil. In Keane's series of 1,400 patients, 53% of diabetic CN III palsies involved the pupil, but only 2% of aneurysms spared the pupil. In diabetics, pupil abnormalities were often bilateral, suggesting autonomic neuropathy. However, only rarely does a complete aneurysmal third nerve palsy spare the pupil. When the pupil is spared, some other functions are usually spared as well. Barton summarized the correct "pupil rule" as follows: complete pupil sparing with otherwise complete and isolated palsy of CN III is never due to an aneurysm. The pupil is usually involved early and prominently with third nerve compression because of uncal herniation (Hutchinson's pupil).

When the ocular sympathetics are involved along with CN III, the pupil may be midposition because the sympathetic denervation prevents the pupil from dilating fully. This occurs most often in cavernous sinus lesions when there is compression of both CN III and the pericarotid sympathetics, leaving the pupil midsize but unreactive. This should not be mistaken for pupil sparing. CN III palsies are sometimes complicated by aberrant reinnervation. This misdirection syndrome may cause abnormal pupil constriction in relation to eye movements that may mimic pupil sparing.

The patient presenting with Adie's pupil (tonic pupil, Holmes-Adie pupil) is typically a young woman who suddenly notes a unilaterally enlarged pupil, with no other symptoms. The pupillary reaction to light may appear absent, although prolonged illumination may provoke a slow constriction. The reaction to near, although slow, is better preserved. Once constricted, the tonic pupil redilates very slowly when illumination is removed or the patient looks back at distance, often causing a transient reversal of the anisocoria. The pathology in Adie's pupil lies in the ciliary ganglion or short ciliary nerves, or both; its precise nature remains unknown. The parasympathetic denervation eventually leads to denervation supersensitivity; the pupil may then constrict to solutions of pilocarpine or methacholine that are too dilute to affect a normal eye. About 20% of patients develop a tonic pupil in the other eye. Adie's syndrome is the association of the pupil abnormality with depressed or absent deep tendon reflexes, particularly in the lower extremities. With the passage of time, the pupil may become smaller. An old Adie's pupil can be a cause of unilateral miosis. The light reaction never recovers.

The term "tectal pupils" refers to the large pupils with light-near dissociation sometimes seen when lesions affect the upper midbrain. Such pupils may accompany the impaired upgaze and convergence/retraction nystagmus of Parinaud's syndrome. The variably dilated, fixed pupils reflecting midbrain dysfunction in a comatose patient carry a bleak prognosis. Glutethimide intoxication, infamous for causing fixed pupils in drug-induced coma, has fortunately become rare. Acute angle closure glaucoma can cause severe frontotemporal headache and a dilated, poorly reactive pupil. A cloudy cornea may provide the clue that the patient does not harbor an aneurysm and needs to quickly see an ophthalmologist rather than a neurologist or a neurosurgeon. Deliberately or accidentally instilled mydriatics will produce a dilated, fixed pupil. Such pharmacologic blockade can be distinguished by the failure to respond to full strength pilocarpine, which promptly constricts a large pupil of any other etiology.

Small Pupils

The pupils in the elderly are normally smaller. Many older patients use pilocarpine eye drops to manage chronic open angle glaucoma. Many systemic drugs, such as opiates, may symmetrically shrink the pupils. Important neurologic conditions causing an abnormally small pupil include Horner's syndrome and neurosyphilis.

HORNER'S SYNDROME

In Horner's syndrome, sympathetic dysfunction produces ptosis, miosis, and anhidrosis. Lack of sympathetic input to the accessory lid retractors results in ptosis and apparent enophthalmos. The ptosis of the upper lid due to denervation of Müller's muscle is only 1 to 3 mm, never as severe as with a complete CN III palsy, although it may simulate partial third nerve palsy. The ptosis can be subtle and is often missed. The lower lid is frequently elevated 1 to 2 mm because of loss of the action of the lower lid accessory retractor that holds the lid down (inverse ptosis). The resulting narrowing of the palpebral fissure causes apparent enophthalmos. Because the fibers mediating facial sweating travel up the external carotid, lesions distal to the carotid bifurcation produce no facial anhidrosis except for perhaps a small area of medial forehead that is innervated by sympathetic fibers traveling with the internal carotid.

The small pupil dilates poorly in the dark. Pupillary asymmetry greater in the dark than in the light generally means Horner's syndrome. Recall that physiologic anisocoria produces about the same degree of pupillary asymmetry in the light and dark. In contrast, third nerve palsy and Adie's pupil cause greater asymmetry in the light because of the involved pupil's inability to constrict. Examining the eyes under light and dark conditions can help greatly in sorting out asymmetric pupils (Figures 14.19 and 14.20). Should the examiner err by having the patient fixate at near during testing, the pupillary constriction in the good eye may lessen the asymmetry and cause the abnormal pupil to be missed. The pupil in Horner's syndrome not only dilates less fully but also dilates less rapidly. In the first few seconds after dimming the lights, the slowness of dilation of the affected pupil may cause the anisocoria to be even more pronounced (dilation lag). There is more anisocoria at 4 to 5 seconds after lights out than at 10 to 12 seconds.

The causes of Horner's syndrome are legion and include the following: brainstem lesions (especially of the lateral medulla), cluster headache, internal carotid artery thrombosis or dissection, cavernous sinus disease, apical lung tumors, neck trauma, and other conditions (Figure 14.21). Horner's syndrome may be an isolated manifestation of syringomyelia. The tiny and minimally reactive pupils seen commonly in pontine hemorrhage may represent acute, severe, bilateral oculosympathetic paresis. The rare condition of reverse Horner's syndrome (Pourfour du Petit syndrome) is unilateral mydriasis, sometimes with facial flushing and hyperhidrosis, because of transient sympathetic overactivity in the early stages of a lesion involving the sympathetic pathways to one eye. In Harlequin syndrome, there is unilateral facial anhidrosis with contralateral flushing and sweating, induced by exercise, heat, and emotion. The condition is usually idiopathic but can occur as a manifestation of serious underlying disorders including brainstem infarction and carotid artery dissection. There are no eye findings.

Pharmacologic testing is occasionally done to help determine whether a miotic pupil is due to Horner's syndrome. In about half the patients with Horner's syndrome, the etiology is apparent from other signs and the history. In the other half, clinical localization is uncertain; pharmacologic testing may help determine the level of the lesion and guide further investigations. Interruption of the sympathetic pathways between the hypothalamus and the spinal cord (e.g., Wallenberg syndrome) causes a first-order Horner's syndrome. The second-order neuron lies

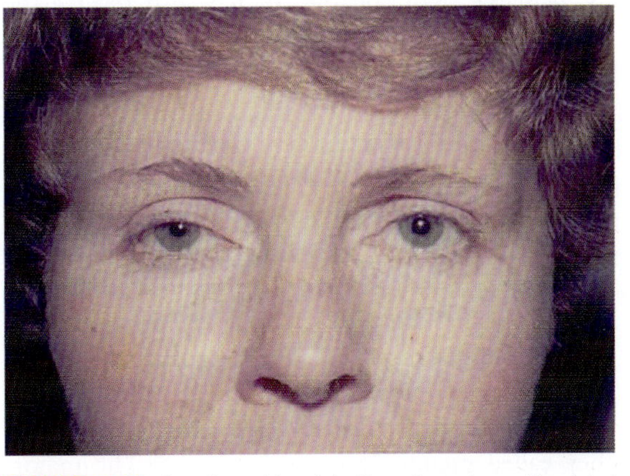

FIGURE 14.21 A patient with a right Horner's syndrome. (Reprinted from Campbell WW. *Clinical Signs in Neurology: A Compendium.* Philadelphia: Wolters Kluwer, 2016, with permission.)

in the ciliospinal center at C8-T2. A lesion involving this portion of the pathway (e.g., syringomyelia, C8 root lesion) causes a second-order Horner's syndrome. The third-order neuron lies in the superior sympathetic ganglion; a lesion at or distal to here (e.g., carotid artery dissection) causes a third-order Horner's syndrome. With a third-order Horner's, the final neuron in the pathway dies and its peripheral processes atrophy and disappear. With first- and second-order Horner's syndrome, the third-order neuron is disconnected but intact, and its terminal connections sound and viable.

Cocaine drops instilled into the eye can confirm the presence of Horner's syndrome, but cannot localize the lesion; hydroxyamphetamine can distinguish a third order from other types of Horner's syndrome. Cocaine blocks the reuptake of norepinephrine from the nerve terminals, increasing its effect. With Horner's syndrome of any type, there is less norepinephrine being released, less accumulates at the pupillodilator, and cocaine will fail to dilate the affected pupil. Hydroxyamphetamine drops cause release of norepinephrine, but only from intact nerve endings. If the third-order neuron is intact, as with first- or second-order Horner's syndrome, the pupil will dilate in response to hydroxyamphetamine. In a third-order Horner's syndrome, there are no surviving nerve endings in the eye to release norepinephrine and the pupil will fail to dilate. Table 14.1 summarizes pupil pharmacologic testing for Horner's syndrome. Apraclonidine, a new selective α_2 agonist used to reduce intraocular pressure, may also be used to demonstrate denervation hypersensitivity and is much more readily available than cocaine. It may also reverse the ptosis. Denervation hypersensitivity may occur as soon as 36 hours after development of the Horner's syndrome.

Other findings in Horner's syndrome include loss of the ciliospinal reflex, ocular hypotony, and increased amplitude of accommodation and vasodilation in the affected distribution. Congenital Horner's syndrome may cause sympathetic heterochromia iridis and other trophic changes of the head and face.

Thompson et al. described a group of patients with unilateral ptosis and miosis of unrelated origin simulating oculosympathetic paresis, which they called pseudo-Horner's syndrome. The majority of patients had simple, physiologic anisocoria accompanied by incidental ptosis because of LDD or blepharochalasis.

Argyll Robertson Pupil

Argyll Robertson pupils (AR pupil; for Argyll Robertson, Scottish ophthalmologist) are small (1 to 2 mm), irregular in outline, and have light-near dissociation. They react poorly or not at all to light, but very well to near. Anterior visual pathway function must be normal. Argyll Robertson pupils are generally bilateral and asymmetric, but may be symmetric and rarely unilateral. Argyll Robertson pupils are the classic eye finding of neurosyphilis and when present they mandate appropriate serologic testing. The lesion lies in the periaqueductal region, pretectal area, and rostral midbrain dorsal to the EW nuclei. Other conditions may cause an AR-like pupil. With the declining incidence of neurosyphilis, AR-like pupils with light-near dissociation are increasingly likely to be of some other etiology. Other causes of light-near dissociation are discussed in the following section.

Pupils with Abnormal Reactions

Disruption of the afferent or efferent limbs of the pupillary reflex arcs, or disease of the brainstem pupil control centers, may alter pupil reactivity to light or near, as may local disease of the iris sphincter (e.g., old trauma). Disease of the retina does not affect pupil reactivity unless there is involvement of the macula severe enough to cause near blindness. Cataracts and other diseases of the anterior segment do not impair light transmission enough to influence the pupil. Because of the extensive side-to-side crossing of pupillary control axons through the posterior commissure, light constricts not only the pupil stimulated (the direct response) but also its fellow (the consensual response). The eye with a severed optic nerve will show no direct response, but will have a normal consensual response to a light stimulus in the other eye, as well as constriction to attempted convergence (amaurotic pupil). Lesser degrees of optic nerve dysfunction can often be detected by checking for an APD (see below). The pupil frozen because of third nerve palsy will have no near response and no direct or consensual light response, but the other eye will exhibit an intact consensual response on stimulation of the abnormal side (Table 14.2).

Light-Near Dissociation

The pupillary reaction to light is normally equal to or greater than the reaction to near. Light-near

TABLE 14.2 Direct and Consensual Light Reaction

Comparison of direct and consensual light reflex and pupillary constriction to the near reflex in the presence of a complete lesion of the right optic nerve versus the right oculomotor nerve. In both instances, the right pupil is frozen to direct light stimulation, and the distinction is made by the other reactions

	Complete Lesion CN II OD		Complete Lesion CN III OD	
	Response OD	**Response OS**	**Response OD**	**Response OS**
Light stimulus OD	No response	No response	No response	Normal
Light stimulus OS	Normal	Normal	No response	Normal
Near reflex	Normal	Normal	No response	Normal

OD, right eye; OS, left eye.

dissociation refers to a disparity between the light and near reactions. The most common form is a poor light response but good constriction with the near response; it is relatively common, and there are a number of causes. The converse, better reaction to light than to near, is rare and most often because of lack of patient effort in attending to the near target. In the routine case, if the pupillary light reaction is normal, there is little to be gained by examining the near reaction.

The fibers mediating the pupillary light reflex enter the dorsal brainstem, but the near response fibers ascend to the EW nucleus from the ventral aspect. Disorders that affect the dorsal rostral brainstem may affect the light reaction but leave the near reaction intact. This anatomical arrangement likely explains many instances of the phenomenon of light-near dissociation of the pupils. Pressure on the pupillary fibers in the region of the pretectum and posterior commissure (e.g., from pinealoma) impairs the light reaction. However, fibers mediating the near response, the EW nucleus, and the efferent pupil fibers are spared, which leaves the near response intact. Causes of light-near dissociation include neurosyphilis, other lesions involving the dorsal rostral midbrain, diabetic autonomic neuropathy (tabes diabetica), Lyme disease, chronic alcoholism, chiasmal lesions (tabes pituitaria), myotonic muscular dystrophy, amyloidosis, Adie's pupil, aberrant regeneration of CN III, sarcoidosis, multiple sclerosis (MS), and severe retinal or optic nerve disease.

Afferent Pupillary Defect

When testing the light reflex, the amplitude of the initial pupillary constriction and subsequent slight escape depend greatly on the specific circumstances of illumination. Therefore, the status of the light reflex must be judged by comparing the two eyes. The importance of the pupil light reflex as an indicator of optic nerve function has been recognized since antiquity; Hippocrates and Galen understood the basic concept. With mild to moderate optic nerve disease, it is difficult to detect any change in pupil reactivity to direct light stimulation. As provocatively pointed out by Landau, Marcus Gunn (in 1902) described pathologic pupillary escape, what he termed secondary dilatation under continued exposure (for 10 to 20 seconds), or the adapting pupillary response, due to optic nerve disease. In 1959, Levitan described looking for the Marcus Gunn pupillary sign by swinging a light back and forth between the two eyes (swinging flashlight test, alternating light test). He thought that moving the light back and forth amplified the asymmetry of the pupillary escape. There seems to be general agreement that the swinging flashlight test is a very useful technique that can quickly and accurately compare the initial constriction and subsequent escape of the two pupils. It is a key clinical technique in the evaluation of suspected optic neuropathy, and it can often detect a side-to-side difference even when the lesion is mild and there is no detectable difference in the direct light reflex when testing each eye individually (Figure 14.22).

There are two techniques for the swinging flashlight test. In the first, the light is held about 1 in from the eye along and just below the visual axis; the light is rapidly alternated, pausing for about one full second on each side. The examiner attends only to the stimulated eye, comparing the amplitude and velocity of the initial constriction in the two eyes. The reaction is relatively weaker when the bad eye is illuminated. In the other technique, the light is allowed to linger a bit longer. With stimulation of the good eye, both pupils constrict smartly because of the direct

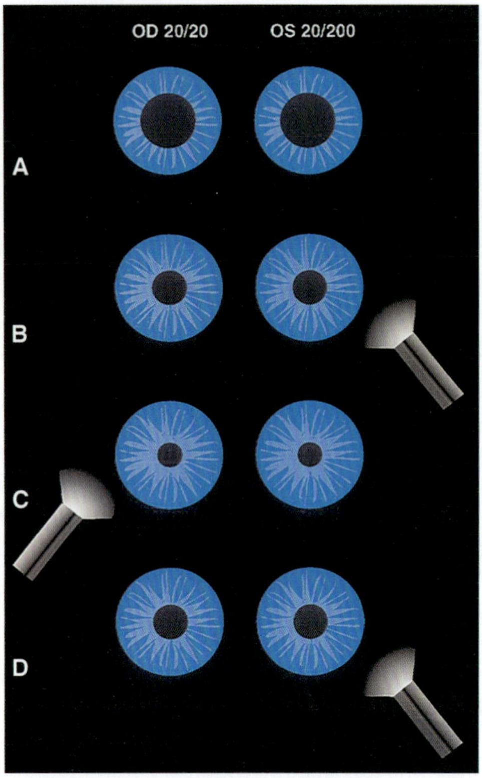

FIGURE 14.22 Relative afferent pupillary defect. Vision on the right 20/20; vision on the left 20/200 because of optic neuropathy. **A.** The pupils in dim light are equal. **B.** Light directed into the left eye results in a partial and sluggish contraction in each eye. **C.** Light directed into the right eye results in a brisk and normal reaction in each eye. **D.** The light quickly redirected into the left eye results in a dilatation of both pupils. Swinging the light back and forth will bring out the dynamic anisocoria. (From Tasman W, Jaeger E. *The Wills Eye Hospital Atlas of Clinical Ophthalmology*. 2nd ed. Baltimore: Lippincott Williams & Wilkins, 2001, with permission.)

reflex in the stimulated eye and the consensual reflex in the opposite eye. After 3 to 5 seconds to allow the pupil to stabilize, the light is quickly swung to the bad eye. With an optic nerve lesion, the brain detects a relative diminution in light intensity and the pupil may dilate a bit in response. The pupil in the other eye dilates as well because the consensual reflex constricting the pupil in the good eye is less active than its direct reflex, but this is not observed. On moving the light back to the good eye, the more active direct response causes the pupil to constrict. On moving back to the bad eye, the pupil dilates because the direct light reflex is weaker than the consensual reflex that had been holding it down. As the light passes back and forth, the pupil of the good eye constricts to direct light stimulation and the pupil of the bad eye dilates to direct light stimulation. It may require several swings to find the optimum speed to bring out the dynamic anisocoria. Over several cycles, it may be striking to see one pupil consistently dilate to the same light stimulus that causes the other to constrict. The weaker direct response or the paradoxical dilation of the light-stimulated pupil is termed an APD, or Marcus Gunn pupil. It is an extremely useful and important neurologic sign. Some modify the term with "relative" (RAPD) to emphasize that the finding depends on the difference between the two eyes—the state of the afferent system and activity of the light reflex in one eye relative to the other eye. The shorter form, APD, is currently in more widespread use. Active hippus may cause difficulty in interpretation. Hippus is random; a true APD will be consistent over multiple trials. Pay attention to the first movement of the pupil; if it is consistently a dilation movement, the patient has an APD and not hippus.

The magnitude of an APD is often graded. In one scheme, a 1+ APD refers to initial constriction followed by escape, 2+ indicates no initial constriction, then dilation, 3+ indicates immediate redilation, and 4+ means an amaurotic pupil. More precise grading is done with neutral density filters. Asking the patient to compare the light intensity in the two eyes provides a subjective estimate of APD severity.

The presence of an APD depends on asymmetry in the afferent signal. A bilateral APD cannot occur, although a severe bilateral afferent defect may cause light-near dissociation or abnormal pupillary escape. An APD can occur with bilateral optic neuropathy only if there is significant asymmetry of involvement. An APD can also occur with asymmetric chiasmal disorders or an optic tract lesion. A pretectal lesion can cause a contralateral APD without visual field loss. Media opacities will not cause an APD. In fact, mature cataract may so scatter the incoming light as to actually increase the light reflex and cause a minor APD in the opposite eye. Only severe retinal or macular disease will cause an APD, and then it will be slight. Maculopathy with 20/200 vision might cause a 1+ APD, whereas optic neuropathy with 20/30 vision would cause a 3+ to 4+ APD. For a demonstration of the swinging flashlight test and a demonstration of an APD, see *RAPD Present* by Dr. Kathleen B. Digre, John A. Moran Eye Center, Neuro-ophthalmology Virtual Education Library [NOVEL], University of Utah, available at **Video Link 14.5**.

BOX 14.2

Unusual Pupillary Abnormalities

Paradoxical pupils constrict in darkness. The phenomenon is seen in congenital retinal and optic nerve disorders; the mechanism is unknown. Springing pupil (benign, episodic pupillary dilation; mydriasis á bascule) is intermittent, sometimes alternating, dilation of one pupil lasting minutes to hours seen in young, healthy women, often followed by headache. Tadpole pupil is a benign condition in which a pupil intermittently and briefly becomes comma shaped because of spasm involving one sector of the pupillodilator; it may be a forme fruste of springing pupil. Periodic unilateral mydriasis has been reported in migraine and as an ictal phenomenon. Scalloped pupils occur in familial amyloidosis. Oval pupils usually portend major intracranial pathology and may be a transient phase in evolving injury to the third nerve nuclear complex. Corectopia iridis (ectopia pupillae, Wilson's sign) is spontaneous, cyclic displacement of the pupil from the center of the iris; it is usually seen in severe midbrain disease.

Unusual Disorders of the Pupil

Some rare pupillary disorders include paradoxical pupils, springing pupil, tadpole pupil, oval pupils, and corectopia (Box 14.2).

OCULAR MOTILITY

The eyes move in the service of vision, bringing objects of regard into the field of vision and following them if they move. Eye movements are divided into ductions (movements of one eye), versions (binocular conjugate movements), and vergences (binocular dysconjugate movements). Vertical movements are sometimes divided into supraductions/versions and infraductions/versions. The different eye movement control systems (e.g., saccade, pursuit, vergence) normally function harmoniously to secure and maintain vision. The globe rotates around one or more of three primary axes that intersect at right angles at the center of rotation, 15.4 mm behind the cornea. Movement takes place perpendicular to the axis of rotation. Abduction and adduction are rotation in the horizontal plane about the vertical axis going from superior to inferior. Elevation and depression are up and down movements around the horizontal axis that runs from medial to lateral across the eye. The third axis runs from anterior to posterior; rotation about this axis is referred to as torsion. Intorsion (incyclotorsion) is movement of the upper pole of the eye toward the nose; extorsion (excyclotorsion) is movement away from the nose.

The eyes are said to be in primary position when gaze is straight ahead and the visual axes of the two eyes are parallel. Because the orbits diverge, primary position must be obtained by precisely adjusted contractions of the extraocular muscles, which are controlled by the cerebral cortex. It is a delicate system. When regarding an object, the extraocular muscles move the eyes so that the visual axes meet at the proper point to ensure that the object's image falls on corresponding points on each macula. The point where the visual axes meet is called the fixation point. Normal eye movements are usually conjugate in order to maintain binocular vision and stereopsis. The MLF coordinates the contractions of the yoked muscles and the relaxation of their antagonists so that the two eyes move together.

During a monocular duction movement, the agonist contracts and the antagonist relaxes. When the medial rectus in one eye contracts, the lateral rectus in the same eye must relax. Sherrington's law describes the balance between the contraction of the agonist and the inhibition of the antagonist. In certain conditions (e.g., Duane's syndrome, Parinaud's syndrome), there is failure of antagonist inhibition resulting in co-contraction of muscles. Co-contraction causes the globe to retract into the orbit rather than moving in a normal manner.

During binocular version movements, the extraocular muscles work as yoked pairs (e.g., the lateral rectus in one eye contracts with the medial rectus in the other eye) (Figure 14.3). The yoke muscles are paired agonists for the binocular movement, and in each eye, their respective antagonists, per Sherrington's law, must be reciprocally inhibited. Hering's law, or the law of equal innervation, states that the same amount of innervation goes to an extraocular muscle and to its yoked fellow. The amount of innervation to the yoked pair is always determined by the fixating eye. Hering's law is important in understanding the topic of primary and secondary deviations.

Patients with diplopia become symptomatic because of visual confusion. The confusion results because of discordant retinal images—one real, one not. Diplopia is usually preceded by blurring of vision. Even when ocular malalignment is obvious, it is common for patients to have nonspecific complaints, such as blurry vision or dizziness, rather than complaining of frank "double vision." Historical details are often helpful in deciphering the cause of diplopia. The first step should be to determine whether the diplopia is binocular or monocular. Surprisingly, few patients have been observant enough to cover one eye and thus answer this question. With binocular diplopia, covering one eye eliminates the visual confusion. Monocular diplopia persists when using the affected eye alone. Monocular diplopia is often considered a nonorganic symptom, but there are many organic causes, primarily ophthalmologic conditions such as cataract, corneal astigmatism, lens subluxation, retinal detachment, and macular disease. Rare patients with cortical lesions will develop polyopia, seeing multiple afterimages with either eye, which can be confused with monocular diplopia.

Observant patients may be able to state whether the diplopia is horizontal or vertical, worse at near or distance, or worse in a particular direction of gaze; all are pertinent observations. Horizontal diplopia usually results from dysfunction of the medial or lateral rectus muscles. Vertical diplopia tends to result from disorders of the oblique muscles, less often of the vertically acting recti. Patients with sixth nerve palsy have difficulty diverging the eyes and tend to have more diplopia at distance. The lateral recti are not active when the eyes are converging for near vision, and patients have less diplopia at near (reading) as compared to distance (driving). Conversely, patients with medial rectus weakness have difficulty converging with more diplopia at near and less at distance. Diplopia is worse with gaze in the direction of the involved muscle. The patient with either a right sixth nerve palsy or a left third nerve palsy will have more diplopia on right gaze. Patients with fourth nerve palsy often describe an obliquity or tilt to the image. A patient with diplopia may keep one eye closed or may tilt or turn the head to minimize the visual confusion (ocular torticollis). An ocular cause of abnormal head position is common in children; the most common causes are congenital nystagmus, superior oblique paresis, dissociated vertical deviation, Brown's syndrome (see below), and refractive errors.

The diplopia of MG varies greatly with time of day and fatigue. Transient diplopia may occur with vertebrobasilar insufficiency. Persistent diplopia of sudden onset suggests a vascular event, with ischemia involving either a specific CN, as in diabetic third nerve palsy, or the brainstem. Ischemic CN palsy tends to resolve in 2 to 3 months. Progressive diplopia raises the possibility of a compressive lesion involving a CN. Trauma to the head or orbit frequently causes diplopia. Patients with a history of congenital strabismus may develop diplopia later in life because of decompensation of the squint and failure of fusion. A history of squint, "lazy eye," wearing glasses, patching one eye, or visits to the eye doctor as a child may all be relevant in the adult patient.

Associated symptoms may be important. Diplopia accompanied by ptosis may occur with third nerve palsy, as well as with MG and other neuromuscular disorders. Pain in the head or eye in association with diplopia suggests such conditions as diabetic third nerve palsy, posterior communicating aneurysm, ophthalmoplegic migraine, Tolosa-Hunt syndrome (painful ophthalmoplegia), and giant cell arteritis.

EXAMINATION OF EYE MOVEMENTS

Assessment of ocular movements should include an assessment of visual acuity. When acuity is impaired, the patient may not be able to adequately fixate. This influences the results of various maneuvers used to assess motility, particularly the cover test. Note the position of the patient's head. Many patients with ocular malalignment will hold their head in an unusual position. Usually, there is a turn or tilt that minimizes the diplopia. Occasional patients will use a different strategy and hold the head in a position that maximizes diplopia in order to make the false image fainter and more easily ignored. Patients with congenital nystagmus typically turn the head to maintain the eyes in a null zone where the nystagmus is least. Note the lid position. Lid asymmetry may accompany vertical strabismus; the appearance depends on which eye is fixing.

Assuming reasonable visual acuity and normal head position, the motility examination begins with an assessment of fixation. A patient with normal acuity can fixate steadily on an object of regard, whether near or distant. Inability to maintain normal steady fixation may occur because of square wave jerks, macro square wave jerks, macrosaccadic oscillations, and other disorders. These conditions cause fixation instability, or saccadic intrusions, transient deviations away from fixation with a quick return. Saccadic intrusion may be more apparent when viewing the fundus. Saccadic intrusions may be mistaken for nystagmus. Although saccadic intrusions can occur in normals, especially the elderly, they are usually a sign of brainstem or cerebellar disease. The patient with nystagmus greater than first degree will also not have normal steady fixation.

In routine cases where there are no eye complaints and the likelihood of abnormality is low, the ocular motility examination is usually limited to assessing versional pursuit movements in the six cardinal positions of gaze, including full lateral gauge to each side, as well as upgaze and downgaze when looking to either side (Figures 14.2 and 14.3). The target should slowly trace a large letter "H" for the patient to follow. Some add primary gaze plus upgaze and downgaze in the center to make nine cardinal positions. Eye movements should remain smooth and conjugate throughout. The six cardinal positions are designed to search for dysfunction of individual muscles or nerves, as well as supranuclear abnormalities of horizontal gaze. Assessment of upgaze and downgaze in primary position assesses the supranuclear vertical gaze mechanisms.

Pursuit versions are done by asking the patient to follow a target held about 0.5 to 1.0 m away, such as an examining light, a pointer, a pen, or the examiner's finger. A linear target should be held perpendicular to the direction of gaze, vertical for testing horizontal gaze, and horizontal for vertical gaze. Use of an examining light adds the ability to assess the corneal reflection, which gives objective evidence of ocular malalignment. The light reflection should be just medial to the center of the pupil and at corresponding points in each eye. The patient should indicate if she sees more than one target at any point. Pursuit movements are normally smooth. In certain disease states with abnormal pursuit, the tracking movements become disrupted by superimposed saccades, creating a ratchety or jerky movement termed saccadic pursuit (cogwheel eye movements). The finding is nonspecific and can occur bilaterally with fatigue, inattention, decreased consciousness, basal ganglia disorders, diffuse hemispheric disease, drug effects, or if the target velocity is too fast. Abnormal pursuit in one direction may indicate an ipsilateral deep occipitoparietal lobe lesion involving the pursuit pathways.

Normally, the eyes can move through a range of about 45 degrees to either side of primary position. In absolute terms, for the normal adult eye, the excursions are about 10 mm for adduction, abduction, and elevation, and about 7 mm for depression. The last 10 degrees of abduction is difficult to maintain and holding there may result in end-point nystagmus, a normal physiologic phenomenon. Patients can normally "bury the limbus" with both eyes in full lateral gaze in each direction, somewhat better on adduction than abduction. In full lateral gaze, the temporal limbus abuts the lateral canthus; in full medial gaze, about the inner third of the nasal limbus is buried. A small rim of sclera showing on extreme abduction is not abnormal. Normally, the amount of scleral show on abduction is symmetric in the two eyes. Greater scleral show on full abduction in one eye than the other may be a subtle sign of abduction impairment. Assessment of upgaze and downgaze is occasionally difficult. Normal aging causes impairment of upgaze, which varies from individual to individual. The best control for assessing normality of upgaze is usually the patient's spouse.

The vergence system comes into play when an object moves toward or away from the observer. Dysconjugate eye movements, convergence or divergence, are required. Testing convergence is not always necessary. However, the central mechanisms subserving adduction of the eyes for convergence are different from the mechanisms for adduction during conjugate gaze. Testing convergence is helpful in some circumstances, such as when the pupillary light reflex is not crisply normal (in order to look for light-near dissociation of the pupils), or when there is anything to suggest an INO.

The saccadic system can be tested by having the patient rapidly refixate between two targets. The patient is instructed to switch gaze between one target, such as the examiner's nose, and an eccentric target, such as the examiner's finger held to one side. The examiner assesses the velocity, magnitude, and accuracy of the saccades and compares adduction and abduction saccades in each eye and saccades in the two eyes. Saccadic velocity may be decreased globally in some conditions, such as MG, or selectively, such as slow adduction saccades in the involved eye in a unilateral INO. Saccades may be hypometric, falling short of target and requiring additional, smaller saccades to attain fixation, or hypermetric, overshooting the target and requiring saccades back in the opposite direction. In some conditions, reflex eye movements may be present when other movements are impaired. VOR movements can be examined by having the patient fix on a target, then passively moving the head from side to side, or up and down.

EVALUATION OF OCULAR MALALIGNMENT

Testing for diplopia and ocular malalignment may be subjective or objective. The subjective tests depend on the patient's observation of images, the objective tests on the examiner's observation of eye movements during certain maneuvers. Common subjective bedside evaluations include the red lens and Maddox rod tests; common bedside objective tests are the corneal light reflex tests and the cover tests (cover-uncover and alternate cover). The objective tests only require the patient to fixate; they do not require any subjective responses or interpretation of the color or separation of images.

Subjective Tests

Subjective tests for diplopia depend on the patient's description of the images seen. These are most helpful soon after the onset of an oculomotor disturbance. With the passage of time, there is compensation and precise delineation of the faulty nerve or muscle becomes more difficult. Testing should be done at a distance of 1 m to avoid any potentially confusing convergence. It may be useful to have the patient hold up both index fingers and demonstrate the separation of images in each position of gaze.

When a patient has diplopia because of extraocular muscle weakness, she sees two images. The real image falls on the macula of the normal eye. The false image falls on the retina beside the macula of the paretic eye. The brain is accustomed to images falling off the macula coming from peripheral vision, so it projects the false image peripherally. The farther away from the macula that the image falls, the farther peripherally the misinterpretation of its origin. As the eye moves in the direction of the paretic muscle, the separation of images increases, and the false image appears to be more and more peripheral. The false image is also usually fainter than the true image because extramacular vision is not as acute. The clarity, however, depends on the visual acuity in the two eyes.

Consider a patient with right lateral rectus weakness gazing to the right. The left eye accurately tracks the target; the right eye does not pass midline. The true image falls on the left macula. The false image falls on the nasal hemiretina of the right eye. The brain interprets the light ray falling on the right nasal hemiretina as coming from the right side of space. The farther onto the right nasal hemiretina the light ray falls, the farther to the right side the brain thinks it came from. These considerations lead to three "diplopia rules" to identify the false object: (a) the separation of images is greatest in the direction of action of the weak muscle, (b) the false image is the more peripheral, and (c) the false image comes from the paretic eye.

The false image may be identified in different ways. The simplest is to move the patient's eyes into the position with the greatest separation of images. Then cover one eye. If the more peripheral image disappears, the covered eye is the paretic eye. Consider a patient with maximal diplopia in right horizontal gaze. The candidate faulty muscles are the right lateral rectus and the left medial rectus. If the examiner then covers the patient's left eye and the image on the patient's left disappears, the diagnosis is right lateral rectus weakness. This is because the image that disappeared was less peripheral; therefore, the true image and the false image must have been arising from the right eye.

The red lens (red glass) and Maddox rod tests are attempts to be more precise. They may be especially useful when the diplopia is mild and the weak muscle or muscles not apparent from examination of ocular versions (Box 14.3). The theory of the red lens test is sound, but often the results of testing in clinical practice are less than clear. One reason is that the red lens breaks fusion just enough to bring out unrelated phorias, which muddy the findings. The results of the red lens test may be drawn to aid interpretation. There should be a notation as to whether the diplopia fields are drawn as seen by the patient or as seen by the examiner (Figure 14.23).

BOX 14.3

Red Lens and Maddox Rod Testing

The red lens is a simple translucent red glass that is placed, by convention, over the patient's right eye. When an examining light is shone into an orthophoric patient's eyes, the patient sees a single pink light in all positions of gaze. A Maddox rod is an array of cylinders in a plastic housing that creates a line, which may be vertical or horizontal depending upon how it is held. The vertical line is used for evaluating horizontal diplopia, the horizontal line for vertical diplopia. The Maddox rod is placed over the right eye. If the instrument is held so as to create a vertical line, the orthophoric patient sees a white light bisected by a red vertical line in all directions of gaze. The red line indicates which image is coming from the patient's right eye.

Consider again the patient with maximal diplopia in right horizontal gaze, with the red lens over the right eye. The patient sees a pink light in primary and left gaze, but a red light and a white light in right lateral gaze. If the red light is more peripheral, the patient has right lateral rectus weakness, because the more peripheral image is coming from the right eye. If the white light is more peripheral, the patient has left medial rectus weakness.

Diplopia may be divided into crossed (heteronymous) and uncrossed (homonymous). If the false image is on the same side as the eye that sees it, there is homonymous diplopia; if the image is on the opposite side, there is heteronymous diplopia. With the red-lens test, if the false image comes from the ipsilateral eye (e.g., red image to the right on right gaze), the diplopia is uncrossed (a line could be drawn directly from the false image to the paretic eye). If the false image comes from the contralateral eye (e.g., white image to the right on right gaze), a line from the false image to the paretic eye would cross a line drawn from the true image to the nonparetic eye and the diplopia is said to be crossed. For the patient with maximal separation of images on right horizontal gaze, uncrossed diplopia would imply right lateral weakness and crossed diplopia left medial rectus weakness. Of course, apparent weakness of any particular extraocular muscle could be simulated by any process that prevents relaxation of the antagonist—such as fibrosis, contracture, infiltrations, entrapment, or co-contraction.

Objective Tests

The corneal light reflex test (Hirschberg's test) depends on observing the reflection of an examining light on the cornea and estimating the amount of ocular deviation depending on the amount of displacement of the reflection from the center of the pupil. The test can only be done at near because distant reflections are too dim, so the confounding effects of the near reflex must be reckoned with. Each millimeter of light displacement from the center indicates 18 degrees of eye deviation.

Cover Tests

An elementary review of strabismus is useful to help understand the cover tests (Box 14.4). The cover tests are predicated on forcing one eye or the other to fixate

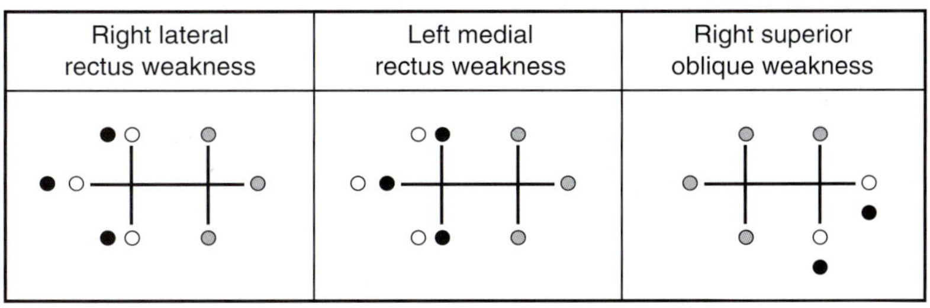

FIGURE 14.23 *Red lens* diplopia fields, drawn as seen by the examiner. The *red lens* is placed over the right eye, and the eyes move through the six cardinal positions of gaze with the patient looking at an examining light. *White circles* depict images coming from the left eye (*white light*); *dark circles*, images from the right eye (*red light*); and intermediate circles, images from both eyes (*pink light*).

BOX 14.4

Strabismus

Strabismus, or squint, means nonconcordance of the visual axes. Strabismus may be paralytic or nonparalytic. Ordinary strabismus, or congenital squint, occurs when the cerebral cortical mechanisms designed to maintain binocular vision fail for some reason, but the eyes are otherwise normal. This variety of strabismus is very common in children. Congenital strabismus is nonparalytic. In acquired strabismus, one or more eye muscles fail to function normally. Acquired strabismus is often paralytic (e.g., from third nerve palsy). There is an ocular malalignment, which is worse in the field of action of the affected muscle or muscles.

Perfect eyes are orthophoric (Gr. orthos "straight") in all fields of gaze; the visual axes are precisely parallel during all versional eye movements, even without a stimulus to fusion. Any deviation from perfection is termed heterophoria or heterotropia, usually shortened to phoria and tropia, respectively. In heterotropia, the malalignment is evident at rest. Esotropia is a manifest medial deviation (convergent or internal strabismus; "cross eye"); exotropia is a manifest lateral deviation (divergent or external strabismus; "wall eye"). Hypertropia is elevation, and hypotropia is depression. Heterophoria is a latent tendency for deviation, which only becomes apparent when the stimulus to fusion fails under certain circumstances, such as fatigue or when binocular fusion is deliberately broken, as by covering one eye. Congenital exophoria is very common. Exophoria may occur with myopia, esophoria with hyperopia. When an eye with exophoria is not fixing, it tends to drift back to its anatomical position of slight abduction.

by occluding its fellow, and determining the drift of the nonfixing eye while it is under cover. Varieties of cover testing include the cover-uncover test and the alternate cover test. The cover-uncover test is used primarily by ophthalmologists to evaluate patients with congenital strabismus where there is an obvious squint. When neurologic patients have an obvious malalignment, its nature is usually apparent. The alternate cover test is used to evaluate more subtle deviations.

A phoria is a latent deviation held in check by fusion. Breaking fusion by covering one eye causes the covered eye to deviate nasally (esophoria) or temporally (exophoria). If the cover is switched to the other eye (alternate cover), the just uncovered eye is forced to move into position to take up fixation. If an adduction movement occurs, it means the eye had been deviated outward under cover (exophoria). An abduction movement means the eye had been deviated inward (esophoria). The magnitude of the deviation can be quantitated by placing base-in or base-out prisms of increasing diopter strength before the involved eye until the refixation movements no longer occur.

COMITANCE

A phoria or tropia may be comitant (concomitant) or incomitant (noncomitant, nonconcomitant). Comitance describes the consistency of the deviation in various fields of gaze (Box 14.5). In neurologic patients, strabismus is typically paralytic and incomitant. Primary and secondary deviations are related to which eye is abnormal and which eye is fixing. In paralytic strabismus, the secondary deviation is greater than the primary deviation.

OPTOKINETIC (OPTICOKINETIC, OPTOMOTOR) NYSTAGMUS

OKN is a normal, physiologic phenomenon sometimes affected by disease. OKN is conjugate nystagmus induced by a succession of moving visual stimuli. OKN occurs whenever the eyes must follow a series of rapidly passing objects, such as telephone poles zipping by a car or train window. Clinical testing entails moving a striped target, a rotating drum, or a cloth tape bearing stripes or squares in front of the patient and requesting that she "count" the stripes or squares. Several OKN applications are available for smartphones and similar devices. Although OKN is more complex, it can be viewed for clinical purposes as testing pursuit ipsilateral to the direction of target movement, and contralateral saccades. The ipsilateral PTOJ mediates pursuit of the acquired stripe via connections that run in the internal sagittal stratum,

BOX 14.5

Comitance and Primary and Secondary Deviation

A comitant strabismus shows the same degree of deviation in all directions of gaze. Congenital, nonparalytic strabismus is typically comitant. Paralytic strabismus, likely to be seen in neurologic patients, is characterized by incomitance; the ocular malalignment as revealed by cover testing varies with the direction of gaze and is greatest in the direction of action of the paretic muscle. A patient with right lateral rectus weakness will have no abnormality on alternate cover testing while looking to the left, because the right lateral rectus has no role to play in left gaze. In primary gaze, the affected eye might drift into esophoria under cover and changing the cover to the normal eye would reveal an abduction refixation movement of the right eye. In right lateral gaze, the right lateral rectus insufficiency would become more obvious. The right eye would drift even more to the left under cover than it did in primary gaze, and uncovering would reveal a larger abduction refixation saccade. The eye deviation thus varies with the direction of gaze, none in left gaze, mild in primary gaze, and moderate in right gaze. This variability is incomitance and is the hallmark of paralytic strabismus.

In paralytic strabismus, the affected eye will be deviated away from the field of action of the involved muscle. With a right cranial nerve (CN) VI palsy, the right eye will be slightly adducted. With equal vision in the two eyes, the noninvolved left eye will fixate so that in primary gaze the left eye is fixing and the right eye is deviated toward the nose. This deviation of the right eye is the primary deviation. If the target is moved into the field of action of the paretic muscle, to the right, and the left eye is covered so that the right eye is forced to fixate, the left medial rectus (the yoke muscle of the right lateral rectus) will receive equal and simultaneous innervation per Hering's law. Because the right lateral rectus is trying mightily to contract in an attempt to fixate, the left medial rectus is simultaneously contracting mightily and, under cover, the left eye is markedly adducting into right lateral gaze. Removal of the cover reveals deviation of the left eye, which is termed the secondary deviation. In summary, the primary deviation is the deviation of the bad eye with the good eye fixing; the secondary deviation is the deviation of the good eye with the bad eye fixing.

deep in the parietal lobe medial to the geniculocalcarine radiations and adjacent to the atrium of the lateral ventricle. When ready to break off, it communicates with the ipsilateral frontal lobe, which then generates a saccadic movement in the opposite direction to acquire the next target. In normal, alert individuals, an OKN stimulus induces brisk nystagmus with the fast phase in the direction opposite tape movement. The response is intensified if the subject looks in the direction of the quick phase. Responses in one direction are compared with responses in the other direction. A vertically moving stimulus can evaluate upgaze and downgaze. For an example of normal and of blunted OKN responses, see **Video Link 14.6**.

Patients with hemianopsias because of occipital lobe disease have a normal OKN response, despite their inability to see into the hemifield from which the tape originates. Because of interruption of the OKN pathways, patients with hemianopsias because of disease of the optic radiations in the deep parietal lobe have abnormally blunted or absent OKN responses. The patient is unable to pursue normally toward the side of the lesion and is unable to generate contraversive saccades into the blind hemifield. The significance of OKN asymmetry lies in the vascular anatomy and the differing pathologies that affect the parietal and occipital lobes. Tumors are rare in the occipital lobe and much more common in the parietal lobe. Furthermore, the OKN pathways in the deep parietal lobe are outside the distribution of the posterior cerebral artery. Therefore, a patient with a hemianopsia and normal OKN responses is more likely to have an occipital lesion, and more likely to have had a stroke. With asymmetric OKNs, the lesion is more likely to reside in the parietal lobe, and more likely to be nonvascular, that is, a tumor (Cogan's rule). An asymmetric OKN response has a positive LR of 5.7 for detecting parietal lobe disease.

The primary clinical utility of OKN testing is investigation of patients with parietooccipital lesions, but the OKN tape has other uses. It may be used to crudely check visual acuity, especially in infants. OKN responses can be elicited beginning at 4 to 6 months of age. OKN may also be useful for estimating visual function in patients with depressed consciousness. It may provide a clue to the presence of psychogenic visual loss. OKN testing can demonstrate the slowed adducting saccades of a subtle INO, and sometimes accentuate the nystagmus in the abducting eye. OKN-forced upward saccades may induce convergence retraction nystagmus in patients with Parinaud's syndrome. OKN abnormalities may be seen early in PSP.

DISORDERED OCULAR MOTILITY

Abnormal eye movements can occur for many reasons. Disorders can be broadly divided into peripheral (infranuclear and nuclear) and central (internuclear and supranuclear). Peripheral disorders involve the extraocular muscles (e.g., MG or ocular myopathy) or the CNs (e.g., fourth nerve compression). Peripheral disorders include things that affect the CN nuclei, fascicles, or peripheral trunks. Although the nuclei and fascicles are "central," the clinical characteristics of conditions involving these structures is much more akin to other infranuclear conditions than to supranuclear disorders. Central disorders can be divided into supranuclear, involving the optomotor control centers; and internuclear, involving the pathways connecting and coordinating the activity of the ocular motor nuclei, primarily the MLF. There are many primary ophthalmologic conditions that can cause abnormal eye movements that can be confused with neurologic disorders (Table 14.3).

PERIPHERAL DISORDERS OF OCULAR MOTILITY

Disturbances of ocular motility may result from processes involving the orbit causing mechanical limitation of eye movement, or from ocular myopathies, neuromuscular transmission disorders, or a palsy of an individual ocular motor nerve.

Orbital Disease

Masses within the orbit may mechanically inhibit movement of the globe, often causing telltale proptosis as well. Following trauma to the orbit, individual extraocular muscles may become caught in fracture fragments, such as entrapment of the inferior rectus by an orbital blowout fracture producing a mechanical limitation of upgaze and vertical diplopia. Other examples of orbital disease causing ocular dysmotility include orbital pseudotumor, lymphoma, and rhabdomyosarcoma. Mechanically limited eye excursions exist for passive as well as active movements. Forced ductions involve pushing or pulling on the anesthetized globe in order to passively move it through the impaired range. An eye affected by ocular muscle

TABLE 14.3 Disorders That May Cause Diplopia Mimicking Cranial Nerve Palsies

Disorder	Condition Mimicked	Distinguishing Feature
Duane's syndrome	Cranial nerve (CN) VI palsy	Globe retraction and narrowing of palpebral fissure on adduction
Brown's tendon sheath syndrome	Inferior oblique palsy	Click on eye elevation
Myasthenia gravis	Any	Fluctuating findings
Thyroid eye disease	Any	Exophthalmos, lid abnormalities, chemosis, history of thyroid disease, abnormal forced ductions
Convergence spasm	CN VI palsy	Pupil constricts on lateral gaze
Medial rectus restriction	CN VI palsy	Abnormal forced ductions
Inferior rectus restriction	Elevator palsy	Abnormal forced ductions
Superior rectus restriction	CN IV palsy	Abnormal forced ductions
Möbius' syndrome	CN VI palsy	Congenital, often bilateral
Divergence insufficiency or paralysis	CN VI palsy	Full ductions, can't diverge
Orbital pseudotumor	Any	Proptosis, abnormal forced ductions
Decompensation of congenital squint	Any	Deviation is comitant

weakness, MG, or an ocular motor nerve palsy moves freely and easily through a full range. An eye affected by restrictive myopathy or an entrapped muscle cannot be moved passively any better than actively. Brown's tendon sheath syndrome is limitation of the free movement of the superior oblique tendon through the trochlea; it is most often congenital. The restriction of movement is analogous to trigger finger and causes an impairment of upgaze in adduction simulating inferior oblique palsy **(Video Link 14.7)**.

Muscle Disease

Primary ocular muscle disease may cause impaired motility because of weakness or because of restriction of movement. A number of myopathies and muscular dystrophies may affect eye muscles. Muscle disorders may be divided into myopathies and restrictive orbitopathies. The most common restrictive orbitopathy is TED, which is an autoimmune disorder that causes deposition of mucopolysaccharide and lymphocytic infiltration in eye muscles, making them bulky, stiff, and unable to relax during contraction of the antagonist. This sort of restrictive myopathy is easily confused with weakness of the antagonist (e.g., restrictive myopathy of the medial rectus simulating weakness of the lateral rectus). Extraocular muscles affected by TED also do not contract normally. Forced ductions are often done to clarify matters. The inferior rectus is the most commonly involved muscle in TED, producing impaired upgaze on the affected side. The possibility of TED must be constantly borne in mind when dealing with ocular motility disturbances.

Ocular myopathies cause weakness of the extraocular muscles, usually accompanied by ptosis and weakness of eye closure because of myopathic involvement of the facial muscles. Weakness of eye closure is strongly suggestive of ocular myopathy or neuromuscular transmission disorder as the cause of eye muscle weakness. Few other conditions affect both eye muscles and facial muscles. The common conditions causing ocular myopathy are chronic progressive external ophthalmoplegia (CPEO) and oculopharyngeal muscular dystrophy (Box 14.6).

Neuromuscular Transmission Disorders

MG, the most common neuromuscular transmission disorder, frequently involves the extraocular muscles, affecting any muscle or combination of muscles. Ocular involvement occurs early in 50% to 70% of patients, and it eventually develops in 90%. Patients typically present with ptosis or diplopia, or both. In some patients, the disease remains limited to the

BOX 14.6

Ocular Myopathies

Chronic progressive external ophthalmoplegia (CPEO) is a syndrome that has numerous etiologies, but it is most often due to mitochondrial myopathy. It causes inexorably progressive ptosis and symmetric eye muscle weakness, eventually leaving the patient with marked ptosis and eyes that are essentially immobile. Patients do not typically have diplopia. Examination shows loss of both voluntary and reflex eye movements; Bell's phenomenon is absent. Muscle biopsy usually shows ragged red fibers. Kearns-Sayre syndrome is a type of CPEO that is associated with pigmentary retinopathy, cardiac abnormalities, particularly conduction block with an increased risk of sudden death, hearing loss, ataxia, severe intellectual disability, endocrine dysfunction, short stature, and increased cerebrospinal fluid (CSF) protein; all with onset before age 20.

Most of the classical muscular dystrophies do not involve the eye muscles. An exception is oculopharyngeal dystrophy, which causes prominent, progressive bilateral ptosis and dysphagia that usually begin in the fifth or sixth decade. The signature of the disease is ocular myopathy accompanied by pharyngeal weakness. Congenital myopathies usually spare the eye muscles. An exception is myotubular myopathy, where there may be early and prominent involvement. Myotonic dystrophy causes prominent ptosis. It can affect the extraocular muscles causing slowed saccades, but major involvement is not a typical feature of the disease. Eyelid myotonia is common but can occur with most of the myotonic disorders, and it is not specific for myotonic dystrophy. Rarely, the extraocular muscles may be affected by inflammatory myositis.

BOX 14.7

Myasthenia Gravis

Having the patient rest with eyes closed for 30 minutes may produce temporary improvement of the ophthalmoparesis (sleep test). Applying a cold pack to the eye may relieve, and a hot pack exacerbate, both the ptosis and ophthalmoparesis. A convenient way to warm the eye is with an electric hair dryer on low setting. Warming just one eye can produce dramatic asymmetries. The edrophonium (Tensilon) or neostigmine (Prostigmin) test can be very helpful when there is a muscle with clear-cut weakness to evaluate before and after the injection. Myasthenia gravis (MG) may induce central adaptive effects to compensate for the extraocular muscle weakness. Because of fatigue during a saccade, the central nervous system may begin to generate an increased signal for a saccadic movement in order for the eye to find the target. Administration of edrophonium may cause the weakness to temporarily resolve, but the central adaption effect persists and saccades suddenly become hypermetric, overshooting the target. The development of hypermetric saccades or macrosaccadic oscillations after edrophonium is highly suggestive, some say diagnostic, of MG. Other useful tests include assay for antiacetylcholine receptor antibodies, repetitive nerve stimulation, and single-fiber electromyography.

eyes (pure ocular myasthenia). Most patients present with ocular involvement and then later develop generalized MG, as the disease affects bulbar and limb muscles. Even in patients with generalized MG, the ocular component usually remains a prominent feature. The hallmark of MG is fatigable weakness. The weakness gets worse with repetitive contraction of the muscle. The ptosis in MG is "fatigable"; it gets progressively worse with prolonged upgaze. The eyelid signs of MG are discussed above. Patients may develop diplopia with sustained eccentric gaze even when not present initially. Fluctuating ptosis and diplopia and worsening symptoms toward the end of the day are characteristic. The ptosis and ophthalmoparesis of MG are usually asymmetric and may vary from minute to minute. During the course of a neurologic examination, the ptosis may switch sides and the diplopia may vary. These features along with accompanying weakness of eye closure are virtually diagnostic. The earliest manifestation of ocular MG is slowing of saccadic movement on rapid refixation.

MG can cause weakness of any muscle or combination of muscles. It is rare but not unheard of to have ophthalmoparesis without ptosis. MG can cause weakness of any isolated muscle and should be considered in the differential diagnosis whenever ophthalmoparesis does not fit any particular pattern. MG can also produce ophthalmoparesis that simulates other conditions. Selective involvement of one medial rectus may produce a "myasthenic pseudo-INO," complete with nystagmus of the abducting eye (Figure 14.15, also see **Video Link 14.8**). Involvement of one lateral rectus can simulate sixth nerve palsy. MG can mimic gaze palsy or the pattern of any individual nerve. It should be considered in the differential diagnosis of virtually any patient with external ophthalmoplegia, but involvement of the pupil excludes MG. Ability to manipulate the myasthenic eye signs helps greatly in diagnosis (Box 14.7).

Except for mild ptosis, Lambert-Eaton syndrome does not usually involve the eyes. Botulism can cause severe ophthalmoparesis, often but not invariably with pupillary involvement. Other unusual neuromuscular disorders, such as marine toxins and congenital myasthenic syndromes, can also produce ophthalmoparesis.

INDIVIDUAL NERVE PALSIES

The same basic processes cause third, fourth, and sixth nerve palsies, but with different frequencies. As many as 25% of cases are idiopathic, and of these, 50% recover spontaneously. Some processes may affect more than one ocular motor nerve. Trauma is the most common cause of fourth nerve palsy and the second most common cause of third and sixth nerve palsy. Microangiopathic vascular disease because of diabetes or hypertension is the most common etiology of nontraumatic third and sixth nerve palsies. Aneurysms are an important etiology of third nerve disease. Increased intracranial pressure may cause third nerve palsies because of uncal herniation and sixth nerve palsies as a nonspecific and nonlocalizing effect. Neoplasms may affect any of these nerves. A third nerve palsy developing after trivial head trauma suggests the possibility of subclinical stretch because of an underlying mass. Basilar meningitis, migraine, viral infection, immunizations, cavernous sinus disease, sarcoid, vasculitis, and Guillain-Barré syndrome are occasional etiologies; the list of rare etiologies is long.

The Oculomotor Nerve

CN III palsy produces varying degrees and combinations of extraocular muscle weakness, ptosis, and pupil involvement. Internal ophthalmoplegia means involvement limited to the pupillary sphincter and ciliary muscle; external ophthalmoplegia means involvement of only the extraocular muscles; complete ophthalmoplegia is both. The most common identifiable etiologies are ischemia, aneurysm, tumor, and trauma; some 20% remain unexplained. Differentiating benign ischemic palsies from those due to aneurysms is a challenge, especially because both can present with painful diplopia; delay in diagnosis increases mortality. Third nerve dysfunction is frequently an ominous sign, especially in the setting of any alteration of consciousness. Uncal herniation from mass effect of any sort may result in compression as the temporal tip crowds through the tentorial hiatus and traps CN III against the sharp edge of the tentorium. Posterior communicating or distal internal carotid aneurysms commonly cause third nerve palsy (Figure 14.5). With third nerve palsy, processes affecting the nucleus or fascicles within the brainstem generally produce accompanying neighborhood signs permitting localization (e.g., Weber's or Benedikt's syndrome). In its long course along the base of the brain, CN III may be affected in isolation. In the cavernous sinus or orbit, accompanying deficits related to involvement of other structures usually permit localization.

Complete paralysis of the third nerve causes severe ptosis of the upper lid; impairment of medial, upward, and downward gaze; and loss of accommodation, with a dilated pupil that does not react to light, directly or consensually, or to near (Figure 14.12). There may be no complaint of diplopia if the lid completely covers the eye. When there is diplopia, the images are often oblique because of the combination of weak muscles. The eye rests in a down and out position because of preservation of the lateral rectus and superior oblique functions.

In a large series, third nerve palsies were complete in only 33%. Incomplete CN III lesions, causing paresis rather than paralysis and affecting certain functions more than others, are more common than complete ones. Ischemic lesions usually spare pupillary function. Lesions involving the midbrain or the course of the nerve after it has split into its superior and inferior divisions are more likely to involve only certain functions (see "Large Pupils," below). Lesions between the interpeduncular fossa and the point of division tend to cause paralysis of all functions, but divisional palsy may occur from a lesion anywhere along the course of the nerve. Very rarely, the only manifestation of a third nerve palsy may be an abnormal pupil. Depending on the etiology, a CN III palsy may show fluctuations, even over a short period of time, especially when there is nerve compression. A third nerve palsy because of uncal herniation may promptly resolve if the herniation can be reversed.

In addition to pupil sparing, the most helpful clinical feature distinguishing ischemic from mechanical, compressive lesions is aberrant reinnervation (misdirection syndrome, oculomotor synkinesis). Aberrant reinnervation is very common after facial nerve lesions (see Chapter 16), and a similar process may involve CN III (Box 14.8). Conditions that mechanically disrupt the nerve may result in regenerating sprouts growing into the wrong tubes and eventually innervating some structure other than the one originally intended. For instance, fibers that originally innervated the medial rectus may reinnervate the levator palpebrae. The common causes are aneurysm and head trauma, less common causes are tumor and neurosyphilis; the condition can occur congenitally. The misdirection syndrome typically emerges about 3 months after the inciting event. Aberrant reinnervation does not occur after ischemic or idiopathic third nerve palsy. For a dramatic example of bilateral third nerve synkinesias because of a midbrain injury, see **Video Link 14.9** (From Taieb et al). The lid changes are the reverse of those seen in Duane syndrome (see Box 14.9).

Localization of Oculomotor Nerve Lesions

CN III palsy can occur because of lesions anywhere along its course from the oculomotor nucleus in the midbrain to the orbit. Common causes are trauma, tumor, diabetes, aneurysm, surgery, and stroke. Midbrain lesions are discussed further in Chapter 21;

BOX 14.8

Aberrant Regeneration of CN III

The third nerve misdirection syndrome has certain characteristic features. The dual innervation of muscles causes a failure of normal reciprocal relaxation of the antagonist, violating Sherrington's law and causing co-contraction and retraction of the globe on certain movements. The clinical picture is stereotyped but may vary in degree. Attempted upgaze causes adduction and retraction because of misdirection of superior rectus fibers to the medial and inferior recti with co-contraction. The upper lid may retract on downgaze (pseudo-Graefe sign) because of inferior rectus fibers aberrantly innervating the levator. The lid retracts on adduction because of synkinesis between the medial rectus and the levator. The lid may droop on abduction because the reciprocal inhibition of the medial rectus causes the levator to relax.

Misdirection may also involve the pupil. The pupillary light reaction typically remains poor to absent, but the pupil constricts on ocular adduction with either convergence or horizontal gaze. The constriction on convergence with an impaired light reaction mimics light-near dissociation (pseudo-Argyll Robertson pupil). The ciliary muscle is about 30 times larger than the iris sphincter; most of the neurons in the ciliary ganglion are devoted to accommodation rather than pupillary function. The great preponderance of ciliary muscle over pupillary sphincter axons make it likely that misdirection will result in accommodation fibers aberrantly innervating the pupil, which causes pupil constriction with any attempt to focus.

they are usually accompanied by neighborhood signs that permit localization. Processes involving the third nerve nucleus may cause characteristic patterns of weakness not seen with lesions at other locations. Because of the contralateral innervation of the superior rectus, a nuclear lesion may cause weakness of the contralateral superior rectus. Involvement of the caudal central subnucleus may cause bilateral ptosis with an otherwise unilateral CN III palsy, or isolated bilateral ptosis. Conversely, patients with midbrain disease may have a lid-sparing third nerve palsy if the central caudal nucleus is not involved. Incomplete lesions involving the third nerve fascicles in the midbrain may cause partial CN III palsies. The pattern of involvement may mimic divisional palsy and suggest disease in the cavernous sinus or orbit (pseudodivisional palsy).

Processes involving the subarachnoid course of the nerve usually produce isolated unilateral CN III palsy with few associated findings to assist in localization. Incomplete involvement mimicking divisional palsy can occur. The most pressing diagnostic consideration in an isolated third nerve palsy is posterior communicating artery or basilar artery aneurysm. Aneurysmal third nerve palsies are typically acute, painful, and involve the pupil.

Ischemic third nerve palsies most often occur because of microvasculopathy related to diabetes and hypertension. Patients with ischemic palsies are typically older than those with aneurysms. Microvascular third nerve palsies are of sudden onset, painful, may spare the pupil, begin to resolve by about 2 months, and do not result in aberrant regeneration.

BOX 14.9

Duane's Syndrome

There are three recognized subtypes of Duane's syndrome; type I accounts for about 80% of cases. The core feature of type I Duane's syndrome is a limitation of abduction with otherwise normal eye movements. It is caused by aplasia or hypoplasia of the sixth nerve nucleus, as occurs in Möbius' syndrome, but accompanied by anomalous innervation of the lateral rectus by CN III. The patient is unable to abduct the eye, and adduction induces co-contraction of the lateral rectus, causing retraction of the globe into the orbit. Dynamic enophthalmos caused by co-contraction makes the palpebral fissure narrow on adduction (pseudoptosis). Aberrant reinnervation of the third nerve causes the palpebral fissure to widen on adduction; Duane's syndrome causes it to narrow.

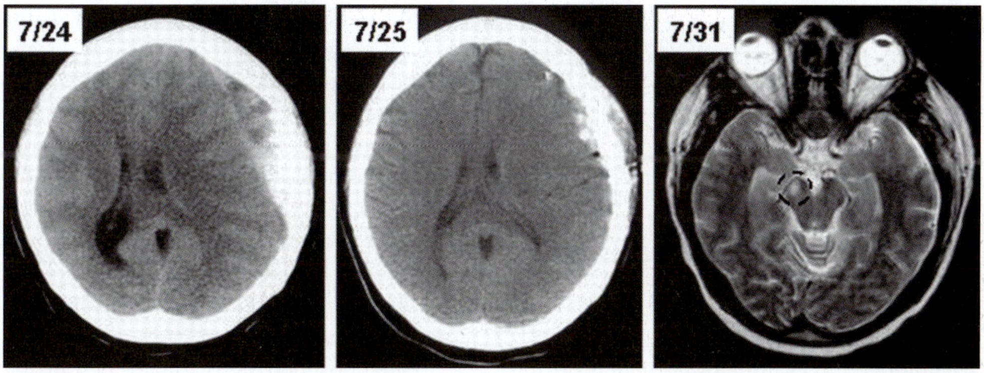

FIGURE 14.24 CT brain scan showed a left subdural hematoma with 1.5 cm midline shift (panel 7/24). After emergency platelet transfusion, the subdural hematoma was evacuated. Brain CT the next day showed resolution of the shift (panel 7/25). Brain MRI a week later showed a cerebral peduncle lesion in the T2-weighted sequence (panel 7/31). There was no history of head trauma.

Traumatic CN III palsy usually occurs only with major head injuries, severe enough to cause loss of consciousness or skull fracture. Increased intracranial pressure with uncal herniation most often compresses the ipsilateral nerve; the earliest sign is usually an abnormal pupil. Compression of the contralateral cerebral peduncle causing a false localizing hemiparesis ipsilateral to the lesion is not uncommon (Kernohan's notch syndrome, Figure 14.24). CN III can be affected bilaterally with lesions in the region of the rostral midbrain, such as central transtentorial herniation with Duret hemorrhages, ischemic top of the basilar syndrome, and basilar tip aneurysm.

Cavernous sinus disease usually affects other structures in addition to CN III, but mononeuropathy can occur. It is important in the evaluation of a complete third nerve palsy to be sure that CN IV is intact by having the patient attempt to look down and medially; look for a slight intorsion movement (best appreciated by observing the conjunctival blood vessels). For an example of a pupil-sparing ischemic CN III palsy with preserved CN IV function, see *3rd nerve palsy with preserved 4th nerve function* from Dr. Daniel R. Gold, Neuro-ophthalmology Virtual Education Library [NOVEL], University of Utah, available at **Video Link 14.10**. If the third nerve palsy is accompanied by involvement of CN IV, the likelihood of cavernous sinus disease is high. Cavernous sinus syndromes are discussed in Chapter 21. Lesions in the anterior cavernous sinus or orbit may selectively involve one of the divisions. A superior division third nerve palsy causes ptosis and impairment of upgaze. An inferior division palsy causes medial and inferior rectus weakness and pupillary dysfunction but with no accompanying ptosis or superior rectus weakness. Lesions involving CN III in the apex of the orbit often involve CN II as well and may cause proptosis.

Other causes of isolated third nerve palsy include nerve sheath tumors, Lyme disease, sarcoidosis, dolichoectatic basilar arteries, ophthalmoplegic migraine, dural arteriovenous malformations, postinfectious syndromes, sphenoid sinusitis or mucocele, nasopharyngeal carcinoma, herpes zoster, and meningeal inflammation or infiltration.

The Trochlear Nerve

CN IV is slender and has a long intracranial course; these two factors increase its vulnerability to injury. The most common etiology of acquired CN IV palsy is head trauma. Nontraumatic cases are usually microvascular, idiopathic, or congenital. A patient with a congenital fourth nerve palsy may decompensate as an adult and present as an apparently new onset condition. Other causes of fourth nerve palsy include meningioma, cavernous sinus syndrome, herpes zoster, Lyme disease, ophthalmoplegic migraine, sarcoidosis, Guillain-Barré syndrome, meningeal disease, and Tolosa-Hunt syndrome.

Patients with fourth nerve palsies may not complain of diplopia, but rather blurry vision or some vague problem when looking down—as when reading a book or descending stairs. The diplopia is vertical or diagonal and maximal in downgaze. Patients may tilt the head to the opposite side to eliminate diplopia, tucking the chin so the affected eye may ride up and into extorsion, out of the field of action of the weak superior oblique. Some fourth nerve palsies, particularly in children, present with head tilt

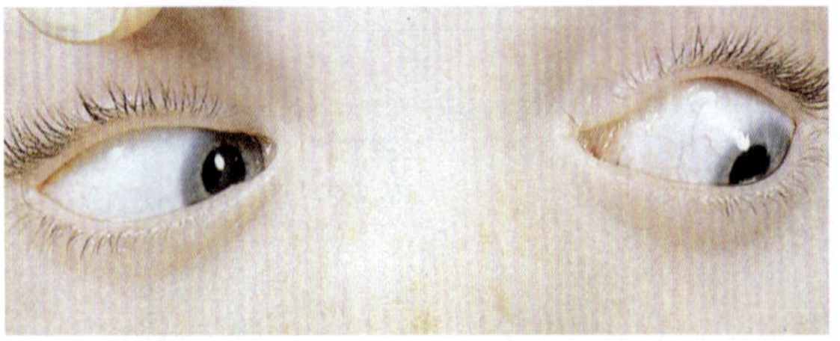

FIGURE 14.25 Right fourth nerve palsy. The patient is unable to depress the adducted eye on attempted downgaze.

rather than diplopia. On examination, there is extorsion and impairment of depression of the adducted eye (Figure 14.25). The involved eye has incomitant hypertropia or hyperphoria; with the patient looking down and in, alternate cover testing shows corrective downward refixations indicating upward drift of the affected eye under cover. The Bielschowsky head tilt test consists of tilting the head to each side, localizing the fourth nerve palsy by the changes in diplopia that result. If diplopia improves with head tilt to the left and worsens with tilt to the right, the patient has a right fourth nerve palsy. Forcing the involved eye to intort worsens the diplopia. For an excellent discussion of the bedside evaluation of vertical diplopia, see Prasad and Volpe. For a demonstration of the head tilt test in a patient with a CN IV palsy, see *Fourth Nerve Palsy* from Dr. Shirley Wray, Neuro-ophthalmology Virtual Education Library [NOVEL], University of Utah, available at **Video Link 14.11**.

Except that a nuclear lesion causes the fourth nerve palsy on the contralateral side, lesions at the nuclear and fascicular level in the midbrain cause the same clinical appearance as lesions involving the nerve proper in the subarachnoid space, cavernous sinus, or orbit. CNs III and IV can be involved together in processes affecting either the midbrain or cavernous sinus.

Superior oblique myokymia (microtremor) is a spasmodic, intermittent contraction of the superior oblique muscle that may cause transient vertical diplopia or monocular oscillopsia. The etiology is unknown but likely related to other conditions that cause focal myokymia. In rare instances, patients may go on to develop weakness of the superior oblique.

The Abducens Nerve

Sixth nerve palsies are common, and many resolve with no explanation. With a complete CN VI palsy, the eye cannot be abducted and often rests in a position of adduction (Figure 14.26). Patients present with horizontal diplopia worse at distance. There may be esotropia in primary position. Examination shows paralytic (noncomitant) strabismus, worse in the direction of action of the involved muscle. Incomplete palsies are common, and mild weakness may show only esophoria on alternate cover testing when the patient looks toward the side of the involved muscle. Neoplasms, trauma, demyelinating disease, and microvascular neuropathy are the most common etiologies. Many cases remain unexplained.

Neighborhood signs usually permit localization when the nerve is involved in the brainstem, cavernous sinus, or orbit. Pontine syndromes are discussed in Chapter 21. Brainstem lesions do not necessarily produce other signs and can cause an apparently isolated sixth nerve palsy. The CN VI nucleus contains both lateral rectus motor neurons and interneurons that project up the MLF, so a lesion involving the nucleus causes an ipsilateral gaze palsy rather than a sixth nerve palsy.

Sixth nerve palsies occur with increased intracranial pressure, after head injury, with structural disease in the middle or posterior fossa, with nasopharyngeal tumors, and for numerous other reasons. CN VI palsies are the most common and classic of all false localizing signs: they are nonspecific and bear no necessary anatomical relationship to the CNS pathology producing them. Elevated intracranial pressure often produces CN VI dysfunction because of stretching of the nerve over the petrous tip as the increased pressure forces the brainstem attachments inferiorly. Sixth nerve palsy is common in pseudotumor cerebri, see *Bilateral 6th nerve palsies due to idiopathic intracranial hypertension* from Dr. Daniel R. Gold, Neuro-ophthalmology Virtual Education Library [NOVEL], University of Utah, available at **Video Link 14.12**.

Gradenigo's syndrome is sixth nerve palsy, facial pain, and V_1 sensory loss because of lesions at the petrous apex (usually neoplastic, traumatic, or inflammatory). Any process in the cavernous sinus can involve CN VI, usually along with other structures. Iatrogenic CN VI palsy may occur after lumbar puncture, myelography, and certain neurosurgical procedures. Other etiologies for CN VI palsy include Möbius' syndrome, herpes zoster, ophthalmoplegic migraine, viral infection, and postviral syndromes. Bilateral sixth nerve palsies are not uncommon. They may occur because of tumors along the clivus, where the two nerves lie close together, with meningeal

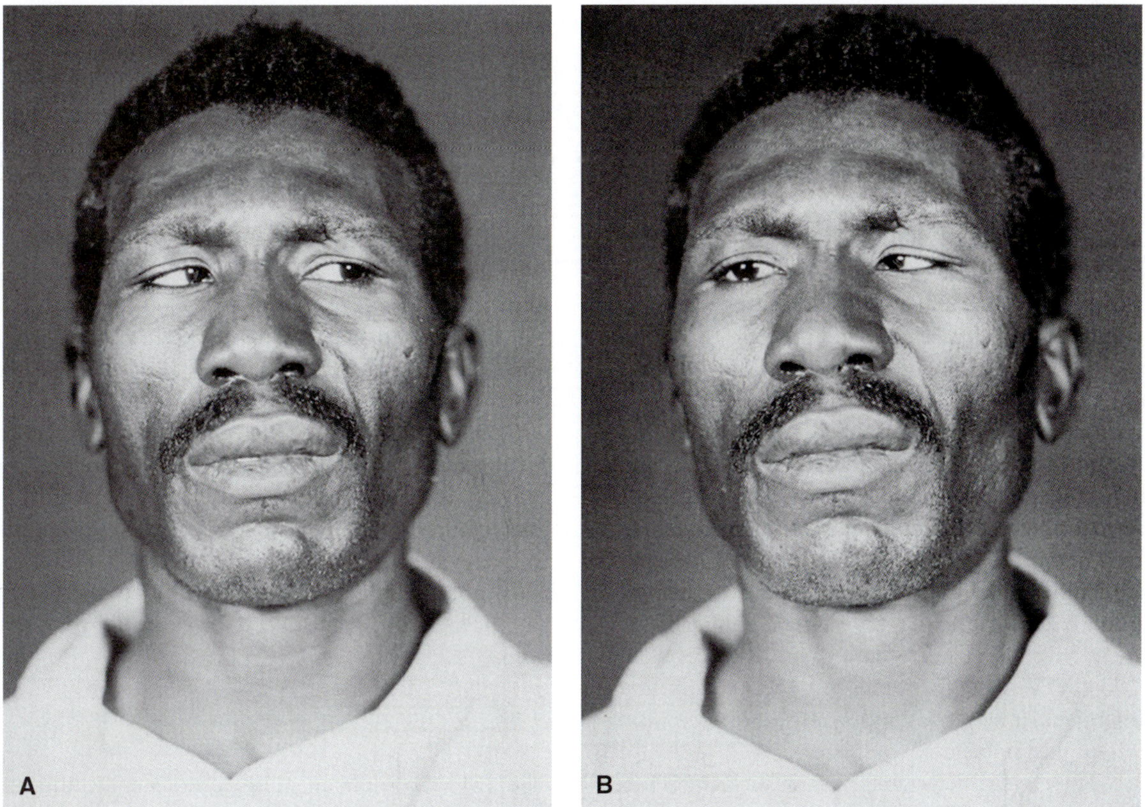

FIGURE 14.26 Paralysis of the right abducens nerve in a patient with a posterior fossa neoplasm. **A.** Patient looking to left. **B.** Patient attempting to look in the direction of action of the paralyzed muscle.

processes such as subarachnoid hemorrhage and meningitis and with increased intracranial pressure.

Other Causes of Abduction Impairment

Not all abduction failure is due to CN VI palsy. Some of the other causes include entrapment of the medial rectus by a medial orbital fracture, TED, MG, convergence spasm, divergence insufficiency, Duane's syndrome, orbital pseudotumor, and Möbius syndrome (Table 14.3).

Duane's retraction syndrome is a common cause of congenital strabismus that can mimic sixth nerve palsy (Box 14.9). Divergence insufficiency and divergence paralysis are conditions in which there is impaired abduction with esotropia when looking at distance, but full abduction on testing ductions. Patients have horizontal, comitant, uncrossed diplopia at far with no abnormality at near. Divergence insufficiency may develop as an isolated, benign, often self-limited abnormality in an otherwise healthy individual, or in patients who have other neurologic findings and underlying disease of the kind that more typically causes sixth nerve palsy.

Convergence spasm causes esotropia on lateral gaze that can mimic a CN VI palsy. The disorder is usually functional and caused by voluntary convergence interrupting normal lateral gaze. As the patient looks laterally, the sudden convergence halts the abducting eye in midflight and simulates weakness of the lateral rectus. The mechanism is betrayed by pupillary constriction accompanying the eye movement that indicates the patient is converging. There is a report of convergence spasm as an isolated finding in a patient with midbrain compression.

CENTRAL DISORDERS OF OCULAR MOTILITY

Central disorders can be divided into supranuclear and internuclear. Supranuclear disorders include those that affect the supranuclear gaze centers in the hemispheres and brainstem, as well as other areas that influence eye movements, such as the basal ganglia and cerebellum. Internuclear disorders affect the connections between the ocular motor nerve nuclei in the brainstem.

Internuclear Ophthalmoplegia

Lesions of the MLF cause an INO (Figure 14.27). The contralateral medial rectus receives no signal to contract when the PPRF and sixth nerve nucleus act to initiate lateral gaze. As a result, gaze to one side results in abduction of the ipsilateral eye, but no adduction of its fellow. Typically, the abducting eye has nystagmus as well, sustained or only a few beats **(Video Link 14.13)**. Failure of the medial rectus to adduct is an isolated abnormality in the affected eye; normality of the lid and pupil distinguish an INO from a third nerve palsy. Some patients have total adduction failure, and some may have exotropia in primary gaze. Patients with bilateral INO and exotropia have been said to have the wall-eyed bilateral INO (WEBINO) syndrome. An INO is commonly accompanied by vertical nystagmus, most commonly gaze-evoked upbeat.

The earliest detectable sign of an INO is often slowness of adducting saccades compared to abducting saccades, demonstrated by rapid refixations or OKNs. By convention, the INO is labeled by the side of the adduction failure; a right INO produces adduction failure of the right eye. Many brainstem lesions can cause an INO, but the common conditions are MS and brainstem stroke. INOs due to MS are usually bilateral and seen in young patients; those due to brainstem vascular disease are more often unilateral and seen in older patients. Conditions such as MG, Wernicke's encephalopathy, TED, or partial third nerve palsy can cause a "pseudo-INO." Wernicke's encephalopathy can occur without mental status changes.

Despite impaired adduction on horizontal gaze, some patients with INO are still able to converge. INOs have been divided into those with and without preservation of convergence. The convergence centers are in the midbrain, and when adduction on convergence is impaired, the INO may be classified as rostral (anterior). When convergence is preserved, the INO may be classified as caudal (posterior). However, many normal individuals have impaired convergence, and the localizing value of convergence ability has not been borne out.

Gaze Palsies and Gaze Deviations

The FEFs move the eyes into contralateral conjugate horizontal gaze. The eyes normally remain straight ahead because of a balance of input from the FEFs in each hemisphere. Seizure activity in one frontal lobe drives the eyes contralaterally. In an adversive

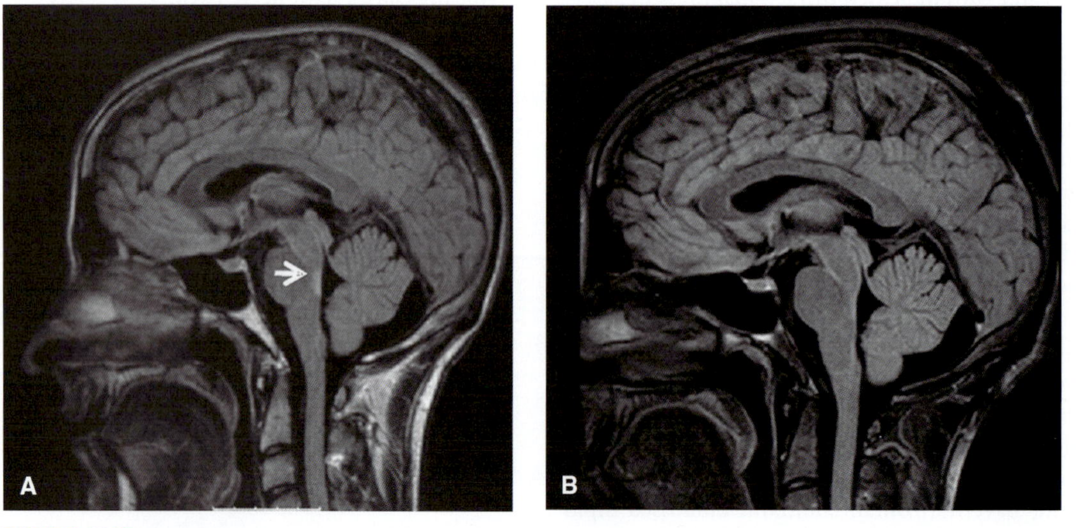

FIGURE 14.27 Sagittal MRI demonstrating a focus of high FLAIR signal change in the medial longitudinal fasciculus within the posterior pons (*white arrows*) in a patient with internuclear ophthalmoplegia, acutely **(A)** and with resolution **(B)**. (Reproduced from Auce P, Rajakulendran S, Nesbitt A, et al. Neurological picture. Internuclear ophthalmoplegia following African tick bite fever. *J Neurol Neurosurg Psychiatry* 2011;82[6]:681, with permission from BMJ Publishing Group Ltd.)

seizure, the eyes and then the head deviate to one side, after which the seizure may generalize. Sustained eye deviation can be a manifestation (rarely the only manifestation) of seizure activity, even of status epilepticus. With destructive frontal lobe lesions, most often ischemic stroke, the patient is unable to move the eyes contralaterally—a gaze palsy, or, if less severe, a gaze paresis. The intact, normal hemisphere maintains its tonic input, the imbalance causing the eyes to move contralaterally, toward the diseased side—a gaze deviation. Patients may have gaze palsy without gaze deviation. The presence of gaze deviation usually means gaze palsy to the opposite side, but it may occasionally signal seizure activity.

Similar considerations apply to disease of the pons. The PPRF governs ipsilateral, conjugate horizontal gaze. The PPRF draws the eyes ipsilaterally, in contrast to the FEFs, which force the eyes contralaterally. Destructive lesions of the PPRF impair the ability to gaze ipsilaterally, resulting in a gaze deviation toward the intact side as the normal PPRF pulls the eyes over (see *Unilateral Horizontal Gaze Palsy* from Dr. Shirley Wray, Neuro-ophthalmology Virtual Education Library [NOVEL], University of Utah, available at **Video Link 14.14**). The PPRF is the final common pathway for horizontal gaze, and pontine gaze palsies that involve the PPRF affect all functions, voluntary and reflex. Even ice water calorics will not move the eyes. Large, bilateral lesions may cause bilateral gaze palsy, and the only preserved eye movements are vertical.

When faced with a patient whose eyes rest eccentrically to one side, the possibilities are (a) frontal lobe seizure activity, (b) frontal lobe destructive lesion, and (c) pontine destructive lesion. Patients with destructive frontal lesions gaze away from the side of the hemiparesis; patients with pontine strokes gaze toward the hemiparesis. Frontal lobe gaze deviations are generally large amplitude, pronounced, and clinically obvious, whereas pontine gaze deviations tend to be subtle and easily missed. Frontal gaze deviations tend to resolve in a few days, pontine deviations persist much longer, sometimes permanently. Epileptogenic gaze deviations are usually betrayed by a component of jerky eye movement and subtle twitches elsewhere.

One-and-a-Half Syndrome

The MLF fibers arising from the CN VI nucleus decussate just after their origin and run in close proximity to the PPRF and sixth nerve nucleus on the opposite side. A medial pontine lesion can affect both the PPRF on one side and the MLF crossing from the contralateral side. Because of the ipsilateral lesion, the patient has a gaze palsy to the same side. Because of the MLF lesion, the patient has an INO on the same side. A lesion of the right pons can then cause a right gaze palsy with a superimposed right INO, which results in complete horizontal gaze palsy to the right and inability to adduct the right eye on left gaze ("half a gaze palsy" to the left). The only eye movement possible is abduction of the left eye, see *One and Half Syndrome* from Dr. Robert Daroff, Neuro-ophthalmology Virtual Education Library [NOVEL], University of Utah, **Video Link 14.15**. Fisher named this constellation of findings the "one-and-a-half syndrome." The most common causes are infarction and demyelinating disease. Paralytic pontine exotropia refers to such patients in the acute phase who have exotropia in primary position because of the preserved abduction in the contralateral eye.

Vertical Gaze Abnormalities

Two common disorders affecting vertical gaze are Parinaud's syndrome and PSP.

Parinaud's Syndrome

The core feature of Parinaud's syndrome (for Henri Parinaud, French neurologist, considered the father of neuro-ophthalmology) is impaired upgaze (Figure 14.18). Patients are unable to look up, and when they attempt it, the eyes may spasmodically converge and retract backward into the orbits (convergence-retraction nystagmus). The convergence-retraction movements readily appear during forced upward saccades in response to a down-moving OKN tape. The retraction movement is best seen from the side. Parinaud's syndrome usually results from a mass lesion involving the region of the posterior third ventricle and upper dorsal midbrain, such as a pinealoma; it is also known as the sylvian aqueduct, dorsal midbrain or pretectal syndrome, or the syndrome of the posterior commissure. Other frequent signs include eyelid retraction (Collier's sign) and abnormal pupils. The pupils in Parinaud's syndrome have a poor, rarely absent, light response, and much better near response (tectal pupils). The pupils tend to be large, partly because young people have larger pupils and lesions in this region tend to occur in younger patients. Sometimes, upgaze paresis is severe enough that the eyes are forced into sustained downgaze with retracted eyelids—the "setting sun sign," seen in children with obstructive hydrocephalus ballooning the posterior third ventricle and rostral aqueduct. Leading causes of the pretectal syndrome in Keane's series were hydrocephalus, stroke, and tumor. For a video showing all the features of Parinaud's syndrome, see **Video Link 14.16**.

Progressive Supranuclear Palsy

In PSP, degenerative changes in the rostral brainstem and thalamus result in impairment first of downgaze, then of upgaze, and eventually in global gaze paresis. Reflex eye movements are preserved until late in the disease. The gaze abnormalities are accompanied by parkinsonian signs and a pronounced tendency to extensor axial rigidity. Patients may have particular difficulty with the antisaccade task.

Other Disorders of Vertical Gaze

Skew deviation is a small, vertical misalignment of the eyes that usually results from a prenuclear lesion involving the brainstem or cerebellum. The deviation is usually comitant, remaining about the same in all directions of gaze, and the lesion is usually on the side of the hypotropic eye. Skew deviation is sometimes associated with an INO, with the lesion on the side of the hypertropic eye. The ocular tilt reaction (OTR) consists of skew deviation with torsion of the eyes and a head tilt; the head and the upper poles of both eyes tilt toward the hypotropic eye (Figure 14.28). It occurs primarily with peripheral vestibular disease, but can be seen in lateral medullary infarction. The OTR can simulate fourth nerve palsy because both cause an unusual head tilt. The pathway responsible for the OTR crosses the midline just above the sixth nerve nucleus and ascends in the contralateral MLF;

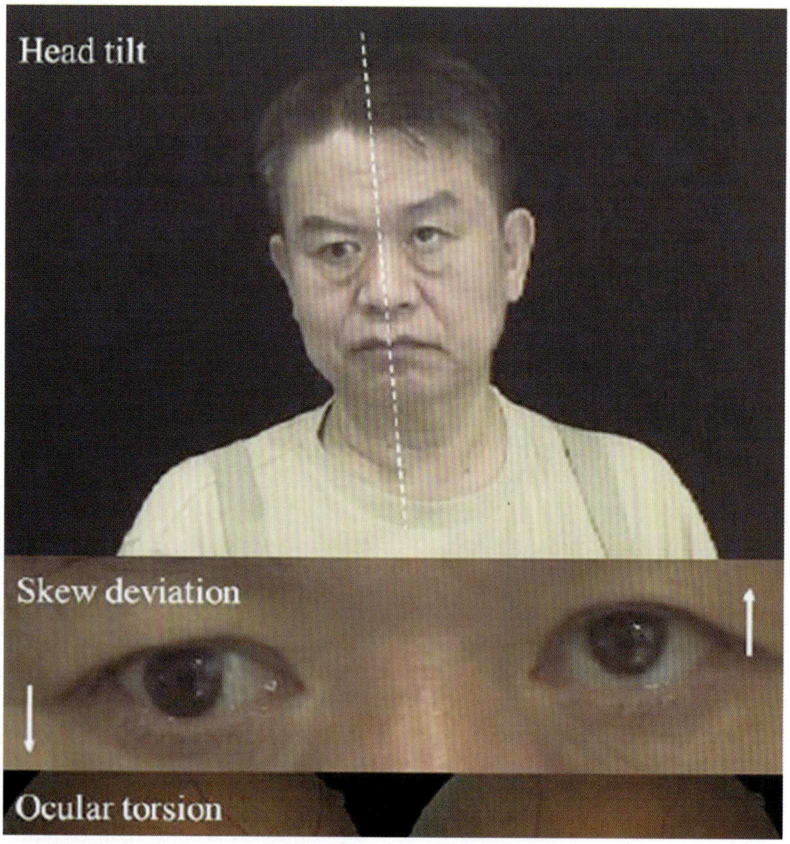

FIGURE 14.28 The ocular tilt reaction refers to the head tilt, ocular torsion, and skew deviation that are ascribed to asymmetry in the otolithic pathway from the utricle. The head tilt and ocular torsion occur toward the hypotropic eye. (Reprinted with permission from Huh YE, Kim JS. Bedside evaluation of dizzy patients. *J Clin Neurol* 2013;9[4]:203–213. Copyright © 2013 Korean Neurological Association.)

lesions in the lower pons cause an ipsilateral OTR; and more rostral lesions cause a contralateral OTR. Cerebellar lesions may cause either an ipsilateral or contralateral OTR depending on the structures involved. Isolated downgaze palsy is rare, but it can occur with small strategically placed lesions in the rostral midbrain. Double elevator palsy is a monocular paresis of elevation involving both the superior rectus and inferior oblique; it may occur with pretectal lesions. A vertical one-and-a-half-syndrome has been described.

Nystagmus and Other Ocular Oscillations

Nystagmus is a rhythmic, biphasic, involuntary movement of the eyes. When faced with a patient with nystagmus or similar-appearing movements, the usual clinical exercises include the following two steps: (a) deciding if the nystagmus indicates neurologic pathology and (b) if so, whether the pathology is central or peripheral. There are normal, physiologic forms of nystagmus. A few beats of nystagmus at the extremes of lateral gaze occur commonly and have no pathologic significance. A whole host of conditions can cause nystagmus, including ocular disease, drug effects, peripheral vestibular disease, and CNS disease. Nystagmus may also be congenital. Schemes have classified nystagmus in many different ways. This discussion focuses on the types of nystagmus commonly encountered in neurologic practice and on the differentiation between nystagmus that likely signifies neurologic disease (neuropathologic) and the kind that does not (nonneuropathologic).

Nystagmus is classified in multiple ways: pendular (both phases of equal amplitude and velocity) versus jerk (a fast phase and a slow phase); central versus peripheral; induced versus spontaneous; and physiologic versus pathologic. Further characterizations include rapid/slow, coarse/fine, manifest/latent, sensory/motor, and horizontal/vertical. Pendular nystagmus is classified by its plane of movement, usually horizontal. Pendular nystagmus only rarely signifies neurologic disease, and this discussion is focused primarily on jerk nystagmus. Jerk nystagmus is classified by the direction of the fast phase. Alexander's law states that jerk nystagmus increases with gaze in the direction of the fast phase. First-degree nystagmus is present only with eccentric gaze (e.g., right-beating nystagmus on right gaze). Second-degree nystagmus is present in primary gaze and increases in intensity with gaze in the direction of the fast component (e.g., right-beating nystagmus in primary gaze increasing with gaze to the right). With third-degree nystagmus, the fast component continues to beat even with gaze in the direction of the slow component (e.g., right-beating nystagmus persisting even with gaze to the left). Dissociated nystagmus is different in the two eyes (e.g., the nystagmus in the abducting eye in INO).

Nonneuropathologic Nystagmus

Nystagmus that does not signify neurologic disease may be physiologic, or because of ocular disease (e.g., poor vision), or other conditions.

Physiologic Nystagmus

Types of physiologic nystagmus include end point, OKN, and induced vestibular. Although these types of nystagmus are normal, they may be altered when disease is present in such a way as to assist in localization.

End-point nystagmus is fine, variably sustained nystagmus at the extremes of lateral gaze, especially with gaze eccentric enough to eliminate fixation by the adducting eye. In some, physiologic end-point nystagmus appears with as little as 30 degrees of deviation from primary position, often with greater amplitude in the abducting eye. End-point nystagmus is typically low amplitude and irregular. Symmetry on right and left gaze, abolition by moving the eyes a few degrees toward primary position, and the absence of other neurologic abnormalities generally serve to distinguish end-point from pathologic nystagmus. End-point nystagmus is the most common form of nystagmus seen in routine clinical practice.

Although OKN is a normal response, its characteristics may be altered in disease. Changes in OKN occur primarily with deep parietal lobe lesions. OKN abnormalities are discussed above (see section on OKN).

Vestibular nystagmus can be induced by rotation (e.g., Barany chair) or by irrigation of the ear with hot or cold water. This complex subject is discussed in more detail in Chapter 17.

Other Forms of Nonneuropathologic Nystagmus

These types of nystagmus are not physiologic, but they do not result from neurologic disease.

Voluntary Nystagmus

Some normal individuals have the ability to saccade very rapidly back and forth horizontally, producing a high frequency, low amplitude, pendular eye movement that is startling but of no consequence (see *Voluntary Nystagmus* from Dr. Robert Daroff, Neuro-ophthalmology Virtual Education Library [NOVEL], University of Utah, available at **Video Link 14.17**). Voluntary nystagmus may alarm the physician who has not previously seen these impressive oscillations. The movements cannot be sustained for long, generally less than 30 seconds.

Drug-Induced Nystagmus

Alcohol, sedative hypnotics, anticonvulsants, and other drugs commonly produce nystagmus. Such drug-induced nystagmus is typically symmetric and gaze evoked horizontally and vertically, especially in upgaze, only rarely in downgaze. Nystagmus more prominent than the commonly seen, few unsustained end-point jerks will usually prove to be a drug effect.

Congenital Nystagmus

A patient with a clear history of nystagmus present because infancy presents no neurologic diagnostic problem. However, occasionally, patients with congenital nystagmus are unaware of its presence; when they present later in life with neurologic complaints, sorting out the significance of the nystagmus may prove difficult. In distinguishing congenital from other types of nystagmus, the following features are helpful. Congenital nystagmus is most often horizontal jerk and remains horizontal even in upgaze and downgaze (i.e., it is not gaze evoked). This pattern is unusual in other forms of nystagmus. Patients often have a null point of least nystagmus intensity and best vision in slightly eccentric gaze. They may adopt a head turn or tilt to maintain gaze in this null zone. The nystagmus typically damps with convergence. The patient with congenital nystagmus characteristically holds reading material extremely close and regards it with a peculiar head tilt and may still have mediocre vision. For video, see *Congenital Nystagmus* from Dr. Shirley Wray, Neuro-ophthalmology Virtual Education Library [NOVEL], University of Utah, available at **Video Link 14.18**. A virtually pathognomonic feature of congenital nystagmus is "inversion" of OKNs. Moving an OKN tape so as to cause an expected summation with the fast phase of the congenital nystagmus produces instead a diminution or a paradoxical reversal of nystagmus direction. Patients with congenital nystagmus are not immune to acquired visual system abnormalities. Eye movement recordings help differentiate it from other nystagmus types. Confirmation that it is long-standing supports the diagnosis.

A form of congenital nystagmus, latent nystagmus occurs only when one eye is covered. This may happen when the examiner blocks the patient's vision during ophthalmoscopic examination, causing jerk nystagmus with the fast component toward the uncovered eye. The nystagmus disappears with binocular fixation. Latent nystagmus may exist in isolation or as a manifestation of typical congenital nystagmus.

Ocular Disease

Patients with very poor vision may develop continuous pendular nystagmus, and nystagmus can occur in otherwise normal individuals who work in perpetually dark environments. Visual-loss–induced nystagmus usually damps with convergence. Pendular nystagmus can develop monocularly in an eye with visual loss. Spasmus nutans is a disorder usually seen in infants between 6 and 12 months of age, but onset can be later. The classic triad is nystagmus, head nodding, and torticollis, but not all patients have all three. Head nodding and nystagmus are the most common manifestations, with head turn in a third. The nystagmus is low amplitude, high frequency, and dysconjugate. The nystagmus may be monocular. The etiology is uncertain, possibly related to sensory deprivation, but the condition is benign and disappears before age 4.

Neuropathologic Nystagmus

Nystagmus is a frequent manifestation of disease of the nervous system. Common types include vestibular, positional, gaze evoked, and gaze paretic nystagmus. Table 14.4 summarizes important but less often encountered types of nystagmus and related movements. Vestibular and positional nystagmus are discussed in Chapter 17. There are many online sources for videos of different types of nystagmus, especially the Neuro-ophthalmology Virtual Education Library at the University of Utah (https://novel.utah.edu) and the Canadian Neuro-Ophthalmology Group (http://www.neuroophthalmology.ca).

Symmetric, equal activity of the vestibular systems on each side normally maintains the eyes in straight-ahead, primary position. Vestibular imbalance causes the eyes to deviate toward the less active side as the normal side overcomes the weakened tonic activity from the hypoactive side. In an alert patient, the FEFs

TABLE 14.4 Nystagmus and Other Abnormal Ocular Movements

Nystagmus Type	Characteristics	Location of Pathology	Possible Disease or Condition
Upbeat nystagmus	Upbeating nystagmus in primary gaze	Cerebellar vermis (if nystagmus increases), or medulla (if it decreases) in upgaze	Cerebellar or medullary lesion; meningitis; WE; rarely, drug intoxication
Downbeat nystagmus	Downbeating nystagmus in primary gaze, maximal in eccentric downgaze gaze ("downbeat in the corners")	Cervicomedullary junction	Arnold-Chiari malformation; basilar invagination; MS; foramen magnum tumor; spinocerebellar degeneration; WE; vascular disease; rarely, drug intoxication
Convergence-retraction nystagmus	Convergence motions and/or simultaneous retraction of globes back into the orbits	Rostral midbrain, pretectum, posterior commissure, posterior third ventricle	Mass lesions, especially pinealoma; vascular disease; upward transtentorial herniation
Rebound nystagmus	Horizontal nystagmus that briefly beats in opposite direction on return to primary position	Cerebellum or cerebellar connections	MS; cerebellar or posterior fossa lesion
Periodic alternating nystagmus	Horizontal nystagmus that beats in one direction for 1–3 min, pauses, then beats in the other direction, cycling continuously	Brainstem or cerebellum	Craniocervical junction abnormality; MS; spinocerebellar degeneration; tumor; cryptococcosis; neurosyphilis; congenital; phenytoin intoxication
Seesaw nystagmus	Pendular nystagmus; one eye rises and intorts, the other falls and extorts; sometimes associated with bitemporal hemianopsia	Anterior third ventricle, parasellar or optic chiasm region	Tumor, especially craniopharyngioma; head trauma; septo-optic dysplasia; congenital
Bruns' nystagmus	Large and coarse in one direction, fine in the opposite direction	Cerebellopontine angle	Tumor
Ocular bobbing	Downward jerk with slow drift back to primary position	Pons (lesion usually massive and patient comatose)	Pontine hemorrhage or infarct; atypical forms occur
Ocular flutter	Intermittent, rapid, back-to-back horizontal saccades causing a quivering or shimmering movement	Cerebellum or brainstem cerebellar connections; dentate nucleus	Same as for opsoclonus (see next page); flutter and opsoclonus are a continuum
Opsoclonus	Continuous, involuntary, random, chaotic saccades in any direction (saccadomania, dancing eyes, lightning eye movements)	Cerebellum or brainstem cerebellar connections; dentate nucleus	In children: occult neuroblastoma (dancing eyes-dancing feet; opsoclonus-myoclonus syndrome, Kinsbourne's syndrome); in adults: occult lung or breast carcinoma; encephalitis; cerebellar disease

Nystagmus is jerk unless otherwise noted.
MS, multiple sclerosis; WE, Wernicke's encephalopathy.

generate a saccade to bring the eyes back toward primary position, creating the fast phase of vestibular nystagmus. When the cortex does not generate a correcting saccade, as in coma, only the tonic deviation develops; the eyes deviate toward the ice-water–irrigated ear.

Degenerative changes in the otoliths frequently produce the syndrome of positional vertigo and nystagmus. Nystagmus occurs after a latency of up to 30 seconds, beats with the fast phase toward the down ear, quickly fatigues despite holding the position, and adapts with repeated attempts to elicit it. Positional nystagmus is a very common condition. Although generally peripheral, it may occur with central disease (tumor, stroke, MS, degenerative disease). See Chapter 17 for further discussion.

Any nystagmus not present in primary gaze but appearing with gaze in any direction with the fast phase in the direction of gaze is referred to as gaze-evoked nystagmus. Normal physiologic end-point nystagmus is gaze evoked, but only present horizontally and at extremes of gaze. Abnormal gaze-evoked nystagmus occurs short of extreme gaze and is more sustained than end point. Drug-induced nystagmus is gaze evoked, usually horizontally and in upgaze. Nystagmus with the same appearance in the absence of drug effects is nonspecific but usually indicates disease of the cerebellum or cerebellar connections. Gaze paretic nystagmus is a form of gaze-evoked nystagmus seen in patients with incomplete gaze palsies. Rather than having an absolute inability to gaze in a particular direction, the patient achieves full lateral gaze transiently but is not able to maintain it. The eyes drift back toward neutral and then spasmodically jerk back in the desired gaze direction.

Other Disorders of Ocular Motility

Other types of abnormal eye movements include ocular bobbing, ocular flutter, and opsoclonus (Table 14.4). Ocular flutter and opsoclonus are types of saccadic intrusions, spontaneous saccades away from fixation; they may be confused with nystagmus. Patients with ocular motor apraxia are unable to generate saccades to look horizontally and develop compensatory blinking or head-thrusting movements to shift gaze. The blinks or head movements help to trigger a saccade. Ataxia telangiectasia may cause similar gaze difficulties. Parkinson's disease can produce a variety of ocular motility disturbances, including hypometric saccades, impaired smooth pursuit, square wave jerks, and lid retraction. Oculogyric crisis refers to attacks of involuntary conjugate upward deviation of the eyes, which may be transient or last for hours. Occasionally, there is also some deviation to one side, or the eyes may be turned downward. Classically associated with postencephalitic parkinsonism, these episodes are now seen as a dystonic reaction from phenothiazines and related drugs. Oculogyric crises from neuroleptic drugs may also occur as a tardive syndrome. In absence seizures, there may be brief spasms of upward gaze. Ocular dysmetria is an over- or undershooting of the eyes on rapid refixation of gaze toward either side or on returning to the primary position that requires corrective saccades; there may also be overshooting in following movements when the object of regard is suddenly stopped.

Video Links

Video Link 14.1. Cogan's lid twitch sign and eyelid hopping. http://neurosigns.org/wiki/Cogan%27s_lid_twitch_and_eyelid_hopping

Video Link 14.2. Curtain sign in myasthenia gravis. http://neurosigns.org/wiki/Curtain_sign_(enhanced_ptosis)

Video Link 14.3. Positive edrophonium test in myasthenia gravis. https://collections.lib.utah.edu/details?id=188589&q=sort_type_t%3A%2AMovingImage%2A+AND+edrophonium&fd=type_t%2Ctitle_t%2Cdescription_t%2Csubject_t%2Ccollection_t&rows=50&sort=sort_title_t+asc&facet_setname_s=ehsl_novel_%2A

Video Link 14.4. Duane's syndrome. https://collections.lib.utah.edu/details?id=180331

Video Link 14.5. Demonstration of APD by swinging flashlight test. https://collections.lib.utah.edu/details?id=180307&q=sort_type_t%3A%2AMovingImage%2A+AND+relative+afferent+pupillary+defect&fd=type_t%2Ctitle_t%2Cdescription_t%2Csubject_t%2Ccollection_t&rows=50&sort=sort_title_t+asc&facet_setname_s=ehsl_novel_%2A

Video Link 14.6. Optokinetic nystagmus. http://neurosigns.org/wiki/Optokinetic_nystagmus

Video Link 14.7. Brown's tendon sheath syndrome. http://www.youtube.com/watch?v=lBdEZU7Vkrs&NR=1

Video Link 14.8. Myasthenic pseudo-INO. http://www.neuroophthalmology.ca/case-of-the-month/eye-movements/intermittent-diplopia-and-trouble-sucking-on-a-straw

Video Link 14.9. Bilateral third nerve synkinesias. http://archneur.jamanetwork.com/multimediaPlayer.aspx?mediaid=2522009

Video Link 14.10. Pupil-sparing ischemic CN III palsy with preserved CN IV function. https://collections.lib.utah.edu/details?id=187726&q=sort_type_t%3A%2AMovingImage%2A+AND+third+nerve&fd=type_t%2Ctitle_t%2Cdescription_t%2Csubject_t%2Ccollection_t&rows=50&sort=sort_title_t+asc&facet_setname_s=ehsl_novel_%2A

Video Link 14.11. Head tilt test in CN IV palsy. https://collections.lib.utah.edu/details?id=188602&q=sort_type_t%3A%2AMovingImage%2A+AND+fourth+nerve+palsy&fd=type_t%2Ctitle_t%2Cdescription_t%2Csubject_t%2Ccollection_t&rows=50&sort=sort_title_t+asc&facet_setname_s=ehsl_novel_%2A

Video Link 14.12. Bilateral 6th nerve palsies due to idiopathic intracranial hypertension. https://collections.lib.utah.edu/details?id=1256233&q=creator_t%3A%22gold%22+AND+curriculum_t%3A%22sixthnervepalsy%22&fd=title_t%2Cdescription_t%2Csubject_t&sort=facet_title_t+asc&facet_setname_s=ehsl_novel_novel

Video Link 14.13. Internuclear ophthalmoplegia. http://neurosigns.org/wiki/Internuclear_ophthalmoplegia

Video Link 14.14. Unilateral horizontal gaze palsy. https://collections.lib.utah.edu/details?id=188642&page=2&q=sort_type_t%3A%2AMovingImage%2A+AND+horizontal+gaze+palsy&fd=type_t%2Ctitle_t%2Cdescription_t%2Csubject_t%2Ccollection_t&rows=50&sort=sort_title_t+asc&facet_setname_s=ehsl_novel_%2A

Video Link 14.15. One-and-a-half syndrome. https://collections.lib.utah.edu/details?id=188473&q=sort_type_t%3A%2AMovingImage%2A+AND+one+and+a+half+syndrome&fd=type_t%2Ctitle_t%2Cdescription_t%2Csubject_t%2Ccollection_t&rows=50&sort=sort_title_t+asc&facet_setname_s=ehsl_novel_%2A

Video Link 14.16. Parinaud's syndrome. http://www.youtube.com/watch?v=u7D1-zj98l8

Video Link 14.17. Voluntary nystagmus. https://collections.lib.utah.edu/details?id=188469&q=sort_type_t%3A%2AMovingImage%2A+AND+%22voluntary+nystagmus%22&fd=type_t%2Ctitle_t%2Cdescription_t%2Csubject_t%2Ccollection_t&rows=50&sort=sort_title_t+asc&facet_setname_s=ehsl_novel_%2A

Video Link 14.18. Congenital nystagmus. https://collections.lib.utah.edu/details?id=188527&q=sort_type_t%3A%2AMovingImage%2A+AND+%22congenital+nystagmus%22&fd=type_t%2Ctitle_t%2Cdescription_t%2Csubject_t%2Ccollection_t&rows=50&sort=sort_title_t+asc&facet_setname_s=ehsl_novel_%2A

BIBLIOGRAPHY

Algahtani H, Shirah B, Algahtani R, et al. Idiopathic harlequin syndrome manifesting during exercise: a case report and review of the literature. *Case Rep Med* 2017; Epub Feb 21.

Auce P, Rajakulendran S, Nesbitt A, et al. Neurological picture. Internuclear ophthalmoplegia following African tick bite fever. *J Neurol Neurosurg Psychiatry* 2011;82:681.

Averbuch-Heller L. Neurology of the eyelids. *Curr Opin Ophthalmol* 1997;8:27–34.

Averbuch-Heller L, Leigh RJ, Mermelstein V, et al. Ptosis in patients with hemispheric strokes. *Neurology* 2002;58:620–624.

Barr D, Kupersmith MJ, Turbin R, et al. Isolated sixth nerve palsy: an uncommon presenting sign of multiple sclerosis. *J Neurol* 2000;247:701–704.

Barton JJS. Neuro-ophthalmology III: eye movements. In: Joynt RJ, Griggs RC, eds. *Baker's Clinical Neurology*. Philadelphia: Lippincott Williams & Wilkins, 2002.

Bhidayasiri R, Plant GT, Leigh RJ. A hypothetical scheme for the brainstem control of vertical gaze. *Neurology* 2000;54: 1985–1993.

Biousse V, Newman NJ. Third nerve palsies. *Semin Neurol* 2000; 20:55–74.

Boricean ID, Ba˘rar A. Understanding ocular torticollis in children. *Oftalmologia* 2011;55:10–26.

Brazis PW. Localization of lesions of the oculomotor nerve: recent concepts. *Mayo Clin Proc* 1991;66:1029–1035.

Brazis PW. Isolated palsies of cranial nerves III, IV, and VI. *Semin Neurol* 2009;29:14–28.

Brazis PW, Masdeu JC, Biller J. *Localization in Clinical Neurology*. 7th ed. Philadelphia: Wolters Kluwer/Lippincott Williams & Wilkins, 2017.

Breen LA, Hopf HC, Farris BK, et al. Pupil-sparing oculomotor nerve palsy due to midbrain infarction. *Arch Neurol* 1991;48:105–106.

Bruce BB, Biousse V, Newman NJ. Third nerve palsies. *Semin Neurol* 2007;27:257–268.

Burde RM, Landau WM. Shooting backward with Marcus Gunn: a circular exercise in paralogic. *Neurology* 1993;43:2444–2447.

Buttner U, Kremmyda O. Smooth pursuit eye movements and optokinetic nystagmus. *Dev Ophthalmol* 2007;40:76–89.

Campbell WW. *Clinical Signs in Neurology: A Compendium*. Philadelphia: Wolters Kluwer Health, 2016.

Choi KD, Lee HS, Bae JW, et al. Teaching Video NeuroImages: positional exophthalmos in orbital varices. *Neurology* 2009;73:e8.

Cox TA. Pupillary escape. *Neurology* 1992;42:1271–1273.

Crippa SV, Borruat FX, Kawasaki A. Pupillary dilation lag is intermittently present in patients with a stable oculosympathetic defect (Horner syndrome). *Am J Ophthalmol* 2007;143:712–715.

Dacso CC, Bortz DL. Significance of the Argyll Robertson pupil in clinical medicine. *Am J Med* 1989;86:199–202.

David NJ. Optokinetic nystagmus. A clinical review. *J Clin Neuroophthalmol* 1989;9:258–266.

Donahue SP, Lavin PJ, Hamed LM. Tonic ocular tilt reaction simulating a superior oblique palsy: diagnostic confusion with the 3-step test. *Arch Ophthalmol* 1999;117:347–352.

Dresner SC, Kennerdell JS. Dysthyroid orbitopathy. *Neurology* 1985;35:1628–1634.

Eggenberger ER, Kaufman DI. Ocular motility review 1996. *J Neuroophthalmol* 1998;18:211–226.

Espinosa PS. Teaching NeuroImage: one-and-a-half syndrome. *Neurology* 2008;70:e20.

Fisher CM. Oval pupils. *Arch Neurol* 1980;37:502–503.

Frohman TC, Galetta S, Fox R, et al. Pearls and Oysters: the medial longitudinal fasciculus in ocular motor physiology. *Neurology* 2008;70:e57–e67.

Galetta SL, Gray LG, Raps EC, et al. Pretectal eyelid retraction and lag. *Ann Neurol* 1993;33:554–557.

Galetta SL, Raps EC, Liu GT, et al. Eyelid lag without eyelid retraction in pretectal disease. *J Neuroophthalmol* 1996;16:96–98.

Gaymard B, Lafitte C, Gelot A, et al. Plus-minus lid syndrome. *J Neurol Neurosurg Psychiatry* 1992;55:846–848.

Hamilton SR. Neuro-ophthalmology of eye-movement disorders. *Curr Opin Ophthalmol* 1999;10:405–410.

Keane JR. Bilateral sixth nerve palsy. Analysis of 125 cases. *Arch Neurol* 1976;33:681–683.

Keane JR. Third nerve palsy: analysis of 1400 personally-examined inpatients. *Can J Neurol Sci* 2010;37:662–670.

Keane JR, Zaias B, Itabashi HH. Levator-sparing oculomotor nerve palsy caused by a solitary midbrain metastasis. *Arch Neurol* 1984;41:210–212.

Kerrison JB, Biousse V, Newman NJ. Isolated Horner's syndrome and syringomyelia. *J Neurol Neurosurg Psychiatry* 2000;69:131–132.

Kline LB, Bajandas FJ. *Neuro-ophthalmology Review Manual*. Thorofare: Slack, Inc., 2000.

Koller HP, Olitsky SE, O'Hara M, et al. Diagnosis and treatment of fourth nerve palsy. *J Pediatr Ophthalmol Strabismus* 2016;53:70–74.

Kremmyda O, Rettinger N, Strupp M, et al. Teaching video neuroimages: unilateral RIMLF lesion: pathologic eye movement torsion indicates lesion side and site. *Neurology* 2009; 73(18):e92–e93.

Landau WM. Clinical neuromythology. I. The Marcus Gunn phenomenon: loose canon of neuro-ophthalmology. *Neurology* 1988;38:1141–1142.

Leigh RJ. Clinical features and pathogenesis of acquired forms of nystagmus. *Baillieres Clin Neurol* 1992;1:393–416.

Leigh RJ, Zee DS. *The Neurology of Eye Movements*. New York: Oxford University Press, 2006.

Levitan P. Pupillary escape in disease of the retina or optic nerve. *Arch Ophthalmol* 1959;62:768–779.

Liu GT, Volpe NJ, Galetta S. *Neuro-ophthalmology: Diagnosis and Management*. 2nd ed. Philadelphia: Saunders Elsevier, 2010.

MacDonald RJ, Stanich PP, Monrad PA, et al. Teaching Video NeuroImages: Wernicke encephalopathy without mental status changes. *Neurology* 2009;73:e97.

Martin TJ, Corbett JJ. *Neuro-ophthalmology*. St. Louis: Mosby, 2000.

Martin TJ, Corbett JJ, Babikian PV, et al. Bilateral ptosis due to mesencephalic lesions with relative preservation of ocular motility. *J Neuroophthalmol* 1996;16:258–263.

McGee S. *Evidence Based Physical Diagnosis*. 3rd ed. Philadelphia: Elsevier/Saunders, 2012.

McMillan HJ, Keene DL, Jacob P, et al. Ophthalmoplegic migraine: inflammatory neuropathy with secondary migraine? *Can J Neurol Sci* 2007;34:349–355.

Miller NR. The ocular motor nerves. *Curr Opin Neurol* 1996; 9:21–25.

Miller NR, Subramanian PS, Patel VR. *Walsh and Hoyt's Clinical Neuro-ophthalmology: The Essentials*. 3rd ed. Philadelphia: Wolters Kluwer, 2016.

Mollan SP, Edwards JH, Price A, et al. Aetiology and outcomes of adult superior oblique palsies: a modern series. *Eye (Lond)* 2009;23:640–644.

Mughal M, Longmuir R. Current pharmacologic testing for Horner syndrome. *Curr Neurol Neurosci Rep* 2009;9(5): 384–389.

Olsen T, Jakobsen J. Abnormal pupillary function in third nerve regeneration (the pseudo-Argyll Robertson pupil). A case report. *Acta Ophthalmol (Copenh)* 1984;62:163–167.

Peters GB III, Bakri SJ, Krohel GB. Cause and prognosis of non-traumatic sixth nerve palsies in young adults. *Ophthalmology* 2002;109:1925–1928.

Prasad S, Volpe NJ. Clinical reasoning: 36-year-old man with vertical diplopia. *Neurology* 2009;72:e93–e99.

Romano LM, Besocke AG. Teaching video neuroimages: recurrent oculomotor neuropathy with isolated ptosis vs ophthalmoplegic migraine. *Neurology* 2009;72(9):e44.

Rucker JC. An update on acquired nystagmus. *Semin Ophthalmol* 2008;23:91–97.

Sadun AA, Thompson HS, Corbett JJ, et al. Swinging flashlight test. *Neurology* 1989;39:154–156.

Saeki N, Yamaura A, Sunami K. Bilateral ptosis with pupil sparing because of a discrete midbrain lesion: magnetic resonance imaging evidence of topographic arrangement within the oculomotor nerve. *J Neuroophthalmol* 2000;20:130–134.

Sakamoto Y, Kimura K, Iguchi Y, et al. A small pontine infarct on DWI as a lesion responsible for wall-eyed bilateral internuclear ophthalmoplegia syndrome. *Neurol Sci* 2012;33:121–123.

Selhorst JB, Hoyt WF, Feinsod M, et al. Midbrain corectopia. *Arch Neurol* 1976;33:193–195.

Shin RK, Cheek AG. Teaching neuroimages: positive apraclonidine test in Horner syndrome. *Neurology* 2011;76:e100.

Shinoda K, Matsushita T, Furuta K, et al. Wall-eyed bilateral internuclear ophthalmoplegia (WEBINO) syndrome in a patient with neuromyelitis optica spectrum disorder and anti-aquaporin-4 antibody. *Mult Scler* 2011;17:885–887.

Singman EL, Matta NS, Silbert DI. Use of the Cogan lid twitch to identify myasthenia gravis. *J Neuroophthalmol* 2011;31: 239–240.

Stahl JS, Leigh RJ. Nystagmus. *Curr Neurol Neurosci Rep* 2001;1:471–477.

Taieb G, Renard D, Jeanjean L, et al. Unusual third nerve synkinesis due to midbrain injury. *Arch Neurol* 2011;68:948–949.

Thompson HS, Corbett JJ, Cox TA. How to measure the relative afferent pupillary defect. *Surv Ophthalmol* 1981;26:39–42.

Thompson BM, Corbett JJ, Kline LB, et al. Pseudo-Horner's syndrome. *Arch Neurol* 2003;39:108–111.

Thurtell MJ. Diagnostic approach to abnormal spontaneous eye movements. *Continuum (Minneap Minn)* 2014;20(4 Neuro-ophthalmology):993–1007.

Thurtell MJ, Leigh RJ. Nystagmus and saccadic intrusions. *Handb Clin Neurol* 2011;102:333–378.

Thurtell MJ, Weber KP, Halmagyi GM. Teaching video NeuroImage: acquired or congenital gaze-evoked nystagmus? *Neurology* 2008;70:e96.

Weber KP, Thurtell MJ, Halmagyi GM. Teaching neuroImage: convergence spasm associated with midbrain compression by cerebral aneurysm. *Neurology* 2008;70:e49–e50.

Yotharak P, Aui-Aree N. Correlation between clinical grading and quantification by neutral density filter of relative afferent pupillary defect (RAPD). *J Med Assoc Thai* 2012;95(Suppl 4):S92–S95.

Zak R, Slamovits T, Burde R. Oculomotor brainstem anatomy: nuclei to fascicles. *J Neurooncol* 1994;18:241–248.

CHAPTER 15

The Trigeminal Nerve

ANATOMY AND PHYSIOLOGY

The trigeminal, or fifth cranial, nerve (CN V) is the largest and one of the most complex CNs. It has a large sensory part (portio major; 170,000 fibers) and a much smaller motor part (portio minor; 7,700 fibers). The sensory component has three divisions: the first or ophthalmic division (CN V_1), the second or maxillary division (CN V_2), and the third or mandibular division (CN V_3). The motor and principal sensory nuclei are located in the mid-pons (Figure 15.1). The spinal tract and nucleus, which subserve pain and temperature, extend from the pons down into the upper cervical spinal cord. The mesencephalic root receives proprioceptive fibers. Trigeminal nuclear structures thus extend from the rostral midbrain to the rostral spinal cord. The sensory portion innervates the face, teeth, oral and nasal cavities, the scalp back to the vertex, the intracranial dura, and the cerebral vasculature, and provides proprioceptive information for muscles of mastication. The motor portion innervates the muscles of mastication. CN V has extensive connections with other CNs. There is a small input to both the mossy and climbing fiber systems of the cerebellum (trigeminocerebellar fibers). Functional magnetic resonance imaging (MRI) using specific sensory stimuli or motor tasks has been used to localize the brainstem nuclei.

The Motor Portion

Upper motor neuron control of trigeminal motor functions arises primarily from the lower third of the contralateral motor cortex, although each trigeminal motor nucleus receives projections from both cerebral hemispheres. Fibers descend in the corticobulbar tract to the pons, where they decussate (Figure 15.2). There is extrapyramidal innervation from the premotor cortex and basal ganglia. The muscles supplied by the trigeminal are derived from the first branchial arch, and the system is special visceral efferent (SVE) or branchial motor. The fibers exit laterally, typical for SVE fibers, but do not form an internal loop as other branchial motor fibers do.

The motor root exits the lateral pons anteromedial to the sensory root. It passes beneath the gasserian ganglion, leaves the skull through the foramen ovale, and then joins the mandibular sensory division briefly before separating to supply the muscles of mastication and associated muscles.

The principal function of the motor root is to innervate the muscles of mastication: masseter, temporalis, and medial and lateral pterygoids. The masseter muscles close the jaw and protrude it slightly; the masseter may be the most powerful muscle in the body. The temporalis muscles close the jaw and retract it slightly. The medial pterygoids acting synchronously close the jaw and protrude it. The lateral pterygoids acting synchronously open the jaw and protrude it. The medial and lateral pterygoids originate from the skull base and extend laterally to insert on the inner aspect of the mandible. When they contract on one side, they pull the mandible contralaterally. When there is unilateral pterygoid weakness, the jaw deviates toward the side of the weak muscles.

Mastication is a complex opening, closing, forward, backward, and lateral movement of the jaw. The motor root of CN V is responsible for all of these intricate motions. CN V also supplies the mylohyoid, anterior belly of the digastric, tensor veli palatini, and tensor tympani muscles. The mylohyoid pulls the hyoid bone upward and forward, raising the floor of the mouth and pressing the base of the tongue against the palate. The anterior belly of the digastric raises and advances the hyoid bone if the jaw is fixed. The tensor veli palatini tenses the soft palate and helps prevent food from escaping from the oro- to the

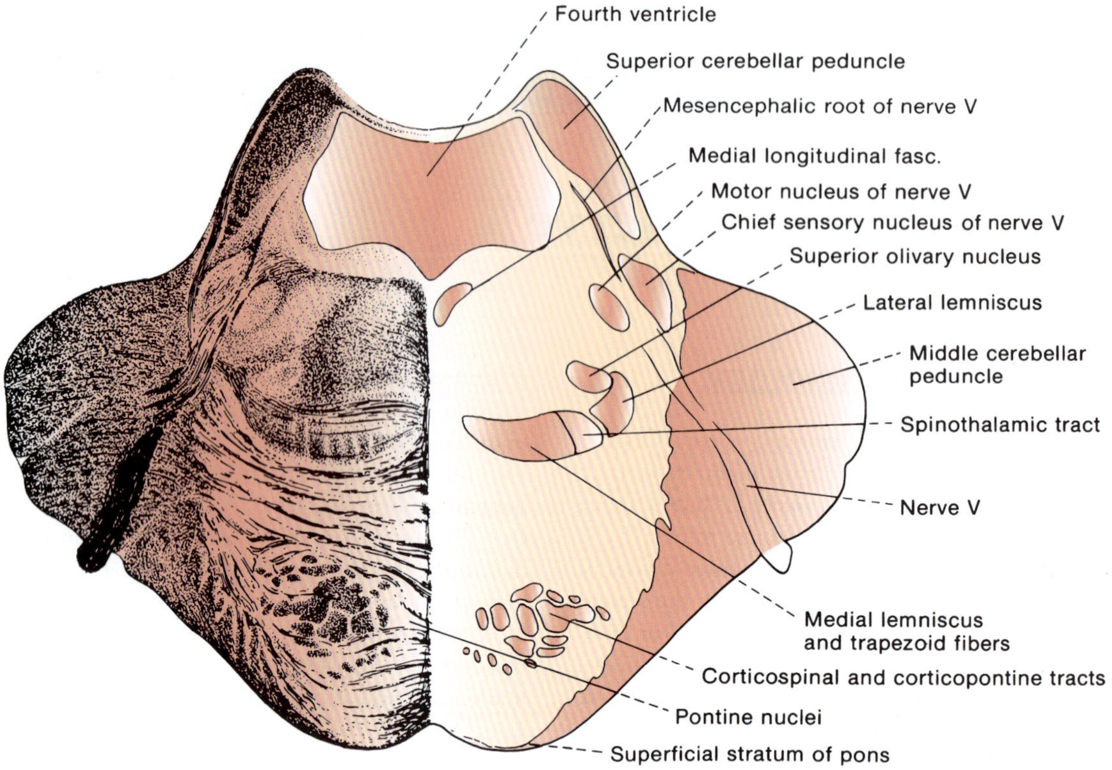

FIGURE 15.1 Section through the pons at the level of the trigeminal nuclei.

nasopharynx; it also dilates the eustachian tube. The tensor tympani, through interaction with CN VIII, tenses the tympanic membrane and helps dampen its excursions in response to sound intensity.

The Sensory Portion

The trigeminal, or gasserian (for J. L. Gasser), ganglion, the largest ganglion in the peripheral nervous system, lies just beside the pons in a shallow depression in the petrous apex called Meckel's cave. The ganglion is crescent shaped, convex anterolaterally, and is also known as the semilunar ganglion. It lies just lateral to the internal carotid artery and the posterior part of the cavernous sinus. The ganglion is analogous to a dorsal root ganglion; it contains unipolar sensory neurons, whose central processes enter the lateral pons through the large sensory root that passes beneath the tentorium to connect the concave side of the ganglion to the brainstem. The sensory root can be compressed by vascular loops, causing trigeminal neuralgia (TN). The peripheral processes subserve sensation to the face and head. There are two types of sensory neurons in the gasserian ganglion. One mediates fine discriminative touch; the other mediates primarily pain and temperature.

Afferent fibers conveying light touch and pressure enter the principal sensory nucleus, which lies in the tegmentum just lateral and posterior to the motor nucleus; most fibers synapse there and give rise to second-order neurons that cross the midline and ascend in the ventral trigeminothalamic tract en route to the ventral posterior medial (VPM) thalamic nucleus (Figure 15.2). Some fibers ascend ipsilaterally in the small dorsal trigeminothalamic tract to VPM. The two sets of trigeminothalamic fibers, both of which run near the medial lemniscus, are sometimes referred to as the trigeminal lemniscus.

Fibers subserving pain and temperature take a much more circuitous route to the thalamus. The spinal tract, or the descending root, of the trigeminal extends from the principal sensory nucleus down through the lower pons and medulla, into the spinal cord as far as C3, or even C4 (Figure 15.2). There the spinal tract becomes continuous with Lissauer's tract. The nucleus of the spinal tract is a cell column that lies just medial to the fiber tract throughout its course. In the cervical cord, the nucleus of the spinal

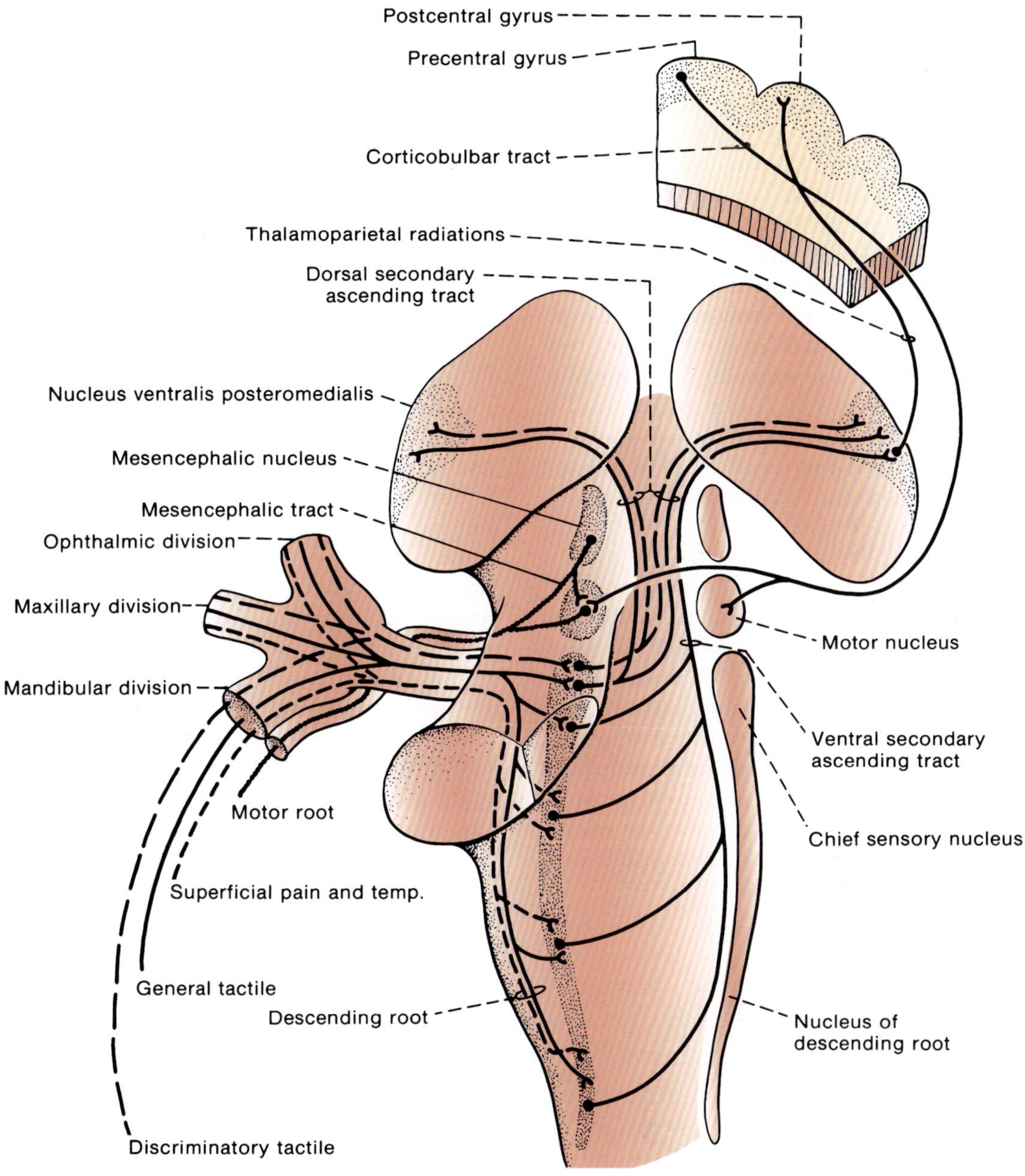

FIGURE 15.2 The trigeminal nerve and its connections.

tract becomes continuous with the substantia gelatinosa of the posterior horn. Fibers conveying pain and temperature enter the spinal tract of the trigeminal and descend to various levels depending on their somatotopic origin, then synapse in the adjacent nucleus of the spinal tract. The axons of second-order neurons cross the midline, aggregate in the ventral trigeminothalamic tract, and ascend to VPM alongside the medial lemniscus and spinothalamic tracts. Fibers arising from the pars caudalis send collaterals to the intralaminar and posterior thalamic nuclei. From VPM, fibers project through the thalamic radiations to the sensory cortex in the postcentral gyrus, where facial sensation occupies the lower third. Some projections from VPM terminate in the precentral gyrus. Fibers from the intralaminar nuclei project well outside the primary sensory cortex. Sensory fibers from CNs VII, IX, and X provide sensation to the region of the external ear canal; these fibers join the trigeminal system centrally.

The somatotopic organization of the nucleus and spinal tract is complex. There are three subnuclei, from above to below—the nuclei (or pars) oralis, interpolaris, and caudalis. The pars oralis extends from mid-pons to the level of the inferior olive, the pars interpolaris from the inferior olive to the obex, and the pars caudalis from there to the upper cervical cord. At one time, it was thought that different divisions of the trigeminal descended to different levels in the spinal tract. This concept was based in part on the alterations in corneal sensation after surgical tractomy of the cervical cord, which is done to treat chronic pain. Current thinking is that all three divisions are represented at all levels of the nucleus, although V_1 may not project as far caudally as V_2 and V_3. Somatotopically, V_1 is represented most anteriorly, and V_2 and V_3 more posteriorly (resembling a small inverted face with the forehead anterior on a typical cross section).

Dejerine, using clinical and pathologic material, demonstrated an "onion skin" somatotopic organization (Figure 15.3). The face is represented as concentric rings from the perioral region to the preauricular region. Fibers from the foreface (upper lip, mouth, and tip of the nose) synapse most rostrally in the nucleus of the spinal tract; those from the hindface synapse more caudally, adjacent to the sensory input from C2 and C3. Because of this organization, there is occasionally sparing, less frequently selective involvement of the perioral region compared to the posterior face (balaclava helmet distribution). The onionskin distribution is important in understanding the patterns of facial sensory loss that may occur with intrinsic brainstem and cervical spinal cord lesions, especially syringomyelia and syringobulbia. Chang reported a clinical demonstration of the onionskin organization in a case of central cord syndrome where facial dysesthesias retreated from the center toward the periphery. Onionskin sensory loss was apparently common in neurosyphilis.

The third sensory component, the mesencephalic root of the trigeminal nerve, runs with the motor root and then extends posteriorly and cephalad from the level of the motor nucleus into the mesencephalon. It carries proprioceptive impulses from the muscles supplied by the trigeminal nerve and probably for the extraocular muscles and the muscles of facial expression as well. Neurons subserving proprioception are unipolar neurons, but they reside inside the brainstem in the mesencephalic nucleus of CN V, making it in essence an ectopic dorsal root ganglion within the central nervous system (CNS). Proprioceptive fibers pass through the gasserian ganglion without synapsing and terminate in the mesencephalic nucleus. The mesencephalic nucleus mediates the jaw jerk reflex. Projections join the trigeminothalamic tracts and ascend to VPM.

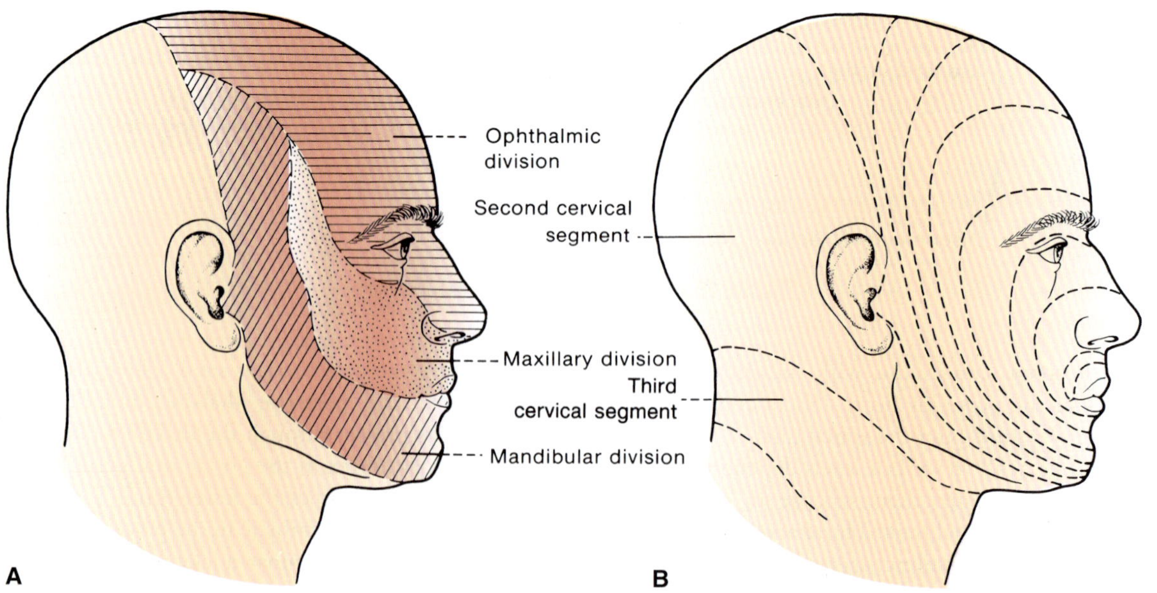

FIGURE 15.3 Cutaneous distribution of the trigeminal nerve. **A.** Peripheral distribution. **B.** Segmental distribution.

The Trigeminal Divisions

The three divisions of CN V arise from the trigeminal ganglion. Each division has a meningeal branch. Disregarding these, the ophthalmic division has three major terminal branches; the other two divisions have four each. The terminal branches of V_1 are the frontal, lacrimal, and nasociliary nerves. The terminal branches of the maxillary division are the infraorbital, zygomatic, superior alveolar, and pterygopalatine. The terminal branches of the mandibular division are the buccal, lingual, inferior alveolar, and auriculotemporal. The cutaneous distribution of the divisions is summarized in Table 15.1.

From the gasserian ganglion, V_1—the smallest of the three divisions—runs forward and enters the cavernous sinus; it lies laterally in the wall of the sinus between the folds of dura (Figure 14.6). A branch is given off to the meninges of the tentorium cerebelli just after leaving the ganglion. CN V_1 runs forward through the superior orbital fissure and divides into its terminal branches. The sensory innervation of V_1 is shown in Figure 15.3. Note that V_1 supplies most of the nose. Sensory loss along the nose because of a lesion of the distal branches of V_2 is shown in Figure 15.5. The sensory fibers to the eye pass through the ciliary ganglion without synapsing and continue as the short ciliary nerves; these convey sensation from the globe and carry postganglionic sympathetic fibers to the pupilloconstrictor muscle. The long ciliary nerves carry sensation from the ciliary body and cornea, as well as sympathetic fibers to the pupillodilator muscle. Proprioceptive fibers from the extraocular muscles travel initially with their respective CNs but join V_1 and proceed to the mesencephalic nucleus.

The maxillary branch gives off the middle, or recurrent, meningeal nerve to the dura of the middle fossa, passes through the lateral wall of the cavernous sinus, and then exits through the foramen rotundum. It crosses the pterygopalatine (sphenopalatine) fossa, where the sensory branches to the palate are given off, after which the nerve splits into the zygomatic and posterior superior alveolar branches. The palatine nerves traverse the sphenopalatine ganglion without synapsing to innervate the hard and soft palate. The nerve enters the orbit via the inferior orbital fissure and transits the infraorbital canal. The middle and anterior alveolar branches arise in the infraorbital canal. The anterior alveolar branch exits through the infraorbital foramen and becomes the infraorbital nerve. Lesions of the infraorbital nerve cause the numb cheek syndrome (see below).

The mandibular division, the largest of the branches, gives off a small meningeal branch, and then exits through the foramen ovale. It runs for a short distance with the motor root, forming a large trunk. This trunk gives off the nervous spinosus and the branch to the medial pterygoid muscle. The nervous spinosus is a recurrent twig that re-enters the skull through the foramen spinosum and runs alongside the middle meningeal artery to innervate the meninges of the anterior and middle fossa. The trunk then divides into a small, anterior, chiefly motor branch and a large, posterior, chiefly sensory branch. The sensory filaments of the anterior branch form the buccal nerve. The posterior branch divides into three large terminal nerves. Two, the lingual and

TABLE 15.1 The Divisions of the Trigeminal Nerve, the Foramina Through Which They Pass, Their Terminal Branches, and Fields of Cutaneous Innervation

Division	Skull Foramen	Terminal Branches	Cutaneous Innervation of Division
Ophthalmic	Superior orbital fissure	Frontal Lacrimal Nasociliary Meningeal	Bridge and side of nose, upper eyelid, forehead, scalp back to vertex, eyeball, lacrimal gland, nasal septum, lateral wall of nasal cavity, ethmoid sinus, tentorium cerebelli
Maxillary	Foramen rotundum	Infraorbital Zygomatic Superior alveolar Pterygopalatine Meningeal	Cheek, lateral forehead, side of nose, upper lip, upper teeth and gums, palate, nasopharynx, posterior nasal cavity, meninges of anterior and middle cranial fossa
Mandibular	Foramen ovale	Buccal Lingual Inferior alveolar Auriculotemporal Meningeal	Inner cheek, temple, lateral scalp, external auditory meatus, tympanic membrane, temporomandibular joint, mandible, lower teeth and gums, anterior two-thirds of tongue, lower lip, chin, meninges of anterior and middle cranial fossa

auriculotemporal, are purely sensory. The third, the inferior alveolar, also carries motor fibers to the mylohyoid and anterior belly of the digastric. The lingual nerve carries somatic sensation from the anterior two-thirds of the tongue. Taste sensation from the same region is carried by the chorda tympani and CN VII. After the origin of the lingual nerve, the nerve enters the mandibular foramen, traverses the mandibular canal, and emerges through the mental foramen as the mental nerve to supply sensation to the chin. Lesions of the mental nerve produce the numb chin syndrome (see below).

Some specifics about the trigeminal sensory innervation are clinically noteworthy. The innervation of the cornea is generally said to be CN V_1, although there is some evidence that the upper cornea may be CN V_1 and the lower cornea CN V_2, at least in some patients. CN V_1 innervates most of the nose, including the nasal septum. CN V_1 territory extends back to the scalp vertex; it does not stop at the hairline. Figure 15.4 demonstrates the territory of the ophthalmic division outlined by post-zoster scarring. CN V_2 innervates the inferior lateral aspect of the nose and the cheek. The cutaneous distribution of CN V_2 is nearly identical to the infraorbital nerve (Figure 15.5). Changes in sensation involving the upper teeth and gums can be helpful in distinguishing a CN V_2 lesion from an infraorbital nerve lesion in patients with the numb cheek syndrome.

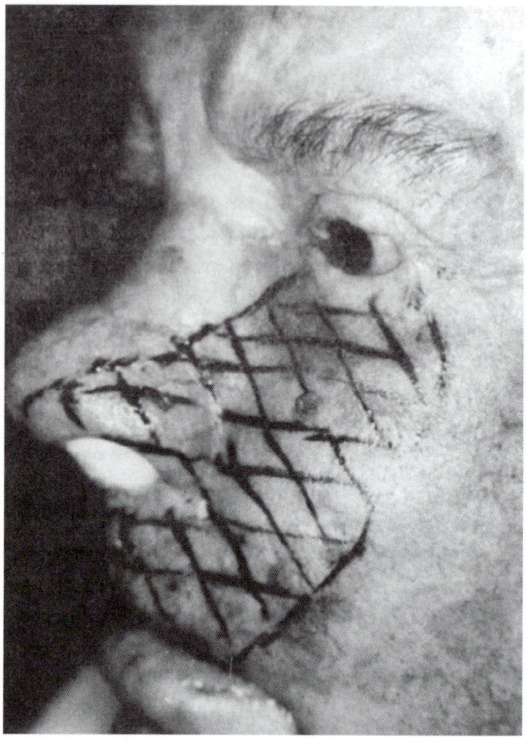

FIGURE 15.5 Patient with infraorbital neuropathy from carcinomatous infiltration. Note that the maxillary division innervates only the side of the nose distally. This patient had numbness of only the anterior teeth and gums, which proved the lesion was at the infraorbital foramen and not intracranial. (Reprinted from Campbell WW. The numb cheek syndrome: a sign of infraorbital neuropathy. *Neurology* 1986;36[3]:421–423, with permission.)

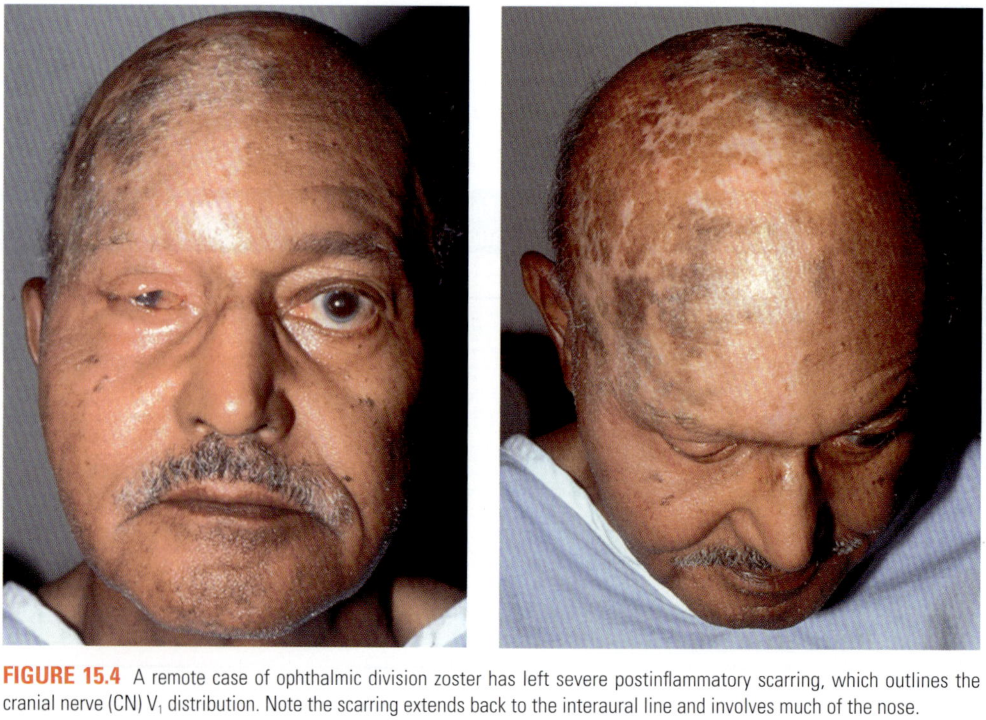

FIGURE 15.4 A remote case of ophthalmic division zoster has left severe postinflammatory scarring, which outlines the cranial nerve (CN) V_1 distribution. Note the scarring extends back to the interaural line and involves much of the nose.

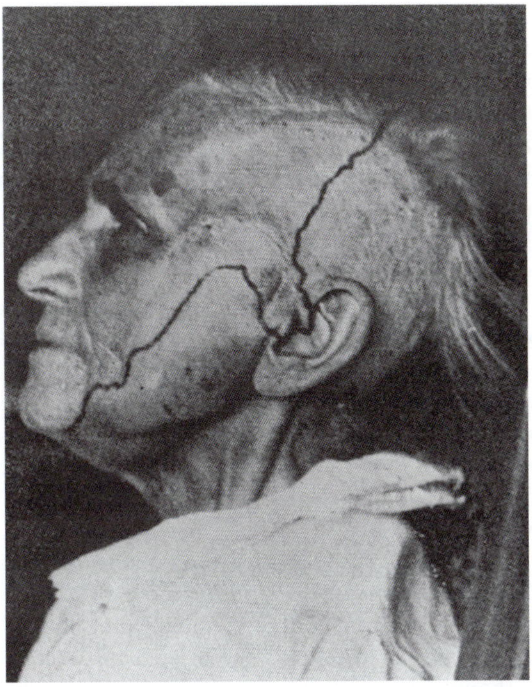

FIGURE 15.6 The distribution of sensory loss following complete section of the trigeminal root. Note the large area at the angle of the jaw that is innervated by C2 through the greater auricular nerve, and the inclusion of the tragus of the ear in the trigeminal distribution.

The major terminal branch of CN V_3 is the mental nerve, which provides sensation to the chin and lower lip. The distribution of CN V_3 does not extend to the jaw line; there is a large "notch" at the angle of the jaw innervated by the greater auricular nerve (C2-C3). This notch of C2-C3 innervation can be surprisingly large (Figure 15.6).

CN V supplies filaments to four ganglia in the head: the ciliary, sphenopalatine, otic, and submaxillary (Box 15.1).

CLINICAL EXAMINATION

Examination of the Motor Functions

Assessment of trigeminal motor function is accomplished by examining the muscles of mastication. Bulk and power of the masseters and pterygoids can be gauged by palpating these muscles as the patient clinches the jaw. An effective technique is to place the examining fingers along the anterior, not lateral, border of the masseters bilaterally. When the jaw is clenched, the fingers will move forward; this movement should be symmetric on the two sides. Unilateral trigeminal motor weakness

BOX 15.1

The Ciliary, Sphenopalatine, Otic, and Submaxillary Ganglia

The ciliary ganglion, located in the posterior orbit, receives sensory fibers from the nasociliary branch of cranial nerve (CN) V_1 (the long root of the ciliary ganglion), parasympathetic fibers from the Edinger-Westphal nucleus through the inferior division of CN III (the short root), and sympathetic fibers from the cavernous sympathetic plexus, running through the long ciliary nerves. Its branches, the short ciliary nerves, supply the ciliary muscle, sphincter and dilator of the pupil, and cornea.

The sphenopalatine ganglion, located in the pterygopalatine fossa, receives sensory fibers from the sphenopalatine branches of CN V_2, parasympathetic fibers from the nervus intermedius via the greater superficial petrosal nerve, and sympathetic fibers from the pericarotid plexus through the deep petrosal nerve. The deep and greater superficial petrosal nerves join to form the vidian nerve, or nerve of the pterygoid canal, before entering the ganglion. The sphenopalatine ganglion sends branches to the posterior ethmoidal and sphenoidal sinuses, the hard and soft palates, tonsils, uvula, nasal mucosa, and nasopharynx. Lacrimal fibers pass along the zygomaticotemporal branch of CN V_2 to the lacrimal branch of CN V_1, then to the lacrimal gland.

The otic ganglion, located in the infratemporal fossa just below the foramen ovale, receives a motor and possibly a sensory branch from CN V_3, parasympathetic and sensory fibers from CN IX through the lesser superficial petrosal nerve, and sympathetic fibers from the plexus surrounding the middle meningeal artery. It sends motor branches to the tensor tympani and tensor veli palatini muscles and secretory fibers to the parotid gland through the auriculotemporal nerve.

The submaxillary ganglion, located near the submaxillary gland, receives sensory fibers from the lingual branch of CN V_3, parasympathetic fibers from the superior salivatory nucleus of CN VII through the chorda tympani, and sympathetic fibers from a plexus around the external maxillary artery. It sends secretory fibers to the submaxillary and sublingual glands and the mucous membrane of the mouth and tongue.

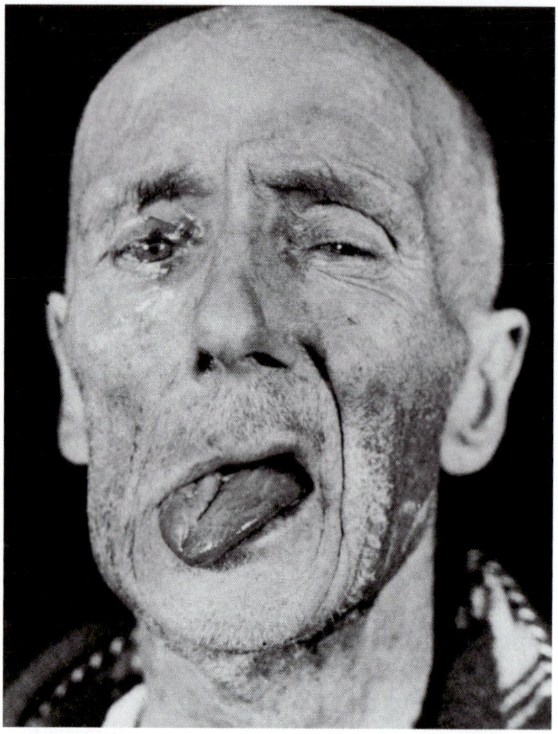

FIGURE 15.7 Infranuclear paralysis of the right trigeminal, facial, and hypoglossal nerves in a patient with metastatic carcinoma, showing deviation of the tongue and mandible to the right.

causes deviation of the jaw toward the weak side on opening, because of the unopposed action of the contralateral lateral pterygoid. The tongue also deviates toward the side of the weakness with CN XII lesions. So, both the tongue and the jaw deviate toward the weakness. Whether this is toward or away from the lesion depends on the specifics of the lesion. Figure 15.7 shows a patient with both tongue and jaw deviation. For a video of a patient with jaw deviation, see **Video Link 15.1.**

Careful observation of jaw opening is often the earliest clue to the presence of an abnormality. It is occasionally difficult to be certain whether the jaw is deviating or not. Note the relationship of the midline notch between the upper and lower incisor teeth; it is a more reliable indicator than lip movement. The tip of the nose and the interincisural notches should line up. A straightedge against the lips can help detect deviation. Another useful technique is to draw a vertical line across the midline upper and lower lips using a felt-tip marker. Failure of the two vertical marks to match when the jaw is opened indicates deviation. If there is any suggestion of a problem, have the patient move the jaw from side to side. With unilateral weakness, the patient is unable to move the jaw contralaterally. To review, weakness of the right pterygoids causes deviation of the jaw to the right on spontaneous opening and inability to move the jaw to the left on command. With facial weakness, there may be apparent deviation of the jaw, and of the tongue, because of the facial asymmetry. Holding up the weak side manually will sometimes eliminate the pseudo-deviation.

Other techniques for examining trigeminal motor function include having the patient protrude and retract the jaw, noting any tendency toward deviation, and having the patient bite on tongue depressors with the molar teeth, comparing the impressions on the two sides and comparing the difficulty of extracting a tongue depressor held by the molar teeth on each side.

Unilateral weakness of CN V–innervated muscles generally signifies a lesion involving the brainstem, gasserian ganglion, or the motor root of CN V zat the base of the skull. Severe bilateral weakness of the muscles of mastication with inability to close the mouth (dangling jaw) suggests motor neuron disease, a neuromuscular transmission disorder, or a myopathy. With significant atrophy of one masseter, a flattening of the jowl on the involved side may be apparent (Figure 15.8). With temporalis atrophy, there may be a hollowing of the temple. Rarely, fasciculations or other abnormal involuntary movements occur. There is no reliable or realistic method for examination of the other muscles supplied by CN V. Paralysis of the tensor tympani may cause difficulty hearing high notes. Because of bilateral innervation, unilateral upper motor neuron lesions rarely cause significant impairment of trigeminal motor function. There may be mild, transitory unilateral weakness. The amount of involvement depends on the extent of decussation. In bilateral supranuclear lesions, there may be marked paresis.

Examination of the Sensory Functions

In testing facial sensation, touch, pain, and occasionally temperature are examined in the same manner as elsewhere on the body (Chapter 32), searching for areas of altered sensation. It is better to ask the patient if the stimuli feel the same on the two sides, rather than suggesting they might feel different. Sensation should be compared in each trigeminal division, and the perioral region compared to the posterior face to exclude an onionskin pattern. Pain

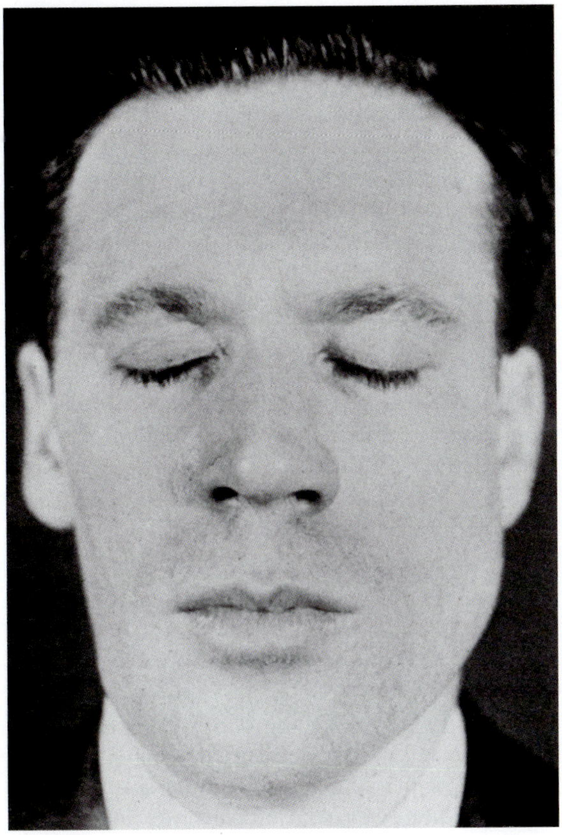

FIGURE 15.8 Infranuclear paralysis of the right trigeminal nerve with atrophy of the muscles of mastication.

or temperature should be compared with touch to exclude dissociated sensory loss (a common finding in lateral medullary syndrome). Sometimes it is useful to examine the nostrils, gums, tongue, and insides of the cheeks. Proprioception cannot be adequately tested, but one can test for extinction and the ability to identify figures written on the skin.

There are three common exercises in evaluating facial sensation: (a) determining whether sensory loss is organic or nonorganic, (b) determining which modalities are involved, and (c) defining the distribution. Complaints of facial numbness are common, and not all are organic. However, real facial sensory loss can be a serious finding, occasionally signifying underlying malignancy. The various methods and tricks for detecting nonorganic sensory loss are not entirely reliable, and this diagnosis should be made with caution. Patients with nonorganic sensory loss may have a demarcation of the abnormal area at the hairline rather than the scalp vertex. On the lower face, functional sensory loss tends to follow the jaw line and involve the notch over the masseter muscle, which is not trigeminal innervated (Figure 15.6). However, patients with intramedullary lesions may have involvement of the angle of the jaw. On the trunk, organic sensory loss typically stops short of midline because of the overlap from the opposite side, and splitting of the midline suggests nonorganicity. This finding is not reliable on the face because there is less midline overlap, so organic facial sensory loss may extend to the midline. The corneal and sternutatory reflexes (see below) should be normal in nonorganic sensory loss. Splitting of vibration along the midline is reputedly a nonorganic sign. Because the frontal bone and mandible are single bones, there should be no difference in vibratory sensibility on either side of midline. Patients who report a difference in vibratory sensibility on testing just to either side of midline may have nonorganic sensory loss. The reliability of this sign has not been validated; it can be misleading. Other signs suggestive of nonorganicity include dissociation between pinprick and temperature, variability from trial to trial, history of hypochondriasis, secondary gain, la belle indifference, nonanatomical sensory loss, and changing boundaries of hypalgesia. Gould et al. have appropriately cautioned about the validity of psychogenic signs and symptoms.

Examination of the Reflexes

The corneal, sternutatory, and jaw reflexes are the reflexes most often assessed in evaluating the trigeminal nerve.

The Jaw, Masseter, or Mandibular Reflex

To elicit the jaw (or jaw muscle) reflex, the examiner places an index finger or thumb over the middle of the patient's chin, holding the mouth open about midway with the jaw relaxed, then taps the finger with the reflex hammer. The response is an upward jerk of the mandible. Other methods to elicit the reflex include tapping the chin directly and placing a tongue blade over the tongue or the lower incisor teeth and tapping the protruding end. All of these cause a bilateral response. A unilateral response may sometimes be elicited by tapping the angle of the jaw or by placing a tongue blade over the lower molar teeth along one side and tapping the protruding end.

The afferent impulses of this reflex are carried through the sensory portion of the trigeminal nerve to the mesencephalic nucleus, with the efferent impulses through its motor portion. In normal individuals, the jaw jerk is minimally active or absent. Its greatest use is in distinguishing limb hyperreflexia because of a cervical spine lesion (where the jaw jerk is normal) from a state of generalized hyperreflexia (where the jaw jerk is increased along with all of the other reflexes). The jaw reflex is exaggerated with lesions affecting the corticobulbar pathways above the motor nucleus, especially if bilateral, as in pseudobulbar palsy or amyotrophic lateral sclerosis (ALS). It is sometimes possible to elicit extra beats or jaw clonus. For a video of a hyperactive jaw reflex see Osama et al. The reflex may be unilaterally depressed in lesions involving the reflex arc.

The Corneal Reflex

The corneal reflex is elicited by lightly touching the cornea with a wisp of cotton or tissue. It is used to assess CN V_1 function. The stimuli should ideally be delivered to the upper cornea, because the lower cornea may be CN V_2 innervated in some individuals. The stimuli should be brought in from below or from the side so the patient cannot see it (Figure 15.9).

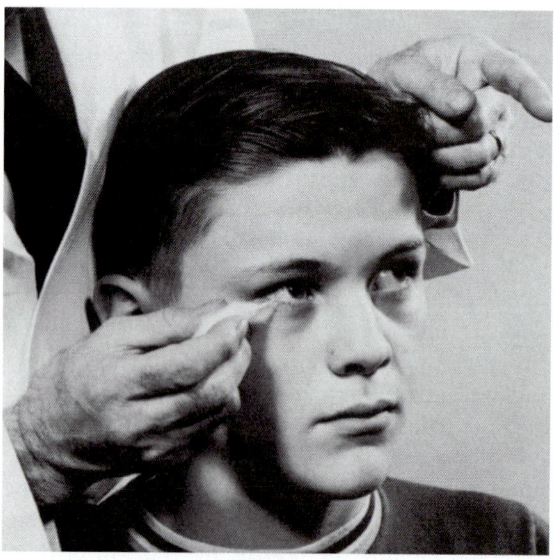

FIGURE 15.9 Eliciting the corneal reflex. The stimulating object should be brought in outside the patient's vision. The patient should look upward as the object is brought in from below, or laterally as the object is brought in from the other side. The stimulus must be applied to the cornea, not the sclera.

The stimulus must be delivered to the cornea, not the sclera. If there is any evidence of eye infection, different pieces of cotton or tissue should be used for the two eyes. Crude stimuli, such as a large blunt object or fingertip, should never be used, even in comatose patients.

In response to the corneal stimulus, there should be blinking of the ipsilateral (direct reflex) and contralateral (consensual reflex) eyes. The afferent limb of the reflex is mediated by CN V_1, the efferent limb by CN VII. The blink reflex is an electrophysiologic test in which an electrical stimulus is delivered to the trigeminal nerve, and a response is recorded from facial muscles. It can provide further information about CN V, CN VII, and the connections between them. For brainstem lesions, electrophysiologic lesion localization corresponds well with imaging findings.

With a unilateral trigeminal lesion both the direct and consensual responses may be absent; neither eye blinks. Stimulation of the opposite eye produces normal direct and consensual responses. With a unilateral CN VII lesion, the direct response may be impaired, but the consensual reflex should be normal. Stimulation of the opposite side produces a normal direct response but an impaired consensual response. These patterns are summarized in Table 15.2. Lesions involving the brainstem polysynaptic trigeminofacial connections may produce impairment of both direct and consensual responses. The corneal reflex may be depressed with lesions of the contralateral hemisphere, especially if there is thalamic involvement. Because of the descent of the spinal tract and nucleus of CN V into the upper cervical cord, lesions there sometimes affect the corneal reflex. Corneal anesthesia can be a complication of cervical tractotomy done for chronic pain. Corneal sensation may be impaired in contact lens wearers, even when the lenses are out.

The Sternutatory (Nasal, Sneeze) Reflex

Stimulation of the nasal mucous membrane with cotton, a spear of tissue, or similar objects causes wrinkling of the nose, eye closure, and often a forceful exhalation resembling a feeble sneeze, as the nose tries to rid itself of the foreign object. The ophthalmic, not the maxillary, division of the trigeminal innervates the nasal septum and the anterior nasal passages.

TABLE 15.2 Patterns of Direct and Consensual Corneal Reflex Abnormality with Trigeminal and Facial Nerve Lesions

		Direct Corneal Reflex	Consensual Corneal Reflex
Complete Trigeminal Nerve Lesion			
	Stimulate involved eye	Absent	Absent
	Stimulate opposite eye	Normal	Normal
Complete Facial Nerve Lesion			
	Stimulate involved eye	Absent	Normal
	Stimulate opposite eye	Normal	Absent

The afferent limb of the reflex arc is carried over CN V_1, the efferent limb over CNs V, VII, IX, X, and the motor nerves of the cervical and thoracic spinal cord. The reflex center is in the brainstem and upper spinal cord. The nasal mucosa may also be stimulated by irritating inhalants; this is a nasal reflex that should not be confused with olfaction (Chapter 12). The primary clinical use of the sternutatory reflex is as a cross-check on the corneal reflex. The ordinary sneeze reflex can obviously be elicited in many ways. An interesting phenomenon is the photic sneeze, photosternutatory, or "ACHOO" (autosomal dominant compelling helio-ophthalmic outburst) reflex—sneezing in response to looking at a bright light, which is seen in many normal individuals. Pryse-Phillips commented, "The acronym is slightly forced, but remains... the best of the decade."

Other Trigeminal Mediated Reflexes

Other reflexes mediated in part by CN V include the nonfocal orbicularis oculi reflex and other trigeminofacial responses (Chapter 16), corneomandibular reflex (Chapter 40), and the snout reflex (Chapter 40). Many other reflexes have been described, but they are of limited value and are seldom used. The afferent limbs of these reflexes are trigeminal mediated. In some, the efferent limb is also trigeminal (e.g., the jaw jerk); in others, the efferent limb is executed through connections with CN III, CN VII, or other pathways.

Disorders of Function

Trigeminal nerve lesions may cause weakness, abnormal involuntary movements, sensory loss or other sensory abnormalities, facial pain, trophic abnormalities, autonomic dysfunction, or abnormalities of the reflexes mediated by the trigeminal nerve. The conditions most commonly seen are facial pain, particularly TN, and facial numbness.

Motor Dysfunction

Because of the bilateral hemispheric innervation, weakness in the trigeminal distribution does not often occur with upper motor neuron lesions, although slight weakness of the contralateral muscles with an exaggerated jaw reflex can occur. Bilateral supranuclear lesions, as in pseudobulbar palsy or ALS, can cause marked weakness, often with a grossly exaggerated jaw reflex. In supranuclear lesions, no atrophy or fasciculations occur.

Significant weakness in the trigeminal motor distribution is most often the result of a neuromuscular transmission disorder or ALS. Patients with myasthenia gravis (MG) may have chewing difficulties with masticatory fatigue, especially when eating difficult-to-chew things such as tough meat. When severe, MG may cause an inability to close the mouth (jaw drop). Patients with severe polymyositis, rarely with other myopathies, may also have difficulty with jaw power. Patients with giant cell arteritis commonly have jaw claudication with focal pain in the masseter when chewing, which can be confused with weakness. ALS commonly causes a jaw drop, often with dysphagia and difficulty swallowing saliva, requiring the patients to constantly keep absorbent materials in their mouth. Jaw drop may also occur in Kennedy's disease. Needle electromyography of trigeminal innervated muscles may demonstrate subclinical involvement. Lesions anywhere along the course of the lower motor neuron can cause weakness accompanied by atrophy, sometimes marked; fasciculations; and a decreased jaw jerk (Figure 15.7).

Abnormal involuntary movements commonly affect the jaw. Oromandibular dystonia produces a variety of abnormal movements: jaw opening, jaw closing, lateral movements, bruxism, and combinations of these (see **Video Link 15.2**). Jaw dystonia may occur as part of an extrapyramidal syndrome due to psychoactive drugs, and abnormal jaw movements are a common manifestation of tardive dyskinesias. Meige's syndrome is oromandibular dystonia and blepharospasm. Chewing movements and grinding of the teeth are sometimes present in psychoses, and chewing or tasting movements in complex partial seizures. Bruxism may occur as a side effect of levodopa. Rarely, a focal seizure limited to the muscles of mastication may cause clenching of the jaws with biting of the tongue or cheeks. Trismus is marked spasm of the muscles of mastication: The teeth are tightly clenched, the muscles hard and firm, and the patient is unable to open his jaws. It is a classical manifestation of tetanus, and sometimes occurs in encephalitis, rabies, acute dystonic reactions due to neuroleptic medications, and tetany. Trismus may occur in Foix-Chavany-Marie syndrome (Chapter 9). Some myopathies, especially polymyositis, may result in fibrosis of the masseters, which causes painless trismus. Trismus may be psychogenic. Patients with Parkinson's disease may have jaw tremor. Hemimasticatory spasm is a syndrome of brief, sometimes painful, involuntary contractions or spasms of the jaw-closing muscles unilaterally. It may eventually result in masseter hypertrophy. Hemimasticatory spasm may be associated with other conditions, including scleroderma and facial hemiatrophy. Neuromyotonia of the jaw muscles may follow cranial irradiation.

Sensory Dysfunction

Supranuclear lesions, particularly of the parietal lobe or sensory radiations, may raise the sensory threshold of the contralateral face; a thalamic lesion may cause facial hypesthesia with hyperpathia or allodynia. Lesions of the principal sensory nucleus in the pons may cause diminished tactile sensation involving both skin and mucous membranes on the involved side, and loss of reflexes in which the afferent arc is mediated by the trigeminal nerve. Lesions of the spinal tract or nucleus cause a disturbance of the pain and temperature modalities, and, possibly to a lesser extent, of tactile sense.

Dissociation of sensation, with different degrees of involvement of light touch as compared to pain and temperature, suggests a lesion in the substance of the brainstem (intramedullary), where the different sensory pathways are running in widely separate locations. Extramedullary lesions are characterized by loss or diminution of all types of exteroceptive sensation, dysesthesias or paresthesias, or spontaneous pain. A lesion central to or at the gasserian ganglion will affect all three divisions; a lesion peripheral to the ganglion, will involve only isolated divisions or branches. There may also be reflex changes, such as absence of the corneal or sternutatory.

Trigeminal nerve lesions may also cause trophic changes. With CN V_1 lesions impaired, corneal sensation may result in corneal ulcerations and other ocular complications. The eye must be scrupulously protected when the cornea is anesthetic. Interaction between the trigeminal and olfactory systems has a powerful influence on the perception of odors, and trophic changes in the nasal mucosa because of a trigeminal lesion may cause a secondary anosmia. Nasal anesthesia may result in disfiguring erosion of the ala nasi. Because of the many connections of CN V with other CNs, particularly CNs VII and IX, a decrease or increase in lacrimal, salivary, and mucous secretion can follow a trigeminal lesion, particularly when the functions are trigeminal-mediated reflex responses. Even taste, not a trigeminal function, may be affected because of taste fibers carried through the lingual nerve to the chorda tympani.

The most common disorder to involve trigeminal sensory function is TN, or tic douloureux. TN causes paroxysms of fleeting but excruciating unilateral facial pain. It usually involves the second or third division, rarely the first (the inverse of herpes zoster [HZ]). Occasional patients have involvement of both CN V_2 and CN V_3. The lancinating pain usually lasts only seconds, occasionally up to 2 minutes, but may occur many times a day. The patient may wince, hence the designation "tic." Stimulation of some specific area, a trigger zone, in the involved nerve distribution will often provoke a paroxysm of pain. Pain may be brought on by activities such as talking, chewing, brushing teeth, exposure to cold, or by wind on the face. Men may present with the trigger zone unshaven, women with it not made up. The patient may be reluctant to allow neurologic examination of the involved area for fear of triggering a paroxysm of pain. Trigger zones are small, sometimes punctate. Stimulus-evoked pain is one of the most striking features of TN and has high diagnostic value. A refractory period lasting seconds or minutes following a provoked paroxysm may occur. TN enters into periods of complete remission in up to 63% of patients.

The most common cause of TN is compression of the sensory root by an ectatic arterial loop off the basilar artery, usually the anterior inferior cerebellar or superior cerebellar. However, advanced imaging studies have shown that some contact between the trigeminal nerve and nearby vessels occurs in asymptomatic individuals. A meta-analysis showed neurovascular contact in 89% of symptomatic nerves, but also in 36% of asymptomatic nerves, indicating high sensitivity but poor specificity. Displacement, distortion, flattening, or atrophy of the nerve roots are sensitive signs of clinically relevant neurovascular compression. MRI in TN is rarely abnormal except for vascular loops or abnormalities related to vascular compression.

Rarely, structural lesions may cause facial pain resembling TN, referred to as secondary or symptomatic TN. These lesions may cause sensory loss in the involved distribution, motor dysfunction, or involve neighboring structures. Examples include multiple sclerosis (MS), tumors involving the gasserian ganglion or its branches, and other tumors in the cerebellopontine angle. Among patients with TN-like symptoms, 6% to 16% are variously reported to harbor an intracranial tumor, such as an acoustic neuroma. The presence of a complaint of numbness, impaired sensation on examination, other neurologic abnormalities, history of symptom progression, and duration of symptoms of less than 1 year increase the likelihood of an abnormal imaging study. Other central processes involving the trigeminal pathways in the brainstem, such as syringobulbia and infarction, may cause pain resembling TN. Facial pain is not uncommon in Wallenberg's lateral medullary syndrome and may rarely resemble TN.

Patients with idiopathic or classical TN have no clinical motor or sensory deficit in the distribution of the involved nerve. Absence of a sensory deficit is one criterion for the diagnosis of classical TN. Subtle sensory changes may be detected with quantitative sensory testing. Reports indicate that about one-third of patients with TN because of tumor or MS have a demonstrable sensory deficit, but the absence of a sensory deficit does not exclude secondary TN.

Occasional patients develop persistent, non-paroxysmal, pain in the involved distribution, frequently described as dull, burning, or tingling. This has been referred to as atypical TN or TN2. The term atypical TN is problematic because of potential confusion with the entity of atypical facial pain. Some have used the term TN2, or atypical TN, in referring to what others would cause atypical facial pain.

TN occurs in MS patients much more commonly than in the general population; it is usually caused by a demyelinating lesion involving the trigeminal root entry zone in the pons, although vascular compression at the root entry zone can occur even in MS patients. TN occurs in 2% to 5% of patients with MS, and MS is found in 2% to 14% of patients presenting with TN. Bilateral TN is especially suggestive of MS. Most TN patients are in the fifth decade or beyond; onset in a young person should prompt consideration of symptomatic TN, especially due to demyelinating disease.

Some published diagnostic guidelines have inadvertently made the classification of TN more difficult. The most recent version of the International Classification of Headache Disorders no longer includes symptomatic or secondary TN as a diagnostic category. Crucco et al. proposed a new classification and diagnostic grading scheme for practice and research. In this scheme, classical TN is defined as a specific category in which MRI demonstrates vascular compression with morphologic changes of the trigeminal nerve root. Secondary TN is that due to a major underlying neurologic disease, such as tumor or MS. The category of idiopathic TN is reserved for the small proportion of patients in which imaging studies are completely normal except for incidental vascular contact. TN with continuous pain refers to those patients who experience nonparoxysmal pain between attacks.

The operative technique of microvascular decompression insulates the nerve from a compressing vessel. Microvascular decompression is widely performed and quite effective. In the past, ablative involvement procedures such as retrogasserian rhizotomy were often performed on the gasserian ganglion or sensory root. These would leave the patient's face numb to various degrees. Sometimes the operation would cause facial numbness but fail to relieve the pain, leaving the patient with a numb but painful face, a condition called anesthesia dolorosa or deafferentation pain. Ablative procedures used currently in resistant cases can also cause anesthesia dolorosa.

Many other craniofacial neuralgias have been described, but most of these syndromes have not withstood the test of time and their existence as real entities remains in doubt. These include Sluder's, or sphenopalatine, neuralgia, vidian neuralgia, Costen's syndrome, and Eagle's syndrome. The term persistent idiopathic facial pain, formerly called atypical facial pain, is used to refer to a syndrome of facial pain that does not have the characteristics of TN. The pain in atypical facial pain is typically constant and not paroxysmal, described as deep and poorly localized, not restricted to a single trigeminal division, not lancinating, and not associated with any trigger zone. No identifiable etiology is usually apparent, and the pain is often attributed to depression or other emotional factors. There is increasing evidence that in some cases it is a neuropathic pain syndrome with objective abnormalities on neurophysiologic testing. Forssell et al. found that 75% of a series of 20 patients with atypical facial pain had either an abnormal electrodiagnostic blink reflex or abnormal thermal quantitative thermal sensory testing. Aching pain in the face may precede the development of TN (preTN).

Unusual facial pain may occur in Gradenigo's syndrome because of gasserian ganglion involvement in lesions at the petrous apex. Affected patients may have pain and sensory disturbances in the V_1 distribution, accompanied by CN VI palsy (Chapter 14). In Raeder's paratrigeminal syndrome (paratrigeminal oculosympathetic syndrome), there is headache, facial pain in the distribution of V_1 and an oculosympathetic paresis. There is no anhidrosis as in Horner's syndrome because those fibers travel via the external carotid artery. There may or may not be demonstrable trigeminal sensory loss. Other CNs may be involved. The responsible lesion lies in the middle cranial fossa near the petrous apex. Headache and oculosympathetic paresis (or Horner's syndrome) may also occur with cluster headache and carotid dissecting aneurysms. CN V_1 or V_2, or both, may be involved in lesions of the cavernous sinus (Chapter 21). In the superior orbital fissure syndrome, there is involvement of V_1 and other structures passing through the fissure (Chapter 21). Only when V_2 is affected can lesions of the cavernous sinus and superior orbital fissure be clinically differentiated. Nurmikko stressed the value of a semi-structured interview, posing a series of specific questions, in the differential diagnosis of facial pain syndromes.

Acute HZ of the trigeminal nerve is extremely painful. It is usually seen in elderly or immunocompromised patients, and affects CN V_1 in 80% of cases, causing pain and vesicles over the forehead, eyelid, and cornea (herpes ophthalmicus). The inflammation causes neuronal loss in the affected ganglion, and a reduction of both axons and myelin in the affected nerve. Cutaneous scarring is common (Figure 15.4). Ophthalmic involvement may lead to keratitis, corneal ulcerations, residual corneal scarring, and sometimes result in blindness. In some patients, only the eye, mainly the cornea, is involved. Zoster may affect any of the trigeminal divisions, and there may be motor involvement (Figure 15.10). Rarely, trigeminal HZ may be complicated by encephalitis or a syndrome of delayed contralateral hemiparesis due to arteritis. Pain without a cutaneous eruption is referred to as zoster sine zoster or zoster sine herpete.

Postherpetic Neuralgia

In some patients with trigeminal HZ, the pain of the acute phase evolves into a dreadful, persistent neuralgic pain syndrome called postherpetic neuralgia (PHN). Pain persisting for more than 3 months after the acute eruption is appropriately labeled as PHN.

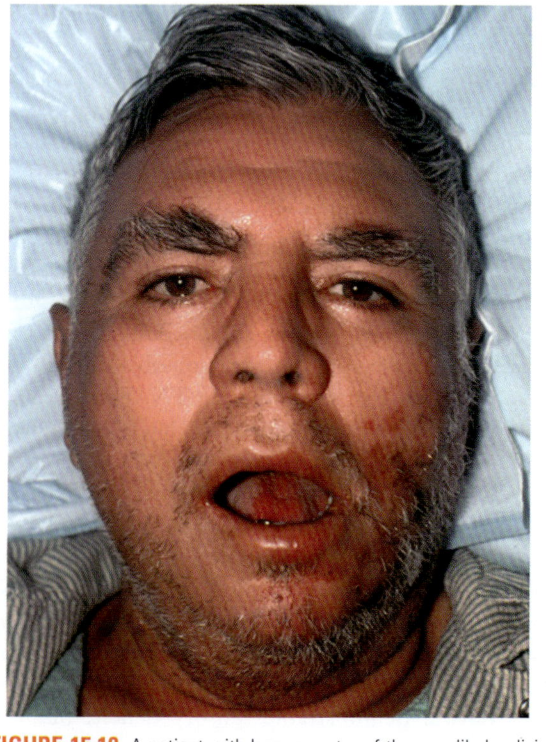

FIGURE 15.10 A patient with herpes zoster of the mandibular division on the left involving the motor root, producing weakness of the pterygoids, and causing deviation of the jaw to the left. The herpetic rash is in the distribution of CN V_3.

The pain is probably related to deafferentation and mediated centrally. It is typically dysesthetic with a burning component, constant but with superimposed paroxysms of lancinating pain that may be provoked by touching certain spots within the affected area. There may be hypesthesia or hyperesthesia in the affected area. Age is an important factor in predisposing to PHN; it develops in only 10% of those less than age 60, but in 40% of those over 60 years.

Facial Numbness

Isolated facial numbness is a common problem. Facial sensory loss may occur with lesions involving the main trigeminal divisions or their distal branches. A number of processes, some ominous, may be responsible. The numb chin syndrome refers to hypesthesia and sometimes paresthesias involving the lower lip and chin, approximately in the distribution of the mental nerve (chin neuropathy, Roger's sign). The numb chin syndrome is often due to a neoplastic process, with metastasis either to the mental foramen of the mandible or to the intracranial meninges or skull base, often from carcinoma of the breast or lung. Lesions of the inferior alveolar nerve may also be responsible. The predilection for involvement of the CN V_3 distribution may reflect the relatively protected position of the other trigeminal divisions in the cavernous sinus, with greater exposure of the third division to neoplastic processes involving the meninges and base of the skull. Possible clues to a skull base or meningeal origin of a numb chin include sensory disturbance extending beyond the chin or involvement of other CNs. Loss of sensation of the anterior teeth and gums suggests a distal process involving the inferior alveolar nerve. Sparing of oral sensation or dissociation of modalities suggests an intraparenchymal CNS lesion. In a series of 42 numb chin patients with cancer, 50% had metastases to the mandible, 22% had neoplastic meningitis and 14% had metastases to the skull base. Non-neoplastic causes include dental procedures, tooth abscess, connective tissue disease, sickle cell disease, tumors or cysts of the mandible, erosion of the mental foramen in edentulous patients, and trauma. In one series, the most common etiology of the numb chin syndrome was dental.

The numb cheek syndrome is similar but usually because of a lesion involving the infraorbital nerve with perineural spread of a tumor (Figure 15.5). When hypesthesia also involves the medial and lateral upper incisors and canine teeth (distribution of the anterior superior alveolar branch), and adjacent gingiva, sparing the more posterior teeth and gums, the pathologic process localizes to the infraorbital foramen and makes involvement of the maxillary division more proximally unlikely. Perineural spread of skin cancer is the most common etiology. The molar and premolar teeth and gums are innervated by the posterior and middle superior alveolar nerves. The numb cheek-limp lower lid syndrome includes weakness involving the distal branches of the facial nerve because of carcinoma infiltrating the infraorbital and facial nerves.

The numb chin or cheek syndrome can be the presenting manifestation of cancer, more often it is due to progression or relapse of a known malignancy. Unusual causes of trigeminal sensory dysfunction include pontine hemorrhage, Wegener's granulomatosis, localized hypertrophic mononeuropathy, and a midbrain lesion affecting the trigeminothalamic fibers. Trauma may involve the distal trigeminal branches. Trumpet player's neuropathy affects musicians, causing pain and numbness of the upper lip because of injury to the anterior superior alveolar nerve.

Trigeminal sensory neuropathy (TSN) refers to a syndrome of isolated facial numbness, usually gradual in onset, which may involve a single division or the entire face; it is occasionally bilateral. Some patients have paresthesias and dysesthesias. The pathology probably involves the ganglion. Some cases are idiopathic, but many underlying diseases, particularly connective tissue disorders, can cause TSN (Table 15.3). Occasionally, TSN is part of a multiple

TABLE 15.3 Some Causes of Trigeminal Sensory Neuropathy

- Idiopathic
- Connective tissue disorder
  - Sjögren's syndrome
  - Scleroderma
  - Mixed connective tissue disorder
  - Other
- Sarcoidosis
- Wegener's granulomatosis
- Giant cell arteritis
- Multiple sclerosis
- Tumor
- Diabetes
- Syringobulbia
- Toxins
  - Trichlorethylene
  - Stilbamidine
  - Mefloquine

cranial neuropathy syndrome, especially in patients with scleroderma. Some patients with idiopathic TSN have shown gadolinium enhancement in the cisternal segment suggesting a similarity to Bell's palsy.

Facial sensory loss is common in brainstem lesions; most are vascular. A frequent cause is the lateral medullary syndrome (Wallenberg's), which classically causes loss of pain and temperature sensation over the ipsilateral face and contralateral body. Variations on this pattern have been well reported, including sensory loss of only $V_{1,2}$ or only $V_{2,3}$. In a series of 50 patients, only 13 (26%) had the classic pattern. Others had bilateral facial sensory loss, contralateral facial sensory loss, only body and limb loss, only facial loss not involving the body, or no sensory signs. When facial sensory loss occurred, it was most often in an onionskin distribution. Intraoral sensation may be spared.

Other Trigeminal Nerve Disorders

Pathology involving the trigeminal nerve and its connections may result in misdirection of nerve fibers, producing unusual and interesting effects. Congenital ocular aberrant innervation syndromes are a complex group of disorders involving abnormal miswiring of the extraocular muscles (Chapter 14). The Marcus Gunn phenomenon, or jaw-winking, occurs in patients with congenital ptosis; opening the mouth, chewing, or lateral jaw movements causes an exaggerated reflex elevation of the ptotic lid, see **Video Link 15.3.** The phenomenon may be the result of proprioceptive impulses from the pterygoid muscles being misdirected to the oculomotor nucleus. Trigemino-abducens synkinesis is due to abnormal communications between CN V and CN VI. Involuntary closure of one eye on mouth opening (reversed Gunn phenomenon, inverse jaw winking, or Marin Amat sign) is a synkinesia because of aberrant regeneration of the facial nerve; it occurs most often following Bell's palsy (Chapter 16). The auriculotemporal (Frey) syndrome produces flushing, warmness, and excessive perspiration over the cheek and pinna on one side following ingestion of spicy food (gustatory sweating). This syndrome is due to misdirection of the secretory fibers to the parotid gland to the sweat glands and vasodilator endings in the auriculotemporal nerve distribution; it usually follows trauma or infection of the parotid gland or local nerve injury.

Migraine may be a neurovascular syndrome related to abnormalities in the trigeminovascular system with serotonin playing an important role. Other trigeminal autonomic cephalgias involve pain in the V_1 distribution and autonomic symptoms. There include cluster headache; paroxysmal hemicrania; and the short-lasting, unilateral, neuralgiform headache with conjunctival injection, and tearing syndrome. In encephalotrigeminal angiomatosis (Sturge-Weber syndrome, or Weber-Dimitri disease), there are congenital nevi or angiomas over one side of the face in the trigeminal distribution with associated ipsilateral leptomeningeal angiomas and intracortical calcifications with attendant neurologic complications (Figure 15.11). Neck-tongue syndrome is a rare disorder involving the trigeminal and upper cervical nerves. Pain and numbness in the distribution of the lingual nerve and C2 root are provoked by sudden head turning. Afferent fibers from the lingual nerve are thought to join the hypoglossal nerve and send filaments to the upper cervical nerves. The symptoms are allegedly caused by minor subluxation of the C2 articulatory process tweaking these nearby structures.

Localization of Trigeminal Nerve Lesions

In reviews of the regional pathology of the trigeminal nerve from an imaging perspective, the common brainstem lesions were neoplasms, vascular disease, and demyelinating processes.

The most common causes in the segment from the brainstem to the skull base—including the cisternal, Meckel cave, and cavernous sinus segments—were neurovascular compression, followed by acoustic or trigeminal schwannoma, meningioma, lymphoma,

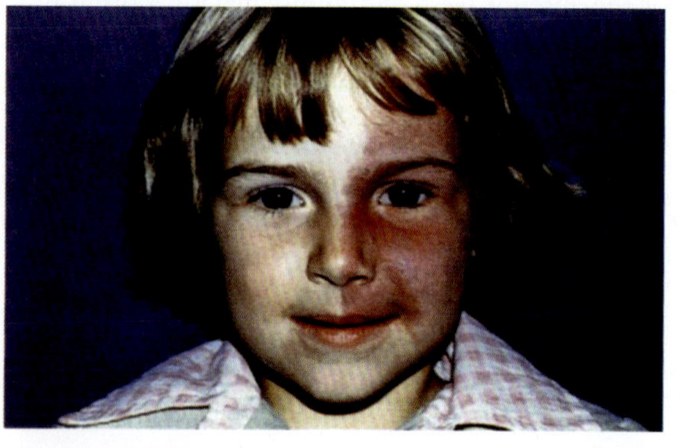

FIGURE 15.11 Child with the Sturge-Weber syndrome, causing the typical port-wine hemangioma of the skin along the distribution of the left trigeminal nerve. (Reprinted from Allingham RR, Damji KF, Shields MB. *Shields' Textbook of Glaucoma.* 6th ed. Philadelphia: Wolters Kluwer Health/Lippincott Williams & Wilkins, 2011, with permission).

epidermoid cyst, lipoma, pituitary adenoma, metastasis, and aneurysm. Skull base abnormalities included chordoma, chondrosarcoma, metastasis, bone dysplasias, and Paget's disease. The peripheral divisions of the trigeminal nerve were commonly involved by adjacent inflammatory disease in the sinuses, perineural spread of malignancy, and schwannoma. Trauma is a common cause of impaired trigeminal sensory dysfunction, because of dental and other surgical procedures, dental anesthetic injections and facial fractures.

Video Links

Video Link 15.1. Jaw deviation. https://www.youtube.com/watch?v=cbW6ki4g0JE

Video Link 15.2. Oromandibular dystonia. http://neurosigns.org/wiki/Oromandibular_dystonia

Video Link 15.3. Marcus Gunn phenomenon (jaw-winking). http://neurosigns.org/wiki/Jaw_winking

BIBLIOGRAPHY

Agostoni E, Frigerio R, Santoro P. Atypical facial pain: clinical considerations and differential diagnosis. *Neurol Sci* 2005;26(Suppl 2):S71–S74.

Akita K, Shimokawa T, Sato T. Positional relationships between the masticatory muscles and their innervating nerves with special reference to the lateral pterygoid and the midmedial and discotemporal muscle bundles of temporalis. *J Anat* 2000;197 (Pt 2):291–302.

Becker M, Kohler R, Vargas MI, et al. Pathology of the trigeminal nerve. *Neuroimaging Clin N Am* 2008;18:283–307.

Bennetto L, Patel NK, Fuller G. Trigeminal neuralgia and its management. *BMJ* 2007;334:201–205.

Boerman RH, Maassen EM, Joosten J, et al. Trigeminal neuropathy secondary to perineural invasion of head and neck carcinomas. *Neurology* 1999;53:213–216.

Bowsher D. Trigeminal neuralgia: an anatomically oriented review. *Clin Anat* 1997;10:409–415.

Brazis PW, Vogler JB, Shaw KE, et al. The "numb cheek-limp lower lid" syndrome. *Neurology* 1991;41:327–328.

Brazis PW, Masdeu JC, Biller J. *Localization in Clinical Neurology*. 7th ed. Philadelphia: Wolters Kluwer/Lippincott Williams & Wilkins, 2017.

Calverly JR, Mohnac AM. Syndrome of the numb chin. *Arch Intern Med* 1963;112:819–821.

Campbell WW Jr. The numb cheek syndrome: a sign of infraorbital neuropathy. *Neurology* 1986;36:421–423.

Campbell WW. *Clinical Signs in Neurology: A Compendium*. Philadelphia: Wolters Kluwer Health, 2016.

Caranci G, Mercurio A, Altieri M, et al. Trigeminal neuralgia as the sole manifestation of an Arnold-Chiari type I malformation: case report. *Headache* 2008;48:625–627.

Caselli RJ, Hunder GG. Neurologic complications of giant cell (temporal) arteritis. *Semin Neurol* 1994;14:349–353.

Catalano PJ, Sen C, Biller HF. Cranial neuropathy secondary to perineural spread of cutaneous malignancies. *Am J Otolaryngol* 1995;16:772–777.

Chang HS. Cervical central cord syndrome involving the spinal trigeminal nucleus: a case report. *Surg Neurol* 1995;44:236–239.

Chang Y, Horoupian DS, Jordan J, et al. Localized hypertrophic mononeuropathy of the trigeminal nerve. *Arch Pathol Lab Med* 1993;117:170–176.

Colella G, Giudice A, Siniscalchi G, et al. Chin numbness: a symptom that should not be underestimated: a review of 12 cases. *Am J Med Sci* 2009;337:407–410.

Cruccu G, Leandri M, Feliciani M, et al. Idiopathic and symptomatic trigeminal pain. *J Neurol Neurosurg Psychiatry* 1990;53:1034.

Cruccu G, Truini A, Priori A. Excitability of the human trigeminal motoneuronal pool and interactions with other brainstem reflex pathways. *J Physiol* 2001;531:559–571.

Cruccu G, Finnerup NB, Jensen TS, et al. Trigeminal neuralgia: new classification and diagnostic grading for practice and research. *Neurology* 2016;87:220–228.

Cruccu G, Bonamico LH, Zakrzewska JM. Cranial neuralgias. *Handb Clin Neurol* 2010;97:663–678.

Currier RD, Giles CL, DeJong RN. Some comments on Wallenberg's lateral medullary syndrome. *Neurology* 1961;11:778–791.

Dean L. ACHOO syndrome. In: Pratt V, McLeod H, Dean L, et al., eds. *Medical Genetics Summaries [Internet]*. Bethesda: National Center for Biotechnology Information, 2012. Available from http://www.ncbi.nlm.nih.gov/books/NBK109193/. Updated on July 27, 2015.

Dillingham TR, Spellman NT, Chang AS. Trigeminal motor nerve conduction: deep temporal and mylohyoid nerves. *Muscle Nerve* 1996;19:277–284.

Ertekin C, Celebisoy N, Uludag B. Trigeminocervical reflexes elicited by stimulation of the infraorbital nerve: head retraction reflex. *J Clin Neurophysiol* 2001;18:378–385.

Evans RW, Agostoni E. Persistent idiopathic facial pain. *Headache* 2006;46:1298–1300.

Finsterer J, Erdorf M, Mamoli B, et al. Needle electromyography of bulbar muscles in patients with amyotrophic lateral sclerosis: evidence of subclinical involvement. *Neurology* 1998;51:1417–1422.

Forssell H, Tenovuo O, Silvoniemi P, et al. Differences and similarities between atypical facial pain and trigeminal neuropathic pain. *Neurology* 2007;69:1451–1459.

Fromm GH, Graff-Radford SB, Terrence CF, et al. Pre-trigeminal neuralgia. *Neurology* 1990;40:1493.

Frontera JA, Palestrant D. Acute trismus associated with Foix-Marie-Chavany syndrome. *Neurology* 2006;66:454–455.

Frucht S. Anterior superior alveolar neuropathy: an occupational neuropathy of the embouchure. *J Neurol Neurosurg Psychiatry* 2000;69:563.

Furukawa T. Numb chin syndrome in the elderly. *J Neurol Neurosurg Psychiatry* 1990;53:173–176.

Gass A, Kitchen N, MacManus DG, et al. Trigeminal neuralgia in patients with multiple sclerosis: lesion localization with magnetic resonance imaging. *Neurology* 1997;49:1142–1144.

Go JL, Kim PE, Zee CS. The trigeminal nerve. *Semin Ultrasound CT MR* 2001;22:502–520.

Goadsby PJ. Raeder's syndrome [corrected]: paratrigeminal paralysis of the oculopupillary sympathetic system. *J Neurol Neurosurg Psychiatry* 2002;72:297–299.

Gonella MC, Fischbein NJ, So YT. Disorders of the trigeminal system. *Semin Neurol* 2009;29:36–44.

Gould R, Miller BL, Goldberg MA, et al. The validity of hysterical signs and symptoms. *J Nerv Ment Dis* 1986;174:593–597.

Govsa F, Kayalioglu G, Erturk M, et al. The superior orbital fissure and its contents. *Surg Radiol Anat* 1999;21:181–185.

Graham SH, Sharp FR, Dillon W. Intraoral sensation in patients with brainstem lesions: role of the rostral spinal trigeminal nuclei in pons. *Neurology* 1988;38:1529–1533.

Hamlyn PJ, King TT. Neurovascular compression in trigeminal neuralgia: a clinical and anatomical study. *J Neurosurg* 1992;76:948.

Hargreaves RJ, Shepheard SL. Pathophysiology of migraine—new insights. *Can J Neurol Sci* 1999;26:S12–S19.

Hummel T, Livermore A. Intranasal chemosensory function of the trigeminal nerve and aspects of its relation to olfaction. *Int Arch Occup Environ Health* 2002;75:305–313.

Kakizawa Y, Seguchi T, Kodama K, et al. Anatomical study of the trigeminal and facial cranial nerves with the aid of 3.0-tesla magnetic resonance imaging. *J Neurosurg* 2008;108:483–490.

Kalladka M, Proter N, Benoliel R, et al. Mental nerve neuropathy: patient characteristics and neurosensory changes. *Oral Surg Oral Med Oral Pathol Oral Radiol Endod* 2008;106:364–370.

Kamel HA, Toland J. Trigeminal nerve anatomy: illustrated using examples of abnormalities. *AJR Am J Roentgenol* 2001;176:247–251.

Katusic S, Beard CM, Bergstralh E, et al. Incidence and clinical features of trigeminal neuralgia, Rochester, Minnesota, 1945–1984. *Ann Neurol* 1990;27:89.

Kehrli P, Maillot C, Wolff MJ. Anatomy and embryology of the trigeminal nerve and its branches in the parasellar area. *Neurol Res* 1997;19(1):57–65.

Kiernan JA, Rajakumar N. *Barr's The Human Nervous System: An Anatomical Viewpoint.* 10th ed. Philadelphia: Wolters Kluwer Health/Lippincott Williams & Wilkins, 2014.

Kim JS. Trigeminal sensory symptoms due to midbrain lesions. *Eur Neurol* 1993;33:218–220.

Kim JS, Choi-Kwon S. Sensory sequelae of medullary infarction: differences between lateral and medial medullary syndrome. *Stroke* 1999;30:2697–2703.

Kim HJ, Jeon BS, Lee KW. Hemimasticatory spasm associated with localized scleroderma and facial hemiatrophy. *Arch Neurol* 2000;57:576–580.

Kim JS, Kang JH, Lee MC. Trigeminal neuralgia after pontine infarction. *Neurology* 1998;51:1511–1512.

Kim JS, Lee MC, Kim HG, et al. Isolated trigeminal sensory change due to pontine hemorrhage. *Clin Neurol Neurosurg* 1994;96:168–169.

Kim JS, Lee JH, Lee MC. Patterns of sensory dysfunction in lateral medullary infarction. Clinical-MRI correlation. *Neurology* 1997;49:1557–1563.

Kodsi S. Marcus Gunn jaw winking with trigemino-abducens synkinesis. *J AAPOS* 2000;4:316–317.

Komisaruk BR, Mosier KM, Liu WC, et al. Functional localization of brainstem and cervical spinal cord nuclei in humans with fMRI. *AJNR Am J Neuroradiol* 2002;23(4):609–617.

Lance JW. Current concepts of migraine pathogenesis. *Neurology* 1993;43:S11–S15.

Lance JW, Anthony M. Neck-tongue syndrome on sudden turning of the head. *J Neurol Neurosurg Psychiatry* 1980;43:97–101.

Lossos A, Siegal T. Numb chin syndrome in cancer patients: etiology, response to treatment, and prognostic significance. *Neurology* 1992;42:1181–1184.

Macaluso GM, De Laat A. H-reflexes in masseter and temporalis muscles in man. *Exp Brain Res* 1995;107(2):315–320.

Majoie CB, Aramideh M, Hulsmans FJ, et al. Correlation between electromyographic reflex and MR imaging examinations of the trigeminal nerve. *AJNR Am J Neuroradiol* 1999;20:1119–1125.

Majoie CB, Hulsmans FJ, Castelijns JA, et al. Symptoms and signs related to the trigeminal nerve: diagnostic yield of MR imaging. *Radiology* 1998;209:557–562.

Majoie CB, Verbeeten B Jr, Dol JA, et al. Trigeminal neuropathy: evaluation with MR imaging. *Radiographics* 1995;15:795–811.

Marsot-Dupuch K, De Givry SC, Ouayoun M. Wegener granulomatosis involving the pterygopalatine fossa: an unusual case of trigeminal neuropathy. *Am J Neuroradiol* 2002;23:312–315.

Matsuka Y, Fort ET, Merrill RL. Trigeminal neuralgia due to an acoustic neuroma in the cerebellopontine angle. *J Orofac Pain* 2000;14:147–151.

May A, Goadsby PJ. The trigeminovascular system in humans: pathophysiologic implications for primary headache syndromes of the neural influences on the cerebral circulation. *J Cereb Blood Flow Metab* 1999;19:115–127.

Meaney JF, Watt JW, Eldridge PR, et al. Association between trigeminal neuralgia and multiple sclerosis: role of magnetic resonance imaging. *J Neurol Neurosurg Psychiatry* 1995;59:253–259.

Mellgren SI, Goransson LG, Omdal R. Primary Sjogren's syndrome associated neuropathy. *Can J Neurol Sci* 2007;34:280–287.

Merello M, Lees AJ, Leiguarda R, et al. Inverse masticatory muscle activity due to syringobulbia. *Mov Disord* 1993;8:359–360.

Mokri B. Raeder's paratrigeminal syndrome. Original concept and subsequent deviations. *Arch Neurol* 1982;39:395–399.

Murphy MA, Szabados EM, Mitty JA. Lyme disease associated with postganglionic Horner syndrome and Raeder paratrigeminal neuralgia. *J Neuroophthalmol* 2007;27:123–124.

Nakamura K, Yamamoto T, Yamashita M. Small medullary infarction presenting as painful trigeminal sensory neuropathy. *J Neurol Neurosurg Psychiatry* 1996;61:138.

Nemzek WR. The trigeminal nerve. *Top Magn Reson Imaging* 1996;8:132–154.

Nurmikko TJ. Altered cutaneous sensation in trigeminal neuralgia. *Arch Neurol* 1991;48:523.

Nurmikko T, Bowsher D. Somatosensory findings in postherpetic neuralgia. *J Neurol Neurosurg Psychiatry* 1990;53:135.

Nurmikko TJ. Recent advances in the diagnosis and management of trigeminal neuralgia. *Int J Pain Palliat Care* 2003;3:2–11.

Nurmikko TJ. Trigeminal neuralgia and other facial neuralgias. *Handb Clin Neurol* 2006;81:573–596.

Ordas CM, Cuadrado ML, Simal P, et al. Wallenberg's syndrome and symptomatic trigeminal neuralgia. *J Headache Pain* 2011;12:377–380.

Orrell RW, Marsden CD. The neck-tongue syndrome. *J Neurol Neurosurg Psychiatry* 1994;57:348–352.

Osama SM, Amin FACP, Shwani SS. Exaggerated Jaw Jerk. Available from http://www.youtube.com/watch?v=ctFvOasAKo0. Accessed on February 10, 2018.

Papanastassiou AM, Schwartz RB, Friedlander RM. Chiari I malformation as a cause of trigeminal neuralgia: case report. *Neurosurgery* 2008;63:E614–E615.

Pavesi G, Macaluso GM, Marchetti P, et al. Trigemino-facial reflex inhibitory responses in some lower facial muscles. *Muscle Nerve* 2000;23:939–945.

Reske-Nielsen E, Oster S, Pedersen B. Herpes zoster ophthalmicus and the mesencephalic nucleus. *Acta Pathol Microbiol Immunol Scand A* 1986;94:263.

Rorick MB, Chandar K, Colombi BJ. Inflammatory trigeminal sensory neuropathy mimicking trigeminal neurinoma. *Neurology* 1996;46:1455–1457.

Seidel E, Hansen C, Urban PP, et al. Idiopathic trigeminal sensory neuropathy with gadolinium enhancement in the cisternal segment. *Neurology* 2000;54:1191–1192.

Shankland WE II. The trigeminal nerve. Part I: an overview. *Cranio* 2000;18(4):238–248.

Shoja MM, Tubbs RS, Ghabili K, et al. Johan Georg Raeder (1889-1959) and paratrigeminal sympathetic paresis. *Childs Nerv Syst* 2010;26:373–376.

Singer PA, Chikarmane A, Festoff BW, et al. Trismus. An unusual sign in polymyositis. *Arch Neurol* 1985;42:1116–1118.

Soeira G, Abd el-Bary TH, Dujovny M, et al. Microsurgical anatomy of the trigeminal nerve. *Neurol Res* 1994;16(4):273–283.

Solomon S. Raeder syndrome. *Arch Neurol* 2001;58:661–662.

Sumner CJ, Fischbeck KH. Jaw drop in Kennedy's disease. *Neurology* 2002;59:1471–1472.

Szewka AJ, Purdy H, Topel J, et al. Teaching neuroimages: numb chin syndrome in an edentulous patient. *Neurology* 2011;77:e38.

ten Hove MW, Glaser JS, Schatz NJ. Occult perineural tumor infiltration of the trigeminal nerve. Diagnostic considerations. *J Neuroophthalmol* 1997;17:170–177.

Warden KF, Parmar H, Trobe JD. Perineural spread of cancer along the three trigeminal divisions. *J Neuroophthalmol* 2009;29:300–307.

Watt-Smith S, Mehta K, Scully C. Mefloquine-induced trigeminal sensory neuropathy. *Oral Surg Oral Med Oral Pathol Oral Radiol Endod* 2001;92:163–165.

Wilson-Pauwels L, Stewart PA, Akesson EJ, et al. *Cranial Nerves: Function and Dysfunction*. 3rd ed. Shelton: People's Medical Publishing House, 2010.

Woolfall P, Coulthard A. Pictorial review: trigeminal nerve: anatomy and pathology. *Br J Radiol* 2001;74:458–467.

CHAPTER 16

The Facial Nerve

ANATOMY AND PHYSIOLOGY

The facial, or seventh, cranial nerve (CN VII) is a predominantly motor nerve that innervates the muscles of facial expression and the muscles of the scalp and ear, as well as the buccinator, platysma, stapedius, stylohyoid, and posterior belly of the digastric. In addition, it carries parasympathetic secretory fibers to the submandibular and sublingual salivary glands, the lacrimal gland, and to the mucous membranes of the oral and nasal cavities. It has some sensory functions; the most important is to mediate taste from the anterior two-thirds of the tongue. It also conveys exteroceptive sensation from the eardrum and external auditory canal, proprioceptive sensation from the muscles it supplies, and general visceral sensation from the salivary glands and mucosa of the nose and pharynx. Anatomically, the motor division of the nerve is separate from the sensory and parasympathetic portions. In its course from its exit from the pons until its terminal arborizations, several important branches are given off in the following order: the greater (superficial) petrosal nerve, the nerve to the stapedius, and the chorda tympani.

The nerve may be understood as a series of segments: a brainstem or intramedullary segment (from the brainstem nuclei to the exit point), a segment from the exit point to the entrance into the internal auditory canal (IAC) or cisternal segment, a meatal or canal segment (course through the IAC) to the entrance to the facial canal, a labyrinthine segment (from there to the geniculate ganglion), a short horizontal segment (from the geniculate ganglion to the pyramidal eminence of the posterior wall of the tympanic cavity), a mastoid segment (from the pyramidal eminence to the stylomastoid foramen), and an extratemporal or peripheral segment (from the stylomastoid foramen to the pes anserinus). These segments are discussed in more detail below. The associated findings in CN VII palsy often allow identification of the involved segment.

The Motor Portion

The supranuclear innervation to the muscles of facial expression arises from the lower third of the contralateral precentral gyrus in the facial area of the motor homunculus. Fibers descend in the corticobulbar tract through the corona radiata, genu of the internal capsule, medial portion of the cerebral peduncles and into the pons, and then decussate to converge on the facial nuclei. The portion of the nucleus that innervates the lower half to two-thirds of the face has predominantly contralateral supranuclear control; the portion that innervates the upper third to half has bilateral control. The muscles of the lower face may also receive more abundant cortical innervation than the muscles of the upper face and forehead. This scheme applies to voluntary facial movements. Unconscious, emotional, involuntary supranuclear control follows a different pathway. Patients with lesions in certain parts of the nervous system may have different degrees of involvement of the voluntary and involuntary systems (see below).

Studies in humans and nonhuman primates show distributed motor control of facial expression with at least five cortical regions involved: the primary motor cortex, the ventral lateral premotor cortex, the supplementary motor area, and the cingulate cortex. Recent investigations confirm the long established paradigm of bilateral control of the upper face and mainly contralateral control of the lower face. The primary motor cortex, the ventral lateral premotor cortex, and the supplementary motor area are essential for voluntary control of facial expressions. The cingulate cortical areas receive input from different structures of the limbic system and are important for emotional facial expression.

Although most corticobulbar fibers to the facial nuclei decussate in or rostral to the pons, some descend in the aberrant pyramidal tract to medullary levels, decussate there, and ascend contralaterally in the dorsolateral medulla to reach the facial nucleus. The aberrant pyramidal tract is a normal descending fiber tract that leaves the pyramidal tract in the crus cerebri and travels in the medial lemniscus to the upper medulla. Involvement of the aberrant pyramidal tract explains the occurrence of ipsilateral upper motor neuron facial palsy in the lateral medullary syndrome.

A study using transcranial magnetic stimulation to investigate the corticofacial projections found that in the majority of patients, the corticofacial fibers traveled in the base of the pons and crossed at the level of the facial nucleus. But in some individuals, corticofacial fibers formed an "aberrant bundle" in a paralemniscal position at the dorsal edge of the pontine base. In other patients, the corticofacial fibers looped down into the ventral upper medulla, crossed the midline, and ascended in the dorsolateral medullary region ipsilateral to the facial nucleus. The findings suggest that facial paresis because of a brainstem lesion may present as contralateral supranuclear facial paresis by a lesion of the cerebral peduncle, pontine base, the aberrant bundle, and the ventral medulla. Supranuclear facial paresis ipsilateral to the lesion side may result from a lesion in the lateral medulla, and facial paresis of the supranuclear type may be imitated by a lesion of the peripheral facial nerve in the dorsolateral medulla with involvement of the lower pons. The facial nuclei also receive bilateral extrapyramidal, basal ganglia, and hypothalamic innervations that are concerned with maintaining facial muscle tone and with automatic and emotional movements.

The facial nucleus is special visceral efferent, or branchiomotor; it innervates the muscles of the second branchial arch. It lies deep in the tegmentum of the caudal pons, anteromedial to the nucleus of the spinal tract of CN V, anterolateral to the nucleus of CN VI, and posterior to the superior olivary nucleus (Figures 11.6 and 14.8). The facial motor nucleus has lateral, medial, and dorsal subnuclei, arranged in columns. The subnuclear innervation pattern is not as well worked out as for the oculomotor nucleus, but the lateral subnucleus is thought to innervate the lower facial muscles and buccinators; the medial subnucleus the posterior auricular, platysma, and occipital muscles, and probably the stapedius; and the dorsal subnucleus the upper facial muscles via the temporal, orbital, and zygomatic branches. Other schemes of organization have been postulated.

Axons of the facial nerve arise from the dorsal surface of the nucleus and travel dorsomedially, moving up and around to encircle the abducens nucleus and forming the internal genu of the facial nerve. The internal loop of CN VII fibers around the CN VI nucleus forms the facial colliculus, a bump in the rhomboid fossa in the floor of the fourth ventricle, a prominent landmark for surgeons working in the area (Figure 11.4). The facial nucleus is in a somewhat aberrant position more anterolaterally than expected, even considering its branchial arch relationships. In embryonic life, the nucleus is more dorsal and medial, near the CN VI nucleus, but with maturation moves to its adult position trailing its axons behind. In their course, the facial nerve axons run in proximity to the nucleus and fibers of CN VI, the pontine paramedian reticular formation, CN V, and CN VIII as well as the descending and ascending long tracts that course through the pons.

The facial nerve has two components, the motor root, which makes up about 70% of the fibers, and the sensory root, which accounts for 30%. The sensory root forms the nervus intermedius (NI) and contains both sensory and autonomic fibers. The autonomic fibers run near the incoming sensory fibers through the pons. The intrapontine filaments of CN VII thus consist of exiting branchiomotor and parasympathetic fibers, and incoming sensory fibers (Figure 16.1).

CN VII exits the pons laterally at the pontomedullary junction, just caudal to the roots of CN V between the olive and the inferior cerebellar peduncle (Figure 11.3). The NI is a small bundle that usually leaves the pons closer to CN VIII than CN VII and runs between the larger trunks across the cerebellopontine angle (CPA). In about 20% of specimens, the NI is not identifiable as a separate structure in the CPA. At the entrance to the IAC, the facial nerve motor root lies in a groove on the anterosuperior surface of the vestibulocochlear nerve, with the NI in between. In this segment, CN VII is a paler white color than CN VIII. The facial nerve at this point lies in close proximity to the anterior inferior cerebellar artery (AICA). In some individuals, the AICA loops down into the IAC. As with the vaginal sheaths of the optic nerve, the subarachnoid space extends along the facial nerve to the geniculate ganglion.

At the bottom or lateral end of the IAC, the nerve pierces the meninges and enters the facial canal, or fallopian aqueduct. The point of entry is the

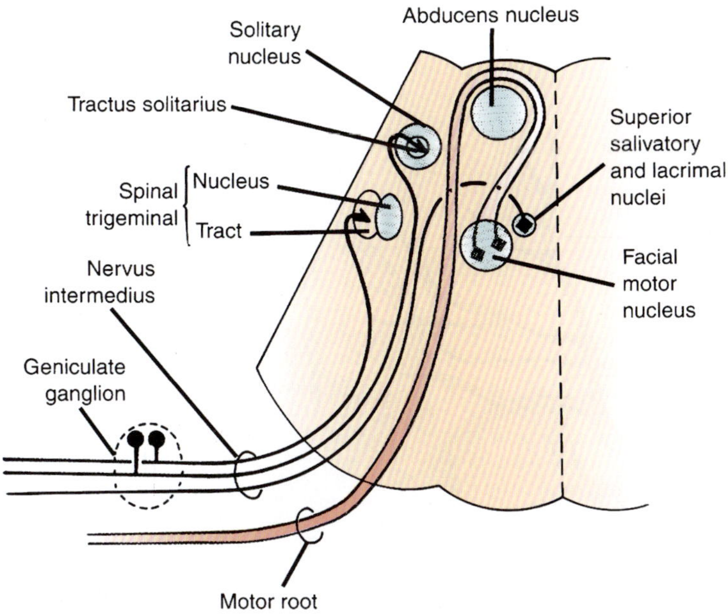

FIGURE 16.1 Components of the facial nerve in the pons. (Modified from Kiernan JA. *Barr's The Human Nervous System: An Anatomical Viewpoint*. 9th ed. Philadelphia: Wolters Kluwer Health/Lippincott, Williams & Wilkins, 2009, with permission.)

narrowest portion of the canal. The facial nerve and the NI merge as the nerve enters the canal. In traversing the facial canal, the nerve makes two abrupt, tortuous turns, creating two external genus. In its course through the petrous bone, from its entrance into the facial canal until its exit from the stylomastoid foramen, the nerve has three segments: labyrinthine, horizontal or tympanic, and mastoid or vertical. The labyrinthine segment lies laterally between the cochlea and vestibule, toward the medial wall of the tympanic cavity, running perpendicularly to the long axis of the petrous pyramid. The labyrinthine segment ends at the first external genu where the geniculate ganglion lies. At this point, the nerve turns abruptly and runs horizontally for about 1 cm (the horizontal or tympanic segment), then turns backward and arches downward behind the tympanic cavity (mastoid or vertical) segment. The branch to the stapedius muscle arises from the distal tympanic or upper end of the mastoid segment. At the end of the tympanic segment, the nerve encounters the second external genu as it makes a 90-degree turn to enter the mastoid segment. The mastoid segment then descends toward the stylomastoid foramen, gives off the chorda tympani about 6 mm before its exit, and emerges from the stylomastoid foramen. The tight confines of the bony canal may make the nerve particularly vulnerable to damage from inflammation and edema, a point of possible significance in some CN VII neuropathies (see below). In patients with Bell's palsy, the involved side usually correlates with the side of the narrower facial canal as determined by high-resolution computed tomography (CT). CN VII runs along with the labyrinthine branch of the AICA, but there is evidence to suggest that it is less well vascularized in its intrapetrous segment, particularly in the labyrinthine segment, than elsewhere along its course. This may also have relevance to the pathologic changes in Bell's palsy.

There may be anatomical variations in the nerve's course through the petrous bone. It may split into two or three strands at or distal to the geniculate ganglion. The more proximal the division into strands, the more bizarre the subsequent course. Facial motor fibers may run in an enlarged chorda tympani, diminishing the distal facial nerve into a tenuous strand exiting through a narrowed stylomastoid foramen.

Just after exit, the posterior auricular, digastric, and stylohyoid branches arise. The posterior auricular branch supplies the occipitalis, posterior auricular, and transverse and oblique auricular muscles. The digastric and stylohyoid branches supply, respectively, the posterior belly of the digastric and the stylohyoid. The nerve turns forward and passes into the parotid gland. Within the substance of the parotid, it divides into temporofacial and cervicofacial divisions at the pes anserinus (intraparotid plexus) in the cleft between the superficial and deep lobes of the gland (Figure 16.2). The temporofacial branch crosses the zygoma about 1 cm anterior to the ear, where it is vulnerable to injury.

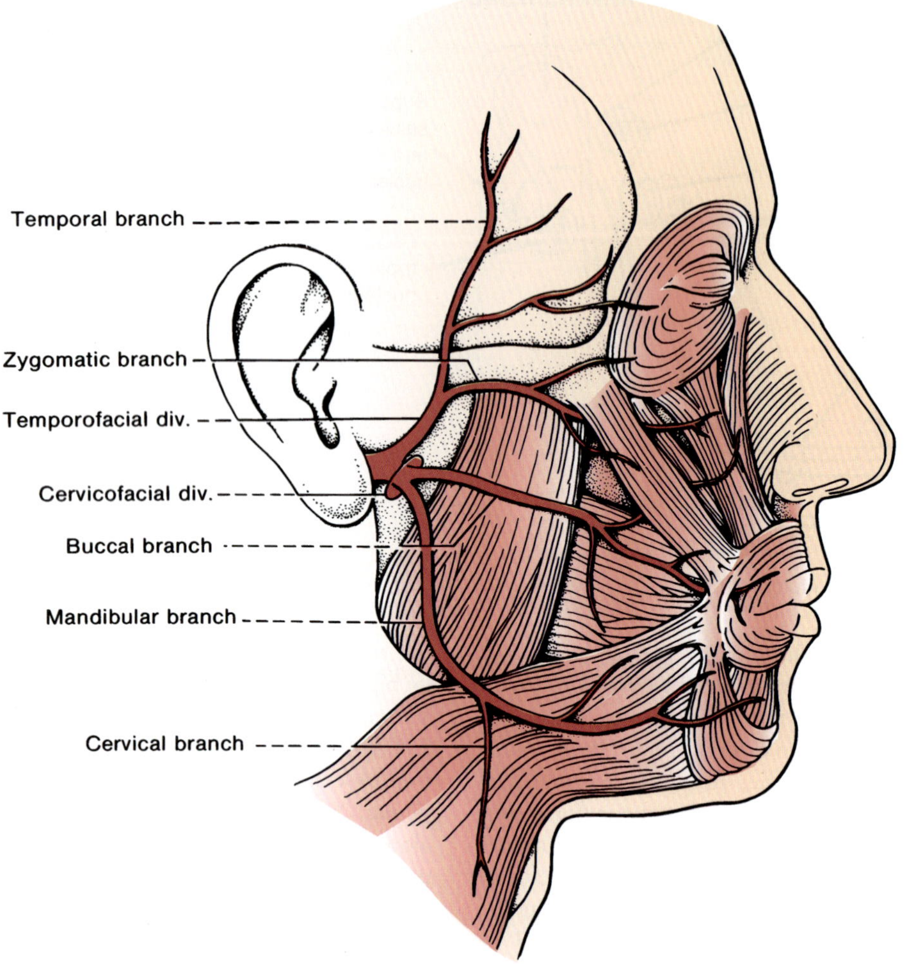

FIGURE 16.2 Branches and distribution of the facial nerve.

The facial nerve supplies all the muscles of facial expression from the scalp and forehead through the platysma, including the extrinsic and intrinsic muscles of the ear. The muscles of facial expression are responsible for all voluntary and involuntary movements of the face except those associated with movement of the jaws and for all play of emotions upon the face. The muscles innervated by the terminal branches are summarized in Table 16.1.

The Nervus Intermedius

The NI is the sensory and autonomic component of the facial nerve. It runs in a position intermediate between CNs VII and VIII across the CPA, moving ever closer to the main facial nerve trunk as it enters the facial canal. At the external first external genu, the NI fuses with the geniculate ganglion. The sensory cells located in the geniculate ganglion are general somatic afferent (GSA) and special visceral afferent (SVA). The GSA fibers carry exteroceptive impulses from the region of the external auditory canal and tympanic membrane. The SVA fibers convey taste from the anterior two-thirds of the tongue. The autonomic component of the NI consists of preganglionic general visceral efferent parasympathetic fibers from the superior salivatory and lacrimal nuclei, which consist of scattered cells in the reticular formation near the caudal end of the motor nucleus. Their axons are bound for the submandibular gland en route to the sublingual and submaxillary glands, the lacrimal glands, and glands in the nasal mucosa.

TABLE 16.1 Muscles of the Face, Their Actions, and Innervations

Nerve Branch	Muscle Innervated	Muscle Action
Temporal branch	Frontalis	Raises eyebrows and skin over the root of the nose; draws scalp forward, throwing forehead into transverse wrinkles
	Corrugator (corrugator supercilii)	Draws eyebrow down and medially, produces vertical wrinkles in the forehead (the frowning muscle)
	Upper part of the orbicularis oculi (orbicularis palpebrarum)	Eyelid sphincter; palpebral portion narrows palpebral fissure and gently closes eyelids; orbital portion draws skin of forehead, temple, and cheek toward medial orbit, pulls eyebrow down, draws skin of cheek up; closes eye firmly
	Occipitalis	Draws scalp backward
	Procerus (pyramidalis nasi)	Draws medial eyebrow downward, produces transverse wrinkles over bridge of nose
Zygomatic	Lower and lateral orbicularis oculi	Eyelid sphincter
Buccal	Orbicularis oculi	Eyelid sphincter
	Buccinator	Compresses cheeks, keeps food under pressure of cheeks in chewing
	Zygomaticus	Draws mouth backward and upward
	Nasalis (compressor nares)	Depresses cartilaginous portion of nose, draws the ala toward septum
	Levator anguli oris (caninus)	Raises angle of mouth
	Levator labii superioris (quadratus labii superioris)	Elevates upper lip, dilates nostril
Mandibular	Lower part of the orbicularis oris	Sphincter of the mouth; closes lips; superficial fibers protrude lips; deep fibers draw lips in and press them against teeth
	Mentalis	Protrudes lower lip, wrinkles skin of chin
	Risorius	Retracts angle of mouth
	Triangularis (depressor anguli oris)	Depresses angle of mouth
	Depressor labii inferioris (quadratus labii inferioris)	Draws lower lip downward and lateralward
Cervical	Platysma	Pulls lower lip and angle of mouth down; depresses lower jaw; raises and wrinkles skin of neck

Course and Branches of the Facial Nerve

The first branch given off in the facial nerve's course is the greater (superficial) petrosal nerve, which carries preganglionic parasympathetic fibers (Figure 16.3). These fibers are conveyed by the NI to the geniculate ganglion. They pass through the ganglion without synapsing into the greater petrosal nerve, which goes forward through the hiatus of the facial canal to join the deep petrosal nerve from the carotid sympathetic plexus to form the vidian nerve, or the nerve of the pterygoid canal, which runs to the sphenopalatine ganglion, from where postganglionic fibers proceed to the lacrimal gland.

Distal to the geniculate ganglion, the facial nerve continues to descend. As above, the nerve to the stapedius arises from the distal tympanic or upper mastoid segment and passes forward through a small canal to reach the muscle. Although there is some variability, the chorda tympani usually leaves the main trunk slightly above the stylomastoid foramen; it carries taste and general visceral afferent (GVA) fibers as well as preganglionic parasympathetics. It runs forward and upward in a minute canal in the posterior wall of the tympanic cavity, acquires a mucous membrane investment, and then enters and crosses the middle ear. It is sometimes visible as a small white cord behind the tympanic membrane on otoscopic examination. The chorda tympani runs downward and forward to exit the skull and join the lingual nerve, a branch of the mandibular division of CN V, on its posterior border.

Fibers carrying somatosensory afferents in the chorda tympani have their cell bodies in the geniculate ganglion. The peripheral processes innervate part of the external auditory canal, the tympanic membrane, lateral surface of the pinna, and a small area

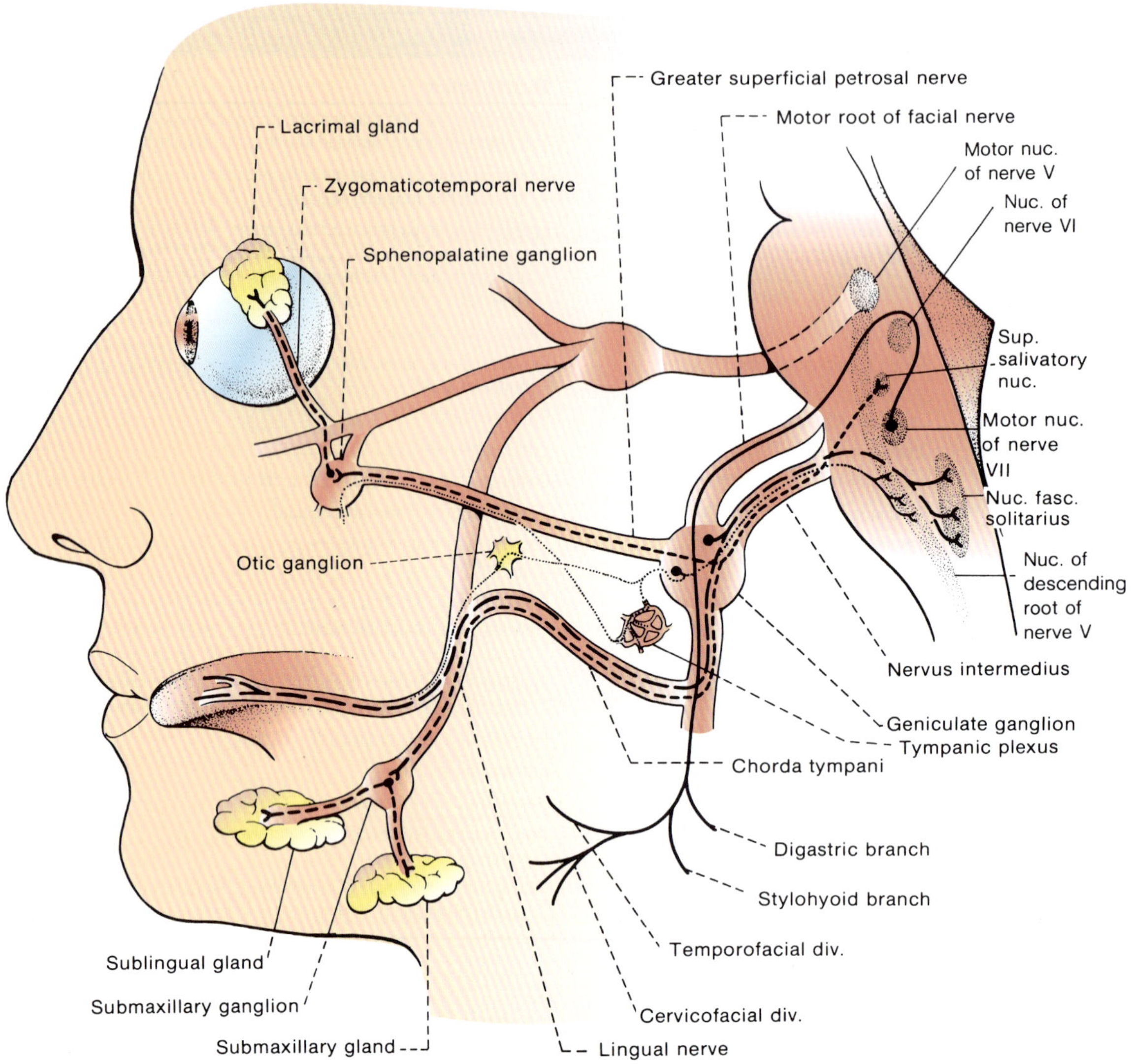

FIGURE 16.3 Course and branches of the facial nerve.

behind the ear and over the mastoid process. There is a marked individual variation in this distribution. Their central processes terminate in the spinal tract and nucleus of the trigeminal, and the central connections are identical with those of the trigeminal nerve. CN VII may also subserve deep pain and deep pressure from the face.

Taste sensation from the anterior two-thirds of the tongue is carried through the lingual nerve to the chorda tympani, then to the geniculate ganglion. CN VII may also carry taste sensation from the mucosa of the soft palate through the sphenopalatine ganglion. Central processes carrying taste and GVA sensation terminate in the nucleus of the solitary tract. The solitary tract sends communications to the superior and inferior salivatory nuclei, which send parasympathetics to the salivary glands. Other fibers synapse in the reticular formation; next order neurons form a component of the reticulospinal tract bilaterally to synapse with sympathetic neurons in the intermediolateral gray column of the upper thoracic spinal cord. These send sympathetic innervation via the superior cervical ganglion to the salivary glands. Fibers subserving taste sensation ascend with the contralateral medial lemniscus to the thalamus. The primary gustatory cortex, located in the anterior insula and the frontal operculum, mediates the perception of taste. Taste fibers also communicate with the hypothalamus and the olfactory system.

The chorda tympani also carries preganglionic parasympathetic fibers to the submandibular ganglion. Postganglionic fibers convey secretory and vasodilator impulses to the submandibular and sublingual salivary glands and mucous membranes of the mouth and tongue (Figure 16.3). These glands also receive sympathetic innervation through the superior cervical ganglion and the carotid plexus. The parasympathetic fibers cause vasodilation and a copious, thin, watery secretion high in enzymes; the sympathetic fibers cause vasoconstriction and a scant, thick, mucoid secretion low in enzyme content.

CLINICAL EXAMINATION

Examination of the Motor Functions

Examination of facial nerve motor functions centers on assessment of the actions of the muscles of facial expression. A great deal can be learned from simple inspection. At rest the face is generally symmetric, at least in young individuals. With aging, the development of character lines may cause asymmetry that does not indicate disease. Distinguishing minor, clinically insignificant, facial asymmetry from subtle facial weakness is sometimes challenging. Note the tone of the muscles of facial expression, and look for atrophy and fasciculations. Note the resting position of the face and whether there are any abnormal muscle contractions. Note the pattern of spontaneous blinking for frequency and symmetry. A patient with parkinsonism may have infrequent blinking and an immobile, expressionless, "masked" face. Facial dystonia causes an abnormal fixed contraction of a part of the face, often imparting a curious facial expression. The procerus sign is seen most characteristically in progressive supranuclear palsy (PSP) and corticobasal degeneration. There is contraction of the forehead muscles, particularly the procerus and corrugator, with knitting of the brows, raised eyebrows, lid retraction, widening of the palpebral fissures, and reduced blinking. The expression is one of surprise, astonishment, perplexity, or consternation (Figure 16.4). Synkinesis causes abnormal contractions of the face, often subtle, synchronous with blinking or mouth movements. Synkinesis suggests remote facial nerve palsy with aberrant regeneration **(Video 16.1)**. Spontaneous contraction of the face may be due to hemifacial spasm (HFS) (see below). Other types of abnormal involuntary movements that may affect the facial muscles include tremors, tics, myoclonic jerks, chorea, and athetosis (see below).

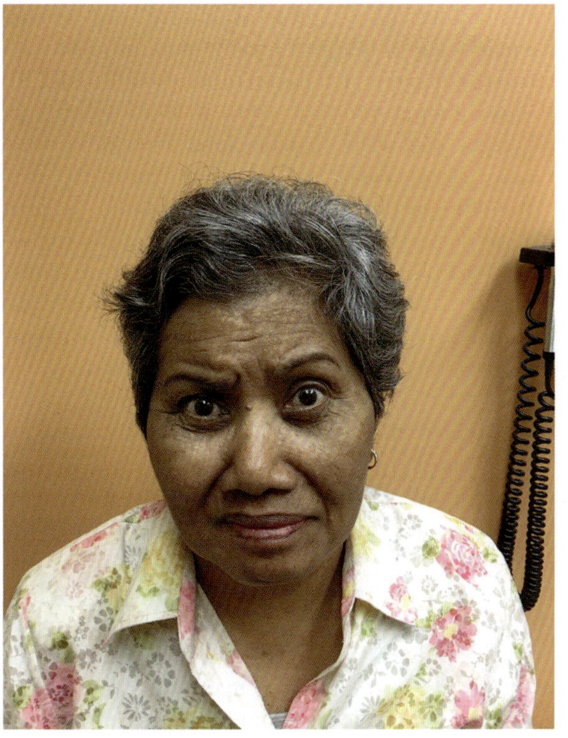

FIGURE 16.4 Procerus sign in a patient with progressive supranuclear palsy.

Observe the nasolabial folds for depth and symmetry and note whether there is any asymmetry in forehead wrinkling or in the width of the palpebral fissures with the face at rest. A flattened nasolabial fold with symmetric forehead wrinkles suggests a central (upper motor neuron) facial palsy; a flattened nasolabial fold with smoothing of the forehead wrinkles on the same side suggests a peripheral (lower motor neuron) facial nerve palsy. Eyelid position and the width of the palpebral fissures often provide subtle but important clinical clues. Eyelid position is discussed further in Chapter 14. A unilaterally widened palpebral fissure suggests a facial nerve lesion causing loss of tone in the orbicularis oculi muscle, the eye closing sphincter; this is sometimes confused with ptosis of the opposite eye. It is a common misconception that facial nerve palsy causes ptosis.

Some diseases cause a characteristic abnormality of facial expression that can sometimes be recognized at a glance, either because of facial immobility or some peculiar facial expression. Examples of primarily neurologic conditions include parkinsonism and related extrapyramidal disorders (masked facies), PSP (facial dystonia, procerus sign), Möbius' syndrome, myotonic dystrophy (hatchet face, myopathic face, Figure 16.5), facioscapulohumeral muscular dystrophy (myopathic face, transverse smile), general paresis (facies paralytica), myasthenia gravis (myasthenic snarl, see below), facial nerve palsy (unilateral or bilateral), and Wilson's disease (risus sardonicus, Chapter 30). There are of course numerous congenital syndromes that cause distinctively dysmorphic facies.

Observe the movements during spontaneous facial expression as the patient talks, smiles, or frowns. Certain upper motor neuron facial palsies are more apparent during spontaneous smiling than when the patient is asked to smile or show the teeth. In infants, facial movements are observed during crying. Have the patient grin, vigorously drawing back the angles of the mouth and baring the teeth. Note the symmetry of the expression, how many teeth are seen on each side and the relative amplitude and velocity of the lower facial contraction. Have the patient close her eyes tightly and note the symmetry of the upper facial contraction. How completely the patient buries the eyelashes on the two sides is a sensitive indicator of orbicularis oculi strength.

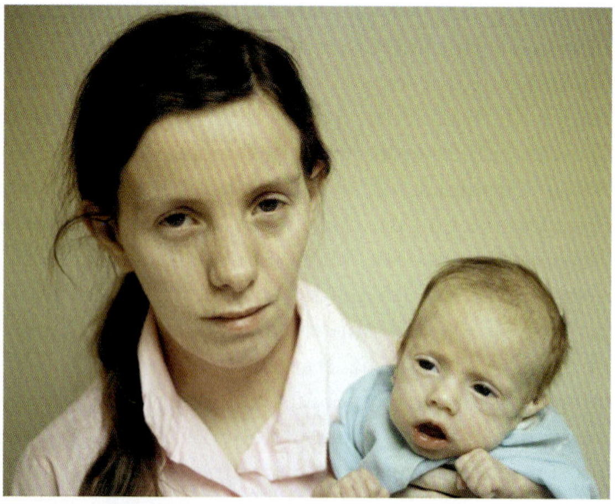

FIGURE 16.5 Myopathic facies in a newly diagnosed young mother with myotonic dystrophy, holding her hypotonic infant, who has the congenital form. The mother has bilateral ptosis, hollowed temporalis, and a slack lower face. The infant has ptosis and the classic "tented upper lip." (Reprinted from Campbell WW. *Clinical Signs in Neurology: A Compendium*. Philadelphia: Wolters Kluwer, 2016, with permission.)

Other useful movements include having the patient raise the eyebrows, singly or in unison, and noting the excursion of the brow and the degree of forehead wrinkling; close each eye in turn; corrugate the brow; puff out the cheeks; frown; pucker; whistle; alternately smile and pucker; contract the chin muscles; and pull the corners of the mouth down in an exaggerated frown to activate the platysma. There is no good command for platysma contraction, and the movement must be demonstrated. The platysma can also be activated by having the patient open the mouth against resistance or clinch the teeth. The patient may smile spontaneously after attempting to whistle, or the examiner may make an amusing comment to assess emotional facial movement. Because of their paucity of facial expression, patients with Parkinson's disease may fail to smile after being asked to whistle: the whistle-smile (Hanes) sign.

Trying to gently push down the uplifted eyebrow may detect mild weakness. It is difficult to pry open the tightly shut orbicularis oculi in the absence of weakness. Vigorously pulling with the thumbs may sometimes crack open a normal eye. If the examiner can force the eye open with her small fingers, then the orbicularis oculi is definitely weak. Likewise, it is difficult to force open the tightly pursed lips in a normal individual. When the orbicularis oris sphincter is impaired, the examiner may be able to force air out of the puffed cheek through the weakened lips. Testing ear and scalp movements is seldom useful, although loss of the ability to wiggle the ear in someone previously able to do so has been cited as a sensitive sign of peripheral facial palsy (PFP). The stylohyoid muscle and posterior belly of the digastric cannot be adequately tested. With stapedius weakness, the patient may complain of hyperacusis, especially for low tones. Other tests of motor function and confirmatory signs of facial paresis are discussed in the following sections. It is important in patients with PFP to examine the ear for vesicles or rash, indicative of zoster infection, and to palpate the parotid to exclude a mass lesion.

Examination of the Reflexes

The corneal and other reflexes mediated largely by CN V are discussed in Chapter 15. Frontal release signs such as the snout, suck, and palmomental reflexes are discussed in Chapter 40. Various other reflexes mediated in large part by CN VII can be

TABLE 16.2 Facial Reflexes

Reflex	Technique
Orbicularis oculi—focal	Best elicited by pulling back, between the thumb and index finger, a fold of skin on the temple lateral to the outer canthus, then briskly tapping the thumb or finger. Sudden stretch of the muscle causes contraction of orbicularis oculi with closing of the eye.
Orbicularis oculi—nonfocal (supraorbital, trigeminofacial, McCarthy's, or nasopalpebral reflex, glabellar tap, Myerson's sign—depending on the site of stimulus)	Tapping over outer aspect of supraorbital ridge, over glabella, or around orbital margin; can sometimes be elicited by tapping the forehead as far back as the hairline. Causes bilateral eye blinking. Response can normally be inhibited; in patients with Parkinson's disease and other conditions, the patient cannot suppress the blinking.
Auditory-palpebral, auro- or acousticopalpebral, cochleo-palpebral, or cochleo-orbicularis reflex	Reflex contraction of the orbicularis oculi causing eye closure, usually bilateral but more marked on the ipsilateral side, in response to a sudden loud noise.
Visuopalpebral, visual orbicularis, opticofacial, blink, or menace reflex	Reflex eye closure in response to a strong light or a sudden visual stimulus.
Palpebro-oculogyric reflex (Bell's phenomenon)	Tight eye closure causes eyeballs to turn upward, a normal response but obvious only when eye closure is weak and the rolling of the eyes is seen through the incompletely closed lids. A method for testing reflex upgaze in patients with upgaze deficits.
Chvostek's sign	A spasm or tetanic, cramp-like contraction, of the ipsilateral facial muscles on tapping over the pes anserinus anterior to the ear; various degrees of response may occur. A sign of tetany, but also occurs with hyperreflexia because of upper motor neuron dysfunction. Likely a motor example of Tinel's sign.

obtained but are of little practical value. Some merit brief discussion. They are summarized in Table 16.2.

Wartenberg wrote at length about the orbicularis oculi reflex, which he considered an important reflex, and the "chaos of nomenclature concerned with this reflex." A reflex contraction of the orbicularis oculi causing an eye blink—the nonfocal orbicularis oculi reflex—can be elicited in different ways **(Video 38.2)**. The threshold for reflex contraction is very low, and the reaction is very quick. Tapping with a finger or percussing with a reflex hammer at many different sites over the forehead and about the eyes may elicit a reflex eye blink. Wartenberg said the muscle "reacts… easily to…a multitude of external stimuli." Different names were given to methods of eliciting the reflex by stimulating different areas, all essentially the same response. The most frequently used version currently is the glabellar tap. Patients with Parkinson's disease are unable to inhibit the reflexive eye blinks (Myerson's sign; not to be confused with Myerson's reflex). Despite the widespread use of the eponym, it is in fact difficult to find any clear reference linking Myerson to the glabellar tap reflex.

A more specific orbicularis oculi reflex is the focal "deep muscle" response elicited from one side by a percussion that stretches the muscle **(Video 38.2)**. A fold of the muscle at the temple is held between the thumb and forefinger and then percussed to stretch it back toward the ear. Wartenberg thought this reflex useful because it may be decreased in PFP in proportion to the severity of the palsy, but it is normal or increased with facial weakness of central origin.

Examination of the Sensory Functions

Testing of CN VII sensory functions is limited to taste. Although Hitselberg described hypesthesia of the posterior wall of the external auditory meatus in proximal facial nerve lesions, there is no reliable way to assess the small sensory contribution the nerve makes to the skin of the external ear region. The peripheral receptors are the taste buds embedded in the tongue epithelium and to a lesser extent in the soft palate and epiglottis. Taste buds respond preferentially, but not solely, to one taste quality. Taste is also carried through CN IX and probably CN X.

There are five primary tastes: bitter, sour, sweet, salty, and umami (delicious or savory). Umami has only recently been added to the list. It is a response to compounds of some amino acids, particularly l-glutamate. Umami is a Japanese term that has no English translation. The many flavors encountered in life are a combination of the primary tastes plus olfaction and oral sensory information ("mouth feel"). Sweet and salty substances are most commonly employed for clinical bedside testing because of their ready availability; sour and bitter are more difficult to come by. Chemosensory referral centers typically use four substances for testing: sucrose (sweet), sodium chloride (salty), quinine (bitter), and citric acid (sour). CN VII only subserves taste on the anterior two-thirds of the tongue. When the tongue is retracted into the mouth, there is rapid dispersion of the test substance outside the area of interest. The tongue must therefore remain protruded throughout testing of an individual substance, and the mouth must be rinsed between tests. If bitter is tested, it should be last because it leaves the most aftertaste.

Some examiners prefer to manually hold the patient's tongue with a piece of gauze to prevent retraction. Because the patient will be unable to speak with the tongue protruded, instructions must be clear in advance. The patient may raise the hand using some signaling system when taste is perceived, point to words written on paper, or make a similar nonverbal response. A damp applicator stick may be dipped into a packet of sugar, artificial sweetener, or salt and coated with the test substance and then placed on one side of the patient's tongue and rubbed around. The patient signals whether she can identify the substance. Most patients will identify the test substance in less than 10 seconds. Taste sensation is less on the tip of the tongue, and the substance is best applied to the dorsal surface at about the junction of the anterior and middle third of the tongue. The sweetness of artificial sweeteners such as saccharine and aspartame is more intense, and they may make better test substances than ordinary sugar. For a demonstration of taste testing technique, see **Video Link 16.1.** More sophisticated methods are available to test for subtle dysfunction in patients who have primary taste and smell complaints. There are many referral centers that specialize in the management of taste and smell disorders (see Chapter 12). There are now commercially available filter paper strips impregnated with sweet, sour, salty, and bitter in different concentrations (taste strips). It is seldom necessary or practical to examine taste on the posterior third of the tongue.

The most common situation calling for assessment of taste is the evaluation of facial nerve palsy. If a patient with a peripheral pattern of facial weakness has impaired taste, the lesion is proximal to the junction with the chorda tympani. A lesion at or distal to the stylomastoid foramen (e.g., in the parotid gland) does not affect taste.

Ageusia is the complete inability to taste. With hypogeusia, taste perception is blunted or delayed. Perversions or abnormal perceptions of taste are parageusias. There is marked individual variation in taste. Complete ageusia is rare unless there is also loss of smell. If there is loss of taste, one should first eliminate the possibility of disease of the tongue. Some causes of disturbed taste are listed in Table 16.3. There are many medications that reportedly alter taste; some commonly used in neurologic practice include the following: carbamazepine, phenytoin, tricyclic antidepressants, dexamethasone, hydrocortisone, penicillamine, lithium, methotrexate, levodopa or levodopa/carbidopa, clozapine, trifluoperazine, baclofen, and dantrolene.

Examination of the Secretory Functions

The secretory functions of CN VII can usually be evaluated by history and observation. Increased tearing is usually apparent; decreased tearing may be

TABLE 16.3 Possible Causes of Disturbed Taste

Oral and perioral infections (e.g., candidiasis, gingivitis, periodontitis)
Bell's palsy
Medications
Dental procedures
Dentures and other dental devices
Age
Nutritional compromise (e.g., vitamin B_{12} deficiency, zinc deficiency, malnutrition, chronic disease)
Lesions involving neural taste pathways
Head trauma
Toxic chemical exposure
Radiation treatment of head and neck
Psychiatric conditions (e.g., depression, anorexia nervosa, bulimia)
Epilepsy (gustatory aura)
Migraine headache (gustatory aura)
Sjögren's syndrome
Multiple sclerosis
Endocrine disorders (e.g., diabetes mellitus, hypothyroidism)

Modified from Bromley SM. Smell and taste disorders: a primary care approach. *Am Fam Physician* 2000;61:427–436, 438.

determined from the history. Tear production may be quantitated with the Schirmer test. Commercially available filter strips are placed in the inferior conjunctival sac and left in place for 5 minutes. The advancing edge of moisture down the strip is proportional to the moisture in the eye; the results are expressed in millimeters. This test is simple and does not require referral to an ophthalmologist.

The lacrimal reflex is tearing, usually bilateral, caused by stimulating the cornea. The nasolacrimal reflex is elicited by mechanical stimulation of the nasal mucosa or by chemical stimulation using irritating substances such as ammonia. Abnormalities of salivation are usually suggested by the history. Otolaryngologists and oral surgeons can use special techniques to quantitate salivary flow.

DISORDERS OF FUNCTION

Motor abnormalities, either weakness or abnormal movements, account for the preponderance of clinical abnormalities of facial nerve function. Changes in sensation, primarily taste, and in secretory function, sometimes occur as a sidebar, but are rarely if ever the major manifestation of disease of CN VII. Changes in these functions can help to localize the lesion along the course of the nerve, although this exercise has little practical value. The major branches in sequence are the greater superficial petrosal, nerve to the stapedius, and chorda tympani, after which the nerve continues to the facial muscles. The mnemonic tear-hear-taste-face may help recall the sequence.

Facial Weakness

There are two types of neurogenic facial nerve weakness: peripheral, or lower motor neuron; and central, or upper motor neuron. PFP may result from a lesion anywhere from the CN VII nucleus in the pons to the terminal branches in the face. Central facial palsy (CFP) is due to a lesion involving the supranuclear pathways before they synapse on the facial nucleus. PFP results from an ipsilateral lesion, whereas CFP, with rare exception, results from a contralateral lesion.

Peripheral Facial Palsy

With PFP, there is flaccid weakness of all the muscles of facial expression on the involved side, both upper and lower face, and the paralysis is usually complete (prosopoplegia). The affected side of the face is smooth; there are no wrinkles on the forehead; the eye is open; the inferior lid sags; the nasolabial fold is flattened; and the angle of the mouth droops (Figure 16.6). The patient cannot raise the eyebrow, wrinkle the forehead, frown, close the eye, laugh, smile, bare the teeth, blow out the cheeks, whistle, pucker, retract the angle of the mouth, or contract the chin muscles or platysma on the involved side. She talks and smiles with one side of the mouth, and the mouth is drawn to the sound side on attempted movement. The cheek is flaccid and food accumulates between the teeth and the paralyzed cheek; the patient may bite the cheek or lip when chewing. Food, liquids, and saliva may spill from the corner of the mouth. The cheek may puff out on expiration because of buccinator weakness. The facial asymmetry may cause an apparent deviation of the tongue (see Chapter 20 and Figure 15.7). A patient with an incomplete PFP may be able to close the eye, but not with full power against resistance. Inability to wink with the involved eye is common. The palpebral fissure is open wider than normal, and there may be inability to close the eye (lagophthalmos). During spontaneous blinking, the involved eyelid tends to lag behind, sometimes conspicuously. Very mild PFP may produce only a slower and less complete blink on the involved side. Attempting to close the involved eye causes a reflex upturning of the eyeball (Bell's phenomenon). The iris may completely disappear upwardly. This is a normal response, but only visible in the patient with orbicularis oculi weakness. To elicit the levator sign of Dutemps and Céstan, have the patient look down, then close the eyes slowly; because the function of the levator palpebrae superioris is no longer counteracted by the orbicularis oculi, the upper lid on the paralyzed side moves upward slightly. Akin to Bell's phenomenon is Negro's sign, where the eyeball on the paralyzed side deviates outward and elevates more than the normal one when the patient raises her eyes (not to be confused with the other Negro's sign, cogwheel rigidity).

A sensitive sign of upper facial weakness is loss of the fine vibrations palpable with the thumbs or fingertips resting lightly on the lids as the patient tries to close the eyes as tightly as possible (Bergara-Wartenberg sign). The platysma sign of Babinski is an asymmetric contraction of the platysma, less on the involved side, when the mouth is opened

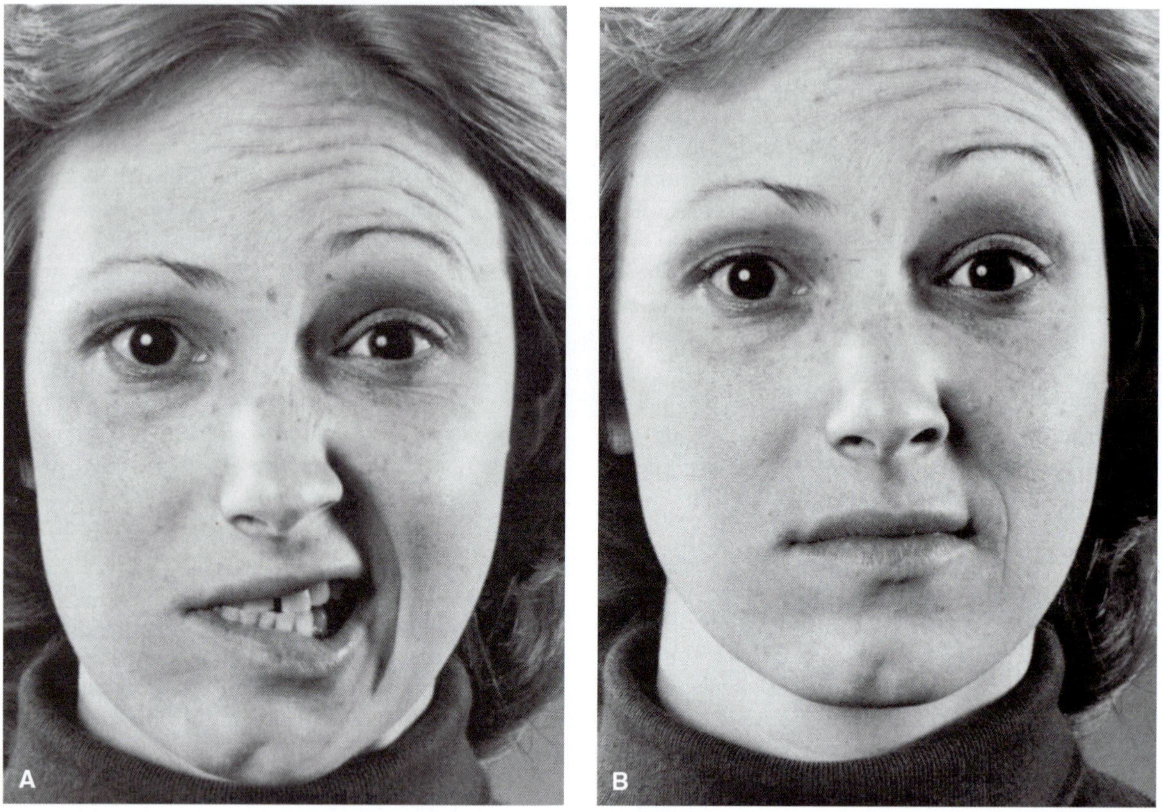

FIGURE 16.6 A patient with a peripheral facial nerve palsy on the right. **A.** The patient is attempting to retract both angles of the mouth. **B.** The patient is attempting to elevate both eyebrows.

(Figure 16.7). Labials and vowels are produced by pursing the lips; patients with peripheral facial weakness have a great deal of difficulty in articulating these sounds. Articulation of labial sounds is discussed further in Chapter 9. The House-Brackmann scale, Burres-Fisch index, and facial nerve function index may be useful to try to quantitate the degree of weakness.

Because of weakness of the lower lid sphincter, tears may run over and down the cheek (epiphora), especially if there is corneal irritation because of inadequate eye protection. A lack of tearing may signal very proximal involvement, above the origin of the greater superficial petrosal nerve. With severe weakness, the eye never closes, even in sleep. The involvement of the intrinsic and extrinsic ear muscles, stylohyoid and posterior belly of the digastric cannot be demonstrated by clinical examination. Electromyographic needle examination can sample some of these muscles, particularly the posterior auricular and posterior belly of the digastric. Denervation in these muscles indicates a very proximal lesion and may be of help in some cases, particularly in distinguishing Möbius' syndrome from birth-related facial nerve trauma. Weakness of the stapedius may produce hyperacusis, especially for low tones that sound louder and higher.

The facial weakness in PFP is obvious on both voluntary and spontaneous contraction. There is no dissociation. With a severe lesion, the passage of time may lead to atrophy of the involved muscles. With PFP, the motor limb of the direct corneal reflex is impaired, but the consensual is intact; in the opposite eye, the direct response is intact and the consensual impaired (Table 15.3); in other words, the involved eye does not blink no matter which side is stimulated, and the normal eye does blink no matter which side is stimulated. The various reflexes that involve motor responses of CN VII supplied muscles are impaired. Some patients with PFP complain of numbness of the face. Sometimes, they are describing the wooden feeling that accompanies immobility, but at other times, patients seem to have slight sensory loss that

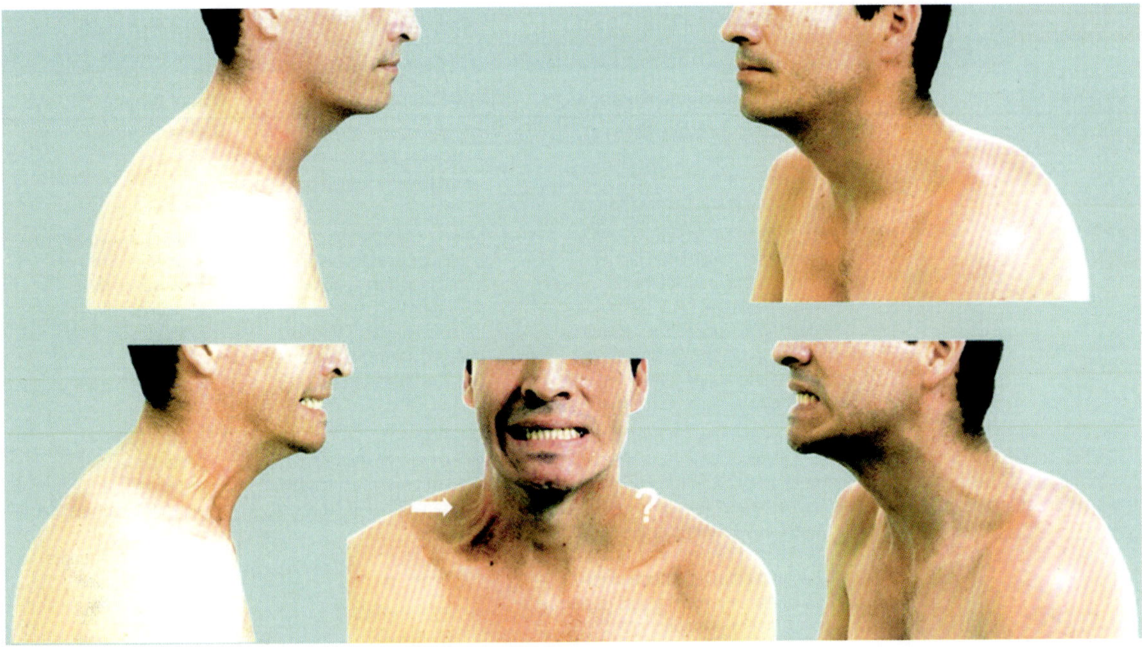

FIGURE 16.7 On the patient's right side, there is a clear difference between the appearance of the platysma muscle at rest (view at *upper left* in composite photograph) and during voluntary effort to retract both corners of the mouth (view at *lower left*). On the patient's left side, there is only minimal contraction (views at *upper and lower right*). In the frontal view, the fully contracting right platysma (*arrow*) can be directly compared with the paretic muscle on the left (*question mark*). Note also the incomplete retraction of the left corner of the mouth. (Reprinted from Leon-Sarmiento FE, Prada LJ, Torres-Hillera M. The first sign of Babinski. *Neurology* 2002;59[7]:1067, with permission.)

is real and more than logically expected for a lesion of a predominantly motor nerve. The cause of this is unclear.

In comatose or otherwise uncooperative patients, facial movements can be elicited by painful pressure over the supraorbital nerves or by other painful stimuli applied to the face to elicit an avoidance response. Pinprick marks on a comatose patient's face are best avoided. The jab of a broken applicator stick is usually sufficient and causes less tissue damage. The groove between the nostrils and the cheek is particularly sensitive for these purposes.

Minimal facial weakness on one side must be differentiated from a facial contracture on the opposite side, which can cause the normal nasolabial fold to appear flattened in comparison. Bona fide facial weakness must also be differentiated from developmental asymmetry, facial hemiatrophy, character lines, and habitual emphasis on the use of one side of the mouth ("Brooklyn facial"). Unequal palpebral fissures from ptosis on one side may be confused with facial weakness on the opposite side causing widening of the fissure; the usual error is the reverse.

Localization of Peripheral Facial Nerve Palsy

PFP can occur from a lesion involving the facial nerve nucleus in the pons or at any point along the infranuclear segment. The weakness of the muscles of facial expression is the same with lesions anywhere along the course of the nerve. Diagnostic localization depends on the associated findings, such as hyperacusis, decreased tearing, impaired taste, and involvement of neural structures beyond CN VII. Table 16.4 summarizes the localization and differential diagnosis of PFP. The most common cause of PFP by far is Bell's palsy.

Bell's Palsy

Most cases of idiopathic facial paralysis (Bell's palsy, for Sir Charles Bell [Box 16.1]) are likely due to Herpes simplex virus activation, but there is no simple method of confirming this mechanism in clinical practice. Polymerase chain reaction (PCR) testing suggests viral reactivation leading to inflammation and demyelination. Herpes zoster, Ramsay

TABLE 16.4 Differential Diagnosis of Lesions of the Facial Nerve

Location of Lesion	Possible Associated Findings	Likely Etiologies	Useful Diagnostic Tests
Nuclear	No localizing associated findings, +/– fasciculations, +/– other evidence of motor neuron disease, dysfunction frequently bilateral	Motor neuron disease, Möbius' syndrome, neoplasm	Needle electromyography
Intrapontine fibers	Normal taste sensation, +/– hyperacusis, +/– decreases lacrimation, facial fasciculations, facial myokymia, ipsilateral CN VI or lateral gaze palsy, ipsilateral weakness of the muscles of mastication, contralateral hemiparesis of arm and leg	Infarction, hemorrhage, neoplasm, syringobulbia, abscess, central pontine myelinolysis, tuberculoma, granuloma, trauma, multiple sclerosis; other demyelinating disorders	MRI, auditory evoked potentials, EMG blink reflex, facial muscle needle electromyography
Cerebellopontine angle or cisternal course, just peripheral to the pons or between the pons and the facial canal	Tinnitus, deafness, and vertigo (CN VIII involvement), facial pain or sensory dysfunction (CN V involvement), loss of taste on the anterior two-thirds of the tongue, decreased salivary and lacrimal secretion (nervus intermedius involvement), hyperacusis (lesion proximal to stapedius branch), ipsilateral ataxia and nystagmus (involvement of the cerebellum or cerebellar connections)	Neoplasm (especially acoustic neuroma), cholesteatoma, head trauma, meningeal inflammation or infiltration	MRI with IAC views, posterior fossa CT myelogram, auditory evoked potentials, EMG blink reflex, facial muscle needle electromyography, CSF examination
Facial canal at the geniculate ganglion	Hyperacusis, loss of taste, decreased tearing, pain in the region of the ear and mastoid, vesicular eruption with Ramsay Hunt syndrome, Battle's sign or raccoon eyes with basilar skull fracture	Bell's palsy, geniculate herpes (Ramsay Hunt syndrome), Guillain-Barré syndrome, petrous bone fracture, neoplasm, diabetes mellitus, sarcoidosis, Lyme disease, HIV infection	MRI (gadolinium may show facial nerve enhancement), EMG blink reflex, needle electromyography, audiogram, acoustic reflex study, CSF examination
Facial canal distal to geniculate ganglion but proximal to origin of nerve to stapedius	Hyperacusis, loss of taste, decreased salivation, normal tearing	Same as previous	Tests same as previous
Facial canal between origin of nerve to stapedius and origin of chorda tympani. Facial canal distal to origin of chorda tympani	No accompanying changes, isolated weakness limited to muscles of facial expression with normal taste, hearing, and tearing	Same as previous	Same as previous
After emergence from stylomastoid foramen	No accompanying findings, involvement may be partial because of selective involvement of a certain division or certain branches of the parotid plexus (pes anserinus) with weakness of some but not all of the muscles of facial expression	Parotid tumor or abscess, trauma	Facial nerve conduction studies, needle electromyography, imaging of parotid

CSF, cerebrospinal fluid; CT, computed tomography; EMG, electromyography; IAC, internal auditory canal; MRI, magnetic resonance imaging.

Hunt syndrome (see below), is probably the second most common viral infection associated with PFP. Other viruses implicated include cytomegalovirus, Epstein-Barr virus, human herpes virus 6, and coxsackie. Unfortunately, antiviral treatment has not proved particularly efficacious. An inactivated intranasal influenza vaccine was associated with an increased incidence of Bell's palsy and subsequently withdrawn from the market. Pathologically, abnormalities are present throughout the bony course of the nerve, but nerve damage is concentrated in the narrow labyrinthine part of the facial canal, probably because of compression related to edema and the tenuous blood supply in that segment. Ischemia has

BOX 16.1

Sir Charles Bell

Bell's palsy is named for Sir Charles Bell, a Scottish surgeon, anatomist, and artist. Early in his career, he published a book on anatomy of facial expression for artists. Among his many contributions (Moritz Romberg proclaimed Bell to be the "Harvey of our century") was a description of the nerve supply to the muscles of the face. He described facial palsy of various etiologies, including one patient who was gored in the face by an ox. He provided the illustrations for his own dissections. It is fitting that the Mona Lisa syndrome refers to the facial synkinesis that sometimes follows Bell's palsy, hypothesized to be the basis for the enigmatic Gioconda half smile in da Vinci's painting.

long been thought to play a role in the development of Bell's palsy. There may be a genetic predisposition in some cases. Bell's palsy is more prevalent in women who are pregnant or have recently given birth. The risk is three times greater during pregnancy, especially in the third trimester or in the first postpartum week.

Certain criteria should be fulfilled to confirm a diagnosis of Bell's palsy. There should be diffuse PFP, onset over a day or 2, paralysis reaching a maximum within 3 weeks, and full or partial recovery within 6 months. A prolonged, progressive course suggests a tumor, as does distal involvement of only some branches or the presence of a parotid mass. Involvement of individual distal branches can also occur from trauma, as by obstetrical forceps.

Symptoms often begin with pain behind the ear, followed within a day or 2 by facial weakness. The pain may rarely precede the paralysis by up to 2 weeks. There is peripheral facial weakness involving both upper and lower face. The paralysis is complete in approximately 70% of patients. Some authorities contend there are often subtle or subclinical abnormalities of other CNs. About 25% of patients report some degree of facial numbness that is often dismissed as an odd sensation related to the immobility. Depending on the relationship of the lesion to the geniculate ganglion, to the takeoff of the chorda tympani, and to the takeoff of the branch to the stapedius, patients may note loss of taste sensation on the ipsilateral anterior two-thirds of the tongue, dryness of the eye, or hyperacusis for low tones. The most common symptoms accompanying Bell's palsy are increased tearing, pain in or around the ear, and taste abnormalities. Trying to localize the lesion by testing taste and lacrimation are not very accurate and of little practical value. In patients studied at surgery, only 6% of lesions were distal to the geniculate ganglion.

Dysgeusia occurs in about 60% of patients, ageusia in about 10%. There may be drooling and difficulty speaking because of the slack facial muscles. Patients are often unable to close the eye, liquids and saliva may drool from the affected corner of the mouth, and tears may spill down the cheek. The majority of patients with Bell's palsy, Lyme disease, and geniculate herpes will show enhancement of the facial nerve on gadolinium magnetic resonance imaging (MRI). Some enhancement may be seen in normals, but enhancement of the distal intrameatal and labyrinthine segments appears specific for facial nerve palsy.

Age-adjusted incidence rates are higher in the elderly. About 1% of cases are bilateral. About 80% of patients recover fully within 6 months; some have persistent synkinesis because of aberrant regeneration, and the rare patient is left with complete permanent paralysis. The prognosis is age related: best in children, worst in patients over 55. The condition may recur in 6% to 7% of patients. Those without enhancement may have a better prognosis.

Aberrant regeneration is common after Bell's palsy and after traumatic nerve injury. Axons destined for one muscle regrow to innervate another, so that there is abnormal twitching of the face outside the area of intended movement. On blinking or winking, the corner of the mouth may twitch. On smiling, the eye may close **(Video 16.1)**. These synkinesis can be prominent in some patients; more often, they are subtle, such as a slight twitch of the orbicularis oris synchronous with blinking of the eye. When misdirection is conspicuous, the main effect of smiling on the involved side of the face may be eye closure. The automatic closure of one eye on opening the mouth, the Marin Amat sign, or inverted or reversed Gunn phenomenon (inverse jaw winking), has been explained as a trigeminofacial associated movement. However, it occurs primarily in patients who have had a peripheral facial paralysis and is probably an intrafacial synkinesis.

Aberrant regeneration may also involve autonomic and taste fibers. The syndrome of crocodile tears is a gustatory-lacrimal reflex, characterized by tearing when eating, especially highly flavored foods. It is due to misdirection of salivary axons to the lacrimal gland. Frey auriculotemporal syndrome is similar, but with sweating and flushing over the cheek rather than lacrimation (Chapter 15). In the chorda tympani syndrome, there is unilateral swelling and flushing of the submental region after eating.

Other Causes of Peripheral Facial Weakness

There are numerous other causes of PFP. Common processes involving the motor neurons of the CN VII nucleus in the pons include motor neuron disease and Möbius' syndrome. Clinical involvement of facial muscles is more likely in progressive bulbar palsy than in classical sporadic amyotrophic lateral sclerosis (ALS); needle electromyography may show subclinical changes. In spinobulbar muscular atrophy (Kennedy's syndrome), facial fasciculations and facial weakness are often prominent. Facial nerve paralysis, unilateral or bilateral, may be congenital. Möbius' syndrome (congenital oculofacial paralysis) is the association of congenital facial nerve palsy with paralysis of the extraocular muscles, especially the lateral rectus because of hypoplasia or aplasia of the CN nuclei (Figure 16.8). For a courageous and dramatic video of Möbius' syndrome by an affected patient, see **Video Link 16.2**. Other CN-innervated muscles may be involved, and there may be other developmental defects. The condition is sporadic. Reportedly, involvement of facial nerve motoneurons can be the only manifestation of an acute attack of paralytic poliomyelitis. PFP has been reported in hereditary neuropathy with liability to pressure palsies.

Lesions involving the facial nerve fibers in the pons may cause PFP. There are usually, but not always, associated findings to indicate the lesion is intramedullary. Fascicular lesions may or may not involve tearing and taste. Many disorders may affect the intrapontine fibers of CN VII (Table 16.4). Ischemic lesions are common. Millard-Gubler syndrome is ipsilateral PFP and contralateral hemiparesis, which may be due to pontine stroke, hemorrhage, or tumor. A CN VI palsy is often but incorrectly included as part of Millard-Gubler syndrome (Chapter 21, Box 21.1). Foville syndrome is ipsilateral PFP and horizontal gaze palsy with contralateral hemiparesis (Chapter 21, Box 21.1). The "eight and a half syndrome" is a one-and-half syndrome (Chapter 14) in association with a facial palsy due to a pontine lesion. Combined PFP and abducens palsy in isolation, without a hemiparesis, has been reported with an infarction of the caudal pontine tegmentum. A PFP has also been reported in Wallenberg's syndrome because of extension of the infarct into the caudal pons.

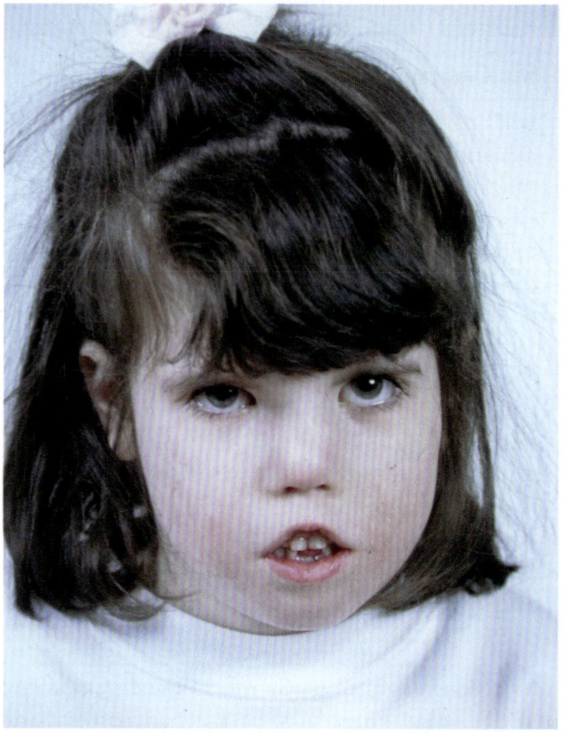

FIGURE 16.8 Child with Moebius syndrome with typical masklike facies and downslanted oral commissures. (Reprinted from Thorne C, Chung KC, Gosain A, et al., eds. *Grabb and Smith's Plastic Surgery*. Philadelphia: Wolters Kluwer Health/Lippincott Williams & Wilkins, 2014, with permission.)

Other processes that may affect CN VII fibers in the pons include abscess, syringobulbia, demyelinating disease, and trauma. Because of the proximity of the nucleus and fibers of CN VII to the nucleus and fibers of CN VI, pontine lesions frequently cause both an ipsilateral facial paralysis and an ipsilateral lateral rectus paralysis. Pontine lesions are discussed further in the Chapter 21.

Mass lesions in the CPA, such as acoustic neuroma and meningioma, commonly extend to involve CN VII, the NI, CN VIII, CN V, the cerebellar peduncles, and the cerebellum. Because of the associated hearing loss, there may not be hyperacusis even though the lesion is proximal to the branch to the stapedius. There is usually hearing loss, facial

BOX 16.2

Ramsay Hunt Syndromes

Other conditions sometimes referred to as Ramsay Hunt syndrome are deep palmar branch ulnar neuropathy, dyssynergia cerebellaris myoclonica, juvenile Parkinson's disease, and dentatorubropallidoluysian atrophy.

sensory changes, ipsilateral ataxia, and nystagmus. CPA syndromes are discussed further in Chapter 17.

In Ramsay Hunt syndrome (herpes zoster oticus, Hunt syndrome, geniculate herpes), the PFP is due to a reactivation of varicella zoster virus (VZV) involving the geniculate ganglion. Geniculate herpes is one of five conditions eponymically tied to James Ramsay Hunt (Box 16.2). Because of the very proximal involvement, the facial weakness is accompanied by taste impairment, hyperacusis, and diminution of salivary and lacrimal secretion. Pain in and behind the ear may be prominent. There may be vesicles on the tympanic membrane, in the external auditory canal, on the lateral surface of the pinna, and in the cleft between the ear and mastoid process (Figure 16.9).

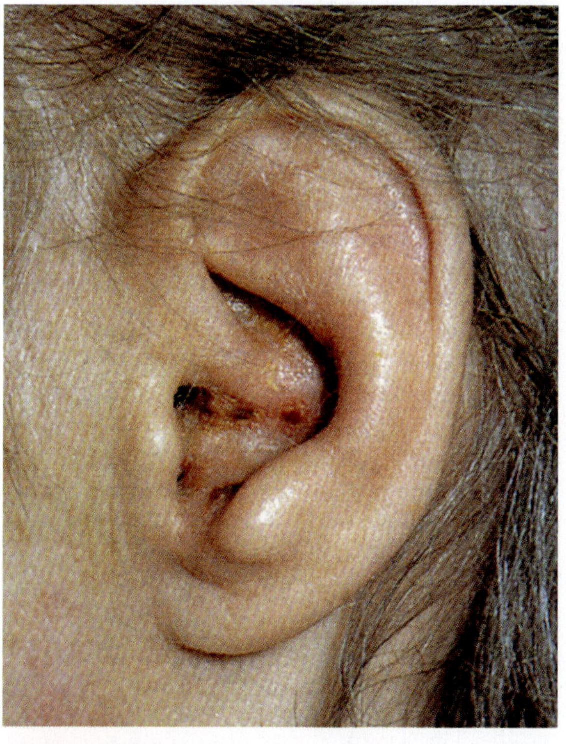

FIGURE 16.9 Vesicles in the external ear canal in a case of geniculate herpes (Ramsay Hunt syndrome).

Occasionally, the herpetic eruption may also involve the anterior faucial pillar of the palate or the neck. Hunt described two types: an otalgic form with pain in the ear and a prosopalgic form with pain deep in the face, primarily in the posterior orbit, palate, and nose. The latter may result from involvement of sensory fibers in the greater superficial petrosal nerve.

Some patients develop facial paralysis without ear or mouth rash but associated with serologic or DNA evidence of VZV infection (zoster sine herpete, zoster sine zoster). Preherpetic neuralgia refers to pain and dysesthesias preceding the development of rash. In one study, 14% of patients developed vesicles only after the onset of facial weakness. It is likely that some patients with Bell's palsy have Ramsay Hunt syndrome without a herpetic eruption. It has been estimated that up to one-third of idiopathic PFP cases may be due to zoster sine herpete. Imaging and virologic studies have shown that extensive viral attack beyond the facial nerve occurs frequently. Tinnitus, hearing loss, nausea, vomiting, vertigo, and nystagmus from involvement of CN VIII are common. Rarely, cochleovestibular symptoms outweigh the PFP, presumably because of VZV reactivation in the ganglia of CN VIII. Other CNs may be affected as well. Compared with Bell's palsy, patients with Ramsay Hunt syndrome often have more severe paralysis at onset and are less likely to recover completely.

Patients with diabetes mellitus have a four- to fivefold increased risk of developing acute PFP, and diabetes is present in about 5% to 10% of patients with PFP. Diabetes is particularly likely in older patients, and those with recurrent or bilateral PFP. Slowly progressive facial weakness can occur with neoplasms involving either the pons or the facial nerve peripherally. Both HIV infection and Lyme disease can occasionally present with facial neuropathy. Lyme disease may cause 10% to 25% of cases of Bell's palsy in hyperendemic areas; there may be no history of tick bite or erythema migrans, and some patients are not seropositive initially. The cerebrospinal fluid (CSF) is often but not invariably normal. PFP because of Lyme disease is particularly prone to be bilateral.

Fractures of the petrous bone because of closed head injury may injure the facial nerve. The fracture may occur longitudinally down the long axis of the petrous pyramid or transversely across it. The facial nerve may be injured in either type. With the more common longitudinal fractures, the facial palsy is usually due to edema, does not occur immediately,

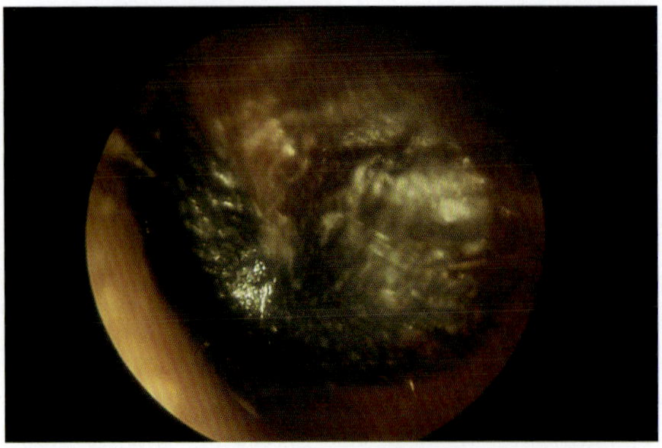

FIGURE 16.10 Hemotympanum due to a left temporal bone fracture. (Reprinted from Chung EK, Atkinson-McEvoy LR, Lai N, et al. *Visual Diagnosis and Treatment in Pediatrics*. 3rd ed. Philadelphia: Wolters Kluwer, 2015, with permission).

and tends to resolve spontaneously. With transverse fractures, the nerve is often lacerated, contused, or severed; the facial palsy comes on immediately and may be permanent. Rupture of the ear drum and bleeding from the ear suggest longitudinal fracture. The tympanic membrane appears bright red, dark red, brown or bluish depending on the color of the fluid in the middle ear (Figure 16.10). CSF otorrhea is more common with transverse fractures (Chapter 17).

Melkersson syndrome (Melkersson-Rosenthal syndrome) is characterized by recurrent attacks of facial palsy, nonpitting facial and lip edema, and a congenitally furrowed and fissured tongue (lingua plicata, scrotal tongue); it is sometimes familial and usually begins in childhood. Its cause is unknown.

Bilateral facial palsy (facial diplegia) refers to bilateral PFP; it is much less common but much more ominous than unilateral PFP. Bilateral facial weakness can also occur because of neuromuscular disorders, including myasthenia gravis, bulbospinal neuronopathy, and muscle disease. Myasthenia gravis may cause marked facial weakness, with difficulty in both closing and opening the eyes. The pattern of perioral muscle involvement is capricious. In some patients, the smile looks like a weak, halfhearted effort, no matter the underlying jocularity, and may be more vertical than horizontal (Figure 16.11). The vertical myasthenic smile may look more like a snarl and is not without social consequences (myasthenic smile, myasthenic snarl). Ectropion, worse in the afternoon and responsive to anticholinesterase agents, is a rare manifestation of myasthenic weakness of the orbicularis oculi

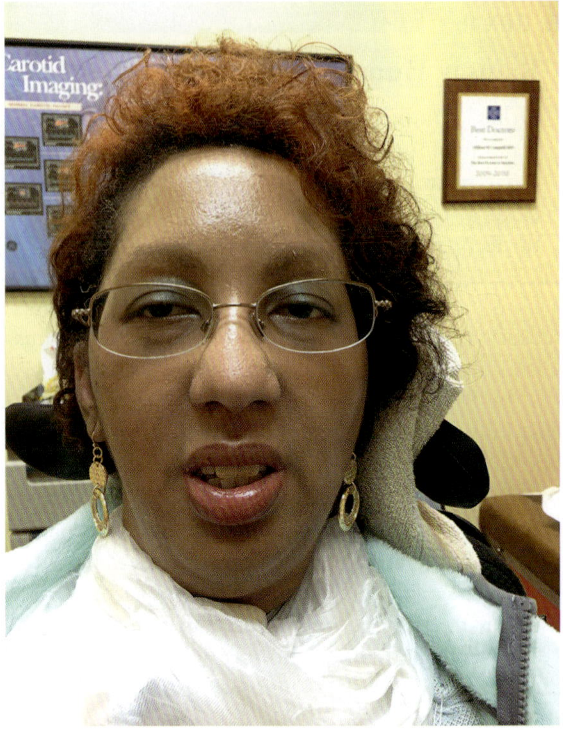

FIGURE 16.11 The vertical myasthenic smile or snarl.

(Figure 16.12). Some myopathies are particularly likely to involve the facial muscles. Myopathic facies are particularly typical of facioscapulohumeral muscular dystrophy (Landouzy-Dejerine syndrome). The eyelids droop, but the eyes cannot be tightly closed. The lips cannot be pursed, but protrude and droop tonelessly, leaving an involuntary protrusion of the upper lip (bouche de tapir). On smiling, the risorius pulls at the angle of the mouth, but the zygomaticus is unable to elevate the lips and the smile is transverse, see **Video Link 16.3**.

In facial hemiatrophy (progressive facial hemiatrophy, Parry-Romberg syndrome, Wartenberg syndrome), there is either congenital failure of development or a progressive atrophy of the skin, subcutaneous fat, and musculature of one half of the face, sometimes with trophic changes in the connective tissue, cartilage, and bone (Figure 16.13). Loss of tongue muscle occurs in some patients. The disorder may be a form of localized scleroderma. Accompanying changes may include trophic changes in the hair, with loss of pigmentation and circumscribed alopecia and vitiligo. The facial atrophy may be accompanied by classic linear scleroderma lesions on the face or elsewhere. Rarely, there is hemihypertrophy instead

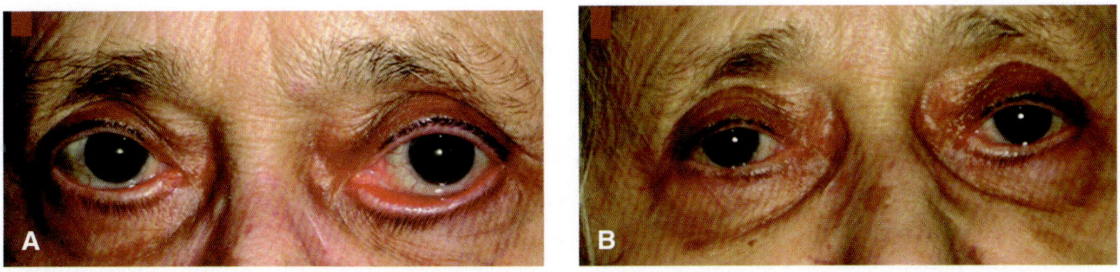

FIGURE 16.12 Myasthenia gravis. **A.** Asymmetric ectropion due to orbicularis oculi weakness. **B.** Improvement after administration of neostigmine. (Reprinted from Solé G, Perez F, Ferrer X. Teaching NeuroImages: reversible ectropion in myasthenia gravis. *Neurology* 2009;73[16]:e83, with permission.)

of hemiatrophy. The disease may be a neural crest migration disorder.

When bilateral facial weakness is due to disease of CN VII, the differential diagnosis includes bilateral Bell's palsy, sarcoidosis, Lyme disease, diabetes, head trauma, HIV infection, Guillain-Barré syndrome, the Fisher variant of Guillain-Barré syndrome, carcinomatous or lymphomatous meningitis, tuberculous or fungal meningitis, pontine tumor, Melkersson-Rosenthal syndrome, pseudotumor cerebri, Möbius' syndrome, and a long list of other conditions. Leprosy may cause bilateral facial paralysis with greater involvement of the upper face. In Keane's series of inpatients with facial diplegia, the most common causes were Bell's palsy, Guillain-Barré syndrome, meningeal tumor, prepontine tumor, idiopathic cranial polyneuropathy, intrapontine tumor, brainstem encephalitis, and syphilis. Bilateral PFP must be differentiated from other causes of bifacial weakness, such as myopathies and myasthenia gravis.

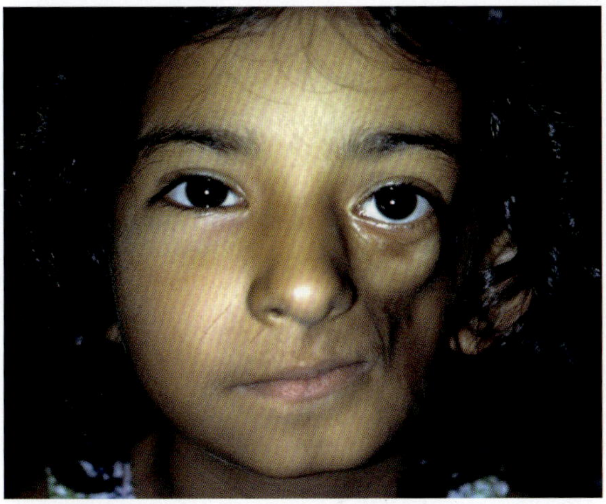

FIGURE 16.13 Facial hemiatrophy (Parry-Romberg syndrome) with atrophy of the skin, subcutaneous fat, and musculature of one half of the face.

In its course across the middle ear, the chorda tympani may be damaged during middle ear surgery. Interestingly, disturbed taste after middle ear surgery is usually transient, even when the chorda tympanis are sectioned bilaterally. However, bilateral chorda tympani lesions may lead to severe and persistent xerostomia because of damage to the autonomic fibers. A syndrome of paroxysmal otalgia because of neurovascular compression of the chorda tympani has been described, with evidence of compression of the nervus intermedius by a branch of the AICA in the IAC demonstrated by magnetic resonance angiography (MRA).

Facial Weakness of Central Origin

In a supranuclear, upper motor neuron or CFP, there is weakness of the lower face, with relative sparing of the upper face. The upper face has both contralateral and ipsilateral supranuclear innervation, and cortical innervation of the facial nucleus may be more extensive for the lower face than the upper. The paresis is rarely complete.

A lesion involving the corticobulbar fibers anywhere prior to their synapse on the facial nerve nucleus will cause a CFP. Lesions are most often in the cortex or internal capsule. Occasionally, a lesion as far caudal as the medulla can cause a CFP because of involvement of the aberrant pyramidal tract. There is considerable individual variation in facial innervation, and the extent of weakness in a CFP may vary from the lower half to two-thirds of the face. The upper face is not necessarily completely spared, but it is always involved to a lesser degree than the lower face. There may be subtle weakness of the orbicularis oculi, the palpebral fissure may be slightly wider on the involved side, and there may be a decrease in palpable lid vibrations. However, involvement of the corrugator and frontalis is unusual, and the patient should be able to elevate the eyebrow and wrinkle the forehead with no more than minimal asymmetry. Inability to independently wink the involved eye may be the only demonstrable deficit. Occasionally, a patient with incompletely developed Bell's palsy will have relative sparing of the upper face, causing confusion with a CFP.

Even if there is some degree of upper facial involvement in a CFP, the patient is always able to close the eye, Bell's phenomenon is absent, the corneal reflex is present, and the orbicularis oculi reflex may be exaggerated. In CFP, the lower face is weak, the nasolabial fold is shallow, and facial mobility is decreased. However, the lower face weakness is never as severe as with a PFP, which suggests that there may be some direct cortical innervation to the lower face as well as the upper. Separating CFP and PFP is rarely difficult. CFP is typically part of a more extensive paralysis because of a lesion of the upper motor neuron pathways. Rarely, it may occur in isolation without other neurologic abnormalities; this pattern has been reported with a lacunar lesion of the contralateral basis pontis.

There are two variations of CFP: (a) volitional, or voluntary; and (b) emotional, or mimetic. In most instances of CFP, the facial asymmetry is present both when the patient is asked to smile or show the teeth, and during spontaneous facial movements such as smiling and laughing. However, spontaneous movements and deliberate, willful movements may show different degrees of weakness (Figure 16.14). When asymmetry is more apparent with one than

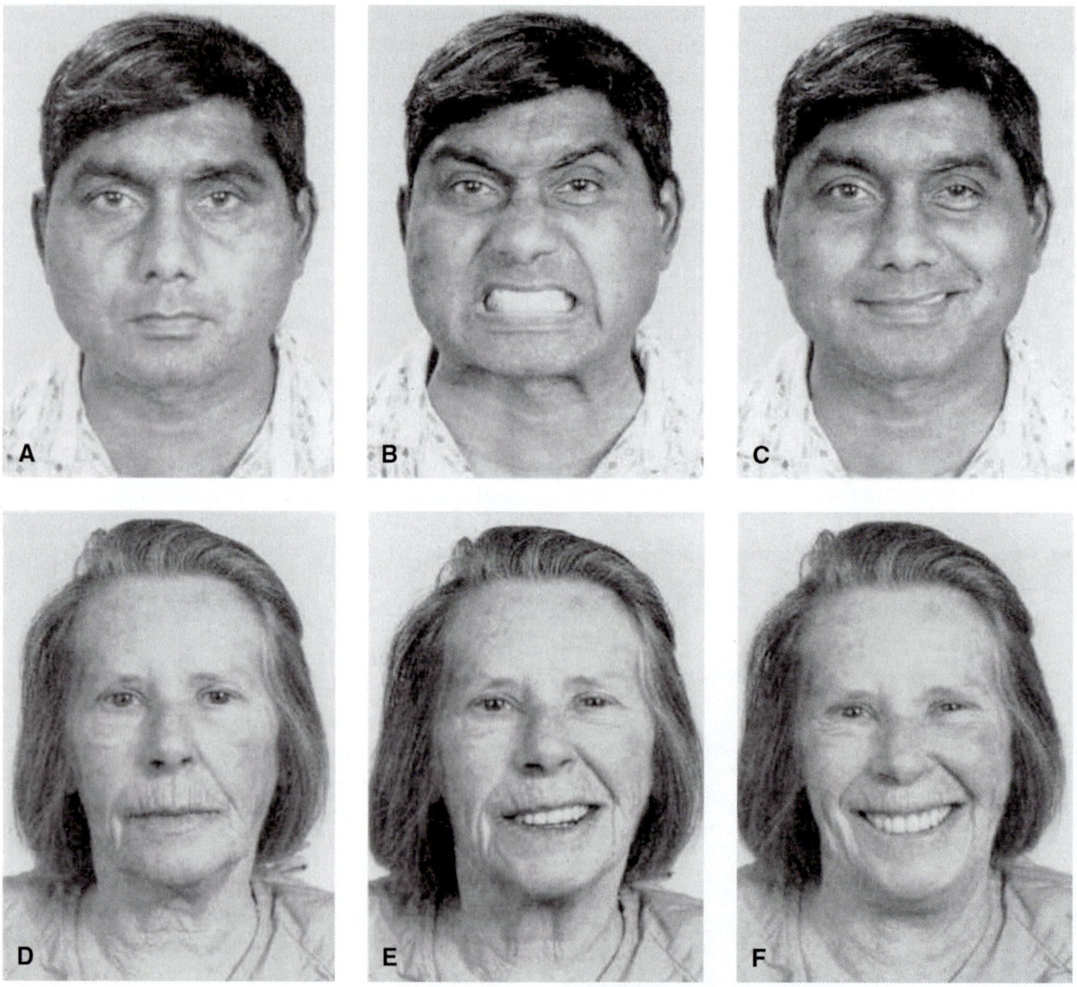

FIGURE 16.14 Patient with left thalamic tumor with face at rest **(A)**, on voluntarily baring the teeth **(B)**, and on reflex smiling **(C)**; there is right facial paresis on smiling but not on voluntary contraction, an emotional facial palsy. Patient with a lesion of the corticobulbar fibers in the genu of the left internal capsule with face at rest **(D)**, on voluntarily baring the teeth **(E)**, and on reflex smiling **(F)**; there is right facial paresis on voluntary contraction but not on smiling, a volitional facial palsy. (From Ross RT, Mathiesen R. Images in clinical medicine. Volitional and emotional supranuclear facial weakness. *N Engl J Med* 1998;338[21]:1515. Copyright © 1998 Massachusetts Medical Society. Reprinted with permission from Massachusetts Medical Society.)

the other, the facial weakness is said to be dissociated. Facial asymmetry more apparent with spontaneous expression, as when laughing, is called a mimetic, emotive or emotional facial palsy (EFP) (see Figure 16.14C); weakness more marked on voluntary contraction, when the patient is asked to smile or bare her teeth, is called a volitional facial palsy (VFP) (see Figure 16.14E). With VFP, automatic or spontaneous movements may not only be preserved, but at times exaggerated. VFP may result from a lesion involving either the cortical center in the lower third of the precentral gyrus that controls facial movements, or the corticobulbar tract. The lesion thus may be either in the cortex or in the subcortical corticobulbar pathways as they go through the internal capsule, the cerebral peduncle, or the pons above the facial nucleus. The dissociation may be due to bilateral supranuclear innervation for lower facial spontaneous, emotional movements not present for volitional movements. In EFP, the weakness is most marked with spontaneous facial movements, and the patient can contract the lower facial muscles on command without difficulty. The anatomical explanation for EFP is unclear. Facial weakness seen only with emotional movements most commonly results from thalamic or striatocapsular lesions, usually infarction, rarely with brainstem lesions. It has been described in lesions of the frontal lobe anterior to the precentral gyrus involving the supplementary motor area. The fibers that mediate the emotional response travel through pathways other than the corticobulbar tracts. Facial asymmetry has been described in patients with temporal lobe seizure foci; the weaker side is usually contralateral to the lesion.

Abnormal Facial Movements

Some conditions involving the face produce abnormal movements rather than weakness. Common disorders causing abnormal facial movements include aberrant regeneration because of facial nerve palsy, blepharospasm, HFS, and facial myokymia.

Hemifacial Spasm

Facial synkinesis may progress to a stage of HFS. More often, HFS arises de novo, because of intermittent compression by an ectatic arterial loop in the posterior circulation, most often a redundant loop of the AICA. The compression is usually near the anterior aspect of the root exit zone. The pathophysiology is similar to that in some cases of trigeminal neuralgia (Chapter 15). The arterial pulsations are thought to cause demyelination and focal nerve damage leading to ephaptic transmission and ectopic excitation. Combined studies using MRI and MRA may demonstrate the neurovascular compression. An MRI study using 3D reconstruction confirmed the AICA as the most common causative vessel, with the posterior inferior cerebellar artery, vertebral artery, internal auditory artery, and veins occasionally causing facial nerve compression at the root entry zone. However, radiographic studies using a 3T MRI has shown that some contact between the facial nerve and nearby vessels, even enough to cause mild nerve deviation, is the rule rather than the exception.

Microvascular decompression is sometimes done and may effectively halt the movements. The lateral spread response is an electrophysiologic phenomenon seen in HFS. Stimulation of the mandibular branch of the facial nerve may cause a compound muscle action potential to appear in the orbicularis oculi. This response does not occur in normals. The lateral spread response is objective evidence of ephaptic transmission from one facial nerve branch to another. During microvascular decompression, the lateral spread response may disappear when the offending vessel is lifted off the nerve, and the status of the response may be used as an indicator of the effectiveness of the decompression. HFS may also occur with other extra-axial or intra-axial lesions, including aneurysm, tumor, multiple sclerosis, or basilar meningitis.

HFS usually develops in older patients, and the condition is twice as common in women than men. Twitching usually begins in the orbicularis oculi, less often in the oris. Initially, the twitching may be subtle and difficult to distinguish from facial synkinesis. HFS may involve the entire facial nerve distribution, or only certain nerve branches; it may propagate from one branch to another. Over months to years, HFS usually spreads to involve all of the facial muscles on one side, but it remains strictly limited to the muscles supplied by the facial nerve. As HFS worsens, it may involve the auricular muscles even when the patient cannot deliberately wiggle the ears; the platysma may also be affected. Fully developed HFS causes repetitive, paroxysmal, involuntary, spasmodic, tonic and clonic contractions of the muscles innervated by the facial nerve on the involved side of the face. The mouth twists to the affected side, the nasolabial fold deepens, the eye closes, and there is contraction of the frontalis muscle **(Video 16.2)**.

The spasms may persist in sleep and are often exacerbated by chewing or speaking. Synkinesis following PFP may cause movements resembling HFS. The essential difference is that synkinesis is provoked by a voluntary movement, whereas HFS is a spontaneous, involuntary contraction. HFS is commonly associated with some degree of facial weakness because of underlying nerve damage. Rare patients may have both HFS and trigeminal neuralgia, with lancinating pain accompanying the facial spasms (tic convulsif). Brissaud-Sicard syndrome is HFS with contralateral hemiparesis because of a lesion in the pons.

Babinski's brow lift sign is seen only in HFS and consists of cocontraction of the frontalis and orbicularis oculi muscles causing simultaneous eye closure and paradoxical elevation of the eyebrow during a spasm. This movement is impossible to execute voluntarily and does not occur in blepharospasm, tic or psychogenic movement disorders. The brow lift sign has been referred to as the "other Babinski sign," but at least nine signs bear Babinski's name and this designation has been used for other signs as well, most notably Babinski's platysma sign.

Blepharospasm (nictitating spasm) causes involuntary twitching that primarily involves the orbicularis oculi and frontalis muscles. Blepharospasm is most often idiopathic or "essential" and is a form of focal dystonia (Chapter 30, **Video 30.5**). Blepharospasm is always bilateral and fairly symmetric. Meige's syndrome is the association of blepharospasm with oromandibular dystonia. Patients with central nervous system (CNS) Whipple's disease may have an oculofacial, more often an oculomasticatory, myorhythmia (see **Video Link 16.4**).

Tic, or habit spasm, can cause a movement resembling HFS or blepharospasm. Tic often causes retraction of the angle of the mouth, contraction of the orbicularis oculi or platysma, or eye blinking. The movements are somewhat more bizarre and purposeful, and other muscles not innervated by CN VII may be brought into action. Bizarre grimacing movements of the face are usually habit spasms. The movements in HFS and essential blepharospasm are stereotyped. The patient with tic can suppress the movements, at least temporarily, while the movements of HFS and blepharospasm are totally beyond volitional control and cannot be suppressed or imitated.

Spastic Paretic Facial Contracture

Instead of spasm, there may be a facial contracture causing a fixed expression with wrinkling of the forehead, narrowing of the palpebral fissure, drawing up or twisting of the angle of the mouth, and increased depth of the nasolabial fold. A facial contracture may give the faulty impression of weakness on the opposite side. Facial contracture may follow a facial paralysis, or occur de novo. Careful testing may reveal that the affected muscles are still paretic, even though in a state of contracture. This type of spastic paretic facial contracture may occur with a progressive lesion of the pons and is suspicious for neoplasm. When facial myokymia and spastic paretic contracture occur together, the likelihood of pontine neoplasm is very high.

Facial Myokymia

Facial myokymia is a continuous, involuntary muscular quivering that has a rippling, wormlike, appearance (Chapter 30). It is usually unilateral. Facial myokymia has been reported with numerous conditions, most intrinsic to the brainstem. It is a classic feature of multiple sclerosis but may also occur with pontine tumor, CPA tumors, Guillain-Barré syndrome, facial nerve compression, rattlesnake envenomation, subarachnoid hemorrhage, meningeal neoplasia, basilar invagination and in association with high titers of voltage-gated K^+ channel antibodies (see **Video Link 16.5**). Facial myokymia may occur after cardiac arrest, even in some patients with brain death. With intraparenchymal lesions, the facial nucleus itself is usually intact, but the process disrupts its connections, possibly disinhibiting some neural generator. Mild, usually fleeting, myokymia is common, especially in the orbicularis oculi, and of no clinical significance. These movements often worsen with fatigue and with hyper caffeinism. Patients often require reassurance.

Other Abnormal Facial Movements

Focal seizures involving the face may occur with seizure foci in the motor cortex. Facial seizures may be part of a versive seizure or Jacksonian march. Disease of the basal ganglia or extrapyramidal system may involve the facial muscles causing hypokinesia or hyperkinesia (Chapter 30). Parkinson's disease causes hypokinesia. Forms of facial hyperkinesias include dyskinesias, choreiform, athetoid, dystonic, grimacing, and myoclonic movements and tremors. Oral-facial dyskinesias are common, most often as a tardive manifestation of psychoactive drug use. Facial muscles, especially the platysma, may sometimes be involved in palatal myoclonus, which is a persistent, rhythmic movement in contrast to other forms of myoclonus (Chapter 30). Facial myoclonus can occur with dolichoectasia of the vertebral artery, with hypocalcemia, serotonin syndrome, and other conditions. Facial fasciculations may occur in any motor neuron disease; perioral and chin fasciculations are frequent in Kennedy's disease.

Sensory Involvement

Except for disturbances of taste, sensory abnormalities are not a common part of facial nerve lesions. Taste may be affected with lesions of the facial nerve proximal to the takeoff of the chorda tympani. Permanent taste disturbances may follow Bell's palsy. Disturbances of taste and smell often occur together. Taste abnormalities are usually due to olfactory dysfunction (Chapter 12). Dysgeusia may be a direct or indirect effect of malignancy. Hypergeusia and parageusias may occur in psychoses and conversion disorder. Gustatory hallucinations may occur with complex partial seizures and with tumors involving the uncus or parietal operculum. Gustatory and olfactory hallucinations often occur together. Elderly patients sometimes develop dysgeusia of obscure origin that may lead to anorexia and weight loss. Increased taste sensitivity occurs in patients with Addison disease, pituitary deficiency, and cystic fibrosis.

Geniculate neuralgia causes paroxysmal pain deep in the ear, sometimes radiating to the face. "Tic douloureux of the chorda tympani" has also been described. Lesions of the lingual nerve may cause loss of taste together with loss of exteroceptive sensation on the involved side of the tongue; there is also usually subjective numbness.

Secretory Changes

CN VII is involved in lacrimation and salivation; lesions of the nerve at or proximal to the geniculate ganglion can cause abnormalities of these functions. Absence of salivation occurs only with bilateral lesions. Central lesions, especially those involving the hypothalamus or the autonomic connections, may cause changes in secretory function. Changes in lacrimal and salivary flow are more often the result of systemic processes. Anticholinergic drugs often cause an unpleasantly dry mouth. Keratoconjunctivitis sicca, which occurs in Sjögren's syndrome and other connective tissue disorders, causes deficient secretion of the lacrimal, salivary, and mucosal glands. This in turn causes dryness of the eyes, mouth, and upper respiratory tract. Sialorrhea (ptyalism) is an excess of saliva. It occurs in Parkinson's disease and when patients are unable to swallow, such as in bulbar involvement with motor neuron disease.

An increase or decrease in lacrimal or salivary secretion may occur on a psychogenic basis. Lacrimation, of course, is most frequently the result of an emotional stimulus. Salivation may occur from the smell, taste, sight, or thought of food. Xerostomia is common in depressed and anxious patients.

Video Links

Video Link 16.1. Demonstration of taste testing technique. http://www.youtube.com/watch?v=ldkpd88KSUA&feature=mfu_in_order&list=UL

Video Link 16.2. Möbius' syndrome. http://www.youtube.com/watch?v=3FJPvBcMNAE

Video Link 16.3. Myopathic facies. http://neurosigns.org/wiki/Myopathic_facies

Video Link 16.4. Oculomasticatory myorhythmia in CNS Whipple's disease. http://neurosigns.org/wiki/Oculomasticatory_myorhythmia

Video Link 16.5. Facial myokymia after rattlesnake bite. https://www.youtube.com/watch?v=KaM3-qy8uqU

BIBLIOGRAPHY

Abboud O, Saliba I. Isolated bilateral facial paralysis revealing AIDS: a unique presentation. *Laryngoscope* 2008;118:580–584.

Adour KK. Mona Lisa syndrome: solving the enigma of the Gioconda smile. *Ann Otol Rhinol Laryngol* 1989;98:196–199.

Agarwal R, Manandhar L, Saluja P, et al. Pontine stroke presenting as isolated facial nerve palsy mimicking Bell's Palsy: a case report. *J Med Case Reports* 2011;5:287.

Baizabal-Carvallo JF, Jankovic J. Distinguishing features of psychogenic (functional) versus organic hemifacial spasm. *J Neurol* 2017;264(2):359–363.

Campos-Benitez M, Kaufmann AM. Neurovascular compression findings in hemifacial spasm. *J Neurosurg* 2008;109:416–420.

Cerrato P, Imperiale D, Bergui M, et al. Emotional facial paresis in a patient with a lateral medullary infarction. *Neurology* 2003;60:723–724.

Cho HJ, Kim HY. Interesting sign of Bell's palsy in an ear wiggler. *Neurol Sci* 2009;30:345–347.

Clement WA, White A. Idiopathic familial facial nerve paralysis. *J Laryngol Otol* 2000;114:132–134.

Compston A. Facial reflexes. *Brain.* 2005;128(Pt 2):235–236.

Croxson G, May M, Mester SJ. Grading facial nerve function: House-Brackmann versus Burres-Fisch methods. *Am J Otol* 1990;11:240–246.

Eggenberger E. Eight-and-a-half syndrome: one-and-a-half syndrome plus cranial nerve VII palsy. *J Neuroophthalmol* 1998;18:114–116.

Evidente VG, Adler CH. Hemifacial spasm and other craniofacial movement disorders. *Mayo Clin Proc* 1998;73:67–71.

Gilchrist JM. AAEM case report #26: seventh cranial neuropathy. *Muscle Nerve* 1993;16:447–452.

Gilchrist JM. Seventh cranial neuropathy. *Semin Neurol* 2009;29:5–13.

Guinand N, Just T, Stow NW, et al. Cutting the chorda tympani: not just a matter of taste. *J Laryngol Otol* 2010;124:999–1002.

Gutmann L. AAEM minimonograph #37: facial and limb myokymia. *Muscle Nerve* 1991;14:1043–1049.

Gutmann L, Tellers JG, Vernino S. Persistent facial myokymia associated with K(+) channel antibodies. *Neurology* 2001;57(9):1707–1708.

Hunt JR. On herpetic inflammations of the geniculate ganglion: a new syndrome and its complications. *J Nerv Ment Dis* 1907;34:73.

James DG. All that palsies is not Bell's. *J R Soc Med* 1996;89:184–187.

Kakizawa Y, Seguchi T, Kodama K, et al. Anatomical study of the trigeminal and facial cranial nerves with the aid of 3.0-tesla magnetic resonance imaging. *J Neurosurg* 2008;108:483–490.

Kanoh N, Nomura J, Satomi F. Nocturnal onset and development of Bell's palsy. *Laryngoscope* 2005;115:99–100.

Karadan U, Manappallil RG, Jayakrishnan C, et al. Pontine haemorrhage disguised as Bell's palsy. *BMJ Case Rep* 2018;5:2018.

Keane JR. Bilateral seventh nerve palsy: analysis of 43 cases and review of the literature. *Neurology* 1994;44:1198–1202.

Kefalidis G, Riga M, Argyropoulou P, et al. Is the width of the labyrinthine portion of the fallopian tube implicated in the pathophysiology of Bell's palsy?: a prospective clinical study using computed tomography. *Laryngoscope* 2010;120:1203–1207.

Kim YH, Choi IJ, Kim HM, et al. Bilateral simultaneous facial nerve palsy: clinical analysis in seven cases. *Otol Neurotol* 2008;29:397–400.

Kinoshita T, Ishii K, Okitsu T, et al. Facial nerve palsy: evaluation by contrast-enhanced MR imaging. *Clin Radiol* 2001;56:926–932.

Krauss JK, Wakhloo AK, Scheremet R, et al. Facial myokymia and spastic paretic facial contracture as the result of anaplastic pontocerebellar glioma. *Neurosurgery* 1993;32:1031–1034.

Kugelberg E. Facial reflexes. *Brain* 1952;75:385.

Kuhweide R, Van de Steene V, Vlaminck S, et al. Ramsay Hunt syndrome: pathophysiology of cochleovestibular symptoms. *J Laryngol Otol* 2002;116:844–848.

Malhotra A. Marin-Amat syndrome: a case of acquired facial synkinesis. *BMJ Case Rep* 2013;18:2013.

Mansoor AM, Sullivan PD. Intrafacial synkinesis. *N Engl J Med* 2016;374(22):e27.

Morris HH, Estes ML. Bilateral facial myokymia following cardiopulmonary arrest. *Arch Neurol* 1981;38:393–394.

Morris AM, Deeks SL, Hill MD, et al. Annualized incidence and spectrum of illness from an outbreak investigation of Bell's palsy. *Neuroepidemiology* 2002;21:255–261.

Müri RM. Cortical control of facial expression. *J Comp Neurol* 2016;524:1578–1585.

Mutsch M, Zhou W, Rhodes P, et al. Use of the inactivated intranasal influenza vaccine and the risk of Bell's palsy in Switzerland. *N Engl J Med* 2004;350:896–903.

Naraghi R, Tanrikulu L, Troescher-Weber R, et al. Classification of neurovascular compression in typical hemifacial spasm: three-dimensional visualization of the facial and the vestibulocochlear nerves. *J Neurosurg* 2007;107:1154–1163.

Nielsen VK. Pathophysiology of hemifacial spasm. I. Ephaptic transmission and ectopic excitation. *Neurology* 1984;34:418.

Patel AA, Tanna N. In: Meyers AD, ed. *Facial Nerve Anatomy.* Available at: http://emedicine.medscape.com/article/835286-overview. Accessed July 11, 2011.

Pavone P, Garozzo R, Trifiletti RR, et al. Marin-Amat syndrome: case report and review of the literature. *J Child Neurol* 1999;14:266–268.

Pryse-Phillips W. *Companion to Clinical Neurology.* 3rd ed. Oxford: Oxford University Press, 2009.

Riaz G, Campbell WW, Carr J, et al. Facial myokymia in syringobulbia. *Arch Neurol* 1990;47:472–474

Roh JK, Kim BK, Chung JM. Combined peripheral facial and abducens nerve palsy caused by caudal tegmental pontine infarction. *Eur Neurol* 1999;41:99–102.

Ronthal M. Bell's palsy: pathogenesis, clinical features, and diagnosis. In: Shefner JM, Eichler AF, eds. *UpToDate.* Available at: www.uptodate.com. Accessed February 28, 2018.

Rowlands S, Hooper R, Hughes R, et al. The epidemiology and treatment of Bell's palsy in the UK. *Eur J Neurol* 2002;9:63–67.

Rubin DI, Matsumoto JY, Suarez GA, et al. Facial trigeminal synkinesis associated with a trigeminal schwannoma. *Neurology* 1999;53:635–637.

Sakas DE, Panourias IG, Stranjalis G, et al. Paroxysmal otalgia due to compression of the intermediate nerve: a distinct syndrome of neurovascular conflict confirmed by neuroimaging. Case report. *J Neurosurg* 2007;107:1228–1230.

Sarwal A, Garewal M, Sahota S, et al. Eight-and-a-half syndrome. *J Neuroimaging* 2009;19:288–290.

Solé G, Perez F, Ferrer X. Teaching NeuroImages: reversible ectropion in myasthenia gravis. *Neurology* 2009;73:e83.

Stamey W, Jankovic J. The other Babinski sign in hemifacial spasm. *Neurology* 2007;69:402–404.

Sweeney CJ, Gilden DH. Ramsay Hunt syndrome. *J Neurol Neurosurg Psychiatry* 2001;71:149–154.

Tzafetta K, Terzis JK. Essays on the facial nerve: part I. Microanatomy. *Plast Reconstr Surg* 2010;125:879–889.

Urban PP, Wicht S, Marx J, et al. Isolated voluntary facial paresis due to pontine ischemia. *Neurology* 1998;50:1859–1862.

Urban PP, Wicht S, Vucorevic G, et al. The course of corticofacial projections in the human brainstem. *Brain* 2001;124(Pt 9):1866–1876.

Valls-Solé J. Facial nerve palsy and hemifacial spasm. *Handb Clin Neurol* 2013;115:367–380.

Varanda S, Rocha S, Rodrigues M, et al. Role of the "other Babinski sign" in hyperkinetic facial disorders. *J Neurol Sci* 2017;378:36–37.

Vrabec JT, Isaacson B, Van Hook JW. Bell's palsy and pregnancy. *Otolaryngol Head Neck Surg* 2007;137:858–861.

Weijnen FG, van der Bilt A, Wokke JH, et al. What's in a smile? Quantification of the vertical smile of patients with myasthenia gravis. *J Neurol Sci* 2000;173:124–128.

Xanthopoulos J, Noussios G, Papaioannides D, et al. Ramsay Hunt syndrome presenting as a cranial polyneuropathy. *Acta Otorhinolaryngol Belg* 2002;56:319–323.

Yamashita M, Yamamoto T. Aberrant pyramidal tract in the medial lemniscus of the human brainstem: normal distribution and pathological changes. *Eur Neurol* 2001;45:75–82.

CHAPTER 17

The Acoustic (Vestibulocochlear) Nerve

The vestibulocochlear, acoustic, or eighth cranial nerve (CN VIII) has two components, the vestibular and the cochlear, blended into a single trunk. The cochlear portion subserves hearing; the vestibular nerve subserves equilibration, coordination, and orientation in space. Both are classified as special sensory afferent nerves. The two components originate in separate peripheral receptors and have distinct central connections. Although they are united along their course through the skull, they differ so greatly both functionally and in their anatomic relationships that they should be considered separately.

THE COCHLEAR NERVE

Anatomy and Physiology

Sound is a form of energy produced by vibrations that create a sinusoidal wave of alternating condensations and rarefactions in a conductive medium such as air. Sound waves converge on the tympanic membrane and are transmitted by the auditory ossicles (malleus, incus, and stapes) to the inner ear, or labyrinth. The labyrinth is a complex of interconnecting cavities, tunnels, ducts, and canals that lies in the petrous portion of the temporal bone (Figure 17.1). The vestibule, cochlea, and semicircular canals form the bony, or osseous, labyrinth, which is made of compact bone and can be dissected free of the cancellous bone that surrounds it (Figure 17.2).

The bony labyrinth is filled with perilymph, a thin watery fluid similar to cerebrospinal fluid. The membranous labyrinth is an arrangement of sacs and ducts that lies within the bony labyrinth, generally follows its outline, and is filled with endolymph (Scarpa's fluid [Antonio Scarpa was an Italian surgeon, anatomist, and artist who first described many structures of the ear]). The membranous labyrinth has two major components: the vestibular apparatus and the cochlear duct (Figure 17.3). The ossicles span the middle ear cavity and transmit the oscillations of the tympanic membrane to the footplate of the stapes, which sits in the oval window (fenestra vestibuli). The ossicles function as an amplifier and help to compensate for the loss of energy as sound waves are transmitted from the air to the perilymph behind the oval window. The tensor tympani muscle, which inserts on the malleus, and the stapedius, which inserts on the stapes, provide reflex protection against sudden, loud noise. The oval window opens into the vestibule of the inner ear, which connects on one side to the cochlea and on the other to the semicircular canals. The cochlea spirals for 2.5 to 2.75 turns to reach its apex. The base of the cochlea faces the internal acoustic meatus and contains myriad fenestrations that admit the filaments of the cochlear nerve. The middle ear cavity acts as an impedance-matching device to transfer sound energy from the low impedance of air to the high impedance of fluid in the cochlea.

The central axis of the cochlea is the modiolus; from it projects a delicate bony shelf, the spiral lamina, which partially divides the cochlear passageway into two parallel channels—the scala tympani and the scala vestibuli. The scala media, or cochlear duct, is part of the membranous labyrinth. It lies in the center of the spirals of the cochlea, completing the partition between the scala tympani and scala vestibuli (Figure 17.4). At the tip of the modiolus, the cochlear duct ends blindly; a narrow slit at the very apex of the cochlea, the helicotrema (Gr. "hole in a helix"), allows for communication and the flow of perilymph between the scala tympani and vestibuli.

The basilar membrane of the cochlear duct projects from the spiral lamina of the modiolus to the outer wall of the cochlea. The spiral ganglion

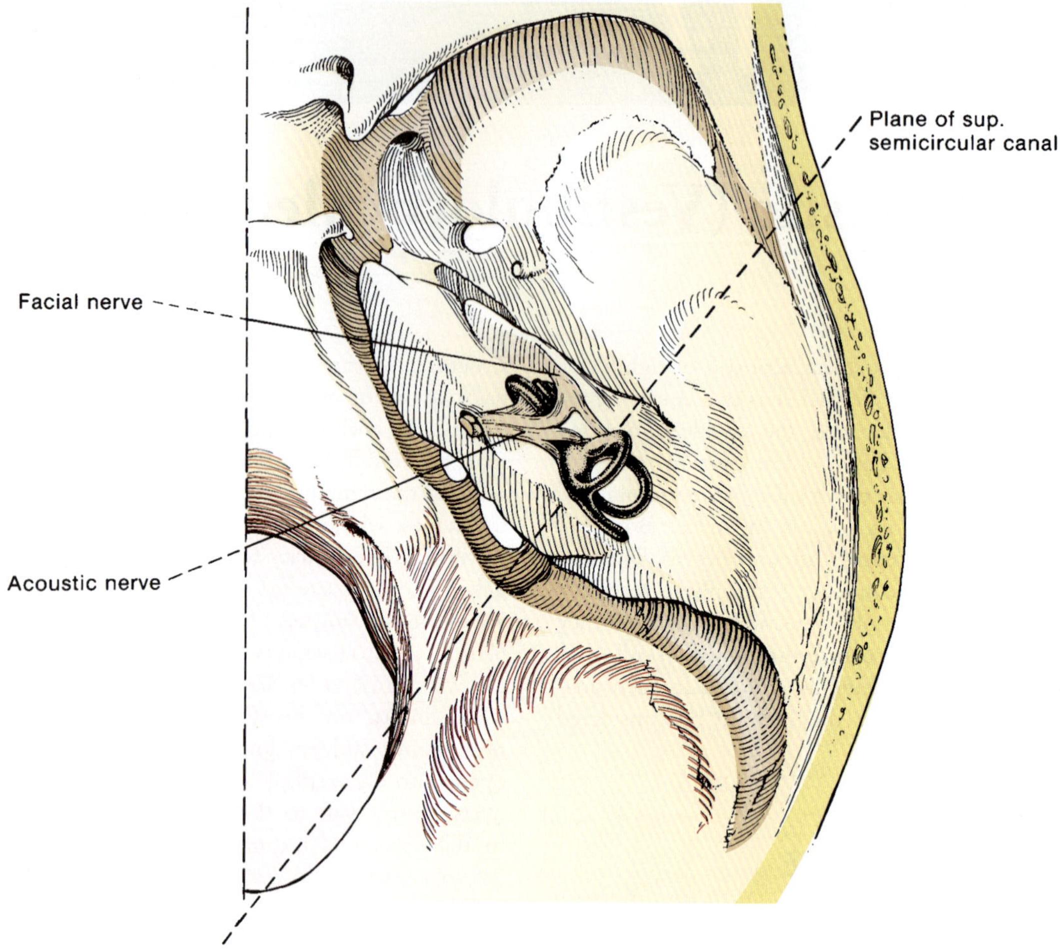

FIGURE 17.1 The right osseous labyrinth in the temporal bone viewed from above.

of the cochlear nerve lies in the spiral canal of the modiolus (Rosenthal's canal). The organ of Corti rests on the basilar membrane and contains inner and outer hair cells. The inner hair cells are the receptors, or end organs, of the cochlear nerve. From the apex of each inner hair cell, a stereocilium extends to just beneath the tectorial membrane (Figure 17.4). Sound waves induce vibrations in the cochlea, which cause movement of the basilar and tectorial membranes. This movement flexes the stereocilia, which activates the hair cell, causing impulses in the spiral ganglion.

Because of the varying width of the basilar membrane, sound of a certain frequency induces harmonic oscillations maximal at a certain point along the cochlear duct, which focally activates certain hair cells and encodes the frequency (Box 17.1). The round window (fenestra cochlea) lies below the oval window (Figure 17.2). It is covered by a delicate membrane, the secondary tympanic membrane, which allows for compliance in the perilymph system and permits the waves of vibration initiated at the oval window to dissipate.

The spiral ganglion consists of type I and type II bipolar neurons that lie in the modiolus. Inner hair cells synapse on type I neurons, which make up 95% of the ganglion. Axons of the spiral ganglion cells form the cochlear nerve, which contains some 30,000 fibers (Figure 17.6). Axons from type I cells are myelinated and form the bulk of the nerve. The type II cells connect with the outer hair cells and modulate the activity of the inner hair cells (Box 17.1).

The acoustic nerve traverses the internal auditory canal (IAC), where it lies lateral and inferior to the facial nerve. It crosses the cerebellopontine angle, passes around the inferior cerebellar peduncle, and

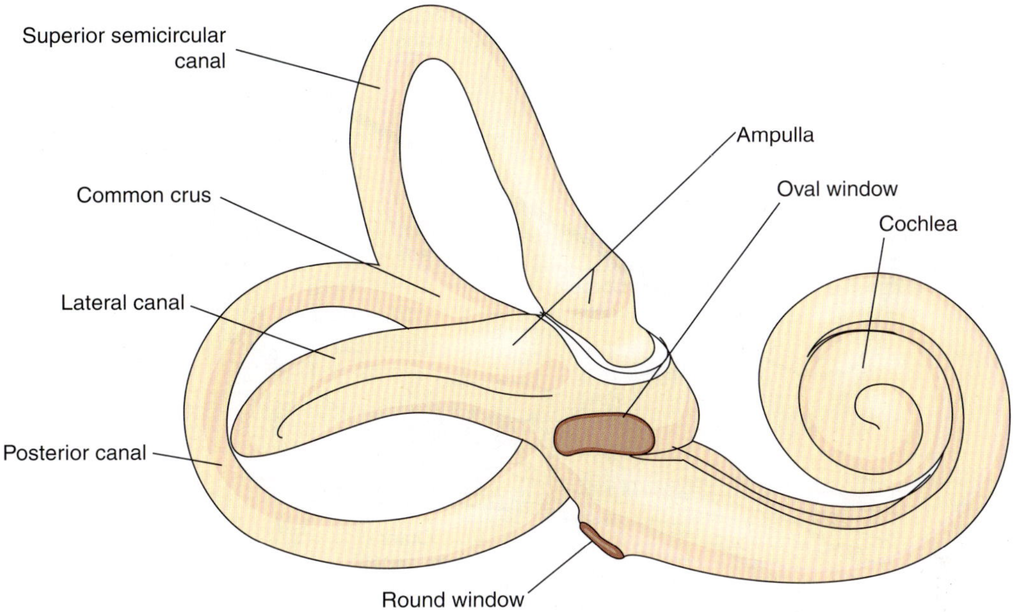

FIGURE 17.2 The right osseous labyrinth, lateral view.

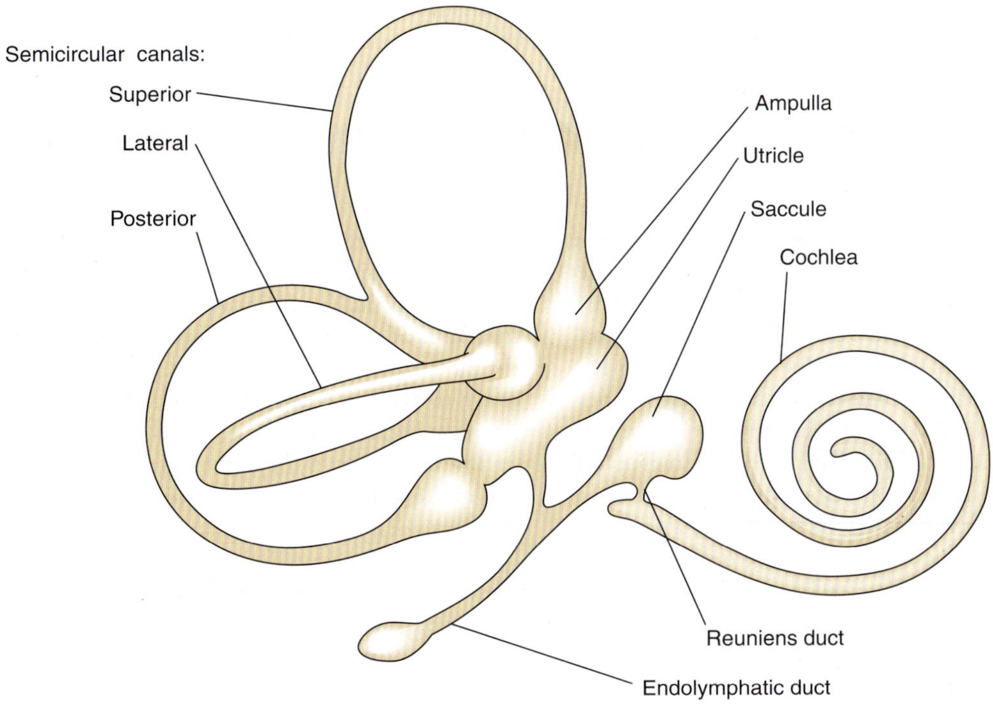

FIGURE 17.3 The membranous labyrinth.

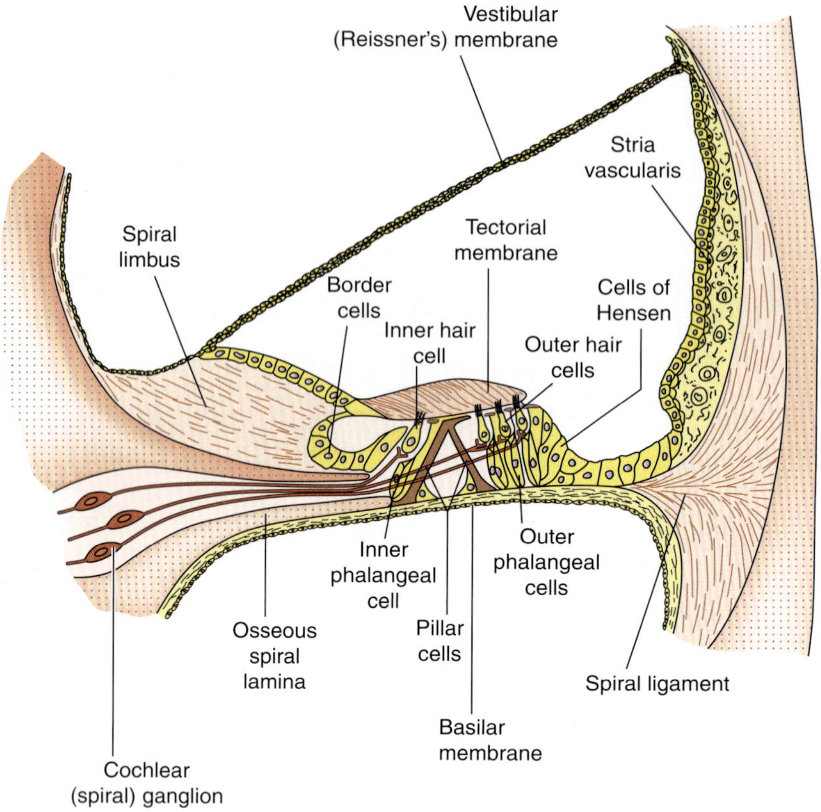

FIGURE 17.4 Structure of the cochlear duct and the spiral organ of Corti. (Modified from Kiernan JA. *Barr's The Human Nervous System: An Anatomical Viewpoint.* 7th ed. Philadelphia: Lippincott-Raven, 1998, with permission.)

BOX 17.1

Tonotopic Organization

The organ of Corti is tonotopically organized. The width of the basilar membrane of the cochlear duct is least at the base of the cochlea, where the spinal lamina of the modiolus extends farthest into the coils of the cochlea. This part of the cochlea is most efficiently activated by high frequencies. Near the apex, the basilar membrane is wider and responds to low-pitched tones. The inner hair cell-spiral ganglion cell complex at a given point along the organ of Corti is frequency dependent, responding best to a particular pitch and coding for that pitch by its discharges in the cochlear nerve. Tonotopic organization continues to varying degrees throughout the auditory system.

Imagine a spiral staircase in the center of a silo—steps winding around a central core, steps wider at the bottom and progressively narrowing, and from each step a cable of violin string extending to the wall of the silo (Figure 17.5). The central core represents the modiolus; the steps, the spiral lamina; and the violin strings, the basilar membrane. A low-tone sounding in the silo would set the long strings near the top of the silo in vibration; a high-pitched tone would affect the short strings near the bottom. Coil the silo into a conch to match the turns in the staircase to complete the resemblance to the cochlear duct.

The stereocilia of the outer hair cells are imbedded in the tectorial membrane and have contractile properties. They help adjust and control the oscillations of the membrane and thereby regulate to some degree the activation of the inner hair cells. The outer hair cells receive innervation from the efferent cochlear, or olivocochlear, bundle, which arises from the superior olivary nucleus in the pons. By controlling the outer hair cells, the olivocochlear bundle helps regulate afferent cochlear traffic and may be involved in attentiveness to auditory stimuli.

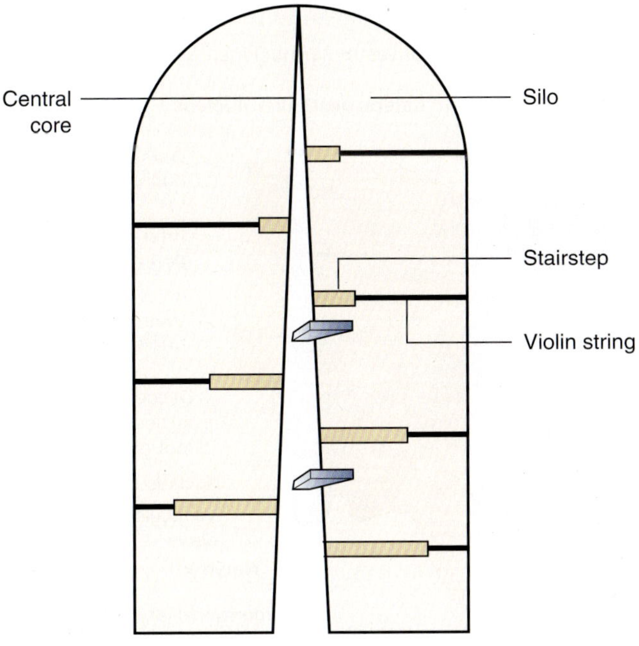

FIGURE 17.5 The cochlear duct and organ of Corti as a spiral staircase in a silo (see Box 17.1).

enters the upper medulla at its junction with the pons near the lateral recess of the fourth ventricle (Figure 17.7). Each entering fiber bifurcates to synapse in both the dorsal (posterior) and ventral (anterior) cochlear nuclei. The ventral nucleus may be divided into anteroventral and posteroventral portions. This dual termination is the beginning of a great deal of redundancy in the auditory system.

Tonotopic organization is maintained in the auditory nuclei and throughout the higher auditory relay centers; the location of fibers is related to their site of origin in the cochlea, which in turn is a reflection of the activating frequency. In the cochlear nuclei, low-frequency tones are processed ventrally and high frequencies dorsally. Second-order neurons in the cochlear nuclei give rise to the dorsal, ventral,

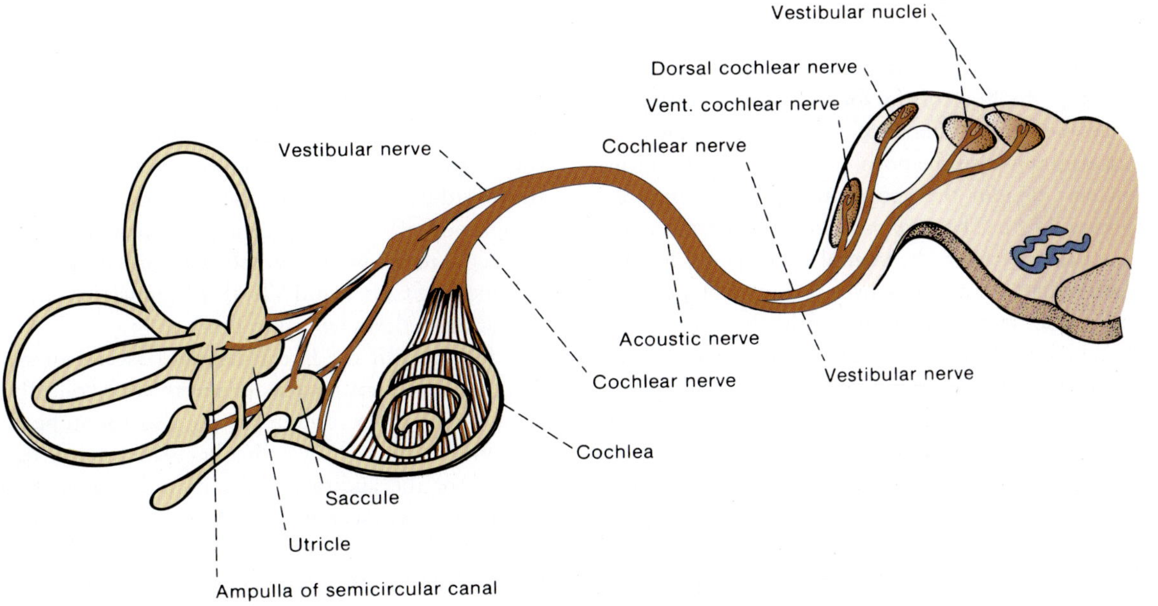

FIGURE 17.6 The acoustic nerve and its connections.

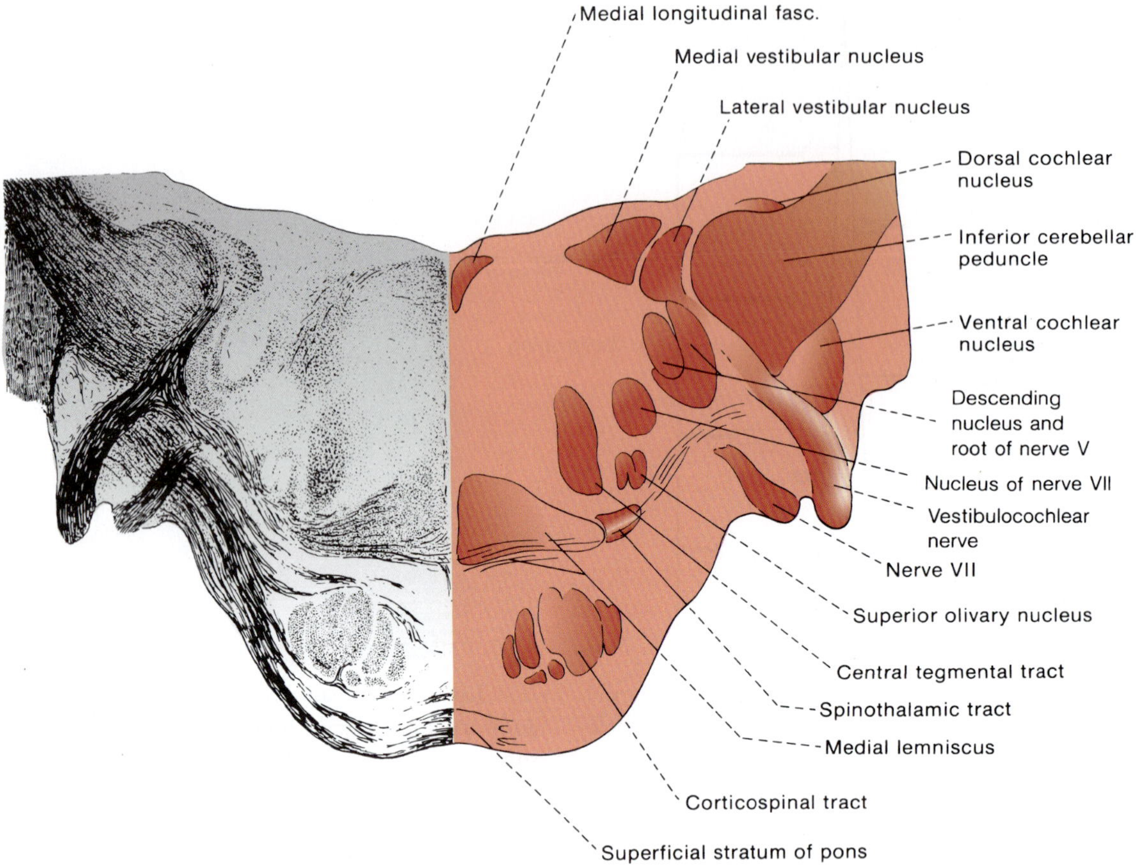

FIGURE 17.7 Section through the junction of the pons and medulla at the level of the cochlear nuclei.

and intermediate acoustic stria. The dorsal acoustic stria consists of fibers from the dorsal cochlear nucleus that pass over the inferior cerebellar peduncle, cross the floor of the fourth ventricle under the striae medullares (fibers of Piccolomini), and then pass ventrally into the pons, near the superior olivary nucleus, to join the contralateral lateral lemniscus (Figure 17.8). The intermediate and ventral acoustic striae arise from the ventral cochlear nuclei. The intermediate stria passes over the inferior peduncle and crosses the tegmentum to join the contralateral lateral lemniscus. Fibers of the ventral stria pass ventral to the peduncle. Some cross the pons as trapezoid fibers to synapse in the contralateral nucleus of the trapezoid body. Others synapse ipsilaterally in the nucleus of the trapezoid body.

Auditory fibers ascend from the trapezoid body as the lateral lemniscus. Fibers in the dorsal and intermediate acoustic stria run to the contralateral inferior colliculus, most directly, some after a relay in the nucleus of the lateral lemniscus. This crossed, monaural auditory pathway primarily carries information about sound frequency. Fibers of the ventral acoustic stria are both crossed and uncrossed and may synapse in the nuclei of the trapezoid body, superior olive, or lateral lemniscus. The binaural pathway, especially the superior olivary complex component, can determine the time difference between the two ears and aid in the localization of sound. Ascending auditory fibers send collaterals to the brainstem reticular formation and to the nuclei of CNs V and VII; these connections mediate various reflexes related to hearing.

Fibers from the lateral lemnisci ascend to synapse in the central nucleus of the inferior colliculus, an auditory reflex center that is also tonotopically organized. The inferior colliculus is the central relay nucleus of the auditory pathway and receives both ascending and descending input. Axons from the inferior colliculus pass through the brachium of the inferior colliculus to the medial geniculate body (MGB), a special sensory nucleus of the thalamus that is the final relay station in the auditory pathway. In the

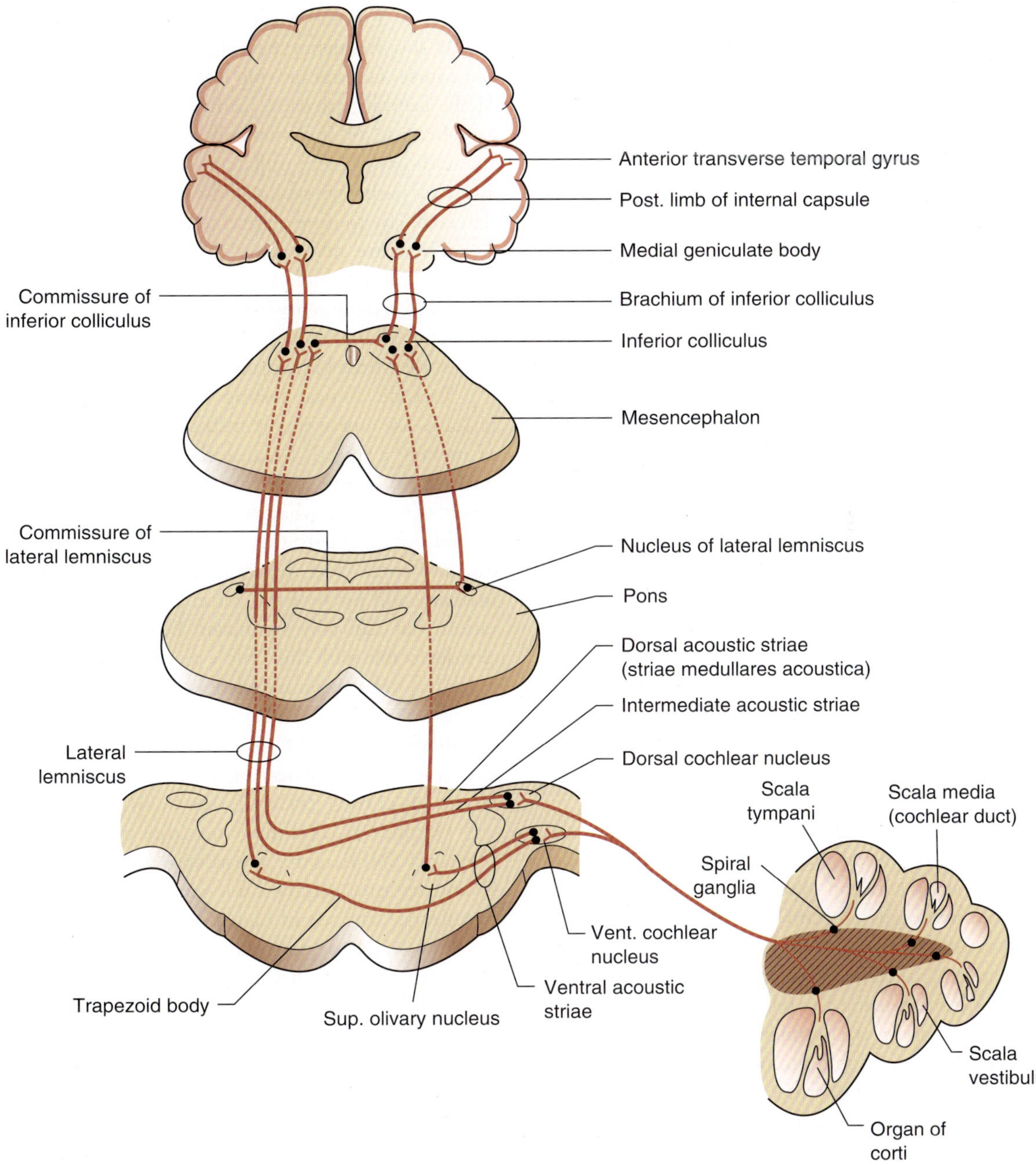

FIGURE 17.8 The cochlear pathway.

MGB, fibers conveying high tones lie medially and low tones laterally. From the MGB, auditory fibers pass through the posterior limb of the internal capsule as the geniculotemporal tract, or auditory radiations, which runs through the sublenticular portion of the internal capsule. The fibers terminate in the cortex of the transverse temporal convolutions (Heschl's gyrus) and the adjacent planum temporale portion of the superior temporal gyrus. The transverse temporal gyri and parts of the planum temporale make up the primary and secondary auditory cortex (Brodmann's areas 41 and 42). The primary auditory cortex is tonotopically organized with high frequencies medial and low frequencies lateral. The auditory association cortex (Wernicke's area in the dominant hemisphere) lies just posterior to the primary auditory cortex.

There is extensive crossing of the central auditory pathways above the level of the cochlear nuclei. Commissures connect the nuclei of the lateral lemniscus (commissure of Probst) and the inferior colliculi (commissure of the inferior colliculus). There are connections through the brachium of the inferior colliculus between the central nucleus of the inferior colliculus on one side and the contralateral MGB. In addition, there is the direct, tonotopically organized auditory pathway, the core projection, and an additional, less-organized pathway, the belt projection. The core system includes the central nucleus of the inferior colliculus, portions of the MGB, and the primary auditory cortex. The belt projection includes the pericentral region of the inferior colliculus, the nonlaminated portion of the MGB, and the secondary auditory cortex. The corpus callosum contains fibers that connect the auditory cortices of the two hemispheres.

Descending auditory projections run parallel to the ascending fibers and are concerned with auditory reflexes. Descending pathways include the corticogeniculate, corticocollicular, geniculocollicular, and collicular efferents. The efferent cochlear bundle projects from the superior olive to the cochlea (Box 17.1).

Clinical Examination

Some information about hearing may be obtained simply by observation and gauging the patient's ability to understand soft and loud tones and low and high pitches; note signs of deafness, such as a tendency to turn the head when listening, lipreading, or speaking with a loud voice. Any history of hearing difficulty, such as trouble using the telephone or hearing conversation in noisy environments, or complaints from family members, should prompt a careful evaluation. Before testing hearing, otoscopic examination should be done to ensure the tympanic membrane is intact and to exclude the presence of wax, pus, blood, foreign bodies, and exudate. The mastoid region should be examined for swelling and tenderness.

Conductive hearing loss (CHL) is that due to impaired conduction of sound to the cochlea and may be due to occlusion of the external auditory canal, middle ear disease (e.g., otitis), or abnormality of the ossicular chain (e.g., otosclerosis). Sensorineural hearing loss (SNHL) is that due to disease of the cochlea (e.g., Ménière's disease) or eighth CN (e.g., acoustic neuroma). As a generality, CHL affects low frequencies and SNHL affects high frequencies. Ménière's disease is a notable exception, causing predominantly low-frequency hearing loss, at least early in the course. Central hearing loss is that due to disease of the central pathways. Central hearing loss is very rare because of the bilaterality and redundancy of the auditory system; unilateral lesions of the central auditory pathways typically do not cause any deficit detectable by routine clinical testing.

There are many ways to assess hearing at the bedside. All are crude compared to the information that can be obtained with a formal audiogram. The subject of audiography is complex. Box 17.2 summarizes some of the basic principles.

Bedside clinical testing of hearing may theoretically use any available instrument that is capable of making a sound. Because the ability to hear and understand speech is the most important functional aspect of audition, whispered voice is useful. Inability to whisper at exactly the same level for testing each ear, and inter- and intraindividual variation in the intensity and pitch of the voice, is a theoretical limitation, but clinically significant hearing loss is usually detectable with this simple technique. Whispered voice has been recommended as an excellent screening test. Inability to perceive a whispered voice has a likelihood ratio (LR) of 6.1 (95% CI, 4.5 to 8.4) for clinically significant hearing loss; normal perception has an LR of 0.03 (95% CI, 0 to 0.24).

Despite its disability for the patient, high-frequency SNHL of the type associated with presbycusis and acoustic trauma is not generally of neurologic significance; the use of high-pitched sounds, such as a ticking watch, seldom provides useful information for neurologic examination purposes. In certain types of deafness, loss of speech discrimination is of clinical significance, even though pure tone and even speech thresholds are normal. Few conditions of neurologic importance cause bilaterally symmetric hearing loss, and an examination designed to detect auditory asymmetry usually suffices. Other useful sounds for bedside testing include finger rub—the noise made by rubbing the thumb and index finger together beside the external auditory meatus—and pure tones created by a tuning fork.

Detailed testing of hearing is done monaurally, ideally while occluding the opposite ear, by pressing the tragus over the canal. For screening purposes in low-yield situations, occlusion of the opposite ear is sometimes omitted, and occasionally, finger rub is done binaurally. In each instance, the patient is asked to compare the sound intensity between the two ears.

BOX 17.2

Audiometry

Detailed assessment of hearing is done with audiometry, which is usually performed as a battery of tests. The range of human hearing is 20 to 20,000 Hz (about 11 octaves). Speech usually falls in the 300- to 3,000-Hz range. There are many different audiologic techniques; those used most commonly for neurologic purposes are pure tone and speech audiometry. An audiogram is a plot of the threshold of audition for short pure tones as a function of frequency on a logarithmic decibel scale. Air conduction (AC), assessed with earphones, tests the entire auditory pathway. Bone conduction (BC) sends a signal directly to the cochlea, bypassing the outer and middle ear structures. The pure tone audiogram displays the severity of any hearing loss in relation to established reference values, and the pattern may suggest the etiology. As with tuning fork testing, a decrease in AC with normal BC, an air-bone gap, indicates conductive hearing loss, and a decrease in both AC and BC indicates sensory or neural loss. The pure tone audiogram is usually normal with lesions involving the central auditory pathways.

Speech audiometry uses spoken words and sentences instead of pure tones. The speech reception threshold is considered the intensity level at which the patient can correctly understand 50% of the material presented. Speech discrimination, or intelligibility, is the proportion of the material the patient can understand when presented at a level that should be easily heard. The loss of discrimination is proportional to the severity of the hearing loss in patients with cochlear lesions. Poor speech discrimination, out of proportion to pure tone hearing loss, is characteristic of a retrocochlear lesion, such as a cerebellopontine angle tumor. In cranial nerve (CN) VIII lesions, discrimination may even paradoxically decline as intensity is raised.

A tympanogram measures the impedance of the tympanic membrane. An abnormal tympanogram is seen in such conditions as otitis media, tympanic membrane perforation, ossicular dislocation, otosclerosis, cerumen impaction, and eustachian tube dysfunction.

The stapedius reflex, or acoustic reflex, measures the change in compliance in response to loud sounds to assess the function of the stapedial muscle. The reflex arc is via CN VIII, brainstem interneurons, and CN VII. In the absence of severe hearing loss, an abnormal stapedius reflex may suggest a lesion of CN VII or VIII or the brainstem.

The AEP, also known as the auditory evoked response, or brainstem auditory evoked potential/response (BAEP/BAER), is a minuscule potential produced by auditory stimuli and recorded using electroencephalogram (EEG) electrodes. The potential is discernible from the much more prominent background EEG activity because it is time locked to the auditory stimuli. This temporal relationship is only apparent after averaging a large number of responses. The background EEG activity is random and not time locked to the stimuli. It tends to cancel itself out if enough auditory stimuli are given, and the signal (the BAER) gradually emerges from the noise (the background EEG activity). The waves that occur in the first 10 ms after an auditory stimulus are short-latency far-field potentials because of electrical activity at various points along the auditory pathway. These are reproducible and reliable wave forms. BAERs are used primarily for evaluating suspected CN VIII and brainstem lesions. There are five to seven waves in the AEP; the correlation of the waveforms with specific anatomic structures is based primarily on animal studies and remains somewhat uncertain. Wave I is the auditory nerve action potential. Wave II is thought to reflect activity in the cochlear nuclei, although it may be generated by the intracranial segment of the auditory nerve. Wave III is thought to come from the superior olive, and waves IV and V are from the inferior colliculus. The origin of waves VI and VII is unclear, but wave VI may come from the medial geniculate body and wave VII from the auditory radiations.

The relationship of the BAER waveforms to the anatomic pathways allows for lesion localization predicated on changes in interpeak latencies and differences in latencies between the two ears. A delay between waves I and III suggests a lesion between the eighth nerve near the cochlea and the lower pons; an interpeak latency delay between waves III and V suggests a lesion between the lower pons and midbrain. The primary clinical applications of BAERs have been in the evaluation of patients with cerebellopontine angle tumors and demyelinating disease and in coma and brain death. It is also of considerable value in newborn and infant hearing assessment.

The examiner may also compare the distance from each ear at which a sound of the same intensity can be heard. An occasionally useful method is to place the earpieces of a stethoscope into the patient's ears. Then, whisper into, scratch softly on, or hold a tuning fork to the chest piece, and ask the patient to compare the sounds heard. One side of the tubing can be occluded to direct the sound into one ear. Ross' method is to stand at a fixed distance (e.g., 6 ft) at a right angle from the patient, have the patient occlude the far ear, and whisper; repeat for the other ear, and compare the auditory acuity on the two sides.

When using whispered voice, certain tones are heard better and at a greater distance than others. Sibilants, and the short vowels such as a, e, and i, are heard at a greater distance than broad consonants such as l, m, n, and r, and such vowels as o and u. "Seventy-six" and "sixty-seven" can be heard at a greater distance than "ninety-nine" and "fifty-three." One key to the effective use of whisper is unpredictability of the stimulus, for example, the numbers "1, 2, 3" in one ear and "7, 8, 9" in the other. Monosyllables are preferable to common stock questions such as "How are you?" in which hearing a small part may enable the patient to "hear" the rest in context. Alternating words and numbers is a challenging test of hearing.

Tuning forks—typically 128, 256, or 512 Hz—are sometimes used to give more specific information and to assess air conduction (AC) and bone conduction (BC). When testing AC, the tuning fork should be kept in gentle motion to avoid null points. The patient may be asked to compare the loudness of the vibrating fork in the two ears, or the examiner may compare the distance on each side at which the fork begins or ceases to be heard. The gradual dampening of the oscillations makes precision difficult. The examiner with good hearing may compare the patient's AC and BC with his own (Schwabach test). In evaluating BC, be certain the patient hears rather than feels the tuning fork. How useful tuning fork tests are for general screening has been questioned. But the primary usefulness of both the Weber and Rinne tests (see below) is not as a screening tool but to make an initial differentiation between SNHL and CHL in a patient complaining of unilateral symptoms of hearing loss or tinnitus.

The Rinne test compares the patient's AC and BC; it can be done in at least two ways. An activated fork may be placed first on the mastoid process and then immediately beside the ear (or vice versa), and the patient is asked which is louder; it should always be louder by the ear. The more time-consuming, traditional method is to place the tuning fork on the mastoid and when no longer heard there move it beside the ear, where it should still be audible. The fork should be heard twice as long by AC as by BC. The Rinne test is normal or positive when AC is better than BC either by subjective assessment of loudness or by the length of time the tuning fork is heard in the two locations. In CHL, BC is better than AC, and the Rinne test is said to be negative. Sound is not conducted normally through the canal or from the tympanic membrane through the ossicular chain to the cochlea, but the sensorineural mechanisms are intact; AC is impaired but BC is preserved. In CHL, BC may even be exaggerated beyond the normal because the middle ear cavity becomes a resonating chamber. In sensorineural deafness, both AC and BC are impaired while retaining their normal relationship of AC better than BC; the Rinne test is positive or normal. With severe sensorineural deafness, BC may be lost whereas slight AC is preserved. Because of inconsistent use of the terms positive and negative, it is preferable to state that AC is better than BC or that the Rinne test is normal.

In the Weber test, a vibrating tuning fork is placed in the midline on the vertex of the skull. It may be placed anywhere in the midline, over the nasal bridge, the forehead, or the maxilla but works best over the vertex. Normally, the sound is heard equally in both ears or seems to resonate somewhere in the center of the head; it is "not lateralized." In CHL, the sound is heard better ("lateralized") to the involved side. A simple way to remember this phenomenon is for the examiner to place a tuning fork over his own vertex and then induce conductive loss by inserting a finger in one ear; the sound will be louder on the side of the occluded canal. In sensorineural deafness, the sound is heard best in the normal ear.

In summary, with unilateral CHL, AC is less than BC (the Rinne test is negative), and the Weber lateralizes to the involved side. In unilateral SNHL, AC is greater than BC (Rinne test positive or normal), and the Weber lateralizes to the normal side (Table 17.1).

Auditory reflex responses are occasionally useful in evaluating hearing in children, patients with altered mental status, and in patients with psychogenic hearing loss or malingering. The auditory-palpebral reflex is a blink or reflex eye closure in response to a loud, sudden noise. The cochleopupillary reflex is pupillary dilatation, or

TABLE 17.1 Rinne and Weber Tests

Normally, the auditory acuity is equal in both ears, air conduction is greater than bone conduction (Rinne test normal or positive) bilaterally, and the Weber test is nonlateralizing (midline). The table depicts the pattern on the involved side with *unilateral* conductive or sensorineural hearing loss.

	Auditory Acuity	Rinne Test	Weber Test
Conductive hearing loss	Decreased	BC > AC (Rinne negative or abnormal)	Lateralizes to the abnormal side
Sensorineural hearing loss	Decreased	AC > BC (Rinne positive or normal)	Lateralizes to the normal side

contraction followed by dilatation, in response to a loud noise. The auditory-oculogyric reflex is eye deviation toward a sound. The general acoustic muscle reflex is a general jerking of the body in response to a loud, sudden noise.

The laboratory evaluation of hearing is done primarily by electronic audiometry and auditory evoked potentials. These are discussed in Box 17.2.

Disorders of Function

Dysfunction of the cochlear nerve and its connections usually causes either diminution or loss of hearing (hypacusis or anacusis), with or without tinnitus. Hyperacusis occurs most often with paralysis of the stapedius muscle in disorders affecting CN VII, but it may occur as an epileptic aura, in migraine (sonophobia or phonophobia), and in certain psychiatric conditions and drug-related disorders. Dysacusis is impairment of hearing that is not primarily a loss of auditory acuity; rather, it is related to dysfunction of the cochlea or central auditory pathways. Diplacusis is a condition in which there is a difference in the pitch or intensity of the same sound as heard in the two ears or when a single sound is heard as having two components; it is usually due to disease of the cochlea. Paracusis is perversion or distortion of hearing. Paracusis of Willis (paracusis Willisii) is an interesting phenomenon in which the ability to hear improves in the presence of loud noises. Thomas Willis described a patient who heard better when a drum was beating loudly nearby. It is a feature of otosclerosis. Disturbances of hearing because of central nervous system (CNS) lesions are rare.

CHL is due to interference with the transmission of sound to the cochlea. SNHL is due to disease of the cochlea or its central connections. In essence, CHL is due to disease external to the oval window, and SNHL is due to disease central to the oval window. With CHL, there is primarily loss of AC; BC is preserved or even exaggerated (Table 17.1). The Weber is referred to the involved side. Low tones are lost, as are some of the broad or flat consonants and vowels such as m, n, l, r, o, and u. Impairment of speech discrimination parallels the loss for pure tones. There is no recruitment, and tone decay is normal. Patients with CHL tend to hear speech better in a noisy background than in a quiet setting. Mixed hearing loss, with elements of both CHL and SNHL, is not uncommon. Some causes of hearing loss are listed in Table 17.2.

With unilateral SNHL, AC and BC are both diminished, but AC remains better than BC (Table 17.1) and the Weber lateralizes to the normal ear. The hearing loss is worse for higher frequencies (Figure 17.9), and there is greater difficulty with sibilants, sharp consonants, and short vowels (e.g., in the words sister, fish, twenty, water, and date). A clearly enunciated whisper is sometimes more easily understood than a loud, indistinct shout.

TABLE 17.2 Causes of Hearing Loss

- Conductive hearing loss
  - External auditory canal obstruction (e.g., cerumen, foreign bodies, water, blood)
  - Perforation of the tympanic membrane
  - Disease of the middle ear
  - Disease of the nasopharynx with obstruction of the eustachian tube
- Sensorineural hearing loss
  - Disease of the cochlea
    - Acoustic trauma
    - Ménière's disease
    - Infections
    - Congenital conditions (e.g., congenital rubella)
    - Presbycusis
  - Disease of the cochlear nerve or nuclei
    - Tumors (e.g., acoustic neuroma)
    - Trauma (e.g., skull fracture)
    - Infection (meningitis, syphilis)
    - Toxins or drugs
    - Presbycusis
    - Nuclear lesions (e.g., vascular, inflammatory, or neoplastic)
- Lesions of the central auditory pathways

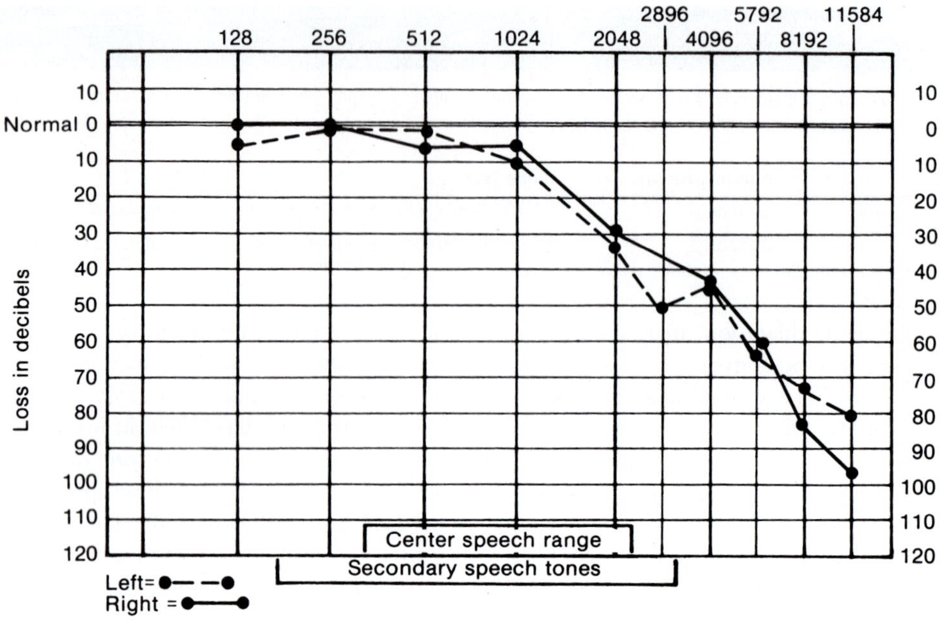

FIGURE 17.9 Audiogram of a patient with sensorineural deafness.

SNHL may be due to disease of the cochlea (end-organ deafness), such as in Ménière's disease, or to disease of CN VIII or more central structures (retrocochlear), as in acoustic neuroma. Typical of cochlear disease is loss of acuity for pure tones with a parallel impairment of speech discrimination, recruitment, and tone decay. Recruitment is an abnormal loudness of sounds because of cochlear dysfunction, which can cause a paradoxical increase in the perception of louder sounds, sometimes accompanied by sound distortion. Recruitment occurs when there is a reduction in the number of hair cells, which causes a loss of the ability to process fine gradations in sound intensity. A small increase in intensity causes an abnormally large recruitment of nerve fibers responding, and the sound is perceived as abnormally loud. Tone decay measures auditory adaption by assessing the ability to maintain the perception of a pure tone continuously. Tone decay does not occur with cochlear lesions. Retrocochlear lesions tend to cause a loss of speech discrimination out of proportion to the loss for pure tones, no recruitment, and abnormal auditory adaptation by tone decay. There is a debate about the existence of a syndrome of purely cochlear Ménière's disease.

SNHL may be bilateral and slowly progressive, as with presbycusis or exposure to ototoxic drugs, for example, aminoglycoside antibiotics or loop diuretics. Gabapentin may cause reversible hearing loss in patients with renal insufficiency. SNHL may be unilateral and progressive, as in Ménière's disease or acoustic neuroma. It may be unilateral and relatively sudden, over hours to days, in vascular disease (e.g., internal auditory artery [IAA] occlusion), viral infection, or autoimmune hearing loss. The syndrome of sudden, unilateral SNHL is due to dysfunction involving the cochlea or CN VIII with variable, often poor, recovery. The pathogenesis is unknown; autoimmunity, viral infection, and vascular disease are suspected etiologies. The IAA may arise from the anterior inferior cerebellar artery (AICA) or directly from the basilar. Isolated IAA ischemia causes hearing loss often associated with vestibular dysfunction. Ischemia in the AICA distribution produces other CNS manifestations (see Chapter 21).

The cochlear and vestibular nerves run together in a common sheath from the brainstem to their respective end organs, and disorders of the eighth nerve between the cochlea and brainstem may cause hearing loss. Some disease processes affect both divisions peripherally (e.g., labyrinthitis) or centrally (e.g., brainstem neoplasm). In its course across the CPA, the most important disorder to affect both divisions is a neoplasm. Acoustic neuroma (acoustic neurinoma, acoustic schwannoma) is most common, but neurofibroma, meningioma, facial nerve schwannoma, cholesteatoma, epidermoid cyst, and other tumors may arise here as well. Acoustic neuromas usually present with insidious, progressive hearing loss; rarely, sudden deafness may occur, sometimes as the presenting manifestation, presumably because of intratumoral hemorrhage or IAA ischemia. Vague disequilibrium and imbalance are more common symptoms than true vertigo. Subsequent manifestations depend on the direction of tumor extension. With anterior extension, CNs V and VI are involved. With inferior extension, CNs IX, X, and XI are involved. CN VII is commonly affected in either case, causing all the signs of a far proximal lesion (see Chapter 16). With medial extension, there is mass effect on the brainstem and cerebellum, often leading to ipsilateral ataxia and evidence of increased intracranial pressure. Other conditions of CN VIII that may cause hearing loss include toxins; superficial siderosis; postinflammatory scarring, as from meningitis; and hereditary conditions. Other conditions that may cause both hearing loss and vertigo include Ménière's disease, labyrinthitis, viral infection (especially herpes), trauma, meningitis, vascular occlusion (internal auditory or anterior inferior cerebellar), Susac's syndrome, Cogan's syndrome, Fabry's disease, perilymphatic fistula, toxins, and drugs.

Lesions of the central auditory pathways (brainstem and central connections) rarely cause clinical loss of hearing, although detailed audiometric testing and BAERs may show abnormalities. However, midbrain lesions or tumors of the posterior third ventricle—or the aqueduct region with compression of either the medial geniculate bodies or the inferior colliculi—may cause bilateral hearing deficits, presumably because the auditory pathways run close together in this region. Impairment of sound localization contralateral to a temporal lobe lesion has been described. Wernicke's aphasia is characterized by the inability to interpret or comprehend spoken words despite normal hearing; it may occur with dominant temporal lobe lesions. Pure word deafness follows bilateral damage to the posterior-superior temporal lobes bilaterally, causing an inability to comprehend speech with intact hearing and reading. Other cortical syndromes involving hearing include auditory agnosia, amusia, and disturbances in the temporal analysis of sounds.

Pseudohypacusis refers to hearing loss in the absence of any organic disease or hearing loss that is exaggerated. It is more common for real hearing loss to be exaggerated in severity than for it to be feigned with entirely normal hearing. The mainstay of diagnosis is inconsistency in the performance on hearing tests and the absence of verifiable abnormalities on objective tests. A diagnosis of pseudohypacusis is easier to establish in children because they are less able to reproduce factitious abnormalities on repeated testing.

Nonorganic hearing loss may be partial or total and unilateral or bilateral. It is often bilateral and total, and the patient makes no attempt to hear what is said or to read the speaker's lips. In most instances, it is a transient symptom related to acute emotional stress. Psychogenic hearing loss may be associated with other nonorganic symptoms, such as mutism and blindness. When there are also nonorganic motor and sensory disturbances, the hearing loss is usually incomplete and on the same side. In malingering, the deafness is usually unilateral and occurs after trauma in the face of potential secondary gain. Organic posttraumatic hearing loss is typically associated with impairment of vestibular function. Normal labyrinthine responses suggest the claimed hearing loss is either simulated or exaggerated. Inconsistent responses on bedside hearing tests suggest nonorganicity. Discrepancies and inconsistencies on repeated audiometric examinations are typical. The BAER is normal.

Patients simulating bilateral deafness do not behave as a deaf person does. Deaf individuals usually raise their voices during conversation and keep their eyes fixed on the speaker's face and lips, watching for any gesture that may help understanding. A deaf man eager to hear will automatically turn his best ear toward the speaker. Experienced lip readers have difficulty with sound-alike words; the dissembler may do better than expected because the words are actually heard. Many tests have been devised for detection of nonorganic deafness. The diagnosis is best made audiometrically.

Tinnitus

Tinnitus is spontaneous noise in the ears originating inside the head. There are many types, and the causes are protean. In many cases, no precise etiology can be established. The most common identifiable cause is noise exposure, either acute or chronic. Objective tinnitus refers to noise audible to both the patient and the examiner, as occurs in carotid stenosis. Most tinnitus is subjective tinnitus. It may vary in pitch and intensity and may be continuous or intermittent. It may be described in many ways, such as ringing, buzzing, blowing, whistling, swishing, or roaring. Tinnitus is commonly associated with deafness. It is common in presbycusis and in other types of SNHL and is a fairly constant feature of otosclerosis. It is caused by the abnormal excitation of the auditory apparatus or its afferent pathways, but the exact mechanism is often unclear. Most cases are due to disease of the cochlea or eighth nerve; some are due to CNS disease. Tinnitus is often more noticeable at night when environmental noises are diminished, and it may interfere with sleep. To the patient, tinnitus may be more distressing than the accompanying deafness, and it may cause depression in elderly individuals.

Pulsatile tinnitus is synchronous with the pulse; it is in reality a bruit. Causes include carotid stenosis; arteriovenous malformations, particularly of the dura; glomus tumors; venous hums; and hypertension. Pulsatile tinnitus is fairly common in pseudotumor cerebri, and it occurs occasionally in increased intracranial pressure of other origins. The perilymphatic duct connects the perilymph-filled spaces of the cochlea and an extension of the subarachnoid space in the region of the jugular foramen. Through this channel, pulsations in the subarachnoid space are transmitted to the cochlea. Vascular tinnitus may occasionally be affected by carotid artery compression. Rhythmic tinnitus not synchronous with the pulse may occur with palatal myoclonus (palatal microtremor). Gaze-evoked tinnitus is tinnitus associated with eye movements; it may be due to abnormal communications between the cochlear and vestibular nuclei.

Other causes of tinnitus include cerumen impaction, medications (particularly ototoxic drugs), Ménière's disease, acoustic neuroma, acute or chronic acoustic trauma, Paget's disease, anemia, labyrinthitis, and Arnold-Chiari malformation. Muscle spasm, contraction of the tensor tympani, nasopharyngeal sounds, and temporomandibular joint clicking may also simulate tinnitus. Tinnitus may be psychogenic. Bizarre types of tinnitus may occur with pontine and cerebral lesions. Auditory hallucinations may occur in lesions of the temporal lobe; these are frequently epileptic auras. More bizarre hallucinations occur in psychotic and drug-induced states. Tinnitus that is unilateral, pulsatile, fluctuating, or associated with vertigo is more likely to indicate a serious underlying condition.

The Vestibular Nerve

The vestibule of the labyrinth connects with five structures that are involved in vestibular function: the utricle, the saccule, and the three semicircular canals. Each of these components lies in the membranous labyrinth, is bathed in endolymph, and contains sensory neuroepithelium. The sensory epithelium consists of cells bearing microvilli, which are referred to as hair cells. The hair cells are the peripheral receptors of the vestibular apparatus. Each hair cell bears a single long kinocilium and an array of shorter stereocilia. The cilia are imbedded in the maculae of the utricle and saccule and in the cupulae of the semicircular canals. Movement of the macula or cupula bends the cilia. Endolymph flows throughout the membranous labyrinth. Changes in endolymph flow in response to external forces or head movement, as well as the effects of gravity and changes in head position, affect neural impulses arising from the areas of sensory epithelium. This is the substrate for vestibular function.

The hair cells function as transducers, converting mechanical deformation of their cilia into receptor potentials. Because of the location of the stereocilia and the kinocilium, each hair cell is structurally polarized. The orientation of each individual hair cell and the arrangement of its microvilli determine its functional response to mechanical stimuli. The cilia contain actin filaments. Bending of the cilia in a specific direction causes the cell to become either depolarized or hyperpolarized. Bending in the opposite direction causes the opposite response. Deformation causes ion fluxes in mechanically sensitive channels in the cilium. Calcium influx because of mechanical deformation depolarizes the cell and causes release of neurotransmitter. A few channels remain open even in the erect cilia, which produces a moderate level of tonic activity in the vestibular system. The receptors send signals by increasing or decreasing this tonic discharge.

The utricle and saccule constitute the otolith organ and are referred to as the static labyrinth. It is designed to detect gravitational effects and linear acceleration and to monitor head position. The utricle is an oblong sac that extends from the posterior-superior portion of the vestibular part of the membranous labyrinth (Figure 17.3). The saccule is a smaller expansion that lies near the opening of the scala vestibuli of the cochlea. The utriculosaccular duct connects the saccule to the utricle and endolymphatic duct, and the ductus reuniens connects it to the cochlea. The osseous ampulla of a semicircular canal is a bulbous expansion at the point where the canal joins the vestibule, and it is about twice the diameter of the rest of the canal (Figure 17.2). The semicircular ducts are membranous labyrinth tubules that follow the semicircular canals in the same way the cochlear duct follows the spirals of the cochlea. The ampullae of the ducts open off the utricle.

The utricle and saccule each contain a macule. Covering the maculae is a gelatinous layer, the otolithic or statoconial membrane. Embedded in the otolithic membrane are millions of crystals, the otoliths (statoliths, otoconia, or statoconia). The utricle and saccule respond to linear acceleration and to gravity because of the mass of the otoliths. They monitor the position of the head and movement of the head in relation to gravity. In the ampulla of each semicircular canal is a gelatinous structure called a cupula. The canals do not respond to gravity because there are no otoliths in the semicircular canals and because the cupula has the same specific gravity as the endolymph. Instead, movement of the head causes endolymph to flow, which displaces the cupula and stimulates or inhibits the hair cells.

The macula of the utricle lies horizontally in the floor of the utricle, parallel to the skull base. The macula of the saccule lies vertically in the wall of the saccule. Hair cells are oriented in every conceivable direction. Bending of the cilia either depolarizes or hyperpolarizes the cell, depending on the direction of movement. Because of the multidirectional orientation of the hair cells and the geometry of the maculae, head movement in any direction can be detected. Because of its orientation, the macula of the utricle responds maximally to head movement in the sagittal plane, whereas the macula of the saccule responds maximally to head movement in the coronal plane.

The semicircular canals are the kinetic or dynamic labyrinth and are designed to detect angular acceleration or rotation. The crista ampullaris, or ampullary crest, is a focal thickening in the membrane lining the ampullae of the semicircular canals. The cristae are covered with the sensory neuroepithelium of the canals. The tips of the cilia of the hair cells are imbedded in the cupula, which forms a dome-shaped cap over the cristae. When rotation of the head occurs, the endolymph lags behind, tilting the cupula and affecting the neural discharges in the hair cells of the cristae.

The semicircular canals are designed to detect rotation. Their orientation in three perpendicular planes and their oval structure guarantee that head movement in any direction will be detected. The three canals are the horizontal (lateral), vertical (anterior or superior), and posterior (inferior). The labyrinth is imbedded deep in the petrous ridge. In turn, the petrous ridge is set at an angle of about 45 degrees from the sagittal plane of the skull. The canals are named because of their anatomical relationships to the labyrinth and to each other, more so than their relationship to the skull. Different names for the same canal compound the difficulty. The following is a useful approximation for the orientation of the canals. The horizontal canal lies horizontally; the anterior and posterior canals stand vertically. The horizontal canal is convex laterally, and it is also called the lateral canal; it actually slants downward from anterior to posterior at an angle of about 30 degrees. The posterior canal arcs posteriorly parallel to the long axis of the petrous bone, toward the base of the petrous pyramid. The anterior canal lies perpendicular to the long axis of the petrous bone, anterior to the other canals, and toward the apex of the petrous bone. In addition, it extends above the other canals and is also known as the superior canal. If the head is placed forward 30 degrees, the lateral canals are horizontal and the vertical canals are vertical.

The canals are maximally stimulated by movement in the plane of their anatomical axis. The horizontal canal best detects rotational head movement in the side-to-side ("no-no") direction (with the chin tucked to bring the canal fully horizontal). The posterior canal best detects movement in the anteroposterior plane ("yes-yes"), and the anterior canal is oriented to detect lateral tilting movement. The canals on the two sides have been said to form functional pairs. The horizontal canals work together. The anterior canal of one side is approximately parallel to the posterior canal on the opposite side, forming a spatial pair. How closely these angles actually match has been questioned.

The hair cells of both the maculae and the cristae produce a tonic discharge in the vestibular nerve. The discharge rate increases and decreases in response to the bending of the hair cells. Endolymph flow toward the utricle is excitatory. Normally, the two labyrinths are in balance, with symmetric activity in the two vestibular nerves and reciprocal changes induced by head movement. When this balance is disturbed, the clinical signs and symptoms of vestibulopathy follow.

Afferent impulses from the hair cells travel centrally via the peripheral processes of bipolar neurons in the vestibular (Scarpa's) ganglion in the internal acoustic meatus. Central processes of the vestibular ganglion cells form the vestibular nerve. There are three peripheral divisions of the vestibular nerve, which arise from different portions of the labyrinth. These join to form the vestibular nerve proper (Figure 17.6). The vestibular component of CN VIII joins the cochlear component in a common sheath; the vestibular component is the larger of the two. The nerve passes through the IAC in company with the facial nerve and the nervus intermedius. It crosses the cerebellopontine angle and enters the brainstem between the inferior cerebellar peduncle and the olive. The cochlear nerve is slightly lateral and caudal to the vestibular component. Within the IAC, CN VIII is lateral and inferior to CN VII. At the pontomedullary junction, CN VIII is slightly lateral and posterior to CN VII.

Entering vestibular fibers pass between the inferior cerebellar peduncle and the spinal tract of CN V. They divide into ascending and descending branches that end primarily in the four vestibular nuclei: lateral, medial, superior, and inferior (Figure 17.10). The vestibular nuclei lie in the rostral medulla and caudal pons. Some fibers form the vestibulocerebellar tract and pass directly to the cerebellum, without synapsing in the vestibular nuclei, in the juxtarestiform body. The medial (Schwalbe's) vestibular nucleus is the largest subdivision of the vestibular nuclear complex, extending from the medulla into the pons. It lies in the floor of the fourth ventricle, beneath the striae medullares. The inferior (descending, spinal, Roller) nucleus lies lateral to the medial, between the medial nucleus and inferior cerebellar peduncle, and descends further inferiorly to reach lower medullary levels. The lateral (Deiters') and superior (Bechterew's) subnuclei are smaller than the medial and inferior. The lateral nucleus is lateral to the rostral end of the medial nucleus. The superior nucleus extends higher into the pons than other subdivisions, forming a cap on the nuclear complex. Vestibular afferents to the superior and medial subnuclei arise predominantly from the semicircular canals and less

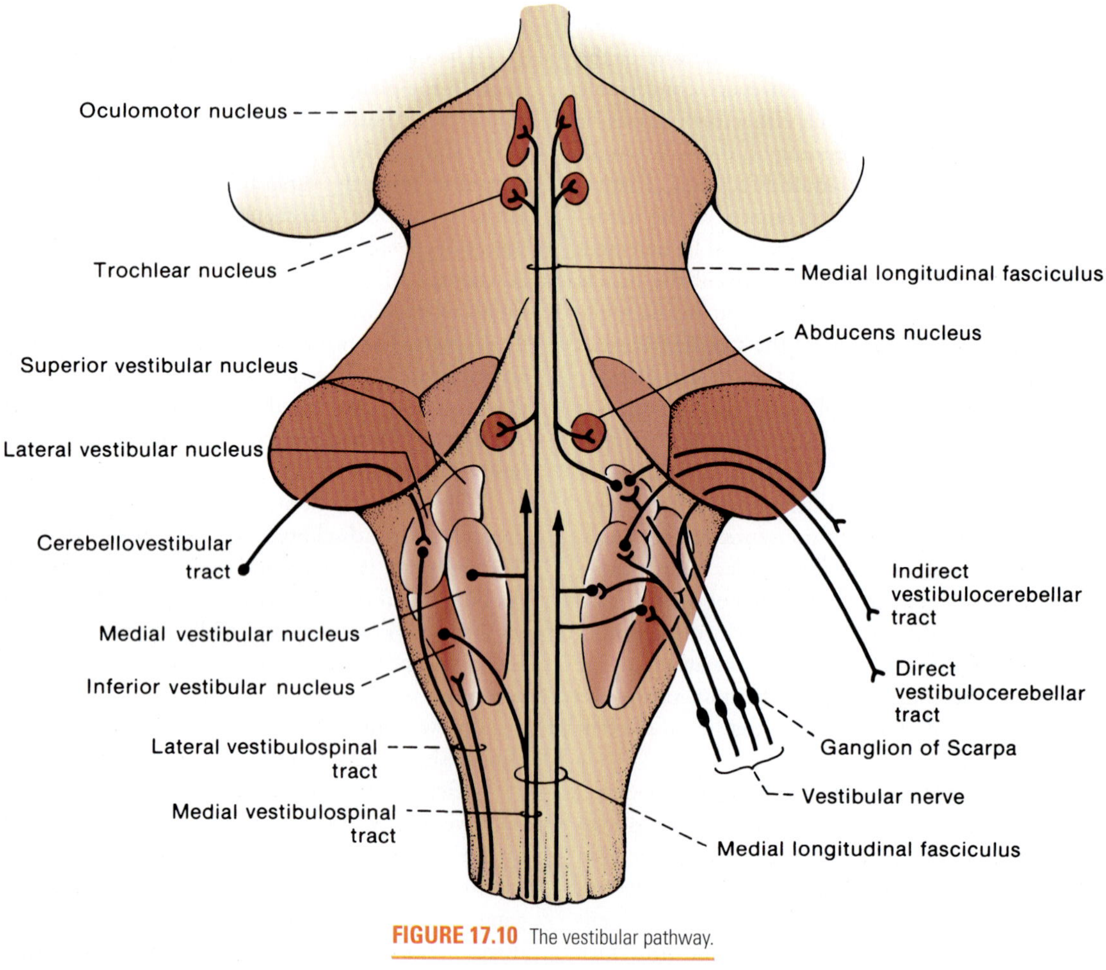

FIGURE 17.10 The vestibular pathway.

so from the otolith organs. Afferents to the lateral and inferior subnuclei arise predominantly from the otolith organs and less so from the semicircular canals. The vestibular nuclei also receive afferent cerebellovestibular fibers through the juxtarestiform body (part of the inferior cerebellar peduncle), primarily from the flocculonodular lobe, as well as afferents from the spinal cord and reticular formation.

The vestibular nuclei make connections with four primary areas: cerebellum, spinal cord, oculomotor system, and cortex. The juxtarestiform body is a collection of fibers medial to the inferior cerebellar peduncle (restiform body). Vestibulocerebellar fibers run through the juxtarestiform body and form part of the mossy fiber input to the cerebellum. The direct (primary) vestibulocerebellar tract bypasses the vestibular nuclei; its fibers terminate primarily in the ipsilateral nodulus, uvula, and fastigial nucleus. The indirect (secondary) vestibulocerebellar fibers arise from the superior, medial, and inferior nuclei and terminate primarily in the flocculus bilaterally and in the same areas that receive the direct vestibulocerebellar input. The vestibular nuclei also receive fibers from the cerebellum. The fastigial nucleus of the cerebellum connects with the vestibular nuclei by the uncinate fasciculus (hook bundle of Russell), which is the major outflow of the fastigial nucleus. The uncinate fasciculus forms a distinctive arc over the superior cerebellar peduncle and then descends in the juxtarestiform body to enter the vestibular nuclei. Multiple areas of the cortex receive vestibular input, and there is probably no primary vestibular cortex.

All four vestibular subnuclei may send fibers into the medial longitudinal fasciculus (MLF), but the vast majority of the ascending fibers arise from the superior and medial nuclei. This pathway, through connections with the nuclei of CNs III, IV, and VI, and the nuclei of CN XI and upper cervical nerves, is important in regulating movements of the eyes, head, and neck in response to stimulation of the semicircular canals. Fibers from the superior and medial nuclei form the indirect vestibulocerebellar pathway, and the medial nucleus receives cerebellar input through cerebellovestibular fibers.

Fibers from the lateral and inferior vestibular nuclei go down the ipsilateral spinal cord as the lateral vestibulospinal tract, which is important in the regulation of muscle tone and posture by increasing extensor muscle tone, particularly of the trunk. Impulses from the medial vestibular nuclei descend to the cervical and upper thoracic spinal cord through the crossed medial vestibulospinal tract. The inferior nucleus sends bilateral projections into the descending MLF and also provides vestibular input to the cerebellum. The vestibular nuclei also have connections with the reticular formation and through this with the dorsal efferent nucleus of the vagus and with the spinal cord. They also send efferent fibers back to the vestibular ganglion. Ascending vestibular connections extend rostrally to the ventrolateral and ventral posterior thalamic nuclei and from the thalamus to the somatosensory cortex to provide conscious perception of head position and movement. There are also projections to the posterior portion of the superior temporal gyrus that are important in vestibulo-ocular function.

Vestibular Physiology

The utricle and saccule respond to linear acceleration, whereas the semicircular canals respond to angular acceleration. These responses are mediated by hair cells and transmitted to the vestibular ganglion and subsequently to the vestibular nuclei. Under normal circumstances, the neural activity in the labyrinths is equal on both sides. It is convenient to visualize the action of each vestibular system as "pushing" toward the opposite side. When the two labyrinths push equally, the system is in balance and function is normal. When one labyrinth is underactive, the opposite labyrinth pushes the eyes, extremities, and body toward the side of underactivity. The clinical manifestations of vestibular dysfunction include vertigo, oscillopsia, nausea, vomiting, nystagmus, past pointing, and lateropulsion.

Nystagmus results from a corrective saccade initiated by the frontal eye fields in response to the deviation of gaze toward the side of the less active labyrinth. The fast component of the nystagmus is therefore in the opposite direction from the hypoactive labyrinth. Without visual information to correct for errors (i.e., with eyes closed), patients with an acutely hypoactive labyrinth will have deviation of their extremities toward the underactive side on finger-to-nose testing. When attempting to walk with eyes closed, they will drift toward the side of the hypoactive labyrinth. On the Unterberger-Fukuda stepping test, they will turn toward the hypoactive side.

When both labyrinths are diseased or malfunctioning, as might occur, for example, with ototoxic drug effects, there is no vestibular imbalance and hence no nystagmus, vertigo, past pointing, and the

TABLE 17.3 Some Causes of "Dizziness"

Symptom Description	Characteristics	Possible Etiologies
Vertigo (spinning, whirling, tilting, falling)	Illusion of motion of self or environment	Dysfunction of the vestibular system, peripheral or central
Disequilibrium (poor balance but not "dizzy")	Impaired balance, unsteady gait	Bilateral vestibular dysfunction; deafferentation (peripheral neuropathy, posterior column disease); brainstem lesion; cerebellar lesion; extrapyramidal disorder; drug effects
Presyncope (light-headed, drunk, woozy, faint)	Light-headedness; often with systemic symptoms (e.g., diaphoresis, nausea, graying of vision) inciting event	Global cerebral hypoperfusion (numerous causes)
Multiple sensory deficits	Elderly patient, vague complaints, difficulty walking	Multiple concurrent problems
Ill defined	Histrionic but vague description and nonspecific complaints	Psychogenic

like. Patients with bilateral labyrinthine disease may nonetheless have great difficulty with balance and equilibrium.

Clinical Examination

Dr. W. B. Matthews said, "There can be few physicians so dedicated...that they do not experience a slight decline in spirits when they learn that their patient's complaint is giddiness." The conditions that may present as dizziness range from trivial to life threatening and are often difficult to evaluate and manage. The nebulousness of the patient's description of dizziness often produces frustration on the part of the clinician, yet in few other conditions are the historical details so pivotal in correct diagnosis. Fortunately, the truly serious conditions that present as dizziness are rare.

Evaluation of the dizzy patient is a very common clinical exercise, and much has been written on the subject. A careful appraisal of the patient's symptoms is often helpful, but even the skilled clinician is sometimes unsure after hearing the patient's complaints. The first step in understanding the symptom is to have the patient describe what he means by "dizziness." Patients use the word dizzy to describe vertigo, as well as a number of other sensations, such as light-headedness or giddiness, sometimes referred to as pseudovertigo. Concomitant dysfunction in several systems may cause dizziness. Conflicting sensory information may certainly cause dizziness; the sensory mismatch from watching a motion picture with dramatic movement in the visual panorama while sitting in a stationary seat illustrates the effect. Simply looking down from a height can cause a sense of dizziness (the subject of the Alfred Hitchcock movie Vertigo). It is important to determine if there are concomitant auditory symptoms; their presence changes the differential diagnosis dramatically.

In a study of 100 dizzy patients in an ambulatory setting, the causes were as follows: vestibulopathy (54), psychiatric disorders (16), multifactorial (13), unknown (8), presyncope (6), disequilibrium (2), and hyperventilation (1). The most common treatable conditions were benign positional, or benign paroxysmal positional vertigo (BPPV), and psychiatric disorders. Other studies have shown a similar distribution. Some of the causes of dizziness are listed in Table 17.3. Table 17.4 lists causes of dizziness because of labyrinthine or vestibular pathway dysfunction. Before discussing vestibular disease, some discussion of nonspecific dizziness is warranted, because patients with such complaints make up a large proportion of the dizzy population.

Cerebral hypoperfusion produces a sensation of light-headedness, drunkenness, or impending syncope without spinning, whirling, or any illusion of environmental motion. Such hypoperfusion may occur under a variety of circumstances, all of which may lead the patient to seek medical

TABLE 17.4 Some Common Causes of Vertigo

- Otologic disorders
  - Benign paroxysmal positional vertigo
  - Ménière's disease
  - Vestibular neuronitis
- Neurologic disorders
  - Migraine-associated vertigo
  - Vertebrobasilar ischemia

attention because of "dizziness." In hyperventilation syndrome, hypocapnia-induced cerebral arterial constriction and the resultant hypoperfusion induce light-headedness along with other symptoms, such as chest pain; headache; numbness and tingling of the hands, feet, and circumoral region; and occasionally outright syncope. Frequently, patients are unaware of their overbreathing, but the high minute volume of respiration produces dryness of the mouth, which the patient may describe spontaneously or respond to on specific questioning. Induced hyperventilation may reproduce the symptom complex. Hyperventilation may also induce nystagmus in patients with acoustic neuroma. Orthostatic hypotension because of drugs, prolonged standing, dehydration, increased vagal tone, or dysautonomia likewise may present as light-headedness or faintness. Accompanying symptoms are few, and only a careful history eliciting the relationship of the dizziness to posture will make the diagnosis. Global cerebral hypoperfusion may also result from decreased cardiac output via any number of mechanisms; arrhythmia is the primary concern.

Elderly patients "deafferented" because of separate disease processes affecting different sensory systems may present with complaints of vague dizziness, unsteadiness, and difficulty with balance, particularly when turning (multiple sensory defect vertigo). Patients can apparently tolerate problems with any one afferent system, but when multiple systems are involved, imbalance and dizziness result. Thus, patients typically will suffer from various combinations of poor vision (e.g., cataracts, macular degeneration), poor hearing (presbycusis), mild peripheral neuropathy, and cervical spondylosis. The term presbylibrium has been applied to poor balance because of aging.

Numerous terms have been employed to describe the clinical phenomenology of vestibular disease; not all are helpful. Vertigo is the sensation of environmental motion (spinning, whirling, lateropulsion, tilt). The term "true vertigo" is sometimes used to describe this symptom. When true vertigo is present, the problem is usually an acute peripheral vestibular disturbance. Objective vertigo creates the sensation that the environment is spinning, whereas subjective vertigo creates the sensation that the patient is spinning. The absence of true vertigo does not exclude peripheral vestibular disease, especially if bilateral pathology exists, such as in ototoxicity because of drugs. Central vertigo is due to CNS disease; peripheral vertigo is due to disease of the peripheral vestibular apparatus or its connections. Patients with CNS lesions may not have true vertigo. Patients with true vertigo, especially when due to a peripheral lesion, often experience vegetative symptoms such as nausea and vomiting, because of projections to the medullary vomiting centers, pallor, and sweating. Acoustic neuroma causes a gradual unilateral loss of vestibular function and is more prone to cause imbalance than true vertigo. Some other serious conditions may present as dizziness without true vertigo, such as cardiac dysrhythmias and dysautonomic orthostasis. Physicians should not make too much of the presence or absence of true vertigo in judging how seriously to take a patient's complaint of dizziness.

Dizziness may be present constantly or intermittently. If intermittent, as in BPPV, one of the most common causes of dizziness, the episodes may occur so frequently that the initial description may lend the impression the symptoms are constant. If the episodes are intermittent, the duration of the attacks is important. Attack duration is one of the most important features in distinguishing between central and peripheral vertigo. In vertigo due to BPPV, the attacks last 10 to 30 seconds; in other peripheral vestibulopathies, such as Ménière's disease, the attacks last hours; and in vertebrobasilar insufficiency, the episodes last for minutes. Exploring the precipitating factors is very helpful. Dizziness may be provoked by head or body movement, standing, or lying down or occur spontaneously. The presence of associated symptoms, such as nausea, vomiting, staggering, deviation of the eyes, oscillopsia, disturbances of balance, prostration, tinnitus, hearing loss, autophony (perception of the reverberation of patient's own voice), or loss of consciousness, is important. Table 3.8 reviews some of the pertinent history to explore in a dizzy patient.

Useful bedside testing of vestibular function includes assessment of vestibulospinal reflexes (past pointing, Romberg, Unterberger-Fukuda stepping test), tests of vestibulo-ocular reflexes (VORs) (oculocephalic reflex, head thrust [head impulse] test, dynamic visual acuity, and caloric responses), and searching for nystagmus (spontaneous, positional, or after head shaking). For vestibular tests of ocular function, patients should wear their customary correction. In recalling the expected pattern of responses to some of these, remember that the vestibular system tends to push (eyes, limbs, and body) to the opposite side; when the system is in balance, the eyes are midline and the limbs and body can accurately find a target. When disease is present, the involved labyrinth is usually hypoactive and the uninvolved labyrinth pushes toward the abnormal side. This can be simulated in a normal volunteer with minicalorics, the instillation of 2 to 5 mL of ice water into one ear. Cold irrigation mimics an acute destructive lesion, and for a brief time thereafter, the subject will display the same clinical findings seen in a patient with an acute peripheral vestibulopathy (APV). The caloric demonstration is a useful teaching exercise for a group of trainees. It is also enlightening to do bilateral cold calorics to demonstrate that when both labyrinths are not functioning, normally the affected individual is still quite impaired, despite the lack of labyrinthine imbalance. The bedside tests of vestibular function are listed in Table 17.5.

A systematic examination of the dizzy patient is in use at Washington University that only requires 10 minutes in experienced hands. The components are (a) observation for spontaneous and gaze-evoked nystagmus and fixation suppression; (b) evaluation of extraocular movement; (c) vestibulo-ocular reflex testing; (d) Dix-Hallpike and static positioning (side-lying) tests; (e) limb coordination, primarily searching for past pointing and ataxia; and (f) gait and Romberg test.

TABLE 17.5 Useful Bedside Tests and Signs to Elicit in the Evaluation of Vestibular Function

Note: Fresnel (or high +) lenses and/or hyperventilation may bring out some of these signs
Observation for spontaneous nystagmus
Evaluation of eye movements
Head thrust test
Dynamic visual acuity
Subjective visual vertical
Vibration-induced nystagmus
Head-shaking nystagmus
Head-tapping test
Past pointing
Dix-Hallpike maneuver
Evaluation of gait, especially tandem
Romberg
Walking straight line, eyes closed
Star walking test
Unterberger-Fukuda stepping test
Calorics

Vestibulospinal Reflexes

Past pointing is a deviation of the extremities caused by either cerebellar or vestibular disease. These two types of past pointing have different patterns **(Video 43.2)**. Testing is usually done with the upper extremities. A quick and effective technique is simply to have the patient close his eyes while doing traditional cerebellar finger-to-nose testing. If past pointing is present, the limb will deviate to the side of the target because of the absence of visual correction. This method will usually bring out past pointing if it is present. The traditional method is to have the patient extend the arm and place his extended index finger on the examiner's index finger; then with eyes closed, raise the arm directly overhead; then bring it back down precisely onto the examiner's finger. With acute vestibular imbalance, the normal (more active) labyrinth will push the limb toward the abnormal (less active) side, and the patient will miss the target. The past pointing will always be to the same side of the target and will occur with either limb. With a cerebellar hemispheric lesion, the ipsilateral limbs have ataxia and incoordination; past pointing occurs only with the involved arm and may be to the side of the lesion or erratically to either side of the target. In vestibulopathy, after a period of compensation, the past pointing disappears and may even begin to occur in the opposite direction.

Romberg's test is described in more detail in Chapter 44. In brief, the Romberg compares balance as the patient stands with eyes open and eyes closed. The feet should be brought as close together as will allow the patient to maintain eyes open balance. A normal individual can stand feet together and eyes open without difficulty, but not all patients can. The critical observation is eyes open versus eyes closed. Inability to maintain balance with eyes open and feet together is not a positive Romberg. In unilateral vestibulopathy, if balance is lost with eyes closed, the patient will tend to fall toward the side of the lesion, as the normal vestibular system pushes him over. If the patient has spontaneous nystagmus because of a vestibular lesion, the fall will be in the direction of the slow phase. In peripheral vestibular disease, the direction of the fall can be affected by changing head position; the patient will fall toward the abnormal ear. With a right vestibulopathy and facing straight ahead, eye closure will cause the patient to fall to the right; looking over his right shoulder, he will fall backward; and looking over his left shoulder, he will fall forward.

The sharpened Romberg (tandem Romberg) test, which is done by having the patient stand tandem with eyes closed, may be useful in some circumstances.

The patient with an acute vestibulopathy may have difficulty with tandem gait with a tendency to fall to the side of the lesion, but normal straightaway walking may appear unimpaired because visual cues compensate for the vestibular abnormality. But straightaway walking with eyes closed may be informative. A normal individual can walk without visual clues well enough to point his index finger at the palm of the examiner's hand, close his eyes, walk along a path of 20 ft or so, and then touch the finger to the examiner's palm. The patient with acute vestibulopathy may drift toward the side of the lesion and end up well off the target, the gait equivalent of past pointing.

The Unterberger-Fukuda stepping test is analogous. The patient, eyes closed, marches in place for 1 minute **(Video 43.2)**. A normal individual will continue to face in the same direction, but a patient with acute vestibulopathy will slowly pivot toward the lesion. In the star walking test, the patient, eyes closed, takes several steps forward then several steps backward, over and over. A normal individual will begin and end oriented approximately along the same line. A patient with acute vestibulopathy will drift toward the involved side walking forward and continue to drift during the backward phase. The resulting path traces out a multipointed star pattern ("star walking"). As with past pointing, the direction of gait drift, pivoting on the stepping test, and similar findings do not reliably indicate the side of the lesion in patients with chronic vestibulopathy after compensation has occurred. These vestibulospinal tests may be abnormal when all other clinical tests of vestibular function are unrevealing.

Vestibulo-Ocular Reflexes

The VOR serves to move the eyes at an equal velocity but in the direction opposite a head movement; this keeps the eyes still in space and maintains visual fixation while the head is in motion (see also Chapter 14). There are several ways to examine the VOR, including the doll's eye test, head thrust test, dynamic visual acuity, and calorics.

Oculocephalic Reflex (Doll's Eye Test)

The oculocephalic response is primarily useful in the evaluation of comatose patients. Turning the head in one direction causes the eyes to turn in the opposite direction. This response indicates that the pathways connecting the vestibular nuclei in the medulla to the extraocular nuclei in the pons and midbrain are functioning and that the brainstem is intact. In an alert patient, visuomotor and ocular fixation mechanisms come into play, limiting the drawing of any conclusions about vestibular function.

Head Thrust Test

The doll's eye test utilizes slow side-to-side head movements in a comatose patient. The head thrust test is done in an awake patient. Abrupt, rapid movements are made in each direction while the patient attempts to maintain fixation straight ahead, as on the examiner's nose (Figure 17.11). The ocular smooth pursuit mechanism cannot compensate for head movements done at such high velocity, but normally, the VOR will maintain fixation and the eyes will hold on target. When the VOR is impaired, the compensatory eye movement velocity is less than the head movement velocity; the eyes lag behind the head movement and a corrective "catch-up" saccade must be made to resume fixation in the eccentric position. For a video of the head thrust test, see **Video Link 17.1**.

Dynamic Visual Acuity

The ability of the VOR to maintain ocular fixation means that a patient can read even while shaking the head to and fro. The dynamic visual acuity test is performed by obtaining a baseline acuity and then determining the acuity during rapid head shaking. Degradation by more than three lines on the Snellen chart suggests impaired vestibular function. One symptomatic corollary of impaired dynamic acuity is oscillopsia, a visual illusion of environmental motion causing jiggling while walking or in a car, and difficulty reading signs while in motion.

Caloric Tests

Robert Bárány was an otologist who pioneered the understanding of vestibular function and disease. He developed caloric testing for vestibular function in 1906; it is still in use over a century later. He did not in fact describe the maneuver to test for positional vertigo, although his name is linked to it.

Caloric responses are frequently used to check for brainstem integrity in comatose patients. Ice water

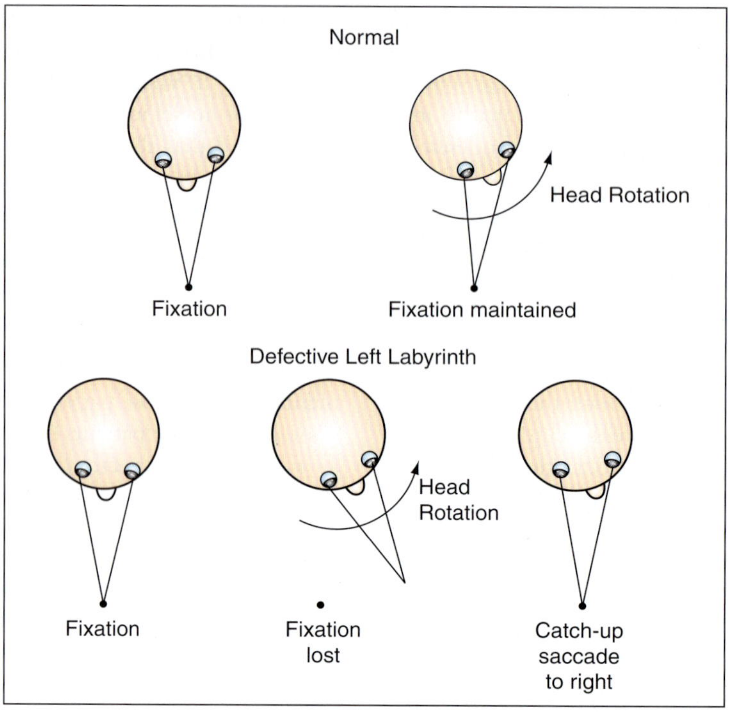

FIGURE 17.11 Head thrust test with a defective left labyrinth. The normal patient maintains fixation throughout. The patient with a defective left labyrinth loses fixation with the rapid head movement and must make a catch-up saccade to the right. (Modified from Barraclough K, Bronstein A. Diagnosis in general practice: vertigo. *BMJ* 2009;339:b3493.)

instilled into one ear canal will abruptly decrease the tonic activity from the labyrinth on the irrigated side. Cold calorics in a comatose patient with an intact brainstem cause tonic deviation of the eyes toward the side of irrigation as the normally active labyrinth pushes the eyes toward the hypoactive, irrigated labyrinth. In an awake patient, cold calorics cause nystagmus with the fast component away from the irrigated side because the cerebral cortex produces a compensatory saccade that jerks in the direction opposite the tonic deviation. The familiar mnemonic "COWS" (cold opposite, warm same) refers to the fast phase of the nystagmus, not to the tonic gaze deviation. Nystagmus is seen only when the cortex is functioning normally. Warm water irrigation has opposite effects. For a video of the normal caloric response, see **Video Link 17.2**. Bilateral simultaneous cold calorics induce tonic downgaze and warm calorics upgaze.

In comatose patients, large volumes of ice water, 30 to 50 mL, are commonly used because it is imperative to elicit the response if it is present. Calorics can also be done to assess vestibular function in dizzy patients, either using much smaller volumes, 2 to 10 mL of an ice and water slush (minicalorics), or larger volumes of water that is less cold. The latency to onset and the duration of the nystagmus elicited are compared on the two sides. A difference of more than 20% in nystagmus duration suggests a lesion on the side of the decreased response.

Whether in comatose or awake patients, the head is positioned so as to bring the horizontal canal into a position to elicit a maximal response. In comatose patients lying supine, this is done with the head flexed 30 degrees to bring the horizontal canal vertical. For awake patients, the same position may be used, or the head may be extended with the seated patient looking at the ceiling.

Nystagmus

Nystagmus is discussed in greater detail in Chapter 14. The characteristics of vestibular nystagmus will be briefly reviewed. Nystagmus because of vestibular disease may occur spontaneously or be produced by various maneuvers. Careful eye observation may reveal other relevant abnormalities, such as fixation instability, for example, because of macro square jerks, or skew deviation (see Chapter 14).

Spontaneous Nystagmus

The slow phase of spontaneous vestibular nystagmus is usually in the direction of the lesion, with the fast phase away, because an acute vestibular lesion typically causes hypoactivity of the labyrinth. The findings are similar to those produced by ice water irrigation of the ear and are due to the normal labyrinth pushing the eyes toward the diseased side with the cortex generating a corrective saccade away from the abnormal side. Because of the influence of the three different semicircular canals, vestibular nystagmus may beat in more than one direction, the summation of which creates an admixed rotatory component rarely seen with other conditions. When evaluating nystagmus, the presence of a torsional component suggests a peripheral origin. The amplitude increases with gaze in the direction of the fast phase.

When nystagmus is only present with gaze in the direction of the fast phase (Alexander's law, Chapter 14), it is termed first degree. Second-degree nystagmus is present in primary gaze. Vestibular nystagmus typically is fine, often present but easily overlooked in primary position. Third-degree nystagmus (fast component opposite to the direction of gaze) rarely occurs with any other nystagmus type. Vertigo, deafness, and tinnitus also help mark nystagmus as vestibular.

Peripheral vestibular nystagmus (i.e., because of disease of the labyrinth or eighth nerve) is markedly inhibited by visual fixation. Inhibiting fixation with Fresnel (Frenzel is a common misspelling) lenses (strongly convex spectacles that block visual fixation) will often make the nystagmus more obvious by both blocking fixation and magnifying the eyes. When Fresnel lenses are used, torsional nystagmus is often more prominent because vertical and horizontal nystagmus are more easily suppressed by visual fixation. Another technique is to have the patient close the eyelids gently and then partially lift one lid and look for abnormal movements of the scleral vessels. For a video of vestibular nystagmus demonstrating Alexander's law, third-degree nystagmus and fixation suppression, see **Video Link 17.3**. The fundoscopic examination may bring out subtle vestibular nystagmus. The dim lighting lessens visual fixation, and the disc is magnified. A rhythmic jerking of the disc to the patient's right indicates left beating nystagmus. Formal eye movement studies are done in darkness with recording of the eye movements by electrodes in order to remove the effects of visual fixation. Failure of visual fixation to suppress nystagmus suggests the nystagmus may be of central origin, usually a cerebellar or brainstem lesion. The spontaneous nystagmus because of a central lesion may be purely horizontal or purely vertical.

Nystagmus can sometimes be induced by having the patient rapidly turn the head back and forth with the eyes closed for about 30 seconds and then opening the eyes (head-shaking nystagmus). No nystagmus occurs in normal individuals, but patients with vestibular imbalance may have brief spontaneous nystagmus beating away from the abnormal side. Alternately, the patient may wear Fresnel lenses while shaking the head. For a video of head-shaking nystagmus, see *Head-Shaking Nystagmus* from Dr. Daniel R. Gold, Neuro-Ophthalmology Virtual Education Library [NOVEL], University of Utah, available at **Video Link 17.4**. Lee et al. recently described a disorder characterized by recurrent spontaneous vertigo and interictal head-shaking nystagmus. Spontaneous nystagmus can occasionally be produced by tapping on the head or by low-frequency vibration applied to the mastoid. Hyperventilation may also help bring out vestibular nystagmus.

Positional Nystagmus

When not present spontaneously, nystagmus can sometimes be elicited by placing the patient's head into a particular position. To perform the Dix-Hallpike (Hallpike or Nylen-Bárány) maneuver, the patient is moved from a seated position to a supine position with the head extended 45 degrees and turned 45 degrees to one side so that one ear is dependent. The patient is returned to sitting and then the maneuver repeated in the opposite direction. The patient should become symptomatic when the affected ear is dependent. For videos of the Dix-Hallpike test, see Barraclough and Bronstein and *Posterior canal BPPV with fixation and with fixation removed* from Dr. Daniel R. Gold, Neuro-Ophthalmology Virtual Education Library [NOVEL], University of Utah, available at **Video Link 17.5**.

If vertigo or nystagmus occurs, the patient is held in the provoking position until the symptoms subside, and then, the movement is repeated to assess its recurrence. The side-lying test may be used in patients unable to extend the neck or tolerate the supine position. The head is turned 45 degrees in one direction, then the patient lies down on the opposite shoulder. In BPPV, nystagmus begins after a latency of about 3 to 10 seconds, occasionally as long as 40 seconds; persists for 20 to 30 seconds, rarely as long as a minute; and then gradually abates (fatigues or habituates) after about 30 seconds, even though the head remains in the provoking position. The nystagmus is commonly torsional with the fast component toward the dependent ear (geotropic). For a video of torsional nystagmus in BPPV, see Barraclough and Bronstein. The response is usually much more dramatic in one particular head position. Typically, the patient will experience whirling, occasionally nausea, and rarely vomiting. With BPPV involving canals other than the posterior one, the Dix-Hallpike maneuver may be negative. The roll test, rolling the head of the supine patient to one side, may provoke a response with horizontal canal BPPV.

In canalithiasis, the response is transient, and repeating the maneuver several times consecutively provokes less of a response each time until eventually the nystagmus and vertigo are nil, adaptability. The term habituation is used to refer to either of these phenomena, which are themselves used inconsistently. After a period of 10 to 15 minutes, the response can be elicited again. In cupulolithiasis, latency and fatigability are absent because the adherent otoconia are in constant contact with the cupula.

Positional nystagmus is most often due to peripheral vestibular disease. Although rare, positional vertigo and nystagmus can occur with a central lesion, especially one near the fourth ventricle, but the characteristics of the nystagmus are different. With a central lesion, there may be no latency, and the nystagmus often begins as soon as the head is placed in the provoking position. Central positional nystagmus is typically vertical (either up- or downbeating), without the rotatory component seen with peripheral lesions. When torsional nystagmus is present, it may be ageotropic, beating away from the ground. In addition, the nystagmus and associated symptoms may persist for a prolonged period, longer than 30 to 40 seconds, sometimes continuing as long as the head position is maintained. With central lesions, there may be a mismatch in the severity of the nystagmus, vertigo, and nausea, in contrast to peripheral lesions where nystagmus, vertigo, and nausea are generally of comparable intensity.

Positional nystagmus can be divided into a paroxysmal type that is fleeting, fatigable, often difficult to reproduce, and associated with prominent vertigo and a static type that does not fatigue, persisting as long as the head is maintained in the provoking position, often with little associated vertigo. The static type can occur with either central or peripheral vestibular lesions, but a lack of visual suppression increases the likelihood of a central lesion. Other potentially useful tests in the dizzy patient include Valsalva maneuver (for perilymphatic fistula, see below), tragal compression, hyperventilation, and attempts to provoke Tullio's phenomenon (see below).

The characteristics of peripheral versus central positional nystagmus and related findings are summarized in Table 17.6.

TABLE 17.6 The Characteristics of Central versus Peripheral Positional Nystagmus on Dix-Hallpike Maneuver

Finding	Peripheral	Central
Latency	Yes, typically 3–10 s, rarely as long as 40 s	No
Fatigability* (habituation)	Yes, individual episode typically lasts 10–30 s, rarely as long as 1 min	No
Adaptability* (fatigability)	Yes, maneuver done several times consecutively provokes less of a response each time	No
Nystagmus direction	Direction fixed, typically mixed rotational upbeating with small horizontal component; quick phase of intorsion movement toward the dependent ear, upbeat toward forehead	Direction changing, variable, often purely vertical (either upbeating or downbeating) or purely horizontal
Suppression of nystagmus by visual fixation	Yes	No
Severity	Severe, marked vertigo, intense nystagmus, nausea	Mild vertigo, less obvious nystagmus, inconspicuous nausea
Consistency (reproducibility)	Less consistent	More consistent
Past pointing	In direction of nystagmus slow phase	May be in direction of fast phase

*Adaptability and fatigability are not used consistently in the literature.

Clinical Investigation

The commonly used quantitative tests for evaluation of vestibular function currently include electronystagmography, rotatory chair testing, and posturography. The tests are summarized in Box 17.3.

Disorders of Function

The primary manifestation of disorders of the vestibular nerve is vertigo and related symptoms such as imbalance. Vertigo will be used in this discussion as a surrogate for all similar symptoms. One of the primary concerns when dealing with a vertiginous patient is to separate central vertigo, because of CNS disease, from peripheral vertigo, because of peripheral vestibular disease. Disease of the peripheral vestibular apparatus or eighth CN produces peripheral vertigo. Disease of the central vestibular connections produces central vertigo. The vestibular nuclei lie within the CNS in the dorsolateral medulla; disease there may act like either peripheral or central forms. Central vertigo is less common than peripheral. Epidemiologic studies indicate that central causes are responsible for about 25% of the dizziness experienced in patients. Some central causes of dizziness include cerebrovascular disorders, migraine, multiple sclerosis (MS), brainstem lesions, global cerebral hypoperfusion, neurodegenerative disorders, and drug effects.

Certain features are helpful in making the distinction. Central vertigo is typically less severe, and other neurologic signs and symptoms are usually present. Peripheral vestibular disorders cause more nausea, vomiting, and autonomic symptoms than do central disorders. Imbalance tends to be more severe with central lesions, and the patients are often unable to stand or walk. Associated symptoms are helpful if present. Aural symptoms (hearing loss, tinnitus, pain or fullness in the ear) suggest a peripheral cause. Facial weakness or numbness occurs with lesions involving the eighth nerve in the cerebellopontine angle. Processes in the brainstem typically cause prominent neighborhood signs; isolated vertigo is rare. Occasionally, vertigo can be a manifestation of disease of the more rostral vestibular pathways, including the temporal lobe.

Distinguishing central from peripheral nystagmus is a common clinical exercise. The most helpful features are of course the presence of aural symptoms and signs in peripheral nystagmus and the presence of CNS symptoms and signs with central nystagmus. Peripheral vestibular nystagmus does not change direction, although it may vary in amplitude depending on the direction of gaze, and is strongly suppressed by visual fixation. Central nystagmus typically changes direction and may not be affected by visual fixation.

Because of the effects of fixation and other compensatory mechanisms, peripheral nystagmus is seldom prominent after the first 12 to 24 hours, but central nystagmus may persist for weeks or months. The vestibular apparatus pushes not only the eyes but also the limbs and the body to the opposite side. With APV, the patient will past point, fall on Romberg, turn on the stepping test, and drift while walking eyes

BOX 17.3

Electronystagmography and Posturography

Electrooculography (EOG) is a quantitative method of recording the direction, amplitude, and velocity of eye movements by measuring changes in the corneoretinal potential with electrodes. EOG done during stimulation of the labyrinth to cause nystagmus is electronystagmography (ENG). Recordings are done in the dark to minimize visual suppression. The horizontal labyrinth may be stimulated by calorics using air or water or by rotation. It is not possible currently to effectively study the vertical canals or the otolith organ. Rotation can be done actively by the patient turning his head to and fro (active head rotation), by the examiner turning the patient's head (passive head rotation), or by sitting in a rotation chair. Rotation testing has some advantages over calorics, but a disadvantage is that both sides are tested simultaneously.

Computerized dynamic posturography is a technique that explores the relative importance of the various sensory inputs critical for balance in patients with complaints of dizziness or imbalance. A force platform measures the compensatory movements of the patient's feet while visual, somatosensory, and vestibular perceptions are manipulated. Posturography is not of use in lesion localization and provides no information about etiology.

closed in the direction of the nystagmus slow phase. Failure to follow these rules (e.g., past pointing in the direction of the fast phase) suggests a central lesion but can occur with a compensated peripheral lesion. Peripheral nystagmus is often positional, and the vertigo and vegetative symptoms are in proportion to the nystagmus. With positional nystagmus, latency to onset, fatigability, and adaptability all support a peripheral process. Minimal vertigo with prominent nystagmus, or lack of latency, fatigability, and adaptability, suggests a central process. Peripheral nystagmus often has a rotary component, and the horizontal nystagmus beats in the same direction in all fields of gaze (may even be third degree). Central nystagmus tends to change directions. Visual fixation inhibits peripheral nystagmus but has no effect on central nystagmus.

Involvement of the vestibular nuclei may cause vertigo that has central features. Common processes that involve the brainstem and that are likely to cause vertigo include ischemia, demyelinating disease, and neoplasms. Less common brainstem lesions causing central vestibular dysfunction include arteriovenous malformation, syringobulbia, hematoma, and spinocerebellar degeneration. Lesions in the cerebellopontine angle affect both the auditory and vestibular portions of CN VIII.

Vertebrobasilar transient ischemic attacks, or "vertebrobasilar insufficiency," commonly cause vertigo, most often along with other signs and symptoms. Rarely, patients may have transient vertigo without accompanying symptoms. A three-step bedside examination is touted as a reliable way to distinguish brainstem stroke from APV: the HINTS—head impulse, nystagmus, test of skew. A syndrome of acute vertigo mimicking labyrinthitis may occur with acute cerebellar infarction or hemorrhage. In acute cerebellar lesions, the patient will tend to fall toward the side of the lesion on Romberg testing; the nystagmus may also be maximal with gaze toward the lesion. As a result, the patient may fall in the direction of the fast phase, opposite the pattern seen in APV.

Dizziness, vertigo, and disequilibrium occur commonly in patients with MS. In one instance, an MS lesion in the medulla caused clinical symptoms mimicking vestibular neuronitis. However, MS patients are not immune from developing the common syndrome of BPPV, and peripheral vestibulopathy may be a more common cause of vertigo in such patients than MS exacerbation.

There is a relationship between migraine and episodic vertigo. Motion sensitivity is common in migraineurs, and episodic vertigo occurs in as many as 25%. Isolated attacks of vertigo have been labeled as a migraine equivalent. Migraine-associated vertigo may be a symptom of migraine or a related disorder (vestibular migraine, migrainous vertigo, or migraine-related vestibulopathy). Epidemiologically, there is a strong link between vertigo and migraine, but whether migraine-associated vertigo exists as a migraine equivalent is unsettled. Migraine-associated vertigo is a separate entity from basilar artery migraine.

Occasionally, migraine patients may also develop cochlear symptoms, perhaps because of spasm of the labyrinthine microvasculature. Migraine can mimic Ménière's disease. In some patients, there may be a channelopathy involved. There is a malignant form of migraine-associated vertigo that can be very disabling.

Disorders of the peripheral vestibular apparatus are the most common causes of vertigo and related symptoms. Table 17.4 lists some of the causes of peripheral vertigo. In BPPV, the most common peripheral vestibulopathy, vertigo is induced by assumption of a particular head position or by rapid head movement. Classically, such patients experience vertigo when first lying down or when rolling over in bed at night, bending over, or looking up. Between paroxysms of vertigo, patients may complain of poor balance or light-headedness. BPPV attacks are brief, generally 10 to 30 seconds, and frequent. BPPV probably results from otoliths that have become detached from the macula of the utricle and formed free-floating debris that settles into one of the semicircular canals (canalithiasis) or becomes adherent to the matrix gel of the cupula (cupulolithiasis). Movement of the debris causes the attacks of vertigo. Otolith movement causes endolymph movement and stimulation of the hair cells of the cupula. The result is vertigo until the otoconia settle to the bottom, hence the brief duration of the attacks. The Dix-Hallpike maneuver causes the debris to move and reproduces the symptoms. The disorder predominantly affects the posterior semicircular canal, the most dependent portion of the vestibular labyrinth, and a movement of the head backward causes vertigo. Between 10% and 30% of cases involve the horizontal canal and about 1% the anterior canal. In a series of 240 patients, the most common identifiable etiologies were head trauma (17%) and viral neurolabyrinthitis (15%). Rarely, patients with posterior fossa tumors have a clinical picture nearly identical to BPPV. In horizontal canal BPPV, there is horizontal nystagmus beating toward the down ear on rapid turning of the head to either side in the supine position. Most cases of horizontal canal BPPV are due to cupulolithiasis rather than canalithiasis.

In vestibular neuronitis (neuritis, neurolabyrinthitis), APV, or labyrinthitis, more severe attacks prostrate the patient for several days. Although often used interchangeably, technically, labyrinthitis is accompanied by cochlear dysfunction with hearing impairment, whereas vestibular neuronitis is purely vestibular. An attack typically causes constant vertigo lasting for days and is accompanied by nausea, vomiting, and sweating. The patient looks and feels extremely ill. The patient will have horizontal-torsional nystagmus in primary gaze and other evidence of vestibular imbalance. During the acute phase, the involved labyrinth may be hyperactive, and after resolution, the involved labyrinth is hypoactive.

The acute phase slowly remits over weeks. Improvement is due to recovery of nerve function and CNS compensation. Mild, brief attacks of vertigo similar to BPPV may plague the patient for months to years after seeming recovery. APV is often a viral or postviral inflammation of the vestibular portion of CN VIII. It may be simulated by hemorrhagic or ischemic disease of the brainstem or cerebellum, MS, or the effects of a drug or toxin. Some instances of apparent labyrinthitis are likely due to IAA ischemia. Ramsay Hunt syndrome (see Chapter 16) may also involve CN VIII and other CNs as well.

In Ménière's disease, the attacks of vertigo typically last minutes to several hours, much longer than the typical symptoms of BPPV but much shorter than with APV. Patients describe other symptoms, either along with the vertigo or independently, including hearing loss (classically fluctuating), tinnitus, and a sensation of vague pain or fullness in the ear. The association of hearing loss and vertigo is classic. Many famous people have been affected, most notably Jonathan Swift (Box 17.4). Some patients have purely vestibular Ménière's; whether there is a purely cochlear form is controversial. Inner ear disease can occasionally cause drop attacks. The distinction between Ménière's disease and Ménière's syndrome is no longer stressed. One of Ménière's original patients suffered a hemorrhage into the labyrinth. It was Hallpike who found endolymphatic hydrops in a patient with Ménière's syndrome, establishing Ménière's disease as an entity. Modern MRI has confirmed the presence of endolymphatic hydrops in patients with Ménière's disease. The cause of the hydrops remains obscure.

Other conditions that may cause vertigo and be confused with CN VIII disease include perilymphatic fistula and superior semicircular canal dehiscence. In perilymphatic fistula, there is an abnormal communication between the inner and middle ear. Patients develop episodic vertigo with or without hearing loss, often provoked by Valsalva or straining. Vertigo and nystagmus may be induced by loud sounds (Tullio's phenomenon) because of physical activation of the vestibular system by sound vibrations. Superior semicircular canal dehiscence is due to a defect of the temporal bone overlying the superior canal, allowing pressure induced by sound to be transmitted to the inner ear. Vertigo and nystagmus may be induced by Valsalva or sound. An otolithic crisis of Tumarkin is a sudden drop to the ground followed by immediate recovery that may occur in Ménière's disease.

BOX 17.4

Ménière's Disease

Well-known affected individuals include Emily Dickinson, Peggy Lee, Alan Shepard, and Vincent Van Gogh. Swift wrote extensively about his "giddiness" and his deafness, which plagued him from an early age. Swift wrote something to the effect that "my friend the giddiness would come to visit, then my friend the hearing loss, and eventually they became such good friends they came to visit together."

Other rare causes of vertigo include seizure disorder, especially partial complex seizures of temporal lobe origin (tornado epilepsy), episodic ataxia, benign paroxysmal vertigo of childhood, hypothyroidism, mal de debarquement (mal de mer), and phobic postural vertigo.

Video Links

Video Link 17.1. Head thrust test. http://neurosigns.org/wiki/Head_impulse_test

Video Link 17.2. Normal caloric responses. http://www.youtube.com/watch?v=H4iQkFUgG6k

Video Link 17.3. Vestibular nystagmus. http://www.youtube.com/watch?v=mghGeKkNBzQ

Video Link 17.4. Head-shaking nystagmus. https://collections.lib.utah.edu/details?id=187675&q=sort_type_t%3A%2AMovingImage%2A+AND+head+shaking+nystagmus&fd=type_t%2Ctitle_t%2Cdescription_t%2Csubject_t%2Ccollection_t&rows=50&sort=sort_title_t+asc&facet_setname_s=ehsl_novel_%2A

Video Link 17.5. The Dix-Hallpike test. https://collections.lib.utah.edu/details?id=187762&q=sort_type_t%3A%2AMovingImage%2A+AND+BPPV&fd=type_t%2Ctitle_t%2Cdescription_t%2Csubject_t%2Ccollection_t&rows=50&sort=sort_title_t+asc&facet_setname_s=ehsl_novel_%2A

BIBLIOGRAPHY

Alpini D, Caputo D, Pugnetti L, et al. Vertigo and multiple sclerosis: aspects of differential diagnosis. *Neurol Sci* 2001;22(Suppl 2): S84–S87.

Armato E, Ferri E, Pinzani A, et al. Cerebellar haemorrhage mimicking acute peripheral vestibulopathy: the role of the video head impulse test in differential diagnosis. *Acta Otorhinolaryngol Ital* 2014;34:288–291.

Asawavichiangianda S, Fujimoto M, Mai M, et al. Significance of head-shaking nystagmus in the evaluation of the dizzy patient. *Acta Otolaryngol Suppl* 1999;540:27–33.

Aw ST, Todd MJ, Aw GE, et al. Benign positional nystagmus: a study of its three-dimensional spatio-temporal characteristics. *Neurology* 2005;64:1897–1905.

Bagai A, Thavendiranathan P, Detsky AS. Does this patient have hearing impairment? *JAMA* 2006;295:416–428.

Baguley D, McFerran D, Hall D. Tinnitus. *Lancet* 2013;382: 1600–1607.

Baloh RW. Approach to the evaluation of the dizzy patient. *Otolaryngol Head Neck Surg* 1995;112:3–7.

Baloh RW. Neurotology of migraine. *Headache* 1997;37:615–621.

Baloh RW. Dizziness: neurological emergencies. *Neurol Clin* 1998;16:305–321.

Baloh RW. Vertigo. *Lancet* 1998;352:1841–1846.

Baloh RW. Differentiating between peripheral and central causes of vertigo. *Otolaryngol Head Neck Surg* 1998;119:55–59.

Baloh RW. Prosper Ménière and his disease. *Arch Neurol* 2001;58:1151–1156.

Baloh RW. Episodic vertigo: central nervous system causes. *Curr Opin Neurol* 2002;15:17–21.

Baloh RW, Honrubia V, Jacobson K. Benign positional vertigo: clinical and oculographic features in 240 cases. *Neurology* 1987;37:371–378.

Baloh RW, Jacobson K, Honrubia V. Horizontal semicircular canal variant of benign positional vertigo. *Neurology* 1993;43:2542–2549.

Baloh RW, Jacobson K, Winder T. Drop attacks with Ménière's syndrome. *Ann Neurol* 1990;28:384–387.

Barraclough K, Bronstein A. Diagnosis in general practice: vertigo. *BMJ* 2009;339:b3493.

Bertholon P, Tringali S, Faye MB, et al. Prospective study of positional nystagmus in 100 consecutive patients. *Ann Otol Rhinol Laryngol* 2006;115:587–594.

Bhupal HK. Ramsay Hunt syndrome presenting in primary care. *Practitioner* 2010;254:33–35, 3.

Brazis PW, Masdeu JC, Biller J. *Localization in Clinical Neurology*. 7th ed. Philadelphia: Wolters Kluwer/Lippincott Williams & Wilkins, 2017.

Brodsky MC. Three dimensions of skew deviation. *Br J Ophthalmol* 2003;87:1440–1441.

Brodsky MC, Donahue SP, Vaphiades M, et al. Skew deviation revisited. *Surv Ophthalmol* 2006;51:105–128.

Casselman JW. Diagnostic imaging in clinical neuro-otology. *Curr Opin Neurol* 2002;15:23–30.

Cha YH, Kane MJ, Baloh RW. Familial clustering of migraine, episodic vertigo, and Meniere's disease. *Otol Neurotol* 2008;29:93–96.

Choi K-D, Kim JS. Hyperventilation-induced nystagmus in peripheral vestibulopathy and cerebellopontine angle tumor. *Neurology* 2007;69:1050–1059.

Cloutier JF, Saliba I. Isolated vertigo and dizziness of vascular origin. *J Otolaryngol Head Neck Surg* 2008;37:331–339.

Cunningham LL, Tucci DL. Hearing loss in adults. *N Engl J Med* 2017;377:2465–2473.

Delaney KA. Bedside diagnosis of vertigo: value of the history and neurological examination. *Acad Emerg Med* 2003;10(12):1388–1395.

Demer JL, Honrubia V, Baloh RW. Dynamic visual acuity: a test for oscillopsia and vestibuloocular reflex function. *Am J Otol* 1994;15:340–347.

Deplanque D, Godefroy O, Guerouaou D, et al. Sudden bilateral deafness: lateral inferior pontine infarction. *J Neurol Neurosurg Psychiatry* 1998;64:817–818.

Derebery MJ. The diagnosis and treatment of dizziness. *Med Clin North Am* 1999;83:163–177.

Dieterich M, Brandt T. Episodic vertigo related to migraine (90 cases): vestibular migraine? *J Neurol* 1999;246:883–892.

Dieterich M, Brandt T, Fries W. Otolith function in man. Results from a case of otolith Tullio phenomenon. *Brain* 1989;112(Pt 5): 1377–1392.

Dix MR, Hallpike CS. The pathology, symptomatology and diagnosis of certain common disorders of the vestibular system. *Proc R Soc Med* 1952;45:341–354.

Drachman DA, Hart CW. An approach to the dizzy patient. *Neurology* 1972;22:323–334.

Dunniway HM, Welling DB. Intracranial tumors mimicking benign paroxysmal positional vertigo. *Otolaryngol Head Neck Surg* 1998;118:429–436.

Epley JM. Human experience with canalith repositioning maneuvers. *Ann N Y Acad Sci* 2001;942:179–191.

Evans RW, Baloh RW. Episodic vertigo and migraine. *Headache* 2001;41:604–605.

Fetter M. Assessing vestibular function: which tests, when? *J Neurol* 2000;247:335–342.

Fife TD, Iverson DJ, Lempert T, et al. Practice parameter: therapies for benign paroxysmal positional vertigo (an evidence-based review): report of the Quality Standards Subcommittee of the American Academy of Neurology. *Neurology* 2008;70:2067–2074.

Froehling DA, Silverstein MD, Mohr DN, et al. The rational clinical examination. Does this dizzy patient have a serious form of vertigo? *JAMA* 1994;271:385–388.

Frohman EM, Zhang H, Dewey RB, et al. Vertigo in MS: utility of positional and particle repositioning maneuvers. *Neurology* 2000;55:1566–1569.

Frohlich AM, Sutherland GR. Epidemiology and clinical features of vestibular schwannoma in Manitoba, Canada. *Can J Neurol Sci* 1993;20:126–130.

Fukuda T. The stepping test. *Acta Otolaryngol* 1959;50:95.

Gilman S, Newman SW. *Manter and Gatz's Essentials of Clinical Neuroanatomy and Neurophysiology*. 10th ed. Philadelphia: FA Davis, 2003.

Giacomini PG, Ferraro S, Di GS, et al. Benign paroxysmal positional vertigo after intense physical activity: a report of nine cases. *Eur Arch Otorhinolaryngol* 2009;266:1831–1835.

Goebel JA. The ten-minute examination of the dizzy patient. *Semin Neurol* 2001;21:391–398.

Gould DJ, Fix JD. *Neuroanatomy*. 5th ed. Philadelphia: Wolters Kluwer Health/Lippincott Williams & Wilkins, 2014.

Grad A, Baloh RW. Vertigo of vascular origin. Clinical and electronystagmographic features in 84 cases. *Arch Neurol* 1989;46:281–284.

Gresty MA, Bronstein AM, Brandt T, et al. Neurology of otolith function. Peripheral and central disorders. *Brain* 1992;115(Pt 3): 647–673.

Grommes C, Conway D. The stepping test: a step back in history. *J Hist Neurosci* 2011;20:29–33.

Halmagyi GM, Curthoys IS. A clinical sign of canal paresis. *Arch Neurol* 1988;45:737–739.

Halmagyi GM, Cremer PD. Assessment and treatment of dizziness. *J Neurol Neurosurg Psychiatry* 2000;68:129–136.

Harner SG, Laws ER Jr. Clinical findings in patients with acoustic neurinoma. *Mayo Clin Proc* 1983;58:721–728.

Hervier B, Bordure P, Masseau A, et al. Auto-immune sensorineural deafness: physiopathology and therapeutic approach. *Rev Med Interne* 2010;31:222–228.

Hillman EJ, Bloomberg JJ, McDonald VP, et al. Dynamic visual acuity while walking in normals and labyrinthine-deficient patients. *J Vestib Res* 1999;9:49–57.

Hoistad DL, Hain TC. Central hearing loss with a bilateral inferior colliculus lesion. *Audiol Neurootol* 2003;8:111–113.

Honaker JA, Boismier TE, Shepard NP, et al. Fukuda stepping test: sensitivity and specificity. *J Am Acad Audiol* 2009;20:311–314.

Honrubia V, Baloh RW, Harris MR, et al. Paroxysmal positional vertigo syndrome. *Am J Otol* 1999;20:465–470.

Hotson JR, Baloh RW. Acute vestibular syndrome. *N Engl J Med* 1998;339:680–685.

Huppert D, Strupp M, Rettinger N, et al. Phobic postural vertigo—a long-term follow-up (5 to 15 years) of 106 patients. *J Neurol* 2005;252:564–569.

Ishiyama G, Ishiyama A, Jacobson K, et al. Drop attacks in older patients secondary to an otologic cause. *Neurology* 2001;57:1103–1106.

Jacobson GP, Newman CW, Safadi I. Sensitivity and specificity of the head-shaking test for detecting vestibular system abnormalities. *Ann Otol Rhinol Laryngol* 1990;99:539–542.

Jani NN, Laureno R, Mark AS, et al. Deafness after bilateral midbrain contusion: a correlation of magnetic resonance imaging with auditory brain stem evoked responses. *Neurosurgery* 1991;29:106–108.

Jeong HS, Oh JY, Kim JS, et al. Periodic alternating nystagmus in isolated nodular infarction. *Neurology* 2007;68:956–957.

Kattah JC, Talkad AV, Wang DZ, et al. HINTS to diagnose stroke in the acute vestibular syndrome: three-step bedside oculomotor examination more sensitive than early MRI diffusion-weighted imaging. *Stroke* 2009;40:3504–3510.

Keane JR. Ocular skew deviation. Analysis of 100 cases. *Arch Neurol* 1975;32:185–190.

Kerber KA, Burke JF, Skolarus LE, et al. A prescription for the Epley maneuver: www.youtube.com? *Neurology* 2012;79:376–380.

Kiernan JA, Rajakumar N. *Barr's The Human Nervous System: An Anatomical Viewpoint.* 10th ed. Philadelphia: Wolters Kluwer Health/Lippincott Williams & Wilkins, 2014.

Kim JS, Lopez I, DiPatre PL, et al. Internal auditory artery infarction: clinicopathologic correlation. *Neurology* 1999;52:40–44.

Kroenke K, Hoffman RM, Einstadter D. How common are various causes of dizziness? A critical review. *South Med J* 2000;93:160–167.

Kroenke K, Lucas CA, Rosenberg ML, et al. Causes of persistent dizziness. A prospective study of 100 patients in ambulatory care. *Ann Intern Med* 1992;117:898–904.

Landau ME, Barner KC. Vestibulocochlear nerve. *Semin Neurol* 2009;29:66–73.

Lanska DJ, Remler B. Benign paroxysmal positioning vertigo: classic descriptions, origins of the provocative positioning technique, and conceptual developments. *Neurology* 1997;48:1167–1177.

Lee H, Kim JS, Chung EJ, et al. Infarction in the territory of anterior inferior cerebellar artery: spectrum of audiovestibular loss. *Stroke* 2009;40:3745–3751.

Lee H, Yi HA, Lee SR, et al. Drop attacks in elderly patients secondary to otologic causes with Meniere's syndrome or non-Meniere peripheral vestibulopathy. *J Neurol Sci* 2005;232:71–76.

Lee SU, Choi JY, Kim HJ, et al. Recurrent spontaneous vertigo with interictal headshaking nystagmus. *Neurology* 2018;90(24): e2135–e2145.

Mathias CJ, Deguchi K, Schatz I. Observations on recurrent syncope and presyncope in 641 patients. *Lancet* 2001;357:348–353.

Matthews WB. *Practical Neurology*. Oxford: Blackwell, 1963.

Mazzola L, Lopez C, Faillenot I, et al. Vestibular responses to direct stimulation of the human insular cortex. *Ann Neurol* 2014;76:609–619.

Meador KJ, Swift TR. Tinnitus from intracranial hypertension. *Neurology* 1984;34:1258–1261.

Mendez MF, Geehan GR Jr. Cortical auditory disorders: clinical and psychoacoustic features. *J Neurol Neurosurg Psychiatry* 1988;51:1–9.

Minor LB. Clinical manifestations of superior semicircular canal dehiscence. *Laryngoscope* 2005;115:1717–1727.

Minor LB, Haslwanter T, Straumann D, et al. Hyperventilation-induced nystagmus in patients with vestibular schwannoma. *Neurology* 1999;53:2158–2168.

Moon IS, Kim JS, Choi KD, et al. Isolated nodular infarction. *Stroke* 2009;40:487–491.

Morelli N, Mancuso M, Cafforio G, et al. Ramsay-Hunt syndrome complicated by unilateral multiple cranial nerve palsies. *Neurol Sci* 2008;29:497–498.

Nascentes SM, Paulo EA, de Andrade EC, et al. Sudden deafness as a presenting symptom of acoustic neuroma: case report. *Braz J Otorhinolaryngol* 2007;73:713–716.

Nedzelski JM, Barber HO, McIlmoyl L. Diagnoses in a dizziness unit. *J Otolaryngol* 1986;15:101–104.

Nelson JR. The minimal ice water caloric test. *Neurology* 1969;19:577–585.

Nodar RH. Tinnitus reclassified; new oil in an old lamp. *Otolaryngol Head Neck Surg* 1996;114:582–585.

Oas JG, Baloh RW. Vertigo and the anterior inferior cerebellar artery syndrome. *Neurology* 1992;42:2274–2279.

Ojala M, Palo J. The aetiology of dizziness and how to examine a dizzy patient. *Ann Med* 1991;23:225–230.

Parnes LS, Agrawal SK, Atlas J. Diagnosis and management of benign paroxysmal positional vertigo (BPPV). *Can Med Assoc J* 2003;169:681–693.

Pierce DA, Holt SR, Reeves-Daniel A. A probable case of gabapentin-related reversible hearing loss in a patient with acute renal failure. *Clin Ther* 2008;30:1681–1684.

Phillips J, Longridge N, Mallinson A, et al. Migraine and vertigo: a marriage of convenience? *Headache* 2010;50:1362–1365.

Ralli G, Atturo F, de FC. Idiopathic benign paroxysmal vertigo in children, a migraine precursor. *Int J Pediatr Otorhinolaryngol* 2009;73(Suppl 1):S16–S18.

Rintelmann WF, Schwan SA, Blakley BW. Pseudohypacusis. *Otolaryngol Clin North Am* 1991;24:381–390.

Saunders JE, Luxford WM, Devgan KK, et al. Sudden hearing loss in acoustic neuroma patients. *Otolaryngol Head Neck Surg* 1995;113:23–31.

Schwartz NE, Venkat C, Albers GW. Transient isolated vertigo secondary to an acute stroke of the cerebellar nodulus. *Arch Neurol* 2007;64:897–898.

Shin SH, Chun YM, Lee HK. A cochlear schwannoma presenting with sudden hearing loss. *Eur Arch Otorhinolaryngol* 2008;265:839–842.

Spoelhof GD. When to suspect an acoustic neuroma. *Am Fam Physician* 1995;52:1768–1774.

Strupp M, Brandt T, Steddin S. Horizontal canal benign paroxysmal positioning vertigo: reversible ipsilateral caloric hypoexcitability caused by canalolithiasis? *Neurology* 1995;45: 2072–2076.

Standring S, ed. *Gray's Anatomy: The Anatomical Basis of Clinical Practice*. 41st ed. New York: Elsevier Limited, 2016.

Tanaka Y, Kamo T, Yoshida M, et al. 'So-called' cortical deafness. Clinical, neurophysiological and radiological observations. *Brain* 1991;114(Pt 6):2385–2401.

Tarnutzer AA, Lee SH, Robinson KA, et al. Clinical and electrographic findings in epileptic vertigo and dizziness: a systematic review. *Neurology* 2015;84:1595–1604.

Torres-Russotto D, Landau WM, Harding GW, et al. Calibrated finger rub auditory screening test (CALFRAST). *Neurology* 2009;72:1595–1600.

Tsunoda A, Komatsuzaki A, Muraoka H, et al. A case with symptoms of vestibular neuronitis caused by an intramedullary lesion. *J Laryngol Otol* 1995;109:545–548.

Verghese J, Morocz IA. Acute unilateral deafness. *J Otolaryngol* 1999;28:362–364.

von Brevern M, Clarke AH, Lempert T. Continuous vertigo and spontaneous nystagmus due to canalolithiasis of the horizontal canal. *Neurology* 2001;56:684–686.

von Brevern M, Lempert T, Bronstein AM, et al. Selective vestibular damage in neurosarcoidosis. *Ann Neurol* 1997;42:117–120.

von Brevern M, Radtke A, Clarke AH, et al. Migrainous vertigo presenting as episodic positional vertigo. *Neurology* 2004;62: 469–472.

Wall M, Rosenberg M, Richardson D. Gaze-evoked tinnitus. *Neurology* 1987;37:1034–1036.

Weber KP, Aw ST. Horizontal head impulse test detects gentamicin vestibulotoxicity. *Neurology* 2009;72:1417–1424.

Yang TH, Oh SY, Kwak K, et al. Topology of brainstem lesions associated with subjective visual vertical tilt. *Neurology* 2014;82:1968–1975.

CHAPTER 18

The Glossopharyngeal and Vagus Nerves

The glossopharyngeal (CN IX) and vagus (CN X) nerves are intimately related and similar in function. Both have motor and autonomic branches with nuclei of origin in the medulla. Both conduct general somatic afferent (GSA) as well as general visceral afferent (GVA) fibers to related or identical fiber tracts and nuclei in the brainstem, and both have a parasympathetic, or general visceral efferent, and a branchiomotor, or special visceral efferent (SVE), component. The two nerves leave the skull together, remain close in their course through the neck, and supply some of the same structures. They are often involved in the same disease processes, and involvement of one may be difficult to differentiate from involvement of the other. For these reasons, the two nerves are discussed together.

THE GLOSSOPHARYNGEAL NERVE

Anatomy and Physiology

The glossopharyngeal, as its name implies, is distributed principally to the tongue and pharynx. It conveys general sensory as well as special sensory (taste) fibers from the posterior third of the tongue. It also provides general sensory innervation to the pharynx, the area of the tonsil, the internal surface of the tympanic membrane, and the skin of the external ear. It conveys GVAs from the carotid body and the carotid sinus. Its skeletomotor neurons innervate the stylopharyngeus muscle, and its parasympathetic component innervates the parotid gland.

Upper motor neuron influences on CN IX arise from the primary motor cortex and descend in the corticobulbar tracts to synapse in the rostral portion of the nucleus ambiguus in the dorsolateral medulla (Figure 18.1). The cortical innervation is bilateral. The cells in the nucleus ambiguus are branchiomotor and innervate muscles derived from the third, fourth, and fifth branchial arches. In keeping with the tendency of SVE axons to create internal loops, the fibers of CN IX first head posteromedially toward the floor of the fourth ventricle and then turn and sweep laterally and forward. The nerve emerges from the medulla as three to six rootlets in the groove between the inferior olive and the inferior cerebellar peduncle, between and in line with the emerging fibers of CN VII above and CN X below (Figure 11.3). These rootlets unite to form a single nerve, which leaves the skull through the jugular foramen.

CN IX exits the skull through the jugular foramen, lateral and anterior to CNs X and XI within a separate dural sheath. After leaving the skull, CN IX enters the carotid sheath, descends between the internal jugular vein and internal carotid artery, dips beneath the styloid process, and then passes between the internal and external carotid arteries. It curves forward, forming an arch on the side of the neck to reach the lateral pharyngeal wall, and then disappears under the hyoglossus muscle to divide into its terminal branches. Two ganglia lie on the nerve just caudal to the jugular foramen: the superior (jugular) and inferior (petrosal) glossopharyngeal ganglia (Figure 18.2). The superior glossopharyngeal ganglion is small, is inconstant, has no branches, and is often fused with the inferior ganglion. CN IX has six terminal branches: (a) the tympanic nerve (Jacobson's nerve), (b) carotid, (c) pharyngeal, (d) muscular, (e) tonsillar, and (f) lingual branches. CN IX has important connections with CNs V, VII, and X and the cervical sympathetics.

The branchiomotor fibers of CN IX go to the pharynx. The muscular branch follows along the posterior border of the stylopharyngeus muscle and then terminates in the belly of the muscle. Most of the pharyngeal muscles are supplied by both CNs IX and X. If CN IX supplies any muscle alone, it is the

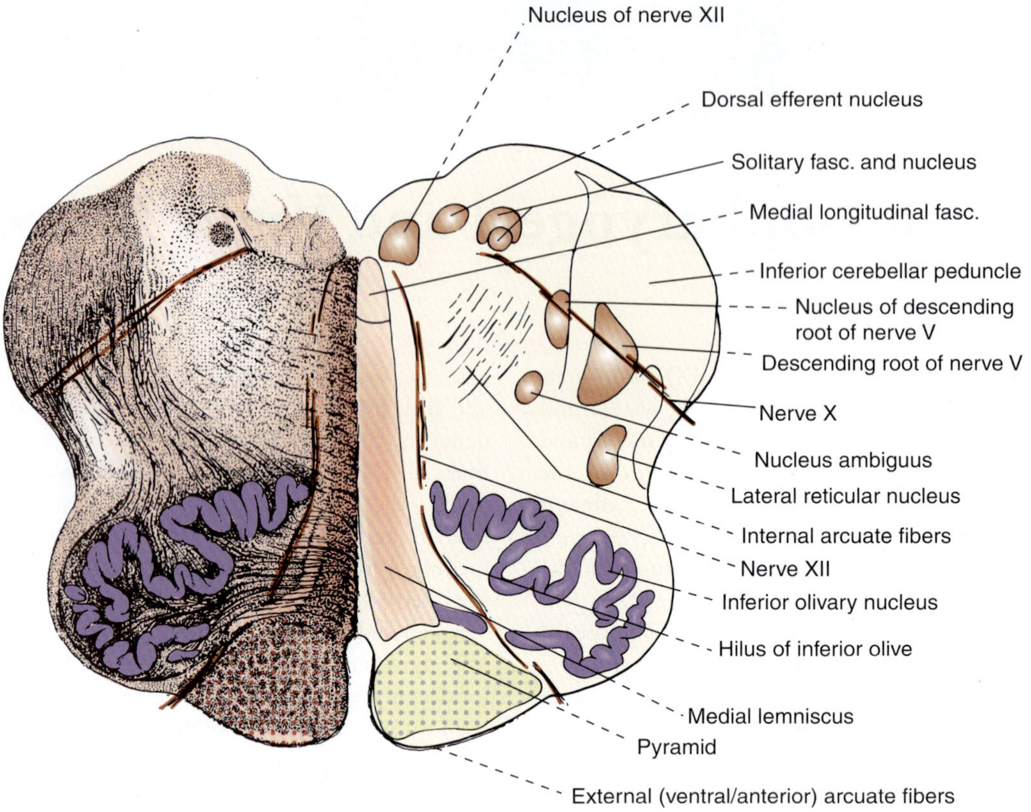

FIGURE 18.1 Section through the medulla at the level of the inferior olivary nucleus.

stylopharyngeus. The actions of the stylopharyngeus are described in Table 18.1.

CN IX supplies parasympathetic innervation to the parotid gland and to the mucous membranes of the posterior-inferior mouth and pharynx (Figure 18.2). The parasympathetic nuclei in the lower brainstem are the superior and inferior salivatory and the dorsal motor nucleus of CN X (DMNX), also known as the dorsal motor or dorsal efferent nucleus of the vagus. The autonomic fibers of CN IX arise primarily from the inferior salivatory nucleus, with some from the DMNX. The parasympathetics pass through the superior and inferior glossopharyngeal ganglia without synapsing. Just below the inferior ganglion, they exit to form the tympanic nerve, which ascends to the tympanic cavity through a small canal on the undersurface of the temporal bone between the carotid canal and the jugular fossa (tympanic canaliculus). The tympanic nerve ramifies in the tympanic cavity to form part of the tympanic plexus. The lesser petrosal nerve is a continuation of the tympanic nerve that leaves the tympanic plexus, enters the middle cranial fossa briefly, and then exits through the foramen ovale to synapse in the otic ganglion. Postganglionic fibers join the auriculotemporal branch of the mandibular division of CN V for distribution to the parotid gland; this is the nerve involved in gustatory sweating (Chapter 15).

Sensory neurons of CN IX are located in the superior and inferior glossopharyngeal ganglia. There are GSA fibers that convey ordinary exteroceptive sensation; GVA fibers that convey information from the carotid body and carotid sinus, as well as visceral sensation from the pharynx; and special visceral afferents that convey taste sensation. The GSA fibers convey exteroceptive sensation from the mucous membranes of the tympanic cavity, mastoid air cells, and auditory canal via the tympanic plexus and tympanic branch. Sensation from the pharynx, tonsil, and posterior third of the tongue travels via the pharyngeal, tonsillar, and lingual branches. Central processes of these cells terminate in the trigeminal nuclei, and their central connections are the same as for other GSA fibers. One of the most important functions of CN IX is

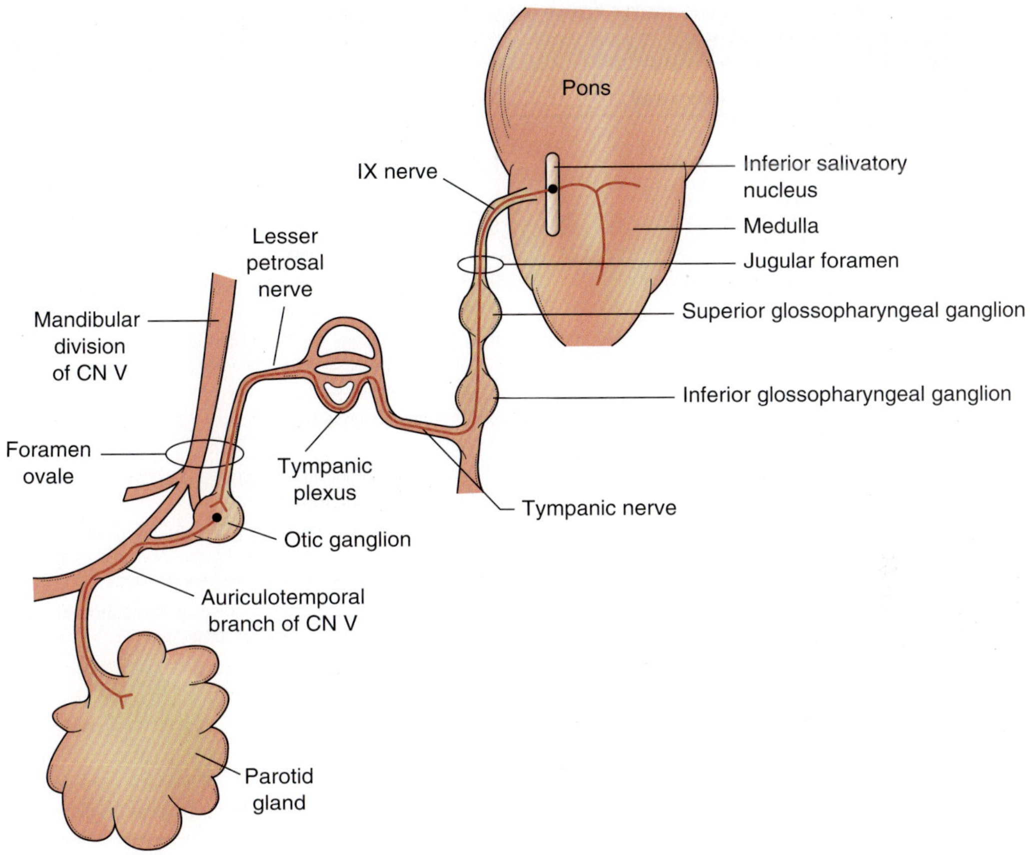

FIGURE 18.2 Peripheral distribution of the parasympathetic branches of the glossopharyngeal nerve.

to carry visceral afferent fibers from the carotid body and sinus involved in the reflex control of heart rate, blood pressure, and respiration. The carotid branch of CN IX (carotid sinus nerve) arises just below the jugular foramen and descends on the internal carotid artery to the carotid sinus and carotid body. It conveys impulses from carotid body chemoreceptors and carotid sinus baroreceptors and terminates centrally on cells in the middle third of the nucleus of the solitary tract. Other fibers carrying visceral afferent fibers from the mucous membranes of the pharynx, soft palate, and posterior third of the tongue pass through the petrous ganglion to terminate in the solitary tract and nucleus. The lingual branches of CN IX carry taste fibers (primarily sour and bitter) from the circumvallate papillae, mucous membranes of the base and taste buds on the posterior third of the tongue, glossoepiglottic and pharyngoepiglottic folds, and lingual surface of the epiglottis. These fibers terminate in the rostral part of the nucleus of the solitary tract (gustatory nucleus). Their central connections are the same as for the taste fibers of CN VII.

Clinical Examination

CN IX is difficult to examine because most or all of its functions are shared by other nerves and because many of the structures it supplies are inaccessible. It is possible to examine pain and touch sensation of the pharynx, tonsillar region and soft palate, and the gag reflex. Bedside testing of taste on the posterior third of the tongue is difficult and seldom attempted. It is not possible to isolate the motor functions from those of the vagus. The small area of cutaneous exteroceptive sensory supply is shared by other nerves. Patients with CN IX lesions might theoretically have detectable sensory loss, but it is not possible to find in patients who have undergone ninth nerve section for glossopharyngeal neuralgia.

The only muscle to receive its motor innervation purely from CN IX is the stylopharyngeus. The only deficit that might be detectable is a slight lowering of the palatal arch at rest on the involved side. Other palatal motor functions are subserved by either CN X or the two nerves working together. The salivary

TABLE 18.1 Branches of the Glossopharyngeal and Vagus Nerves, the Muscles Innervated, and Their Actions

Nerve Branch	Muscle Innervated	Muscle Action
CN IX		
Muscular branch	Stylopharyngeus	Raises and dilates the pharynx
CN X		
Pharyngeal branch	Musculus uvulae	Shortens and bends the uvula backward; helps to block off the nasal passages in swallowing
	Levator veli palatini	Raises the soft palate and pulls it backward; blocks off the nasal passages in swallowing
	Palatopharyngeus	Pulls the pharynx and the thyroid cartilage upward and depresses the soft palate; draws the pharyngopalatine arches together and closes faucial orifice
	Salpingopharyngeus	Blends with palatopharyngeus, raises upper and lateral portion of the pharynx
	Palatoglossus	Elevates posterior part of the tongue and narrows the fauces; depresses the soft palate
	Superior, middle, and inferior constrictors of the pharynx	Flattens and contracts the pharynx in swallowing; forces food into the esophagus in the final act of deglutition; affects speech by changing the shape of the pharyngeal resonator
Superior laryngeal nerve	Cricothyroid	Chief tensors of the vocal cords; elongate the cords by increasing the distance between the vocal processes and the angle of the thyroid
Recurrent laryngeal nerve	Posterior cricoarytenoids	Chief abductors; separate vocal cords and open the glottis by rotating the arytenoids cartilages outward
	Lateral cricoarytenoids	Chief adductors; close the glottis by rotating the arytenoids cartilages inward
	Thyroarytenoids (vocalis)	Pull arytenoids forward to shorten and relax the vocal cords
	Arytenoid	Unpaired; slides arytenoids together and closes the glottic rim

reflex is flow of saliva from the parotid duct after gustatory stimuli. The afferent limb is through taste fibers and the efferent through the parasympathetic outflow of the superior and interior salivatory nuclei.

The gag reflex is elicited by touching the pharynx or palate. Some sources make a distinction between the pharyngeal reflex and the palatal reflex, referring only to the former as the gag reflex. In common clinical usage, no distinction is made between these two and either is referred to as the gag reflex. The reflex is elicited by touching the lateral oropharynx in the region of the anterior faucial pillar with a tongue blade, applicator stick, or similar object (pharyngeal reflex), or by touching one side of the soft palate or uvula (palatal reflex). The pharyngeal reflex is the more active of the two. The reflex also occurs with touching the base of the tongue or posterior pharyngeal wall. The afferent limb of the reflex is mediated by CN IX and the efferent limb through CNs IX and X. The reflex center is in the medulla. The motor response is constriction and elevation of the oropharynx. This causes the midline raphe of the palate and the uvula to elevate and the pharyngeal constrictors to contract. The activity on the two sides is compared. The gag reflex is protective; it is designed to prevent noxious substances or foreign objects from going beyond the oral cavity. There are three motor components: elevation of the soft palate to seal off the nasopharynx, closure of the glottis to protect the airway, and constriction of the pharynx to prevent entry of the substance.

When unilateral pharyngeal weakness is present, the raphe will deviate away from the weak side and toward the normal side. This movement is usually dramatic (see **Video Link 18.1**). Minor movements of the uvula and trivial deviations of the midline raphe are not of clinical significance. In normal adults, both palatal and pharyngeal reflexes are usually present, but there may be inter- and intraindividual variation in the intensity of the stimulus required. The gag reflex may be bilaterally absent in some normal individuals. Unilateral absence signifies a lower motor neuron lesion. Like most bulbar muscles, the pharynx receives bilateral supranuclear innervation, and a unilateral cerebral lesion does not cause detectable weakness.

The gag reflex is often used to predict whether or not a patient will be able to swallow. A poor gag reflex in an awake patient with an acute deficit may be a predictor of swallowing difficulties. In fact, the gag reflex has little to do with normal swallowing. Normal deglutition is a smooth coordinated sequence of muscle contractions that propel a bolus of food from the mouth into the esophagus. A normal swallow bears little resemblance to the chaos of a gag reflex. Higher cortical centers have to inhibit the gag response during normal swallowing. The gag reflex is useful but limited in assessing airway protection. A decreased gag reflex in a patient with depressed consciousness may portend inadequate guarding of the airway and increased aspiration risk, but the status of the gag reflex is not a completely reliable indicator. Patients with an apparently intact gag reflex may still aspirate, and a patient with a depressed gag reflex may not.

Davies et al. found that the gag reflex is absent in 37% of normals, which may explain its low predictive value in the assessment of aspiration risk. Leder and Espinosa concluded that the clinical examination, a major component of which is the status of the gag reflex, underestimated the probability of aspiration in patients who were at risk and overestimated it in patients who were not. The trigeminal nerve contributes to palatal sensation and may allow for paradoxical preservation of the gag reflex in the face of a CN IX lesion. The gag reflex may be hyperactive in some normal individuals, even to the point of causing retching and vomiting. A hyperactive gag reflex may occur with bilateral cerebral lesions, as in pseudobulbar palsy and amyotrophic lateral sclerosis (ALS).

Disorders of Function

Unilateral supranuclear lesions cause no deficit because of the bilateral corticobulbar innervation. Bilateral supranuclear lesions may cause pseudobulbar palsy (Chapter 21).

Isolated lesions of CN IX are extremely rare if they ever occur. In all instances, the nerve is involved along with other CNs, especially CN X. Nuclear and infranuclear processes that may affect CN IX include intramedullary and extramedullary neoplasms and other mass lesions (e.g., glomus jugulare tumor), trauma (e.g., basilar skull fracture or surgical dissection), motor neuron disease, syringobulbia, retropharyngeal abscess, demyelinating disease, birth injury, and brainstem ischemia. Surgical section or other trauma to the carotid branch may cause transient or sustained hypertension. Involvement of CN IX may be related to the cardiovascular dysautonomia that sometimes accompanies Guillain-Barré syndrome. CN IX may be involved along with other CNs in lesions of the skull base, for example, the jugular foramen syndrome (Chapter 21).

Perhaps, the most important lesion of the ninth nerve is glossopharyngeal (or vagoglossopharyngeal) neuralgia or "tic douloureux of the ninth nerve." In this condition, the patient experiences attacks of severe lancinating pain originating in one side of the throat or tonsillar region and radiating along the course of the eustachian tube to the tympanic membrane, external auditory canal, behind the angle of the jaw, and adjacent portion of the ear. As in trigeminal neuralgia, there may be trigger zones; they are usually in the pharyngeal wall, fauces, tonsillar regions, or base of the tongue. The pain may be brought on by talking, eating, swallowing, or coughing. It can lead to syncope, convulsions, and rarely cardiac arrest because of stimulation of the carotid sinus reflex. Glossopharyngeal neuralgia must be differentiated from other craniofacial neuralgias and from pain because of a structural lesion of the nerve. Some authorities differentiate between glossopharyngeal neuralgia, in which the pain radiates from the throat to the ear, and Jacobson's neuralgia, in which the pain is limited to the ear and eustachian tube. Glossopharyngeal neuralgia is most often idiopathic but has been reported with lesions involving the peripheral distribution of the nerves. Multiple sclerosis only rarely causes glossopharyngeal neuralgia, although it is commonly associated with trigeminal neuralgia.

Carotid sinus hypersensitivity is due to inadvertent activation of the baroreceptors in the carotid sinus causing bradycardia and hypotension. Identifiable etiologies may include constriction around the neck (e.g., tight collar) or a mass in the neck impinging on the sinus, but many cases are idiopathic.

THE VAGUS NERVE

Anatomy and Physiology

The vagus (L. "wandering," because of its wide distribution) is the longest and most widely distributed

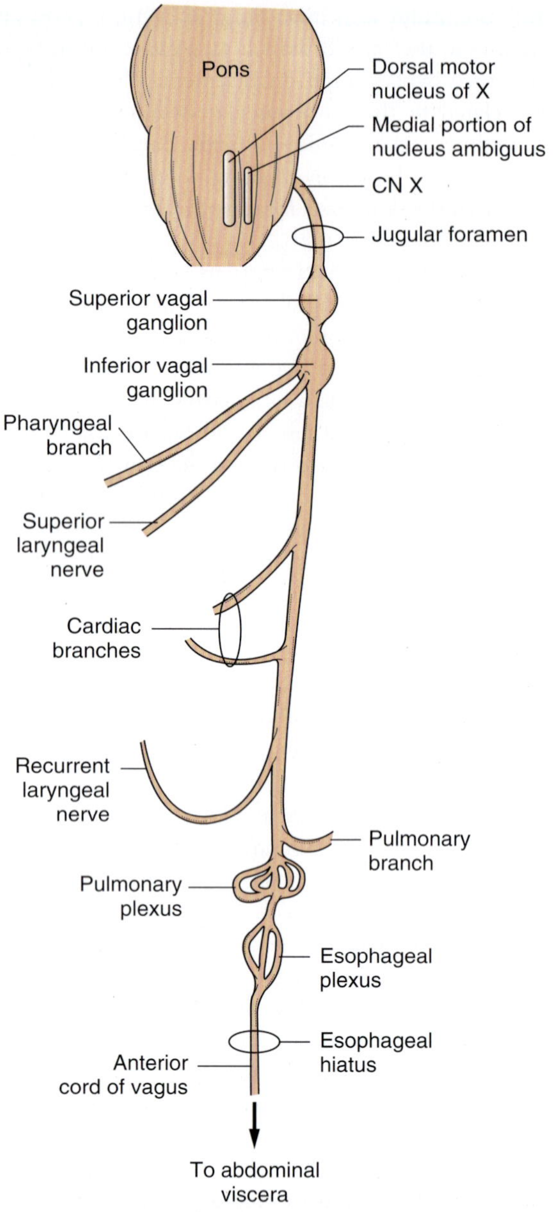

FIGURE 18.3 Peripheral distribution of the branches of the vagus nerve.

CN (Figure 18.3). Some of the nuclei of origin are the same as for CN IX, and it shares many functions with CN IX. It connects with four brainstem nuclei: the nucleus ambiguus, the DMNX, the nucleus of the spinal tract of CN V, and the nucleus of the solitary tract. It conveys exteroceptive GSA sensation from the pharynx, larynx, ear, and meninges and GVA fibers from the larynx, viscera of the thorax and abdomen, and receptors in the aorta. CN X carries skeletomotor axons from the nucleus ambiguus to the pharynx and larynx and parasympathetic axons from the DMNX to the smooth muscles and glands of the pharynx and larynx and to the thoracic and abdominal viscera. Its terminal ramifications reach the splenic flexure of the colon.

The vagus emerges from the medulla as a series of rootlets just below those of the glossopharyngeal. CN X leaves the skull through the jugular foramen in the same neural sheath as the cranial root of CN XI and behind CN IX. In the jugular foramen, the nerve lies close to the jugular bulb, a dilatation of the internal jugular vein that houses the glomus jugulare (tympanic body). The glomus jugulare has functions similar to the carotid body. CN X descends the neck in the carotid sheath, lying between the carotid artery and internal jugular vein to the upper border of the thyroid cartilage and then between the vein and common carotid to the base of the neck. Branches leave in the jugular foramen to supply the meninges and ear; other branches leave distal to the foramen to supply the pharynx and larynx. The major portion of the nerve enters the thorax. The vagus has two sensory ganglia. The superior (jugular) vagal ganglion is located in the jugular fossa of the temporal bone; the inferior (nodose) ganglion is located just distal to the jugular foramen. There are 10 major terminal branches that arise at different levels: (a) meningeal, (b) auricular, (c) pharyngeal, (d) carotid, (e) superior laryngeal, (f) recurrent laryngeal, (g) cardiac, (h) esophageal, (i) pulmonary, and (j) gastrointestinal. The terminal branches are summarized in Table 18.2.

The Motor Portion

The cortical center regulating vagus function lies in the lower portion of the precentral gyrus; the supranuclear innervation is bilateral but primarily crossed. Fibers descend in the corticobulbar tracts to synapse in the nucleus ambiguus. The vagal branchiomotor fibers follow the same looping intramedullary course as the fibers of CN IX. There are three major branchiomotor branches: pharyngeal, superior laryngeal, and recurrent laryngeal. The actions of the muscles innervated by the vagus are summarized in Table 18.1.

The pharyngeal branch runs between the internal and external carotid arteries and enters the pharynx, where it ramifies to form the pharyngeal plexus. The plexus also receives fibers from the external laryngeal branch, CN IX, and the sympathetic trunk. The vagus, with a contribution from the bulbar portion of CN XI, supplies all the striated muscles of the

TABLE 18.2 The Terminal Branches of the Vagus Nerve

Nerve	Anatomy
Meningeal branch	Arises from jugular ganglion; recurrent course upward through the jugular foramen; supplies dura of the posterior fossa
Auricular branch	Arises from superior vagal ganglion; receives filament from the inferior ganglion of CN IX; supplies GSA fibers to posterior part of the tympanic membrane, external acoustic meatus, and the skin of the posterior pinna; communicates with posterior auricular branch of CN VII
Pharyngeal branch	Arises from the inferior vagal ganglion; passes across internal carotid artery to the upper border of the middle pharyngeal constrictor; divides into numerous filaments that join branches of CN IX, superior laryngeal nerves and sympathetic nerves to form pharyngeal plexus. Motor innervation to all muscles of the soft palate and pharynx except for stylopharyngeus and tensor veli palatini; sensory innervation to mucous membrane of the pharynx
Carotid body branches	Arise from the inferior vagal ganglion, carry impulses from baro- and chemoreceptors to middle third of the nucleus of the solitary tract; form plexus with branches of CN IX
Superior laryngeal branch	Arises from the inferior vagal ganglion; divides into external and internal branches. Smaller external branch innervates cricothyroid muscle and sends branches to pharyngeal plexus. Internal branch provides sensory innervation to internal surfaces of the larynx as far down as the vocal folds
Recurrent laryngeal nerves	Arise in the thorax and ascend back to the larynx; on the right, winds backward around subclavian artery; on the left, loops around aortic arch; both ascend between the esophagus and trachea, behind common carotid artery and thyroid gland to the larynx; distributed to all muscles of the larynx except the cricothyroid; supply sensation to the mucous membrane of the larynx below the vocal folds
Cardiac branches	Superior and inferior branches; superior arises from the vagus; inferior arises from the trunk of the vagus and recurrent laryngeal on the right, on the left from the recurrent laryngeal only; communicates with cardiac branches of the sympathetic nervous system to form the cardiac plexus
Pulmonary branches	Arise in the thorax; communicate with filaments from the sympathetic division to form the pulmonary plexuses
Esophageal branches	Arise in the thorax; join filaments from the splanchnic nerves and thoracic sympathetics to form esophageal plexus
Gastrointestinal branches	Arise in the abdomen; form gastric, celiac, and hepatic plexuses

soft palate, pharynx, and larynx except for the stylopharyngeus (CN IX) and tensor veli palatini (CN V).

The superior laryngeal nerve arises distal to the pharyngeal branch and divides into an internal and external branch. The internal branch is primarily sensory. The external branch supplies the cricothyroid. All of the other intrinsic laryngeal muscles are supplied by the recurrent nerves, except for the arytenoid, which may receive some fibers from the internal branch of the superior laryngeal. The recurrent laryngeal nerves both descend deep into the thorax and then loop back to the larynx. On the right, the recurrent laryngeal arches around the subclavian artery and on the left around the aortic arch. Each nerve gives off cardiac, tracheal, and esophageal branches, ending on each side as the inferior laryngeal nerve to supply the intrinsic muscles of the larynx.

The Parasympathetic Portion

The parasympathetic component of CN X arises from the DMNX, a long cell column just dorsolateral to the hypoglossal nucleus extending from the upper pole of the inferior olive to the lower portion of the medulla. Some parasympathetic neurons lie immediately adjacent in the medial part of the nucleus ambiguus. The neurons in the nucleus ambiguus innervate the heart, and those in DMNX supply the other vagally innervated viscera. The fibers stream ventromedially and merge with the branchiomotor fibers coming from the nucleus ambiguus. The autonomic fibers leave the medulla as preganglionic fibers of the craniosacral division of the autonomic nervous system. They terminate in ganglia close to the viscera they supply and send short postganglionic fibers directly to the muscular and glandular structures they innervate. The vagus is the longest parasympathetic nerve in the body and mediates many important functions, which are discussed in Chapter 45. In brief, a vagal discharge causes bradycardia, hypotension, bronchoconstriction, bronchorrhea, increased peristalsis, increased gastric secretion, and inhibition of adrenal function. The vagal centers in the medulla that control these functions are themselves under the control of higher centers in the cortex and hypothalamus. Inhibition of vagal function produces the opposite effects.

In its course through the thorax, the right vagus nerve gives off pulmonary and esophageal branches, passes through the esophageal opening in the diaphragm posterior to the esophagus, and then divides into gastric and celiac branches. The left vagus also gives off pulmonary and esophageal branches and then enters the abdomen anterior to the esophagus and divides into several gastric branches.

The Sensory Portion

The superior vagal ganglion is located in the upper part of the jugular foramen. It communicates through several delicate branches with the cranial portion of CN XI and with the petrous ganglion of CN IX, with CN VII, and with the superior cervical ganglion. The inferior vagal ganglion lies just beneath the jugular foramen. The cranial root of the CN XI passes through it to join CN X. The inferior ganglion also communicates with CN XII, the superior cervical ganglion, and the loop between C1 and C2. Both vagal ganglia are sensory, containing unipolar neurons that mediate general somatic, special visceral, and general visceral afferents. The branchiomotor and parasympathetic axons pass through the ganglia without synapsing. The superior ganglion primarily conveys somatic sensation, and most of its communication is with the auricular nerve. The inferior ganglion relays general visceral sensation and taste.

The somatic sensory portion of the vagus conveys pain, temperature, and touch sensation from the pharynx, larynx, ear canal, external surface of the tympanic membrane, and meninges of the posterior fossa. In the larynx, GSA fibers from above the vocal folds travel in the internal laryngeal branch of the superior laryngeal nerve; fibers from below the vocal folds travel with the recurrent laryngeal nerve. Visceral afferents follow the same pathways. General sensory fibers from the region of the ear, ear canal, and tympanic membrane travel in the auricular branch (nerve of Arnold). Stimulation of the auricular branch, as by tickling the ear canal, can produce reflex activation of DMNX with coughing, vomiting, and even syncope (mitempfindung; see Chapter 31). The GSA fibers in CN X synapse in the nucleus of the spinal tract of CN V and are relayed to the thalamus and to the sensory cortex.

Fibers carrying GVAs from the pharynx, larynx, vagally innervated viscera, and baroreceptors and chemoreceptors in the aorta travel over the peripheral processes of neurons in the inferior vagal ganglion. The central processes terminate in the caudal portion of the solitary tract. Collaterals to the reticular formation, DMNX, and other CN nuclei mediate important visceral reflexes and are involved in the regulation of cardiovascular, respiratory, and gastrointestinal function. There are some taste fibers from the region of the epiglottis and arytenoids, which travel with the taste fibers of CN IX to terminate in the rostral solitary tract.

Normal Functions

Normal functions mediated by CNs IX and X include swallowing, phonation, and airway protection and modulation. The complex process of swallowing is divided into two stages, controlled primarily by CNs IX, X, and XII. In the first stage, the food bolus is driven back into the fauces by tongue action. During the second stage, the epiglottis closes over the entrance to the larynx, and the bolus glides along its posterior surface. The muscles of the soft palate and nasopharynx close above the bolus to prevent passage into the nasopharynx. The bolus is directed downward and backward into the pharynx, and then the constrictors contract to propel it downward into the esophagus.

The larynx is composed of several cartilages. The thyroid and cricoid cartilages form part of the outer casing. The arytenoids are paired cartilages lying in the interior; they have a muscular process and a vocal process. The true vocal cords are mucous membranes that cover the vocal ligaments, which extend from the vocal processes of the arytenoids to the thyroid cartilage. The larynx is controlled by myriad small muscles. The arytenoids may either slide or pivot; either action changes the configuration of the vocal cords. The glottic rim is the passageway between the vocal cords. Contraction and relaxation of the intrinsic laryngeal muscles change the tension or shape of the vocal cords and alter the aperture of the glottic rim. The muscles of the larynx perform three basic functions: They abduct and open the glottic rim to allow air entry and exit, they adduct and close the glottic rim to protect the airway during swallowing, and they regulate the tension on the vocal cords to allow phonation. The cricothyroids, posterior and lateral cricoarytenoids, and thyroarytenoids are paired muscles. The arytenoid muscle is unpaired. The actions of the intrinsic laryngeal muscles are summarized in Table 18.1 and Figure 18.4.

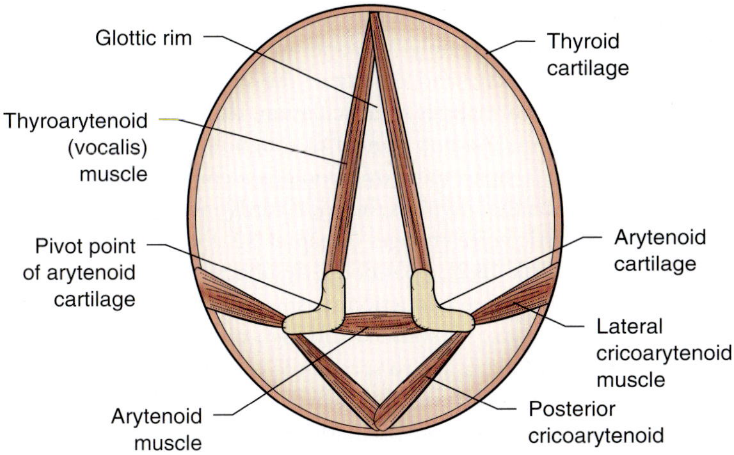

FIGURE 18.4 The cricothyroid muscles (not shown) tilt the thyroid cartilage forward on the cricoid cartilage, tensing the vocal cords. The thyroarytenoid muscles run from the thyroid cartilage to the arytenoid cartilages; contraction tenses the vocal cords. The other muscles attach to the cricoid cartilage. The paired arytenoids may either slide or pivot. Contraction of the arytenoid muscle pulls the arytenoid cartilages together, adducting the cords and closing the glottic rim. The lateral cricoarytenoid muscle causes the vocal process of the arytenoid to pivot medially, adducting the cords. The posterior cricoarytenoid causes the vocal process to rotate laterally, abducting the cords.

Clinical Examination

Despite its size and importance, CN X is difficult to evaluate at the bedside. Formal autonomic function assessment can sometimes provide useful information.

Examination of the Motor Functions

The motor branches of CN X supply the soft palate, pharynx, and larynx in the same distribution as for CN IX and are examined in the same manner. The gag reflex is discussed in the section on CN IX.

The character of the voice and the ability to swallow provide information about the branchiomotor functions of the vagus. With acute unilateral lesions, the speech may have a nasal quality and dysphagia is often present; this is more marked for liquids than solids, with a tendency to nasal regurgitation because of velopharyngeal insufficiency. Examination of the soft palate includes observation of the position of the palate and uvula at rest and during quiet breathing and phonation. The median raphe of the palate rises in the midline on phonation. With a unilateral lesion of the vagus, there is weakness of the levator veli palatini and musculus uvulae, which causes a droop of the palate and flattening of the palatal arch (Figure 18.5). Preserved function of the tensor veli palatini (innervated by CN V) may prevent marked drooping of the palate. On phonation, the median raphe deviates toward the normal side. The palatal gag reflex may be lost on the involved side because of interruption of the motor rather than sensory path.

With bilateral vagus involvement, the palate cannot elevate on phonation; it may or may not droop, depending on the function of the tensor veli palatini. The palatal gag reflex is absent bilaterally. The tendency toward nasal speech and nasal regurgitation of liquids is pronounced. The speech is similar to that of a patient with cleft palate (Chapter 9).

Weakness of the pharynx may also produce abnormalities of speech and swallowing. With pharyngeal weakness, dysarthria is usually minimal

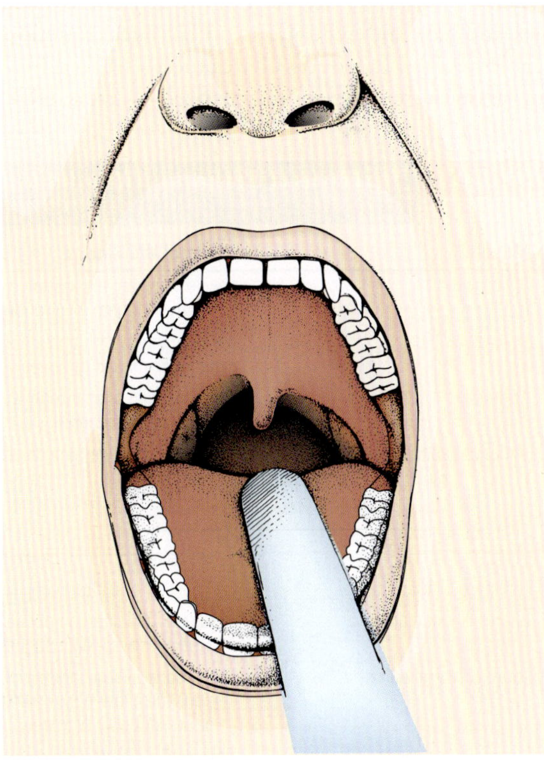

FIGURE 18.5 Unilateral paralysis of the soft palate.

unless there is also weakness of the soft palate or larynx. Spontaneous coughing and the cough reflex may be impaired. Dysphagia may occur but without the tendency to greater difficulty with liquids and to nasal regurgitation that occurs with palatal weakness. Dysphagia is marked only in acute unilateral or in bilateral lesions. Examination of the pharynx includes observation of the contraction of the pharyngeal muscles on phonation, notation of the elevation of the larynx on swallowing, and testing the pharyngeal gag reflex. Unilateral weakness of the superior pharyngeal constrictor may cause a "curtain movement" (Vernet's rideau phenomenon), with motion of the pharyngeal wall toward the nonparalyzed side on testing the gag reflex or at the beginning of phonation. The normal elevation of the larynx may be absent on one side in unilateral lesions and on both sides in bilateral lesions.

CN X innervates the vocal cords. Normal movement of the vocal cords is necessary for three vital functions: breathing, coughing, and talking. During inspiration and expiration, the cords abduct to allow for free airflow; when speaking, the cords adduct and vibrate to accomplish phonation. The cords are also adducted when coughing. Movements of the many small muscles that control the larynx are complex and have different effects on laryngeal function (Table 18.1). The effects of weakness of the different laryngeal muscles are summarized in Table 18.3. A unilateral lesion of the vagus may cause cord weakness or paralysis. Vocal cord dysfunction alters the character and quality of the voice and may produce abnormalities of articulation, difficulty with respiration, and impairment of coughing.

Spasmodic dysphonia is a common focal dystonia that involves the vocal cords and causes characteristic voice changes (Chapter 30; for video, see **Video Link 18.2**). Spasmodic dysphonia most often causes abnormal adduction spasms of both vocal cords, and the voice is strained and high-pitched. Abductor dysphonia is due to spasmodic contraction of the posterior cricoarytenoid, which causes a failure of normal adduction on phonation; the voice is breathy and hoarse. This type of spasmodic dysphonia is most likely to be confused with a lesion of CN X. Direct and indirect laryngoscopy and videostroboscopy are valuable adjuncts to the routine examination.

The most common cause of vocal cord paralysis is a lesion of one recurrent laryngeal nerve. The paralysis may evolve from mild abduction impairment because of isolated involvement of the posterior cricoarytenoid to complete paralysis with the cord in the cadaveric position. With slight weakness of the vocal cords or pharynx, hoarseness and dysphagia may be apparent only when the head is turned to either side. Occasionally, even severe weakness of a vocal cord causes little appreciable effect on the voice because of preserved movement of the normal cord.

TABLE 18.3 The Effects of Weakness of Muscles of the Larynx

Muscle	Effect of Weakness
Cricothyroid	Loss of tension; elongation of the vocal cord in phonation; loss of high tones; voice deep, hoarse, and easily fatigued; inspiration normal with either dyspnea or stridor
Thyroarytenoid	Little difficulty with abduction, but adduction slightly impaired; with bilateral paralysis, the glottis has an oval instead of linear appearance on phonation; voice hoarse; no dyspnea or stridor
Arytenoid	Glottis closed only anteriorly; the larynx shows a small triangular slit posteriorly during phonation; inspiration is normal
Unilateral abductors	The cord lies close to midline; cannot be abducted on inspiration; voice hoarse, but phonation and coughing little affected (adduction is normal); dyspnea uncommon because normal cord abducts on inspiration, but inspiratory stridor may occur
Bilateral abductors	Both cords close to the midline and cannot be abducted; voice hoarse, but phonation little affected and coughing normal because adduction preserved; severe dyspnea with inspiratory stridor
Unilateral adductors	Paralysis of one lateral cricoarytenoid; hoarseness and impairment of coughing
Bilateral adductors	Cords not adducted on phonation and voice either lost or reduced to whisper; inspiration normal without stridor or dyspnea; coughing normal
Total unilateral palsy	Both adduction and abduction affected; involved cord lies in cadaveric position, motionless in midabduction; voice low-pitched and hoarse; difficulty coughing; little or no dyspnea; inspiratory stridor absent or present only with deep inspiration
Total bilateral palsy	Both cords in cadaveric position; phonation and coughing lost; marked dyspnea with stridor, especially on inspiration

Examination of the Autonomic Functions

The autonomic functions of CN X are summarized above and are discussed in more detail in Chapter 45.

Examination of the Sensory Functions

The somatic sensory elements of CN X are discussed above. They are not clinically important and cannot be adequately tested.

Examination of the Reflexes

CN X plays a part in several autonomic, or visceral, reflexes; loss of these reflexes may follow a lesion of the tenth nerve. In some of these reflexes, such as the sternutatory, sucking, and yawning, the vagus plays a supportive role. The nasal, sneeze, or sternutatory reflex is discussed in Chapter 15. Afferent impulses are carried over CN V to the reflex center in the brainstem and upper spinal cord, with efferent impulses primarily by CN VII with some overflow to CNs IX and X and the phrenic nerve. In other reflexes, such as swallowing, vomiting, and coughing, the vagus is central. These are discussed in Box 18.1.

Disorders of Function

A unilateral vagal lesion causes weakness of the soft palate, pharynx, and larynx. Acute lesions may produce difficulty swallowing both liquids and solids

BOX 18.1

Vagally Mediated Reflexes

The oculocardiac reflex is bradycardia caused by pressure on the eyeball. It may also be induced by painful stimulation of the skin on the side of the neck. The afferent limb is carried by cranial nerve (CN) V and the efferent by CN X. The reflex is inconstant, unstandardized, and influenced by emotion. Usually, the pulse is not slowed more than 5 to 8 beats per minute. The slowing may be accompanied by extrasystoles. The oculocardiac reflex may be absent in lesions involving CN X. It is sometimes used to slow an excessively rapid heart rate, as in tachyarrhythmias.

The vomiting reflex produces reverse peristalsis in the esophagus and stomach, with forceful ejection of material from the stomach. The reflex center is in the region of the dorsal efferent nucleus. Vomiting occurs for many reasons. Stimulation of the pharynx, palate, esophagus, stomach, duodenum, or lower gastrointestinal tract may activate the reflex. The afferent limb is carried by CN X, probably to the solitary tract; from there, the impulse is relayed to the dorsal efferent nucleus and also down the spinal cord to contract the diaphragm and abdominal muscles, relax the cardiac sphincter, and contract the pyloric sphincter. The swallowing reflex is caused by stimulation of the pharyngeal wall or back of the tongue. Afferent impulses travel through CNs V, IX, and X and efferent impulses through CNs IX, X, and XII. The cough reflex is activated by stimulation of the mucous membrane of the pharynx, larynx, trachea, or bronchial tree. Stimulation of the tympanic membrane or external auditory canal can also elicit a cough response (mitempfindung). The afferent limb of the reflex is carried through CNs IX and X to the solitary tract, and the efferent impulses descend to the pharyngeal muscles, tongue, palate, and larynx and to the diaphragm, chest, and abdominal muscles.

Hiccup (singultus) is a sudden reflex contraction of the diaphragm causing a forceful inspiration. Associated laryngeal spasm causes the glottis to snap shut, causing sudden arrest of the inspiration and the characteristic sound. The phrenic nerves are the major pathway, but CN X contributes. Yawning is a complex respiratory reflex with deep, prolonged inspiration, usually involuntary, through the open mouth. It typically occurs during sleepiness and fatigue but may also be brought on by suggestion or boredom. Yawning can occur in neurologic disease as well.

The carotid sinus reflex is produced by stimulation of the carotid sinus or the carotid body by pressure at the carotid bifurcation. It causes slowing of the heart rate, a fall in blood pressure, a decrease in cardiac output, and peripheral vasodilatation. When the response is exaggerated, there may be syncope. The afferent limb of the reflex is carried over CN IX and the efferent over CN X. The carotid sinus reflex is discussed further under CN IX.

and hoarseness or a nasal quality to the voice. The only definite sensory change is anesthesia of the larynx because of involvement of the superior laryngeal nerve. It is seldom possible to demonstrate loss of sensation behind the pinna and in the external auditory canal. The gag reflex is absent on the involved side. Autonomic reflexes (vomiting, coughing, and sneezing) are not usually affected. Tachycardia and loss of the oculocardiac reflex on the involved side may occur, but usually there are no cardiac symptoms. Gastrointestinal disturbances are inconspicuous. Bilateral complete vagal paralysis is incompatible with life. It causes complete paralysis of the palate, pharynx, and larynx, with marked dysphagia and dysarthria; tachycardia; slow, irregular, respiration; vomiting; and gastrointestinal atonia. Lesions of individual vagal branches are rare except for involvement of the recurrent laryngeal nerve.

The primary effect of increased vagal activity is bradycardia. The term vasovagal refers to the effects of the vagus nerve on the blood vessels. Vasovagal attacks (fainting, syncope) are characterized by bradycardia, hypotension, peripheral vasoconstriction, and faintness, sometimes with loss of consciousness. Vasovagal attacks are typically induced by strong emotion or pain. The bradycardia and projectile vomiting that occur with increased intracranial pressure may be vagally mediated. Cheyne-Stokes, Biot, and Kussmaul breathing; respiratory tics; forced yawning; and other abnormalities of breathing may be vagally mediated as well. Spasm of pharyngeal muscles can occur in certain central nervous system disorders. Other conditions in which there is increased activity in the vagal system are seldom of primary neurologic origin.

Rhythmic movements of the palate (palatal myoclonus, palatal microtremor, or palatal nystagmus) can occur with a lesion of the brainstem, usually vascular **(Video 30.7)**. The movements are mediated by CN X. Palatal myoclonus is discussed further in Chapter 30. The very rare syndrome of superior laryngeal neuralgia causes lancinating pains that radiate from the larynx to the ear.

Unilateral supranuclear lesions generally cause no dysfunction because of bilateral innervation; dysphagia from a unilateral lesion can occur but is rare. Bilateral supranuclear lesions, as from pseudobulbar palsy, cause dysphagia and dysarthria (Chapter 21). Extrapyramidal disorders may produce difficulty with swallowing and talking. Patients with Parkinson's disease typically have a hypokinetic dysarthria (Chapter 9). Laryngeal spasm with stridor may occur in Parkinson's disease and other extrapyramidal disorders. The voice is commonly affected by essential tremor.

Nuclear lesions of the nucleus ambiguus can occur with any intrinsic brainstem disease. A slowly progressive nuclear lesion, such as in bulbar ALS, syringomyelia, and some neoplasms, may cause fasciculations in the palatal, pharyngeal, and laryngeal muscles. The speech disturbances are discussed in Chapter 9. Lesions of the nucleus ambiguus or intramedullary fibers of CNs IX and X commonly occur with vascular disease, for example, lateral medullary (Wallenberg) syndrome. Nuclear lesions are usually associated with involvement of other CN nuclei and long motor or sensory tracts. Because of the somatotopic organization, lesions limited to the rostral portion of the nucleus ambiguus may produce only weakness of the palate and pharynx, sparing laryngeal functions.

Infranuclear involvement may occur with lesions at the base of the brain, in the cerebellopontine angle, in the jugular foramen, or along the course of the vagus nerves. Extramedullary, intracranial involvement can occur in processes involving the meninges, extramedullary tumors, aneurysms, trauma, sarcoidosis, and skull fractures. Other lower CNs are usually involved as well (Chapter 21). Lesions at the jugular foramen or in the retroparotid space usually involve some combination of CNs IX, X, XI, and XII and the cervical sympathetics. These lower CN syndromes are discussed in Chapter 21. Isolated or multiple lower CN palsies can be a manifestation of dissecting aneurysm of the cervical internal carotid artery or occur as a complication of carotid endarterectomy. Isolated CN IX palsy has been reported as a complication of traumatic internal maxillary artery dissection.

The main trunk of the vagus may be injured in the neck or thorax by trauma, carotid aneurysms, or other mass lesions. Vocal cord and diaphragmatic weakness occur in some forms of Charcot-Marie-Tooth disease. Individual vagal branches may be involved by disease processes in the neck, upper mediastinum, thorax, and abdomen. The recurrent laryngeal nerve is the most frequently affected; the left is more often damaged than the right because of its longer course. The recurrent laryngeals may be damaged by tumors in the neck, especially carcinoma of the thyroid, cervical adenopathy, metastatic lesions, Hodgkin disease, lymphosarcoma, aortic aneurysms, mitral stenosis with enlargement of the left atrium, pericarditis, mediastinal and apical tumors, stab wounds in the neck, or accidental trauma during a thyroidectomy or other surgical procedure. Recurrent laryngeal weakness causes a flaccid dysphonia with breathiness and mild inspiratory stridor; palatopharyngeal functions are preserved. Diplophonia may occur because of unbalanced vocal cord vibration frequency. Compression of the left recurrent laryngeal nerve between the aorta and the pulmonary artery because of a variety of cardiovascular disorders may cause hoarseness (cardiovocal or Ortner's syndrome). Bilateral recurrent laryngeal palsies cause abduction impairment and leave the vocal cords approximating each other in the midline; the most common cause is thyroid surgery. This results in dyspnea and inspiratory stridor. The superior laryngeal and pharyngeal branches may be involved in trauma, or in neoplasms or abscesses in the neck, but clinical dysfunction is scant because of the primarily sensory function of the nerve; there may be mild hoarseness because of weakness of the cricothyroid muscle. Metastatic breast cancer infiltrating behind the carotid sheath at C6 has been reported to produce a combination of recurrent laryngeal and phrenic nerve dysfunction with an accompanying Horner syndrome. Hoarseness and voice fatigue because of laryngeal involvement may be prominent in rare patients with myasthenia gravis.

Syncope, sometimes associated with paroxysmal neck pain, may occur because of neoplasms involving the carotid sinus nerve. The mechanism is probably similar to that seen in syncope due to glossopharyngeal neuralgia. Swallow syncope results from dysfunction, usually because of metastatic disease, of CNs IX and X. The patient develops bradycardia and hypotension because of involvement of the baroreceptor nerves.

Video Links

Video Link 18.1. Palatal deviation. http://neurosigns.org/wiki/Palatal_deviation

Video Link 18.2. Spasmodic dysphonia. http://neurosigns.org/wiki/Spasmodic_dysphonia

BIBLIOGRAPHY

Aguiar PH Jr, Tella OI Jr, Pereira CU, et al. Chiari type I presenting as left glossopharyngeal neuralgia with cardiac syncope. *Neurosurg Rev* 2002;25:99–102.

Ahn JY, Chung YS, Chung SS, et al. Traumatic dissection of the internal maxillary artery associated with isolated glossopharyngeal nerve palsy: case report. *Neurosurgery* 2004;55:710.

Arnold RW, Dyer JA Jr, Gould AB Jr, et al. Sensitivity to vasovagal maneuvers in normal children and adults. *Mayo Clin Proc* 1991;66:797–804.

Arts HA, Fagan PA. Vagal body tumors. *Otolaryngol Head Neck Surg* 1991;105:78–85.

Barbash GI, Keren G, Korczyn AD, et al. Mechanisms of syncope in glossopharyngeal neuralgia. *Electroencephalogr Clin Neurophysiol* 1986;63:231–235.

Bindoff LA, Heseltine D. Unilateral facial pain in patients with lung cancer: a referred pain via the vagus? *Lancet* 1988;1:812–815.

Bleach NR. The gag reflex and aspiration: a retrospective analysis of 120 patients assessed by videofluoroscopy. *Clin Otolaryngol* 1993;18:303–307.

Blumenfeld A, Nikolskaya G. Glossopharyngeal neuralgia. *Curr Pain Headache Rep* 2013;17:343.

Brazis PW, Masdeu JC, Biller J. *Localization in Clinical Neurology*. 7th ed. Philadelphia: Wolters Kluwer/Lippincott Williams & Wilkins, 2017.

Buchholz DW, Neumann S. Gag reflex and dysphagia. *Dysphagia* 1997;12:101–102.

Ceylan S, Karakus A, Duru S, et al. Glossopharyngeal neuralgia: a study of 6 cases. *Neurosurg Rev* 1997;20:196–200.

Chester AC. Referred vagal reflexes. *Ann Intern Med* 1992;117:444.

Davies AE, Kidd D, Stone SP, et al. Pharyngeal sensation and gag reflex in healthy subjects. *Lancet* 1995;345:487–488.

De SR, Ranieri A, Bilo L, et al. Cranial neuralgias: from physiopathology to pharmacological treatment. *Neurol Sci* 2008;29(Suppl 1):S69–S78.

Erman AB, Alexandra E, Kejner BS, et al. Disorders of cranial nerves IX and X. *Semin Neurol* 2009;29:85–92.

Flowers RH III, Kernodle DS. Vagal mononeuritis caused by herpes simplex virus: association with unilateral vocal cord paralysis. *Am J Med* 1990;88:686–688.

Gaul C, Hastreiter P, Duncker A, et al. Diagnosis and neurosurgical treatment of glossopharyngeal neuralgia: clinical findings and 3-D visualization of neurovascular compression in 19 consecutive patients. *J Headache Pain* 2011;12:527–534.

Hammond RR, Ebers GC. Chronic cough following cardiac transplantation: vagal Mitempfindung? *J Neurol Neurosurg Psychiatry* 1992;55:723–724.

Hayden MG, Tornabene SV, Nguyen A, et al. Cerebellopontine angle cyst compressing the vagus nerve: case report. *Neurosurgery* 2007;60:E1150.

Horner J, Buoyer FG, Alberts MJ, et al. Dysphagia following brain-stem stroke. Clinical correlates and outcome. *Arch Neurol* 1991;48:1170–1173.

Hughes TA, Wiles CM. Palatal and pharyngeal reflexes in health and in motor neuron disease. *J Neurol Neurosurg Psychiatry* 1996;61:96–98.

Irioka T, Ohta K, Machida A, et al. Vagus nerve palsy caused by varicella zoster virus infection without rash. *J Neurol* 2007;254:1750–1751.

Jacobs CJ, Harnsberger HR, Lufkin RB, et al. Vagal neuropathy: evaluation with CT and MR imaging. *Radiology* 1987;164:97–102.

Katusic S, Williams DB, Beard CM, et al. Incidence and clinical features of glossopharyngeal neuralgia, Rochester, Minnesota, 1945–1984. *Neuroepidemiology* 1991;10:266–275.

Kobata H, Kondo A, Iwasaki K, et al. Combined hyperactive dysfunction syndrome of the cranial nerves: trigeminal neuralgia, hemifacial spasm, and glossopharyngeal neuralgia: 11-year experience and review. *Neurosurgery* 1998;43:1351–1361.

Leder SB. Gag reflex and dysphagia. *Head Neck* 1996;18:138–141.

Leder SB, Espinosa JF. Aspiration risk after acute stroke: comparison of clinical examination and fiberoptic endoscopic evaluation of swallowing. *Dysphagia* 2002;17:214–218.

Levin B, Posner JB. Swallow syncope. Report of a case and review of the literature. *Neurology* 1972;22:1086–1093.

Lim YM, Lee SA, Kim DK, et al. Aneurysm of the extracranial internal carotid artery presenting as the syndrome of glossopharyngeal pain and syncope. *J Neurol Neurosurg Psychiatry* 2002;73:87–88.

Martino R, Foley N, Bhogal S, et al. Dysphagia after stroke: incidence, diagnosis, and pulmonary complications. *Stroke* 2005;36:2756–2763.

Minagar A, Sheremata WA. Glossopharyngeal neuralgia and MS. *Neurology* 2000;54:1368–1370.

Moussouttas M, Tuhrim S. Spontaneous internal carotid artery dissection with isolated vagus nerve deficit. *Neurology* 1998;51:317–318.

Mulpuru SK, Vasavada BC, Punukollu GK, et al. Cardiovocal syndrome: a systematic review. *Heart Lung Circ* 2008;17:1–4.

Myssiorek D. Recurrent laryngeal nerve paralysis: anatomy and etiology. *Otolaryngol Clin North Am* 2004;37:25–44, v.

Nusbaum AO, Som PM, Dubois P, et al. Isolated vagal nerve palsy associated with a dissection of the extracranial internal carotid artery. *AJNR Am J Neuroradiol* 1998;19:1845–1847.

Reddy GD, Viswanathan A. Trigeminal and glossopharyngeal neuralgia. *Neurol Clin* 2014;32:539–552.

Schmall RJ, Dolan KD. Vagal schwannoma. *Ann Otol Rhinol Laryngol* 1992;101:360–362.

Schott GD. Distant referral of cutaneous sensation (Mitempfindung). Observations on its normal and pathological occurrence. *Brain* 1988;111:1187–1198.

Sellars C, Campbell AM, Stott DJ, et al. Swallowing abnormalities after acute stroke: a case control study. *Dysphagia* 1999;14:212–218.

Smithard DG. Percutaneous endoscopic gastrostomy feeding after acute dysphagic stroke. Gag reflex has no role in ability to swallow. *BMJ* 1996;312:972.

Sturzenegger M, Huber P. Cranial nerve palsies in spontaneous carotid artery dissection. *J Neurol Neurosurg Psychiatry* 1993;56:1191–1199.

Sweasey TA, Edelstein SR, Hoff JT. Glossopharyngeal schwannoma: review of five cases and the literature. *Surg Neurol* 1991;35:127–130.

Tang SC, Jeng JS, Liu HM, et al. Isolated vagus nerve palsy probably associated with herpes simplex virus infection. *Acta Neurol Scand* 2001;104:174–177.

Vaghadia H, Spittle M. Newly recognized syndrome in the neck. *J R Soc Med* 1983;76:799.

Yanagisawa K, Kveton JF. Referred otalgia. *Am J Otolaryngol* 1992;13:323–327.

CHAPTER 19

The Spinal Accessory Nerve

ANATOMY AND PHYSIOLOGY

The spinal accessory (SA) nerve, cranial nerve XI (CN XI), is actually two nerves that run together in a common bundle for a short distance. The smaller cranial portion (ramus internus) is a special visceral efferent (SVE) accessory to the vagus. Arising from cells within the caudal nucleus ambiguus, with some contribution from the dorsal motor nucleus of the vagus, it emerges from the medulla laterally as four or five rootlets caudal to the vagal filaments. The cranial root runs to the jugular foramen and unites with the spinal portion, traveling with it for only a few millimeters to form the main trunk of CN XI. The cranial root communicates with the jugular ganglion of the vagus and then exits through the jugular foramen separately from the spinal portion. It passes through the ganglion nodosum and then blends with the vagus (Figure 19.1). It is distributed principally with the recurrent laryngeal nerve to sixth branchial arch muscles in the larynx, and its contribution is indistinguishable from that of the vagus except there is no CN XI contribution to the cricothyroid muscle. A few fibers that originate in the dorsal motor nucleus may contribute parasympathetic fibers to the cardiac branches of the vagus. Lachman et al. have questioned whether the cranial root of the SA nerve even exists.

The major part of CN XI is the spinal portion (ramus externus). Its function is to innervate the sternocleidomastoid (SCM) and trapezius muscles. The fibers of the spinal root arise from SVE motor cells in the SA nuclei in the ventral horn from C2 to C5, or even C6. The cell column of the SA nucleus lies in a position analogous to the nucleus ambiguus in the medulla. The cell column making up the SA nucleus is somatotopically organized. The upper spinal cord portion innervates primarily the ipsilateral SCM; the lower spinal portion innervates primarily the ipsilateral trapezius. In keeping with the tendency of branchial arch–related nerves to make internal loops, its axons arch posterolaterally through the lateral funiculus and emerge as a series of rootlets laterally between the anterior and posterior roots. These unite into a single trunk, which ascends between the denticulate ligaments and the posterior roots. The nerve enters the skull through the foramen magnum, ascends the clivus for a short distance, and then curves laterally. The spinal root joins the cranial root for a short distance, probably receiving one or two filaments from it. It exits through the jugular foramen in company with CNs IX and X.

CN XI emerges from the skull posteromedial to the styloid process and then descends in the neck near the internal jugular vein, behind the digastric and stylohyoid muscles, to enter the deep surface of the upper part of the SCM muscle. It passes through the SCM, sending filaments to it, and then emerges at its posterior border near the midpoint, coursing near the great auricular nerve. CN XI then runs obliquely across the posterior triangle of the neck on the surface of the levator scapula muscle, superficially and in close proximity to the lymph nodes of the posterior cervical triangle. About three fingerbreadths above the clavicle, the nerve enters the deep surface of the anterior border of the upper trapezius muscle. In the neck, the SA contributes fibers to the cervical plexus, rami trapezii, and then courses to the caudal aspect of the trapezius. Most of the communications with C2 through C4 are conveying proprioceptive information from CN XI, which will enter the spinal cord in the upper cervical segments. The innervation of the SCM may be more complex than is to be found in most anatomical texts, possibly including fibers from CN X. Over half of the patients undergoing division of the SA nerve and the upper cervical motor roots as treatment for cervical dystonia had residual SCM activity of sufficient magnitude to make further surgery necessary before the muscle was effectively paralyzed.

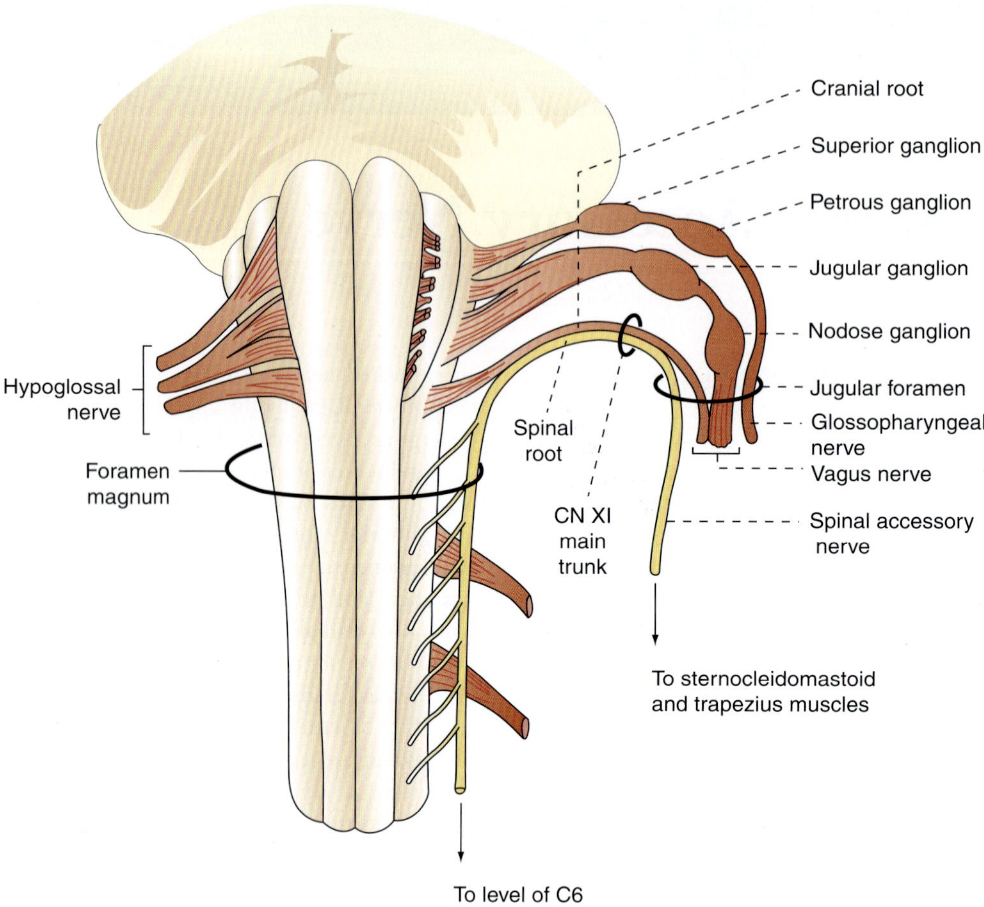

FIGURE 19.1 Relationship of the cranial and spinal portions of the accessory nerve to the vagus and glossopharyngeal nerves.

The innervation of the trapezius shows some individual variability. The SA nerve is the primary innervation to the upper trapezius, but Soo et al. have shown that the cervical plexus may contribute motor fibers, especially to the middle and lower trapezius. The neurons of the spinal portion of XI communicate with the oculomotor, trochlear, abducens, and vestibular nuclei through the medial longitudinal fasciculus. These connections are important in controlling conjugate deviation of the head and eyes in response to auditory, vestibular, and other stimuli.

The supranuclear innervation of CN XI arises from the lower portion of the precentral gyrus. Fibers from the lateral corticospinal tract in the cervical spinal cord communicate with the SA nucleus. There is some controversy, but the bulk of current evidence indicates that both the SCM and trapezius receive bilateral supranuclear innervation. However, the input to the SCM motor neuron pool is predominantly ipsilateral and that to the trapezius motor neuron pool is predominantly contralateral (Box 19.1). The SCM turns the head to the opposite side, and its supranuclear innervation is ipsilateral. Therefore, the right cerebral hemisphere turns the head to the left.

The SCM muscles function with the other cervical muscles to flex the head and turn it from side to side. When one SCM contracts, the head is drawn toward the ipsilateral shoulder and rotates so that the occiput is pulled toward the ipsilateral shoulder, while the face turns in the opposite direction and upward. Acting together, the two muscles flex the neck and bring the head forward and downward. With the head fixed, the two muscles assist in elevating the thorax in forced inspiration.

The trapezius retracts the head and draws it ipsilaterally. It also elevates, retracts, and rotates the scapula and assists in abducting the arm above horizontal. When one trapezius contracts with the

BOX 19.1

Cortical Innervation of the Sternocleidomastoid Muscle

The sternocleidomastoid (SCM) may be an exception to the general scheme of contralateral hemispheric innervation. Authorities debate whether the SCMs receive ipsilateral, contralateral, or bilateral cortical innervation. Studying the function of the SCM muscles during intracarotid injection of amytal (Wada testing), DeToledo et al. demonstrated weakness of the right SCM after injection into the right internal carotid artery in some patients and little to no weakness in others. This suggested that the SCMs receive bilateral hemispheric innervation with the maximal input from the ipsilateral hemisphere. They proposed that the SA nucleus has rostral and caudal portions and that the rostral (SCM) portion receives bihemispheric projections, but the innervation of the caudal (trapezius) portion is predominantly contralateral. This would be analogous to the supranuclear innervation of the facial nerve nucleus, bilateral to the rostral portions but contralateral to the caudal portions. Transcranial stimulation studies concluded projections to the SCM were bilateral but predominantly contralateral, and those to the trapezius exclusively contralateral. Some have contended the nerve double decussates, but this remains unproven.

shoulder fixed, the head is drawn to that side. When both contract, the head is drawn backward and the face deviated upward. When the head is fixed, the upper and middle fibers of the trapezius elevate, rotate, and retract the scapula and shorten the distance between the occiput and the acromion. The lower fibers depress the scapula and draw it toward the midline. The SCM and trapezius muscles thus act together to rotate the head from side to side and to flex and extend the neck.

CLINICAL EXAMINATION

The functions of the cranial portion of CN XI cannot be distinguished from those of CN X, and examination is limited to evaluation of the functions of the spinal portion. A complex array of many muscles is involved in moving the head, including the scaleni, splenii and obliqui capitis, recti capitis, and longi capitis and colli. With bilateral paralysis of CN XI–innervated muscles, there is diminished but not absent neck rotation, and the head may droop or even fall backward or forward, depending upon whether the SCMs or the trapezii are more involved.

One SCM acts to turn the head to the opposite side or to tilt it to the same side. Acting together, the SCMs thrust the head forward and flex the neck. The muscles should be inspected and palpated to determine their tone and volume. The contours are distinct even at rest. With a nuclear or infranuclear lesion, there may be atrophy or fasciculations.

To assess SCM power, have the patient turn the head fully to one side and hold it there, and then try to turn the head back to midline, avoiding any tilting or leaning motion. The muscle usually stands out well, and its contraction can be seen and felt (Figure 19.2). Significant weakness of rotation can be detected if the patient tries to counteract firm resistance. Unilateral SCM paresis causes little change in the resting position of the head. Even with complete paralysis, other cervical muscles can perform some degree of rotation and flexion; only occasionally is there a noticeable head turn. The two SCM muscles can be examined simultaneously by having the

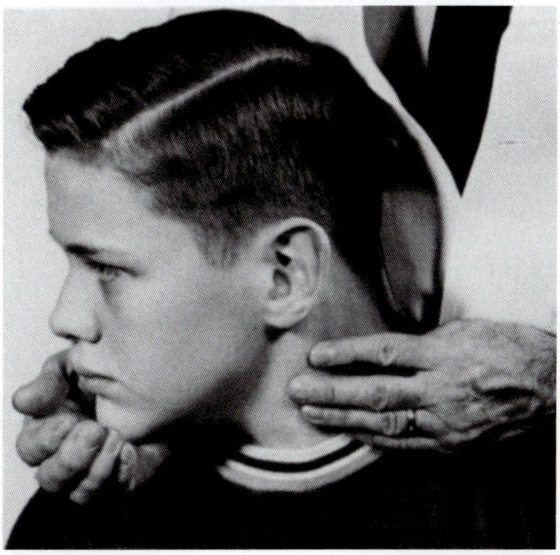

FIGURE 19.2 Examination of the sternocleidomastoid (SCM) muscle. When the patient turns his head to the right against resistance, the contracting muscle can be seen and palpated.

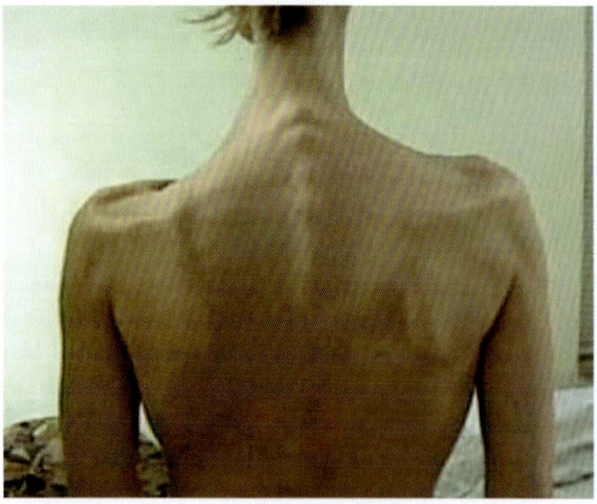

FIGURE 19.3 Paralysis of the left trapezius muscle. There is a depression in the shoulder contour with downward and lateral displacement of the scapula. (Reprinted with permission from Kelley MJ, Kane TE, Leggin BG. Spinal accessory nerve palsy: associated signs and symptoms. *J Orthop Sports Phys Ther* 2008;38(2):78–86. https://doi.org/10.2519/jospt.2008.2454. Copyright © Journal of Orthopaedic & Sports Physical Therapy®.)

patient flex his neck while the examiner exerts pressure on the forehead or by having the patient turn the head from side to side. Flexion of the head against resistance may cause deviation of the head toward the paralyzed side. With unilateral paralysis, the involved muscle is flat and does not contract or become tense when attempting to turn the head contralaterally or to flex the neck against resistance. Weakness of both SCMs causes difficulty in anteroflexion of the neck, and the head may assume an extended position. The SCM reflex may be elicited by tapping the muscle at its clavicular origin. Usually, there is a prompt contraction. The reflex is mediated by the accessory and upper cervical nerves, but has little significance in neurologic diagnosis.

With trapezius atrophy, the outline of the neck changes, with depression or drooping of the shoulder contour and flattening of the trapezius ridge (Figure 19.3). Severe trapezius weakness causes sagging of the shoulder, and the resting position of the scapula shifts downward. The upper portion of the scapula tends to fall laterally, while the inferior angle moves inward. This scapular rotation and displacement are more obvious with arm abduction.

The strength of the trapezius is traditionally tested by having the patient shrug the shoulders against resistance (Figure 19.4). However, much of shoulder shrugging is due to the action of the levator scapulae. A better test of the upper trapezius is resisting the patient's attempt to approximate the occiput to the acromion. The movement may be observed and the contraction seen and palpated. To examine the middle and lower trapezius, place the patient's abducted arm horizontally, palm up, and attempt to push the elbow forward. Muscle power should be compared on the two sides. In unilateral weakness of the trapezius, these movements are impaired.

The trapezius is one of several muscles that act to stabilize the scapula and create a platform for movements of the humerus. The serratus anterior protracts

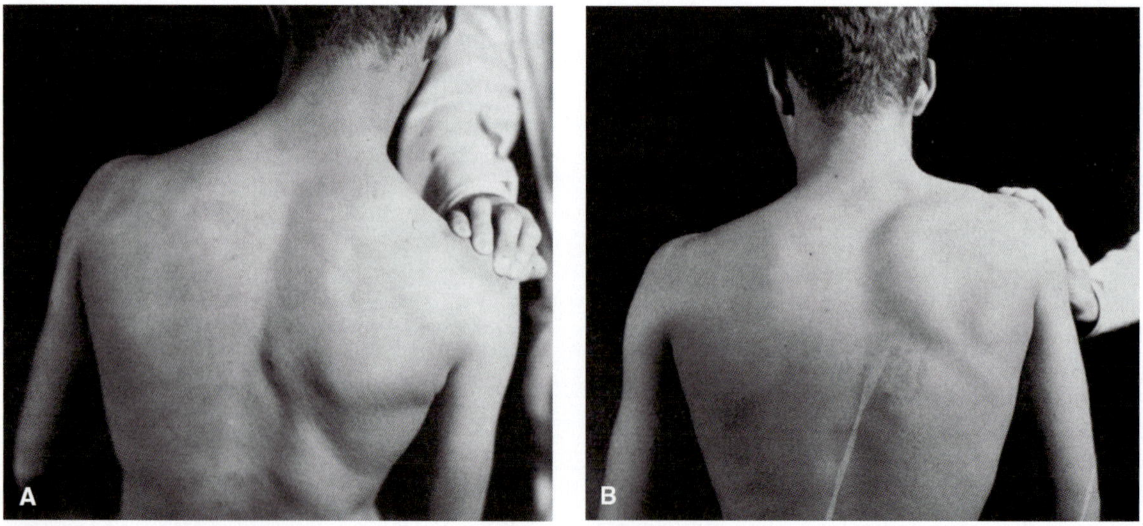

FIGURE 19.4 Examination of the trapezius muscle. **A.** Examiner pressing the shoulder down against patient's resistance. **B.** Patient attempting to elevate shoulder against examiner's resistance.

the scapula, moving it forward as in a boxing jab. The trapezius is a synergist to the main mover, the rhomboids, in retracting the scapula. The trapezius and serratus anterior act in concert to rotate the scapula when the arm is abducting. The trapezius brings the glenoid fossa progressively more cephalad so that the abduction motion is unrestricted. In addition, contraction of the upper trapezius adds the final few degrees of abduction, after the glenohumeral and acromioclavicular ranges of motion are exhausted, so that the arm can be brought directly overhead (Figure 27.4).

Weakness of the trapezius disrupts the normal scapulohumeral rhythm and impairs arm abduction. Impairment of upper trapezius function causes weakness of abduction beyond 90 degrees. Weakness of the middle trapezius muscle causes winging of the scapula. The winging because of trapezius weakness is more apparent on lateral abduction in contrast to the winging due to serratus anterior weakness, which is greatest with the arm held in front. In fact, with winging due to trapezius weakness, the jutting of the inferior angle lessens when the arm is raised anteriorly; in winging due to serratus anterior weakness, it worsens. Scapular winging is discussed further in Chapter 27. For videos of scapular winging, see **Video Links 19.1** and **19.2**.

When the trapezius is weak, the arm hangs lower on the affected side, and the fingertips touch the thigh at a lower level than on the normal side. Placing the palms together with the arms extended anteriorly and slightly below horizontal shows the fingers on the affected side extending beyond those of the normal side. The drooping of the arm and shoulder caused by trapezius weakness may lead to pain and subjective sensory complaints in the extremity because of traction on musculoligamentous structures and possibly sensory nerves. Loss of shoulder mobility may result in a secondary adhesive capsulitis, which further restricts motion.

The two trapezius muscles can be examined simultaneously by having the patient extend his neck against resistance. Bilateral paralysis causes weakness of neck extension. The patient cannot raise his chin, and the head may tend to fall forward (Dropped Head Syndrome, see below). The shoulders look square or have a drooping, sagging appearance because of atrophy of both muscles. The relationship of the trapezius muscle to the movements of the shoulder girdle and the examination of the functions of its lower fibers are discussed in Chapter 27.

DISORDERS OF FUNCTION

Weakness of the muscles supplied by CN XI may be caused by supranuclear, nuclear, or infranuclear lesions. Supranuclear involvement usually causes at worst moderate loss of function because innervation is at least partially bilateral in most patients. In hemiplegia, there is usually no head deviation, but testing may reveal slight, rarely marked, weakness of the SCM, with difficulty turning the face toward the involved limbs. When significant SCM paresis is present, the head may be turned away from the weak limbs, indicating weakness of the SCM ipsilateral to the lesion with the preserved SCM turning the head toward the lesion. This occurs with lesions involving the corticobulbar fibers at any level from the cortex to the brainstem. There may be depression of the shoulder resulting from trapezius weakness on the affected side.

Irritative supranuclear lesions may cause head turning away from the discharging hemisphere. This turning of the head (or head and eyes) may occur as part of a contraversive, ipsiversive, or jacksonian seizure and is often the first manifestation of the seizure. Extrapyramidal lesions may also involve the SCM and trapezius muscles, causing rigidity, akinesia, or hyperkinesis (Chapter 30). Abnormal involuntary movements of the head and neck are seen in chorea, athetosis, dystonia musculorum deformans, and other dyskinesias. The SCM and trapezius are frequently involved in cervical dystonia, a common focal dystonia causing torticollis, anterocollis, or retrocollis (Chapter 30). Cervical dystonia occasionally causes hypertrophy of the SCM (Figure 19.5).

Lesions of the lower brainstem or upper cervical spinal cord may cause dissociated weakness of the SCM and trapezius muscles depending on the exact location. Nuclear involvement of the SA nerve may occur in motor neuron disease, syringobulbia, and syringomyelia. In nuclear lesions, the weakness is frequently accompanied by atrophy and fasciculations.

Infranuclear or peripheral lesions—either extramedullary but within the skull, in the jugular foramen, or in the neck—are the most common causes of impairment of function of the SA nerve. Tumors in the foramen magnum or along the clivus can compress CN XI, usually with concomitant CNs IX and X involvement. Lesions of the cerebellopontine angle occasionally extend caudal toward the foramen

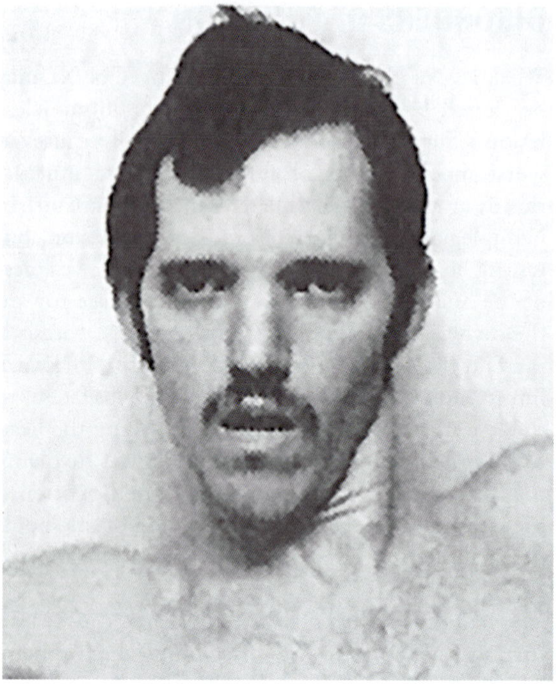

FIGURE 19.5 Marked hypertrophy of the left sternocleidomastoid because of cervical dystonia. (Modified from Jankovic J, Tolosa E. *Parkinson's Disease & Movement Disorders*. 6th ed. Philadelphia: Wolters Kluwer, 2015, with permission.)

magnum and involve CN XI. Tumors more caudal may extend upward; most common are neurinomas of the hypoglossal nerve. Neurinomas involving CN IX or X may extend to involve CN XI. Other intracranial, extramedullary neoplasms include meningiomas and neurofibromas, which may extend through the jugular foramen in dumbbell fashion. Basal skull fractures, meningitis, or processes at or just distal to the skull base give rise to a number of syndromes reflecting involvement of the lower CNs (Chapter 21). The most common is the jugular foramen syndrome, in which the SA nerve is involved along with CNs IX and X (Chapter 21). Such conditions affect both the SCM and the trapezius.

In the posterior triangle of the neck, the SA nerve is very vulnerable, because it lies superficially, covered only by skin and subcutaneous tissue. The nerve may be affected by severe cervical adenopathy, neoplasms, trauma, or abscesses. These lesions are generally distal to the SCM and affect only trapezius function. The most common cause of SA neuropathy in the posterior triangle is trauma, often iatrogenic. Surgical trauma may be unavoidable, as in radical neck dissection, or inadvertent, as in lymph node biopsy. The procedures most commonly implicated are lymph node biopsy and carotid endarterectomy. Intraoperative traction on the SCM may stretch the branch to the trapezius. Intraoperative monitoring may decrease the likelihood of injury. In one series of 111 patients with SA injury, 93% were iatrogenic and 80% of those injuries were from lymph node biopsy.

Traction injury may occur when the shoulder is pulled down and the head turned in the opposite direction. Carrying heavy loads on the shoulder may cause SA injury because of local trauma or stretch. Other causes of SA neuropathy include jugular vein cannulation, upper cervical spine hyperextension injury, cervical internal carotid artery dissection, neuralgic amyotrophy (Parsonage-Turner syndrome), radiotherapy, coronary artery bypass surgery, human bites to the neck, shoulder dislocation, attempted hanging, mononeuritis multiplex, and nerve tumors such as schwannoma or neurinoma.

Spontaneous, idiopathic cases of isolated SA palsy, often benign and self-limited, are likely comparable to similar focal neuropathies, such as Bell's palsy or long thoracic nerve palsy, or may represent a restricted type of neuralgic amyotrophy. In these cases, the onset is typically sudden with pain in the posterior triangle, which resolves and is followed by SA palsy.

Neuromuscular disorders that affect the SCM and trapezius muscles include anterior horn cell disease, myasthenia gravis, inflammatory myopathies, and facioscapulohumeral dystrophy. Atrophy and weakness of both SCM muscles is a prominent feature of myotonic dystrophy (Figure 19.6). The "dropped head syndrome," characterized by severe neck extensor weakness and an inability to hold the head up, occurs in a variety of neuromuscular disorders (Box 19.2, Figure 19.7).

Patients with traumatic SA neuropathies generally have poorer long-term outcomes than those with neuropathies of other etiologies. Dominant limb involvement, impaired arm abduction, and scapular winging are all associated with a poor outcome. Trapezius weakness may lead to drooping of the shoulder with resultant compression of the neurovascular bundle at the thoracic outlet.

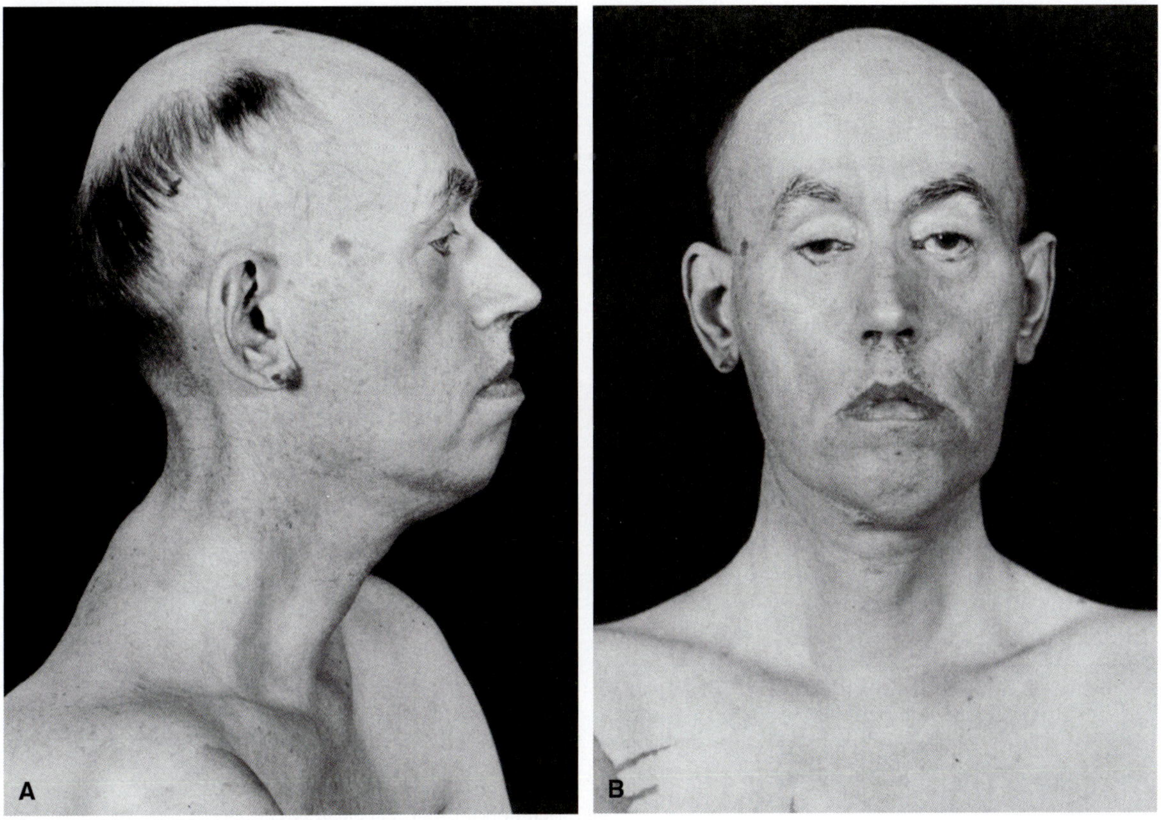

FIGURE 19.6 A patient with myotonic dystrophy. There is atrophy of the SCM muscles.

BOX 19.2

Dropped Head Syndrome

Severe weakness of the neck extensors leads to an inability to hold the head up. The most common causes of the dropped head syndrome (head ptosis, floppy head, camptocormia) are inflammatory myopathy, ALS, and myasthenia gravis. In these conditions, posterior paraspinal muscle weakness can occur early and selectively, and head drop may be the presenting manifestation of the disease. It is common in the later stages of facioscapulohumeral dystrophy and some forms of spinal muscular atrophy. Some cases are due to a relatively benign isolated neck extensor myopathy, an idiopathic restricted noninflammatory myopathy. The "bent spine syndrome," related to thoracic paraspinal weakness, may cause a similar head posture.

Rare causes include adult-onset acid maltase deficiency, chronic inflammatory demyelinating polyneuropathy, desmin myopathy, nemaline myopathy, mitochondrial myopathy, hypothyroid myopathy, hyperparathyroidism, Lambert-Eaton syndrome, myasthenia gravis, and myotonic dystrophy. Dropped head syndrome from neck extensor weakness may be confused with anterocollis because of cervical dystonia. This flexed neck posture is also common in Parkinson's disease, but neck extension strength is unimpaired. Dropped head syndrome has also been reported in syringomyelia.

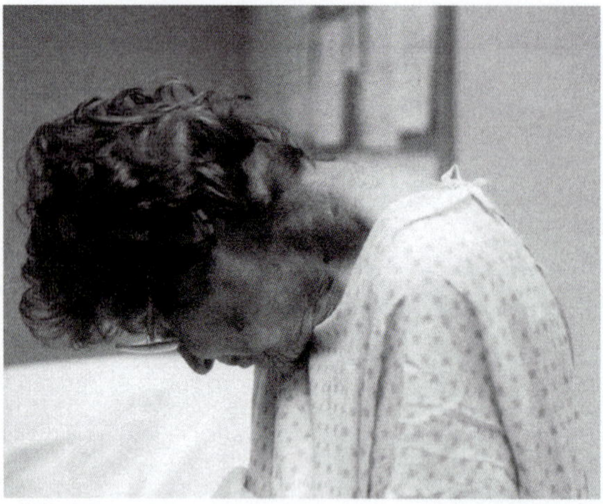

FIGURE 19.7 Dropped head syndrome due to isolated neck extensor myopathy. (From Katz JS, Wolfe GI, Burns DK, et al. Isolated neck extensor myopathy: a common cause of dropped head syndrome. *Neurology* 1996;46[4]:917–921.)

Video Links

Video Link 19.1. Scapular winging. http://www.youtube.com/watch?v=dfTe0nPclDE

Video Link 19.2. Scapular winging. http://neurosigns.org/wiki/Scapular_winging

BIBLIOGRAPHY

Al-Shekhlee A, Katirji B. Spinal accessory neuropathy, droopy shoulder, and thoracic outlet syndrome. *Muscle Nerve* 2003;28:383–385.

Askmark H, Olsson Y, Rossitti S. Treatable dropped head syndrome in hypothyroidism. *Neurology* 2000;55:896–897.

Barbagallo G, Arabia G, Valentino P, et al. Anti-GAD-associated inflammatory myopathy presenting with dropped head syndrome. *Neurol Sci* 2015;36:1517–1519.

Berardelli A, Priori A. Corticobulbar and corticospinal projections to neck muscle motoneurons in man. A functional study with magnetic and electric transcranial brain stimulation. *Exp Brain Res* 1991;87:402–406.

Berry H, Ea M, Mrazek AC. Accessory nerve palsy: a review of 23 cases. *Can J Neurol Sci* 1991;18:337.

Brazis PW, Masdeu JC, Biller J. *Localization in Clinical Neurology*. 7th ed. Philadelphia: Wolters Kluwer/Lippincott Williams & Wilkins, 2017.

D'Amelio M, Di Benedetto N, Ragonese P, et al. Dropped head as an unusual presenting sign of myasthenia gravis. *Neurol Sci* 2007;28:104–106.

DeToledo JC, David NJ. Innervation of the sternocleidomastoid and trapezius muscles by the accessory nucleus. *J Neuroophthalmol* 2001;21:214–216.

DeToledo JC, Dow R. Sternomastoid function during hemispheric suppression by amytal: insights into the inputs to the spinal accessory nerve nucleus. *Mov Disord* 1998;13:809–812.

Dominick J, Sheean G, Schleimer J, et al. Response of the dropped head/bent spine syndrome to treatment with intravenous immunoglobulin. *Muscle Nerve* 2006;33:824–826.

Fitzgerald T. Sternomastoid paradox. *Clin Anat* 2001;14:330–331.

Friedenberg SM, Zimprich T, Harper CM. The natural history of long thoracic and spinal accessory neuropathies. *Muscle Nerve* 2002;25:535–539.

Gandevia SC, Applegate C. Activation of neck muscles from the human motor cortex. *Brain* 1988;111:801–813.

Goh KJ, Wong KT, Tan CT. Myopathic dropped head syndrome: a syndrome of mixed aetiology. *J Clin Neurosci* 2000;7:334–336.

Hayward R. Observations on the innervation of the sternomastoid muscle. *J Neurol Neurosurg Psychiatry* 1986;49:951–953.

Kastrup A, Gdynia HJ, Nagele T, et al. Dropped-head syndrome due to steroid responsive focal myositis: a case report and review of the literature. *J Neurol Sci* 2008;267:162–165.

Katz JS, Wolfe GI, Burns DK, et al. Isolated neck extensor myopathy: a common cause of dropped head syndrome. *Neurology* 1996;46:917–921.

Kierner AC, Zelenka I, Heller S, et al. Surgical anatomy of the spinal accessory nerve and the trapezius branches of the cervical plexus. *Arch Surg* 2000;135:1428–1431.

Kim DH, Cho YJ, Tiel RL, et al. Surgical outcomes of 111 spinal accessory nerve injuries. *Neurosurgery* 2003;53:1106–1112.

Lachman N, Acland RD, Rosse C. Anatomical evidence for the absence of a morphologically distinct cranial root of the accessory nerve in man. *Clin Anat* 2002;15:4–10.

London J, London NJ, Kay SP. Iatrogenic accessory nerve injury. *Ann R Coll Surg Engl* 1996;78:146–150.

Lu L, Haman SP, Ebraheim NA. Vulnerability of the spinal accessory nerve in the posterior triangle of the neck: a cadaveric study. *Orthopedics* 2002;25:71–74.

Manon-Espaillat R, Ruff RL. Dissociated weakness of sternocleidomastoid and trapezius muscles with lesions in the CNS. *Neurology* 1988;38:796–797.

Massey EW. Spinal accessory nerve lesions. *Semin Neurol* 2009;29:82–84.

Matz PE, Barbaro NM. Diagnosis and treatment of iatrogenic spinal accessory nerve injury. *Am Surg* 1996;62:682–685.

Midwinter K, Willatt D. Accessory nerve monitoring and stimulation during neck surgery. *J Laryngol Otol* 2002;116:272–274.

Mokri B, Silvert PL, Schievink WI, et al. Cranial nerve palsy in spontaneous dissection of the extracranial internal carotid artery. *Neurology* 1996;46:356–359.

Nalini A, Ravishankar S. "Dropped head syndrome" in syringomyelia: report of two cases. *J Neurol Neurosurg Psychiatry* 2005;76:290–291.

Nori S, Soo KC, Green RF, et al. Utilization of intraoperative electroneurography to understand the innervation of the trapezius muscle. *Muscle Nerve* 1997;20:279–285.

Ortiz O, Reed L. Spinal accessory nerve schwannoma involving the jugular foramen. *AJNR Am J Neuroradiol* 1995;16:986–989.

Parent A. *Carpenter's Human Neuroanatomy*. 9th ed. Baltimore: Williams & Wilkins, 1996.

Patten C, Hillel AD. The 11th nerve syndrome. Accessory nerve palsy or adhesive capsulitis? *Arch Otolaryngol Head Neck Surg* 1993;119:215–220.

Pierre PA, Laterre CE, Van den Bergh PY. Neuralgic amyotrophy with involvement of cranial nerves IX, X, XI and XII. *Muscle Nerve* 1990;13:704–707.

Rescigno JA, Felice KJ. Spinal accessory mononeuropathy following posterior fossa decompression surgery. *Acta Neurol Scand* 2002;105:326–329.

Rymanowski JV, Twydell PT. Treatable dropped head syndrome in hyperparathyroidism. *Muscle Nerve* 2009;39:409–410.

Sweeney PJ, Wilbourn AJ. Spinal accessory (11th) nerve palsy following endarterectomy. *Neurology* 1992;42:674–675.

Takeshi Y, Mai Y, Kinjo M, et al. Dropped head syndrome and the presence of rimmed vacuoles in a muscle biopsy in scleroderma-polymyositis overlap syndrome associated with anti-Ku antibody. *Intern Med* 2018;57(6):887–891.

Ueda T, Kanda F, Kobessho H, et al. "Dropped head syndrome" caused by Lambert-Eaton myasthenic syndrome. *Muscle Nerve* 2009;40:134–136.

Uemura M, Kosaka T, Shimohata T, et al. Dropped head syndrome in amyotrophic lateral sclerosis. *Amyotroph Lateral Scler Frontotemporal Degener* 2013;14:232–233.

Umapathi T, Chaudhry V, Cornblath D, et al. Head drop and camptocormia. *J Neurol Neurosurg Psychiatry* 2002;73:1–7.

Vengalil S, Preethish-Kumar V, Polavarapu K, et al. Fatty acid oxidation defects presenting as primary myopathy and prominent dropped head syndrome. *Neuromuscul Disord* 2017;27:986–996.

Willoughby EW, Anderson NE. Lower cranial nerve motor function in unilateral vascular lesions of the cerebral hemisphere. *Br Med J* 1984;289:791–794.

Wills AJ, Sawle GV. Accessory nerve palsies. *Pract Neurol* 2010;10:191–194.

Wilson-Pauwels L, Akesson EJ, Stewart PA, et al. *Cranial Nerves in Health and Disease.* 2nd ed. Toronto: BC Decker, 2002.

Pestronk A. Neuromuscular home page. Available at: http://neuromuscular.wustl.edu

CHAPTER 20

The Hypoglossal Nerve

ANATOMY AND PHYSIOLOGY

The hypoglossal nerve (CN XII) is a purely motor nerve, supplying the tongue. Its cells of origin are in the hypoglossal nuclei, which are upward extensions of the anterior gray columns of the spinal cord; they consist of large, multipolar cells, similar to the anterior horn motoneurons. The paired nuclei extend almost the entire length of the medulla just beneath the floor of the fourth ventricle, close to the midline, under the medial aspect of the hypoglossal trigone (Figure 20.1). The nucleus is somatotopically organized, with different cell groups innervating different tongue muscles. From rostral to caudal, the innervation is intrinsic tongue muscles, then genioglossus, hyoglossus, and styloglossus. Numerous fibers connect the nuclei of the two sides. The axons stream ventrolaterally through the reticular formation, just lateral to the medial longitudinal fasciculus and medial lemniscuses, and the nerve emerges from the medulla in the sulcus between the pyramid and inferior olive (preolivary or ventrolateral sulcus) as a series of 10 to 15 rootlets on each side, anterior to the rootlets of CNs IX, X, and XI (see Figures 11.3 and 11.11).

The hypoglossal fibers gather into two bundles, which perforate the dura mater separately, pass through the hypoglossal canal, and then unite. The nerve descends through the neck to the level of the angle of the mandible and then passes forward under the tongue (hence its name) to supply its extrinsic and intrinsic muscles (Figure 20.2). In the upper portion of its course, the nerve lies beneath the internal carotid artery and internal jugular vein and near the vagus nerve. It passes between the artery and vein, runs forward above the hyoid bone, between the mylohyoid and hypoglossus muscles, and breaks up into a number of fibers to supply the various tongue muscles. The nerve sends communicating branches to the inferior vagal ganglion and to the pharyngeal plexus. At the base of the tongue, it lies near the lingual branch of the mandibular nerve, which provides touch sensation to the anterior two-thirds of the tongue.

The branches of the hypoglossal nerve are the meningeal, descending, thyrohyoid, and muscular. The meningeal branches send filaments derived from communicating branches with C1 and C2 to the dura of the posterior fossa. The descending ramus joins with fibers from C1, sends a branch to the omohyoid, and then joins a descending communicating branch from C2 to C3 to form the ansa cervicalis (Figure 20.2), which supplies the omohyoid, sternohyoid, and sternothyroid muscles. The thyrohyoid branch supplies the thyrohyoid muscle. The descending and thyrohyoid branches carry hypoglossal fibers but are derived mainly from the cervical plexus.

The muscular, or lingual, branches constitute the real distribution of the hypoglossal nerve. The tongue has extrinsic and intrinsic muscles. CN XII supplies the intrinsic muscles, and all of the extrinsic muscles of the tongue except the palatoglossus, and possibly the geniohyoid muscle. The paired extrinsic muscles (genioglossus, styloglossus, hyoglossus, and chondroglossus) pass from the skull or hyoid bone to the tongue. The genioglossus is the largest and most important of the extrinsic tongue muscles. It originates from the chin (Gr. geneion "chin") and inserts into the tongue. The intrinsic muscles (superior and inferior longitudinales, transversus, and verticalis) arise and end within the tongue. The extrinsic muscles protrude and retract the tongue and move the root up and down. The intrinsic muscles change the length, the width, and the curvature of the dorsal surface and turn the nonprotruded tip from side to side. The actions of the tongue muscles are summarized in Table 20.1.

The cerebral center regulating tongue movements lies in the lower portion of the precentral gyrus near and within the sylvian fissure. The cortical

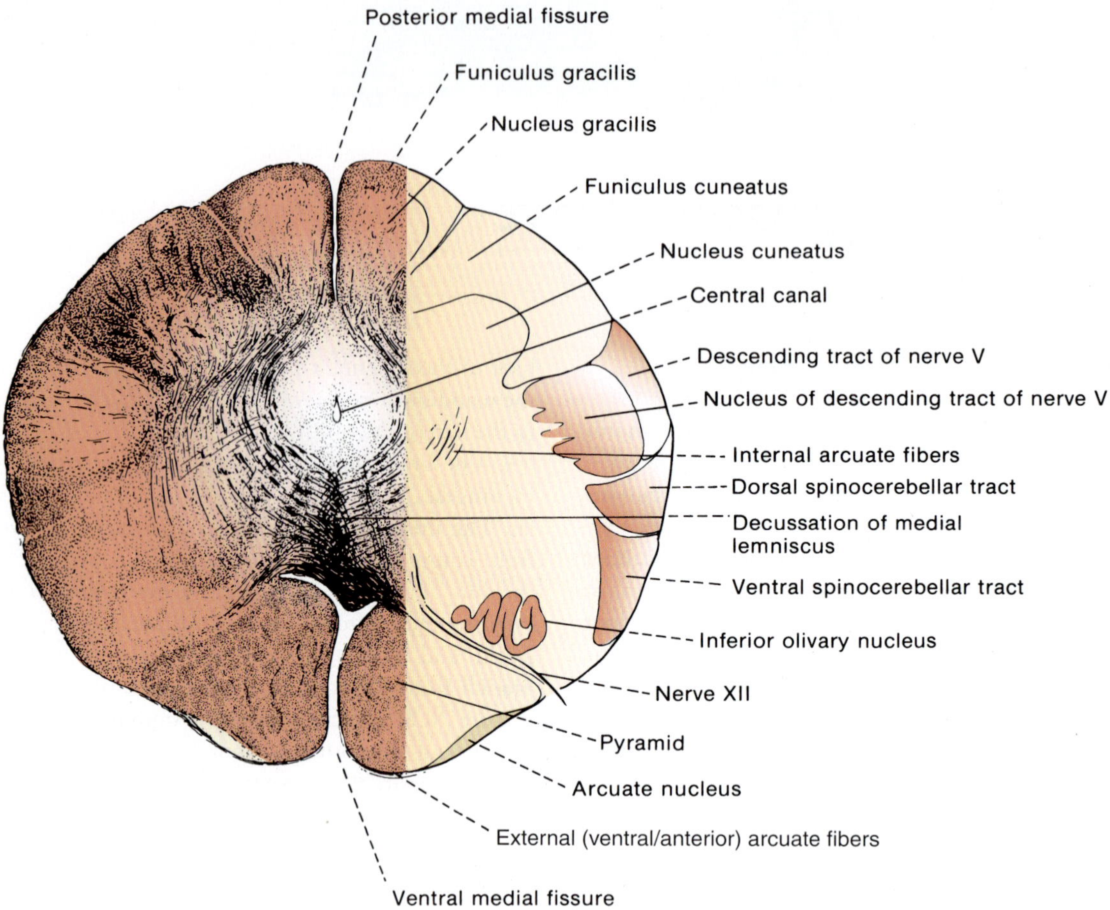

FIGURE 20.1 Section through the medulla at the level of the decussation of the medial lemniscus.

representation of the tongue in humans is huge compared with other mammals and even other primates. In a patient with a small cortical lesion causing obvious tongue deviation, the lesion by magnetic resonance imaging (MRI) was located lateral to the precentral knob, a reliable anatomical landmark for the motor hand area. Therefore, the lesion involved the most lateral part of the precentral gyrus, lateral to the precentral knob.

The supranuclear fibers run in the corticobulbar tract through the genu of the internal capsule and through the cerebral peduncle. Some corticolingual fibers shift to the medial lemniscus in the pons. Other fibers leave the main ventral pyramidal tract and cross the midline at the pontomedullary junction to enter the hypoglossal nucleus from the lateral aspect. Supranuclear control to the genioglossus muscle is primarily crossed; supply to the other muscles is bilateral but predominantly crossed. Some authorities feel the entire supranuclear pathway is crossed.

The suprahyoid muscles also influence tongue movement by changing the position of the hyoid bone. The geniohyoid is supplied by C1 fibers traveling in the hypoglossal nerve. The other suprahyoid muscles are the mylohyoid and anterior belly of the digastric, innervated by CN V, and the stylohyoid and posterior belly of the digastric, innervated by CN VII.

Afferents in the hypoglossal nerve are primarily proprioceptive, but there may be some lingual somatic afferents present as well. The neck-tongue syndrome, consisting of pain in the neck and numbness or tingling in the ipsilateral half of the tongue on sharp rotation of the head, has been attributed to damage to lingual afferent fibers traveling in the hypoglossal nerve to the C2 spinal roots through the atlantoaxial space.

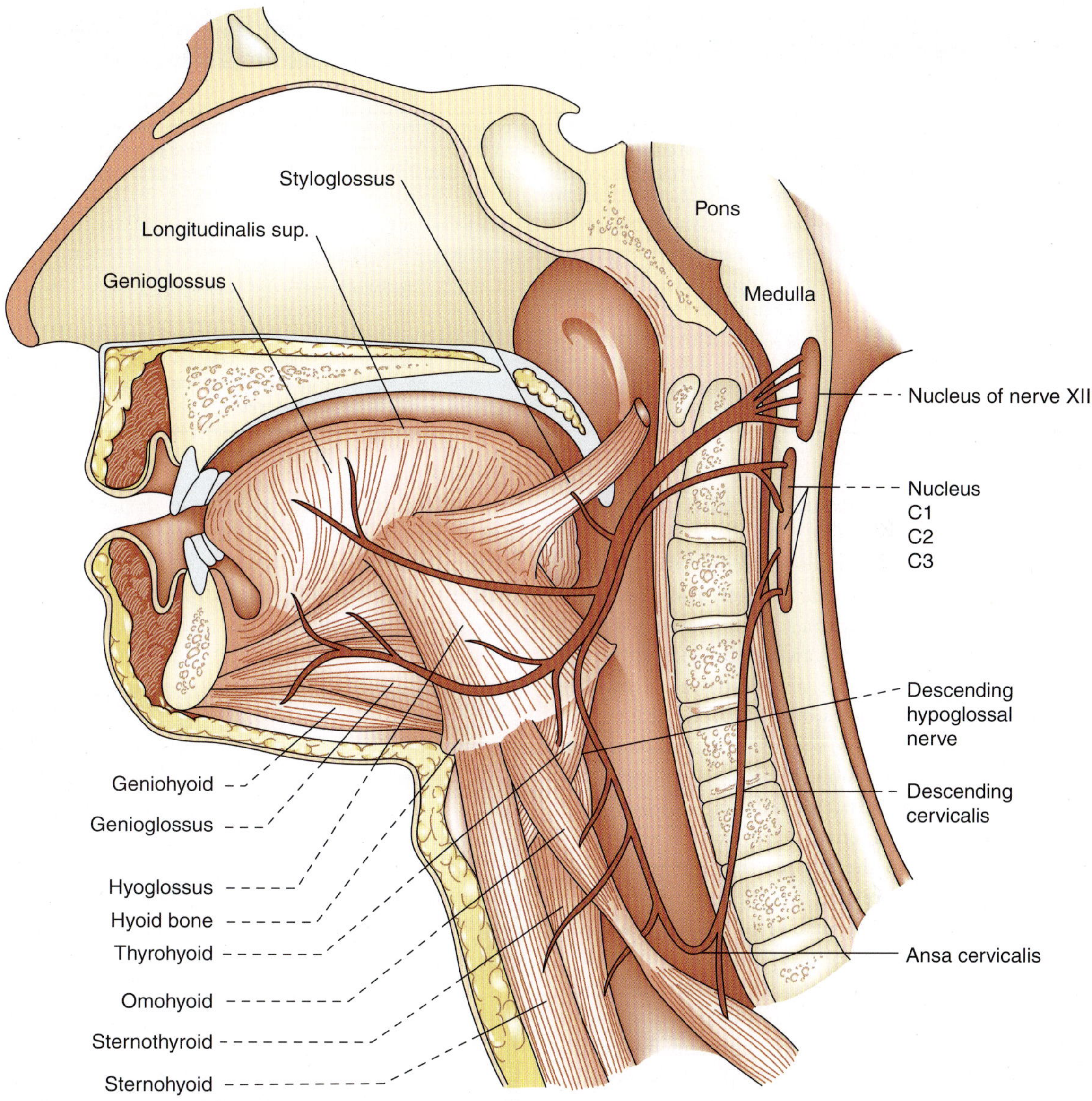

FIGURE 20.2 Ansa cervicalis (hypoglossi) and muscles supplied by the hypoglossal nerve.

CLINICAL EXAMINATION

The clinical examination of hypoglossal nerve function consists of evaluating the strength, bulk, and dexterity of the tongue—looking especially for weakness, atrophy, abnormal movements (particularly fasciculations), and impairment of rapid movements. For a video of tongue fasciculations from the NEJM, see **Video Link 20.1**. After noting the position and appearance of the tongue at rest in the mouth, the patient is asked to protrude it, move it in and out, from side to side, and upward and downward, both slowly and rapidly. Tongue dexterity can be tested by having repeat lingual sounds, as in la-la-la, or use words with the t or d phoneme. For a demonstration of slow tongue movements and difficulty with labials in a case of pseudobulbar palsy, see **Video Link 20.2**. Motor power can be tested by having the patient press the tip against each cheek as the examiner tries to dislodge it with finger pressure. The normal tongue is powerful and cannot be moved. For more precise testing, press firmly with a tongue blade

TABLE 20.1 Actions of the Extrinsic and Intrinsic Tongue Muscles

Muscle	Action
Genioglossi	Posterior fibers draw root of the tongue forward and protrude the tip; anterior fibers depress and retract the tongue and draw it back into the mouth; anterior and posterior fibers together draw the tongue downward and make its superior surface concave from side to side; posterior fibers on one side push the tongue toward the opposite side
Hypoglossi	Retract the tongue and depress its sides; make the superior surface convex
Chondroglossi	Depressor and retractor, sometimes described as part of hypoglossi
Styloglossi	Aids in drawing root of the tongue upward; may be classified as an extrinsic tongue muscle but is more closely related to the muscles of the soft palate; innervated by the vagus nerve
Intrinsic muscles (superior and inferior longitudinales, transversus, verticalis)	Mainly concerned with altering the tongue's shape; causing it to shorten, narrow, or curve in different directions. Both longitudinales shorten the tongue; superior longitudinalis turns the tip, pulls the tip up, and makes the dorsum concave; inferior longitudinalis pulls the tip down and makes the dorsum convex; transversus narrows and elongates the tongue; verticalis flattens and broadens it

against the side of the protruded tongue, comparing the strength on the two sides.

When unilateral weakness is present, the tongue deviates toward the weak side on protrusion because of the action of the normal genioglossus, which protrudes the tongue by drawing the root forward (Figure 20.3). The tongue always deviates toward the weak side (see **Video Link 20.3**). Whether this is toward or away from the side of the lesion depends on the specifics of the lesion. There is impairment of the ability to deviate the protruded tongue toward the opposite side. The patient cannot push the tongue against the cheek on the normal side but is able to push it against the cheek on the side toward which it deviates. At rest, it may deviate or curl slightly toward the healthy side because of unopposed action of the styloglossus, which draws the tongue upward and backward. There is impairment of the ability to deviate the protruded tongue toward the nonparetic side and of the ability to push it against the cheek on the sound side, but the patient is able to push it against the cheek on the paralyzed side. Lateral movements of the tip of the nonprotruded tongue, controlled by the intrinsic tongue muscles, may be preserved. Because of the extensive interlacing of muscle fibers from side to side, the functional deficit with unilateral tongue weakness may be minimal except for difficulty manipulating food in the mouth and an inability to remove food from between the teeth and the cheeks on either side. Either weakness or incoordination may impair rapid tongue movements.

Facial muscle weakness or jaw deviation makes it difficult to evaluate deviation of the tongue. Patients with significant lower facial weakness often have distortion of the normal facial appearance that can produce the appearance of tongue deviation when none is present. Protruding the tongue may cause an appearance of deviation toward the side of the facial weakness. Because of the lack of facial mobility, the corner of the mouth does not move out of the way

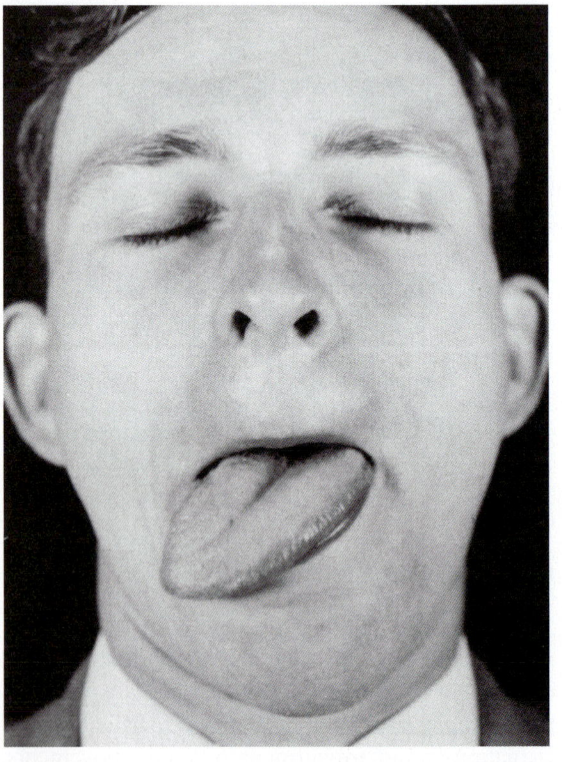

FIGURE 20.3 Infranuclear paralysis of muscles supplied by the hypoglossal nerve: unilateral atrophy and deviation of the tongue following a lesion of the right hypoglossal nerve. (Modified from: https://library.med.utah.edu/neurologicexam/html/cranialnerve_abnormal.html#25, by Dr. Paul D. Larsen.)

and the protruded tongue lies tight against it, making it look as though the tongue has deviated. Manually pulling up the weak side of the face eliminates the "deviation." It may help to gauge tongue position in relation to the tip of the nose or the notch between the upper incisors.

If the paralysis is not accompanied by atrophy, the tongue may appear to bulge slightly and to be higher and more voluminous on the paralyzed side. When atrophy supervenes, the loss of bulk is first apparent along the borders or at the tip, and the tongue may take on a scalloped appearance (Figure 20.4). The normal slight midline groove may become accentuated. With advanced atrophy, the tongue is wrinkled, furrowed, and obviously smaller. The epithelium and mucous membrane on the affected side are thrown into folds. As the paralyzed side becomes wasted, the protruded tongue may curve strikingly toward the atrophic side, assuming a sickle shape. In bilateral paralysis, the patient can protrude the tongue only slightly or not at all. Unilateral tongue atrophy can sometimes be confirmed by palpation.

Progressive bulbar palsy and advanced amyotrophic lateral sclerosis (ALS) may cause atrophy so severe the tongue cannot be protruded and lies inert on the floor of the mouth (glossoplegia). Atrophy may be accompanied by fasciculations, especially in motor neuron disease. In long-standing myasthenia gravis (MG), tongue atrophy may develop and lead to a triple furrowed appearance with grooves paralleling the median sulcus on each side (trident tongue, see **Video Link 20.4**). With bilateral suprasegmental lesions, for example, primary lateral sclerosis, the tongue may be of normal bulk but move slowly.

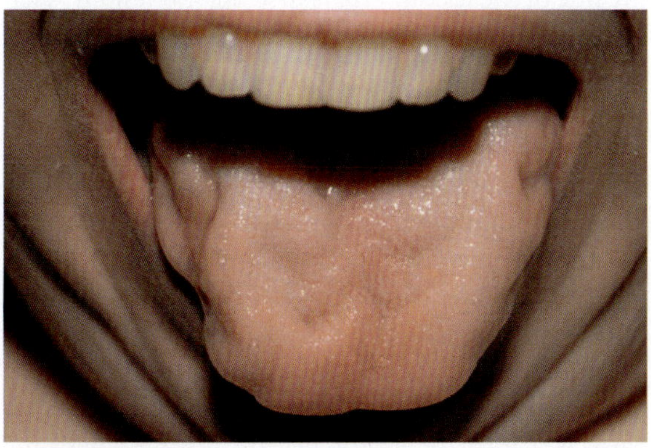

FIGURE 20.4 Tongue atrophy in ALS. (Reprinted from Louis ED, Mayer SA, Rowland LP. *Merritt's Neurology*. 13th ed. Philadelphia: Wolters Kluwer, 2016, with permission.)

In some patients, the tongue is tremulous, and it may be difficult to distinguish these fine, rapid tremors from fasciculations, especially when the tongue is protruded. Tremors will usually disappear when the tongue is lying at rest in the mouth, whereas fasciculations persist. Profuse fasciculations may cause the tongue to have a "bag of worms" appearance.

In addition to fasciculations, other abnormal movements of the tongue sometimes occur. Tremors are usually accentuated by protrusion of the tongue or by talking. Coarse tremors of the tongue can occur in parkinsonism, alcoholism, and general paresis; a fine tremor can occur in thyrotoxicosis. Chorea may cause irregular, jerky movements of the tongue, and often the patient is unable to keep the tongue protruded (snake, trombone, or fly-catcher tongue). Athetosis, dystonia, habit spasms, and tics may involve the tongue; lingual spasm has been described in tetanus. The tongue is often prominently involved in orofacial or buccolingual dyskinesias, which usually occur as a type of tardive dyskinesia following the use of phenothiazines and other psychotropic drugs. Similar dyskinesias may also occur in patients with Parkinson's disease related to the use of levodopa and dopamine agonists and in Meige's syndrome. The bonbon sign is a dystonic or dyskinetic movement of the tongue characterized by protrusion or lateral tongue movements within the mouth producing a bulge in the cheek as if the patient were storing a piece of candy there. It is reportedly helpful in distinguishing tardive dyskinesias, where it is present, from chorea, where it is not.

Morphologic changes in the tongue may be of diagnostic significance in many medical conditions. Some disorders of neurologic interest include the following. Ankyloglossia (tongue-tie) may simulate paresis. A neoplasm involving one side of the tongue may hinder muscle contraction and cause the tongue to deviate. Macroglossia may occur in hypothyroidism, Down's syndrome, amyloidosis, acromegaly, neurofibromatosis, sarcoidosis, GM1 gangliosidosis, glycogen storage diseases, Duchenne's muscular dystrophy, some forms of limb girdle muscular dystrophy, polymyositis, mucopolysaccharidosis, and with local conditions involving the tongue, such as angioma, hamartomas, and lymphoma. Macroglossia can also occur in posterior fossa disease and after posterior fossa surgery. Rarely, ALS may cause macroglossia because of fatty infiltration. Tongue hypertrophy can result from conditions causing excessive movement, such as lingual dyskinesias. Tongue pseudohypertrophy because of denervation has been reported.

The term atrophic glossitis refers to atrophy of the epithelium and papillae, causing a smooth, glistening, often reddened tongue. There may be punctate, erythematous lesions from atrophic, hyperemic papillae. There is no neurogenic atrophy of the musculature. When advanced, atrophic glossitis may cause pain and swelling. Atrophic glossitis occurs in certain deficiency states, especially vitamin B_{12}, folate, other B vitamins, and iron. In pernicious anemia, the tongue is smooth, slick, and translucent, with atrophy of the fungiform and filiform papillae. In some stages, the tongue is pale; in others, it is red. In pellagra and niacin deficiency, the tongue is smooth and atrophic; acutely, it is scarlet red and swollen and may have ulcerations. In riboflavin deficiency, the tongue may be a purplish or magenta hue, with prominent, edematous fungiform and filiform papillae that resemble cobblestones.

Fusion and atrophy of the papillae and fissuring may cause a geographic, or scrotal, tongue. Melkersson-Rosenthal syndrome causes facial nerve palsy and scrotal tongue. Geographic tongue also occurs as a benign curiosity of unknown etiology. Burning tongue (glossodynia, glossalgia) with no visible lesions may occur from early glossitis, tobacco abuse, heavy metal intoxication, as a menopausal symptom, and in pellagra. Xerostomia and local irradiation may make the tongue dry and sore. Longitudinal lingual fissuring occurs in syphilitic glossitis. Ulcerations of the tongue may be seen in primary syphilis (lingual chancre) and in Behçet's disease. The tongue is often bitten during generalized tonic-clonic seizures.

DISORDERS OF FUNCTION

Lesions of CN XII or its central connections may cause weakness of the tongue. There are no sensory changes. Unilateral weakness may cause few symptoms; speech and swallowing are little affected. With severe bilateral weakness, the tongue cannot be protruded or moved laterally; the first stage of swallowing is impaired; and there is difficulty with articulation, especially for linguals. Rarely, the tongue tending to slip back into the throat may cause respiratory difficulty.

Tongue weakness may result from a supranuclear, nuclear, or infranuclear lesion. Supranuclear lesions cause weakness but no atrophy, and the weakness is rarely severe. Because the genioglossus—the principal protractor of the tongue—has mainly crossed supranuclear innervation, the tongue protrudes toward the weak side but to the side opposite the supranuclear lesion. Supranuclear tongue weakness may occur with a destructive lesion of the cerebral cortex or the corticobulbar tract in the internal capsule, cerebral peduncle, or pons. Pontine lesions may cause supranuclear tongue weakness depending on the relationship to the decussating corticolingual fibers. Medial pontine lesions tend to cause contralateral tongue weakness, whereas lateral pontine lesions cause ipsilateral tongue weakness. Medullary lesions may interrupt ipsilateral corticolingual fibers. In a large series of patients with acute unilateral ischemic strokes above the lower brainstem, tongue deviation occurred in 29%, always toward the side of limb weakness; it occurred most commonly in patients with cortical or large subcortical infarctions who also had facial and prominent upper extremity weakness.

Supranuclear lesions may cause dysarthria because of tongue weakness and incoordination (spastic tongue). The dysarthria is spastic and tongue movements are slow and irregular. Isolated dysarthria has been reported as a manifestation of lacunar infarction involving the supranuclear corticolingual pathways. Pseudobulbar palsy because of bilateral upper motor neuron disease may cause bilateral tongue weakness; the tongue may appear small and the patient may be unable to protrude it beyond the teeth. Patients with hemispheric lesions may have apraxia of tongue movements and are often unable to protrude it on command. Extrapyramidal disorders may cause slowing of tongue movements, with thickness of speech and difficulty in protrusion.

In addition to weakness, nuclear and infranuclear lesions cause atrophy of the involved side. The tongue protrudes toward the weak side, which is also the side of the lesion. Progressive nuclear lesions, such as motor neuron disease, often cause fasciculations in addition to weakness. Any accompanying dysarthria is flaccid with particular difficulty with lingual consonants. Common disorders that may involve the hypoglossal nucleus include neoplasms, vascular lesions, and motor neuron disease. Rare disorders include syringobulbia, abscess, granuloma, syphilis, polioencephalitis or postpolio syndrome, and infectious mononucleosis. Nuclear lesions may involve contiguous structures, such as the ascending sensory or descending motor pathways. Progressive bulbar palsy is a form of motor neuron disease where the disease begins in the bulbar motor nuclei; hypoglossal involvement is common. In X-linked bulbospinal muscular atrophy (Kennedy's disease), the bulbar muscles are prominently affected. There are rare forms of bulbar motor neuron disease in childhood (e.g., Fazio-Londe disease).

Infranuclear lesions may involve the intramedullary fibers between the nucleus and the point of exit. Except for motor neuron disease and similar conditions, causes are generally the same as for nuclear lesions. In the medial medullary (Dejerine's, anterior bulbar) syndrome, or inferior alternating hemiplegia, the lesion involves the exiting hypoglossal fibers and the neighboring medullary pyramid, causing tongue weakness and contralateral hemiparesis (Chapter 21, Box 21.1). A patient has been reported with contralateral glossoplegia due to a ventromedial lesion of the upper medulla. Lesions of the medullary tegmentum may involve CNs X, XI, and XII (Jackson's syndrome [Chapter 21]). In Keane's series of 578 cases with bilateral involvement of a single CN, hypoglossal palsy accounted for only 5 (0.9%); of these, 2 were due to tumor, 1 was vascular, and 1 was due to infection. But in a series of 100 cases of hypoglossal palsy, the nerve was involved bilaterally in one-third; tumor and trauma accounted for the majority.

Processes involving the extramedullary, intracranial course of the nerve include disorders involving the meninges, such as infectious and neoplastic meningitis, subarachnoid hemorrhage, neoplasms and other mass lesions (e.g., schwannoma), inflammation, and trauma. Processes involving the skull base—such as basal skull fractures, basilar impression, platybasia, Chiari malformation, impaction of the medulla into the foramen magnum by increased intracranial pressure, or dislocation of the upper cervical vertebrae—may affect the nerve before it leaves the skull. Lesions along the clivus may cause bilateral hypoglossal palsies. Combined CN VI and XII palsies are usually due to a lesion of the clivus, typically malignant, or to nasopharyngeal carcinoma. Lesions within the hypoglossal canal are rare. Inflammatory, neoplastic or traumatic lesions in the region of the occipital condyle may cause isolated hypoglossal palsy and a characteristic pain pattern (occipital condyle syndrome); it is most often due to metastatic disease to the skull base. Bilateral hypoglossal nerve injury may occur with occipital condylar fracture.

Processes involving the extracranial course of the nerve include trauma of various types, especially penetrating wounds (including surgery on the neck, mouth, or tongue), carotid aneurysms (especially dissections), vascular entrapment by the vertebral artery, tumors or infections in the retroparotid or retropharyngeal spaces, deep cervical adenopathy, cranial irradiation, and tumors involving the neck, tongue base, or salivary glands. Hypoglossal nerve palsy can also occur as an idiopathic, benign syndrome that resolves spontaneously. Mechanical lesions may result in aberrant regeneration, which causes progressive difficulty with coordinated tongue movements. Rarely, primary neural tumors involve CN XII extracranially. CN XII may be involved with other lower CNs and the cervical sympathetics in lesions in the retroparotid space (Collet-Sicard or Villaret syndromes, Chapter 21). CN XII may be involved unilaterally or bilaterally in Guillain-Barré syndrome, hereditary neuropathy with liability to pressure palsies, and related polyneuropathies. Tongue involvement can occur in Lewis-Sumner syndrome and multifocal motor neuropathy, causing confusion with ALS.

Except for MG, neuromuscular junction disorders and myopathies rarely involve the tongue to any clinically significant degree. Tongue weakness and fatigability may occur in MG but generally only with severe involvement. The triple furrowed appearance is characteristic (see above). It is often difficult to separate bulbar weakness because of MG from that due to early motor neuron disease.

The tongue may be involved in myotonic disorders, although it rarely causes any symptoms. One way to test for myotonia is to place the edge of a tongue blade across the tongue and then percuss it sharply. Myotonia may cause a temporary focal contraction along the line of percussion, causing the tongue to narrow sharply at that point (see **Video Link 20.5**). The appearance of the resulting constriction has been referred to as the napkin ring sign.

Seizures may involve the tongue, either as part of a jacksonian seizure or rarely in isolation. Paroxysmal, rhythmic tongue movements have been described as a manifestation of subcortical seizures. The tongue may participate in the rhythmic movements of palatal myoclonus. Unusual episodic, rhythmic tongue movements may occur after head and neck trauma (galloping tongue). Serpentine tongue refers to a dyskinesia producing incessant writhing movements (see Sheehy et al. for video). Tongue myokymia may follow cranial radiotherapy (see Rison and Beydoun for video).

Video Links

Video Link 20.1. Tongue fasciculations in ALS. https://www.youtube.com/watch?v=xuwdvBXcr30

Video Link 20.2. Slow tongue movements in pseudobulbar palsy. http://neurosigns.org/wiki/Pseudobulbar_palsy

Video Link 20.3. Tongue deviation. http://neurosigns.org/wiki/Tongue_deviation

Video Link 20.4. Triple-furrowed tongue in myasthenia gravis. http://neurosigns.org/wiki/Triple_furrow_tongue_in_myasthenia_gravis

Video Link 20.5. Myotonia of the tongue (napkin ring sign). http://www.nejm.org/doi/full/10.1056/NEJMicm1014605

BIBLIOGRAPHY

Aladdin Y, Siddiqi ZA, Khan K, et al. Hypoglossal-vertebral entrapment syndrome. *Neurology* 2008;71:461.

Axelsson G, Liedholm LJ. Multifocal motor neuropathy—unusual cause of hypoglossal palsy. *Lakartidningen* 2002;99:1448–1450.

Benito-Leon J, Alvarez-Cermeno JC. Isolated total tongue paralysis as a manifestation of bilateral medullary infarction. *J Neurol Neurosurg Psychiatry* 2003;74:1698–1699.

Brazis PW, Masdeu JC, Biller J. *Localization in Clinical Neurology*. 7th ed. Philadelphia: Wolters Kluwer/Lippincott Williams & Wilkins, 2017.

Burch J, Warren-Gash C, Ingham V, et al. Myasthenia gravis—a rare presentation with tongue atrophy and fasciculation. *Age Ageing* 2006;35:87–88.

Capobianco DJ, Brazis PW, Rubino FA, et al. Occipital condyle syndrome. *Headache* 2002;42:142–146.

Chang D, Cho SH. Medial medullary infarction with contralateral glossoplegia. *J Neurol Neurosurg Psychiatry* 2005;76:888.

Chauvet E, Sailler L, Carreiro M, et al. Symptomatic macroglossia and tongue myositis in polymyositis: treatment with corticosteroids and intravenous immunoglobulin. *Arthritis Rheum* 2002;46:2762–2764.

Combarros O, Alvarez de Arcaya A, Berciano J. Isolated unilateral hypoglossal nerve palsy: nine cases. *J Neurol* 1998;245:98–100.

Galassi G, Albertini G, Valzania F, et al. Cranial nerve involvement as presenting sign of multifocal motor neuropathy. *J Clin Neurosci* 2012;19:1733–1735.

Gelfand AA, Johnson H, Lenaerts ME, et al. Neck-tongue syndrome: a systematic review. *Cephalalgia* 2018;38:374–382.

Giuffrida S, Lo Bartolo ML, Nicoletti A. Isolated, unilateral, reversible palsy of the hypoglossal nerve. *Eur J Neurol* 2000;7:347–349.

Holle D, Kastrup O, Sheu SY, et al. Neurological picture. Tongue pseudohypertrophy in idiopathic hypoglossal nerve palsy. *J Neurol Neurosurg Psychiatry* 2009;80:1393.

İnan R, Barut BÖ, Serim A, et al. Hypoglossal nerve involvement in Lewis-Sumner syndrome: a case report. *Acta Neurol Belg* 2018;118(2):323–325.

Keane JR. Galloping tongue: post-traumatic, episodic, rhythmic movements. *Neurology* 1984;34:251–252.

Keane JR. Twelfth-nerve palsy. Analysis of 100 cases. *Arch Neurol* 1996;53:561–566.

Keane JR. Combined VIth and XIIth cranial nerve palsies: a clival syndrome. *Neurology* 2000;54:1540–1541.

Keane JR. Bilateral involvement of a single cranial nerve: analysis of 578 cases. *Neurology* 2005;65:950–952.

Laigle-Donadey F, Taillibert S, Martin-Duverneuil N, et al. Skull-base metastases. *J Neurooncol* 2005;75:63–69.

Lam CH, Stratford J. Bilateral hypoglossal nerve injury with occipital condylar fracture. *Can J Neurol Sci* 1996;23:145–148.

Lance JW, Anthony M. Neck-tongue syndrome on sudden turning of the head. *J Neurol Neurosurg Psychiatry* 1980;43:97–101.

Lin HC, Barkhaus PE. Cranial nerve XII: the hypoglossal nerve. *Semin Neurol* 2009;29:45–52.

Matsuda C, Shimizu T, Nakayama Y, et al. Macroglossia in advanced amyotrophic lateral sclerosis. *Muscle Nerve* 2016;54:386–390.

McKee HR, Escott E, Damm D, et al. Macroglossia in amyotrophic lateral sclerosis. *JAMA Neurol* 2013;70:1432–1435.

Moris G, Roig C, Misiego M, et al. The distinctive headache of the occipital condyle syndrome: a report of four cases. *Headache* 1998;38:308–311.

Orrell RW, Marsden CD. The neck-tongue syndrome. *J Neurol Neurosurg Psychiatry* 1994;57:348–352.

Parano E, Giuffrida S, Restivo D, et al. Reversible palsy of the hypoglossal nerve complicating infectious mononucleosis in a young child. *Neuropediatrics* 1998;29:46–47.

Quijano-Roy S, Galan L, Ferreiro A, et al. Severe progressive form of congenital muscular dystrophy with calf pseudohypertrophy, macroglossia and respiratory insufficiency. *Neuromuscul Disord* 2002;12:466–475.

Riggs JE. Distinguishing between extrinsic and intrinsic tongue muscle weakness in unilateral hypoglossal palsy. *Neurology* 1984;34:1367.

Rison RA, Beydoun SR. Teaching video NeuroImages: tongue myokymia following head and neck radiotherapy for nasopharyngeal carcinoma. *Neurology* 2009;72:e65.

Sheehy SH, Lawrence T, Thevathasan AW. Serpentine tongue: a lingual dyskinesia. *Neurology* 2008;70:e87.

Srivastava T, Singh S, Goyal V, et al. Hypoglossal nerve paralysis caused by high cervical epidural abscess. *Neurology* 2006;66:522.

Stricker T, Steinlin M, Willi UV, et al. Hypoglossal nerve palsy associated with deep cervical lymphadenopathy. *Neurology* 1998;50:1926–1927.

Umapathi T, Venketasubramanian N, Leck KJ, et al. Tongue deviation in acute ischaemic stroke: a study of supranuclear twelfth cranial nerve palsy in 300 stroke patients. *Cerebrovasc Dis* 2000;10:462–465.

Urban PP, Hopf HC, Connemann B, et al. The course of cortico-hypoglossal projections in the human brainstem. Functional testing using transcranial magnetic stimulation. *Brain* 1996;119:1031–1038.

Urban PP, Wicht S, Hopf HC, et al. Isolated dysarthria due to extracerebellar lacunar stroke: a central monoparesis of the tongue. *J Neurol Neurosurg Psychiatry* 1999;66:495–501.

Weiss MD, Oakley JC, Meekins GD. Hypoglossal neuropathy in Lewis-Sumner syndrome masquerading as motor neuron disease. *Neurology* 2006;67:175–176.

Williams JM, Fox JL. Neurinoma of the intracranial portion of the hypoglossal nerve. Review and case report. *J Neurosurg* 1962;19:248–250.

Wilson JR, Sumner AJ, Eichelman J. Aberrant reinnervation following hypoglossal nerve damage. *Muscle Nerve* 1994;17:931–935.

Winter WC, Juel VC. Hypoglossal neuropathy in hereditary neuropathy with liability to pressure palsy. *Neurology* 2003;61:1154–1155.

Yoon SS, Park KC. Neurological picture. Glossoplegia in a small cortical infarction. *J Neurol Neurosurg Psychiatry* 2007;78:1372.

CHAPTER 21

Brainstem and Multiple Cranial Nerve Syndromes

The brainstem is a compact structure, with cranial nerve (CN) nuclei, nerve fascicles, and long ascending and descending tracts all closely juxtaposed. Structures and centers in the reticular formation control many vital functions. Brainstem diseases are serious and often life threatening. Involvement of the intricate network of neural structures often causes a plethora of clinical findings. Brainstem syndromes typically involve dysfunction of one or more CNs. Deficits due to dysfunction of individual nerves are covered in the preceding chapters. This chapter discusses conditions that cause dysfunction beyond the distribution of a single CN, involving more than one CN, or conditions that involve brainstem structures in addition to the CN nucleus or fascicles. The first part covers intramedullary disorders of the brainstem, and the second part covers disorders that involve multiple CNs in their extramedullary course.

Some may argue it is sufficient to recognize that a brainstem disorder exists and to define the process more precisely with an imaging study. However, some important clinical conditions may cause major brainstem dysfunction without dramatically changing the appearance of the imaging study. Examples of processes easily missed radiographically include Wernicke's disease, progressive bulbar palsy (PBP), progressive supranuclear palsy, basilar artery migraine, Whipple's disease, syringobulbia, olivopontocerebellar atrophy, and Gerstmann-Sträussler-Scheinker syndrome. With disorders causing multiple CN deficits, the imaging studies are often not helpful.

BRAINSTEM SYNDROMES

In the brainstem, descending motor tracts prior to decussation, as well as ascending sensory pathways that have already crossed, lie in intimate relation to the lower motor neurons of the CN nuclei. With a few exceptions, CNs innervate structures of the head and neck ipsilaterally. A process affecting the brainstem long tracts on one side causes clinical abnormalities on the opposite side of the body. For this reason, focal brainstem lesions are characterized by "crossed" syndromes of ipsilateral CN dysfunction and contralateral long motor or sensory tract dysfunction. For instance, in the right side of the pons, the nuclei for CNs VI and VII lie in proximity to the right corticospinal tract, which is destined to decussate in the medulla to innervate the left side of the body. The patient with a lesion in the right pons will have CN findings on the right, such as a sixth or seventh nerve palsy, and a hemiparesis on the left.

This crossed deficit will often be associated with symptoms reflecting dysfunction of other brainstem structures or their connections. Because of the rich vestibular and cerebellar connections, patients with brainstem disease often have dizziness or vertigo, unsteadiness, imbalance, incoordination, difficulty walking, nausea, and vomiting. Pharyngeal and laryngeal muscles are innervated by neurons in the brainstem, and patients often have dysarthria or dysphagia. Dysfunction of CNs III, IV, and VI or their connections may cause ocular motility abnormalities. Unless the process has impaired the reticular activating system, these patients are normal mentally—awake, alert, able to converse (though perhaps dysarthric), not demented, not confused, and not aphasic. The fourth ventricle and cerebral aqueduct lie nearby; if these are involved, patients may develop obstructive hydrocephalus. Although most pathologic processes that involve the brainstem occur in other parts of the brain, some disorders are characterized by primarily brainstem involvement (e.g., central pontine myelinolysis, medulloblastoma, and olivopontocerebellar atrophy). With vascular lesions, the clinical deficit depends on whether the occlusive process has involved the paramedian perforating, short circumferential, or long circumferential branches of the basilar artery.

From an anatomical standpoint, brainstem syndromes may be localized by considering the rostral to caudal level and the medial to lateral level. The rostral to caudal localization is determined by the CN involvement. Abnormality of CN III or IV, or a vertical gaze abnormality, indicates a midbrain lesion; CN VI or VII, or a horizontal gaze palsy—a pontine lesion; CN VIII—a pontomedullary junction lesion; and CNs IX, X, XI, or XII—a medullary lesion. Because of the vast longitudinal extent of the spinal tract of CN V, facial sensory abnormalities can occur with lesions anywhere from the pons to the cervical spinal cord.

The long motor tracts tend to lie medial, and the long sensory tracts lateral, in the brainstem. Somatic motor nuclei (extraocular and hypoglossal) are paramedian; branchiomotor nuclei are more lateral. Involvement of descending motor tracts or somatic motor nuclei indicates medial lesions; involvement of long sensory tracts, branchiomotor nuclei, and special sensory nuclei indicates lateral lesions. The cerebellar peduncles also lie laterally. The alar plate–derived sensory nuclei lie laterally and are separated from the basal plate–derived motor nuclei by the sulcus limitans (Figures 11.2 and 11.4). Paramedian perforators from the basilar artery perfuse the midline structures; circumferential arteries perfuse the lateral structures. There are therefore medial and lateral medullary syndromes; medial and lateral inferior, middle, and superior pontine syndromes; and the midbrain syndromes. The posterior inferior cerebellar artery (PICA) supplies the lateral medulla; the anterior inferior cerebellar artery (AICA) supplies the inferior lateral pons; and the superior cerebellar artery (SCA) supplies the superior lateral pons. Paramedian lesions are typically lacunar; lateral lesions are more often from disease of the larger circumferential vessels. The lateral medullary and pontine syndromes are often referred to by their vascular territory designations: PICA, AICA, and SCA.

Occlusion of medial pontine branches of the basilar artery may cause involvement of the nuclei of CNs VI and VII or their emerging fibers, the medial longitudinal fasciculus (MLF), the corticospinal tract, the medial lemniscus, and the pontine paramedian reticular formation. Clinical manifestations may include ipsilateral facial nerve palsy, abducens palsy, horizontal gaze palsy, internuclear ophthalmoplegia (INO), or impaired taste, with contralateral corticospinal weakness and impaired lemniscal sensation. Thrombosis of the lateral pontine branches of the basilar artery produces ischemia that may involve the middle and superior cerebellar peduncles, the vestibular and cochlear nuclei, the facial and trigeminal motor nuclei, the trigeminal sensory nucleus, and the spinothalamic tract. Findings may include ipsilateral cerebellar ataxia and dysfunction of CNs V, VII, and VIII, with contralateral loss of pain and temperature sensation on the trunk and extremities. Occlusion of the internal auditory artery causes unilateral deafness and impaired vestibular function.

CLASSICAL BRAINSTEM SYNDROMES

Many of the early neurologic pioneer clinicians described the clinical findings due to a focal process affecting the brainstem. These physicians practiced in an era when disorders such as tuberculoma, syphilitic gumma, and tumor were seen much more often than today. Many of the classical brainstem syndromes as originally described were not due to ischemia, and the effects of tuberculoma, gumma, and similar lesions are not limited to vascular distributions. Some degree of mismatch has therefore resulted between the classic descriptions and the current environment when most brainstem syndromes are due to ischemia. There has also been significant drift of many of the eponymic syndromes through failure to honor precisely the original descriptions. Liu et al. pointed out the variability in textbook descriptions of Claude's, Benedikt's, and Nothnagel's syndromes and noted the difference in textbook descriptions compared to the original papers. Box 21.1 contains a discussion of the classical eponymic brainstem syndromes, largely from a historical perspective, and Table 21.1 summarizes the clinical features.

Wallenberg described the lateral medullary syndrome (LMS), the most common form of brainstem stroke. Wallenberg's original patient had an occlusion of the PICA, but LMS is most often due to ischemia in the PICA distribution because of vertebral artery occlusion (Figure 21.1). Typical manifestations include vertigo, nausea and vomiting, nystagmus, hoarseness, dysphagia, dysphonia, singultus, ipsilateral hemiataxia, and numbness of the ipsilateral face and contralateral body. Occipital headache or pain in the back of the neck may occur at the onset; promi-

BOX 21.1

Classical Brainstem Syndromes

Midbrain Syndromes

Weber described a patient with a hematoma of one cerebral peduncle, which damaged the corticospinal and corticobulbar tracts and the exiting third nerve. The patient had a contralateral hemiparesis involving face, arm, and leg and an ipsilateral complete third nerve palsy. Benedikt described one patient with a similar peduncular lesion due to a midbrain tuberculoma, which extended further into the tegmentum and involved the regions of the substantia nigra and red nucleus, causing tremor and involuntary movements of the hemiparetic limbs. Two clinically similar patients were not studied pathologically; one probably had meningovascular syphilis. Claude described a patient with a midbrain infarction in whom the corticospinal pathways were not involved; the clinical picture was ipsilateral third nerve palsy and contralateral cerebellar ataxia due to involvement of the superior cerebellar peduncle. Debate remains about how much red nucleus involvement occurs in Claude's and Benedikt's syndrome. Seo concluded on the basis of clinical and magnetic resonance imaging (MRI) studies that the lesion usually lies just caudal and medial to the red nucleus and that the tremor and ataxia are due to involvement of the cerebellar outflow pathways in the superior cerebellar peduncle.

These three midbrain syndromes are variations on a theme. The lesion is anterior—in the cerebral peduncle—in Weber's syndrome, causing hemiparesis. It is more posterior—in the tegmentum—in Claude's syndrome, causing hemiataxia. In Benedikt's syndrome, the lesion is more extensive, involving both the tegmentum and the peduncle, causing hemiparesis with tremor and ataxia of the involved limbs; Benedikt's is essentially Weber's + Claude's. Because the fascicles of cranial nerve (CN) III are scattered in their course through the midbrain, the third nerve palsy in any of these syndromes may be partial.

Nothnagel's (ophthalmoplegia-ataxia) syndrome is different; it is more a variant of Parinaud's syndrome, with unilateral or bilateral third nerve palsy and ataxia accompanied by vertical gaze deficits and other neurologic signs. The lesion affects the midbrain tectum and is often neoplastic. Nothnagel's original patient had a pineal sarcoma.

Pontine Syndromes

Millard and Gubler separately described patients with an ipsilateral lower motor neuron facial nerve palsy and contralateral hemiparesis due to a lesion involving the pons. Gubler's cases included three with a tumor, one with a stroke, and one with a brownish softening. Millard reported one case due to pontine hemorrhage as a letter to the editor in the journal where Gubler reported his cases. In all cases, the lesion lay in the lateral pons and did not involve CN VI; the patients had no ocular motility disturbance. Nevertheless, it is common to see sixth nerve palsy included in textbook descriptions of Millard-Gubler syndrome. Gubler was a senior clinician reporting several cases; Millard had just graduated from medical school, was essentially a resident, and reported only one. Gubler instructed the journal editor to give Millard precedence, hence the eponym.

Foville described a patient with an ipsilateral lower motor neuron facial palsy and a horizontal gaze palsy, with a contralateral hemiparesis; there was no pathology but the onset was apoplectic. Landry, in a letter commenting on Foville's case, described a patient with sixth nerve palsy and contralateral hemiplegia, including the face, due to pontine ischemia in a patient with syphilis. Yelloly had described a case of abducens palsy with contralateral hemiplegia 50 years previously. Raymond described a patient with sixth nerve palsy and contralateral hemiplegia, but it is not clear that the hemiplegia was of pontine origin.

Medullary Syndromes

There are two primary medullary syndromes, the lateral (Wallenberg) and the medial (Dejerine). The rare medial medullary syndrome is summarized in Table 21.1. In a study of clinical magnetic resonance imaging (MRI) correlation in medial medullary infarction, classical Dejerine's syndrome (ipsilateral tongue weakness with contralateral hemiparesis and lemniscal sensory loss) was seen in 64% of patients; the remainder had

(continued)

BOX 21.1

Classical Brainstem Syndromes *(Continued)*

partial lesions, which may be less readily recognized. In a series of 18 patients, the most common manifestation of medial medullary stroke was a unilateral sensorimotor deficit. The extremely rare bilateral medial medullary syndrome causes quadriparesis and other abnormalities. Isolated tongue weakness has been reported because of bilateral medullary infarction. Other syndromes of the medulla (Avellis's, Jackson's, Schmidt's, Céstan-Chenais, and Babinski-Nageotte) are described in Table 21.1. Except for the occasional upper motor neuron facial palsy in Wallenberg's syndrome, there is sparing of facial motor function in all of the medullary syndromes.

nent pain raises the possibility of vertebral artery dissection. The patient may be unable to talk and swallow initially. Clinical findings are summarized in Table 21.1.

In a series of MRI-verified LMS, the most common findings were ipsilateral Horner's syndrome and ataxia and contralateral body hypalgesia. The spontaneous nystagmus is usually horizontal or mixed horizontal-torsional. Horizontal nystagmus beats away from the side of the lesion and may be second or third degree. Torsional nystagmus with the upper poles beating away from the side of the lesion is also common. The nystagmus is influenced by head and eye position and by fixation. Dysphagia is common. It is often more severe than would be expected simply from a lesion of the nucleus ambiguus, and disruption of connections to a premotor swallowing center in the dorsolateral medulla has been postulated. Partial resolution and survival is the rule; the ability to swallow and talk returns, although residual hoarseness, persistent ataxia, and sensory changes may remain. Aspiration is a major threat. The presence of dysphonia, soft palate dysfunction, or facial sensory loss suggests an increased risk. Although LMS is usually ischemic, it has also been described with aneurysm, abscess, hematoma, arteriovenous malformation, demyelinating disease, and metastatic neoplasm. The LMS may have many unusual manifestations (Box 21.2).

ANATOMIC BRAINSTEM SYNDROMES

The other approach to organizing brainstem syndromes is by the anatomical area or the major blood vessel involved. The midbrain syndromes are variations and combinations of an ipsilateral third nerve palsy and weakness, ataxia, or tremor of the contralateral limbs; this is due to ischemia in the distribution of paramedian penetrating vessels from the rostral basilar artery. The LMS is discussed in the previous section, and the medial medullary syndrome is discussed in Box 21.1.

The vascular pontine syndromes can be divided into medial and lateral and into superior, middle, and inferior. The medial pontine syndromes are due to disease of the paramedian perforators; the lateral pontine syndromes are due to disease of the circumferential arteries. The AICA supplies the lateral inferior pons and upper medulla, whereas the SCA supplies the lateral upper pons. The midpons is supplied by a short circumferential artery. Just as PICA ischemia causes the LMS, ischemia in the AICA distribution causes the lateral inferior pontine syndrome; and ischemia in the SCA distribution causes the lateral superior pontine syndrome. The generally recognized pontine syndromes are therefore the medial inferior pontine, lateral inferior pontine (AICA), medial and lateral midpontine, medial superior pontine, and lateral superior pontine (SCA). The vascular pontine syndromes are summarized in Table 21.2. In a series of patients with lesions involving the AICA distribution, only 29% had the complete AICA syndrome. Partial syndromes were characteristic of small vessel disease; more widespread involvement indicated basilar artery occlusive disease. The SCA syndrome is also often partial. Basilar branch occlusion may involve any of the branches of the basilar artery. The mechanism is atherothrombotic occlusion at the point of origin of the branch, and the infarction typically extends to the ventral surface of the pons.

Vertebrobasilar transient ischemic attacks (vertebrobasilar insufficiency, VBI) are episodes of brainstem ischemia due to occlusive disease involving the posterior circulation. Symptoms depend upon which region of the brainstem is ischemic. The clinical manifestations of an attack of VBI are typically bilateral, with varying degrees of weakness, numbness, and CN

TABLE 21.1 Summary of the Classical Named Brainstem Syndromes

Syndrome	Lesion Location	Structures Involved	Clinical Findings	Comment
Parinaud's	Midbrain dorsum	Quadrigeminal plate region; pretectum; periaqueductal gray matter	Impaired upgaze; convergence retraction nystagmus; dilated pupils with light near dissociation	Usually due to mass lesion in the region of the posterior third ventricle, most often pinealoma, or due to midbrain infarction
Weber's	Midbrain base	CN III fibers; cerebral peduncle	Ipsilateral CN III palsy; contralateral hemiparesis	Usually vascular
Benedikt's	Midbrain tegmentum	CN III fibers; red nucleus; CST	Ipsilateral CN III palsy; contralateral hemiparesis with ataxia, hyperkinesia, and tremor ("rubral tremor")	Usually vascular
Claude's	Midbrain tegmentum	CN III fibers; red nucleus; SCP	Ipsilateral CN III palsy; contralateral ataxia and tremor ("rubral tremor")	Usually vascular
Nothnagel's	Midbrain tectum	Ipsilateral or bilateral CN III	Oculomotor palsies; ataxia	Usually neoplastic
Millard-Gubler	Pons	CN VII; CST	Ipsilateral peripheral facial palsy; contralateral hemiparesis	Usually vascular; CN VI not involved; usage is inconsistent
Foville's (Raymond-Foville)	Pons	CN VII; lateral gaze center, CST	Ipsilateral facial palsy and horizontal gaze palsy; contralateral hemiparesis	Usually vascular; usage is inconsistent
Raymond's (Yelloly, Landry)	Pons	CN VI; CST	Ipsilateral abducens palsy; contralateral hemiparesis	Usually vascular, often lumped with Foville's syndrome; usage is inconsistent
Wallenberg's (lateral medullary syndrome)	Lateral medullary tegmentum	Spinal tract of CN V and its nucleus; nucleus ambiguus; emerging fibers of CNs IX and X; LST; descending sympathetic fibers; vestibular nuclei; inferior cerebellar peduncle; afferent spinocerebellar tracts; lateral cuneate nucleus	Loss of pain and temperature of ipsilateral face and contralateral body; decreased ipsilateral corneal reflex; weakness of ipsilateral soft palate; loss of ipsilateral gag reflex; paralysis of ipsilateral vocal cord; ipsilateral central Horner's syndrome; nystagmus; cerebellar ataxia of ipsilateral limbs; lateropulsion	Several variants recognized; occasional ipsilateral upper motor neuron facial palsy due to involvement of aberrant CST; facial sensation sometimes preserved; ischemia in PICA distribution but more often due to vertebral artery occlusion
Avellis' syndrome	Medullary tegmentum	CN X; LST; nucleus ambiguus	Ipsilateral palatal and vocal cord weakness; loss of pain and temperature of contralateral body	Usually due to vertebral artery thrombosis; occasional involvement of ML and ST with loss of touch and proprioception of contralateral body; occasional ipsilateral Horner's syndrome occasional contralateral hemiparesis
Jackson's syndrome	Medullary tegmentum	CN X fibers or nucleus ambiguus; CNs XI and XII	Ipsilateral flaccid paralysis of the soft palate, pharynx, and larynx; flaccid weakness and atrophy of SCM and trapezius (partial) and of the tongue	Also known as vago-accessory-hypoglossal paralysis; more likely due to extramedullary multiple cranial nerve palsy
Schmidt's	Lower medullary tegmentum	Nucleus ambiguus; bulbar and spinal nuclei of CN XI and/or their radicular fibers	Ipsilateral paralysis of soft palate, pharynx, and larynx; flaccid weakness and atrophy of SCM and trapezius (partial)	Also known as vago-accessory syndrome; more likely due to extramedullary multiple cranial nerve palsy

(continued)

TABLE 21.1 Summary of the Classical Named Brainstem Syndromes *(Continued)*

Syndrome	Lesion Location	Structures Involved	Clinical Findings	Comment
Céstan-Chenais	Medullary tegmentum	Nucleus ambiguus; ICP; sympathetics; CST; ML	Ipsilateral weakness of soft palate, pharynx, and larynx; cerebellar ataxia; Horner's syndrome; contralateral hemiparesis with loss of posterior column function	Due to vertebral artery occlusion below the origin of the PICA; differs from Wallenberg's because of CST and ML involvement and absence of changes in pain and temperature
Babinski-Nageotte (hemi-medullary syndrome)	Medial and lateral medulla	Nucleus ambiguus; solitary tract; spinal tract of V; ICP; sympathetics; CST; ML; +/–XII	Ipsilateral paralysis of soft palate, pharynx, larynx, +/– tongue; loss of taste on posterior third of tongue; impaired facial pain and temperature; ataxia; Horner's syndrome; contralateral hemiparesis; impaired posterior column function; +/– impaired pain and temperature	Caused by multiple or scattered lesions, chiefly in the distribution of the vertebral artery; similar to, perhaps the same as, Céstan-Chenais
Medial medullary syndrome (Dejerine's anterior bulbar syndrome, pyramid-hypoglossal syndrome, alternating hypoglossal hemiplegia)	Medial medulla	XII nucleus or fibers; medullary pyramid (at/near decussation); +/–ML	Ipsilateral tongue weakness; contralateral hemiparesis (sparing the face); +/– impairment of posterior column function; LST functions spared	Due to ischemia in the distribution of paramedian perforator or the anterior spinal artery, findings may be bilateral and of variable laterality because of involvement of the pyramidal decussation and variations in the anatomy of the anterior spinal artery

CN, cranial nerve; CST, corticospinal tract; ICP, inferior cerebellar peduncle; LST, lateral spinothalamic tract; ML, medial lemniscus; PICA, posterior inferior cerebellar artery; SCM, sternocleidomastoid; SCP, superior cerebellar peduncle; ST, solitary tract.

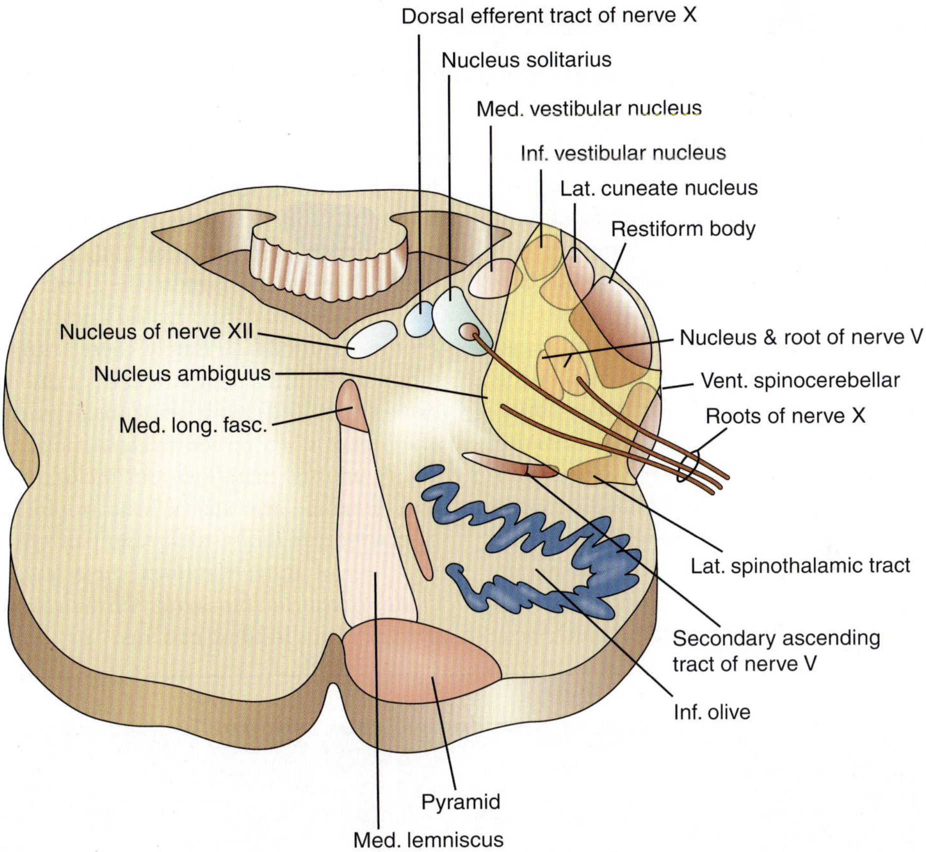

FIGURE 21.1 Cross section of the medulla illustrating the lesion in the lateral medullary syndrome.

dysfunction. Accompanying symptoms indicative of brainstem dysfunction include diplopia, dysarthria, dysphagia, vertigo, nausea, and vomiting. There may be impaired vision due to ischemia in the posterior cerebral artery distribution. Bilateral sensory complaints are common, especially circumoral paresthesias. Attacks usually last from a few minutes to half an hour, sometimes longer.

Basilar artery occlusion may have a gradual onset or a fluctuating course with prodromata, but often, the symptoms appear apocalyptically; death may occur within a short period of time. When the onset is acute, there is sudden loss of consciousness with gradually increasing coma and flaccid extremities or decerebrate rigidity. The onset may be subacute with prodromal vertigo, nausea, headache, and paresthesias, which may occur up to 2 weeks before the stroke, followed by bilateral CN and long tract abnormalities (progressive basilar thrombosis). Fisher described a "herald hemiparesis" in basilar artery thrombosis, frequently present at an early stage, when brainstem signs are absent or inconspicuous, followed within a few hours by bilateral hemiplegia and coma or a locked-in state (Chapter 51). With total occlusion, there is either hemiplegia on one side and partial hemiplegia on the other, or quadriplegia. Involvement of ascending sensory pathways causes a disturbance of both deep and superficial sensations on the body, the extremities, and sometimes the face. The pupils are usually miotic and poorly reactive. Ocular bobbing and palatal myoclonus may occur. The neurologic signs are characteristically variable and complex. Coma and decerebrate rigidity with respiratory and circulatory instability are common.

Patients with coma at the outset have a grave prognosis. The site of occlusion is usually in the lower third of the basilar artery. The outcome with severe brainstem ischemic disease is usually poor. Death is a common outcome of complete basilar artery occlusion. Patients may be left in a locked-in state (Chapter 51).

BOX 21.2

Unusual Manifestations of Lateral Medullary Syndrome

Patients may have an ipsilateral upper motor neuron facial palsy due to involvement of Dejerine's aberrant pyramidal tract (see facial nerve chapter). In the series of Sacco et al., mild ipsilateral facial weakness was present in 42% of patients, usually limited to the lower face. The hypalgesia may involve only the ipsilateral face or only the contralateral body; the classical crossed pattern occurs only in a minority. Other patterns of sensory loss are discussed in Chapter 15. Ocular motor abnormalities are common, including skew deviation with ipsilateral hypotropia, ocular tilt reaction, bizarre environmental tilt illusions including world inversion (floor on ceiling phenomenon), ipsilateral gaze deviation with impaired contralateral pursuit, saccadic abnormalities, seesaw nystagmus, and eyelid nystagmus. Ocular abnormalities and facial weakness are common and do not imply extension of the lesion beyond the lateral medulla. There may be contralateral hemiparesis due to inferior extension of the zone of ischemia to the medullary pyramid prior to decussation or ipsilateral hemiparesis due to inferior extension to the lateral funiculus of the rostral spinal cord (Opalski's submedullary syndrome, Figure 21.2). Rarely, there is impaired sensation of the ipsilateral arm and leg due to inferior extension to the gracile and cuneate nuclei, ipsilateral loss of taste, or contralateral facial hypalgesia. Other unusual manifestations include wild unilateral, proximal arm ataxia; neurotrophic ulceration of the face; inability to sneeze; paroxysmal sneezing; loss of taste; Ondine's curse; and weakness of the sternocleidomastoid. Chronic central facial pain develops in some patients.

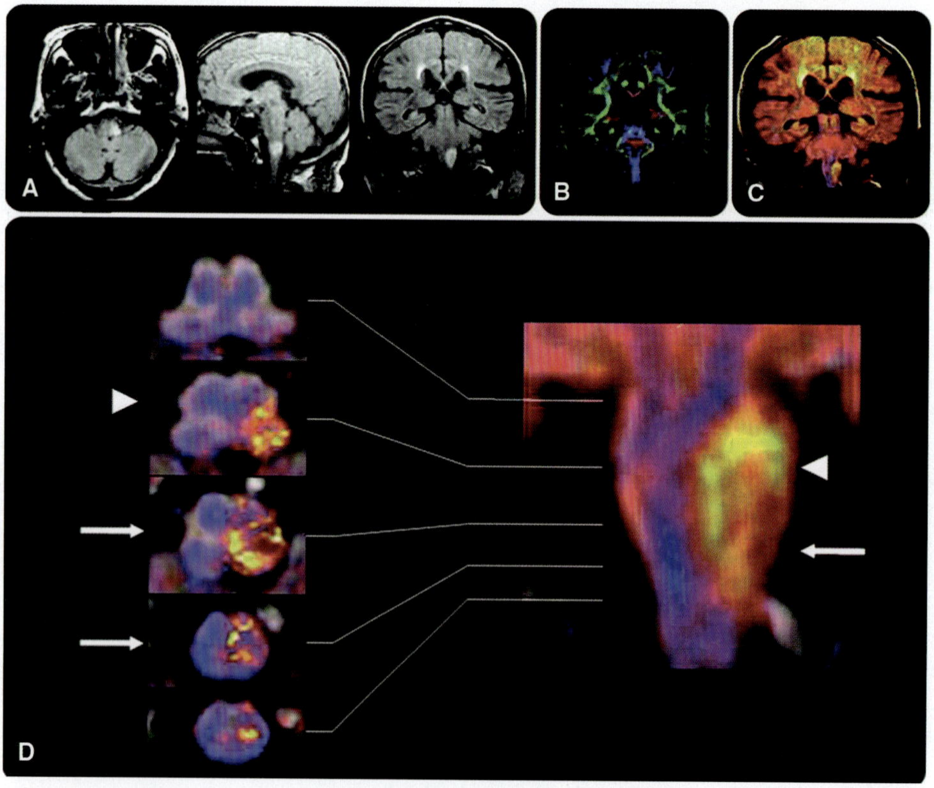

FIGURE 21.2 Imaging features of Opalski syndrome. Fluid-attenuated inversion recovery MRI. **A.** Directionally encoded map with hues reflecting tensor orientation. **B.** Superimposed images. **C,D.** A *yellow halo* represents the infarct and *blue lines* represent the pyramidal tracts (coronal); the tracts fuse at the decussation (transverse). Caudal extension of the lesion involves the ipsilateral corticospinal tract (*arrows*) after the decussation (*arrowheads*). (Reprinted from Nakamura S, Kitami M, Furukawa Y. Opalski syndrome: ipsilateral hemiplegia due to a lateral-medullary infarction. *Neurology* 2010;75[18]:1658, with permission.)

TABLE 21.2 Summary of the Vascular Pontine Syndromes Organized by Anatomical Region and Blood Vessel Involved

Syndrome	Structures Involved	Clinical Findings	Comment
Medial inferior pontine	PPRF; CN VI nucleus or fibers; MCP; CST; ML	Ipsilateral CN VI or horizontal gaze palsy; ataxia. Paresis and impaired lemniscal sensation of contralateral limbs	Due to occlusion of paramedian perforating vessel
Lateral inferior pontine (AICA syndrome)	CN VII nucleus or fibers; CN VIII nuclei; MCP; ICP; CST; principal and spinal nucleus of CN V; LST; ST; flocculus and inferior surface of cerebellar hemisphere	Ipsilateral cerebellar ataxia; loss of pain and temperature sensation and diminished light touch sensation of face; impaired taste sensation; central Horner's syndrome; deafness; peripheral type of facial palsy. Loss of pain and temperature sensation of contralateral limbs	Due to occlusion of AICA
Medial midpontine	MCP; CST; ML	Ipsilateral ataxia. Contralateral weakness of arm, leg, and face; gaze deviation; +/– impaired lemniscal sensation	Due to occlusion of paramedian perforating vessel
Lateral midpontine	MCP; CN V motor and sensory nuclei or fibers	Ipsilateral ataxia; weakness of muscles of mastication; impaired facial sensation	Due to occlusion of short circumferential artery
Medial superior pontine	SCP and/or MCP; MLF, CTT; CST; ML	Ipsilateral ataxia; INO. Contralateral weakness of arm, leg, and face; +/– impaired lemniscal sensation. Palatal myoclonus	Due to occlusion of paramedian perforating vessel
Lateral superior pontine (SCA syndrome, Mills' syndrome)	SCP and MCP; LST; lateral part of ML; superior cerebellar hemisphere	Ipsilateral ataxia; Horner's syndrome; skew deviation. Contralateral impairment of pain, temperature, and lemniscal sensation. Vertigo; dysarthria; lateropulsion to side of lesion	Due to occlusion of superior cerebellar or distal basilar artery

AICA, anterior inferior cerebellar artery; CN, cranial nerve; CST, corticospinal tract; CTT, central tegmental tract; ICP, inferior cerebellar peduncle; INO, internuclear ophthalmoplegia; LST, lateral spinothalamic tract; MCP, middle cerebellar peduncle; ML, medial lemniscus; MLF, medial longitudinal fasciculus; PPRF, pontine paramedian reticular formation; SCA, superior cerebellar artery; SCP, superior cerebellar peduncle; ST, solitary tract.

The "top of the basilar" syndrome is caused by ischemia in the distribution of the distal basilar artery, usually embolic, involving the rostral brainstem, thalamus, and portions of the cerebral hemispheres fed by the posterior cerebral arteries. A variety of oculomotor and pupillary abnormalities may occur, along with visual and behavioral abnormalities, often without significant extremity weakness.

Patients with pontine hemorrhage have a clinical picture similar to basilar artery occlusion, but warning symptoms are less apt to occur. They are comatose and quadriplegic and have bilateral facial paralysis, bilateral horizontal gaze palsies, and pinpoint poorly reactive pupils. Hyperthermia is common. Imaging studies often show a large hematoma in the midpons. Few patients survive such an event. The initial level of consciousness and the size of the hematoma are strongly related to the outcome.

Pressure on the brainstem due to supratentorial mass effect can cause either lateral transtentorial herniation (uncal syndrome), with third nerve involvement and signs of lateral midbrain compression, or central transtentorial herniation, with constricted pupils, Cheyne-Stokes respirations, bilateral corticospinal tract signs, decorticate rigidity, and progressive impairment of diencephalic, midbrain, pontine, and medullary function. Because of the patterns of venous drainage, increased intracranial pressure and herniation at either the foramen magnum or the tentorium may cause secondary bleeding into the midbrain, pons, or medulla. Duret hemorrhages are secondary hemorrhages into the upper brainstem that occur with increased intracranial pressure and descending transtentorial herniation. Brainstem hemorrhage may cause hyperthermia, respiratory abnormalities, coma, and finally death in patients with brain tumors, subarachnoid hemorrhage, cerebral hemorrhage, trauma, rapidly expanding supratentorial mass lesions, or similar conditions causing an increase in intracranial pressure. Affected patients rarely survive; Stiver et al. reported an exception in a young adult traumatic brain injury patient.

When increased intracranial pressure causes tonsillar herniation, the cerebellar tonsils and lower medulla are forced downward through the foramen magnum. Although tonsillar herniation is a feared complication of lumbar puncture done in the face of increased intracranial pressure, it is in fact rare.

BOX 21.3

Other Brainstem Syndromes

The one-and-a-half syndrome is a horizontal gaze palsy and ipsilateral internuclear ophthalmoplegia, or INO (Chapter 14). The association of an ipsilateral lower motor neuron facial nerve palsy and a one-and-a-half syndrome has been termed the eight-and-a-half syndrome. The Brissaud-Sicard syndrome is ipsilateral hemifacial spasm and contralateral hemiparesis due to a pontine lesion. The lateral pontomedullary syndrome consists of the findings of the lateral medullary syndrome with additional involvement of CNs VII and VIII consistent with extension of the lesion to the inferior pons. Raymond-Cestan syndrome is horizontal or vertical gaze palsy, contralateral hemiparesis or quadriparesis, hemianesthesia, and athetosis due to basilar branch occlusion. Rasdolsky's syndrome is contracture and paresis of the masseter and facial muscles due to neoplasm of ipsilateral pontine tegmentum. Marie-Foix syndrome is contralateral hemiparesis and hypalgesia with ipsilateral cerebellar ataxia due to a lesion involving the lateral pons. Other unusual manifestations of brainstem disease include pontine anosognosia, cognitive dysfunction, painful isolated Horner's syndrome, head shaking nystagmus, jaw opening dystonia, hemidystonia, facial pain syndromes, a sensory level on the trunk, unilateral hyper- or hypohidrosis, upside-down reversal of vision, tonic seizures, and convulsive-like movements.

Medullary compression causes profound impairment of all vital functions, with bradycardia, either a fall or rise in blood pressure, slow or rapid respirations, soaring temperature, convulsions, unconsciousness, and death. The Cushing (vasopressor) reflex (response, reaction, or effect) is hypertension, increased pulse pressure, bradycardia, and slow, irregular respirations seen in patients with increased intracranial pressure and brainstem compression. The full triad occurs in only about one-third of cases, and some patients may have isolated hypertension. On postmortem examination, a pressure cone may be seen on the medulla.

Aneurysms of the basilar or vertebral arteries or their branches, and hemangiomas, may cause extramedullary compression and CN involvement. Arteriovenous malformations may cause intramedullary or extramedullary dysfunction, depending on their extent and location. Extravasation of blood about the base of the brain from subarachnoid or intracerebral hemorrhage may affect the CNs as they leave the skull.

Lacunes are small, deep infarctions in the territory of a deep penetrating arteriole. Hypertension is the major predisposing factor. The brainstem, particularly the pons, is a common location for lacunar infarction. Brainstem lacunar syndromes include pure motor stroke, dysarthria–clumsy hand syndrome, and ataxic hemiparesis (homolateral ataxia and crural paresis). Pure motor stroke is the most common lacunar syndrome. Although lacunar syndromes, especially pure sensory stroke and ataxic hemiparesis, are highly predictive of lacunar infarction, in about one in four patients the etiology involves a nonlacunar mechanism.

Other unusual, typically vascular, brainstem syndromes are briefly described in Box 21.3.

Nonvascular Brainstem Disorders

Brainstem gliomas are astrocytomas that diffusely infiltrate the brainstem. Most involve the pons, but they may affect any level of the brainstem, typically causing a combination of multiple cranial nerve palsies (MCNPs), gaze palsy, long tract signs, and ataxia. Because of the slow evolution, there is sometimes a paucity of neurologic signs in spite of the size of the tumor. Ventricular obstruction may produce hydrocephalus and increased intracranial pressure. Ependymomas and medulloblastomas may also involve the brainstem. Extramedullary tumors (neurofibromas, schwannomas, meningiomas, hemangiomas, metastases) may cause pressure effects. The course of a brainstem neoplasm is progressive. Increased intracranial pressure may appear late, particularly in brainstem gliomas. Extrinsic metastases and neoplasms that spread by direct extension from the nasopharynx and neighboring sites may cause widespread CN involvement and bone erosion with signs of brainstem compression. Tuberculomas, sarcoidosis, and other granulomas may produce a picture similar to neoplasms.

Brainstem encephalitis (Bickerstaff's encephalitis) is a clinical syndrome of acute diffuse or multifocal brainstem dysfunction with cerebrospinal fluid (CSF) pleocytosis and increased protein. Actual viral infection has seldom, if ever, been documented, and the disease is usually immunologically mediated. Patients develop ophthalmoplegia and ataxia followed by gradual brainstem dysfunction and altered consciousness. The illness is usually preceded by a viral infection. Some patients have serum anti-GQ1b IgG autoantibodies, the same antibody found in Miller Fisher syndrome (ophthalmoplegia, ataxia, and areflexia). Bickerstaff's brainstem encephalitis is not to be confused with Bickerstaff's (basilar artery) migraine (see below). Brainstem encephalitis may be paraneoplastic. Rhombencephalitis refers to inflammatory disease affecting the hindbrain (brainstem and cerebellum). It has a wide variety of etiologies, including multiple sclerosis (MS), Behcet's disease, paraneoplastic syndrome, lupus, and viral and tuberculous infection. Listeria monocytogenes is particularly likely to cause rhombencephalitis; it accounted for 9% of cases in one series.

Demyelinating disease frequently involves the brainstem. INO due to a demyelinating lesion involving the MLF is a very common clinical manifestation of MS. MS can cause lesions elsewhere in the brainstem and can occasionally simulate one of the vascular syndromes. Acute disseminated encephalomyelitis may affect the brainstem, and the involvement is occasionally limited to the brainstem.

In central pontine myelinolysis (osmotic demyelination syndrome), there is widespread, symmetric myelin loss in the central portion of the pons. Lesions commonly occur in other sites as well (extrapontine myelinolysis). Central pontine myelinolysis occurs especially in alcoholics or other malnourished or debilitated individuals and after correction of severe hyponatremia. It typically begins with diplopia, dysphagia, dysarthria, and other evidence of brainstem dysfunction, followed by quadriplegia, mutism, and extensor rigidity. Central pontine myelinolysis runs a fulminating course and is often fatal.

Developmental or congenital anomalies of the craniocervical junction are frequently associated with brainstem dysfunction. The bony walls of the foramen magnum and upper spinal canal lie in close anatomic relationship to the lower brainstem, upper spinal cord, and cerebellum. Neurologic abnormalities may be produced by mechanical compression by the bony abnormality, but often the bony abnormality and the neural abnormality are part of the same process. Platybasia, basilar impression, occipitalization of the atlas, and cervical spina bifida are examples of primary bony abnormalities. Klippel-Feil syndrome is the congenital fusion of two or more cervical vertebrae. There may be accompanying craniocervical junction abnormalities. The associated neurologic abnormalities may include myelopathy, radiculopathy, syringomyelia, and mirror movements.

Arnold-Chiari (or simply Chiari, who made the greater contribution) malformation is a congenital maldevelopment of the brainstem and cerebellum. The cerebellar tonsils are herniated or displaced down into the upper cervical spinal canal. With more severe maldevelopment, the inferior vermis, lower medulla, and fourth ventricle may also be displaced below the foramen magnum. Clinical manifestations include headache, cerebellar ataxia, nystagmus (typically downbeat), and other brainstem deficits. Three varieties commonly occur. Type 1 is the hindbrain malformation only; it can present in adulthood. Mild type 1 Chiari malformations are not uncommonly found on MRI imaging done for other reasons and may be totally asymptomatic. Type 2 is a more severe hindbrain defect usually associated with a lumbar meningomyelocele. Type 3 is the same as type 2 except that the meningomyelocele or encephalocele occurs in the occipitocervical region. The Dandy-Walker syndrome is agenesis of the cerebellar vermis with a massively dilated fourth ventricle forming a cystic structure that occupies most of the posterior fossa.

Syringobulbia is a slit-like cavity in the brainstem. A brainstem syrinx is usually a rostral extension of a syringomyelic cavity from the cervical spinal cord in a patient with a Chiari malformation, but syringobulbia may rarely occur de novo. In syringobulbia, the syrinx most often involves the lateral medullary tegmentum. The cavity is usually restricted to the lower brainstem but may extend to the pons and rarely higher. The cavity and the resultant clinical picture are typically asymmetric, with lower CN dysfunction, facial numbness, and nystagmus. The facial sensory loss may be in an onion-skin distribution, initially sparing the nasal tip and perioral region. Hypoglossal weakness and atrophy may occur. Facial myokymia is an unusual feature. There may be autonomic involvement and respiratory compromise.

A strategically placed lesion involving the pyramidal decussation may cause unusual patterns of weakness. The corticospinal fibers innervating the upper extremities are thought to decussate more rostrally and medially than the fibers innervating the lower extremities, although this concept has been questioned (Figure 11.12). The term cruciate paralysis is used in two ways. One refers to weakness of both arms, brachial diplegia, with relative sparing of the legs, due to a lesion involving the rostral portion of the pyramidal decussation. The findings are similar to those of a central cord syndrome of the cervical spine or the man-in-the-barrel syndrome because of watershed cerebral infarction. Most cases are due to trauma. The other use refers to corticospinal paralysis of one arm and the opposite leg (cruciate hemiplegia, pyramidal decussation syndrome). This may occur because a lesion involves arm fibers that have already decussated but leg fibers that have not, which causes a crossed pattern of weakness. Triparesis, with weakness of one arm and both legs, has been reported after unilateral medial medullary infarction.

Gerstman-Sträussler-Schinker (GSS) syndrome is a rare autosomal dominant spongiform encephalopathy due to a mutation of the prion protein gene. It begins in midlife and runs a progressive course with ataxia, spasticity, dysarthria, nystagmus, and dementia. GSS is genetically and phenotypically heterogeneous; among the different prion diseases, it has the longest clinical course and the potential to mimic other neurologic disorders, such as cerebellar degeneration and demyelinating disease.

Basilar artery (Bickerstaff's, basilar type, vertebrobasilar, posterior fossa) migraine is an unusual type of complicated migraine with prominent brainstem symptoms similar to those of VBI. The disorder occurs primarily in young females and is usually followed by an occipital headache.

The foramen magnum syndrome can cause some unusual and puzzling clinical deficits. Lesions in the region of the foramen magnum are typically compressive extramedullary mass lesions (e.g., meningioma). Patients may have crossed hemiparesis, involving one arm and the opposite leg, because of involvement of the pyramidal decussation (see above). There may be weakness and wasting of the small hand muscles for reasons that remain unclear. Such hand muscle wasting may also occur as a false localizing sign in upper cervical spinal cord compression. Downbeat nystagmus in primary gaze is suggestive of a lesion at the cervicomedullary junction, and the nystagmus is often greatest in eccentric downgaze. Other symptoms suggestive of a foramen magnum lesion include occipital headache, neck pain, and stiffness; Lhermitte's sign; C2 sensory loss; and shawl distribution upper extremity sensory loss. Tumors are generally histologically benign and often become large before the diagnosis is made. Masses usually intrude from posteriorly, so that posterior column signs, including pseudoathetosis, are common. Lower CN palsies are uncommon. There may be a fluctuating course simulating MS.

Bulbar Palsy

There are two principal types of bulbar palsy: PBP and pseudobulbar palsy. In both, the outstanding symptoms are dysphagia and dysarthria; both run a chronic course. Despite the similarities, the etiologies are different.

PBP is a form of motor neuron disease involving bulbar innervated muscles, causing weakness and atrophy of muscles supplied by the lower CNs, often accompanied by fasciculations. It is closely related to progressive spinal muscular atrophy, in which the process is limited to the anterior horn cells of the spinal cord, and amyotrophic lateral sclerosis (ALS), in which there is involvement of the bulbar nuclei, the anterior horn cells, and the pyramidal cells in the motor cortex.

In PBP, there is a relentlessly progressive degeneration of the neurons of the brainstem motor nuclei, primarily those in the medulla. It usually occurs in late adult life with onset in the sixth and seventh decades. The disease usually starts in the nucleus of the CN XII and ascends. Typical initial manifestations are atrophy, weakness, and fasciculations of the tongue. Involvement is bilateral from the outset. In advanced cases, the patient may be unable to protrude the tongue or to manipulate food in the mouth. The lingual involvement is followed or accompanied by dysphagia and dysarthria. Nasal regurgitation of liquids is common and may lead to choking and aspiration. Involvement of the soft palate, larynx, and tongue causes flaccid dysarthria. Early, the most pronounced difficulty is with pronunciation of linguals and velars; later, the labials are affected. In advanced cases, speech is reduced to unintelligible laryngeal noises. There is often marked drooling of saliva. Patients may keep a tissue or rag at the chin to absorb unswallowed secretions. Sometimes, atrophy and fasciculations extend to the palate and pharynx, and the condition may eventually ascend to involve the facial and trigeminal motor nuclei. Occasionally, the sternocleidomastoid and trapezius muscles are affected. There may be autonomic involvement with tachycardia. The palatal and pharyngeal gag reflexes disappear early. There are no sensory changes. PBP is aggressive and relentless, with death usually caused by aspiration pneumonia. PBP may be the first manifestation of ALS. When ALS causes prominent bulbar weakness, it is referred to as bulbar ALS. In bulbar palsy due to ALS, there are also corticospinal tract manifestations. In a series of 32 patients with PBP, all but two progressed to ALS, regardless of the presence of upper motor signs or generalized denervation on limb electromyography (EMG). The other two died at the PBP stage.

Severe bulbar involvement occurs in other motor neuronopathies. It is often the terminal aspect of Werdnig-Hoffmann disease (hereditary spinal muscular atrophy type 1). Fazio-Londe disease is PBP occurring in children. Kennedy's disease (X-linked recessive bulbospinal neuronopathy) causes a clinical picture resembling ALS but with slow progression and other atypical features; dysphagia or dysarthria may be prominent late in the course. Bulbar polioencephalitis may occur as part of paralytic poliomyelitis, causing paralysis of the throat, tongue, and respiratory muscles. Creutzfeldt-Jakob disease may present as bulbar palsy.

Pseudobulbar palsy also causes marked difficulty with bulbar function, especially speech and swallowing. Although the clinical manifestations are similar, the underlying mechanism is entirely different. Pseudobulbar palsy is caused by bilateral supranuclear lesions, which involve the corticobulbar pathways to the bulbar nuclei. PBP and bulbar ALS cause lower motor neuron weakness; pseudobulbar palsy causes upper motor neuron weakness. In patients with bulbar ALS, both processes may be at work. Because of bilateral supranuclear innervation, unilateral lesions of the corticobulbar tract rarely cause significant bulbar dysfunction. But with bilateral supranuclear lesions, the bulbar dysfunction may be severe. It is usually accompanied by other upper motor neuron signs. There may be weakness and spasticity of the muscles of mastication, an exaggerated jaw jerk, and frontal release signs such as snout and suck reflexes. Difficulty with emotional control causing spontaneous, unprovoked laughing and crying (pseudobulbar affect, emotional incontinence) is common. Pathologic laughing ("fou rire prodromique") and crying have also been reported with brainstem lesions. Some patients have paresis of the muscles of facial expression causing masking of the facies. There are typically significant neurologic abnormalities beyond the distribution of the CN nuclei, with bilateral cortical spinal tract signs.

The most common cause of pseudobulbar palsy is multiple cerebral infarctions. The syndrome may also occur in encephalitis, MS, trauma, cerebral anoxia, primary lateral sclerosis, or other disease processes that cause bilateral corticobulbar tract lesions. The lesions may be in the cortex or in the corona radiata, internal capsule, cerebral peduncles, or brainstem rostral to the nuclear centers. Speech is thick and slurred but may have an explosive quality. There may be dysphagia, nasal regurgitation, choking, and drooling. Patients may keep food in the mouth for prolonged periods. There is less of a tendency to choke than in true bulbar palsy because the gag reflexes are intact and may be hyperactive. Although the tongue may be strikingly immobile, atrophy and fasciculations do not develop. The prognosis in pseudobulbar palsy is no more favorable than in PBP. The eventual outcome in both conditions is death, often because of aspiration. Two types of pseudobulbar palsy have been described; one is due to lesions affecting the corticobulbar fibers, and the other is due to involvement of the basal ganglia or extrapyramidal pathways. In striatal pseudobulbar palsy, there are additional signs of basal ganglia involvement, including rigidity, hyperkinesias, and a parkinsonian picture.

Other conditions that may cause prominent weakness of bulbar muscles or other evidence of brainstem dysfunction include neuromuscular transmission disorders, some neuropathies and myopathies, and certain rare neurologic conditions. The dysarthria and dysphagia of myasthenia gravis (MG) may resemble bulbar palsy. Early in the course, it may be difficult to distinguish bulbar ALS or PBP from MG. The characteristic eye signs of MG are not always present. Bulbar signs and symptoms similar to those of MG can occur in botulism and Lambert-Eaton syndrome.

Patients with MUSK antibody MG tend to have prominent bulbar dysfunction, neck and shoulder girdle weakness, and respiratory symptoms and may develop muscle atrophy. Bulbar muscle weakness can occur in muscular dystrophies, especially oculopharyngeal dystrophy, and other myopathies. Bulbar weakness may complicate Guillain-Barré syndrome and other polyneuropathies. CN involvement is characteristic of diphtheritic polyneuropathy. In tetanus, pharyngeal spasms may accompany trismus. In rabies, spasmodic contractions of the muscles occur on attempts to swallow. Whipple's disease involving the central nervous system (CNS) may have prominent brainstem findings. Oculomasticatory myorhythmia, a striking movement disorder involving the eyes and jaw, is characteristic, perhaps pathognomonic, of CNS Whipple's disease. Brainstem involvement may be a striking feature of Leigh's disease (subacute necrotizing encephalomyopathy). The brainstem can also be damaged by radiation.

MULTIPLE CRANIAL NERVE PALSIES

Intracranial-extramedullary or extracranial processes may involve more than one CN. A disease may involve homologous nerves on the two sides (e.g., bilateral facial palsy) or different nerves on the same or opposite sides. In some conditions, a cluster of nerves is involved in a discrete anatomical region. The progression may follow some anatomical pattern or appear capricious. Multiple CNs may be affected from the outset, or the process may begin with one nerve and progress to involve others. Pain may or may not be present. Table 21.3 lists some conditions that may cause MCNPs. Table 21.4 covers some of the named multiple CN syndromes.

In Keane's series of 979 patients with MCNP, the most commonly involved nerves were CNs VI, VII, V, and VIII. The most common combinations were involvement of CNs III and IV, V and VI, and V and VII. The most common locations were cavernous sinus, brainstem, and individual nerve trunks. The most common causes were neoplasm, vascular disease, trauma, infection, and the Guillain-Barré and Miller Fisher syndromes. A MCNP variant of Guillain-Barré has been described. The most common causes of recurrent cranial neuropathies were diabetes and idiopathic.

A major consideration when there is MCNP is some process affecting the meninges at the base of the skull. Although infectious and inflammatory conditions are possible, the major consideration when there is painless dysfunction of several CNs over a period of days to weeks is neoplastic meningitis, which can be either carcinomatous or lymphomatous (meningeal carcinomatosis or lymphomatosis). Neoplastic meningitis occurs in as many as 15% of patients with systemic malignancy and may be the presenting manifestation in 5% to 10%. The most common neoplastic processes to involve the meninges are small cell carcinoma of the lung, melanoma, and myeloblastic leukemia. Carcinoma of the breast seldom spreads to the meninges but is a common cause of meningeal neoplasia because of its frequency.

Patients with neoplastic meningitis typically have accompanying headache, meningeal signs, and evidence of increased intracranial pressure. Facial numbness in association with a multiple lower CN palsy syndrome is ominous. A combination of CNs VI and XII palsies is particularly suggestive of a neoplastic

TABLE 21.3 Some Disease Processes That May Involve Multiple Cranial Nerves (CNs)

Acute infectious meningitis
Chronic infectious meningitis
Syphilis
Lyme disease
Viral infection (Herpes zoster, herpes simplex, EBV, HIV, HTLV-1, CMV)
Meningeal neoplasia (leptomeningeal metastases, carcinomatous meningitis, lymphomatous meningitis, primary leptomeningeal lymphoma, neurolymphomatosis)
Pituitary apoplexy
Nasopharyngeal carcinoma (Schmincke tumor)
Primary clivus or skull base neoplasm (glomus tumor, meningioma, chordoma, others)
Metastatic clivus or skull base neoplasm (prostate, breast, lung, head, and neck tumors)
Cavernous sinus disease (Tolosa-Hunt syndrome, mass lesion, others)
Sarcoidosis (special predilection for CNs II, VII, and VIII)
Granulomatosis with polyangiitis (Wegener's granulomatosis)
Vasculitis (polyarteritis nodosa, Churg-Strauss, lymphomatoid granulomatosis, giant cell arteritis, granulomatous angiitis)
Connective tissue disease (systemic lupus erythematosis, Sjögren's syndrome, scleroderma, mixed connective tissue disease)
Cryoglobulinemia
Prepontine mass lesion
Skull base trauma
Aneurysm (carotid dissection, fusiform basilar)
Carotid endarterectomy
Bony disease of skull base (Paget's disease, osteopetrosis)
Diabetes mellitus
Guillain-Barré syndrome
Miller Fisher syndrome
Polyneuritis cranialis
Amyloidosis
Craniocervical junction anomalies
Cranial irradiation
Idiopathic cranial polyneuropathy
Idiopathic hypertrophic cranial pachymeningitis

CMV, cytomegalovirus; EBV, Epstein-Barr virus; HTLV-1, human T-cell lymphocytotrophic virus.

TABLE 21.4 Summary of Syndromes with Involvement of Multiple CNs*

Syndrome	Lesion Location	Structures Involved	Clinical Findings	Comment
Superior orbit fissure (Rochon-Duvigneau)	Superior orbital fissure	CNs III; IV; VI; V_1	Weakness of CNs III, IV, VI; sensory loss in V_1 distribution; +/– proptosis	Usually due to tumor or carotid aneurysm
Orbital apex	Orbital apex	Same as superior orbital fissure plus CN II	Same as superior orbital fissure plus visual impairment due to CN II involvement	Usually due to tumor, aneurysm, or inflammatory process (orbital pseudotumor)
Orbital floor (Dejean's)	Orbital floor	Ocular motor nerve or extraocular muscle, V_2	Diplopia, V_2 sensory loss, exophthalmos	Mass lesion or blowout fracture of floor of orbit
Cavernous sinus (Foix-Jefferson)	Cavernous sinus	CNs III; IV; VI; V_1, +/–V_2; pericarotid sympathetics	Weakness of CNs III, IV, VI; sensory loss in V_1 distribution; +/– proptosis	Common causes include granulomatous inflammation (Tolosa-Hunt syndrome), tumor, and aneurysm
Retrosphenoid space (Negro-Jacod)	Retrosphenoid space	CNs II; III; IV; V, VI	Dysfunction of listed nerves	Usual cause is large middle fossa neoplasm
Petrous apex (Gradenigo's)	Apex of the petrous bone	CNs V; VI	Sixth nerve palsy and facial pain and/or numbness	Usual causes are inflammation (*apex petrositis*) and tumor
Cerebellopontine angle	Cerebellopontine angle	CN VIII; +/–VII; +/–V; +/– cerebellar hemisphere	Hearing loss; imbalance; facial sensory loss; large tumors may cause facial weakness, ataxia, increased ICP	Usual cause is acoustic neuroma; other mass lesions may produce the same picture (e.g., meningioma)
Jugular foramen (Vernet's)	Jugular foramen	CN IX; X; XI	Weakness in the distribution of involved nerves	Usual causes are tumor of jugular bulb, aneurysm, and trauma (e.g., basilar skull fracture)
Collet-Sicard (MacKenzie, Lannois-Jouty)	Posterior lateral condylar space	CN IX; X; XI; XII	Weakness in the distribution of involved nerves	Usually due to neoplasm of the skull base, especially glomus jugulare tumor; occasionally carotid aneurysm (including dissection)
Villaret's	Retropharyngeal space	CNs IX; X; XI; XII; carotid sympathetics	Weakness in the distribution of involved nerves; Horner's syndrome	Usually due to neoplasm of the skull base, especially glomus jugulare tumor, occasionally carotid aneurysm (including dissection)
Tapia's	Retroparotid space	CNs X; XII; +/–XI; carotid sympathetics	Weakness in the distribution of involved nerves; Horner's syndrome	Usually due to tumor of parotid or skull base; occasionally carotid aneurysm (including dissection)
Garcin's (half-base)	Skull base	Variable CNs III–XII	Unilateral paralysis of all or most of the cranial nerves; occasionally bilateral	Usually due to tumor of the skull base, nasopharynx, or retropharyngeal space; can be due to granuloma or infection

*Most are due to disease extracranially in the region of the skull base. Some are more commonly known by their anatomic description (e.g., jugular foramen syndrome) and some by their eponym (e.g., Collet-Sicard syndrome). In some instances, the anatomic designation is reasonably precise and appropriate (e.g., cavernous sinus syndrome). In others, the anatomical description is cumbersome or obscure, and the eponym is more convenient. The table lists the usage likely to be most familiar to most readers first.

CN, cranial nerve; ICP, increased intracranial pressure.

process involving the clivus. Leptomeningeal metastatic disease from solid tumors is more likely to present with spinal cord or radicular involvement. Diffuse meningeal involvement from hematologic malignancies is more likely to present with MCNP. Obtaining CSF cytologic confirmation is often difficult initially; biochemical markers may be helpful.

Other neoplastic processes and mass lesions at the base of the skull may also produce an MCNP syndrome. A skull base neoplasm accounted for 13% of cases in Keane's MCNP series. Nasopharyngeal carcinomas (NPCs), such as lymphoepithelioma (Schmincke tumor), occur in younger patients than do other head and neck cancers; there may be an association with Epstein-Barr virus infection. NPC often arises in Rosenmuller's fossa and spreads laterally to the paranasopharyngeal space and then to the skull base. The tumor may infiltrate the pterygopalatine fossa, and the maxillary nerve, and may spread to involve the cavernous sinus. About 20% of patients have CN involvement at the time of the diagnosis of NPC. Radiotherapy for the tumor may itself cause cranial neuropathy, particularly of CN XII. Distinguishing radiation-induced neuropathy from tumor recurrence may be difficult.

NPCs may erode the clivus. Other tumors involving the clivus may also cause MCNP. A chordoma, a rare primary bone tumor, usually presents in males in the sixth decade. The tumor is histologically benign but locally invasive and destructive. When it extends posteriorly, it may cause CN palsies or brainstem compression. Other skull base neoplasms include metastasis, meningiomas, lymphoma, myeloma, histiocytosis, neurinoma, giant cell tumor, hemangiopericytoma, and various primary bone tumors. Osteopetrosis (Albers-Schonberg or marble bone disease) causes a generalized increase in bone density and can narrow exit foramina, causing MCNP. Other bone disorders that may behave similarly include Paget's disease, fibrous dysplasia, and hyperostosis cranialis interna.

Mass lesions lying along the clivus, even though not arising from it directly, may cause MCNP. Vertebrobasilar dolichoectasia may cause cranial neuropathies because of compression or ischemia. Patients with a tortuous basilar artery of normal caliber are more likely to have isolated cranial neuropathy; those with basilar artery ectasia or with fusiform, giant aneurysm are more likely to have MCNP. Rarely, hematoma lying along the clivus in the prepontine region affects multiple CNs. Other processes that may affect the prepontine region include exophytic glioma and dermoid, epidermoid, and other cystic lesions.

Infectious disease accounted for 10% of Keane's MCNP cases. Conditions particularly prone to cause cranial neuropathy include Lyme disease, tuberculosis, neurosyphilis, cryptococcosis, and HIV.

The nervous system is involved in 5% to 15% of patients with sarcoidosis. The disease may present neurologically and rarely remains confined to the nervous system. About half of the patients with neurosarcoidosis have CN involvement. The CNs most commonly involved are II, VII, and VIII. A peripheral facial palsy is the most common manifestation. About half of the patients with CN involvement have a cranial polyneuropathy, most commonly bilateral facial nerve palsy. Other common neurologic complications include chronic meningitis, hydrocephalus, hypothalamic-pituitary dysfunction, myelopathy, myopathy, and peripheral neuropathy. Neurologic involvement occurs in as many as 20% of patients with Behcet's disease, including MCNP due to meningeal or brainstem lesions. The most commonly involved nerves are CN II and CN VIII.

Several forms of systemic vasculitis may cause MCNP; the most common is granulomatosis with polyangiitis (Wegener's granulomatosis). In one series, cranial neuropathies were the most common neurologic abnormality. Giant cell arteritis may cause the combination of optic and extraocular neuropathies. Other vasculitic processes of concern include lymphomatoid granulomatosis, a lymphoreticular malignancy, and vasculitis due to connective tissue disease, especially polyarteritis nodosa.

Polyneuritis cranialis is an MCNP syndrome that may represent a variant of Guillain-Barré syndrome involving the lower CNs. An acute, painful, steroid-responsive MCNP syndrome that may be on a continuum with Tolosa-Hunt syndrome (see section on Cavernous Sinus Syndrome) but involving nerves outside the cavernous sinus has been described (idiopathic cranial polyneuropathy). Bannwarth's syndrome (meningopolyradiculitis) refers to MCNP and painful polyradiculopathies due to Lyme disease. Most patients have an acute peripheral facial paresis with additional involvement of other nerves and spinal roots.

CN palsy occurs occasionally in carotid artery dissection; rarely, it is the dominant or only manifestation. Ipsilateral headache, Horner's syndrome, and lower CN palsy are suggestive of carotid dissection even in the absence of cerebral ischemic symptoms. CN XII is invariably affected, and in some patients, other CNs may be involved as well. The etiology is not certain. There may be compression or stretching by the aneurysmal dilatation or ischemia due to involvement of the segmental arteries supplying the nerves, particularly the ascending pharyngeal artery. CN palsy also occurs as a complication of carotid endarterectomy.

Trauma accounted for 12% of MCNP cases in Keane's series. Blunt trauma, such as MVA or falling, is twice as common as penetrating trauma. Iatrogenic trauma accounts for a significant minority, especially radical head or neck dissections.

DISORDERS OF CRANIAL NERVE GROUPS

In some locations, two or more CNs are bundled in a common anatomical space, such as the cavernous sinus or jugular foramen. A focal disease process may involve the entire cluster of nerves. Intradural, extramedullary pathology involves the nerves after they exit the brainstem but before they exit the skull (e.g., in the cerebellopontine angle [CPA]). Extracranial pathology involves a group of nerves just after they exit the skull but before they disperse (e.g., in the retroparotid space). As with brainstem syndromes, the many syndromes that involve multiple CNs carry an eponym and an anatomical description. The anatomical regions involved are often so arcane that the eponym serves just as well. Table 21.4 summarizes these syndromes. Most of the disorders affecting CN groups are due to mass effect. The mass is often neoplastic. Primary neural tumors, such as schwannoma or neurofibroma, arising from one CN may cause compression of adjacent nerves. Many of these syndromes are rare in neurologic practice. The relatively common ones are the cavernous sinus, CPA, and jugular foramen syndromes.

Cavernous Sinus Syndrome

The cavernous sinuses are complex venous channels that lie on either side of the sphenoid bone and sella turcica, extending from the superior orbital fissure to the apex of the petrous temporal bone (Figure 21.3). The two sides are connected by an anterior and posterior intercavernous sinus. A thin layer of dura, the pituitary capsule, forms the medial wall of the cavernous sinus. The internal carotid artery with its pericarotid sympathetic plexus runs through the sinus. CNs III, IV, and V lie in the wall of the sinus from above to below. CN VI lies free in the lumen of the sinus inferolateral to the carotid artery. The ophthalmic division of CN V traverses the sinus; the maxillary division runs for a short distance through its posterior-inferior part.

Conditions of the cavernous sinus were recognized by Gowers in 1888, but some years later, the writings of C. Foix (French neurologist) and

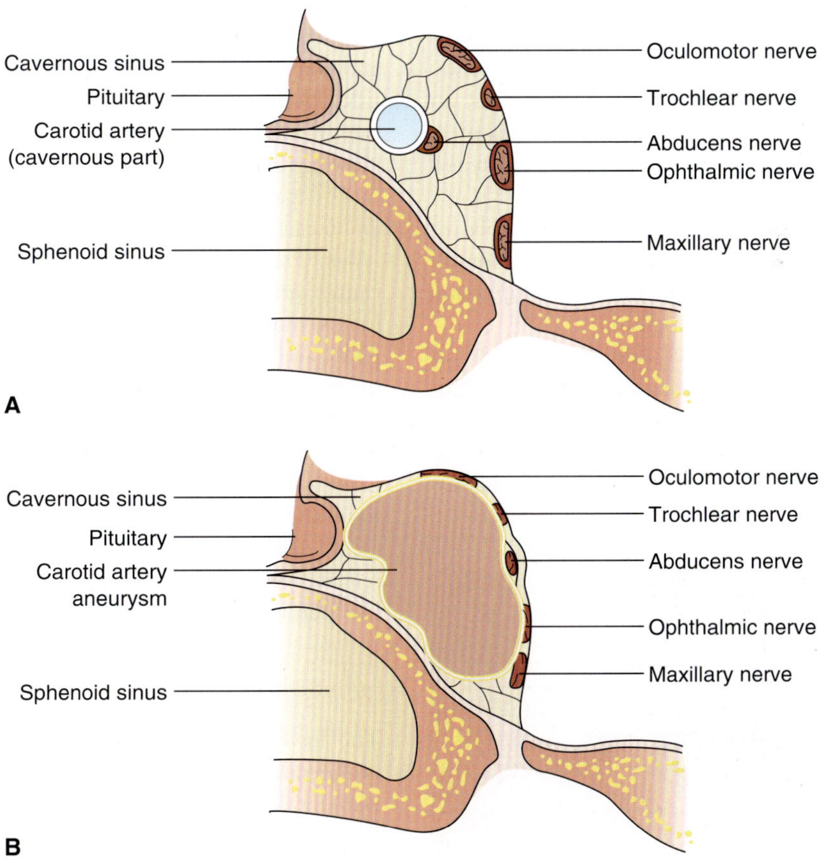

FIGURE 21.3 **A.** The cavernous sinus lies just lateral to the sella turcica. Within it lie the carotid artery and cranial nerves (CNs) III, IV, and VI and branches of CN V. **B.** Pathologic findings involving the cavernous sinus are not rare and can usually be recognized by the pattern of CN involvement.

G. Jefferson (English neurosurgeon, best known for describing C1 fracture) brought wide recognition to the existence of the cavernous sinus syndrome. The cavernous sinus may be involved by tumor, thrombosis (bland or septic), carotid aneurysm, carotid-cavernous fistula, inflammation, infection, and other processes. There is variable involvement of the CNs crossing the sinus. Severe processes may affect all of the nerves, but isolated sixth nerve palsy also occurs. In Keane's series of 151 patients, the most common etiologies were tumor, trauma, self-limited inflammation, carotid aneurysms and fistulas, and infection. These accounted for 88% of the cases. Other causes of cavernous sinus syndrome include pituitary apoplexy, metastasis, lymphoma or leukemia, myeloma, neuroblastoma, mucormycosis, aspergillosis, tuberculosis, carotid-cavernous fistula, trauma, and sarcoidosis.

Intracavernous carotid aneurysms may compress and distort the contents of the cavernous sinus (Figure 21.3B). A carotid-cavernous fistula is a communication between the carotid artery and the cavernous sinus. Fistulas may be traumatic or develop spontaneously because of rupture of an intracavernous carotid aneurysm. In addition to CN palsies, patients may have pulsatile proptosis, chemosis, an ocular bruit, and evidence of increased venous pressure in the eye. Dilated, arteriolized conjunctival and episcleral blood vessels with a tortuous, corkscrew shape are characteristic (Figure 21.4). Neoplasms commonly involve the cavernous sinus. Common tumor types include NPC, metastases, lymphoma, pituitary adenoma, and meningioma.

Two neurosurgeons, E. S. Tolosa (Spanish) and W. E. Hunt (American), described indolent, idiopathic, granulomatous inflammation of the cavernous sinus causing pain and ophthalmoplegia. Pathologically, there is noncaseating, granulomatous inflammation similar to that seen in orbital pseudotumor. Patients present with severe periorbital headache and dysfunction of one or more of the intracavernous CNs. Tolosa-Hunt syndrome is exquisitely responsive to even small doses of steroids, and steroid responsiveness has been used as a diagnostic criterion. However, other conditions involving the cavernous sinus, including tumors, infection, and aneurysm, may also improve with steroids. MRI may show T2 isointense tissue that enhances with gadolinium. Another condition related to cavernous sinus syndrome is Raeder's paratrigeminal (or the paratrigeminal oculosympathetic) syndrome (Chapter 15).

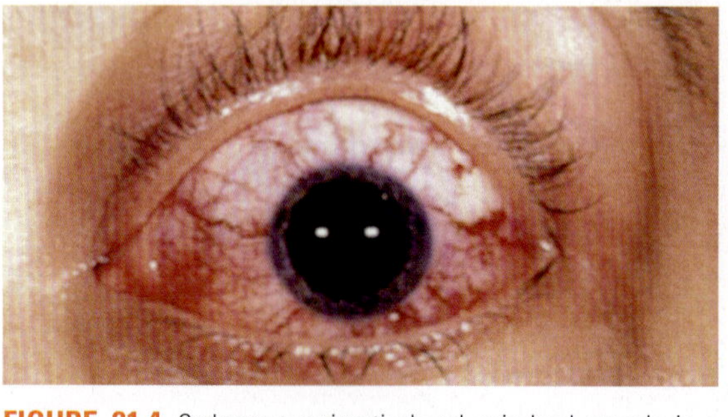

FIGURE 21.4 Corkscrew conjunctival and episcleral vessels in a patient with a carotid-cavernous fistula.

Cerebellopontine Angle Syndrome

A mass lesion in the CPA is usually an acoustic neuroma, but other tumors and masses may arise in the region (Chapter 17). An acoustic neuroma usually arises from the vestibular portion of CN VIII within the internal auditory meatus. The initial symptoms are usually hearing loss and tinnitus. Examination early in the course shows sensorineural hearing loss and impaired labyrinthine function on the involved side. Vertigo is unusual because the tumor grows slowly and the vestibular system compensates, although patients may have impaired balance. As the mass expands, compression of CN V causes ipsilateral facial sensory loss and impairment of the corneal reflex. Pressure on the cerebellum or its peduncles causes ataxia and incoordination. There may be involvement of CN VII, with a peripheral facial palsy, and of CNs VI, IX, and X. Late in the course, increased intracranial pressure may cause headache, papilledema, and occasional loss of consciousness. Nystagmus is common; it may be coarse and slow on gaze toward the side of the lesion (gaze paretic nystagmus) and fine and rapid on gaze away from the lesion (vestibular nystagmus). This unusual combination is referred to as Bruns' nystagmus (for Ludwig Bruns, German neurologist, see **Video Link 21.1**).

Lower Cranial Nerve Syndromes

The lower CN syndromes involve CNs IX to XII unilaterally in various combinations. These nerves exit the skull just above the foramen magnum. CNs IX, X, and XI exit through the jugular foramen along with the jugular vein. CN XII exits through the hypoglossal canal just inferiorly. CNs IX to XII lie close together in their initial course, near the carotid artery, with its pericarotid sympathetic plexus, and the jugular vein in the upper neck. The prototype lower CN syndrome is the jugular foramen syndrome (JFS) characterized by ipsilateral paralysis of CNs IX, X, and XI. JFS is caused by a lesion at the jugular foramen or in the retroparotid space. Collet-Sicard syndrome is the additional involvement of CN XII. Villaret's syndrome is Collet-Sicard with the addition of Horner's syndrome (Table 21.4). Sometimes, the term JFS is used to refer to any combination of palsies affecting the last four CNs.

Glomus tumors (paragangliomas, chemodectomas) arise from the glomera of the chemoreceptor system. They commonly arise in the jugular bulb (glomus jugulare), the middle ear (glomus tympanicum), and the nodose ganglion of the vagus nerve (glomus vagale). On examination, a vascular polyp may be found in the auditory canal or behind the tympanic membrane. Glomus jugulare tumors are a common cause of JFS. These tumors grow slowly, may erode bone, and may extend intracranially. Glomus tumors are much more difficult to manage when there is intracranial extension, and the presence of JFS indicates 50% likelihood that the tumor has invaded the posterior fossa. Involvement of CN XII increases the probability to 75%. Other reported causes of JFS include metastasis, trauma, meningioma, ectopic glioma, hydatid cyst, plasmacytoma, chordoma, malignant external otitis, retroparotid abscess, giant cell arteritis, cephalic herpes zoster, and thrombosis of the jugular bulb. The lower four CNs also run close together just prior to their exit from the skull and may be involved in intracranial processes such as schwannoma, ependymoma, and meningioma.

Video Links

Video Link 21.1. Bruns' nystagmus. http://www.neuroophthalmology.ca/case-of-the-month/eye-movements/diplopia-and-an-unusual-nystagmus

BIBLIOGRAPHY

Agrawal A, Timothy J, Cincu R, et al. Bradycardia in neurosurgery. *Clin Neurol Neurosurg* 2008;110:321–327.

Amarenco P, Hauw J-J. Cerebellar infarction in the territory of the anterior and inferior cerebellar artery. A clinicopathological study of 20 cases. *Brain* 1990;113:139.

Amarenco P, Hauw J-J. Cerebellar infarction in the territory of the superior cerebellar artery. A clinicopathological study of 33 cases. *Neurology* 1990;40:1383–1390.

Amato AA, Prior TW, Barohn RJ, et al. Kennedy's disease: a clinicopathologic correlation with mutations in the androgen receptor gene. *Neurology* 1993;43:791–794.

Arboix A, Padilla I, Massons J, et al. Clinical study of 222 patients with pure motor stroke. *J Neurol Neurosurg Psychiatry* 2001;71:239–242.

Arboix A, Grivé E, Sánchez MJ. Pure motor hemiparesis due to occlusion of the internal carotid artery. *Acta Neurol Belg* 2017;117:337–339.

Asmaro K, Pabaney AH, Rammo R, et al. Man-in-the-barrel syndrome: case report of ventral epidural abscess and review of the literature. *Surg Neurol Int* 2018;9:8.

Balm M, Hammack J. Leptomeningeal carcinomatosis: presenting features and prognostic factors. *Arch Neurol* 1996;53:626–632.

Bassetti C, Bogousslavsky J, Mattle H, et al. Medial medullary stroke: report of seven patients and review of the literature. *Neurology* 1997;48:882–890.

Beal MF. Multiple cranial nerve palsies—a diagnostic challenge. *N Engl J Med* 1990;322:461–463.

Bell HS. Paralysis of both arms from injury of the upper portion of the pyramidal decussation: "cruciate paralysis." *J Neurosurg* 1970;33:376–380.

Bone I, Hadley DM. Syndromes of the orbital fissure, cavernous sinus, cerebello-pontine angle, and skull base. *J Neurol Neurosurg Psychiatry* 2005;76(Suppl 3):iii29–iii38.

Brandt T. Diagnosis and thrombolytic therapy of acute basilar artery occlusion: a review. *Clin Exp Hypertens* 2002;24:611–622.

Brazis PW. Ocular motor abnormalities in Wallenberg's lateral medullary syndrome. *Mayo Clin Proc* 1992;67:365–368.

Brazis PW, Masdeu JC, Biller J. *Localization in Clinical Neurology*. 7th ed. Philadelphia: Wolters Kluwer/Lippincott Williams & Wilkins, 2017.

Caplan LR. Migraine and vertebrobasilar ischemia. *Neurology* 1991;41:55–61.

Carroll CG, Campbell WW. Multiple cranial neuropathies. *Semin Neurol* 2009;29:53–65.

Chamberlain MC. Neoplastic meningitis. *Oncologist* 2008;13:967–977.

Chamberlain MC. Lymphomatous meningitis as a presentation of non-Hodgkin lymphoma. *Clin Adv Hematol Oncol* 2011;9:419–420.

Chan DK, Silver FL. Basilar artery stenosis mimicking the lacunar syndrome of pure motor hemiparesis. *Can J Neurol Sci* 2003;30:159–162.

Charles N, Froment C, Rode G, et al. Vertigo and upside down vision due to an infarct in the territory of the medial branch of the posterior inferior cerebellar artery caused by dissection of a vertebral artery. *J Neurol Neurosurg Psychiatry* 1992;55:188–189.

Colnaghi S, Versino M, Marchioni E, et al. ICHD-II diagnostic criteria for Tolosa-Hunt syndrome in idiopathic inflammatory syndromes of the orbit and/or the cavernous sinus. *Cephalalgia* 2008;28:577–584.

Connolly B, Turner C, DeVine J, et al. Jefferson fracture resulting in Collet-Sicard syndrome. *Spine* 2000;25:395–398.

Currier RD, Bebin J. A medullary syndrome characterized by wild arm ataxia. *Neurology* 1999;53:1608–1609.

Currier RD, DeJong RN. The lateral medullary (Wallenberg's) syndrome. *Med Bull (Ann Arbor)* 1962;28:106–113.

deSouza RM, Zador Z, Frim DM. Chiari malformation type I: related conditions. *Neurol Res* 2011;33:278–284.

Dhamoon SK, Iqbal J, Collins GH. Ipsilateral hemiplegia and the Wallenberg syndrome. *Arch Neurol* 1984;41:179–180.

Dickman CA, Hadley MN, Pappas CT, et al. Cruciate paralysis: a clinical and radiographic analysis of injuries to the cervicomedullary junction. *J Neurosurg* 1990;73:850–858.

Eshbaugh CG, Siatkowski RM, Smith JL, et al. Simultaneous, multiple cranial neuropathies in diabetes mellitus. *J Neuroophthalmol* 1995;15:219–224.

Evyapan D, Kumral E. Pontine anosognosia for hemiplegia. *Neurology* 1999;53:647–649.

Ferbert A, Bruckmann H, Drummen R. Clinical features of proven basilar artery occlusion. *Stroke* 1990;21:1135–1142.

Field TS, Benavente OR. Penetrating artery territory pontine infarction. *Rev Neurol Dis* 2011;8(1–2):30–38.

Fisher CM. A. lacunar stroke. The dysarthria-clumsy hand syndrome. *Neurology* 1967;17:614–617.

Fisher CM. Ataxic hemiparesis. A pathologic study. *Arch Neurol* 1978;35:126–128.

Fisher CM. The "herald hemiparesis" of basilar artery occlusion. *Arch Neurol* 1988;45:1301–1303.

Fisher M, Recht LD. Brain tumor presenting as an acute pure motor hemiparesis. *Stroke* 1989;20:288–291.

Fitzek S, Baumgartner U, Fitzek C, et al. Mechanisms and predictors of chronic facial pain in lateral medullary infarction. *Ann Neurol* 2001;49:493–500.

Fodstad H, Kelly PJ, Buchfelder M. History of the cushing reflex. *Neurosurgery* 2006;59:1132–1137.

Fung HC, Chen ST, Tang LM, et al. Triparesis: MRI documentation of bipyramidal medullary infarction. *Neurology* 2002;58:1130–1131.

Gan R, Sacco RL, Kargman DE, et al. Testing the validity of the lacunar hypothesis: the Northern Manhattan Stroke Study experience. *Neurology* 1997;48:1204–1211.

Garrard P, Bradshaw D, Jager HR, et al. Cognitive dysfunction after isolated brainstem insult. An underdiagnosed cause of long-term morbidity. *J Neurol Neurosurg Psychiatry* 2002;73:191–194.

George TM, Higginbotham NH. Defining the signs and symptoms of Chiari malformation type I with and without syringomyelia. *Neurol Res* 2011;33:240–246.

Georgiadis D, Schulte-Mattler WJ. Cruciate paralysis or man-in-the-barrel syndrome? Report of a case of brachial diplegia. *Acta Neurol Scand* 2002;105:337–340.

Gil Polo C, Castrillo Sanz A, Gutiérrez Ríos R, et al. Opalski syndrome: a variant of lateral-medullary syndrome. *Neurologia* 2013;28:382–384.

Giroud M, Creisson E, Fayolle H, et al. Homolateral ataxia and crural paresis: a crossed cerebral-cerebellar diaschisis. *J Neurol Neurosurg Psychiatry* 1994;57:221–222.

Gladstone JP. An approach to the patient with painful ophthalmoplegia, with a focus on Tolosa-Hunt syndrome. *Curr Pain Headache Rep* 2007;11:317–325.

Glenn SA, Ross MA. Delayed radiation-induced bulbar palsy mimicking ALS. *Muscle Nerve* 2000;23:814–817.

Goel A. Basilar invagination, Chiari malformation, syringomyelia: a review. *Neurol India* 2009;57:235–246.

Gondim FA, Parks BJ, Cruz-Flores S. "Fou rire prodromique" as the presentation of pontine ischaemia secondary to vertebrobasilar stenosis. *J Neurol Neurosurg Psychiatry* 2001;71: 802–804.

Gondim FA, Thomas FP, Oliveira GR, et al. Fou rire prodromique and history of pathological laughter in the XIXth and XXth centuries. *Rev Neurol (Paris)* 2004;160:277–283.

Gordon PH, Cheng B, Katz IB, et al. Clinical features that distinguish PLS, upper motor neuron-dominant ALS, and typical ALS. *Neurology* 2009;72:1948–1952.

Gullapalli D, Phillips LH II. Neurologic manifestations of sarcoidosis. *Neurol Clin* 2002;20:59–83.

Hellmann MA, Djaldetti R, Luckman J, et al. Thoracic sensory level as a false localizing sign in cervical spinal cord and brain lesions. *Clin Neurol Neurosurg* 2013;115:54–56.

Hersch M. Loss of ability to sneeze in lateral medullary syndrome. *Neurology* 2000;54:520–521.

Hoitsma E, Faber CG, Drent M, et al. Neurosarcoidosis: a clinical dilemma. *Lancet Neurol* 2004;3:397–407.

Hopkins B, Khanna R, Dahdaleh NS. Revisiting cruciate paralysis: a case report and systematic review. *J Craniovertebr Junction Spine* 2016;7:265–272.

Ibrahim AG, Crockard HA. Basilar impression and osteogenesis imperfecta: a 21-year retrospective review of outcomes in 20 patients. *J Neurosurg Spine* 2007;7:594–600.

Iizuka O, Hosokai Y, Mori E. Trigeminal neuralgia due to pontine infarction. *Neurology* 2006;66:48.

Inamasu J, Hori S, Ohsuga F, et al. Selective paralysis of the upper extremities after odontoid fracture: acute central cord syndrome or cruciate paralysis? *Clin Neurol Neurosurg* 2001;103:238–241.

Ito M, Kuwabara S, Odaka M, et al. Bickerstaff's brainstem encephalitis and Fisher syndrome form a continuous spectrum: clinical analysis of 581 cases. *J Neurol* 2008;255:674–682.

Jickling GC, Stamova B, Ander BP, et al. Profiles of lacunar and nonlacunar stroke. *Ann Neurol* 2011;70(3):477–485.

Karam C, Scelsa SN, Macgowan DJ. The clinical course of progressive bulbar palsy. *Amyotroph Lateral Scler* 2010;11: 364–368.

Karmon Y, Kurzweil A, Lindzen E, et al. Gerstmann-Straussler-Scheinker syndrome masquerading multiple sclerosis. *J Neurol Sci* 2011;309:55–57.

Kataoka S, Miaki M, Saiki M, et al. Rostral lateral pontine infarction: neurological/topographical correlations. *Neurology* 2003;61:114–117.

Keane JR. Bilateral seventh nerve palsy: analysis of 43 cases and review of the literature. *Neurology* 1994;44:1198–1202.

Keane JR. Cavernous sinus syndrome. Analysis of 151 cases. *Arch Neurol* 1996;53:967–971.

Keane JR. Combined VIth and XIIth cranial nerve palsies: a clival syndrome. *Neurology* 2000;54:1540–1541.

Keane JR. Multiple cranial nerve palsies: analysis of 979 cases. *Arch Neurol* 2005;62:1714–1717.

Kim JS. Sensory symptoms in ipsilateral limbs/body due to lateral medullary infarction. *Neurology* 2001;57:1230–1234.

Kim JS, Kim HG, Chung CS. Medial medullary syndrome. Report of 18 new patients and a review of the literature. *Stroke* 1995;26:1548–1552.

Kim JS, Lee JH, Im JH, et al. Syndromes of pontine base infarction. A clinical-radiological correlation study. *Stroke* 1995;26:950–955.

Kim H, Chung CS, Lee KH, et al. Aspiration subsequent to a pure medullary infarction: lesion sites, clinical variables, and outcome. *Arch Neurol* 2000;57:478–483.

Kinjo Y, Suda S, Sakamoto Y, et al. Ataxic hemiparesis associated with cortical infarct localized in the postcentral gyrus. *Intern Med* 2017;56:2503–2505.

Kleinschmidt-DeMasters BK, Rojiani AM, Filley CM. Central and extrapontine myelinolysis: then…and now. *J Neuropathol Exp Neurol* 2006;65:1–11.

Klimo P Jr, Rao G, Brockmeyer D. Congenital anomalies of the cervical spine. *Neurosurg Clin N Am* 2007;18:463–478.

Krasnianski M, Muller T, Stock K, et al. Between Wallenberg syndrome and hemimedullary lesion: Cestan-Chenais and Babinski-Nageotte syndromes in medullary infarctions. *J Neurol* 2006;253:1442–1446.

Kumar S, Fowler M, Gonzalez-Toledo E, et al. Central pontine myelinolysis, an update. *Neurol Res* 2006;28:360–366.

Kumral E, Afsar N, Kirbas D, et al. Spectrum of medial medullary infarction: clinical and magnetic resonance imaging findings. *J Neurol* 2002;249:85–93.

Kushner MJ, Bressman SB. The clinical manifestations of pontine hemorrhage. *Neurology* 1985;35:637–643.

Laigle-Donadey F, Doz F, Delattre JY. Brainstem gliomas in children and adults. *Curr Opin Oncol* 2008;20:662–667.

Landau WM. Cruciate paralysis. *J Neurosurg* 1992;77:329–330.

Lee H, Sohn CH. Axial lateropulsion as a sole manifestation of lateral medullary infarction: a clinical variant related to rostral-dorsolateral lesion. *Neurol Res* 2002;24:773–774.

Leon-Carrion J, van Eeckhout P, Dominguez-Morales Mdel R, et al. The locked-in syndrome: a syndrome looking for a therapy. *Brain Inj* 2002;16:571–582.

Liu GT, Crenner CW, Logigian EL, et al. Midbrain syndromes of Benedikt, Claude, and Nothnagel: setting the record straight. *Neurology* 1992;42:1820–1822.

Lleo A, Sanahuja J, Serrano C, et al. Acute bulbar weakness: thyrotoxicosis or myasthenia gravis? *Ann Neurol* 1999;46:434–435.

Loher TJ, Krauss JK. Dystonia associated with pontomesencephalic lesions. *Mov Disord* 2009;24:157–167.

Love S. Demyelinating diseases. *J Clin Pathol* 2006;59:1151–1159.

Lyu RK, Chen ST. Acute multiple cranial neuropathy: a variant of Guillain-Barré syndrome? *Muscle Nerve* 2004;30:533–536.

MacGowan DJ, Janal MN, Clark WC, et al. Central poststroke pain and Wallenberg's lateral medullary infarction: frequency, character, and determinants in 63 patients. *Neurology* 1997;49:120–125.

Malik NN, Day AC, Clifton A, et al. Weber's syndrome as the presenting sign of multiple sclerosis. *Neuroophthalmology* 2007;31:15–17.

Manni JJ, Scaf JJ, Huygen PL, et al. Hyperostosis cranialis interna. A new hereditary syndrome with cranial-nerve entrapment. *N Engl J Med* 1990;322:450–454.

Markus HS, van der Worp HB, Rothwell PM. Posterior circulation ischaemic stroke and transient ischaemic attack: diagnosis, investigation, and secondary prevention. *Lancet Neurol* 2013;12:989–998.

Matsumoto S, Okuda B, Imai T, et al. A sensory level on the trunk in lower lateral brainstem lesions. *Neurology* 1988;38:1515–1519.

Mattle HP, Arnold M, Lindsberg PJ, et al. Basilar artery occlusion. *Lancet Neurol* 2011;10:1002–1014.

Milhorat TH, Chou MW, Trinidad EM, et al. Chiari I malformation redefined: clinical and radiographic findings for 364 symptomatic patients. *Neurosurgery* 1999;44:1005–1017.

Mittal M, Hammond N, Husmann K, et al. Creutzfeldt-Jakob disease presenting as bulbar palsy. *Muscle Nerve* 2010;42:833–835.

Miwa H, Koshimura I, Mizuno Y. Recurrent cranial neuropathy as a clinical presentation of idiopathic inflammation of the dura mater: a possible relationship to Tolosa-Hunt syndrome and cranial pachymeningitis. *J Neurol Sci* 1998;154:101–105.

Mokri B, Silbert PL, Schievink WI, et al. Cranial nerve palsy in spontaneous dissection of the extracranial internal carotid artery. *Neurology* 1996;46:356–359.

Moragas M, Martinez-Yelamos S, Majos C, et al. Rhombencephalitis: a series of 97 patients. *Medicine (Baltimore)* 2011;90:256–261.

Morosini A, Burke C, Emechete B. Polyneuritis cranialis with contrast enhancement of cranial nerves on magnetic resonance imaging. *J Paediatr Child Health* 2003;39:69–72.

Moulin T, Bogousslavsky J, Chopard JL, et al. Vascular ataxic hemiparesis: a re-evaluation. *J Neurol Neurosurg Psychiatry* 1995;58:422–427.

Murata Y, Yamaguchi S, Kajikawa H, et al. Relationship between the clinical manifestations, computed tomographic findings and the outcome in 80 patients with primary pontine hemorrhage. *J Neurol Sci* 1999;167:107–111.

Nadeau SE. Neurologic manifestations of systemic vasculitis. *Neurol Clin* 2002;20:123–150.

Nadeau SE. Neurologic manifestations of connective tissue disease. *Neurol Clin* 2002;20:151–178.

Nakamura S, Kitami M, Furukawa Y. Opalski syndrome: ipsilateral hemiplegia due to a lateral-medullary infarction. *Neurology* 2010;75:1658.

Nicolao P, Zoccarato M, Dalsasso M, et al. Bickerstaff's brainstem encephalitis: case report and Tc99m brain SPECT findings. *Neurol Sci* 2011;32:1153–1156.

Nishino H, Rubino FA, DeRemee RA, et al. Neurological involvement in Wegener's granulomatosis: an analysis of 324 consecutive patients at the Mayo Clinic. *Ann Neurol* 1993;33:4–9.

Nogues M, Lopez L, Meli F. Neuro-ophthalmologic complications of syringobulbia. *Curr Neurol Neurosci Rep* 2010;10:459–466.

van Oostenbrugge RJ, Twijnstra A. Presenting features and value of diagnostic procedures in leptomeningeal metastases. *Neurology* 1999;53:382–385.

Parizel PM, Makkat S, Jorens PG, et al. Brainstem hemorrhage in descending transtentorial herniation (Duret hemorrhage). *Intensive Care Med* 2002;28:85–88.

Piradov MA, Pirogov VN, Popova LM, et al. Diphtheritic polyneuropathy: clinical analysis of severe forms. *Arch Neurol* 2001;58:1438–1442.

Polo A, Manganotti P, Zanette G, et al. Polyneuritis cranialis: clinical and electrophysiological findings. *J Neurol Neurosurg Psychiatry* 1992;55:398–400.

Pryse-Phillips W. *Companion to Clinical Neurology*. 3rd ed. Oxford: Oxford University Press, 2009.

Riaz G, Carr J, Campbell WW. Facial myokymia in syringobulbia. *Arch Neurol* 1990;47:472–474.

Ropper AH, Samuels MA, Klein J. *Adams and Victor's Principles of Neurology*. 10th ed. New York: McGraw-Hill Education Medical, 2014.

Sacco RL, Freddo L, Bello JA, et al. Wallenberg's lateral medullary syndrome. Clinical-magnetic resonance imaging correlations. *Arch Neurol* 1993;50:609–614.

Sacco S, Sara M, Pistoia F, et al. Management of pathologic laughter and crying in patients with locked-in syndrome: a report of 4 cases. *Arch Phys Med Rehabil* 2008;89:775–778.

Saposnik G, Caplan LR. Convulsive-like movements in brainstem stroke. *Arch Neurol* 2001;58:654–657.

Savitz SI, Caplan LR. Vertebrobasilar disease. *N Engl J Med* 2005;352:2618–2626.

Schonewille WJ, Tuhrim S, Singer MB, et al. Diffusion-weighted MRI in acute lacunar syndromes. A clinical-radiological correlation study. *Stroke* 1999;30:2066–2069.

Schwartz MA, Selhorst JB, Ochs AL, et al. Oculomasticatory myorhythmia: a unique movement disorder occurring in Whipple's disease. *Ann Neurol* 1986;20:677–683.

Seijo-Martinez M, Varela-Freijanes A, Grandes J, et al. Sneeze related area in the medulla: localisation of the human sneezing centre? *J Neurol Neurosurg Psychiatry* 2006;77:559–561.

Sekula RF Jr, Arnone GD, Crocker C, et al. The pathogenesis of Chiari I malformation and syringomyelia. *Neurol Res* 2011;33:232–239.

Seo SW, Heo JH, Lee KY, et al. Localization of Claude's syndrome. *Neurology* 2001;57:2304–2307.

Sham JS, Cheung YK, Choy D, et al. Cranial nerve involvement and base of the skull erosion in nasopharyngeal carcinoma. *Cancer* 1991;68:422–426.

Shono Y, Koga M, Toyoda K, et al. Medial medullary infarction identified by diffusion-weighted magnetic resonance imaging. *Cerebrovasc Dis* 2010;30:519–524.

Silverman IE, Liu GT, Volpe NJ, et al. The crossed paralyses. The original brain-stem syndromes of Millard-Gubler, Foville, Weber, and Raymond-Cestan. *Arch Neurol* 1995;52:635–638.

Siva A, Altintas A, Saip S. Behcet's syndrome and the nervous system. *Curr Opin Neurol* 2004;17:347–357.

Smith JS, Shaffrey CI, Abel MF, et al. Basilar invagination. *Neurosurgery* 2010;66(3 Suppl):39–47.

Spengos K, Wohrle JC, Tsivgoulis G, et al. Bilateral paramedian midbrain infarct: an uncommon variant of the "top of the basilar" syndrome. *J Neurol Neurosurg Psychiatry* 2005;76:742–743.

Steele JC, Richardson JC, Olszewski J. Progressive supranuclear palsy: a heterogeneous degeneration involving the brain stem, basal ganglia and cerebellum with vertical gaze and supranuclear palsy, nuchal dystonia, and dementia. *Arch Neurol* 1964;10:333.

Stiver SI, Gean AD, Manley GT. Survival with good outcome after cerebral herniation and Duret hemorrhage caused by traumatic brain injury. *J Neurosurg* 2009;110:1242–1246.

Stracciari A, Guarino M, Ciucci G, et al. Acute upside down reversal of vision in vertebrobasilar ischaemia. *J Neurol Neurosurg Psychiatry* 1993;56:423.

Suthar PP, Rana PJ, Mehta C, et al. Top of basilar artery syndrome. *J Clin Diagn Res* 2015;9:TJ01.

Taieb G, Renard D, Jeanjean L, et al. Wallenberg syndrome and "neurotrophic" ulcerations. *Acta Neurol Belg* 2014;114:143–144.

Tan EK, Chan LL, Auchus AP. Hemidystonia precipitated by acute pontine infarct. *J Neurol Sci* 2005;234:109–111.

Thwaites GE, Tran TH. Tuberculous meningitis: many questions, too few answers. *Lancet Neurol* 2005;4:160–170.

Vinas FC, Rengachary S. Diagnosis and management of neurosarcoidosis. *J Clin Neurosci* 2001;8:505–513.

Wang Q, Xiang Y, Yu K, et al. Multiple cranial neuropathy variant of Guillain-Barré syndrome: a case series. *Muscle Nerve* 2011;44:252–257.

Yamamoto R, Johkura K, Nakae Y, et al. The mechanism of ipsilateral ataxia in lacunar hemiparesis: SPECT perfusion imaging. *Eur Neurol* 2015;73:106–111.

Yuki N, Susuki K, Hirata K. Ataxic Guillain-Barré syndrome with anti-GQ1b antibody: relation to Miller Fisher syndrome. *Neurology* 2000;54:1851–1853.

SECTION E The Motor System

CHAPTER 22

Overview of the Motor System

Examination of motor functions includes the determination of muscle power, evaluation of muscle tone and bulk, and observation for abnormal movements. Examination of coordination and gait is closely related to the motor examination. Coordination is often viewed as a cerebellar function, but integrity of the entire motor system is essential for normal coordination and control of fine motor movements. Examination of cerebellar function is discussed in Chapter 43. Station (standing) and gait (walking) are complex and involve much more than motor function; they are usually assessed separately from the motor examination (Chapter 44).

Both the peripheral and central nervous systems participate in motor activity, and various functional components have to be evaluated individually. Our motor systems move our bodies in space, move parts of the body in relation to one another, and maintain postures and attitudes in opposition to gravity and other external forces. All movements, except those mediated by the autonomic nervous system, are effected by contractions of striated muscles through the control of the nervous system.

LEVELS OF MOTOR ACTIVITY

The intricate organization of the motor system and its evolutionary development from the simple responses of unicellular organisms to the patterns of behavior of animals and man account for the complexity of motor function. From anatomic and functional standpoints, there are certain phylogenetic motor levels, or stages of development, which increase in complexity with evolution. In lower vertebrates, motor activities are effected through subcortical centers, but with the greater development of the cerebral cortex in higher mammals, some of these functions are significantly altered. The more primitive centers retain some of their original functions, although modified by cortical control. They are not replaced but are incorporated into an elaborate motor system, subordinate to the cortex. The phylogenetically old and new systems work together, and the efficiency of each depends upon collaboration with the other.

The evolutionary development of motor function from simple to complex movements is duplicated to a certain extent in the maturation of motor skills in man. At the time of birth, simple spinal and brainstem reflexes are already present. A newborn held supported will take rudimentary steps (walking reflex). More complex postural and righting reflexes appear during the first few weeks of life. With maturation of the cortex and commissural pathways, acts requiring associated sensory functions (grasping and groping) are possible, followed by volitional control of movement. Finally, the ability to perform skilled acts with a high degree of precision emerges.

Complex mechanisms underlie even the simplest discrete voluntary movement. All of the levels of motor integration contribute to the precision of movement. Initiation of contraction of the agonist (prime mover) must be accompanied by graded relaxation or contraction of the antagonists and synergists.

Smooth, accurate movement requires the ability for the movement to be stopped at any point, reversed, and started again at a different degree of contraction or in a different direction. Stereotyped and patterned movements, integrated at lower levels, may be part of the act. Postures must be assumed that can be modified or shifted easily and instantly for adjustment to the next movement. Throughout all of this, the volitional elements and purposeful aspects of the act are of paramount importance.

Knowing the structure and function of the different levels of motor control, the relationships between the motor systems, and the changes in motor activity that occur in disease helps in understanding disorders of the motor system. Many neuroscientists over the years have envisioned various hierarchical schemes with different levels of complexity of motor activity. In this text, we consider the following levels: the motor unit (lower motor neuron, final common pathway) and the segmental (spinal cord), brainstem, cerebellar, extrapyramidal, and pyramidal levels.

The lowest echelon of motor activity is the motor unit, which consists of an alpha motor neuron in the spinal cord or brainstem, its axon, and all of the muscle fibers it innervates. The segmental or spinal cord level mediates simple segmental reflexes, such as the withdrawal reflex, and includes the activity of many motor units and elements of both excitation and inhibition involving agonists, synergists, and antagonists. Various descending suprasegmental motor systems modulate the activity that occurs at the segmental level (Figure 22.1). The pyramidal (corticospinal) system arises from the primary motor cortex in the precentral gyrus. The corticospinal system is the primary, overarching suprasegmental motor control mechanism. The function of the corticospinal system is modulated and adjusted by the activity of the extrapyramidal and cerebellar systems. The extrapyramidal system arises primarily in the basal ganglia. Centers in the brainstem that give rise to the vestibulospinal, rubrospinal, and related pathways are of importance in postural mechanisms and standing and righting reflexes. The psychomotor, or cortical associative, level has to do with memory, initiative, and conscious and unconscious control of motor activity that arises primarily from the motor association cortex anterior to the motor strip.

These levels are not individual motor systems and do not normally act individually or separately. Anatomists continue to have difficulty in even defining the constituents of some of these levels (e.g., the corticospinal or pyramidal vs. the basal ganglion or extrapyramidal). These levels are components of the motor system as a whole; each is part of the complex motor apparatus. Each contributes its share to control of the lower motor neuron on which, as the final common pathway, all motor control systems converge. Disease at each of these levels causes characteristic signs and symptoms (Table 22.1). Some disorders of the motor system may involve more than one level. In addition, all purposeful movements are guided by a constant stream of afferent impulses that impinge on various levels of the motor system. Sensory and motor functions are interdependent in the performance of volitional movement, and it is not possible to consider the motor system apart from the sensory system. Impairment of sensation may affect all aspects of motion—volitional, reflex, postural, tonic, and phasic.

A brief sketch of the organization of the motor system may help to lay a foundation before discussing each level in detail (Figures 22.1 and 22.2). The premotor and supplementary cortices control the planning and preliminary preparation for movements, which the primary motor cortex in the precentral gyrus then executes. The primary motor cortex also receives input from the basal ganglia and the cerebellum (Figure 22.2). The corticospinal (pyramidal) and corticobulbar tracts arise from the precentral gyrus, descend through the corona radiata, and enter the posterior limb of the internal capsule. The internal capsules merge in their descent with the cerebral peduncles, which form the base of the midbrain. Corticobulbar fibers terminate in the lower brainstem on cranial nerve nuclei and other structures. Corticospinal fibers aggregate into compact bundles, the pyramids, in the medulla. At the level of the caudal medulla, 90% of the pyramidal fibers decussate to the opposite side and descend throughout the spinal cord as the lateral corticospinal tract. About 10% of the corticospinal fibers descend ipsilaterally in the anterior corticospinal tract and decussate at the level of the local spinal synapse. Pyramidal fibers preferentially innervate certain lower motor neuron groups.

Descending motor system fibers send collaterals to other structures to help control and coordinate movement. These structures in turn project back to the cortex to form feedback loops that ensure coordinated interactions between the suprasegmental motor systems (Figure 22.2). The thalamus, especially the ventral lateral (VL) and the ventral anterior (VA) nuclei, serves as the relay station for projections from

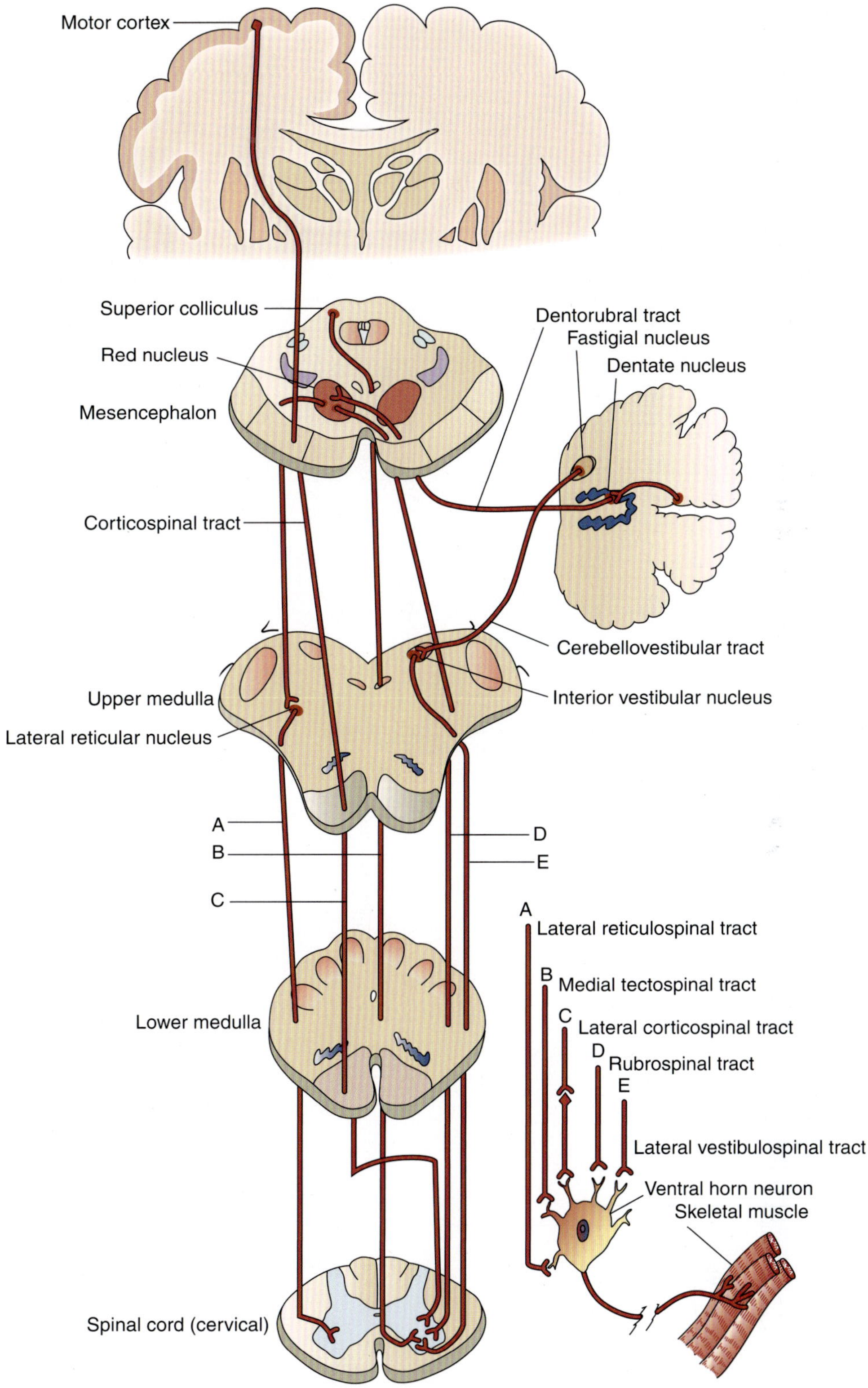

FIGURE 22.1 The most important descending pathways that act upon the anterior horn cell of the spinal cord (final common pathway).

TABLE 22.1 Changes in Motor Function

Level	Weakness	Tone	Volume and Contour	Fasciculations	Ataxia	Deep Tendon Reflexes	Abnormal Movements	Pathologic Associated Movements
Motor Unit Lesions								
a. Lower motor neuron	Focal or segmental, bulbar	Flaccid	Atrophy common	Common	Absent	Focally decreased	None except fasciculations	Absent
b. Nerve root, plexus, peripheral nerve	Focal or segmental	Flaccid	Atrophy common	Occasional	Absent	Decreased or absent	None except rare fasciculations	Absent
c. Neuromuscular junction	Diffuse or proximal, bulbar	Usually normal	Usually no change	Sometimes present because of anticholinesterase therapy	Absent	Usually normal	None	Absent
d. Muscle	Diffuse, proximal, or distal	Normal or flaccid	Normal, atrophy, hypertrophy, or pseudohypertrophy	None	Absent	Normal unless weakness is very severe	None	Absent
Corticospinal tract lesion	Mono-, hemi-, para-, quadriparesis, often incomplete (pyramidal distribution)	Spastic	Normal	None	Absent	Increased unless process is acute	None	Present
Extrapyramidal lesion	None or mild	Rigid	Normal	None	Absent	Normal	Present	Absent
Cerebellar lesion	None; ataxia may simulate weakness	Hypotonic	Normal	None	Present	Pendular or normal	None except intention tremor	Absent
Nonorganic disorder	Bizarre, breakaway, no true loss of power, may simulate any type	Normal or variable, often factitiously increased	Normal	None	Absent, but incoordination may simulate ataxia	Normal, may have poor relaxation and erratic, sham jerkiness	May be present	Absent

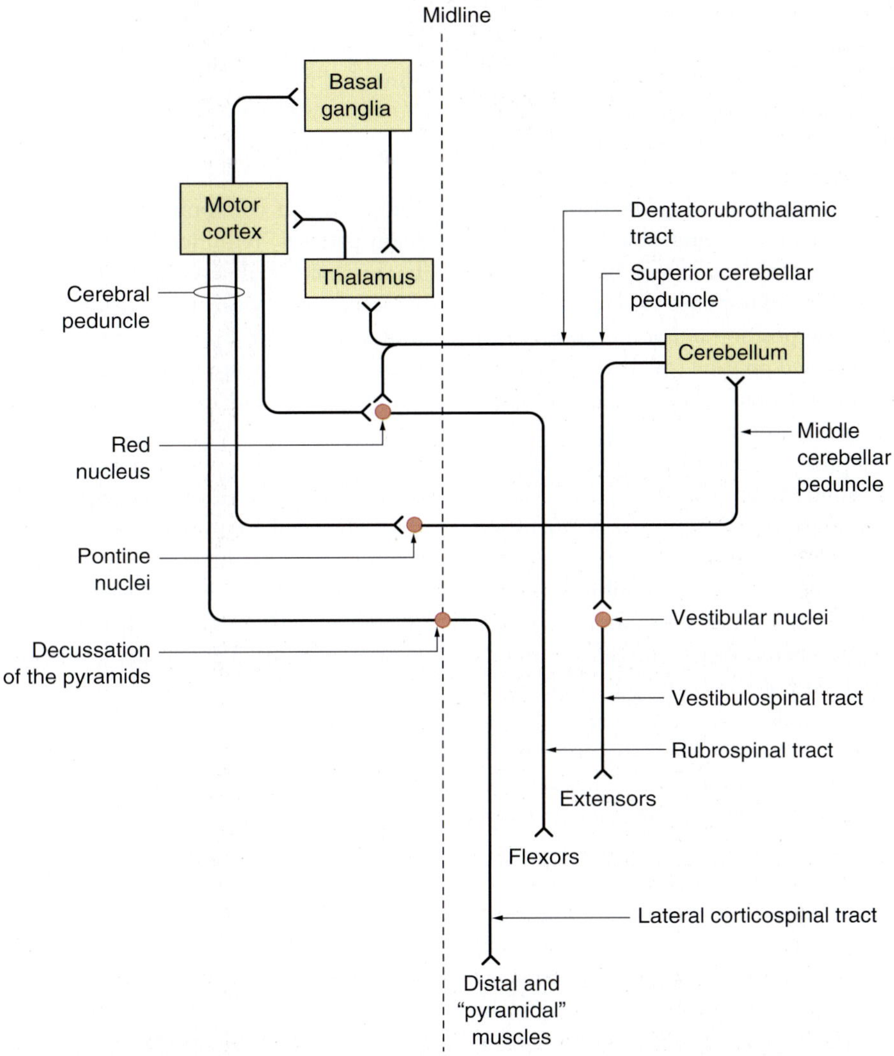

FIGURE 22.2 Major connections of the motor system. Note feedback loops between cortex and cerebellum and cortex and basal ganglia. (Modified from Campbell WW, Pridgeon RP. *Practical Primer of Clinical Neurology.* Philadelphia: Lippincott Williams & Wilkins, 2002, with permission.)

the other centers back to the cortex. The VL projects predominantly to the primary motor cortex and the VA to the premotor regions.

As fibers from the motor cortex run downward through the internal capsule, they send collaterals to the basal ganglia. Fibers from the basal ganglia project to VA and VL, which in turn project to the cortex, creating a feedback loop. The substantia nigra also projects to the striatum and influences its activity. The motor cortex and cerebellum are also part of a circuit. The pontine nuclei lie scattered among the descending motor and crossing pontocerebellar fibers in the basis pontis. Corticopontine fibers synapse on pontine nuclei, which then give rise to pontocerebellar fibers that project across the midline to the contralateral cerebellar hemisphere through the middle cerebellar peduncle. The cerebellum in turn projects to the contralateral VL via the superior cerebellar peduncle, which decussates in the midbrain. The VL nucleus in turn projects to the motor cortex to complete the circuit. The cerebellum also receives unconscious proprioception from muscle spindles and Golgi tendon organs via the spinocerebellar and cuneocerebellar tracts. The cerebellum also projects to the ipsilateral vestibular nuclei, which give rise to the vestibulospinal tracts. The lateral vestibulospinal tract descends from the lateral vestibular nucleus to the spinal cord, where it facilitates ipsilateral extensor muscle tone of the trunk and extremities. As they descend, corticospinal fibers send collaterals to the ipsilateral red nucleus. The rubrospinal tract arises from the red nucleus and then immediately decussates and descends to facilitate flexor muscle tone, primarily in the upper extremities. The tectospinal tract arises from the superior colliculus, crosses in the dorsal tegmental decussation, and descends to influence muscles of the neck and upper back. It functions to move the head in response to external stimuli and to maintain head position in relation to the body position. The uncrossed pontine (medial) reticulospinal tract arises from the oral and caudal pontine reticular nuclei and facilitates extensor muscles, especially of the trunk and proximal extremities. The medullary (lateral) reticulospinal tract arises from the gigantocellular reticular nucleus and is primarily uncrossed but with a small crossed component. It travels just anterior to the rubrospinal tract. It inhibits antigravity muscles and is involved with autonomic functions.

The cerebellar hemispheres influence muscles on the ipsilateral side of the body. The cerebellum projects to the contralateral red nucleus, and the rubrospinal tract then crosses back. Because of the "double decussation," the rubrospinal tract controls muscles ipsilateral to the cerebellar hemisphere where the impulse originated. The vestibulospinal system remains ipsilateral throughout. The cerebral motor cortex on one side and the cerebellar hemisphere on the opposite side act in concert to control the arm and leg on a particular side of the body. Their actions are coordinated by projections from the cerebrum to the pontine nuclei, which send fibers to the contralateral cerebellum, which in turn projects back to the thalamus and cerebrum on the original side via the decussation of the dentatothalamic tract. Consider the right cerebellar hemisphere, it receives input from the left cerebral cortex via the middle cerebellar peduncle and projects back to the left thalamus and motor cortex via the superior cerebellar peduncle. So, both the left cerebral hemisphere and the right cerebellar hemisphere control movements on the right side of the body.

OVERVIEW OF CLINICAL MANIFESTATIONS OF DISEASE OF THE MOTOR SYSTEM

The most common manifestation of motor system disease is weakness. Other abnormalities include alterations in muscle tone, changes in muscle size and shape, abnormal involuntary movements, and defective coordination. Subsequent chapters deal with abnormal motor functions in more detail.

Motor Strength and Power

Weakness is a common abnormality and can follow many patterns. Terminology may become problematic. For instance, weakness may be generalized or localized, symmetric or asymmetric, proximal or distal, or upper motor neuron or lower motor neuron. The term focal is often used to imply asymmetry; a patient with a hemiparesis is said to have a focal examination. The term generalized is often used to imply symmetry, even though the weakness may not truly be generalized. A disease may cause weakness in a particular distribution that is bilaterally symmetric (e.g., the scapuloperoneal syndromes), but these are not generally regarded as focal even though the involvement is very localized. A patient with bilateral carpal tunnel syndrome or bilateral peroneal nerve palsies would most properly be described as having a multifocal pattern of weakness, even though the weakness is bilateral and symmetric. The term nonfocal is often used to describe a patient's neurologic examination, particularly by nonneurologists. The implication is usually that the examination is normal or at least that there is no asymmetry. It is a poor and not very helpful term. A patient with Guillain-Barré syndrome causing generalized weakness and impending respiratory failure would have a nonfocal examination, yet be critically ill.

Focal weakness may follow the distribution of some structure in the peripheral nervous system, such as a peripheral nerve or spinal root. It may affect one side of the body in a hemidistribution. A hemidistribution may affect the arm, leg, and face equally on one side of the body, or one or more areas may be more involved than others. Muscle groups preferentially innervated by the corticospinal tract are often selectively impaired. When weakness is nonfocal, it may be generalized, predominantly proximal, or predominantly distal. These various patterns have differential diagnostic and localizing significance. Identification of the process causing weakness is further aided by accompanying signs, such as reflex alterations and sensory loss (Table 21.1).

Generalized Weakness

Weakness may involve both sides of the body, more or less symmetrically. With truly generalized weakness, bulbar motor functions are also impaired. When the bulbar functions are intact and there is weakness of both arms and both legs, the patient is said to have quadriparesis—if only the legs, then paraparesis. When weakness affects all four extremities, the likely causes include myelopathy, peripheral neuropathy, a neuromuscular junction disorder, or a myopathy.

When myelopathy is the culprit and the deficit is incomplete, more severe involvement of those muscles preferentially innervated by the corticospinal tract can frequently be discerned. Reflexes are usually increased (though in the acute stages, they may be decreased or absent); there is usually some alteration of sensation, sometimes a discrete spinal sensory "level"; superficial reflexes disappear; and there may be bowel and bladder dysfunction. Generalized peripheral nerve disease tends to predominantly involve distal muscles. There is no preferential involvement of corticospinal innervated muscles, reflexes are usually decreased, sensory loss is frequently present, and bowel and bladder functions are not disturbed. With a neuromuscular junction disorder, the extremity weakness is likely to be worse proximally, sensation is spared, reflexes are normal, and there is usually involvement of bulbar muscles. With myopathy, weakness is usually more severe proximally, reflexes are normal, sensation is normal, and, with a few exceptions, bulbar function is spared except for occasional dysphagia. These are generalizations. Some neuropathies may cause proximal weakness, and some myopathies may affect distal muscles; not all patients with a neuromuscular transmission disorder have bulbar involvement.

Localized Weakness

When the arm and leg on one side of the body are weak, the patient is said to have a hemiparesis. This may range in severity from very mild, manifest only as pronator drift and impairment of fine motor control, to total paralysis. Monoparesis is weakness of only one extremity, such as the leg contralateral to an anterior cerebral artery stroke. Reflexes—typically increased unless the process is acute—and accompanying sensory loss help identify such focal weakness as central in origin.

A mononeuropathy, such as a radial nerve palsy, or a spinal root lesion, such as from a herniated disc, causes weakness limited to the distribution of the involved nerve or root. A plexopathy may cause weakness of the entire limb or weakness only in the distribution of certain plexus components. With such lower motor neuron pathology, reflexes are typically decreased, and there is often accompanying sensory loss. Localization of focal weakness due to root, plexus, and peripheral nerve pathology requires intimate familiarity with peripheral neuroanatomy.

Motor neuron disease is a special case. Amyotrophic lateral sclerosis (ALS) characteristically involves both the upper and lower motor neurons. It produces a clinical picture of weakness and wasting due to involvement of the lower motor neurons in the anterior horn of the spinal cord, combined with weakness and hyperreflexia due to involvement of the upper motor neurons in the cerebral cortex that give rise to the corticospinal tract. There is upper motor neuron weakness (cerebral cortex pathology) superimposed on lower motor neuron weakness (spinal cord pathology). ALS usually begins with focal weakness, often involving one hand or one foot.

A multinerve, multiroot distribution of weakness, normal or increased reflexes, and a lack of sensory loss are usually the earliest suggestions as to the nature of the problem. In ALS, the weakness early tends to be asymmetric and associated with hyperreflexia. An extremity that is both atrophic and hyperreflexic is characteristic. As the condition progresses, the clinical picture evolves into one of generalized weakness.

It is very rare for a myopathy or neuromuscular junction disorder to cause focal weakness, although these disorders may have a predilection for certain muscles, such as the extraocular muscles in myasthenia gravis or the thigh muscles in quadriceps myopathy.

Other Motor System Abnormalities

Muscle tone may be increased (hypertonia) or decreased (hypotonia). Hypertonia comes in two common variants: rigidity and spasticity. When the increased tone occurs to more or less the same degree throughout the range of passive motion of a limb, and is independent of the speed of the movement, it is referred to as rigidity. When the hypertonia is most marked near the middle of the range of motion and is more apparent with fast than with slow passive movement, it is referred to as spasticity. One of the key characteristics of spasticity is that the hypertonus is velocity dependent, most evident with rapid movements. In lead pipe (plastic) rigidity, there is smooth resistance throughout the range independent of the rate of movement. Gegenhalten (paratonia) is an increase in tone in a limb more or less proportional to the examiner's attempt to move it. In cogwheel rigidity, there is ratchety, jerky, tremulous variation in the hypertonia, due primarily to superimposed tremor. Spastic hypertonia is typically associated with increased deep tendon reflexes, loss of superficial reflexes, and Babinski signs. Cogwheel rigidity occurs in Parkinson's disease and related conditions. Gegenhalten is usually associated with other abnormal neurologic signs depending on the etiology. The term dystonia refers to transient or sustained hypertonic conditions that do not fit into the other categories. Hypotonia occurs in two primary settings in the adult: myopathies and cerebellar disease. Infantile hypotonia (floppy baby) is a common clinical problem. The differential diagnosis of infantile hypotonia is extensive, and the workup of a floppy baby is a frequent exercise in pediatric neurology.

Muscle Volume and Contour

Muscle mass or volume may be decreased (atrophy) or increased (hypertrophy). Neurogenic atrophy results from a lesion involving the anterior horn cells, nerve root, or peripheral nerve innervating a muscle; it may be severe. Muscle diseases usually cause only mild to moderate atrophy of the involved muscles. Disuse atrophy occurs after immobilization, as when a limb is in a cast, and is usually mild to moderate in severity and recovers quickly with resumption of use.

True muscle hypertrophy results from an increase in the size of the muscle. It is most often physiologic hypertrophy from heavy use, but it can occur in certain neuromuscular disorders. Pseudohypertrophy refers to apparent muscle enlargement due to replacement of diseased muscle by fat and fibrous tissue. Enlarged calf muscles in patients with Duchenne muscular dystrophy are a classic example of muscle pseudohypertrophy.

Abnormal Movements

Abnormal involuntary movements occur in a host of neurologic conditions. They come in many forms, ranging from tremor to chorea to muscle fasciculations to myoclonic jerks. The only common characteristic is that the movements are spontaneous and not under volitional control. Involuntary movements may be rhythmic or random, fleeting or sustained, and predictable or unpredictable. They may occur in isolation or be accompanied by other neurologic signs. Common types include tremor, chorea, athetosis, hemiballismus, dystonia, tics, and dyskinesias.

Coordination

Coordination and control of fine motor movements are delicate functions that require smooth interactions between the different components of the motor system as well as normal sensory function. The cerebellum is a critical component, and disease of the cerebellum frequently causes impaired coordination in the absence of weakness or other motor abnormalities. But poor coordination may also be a manifestation of corticospinal tract or extrapyramidal disorders.

BIBLIOGRAPHY

Campbell WW, Pridgeon RP. *Practical Primer of Clinical Neurology*. Philadelphia: Lippincott Williams & Wilkins, 2002.

Gilman S, Newman SW. *Manter and Gatz's Essentials of Clinical Neuroanatomy and Neurophysiology*. 10th ed. Philadelphia: FA Davis, 2003.

Gould DJ, Fix JD. *Neuroanatomy*. 5th ed. Philadelphia: Wolters Kluwer Health/Lippincott Williams & Wilkins, 2014.

Kiernan JA, Rajakumar N. *Barr's The Human Nervous System: An Anatomical Viewpoint*. 10th ed. Philadelphia: Wolters Kluwer Health/Lippincott Williams & Wilkins, 2014.

Parent A. *Carpenter's Human Neuroanatomy*. 9th ed. Baltimore: Williams & Wilkins, 1996.

Standring S, ed. *Gray's Anatomy: The Anatomical Basis of Clinical Practice*. 41st ed. New York: Elsevier Limited, 2016.

CHAPTER 23

The Motor Unit Level

The motor unit consists of an alpha motor neuron (lower motor neuron), its axon, and all its subject muscle fibers; it is the final common pathway for all motor activity, both voluntary and involuntary (Figure 23.1). Clinical disorders may affect any portion of the motor unit (cell body, nerve root, plexus, peripheral nerve, neuromuscular junction [NMJ], or muscle), and diseases at different sites have different clinical features. Sensory dysfunction—such as pain and paresthesias—may accompany lesions involving the nerve root, plexus, and peripheral nerve portions of the motor unit. Nevertheless, the motor unit remains a useful conceptual framework for understanding disorders involving the peripheral neuromuscular apparatus.

THE MOTOR UNIT

Alpha motor neurons reside in the anterior horn of the spinal cord and the brainstem motor nuclei. The axon traverses the anterior root and the peripheral nerve en route to the muscle. The peripheral nerve enters the muscle at the motor point and divides into intramuscular branches. These arborize within a muscle fascicle and terminate as fine twigs, which end as axon boutons. Terminal boutons abut the motor end plates of individual muscle fibers across a synaptic cleft, forming NMJs. Each muscle fiber has only a single end plate.

Terminal axonal twigs ramify in the muscle and innervate widely dispersed muscle fibers. A motor unit may have anywhere from a handful of muscle fibers to more than a thousand. The innervation ratio refers to the number of muscle fibers in a motor unit. A low innervation ratio means few muscle fibers are innervated by a single axon and is characteristic of muscles under precise and finely graded voluntary control, such as extraocular or laryngeal muscles. A muscle performing a gross motor movement may have several hundred muscle fibers per motor unit. The gastrocnemius has about 2,000. The innervation ratios for the brachial biceps, tibialis anterior, and deltoid are 209, 329, and 239 fibers, respectively. The anatomical scatter of fibers belonging to the same motor unit may vary from muscle to muscle. Electrophysiologic motor unit counting techniques estimate that an intrinsic hand muscle has about 100 motor units. Beyond the age of 60 years, there is a decline in the number of functioning motor units.

Motor units vary by size within a muscle. Smaller motoneurons have smaller motor unit territories. To produce a smoothly graded muscle contraction, motor units are recruited, more or less, in order of increasing size. Small motoneurons are first recruited, and increasing force of contraction calls forth activity from increasingly larger motoneurons: the size principle.

Motor units are classified as type 1 or type 2. Muscles were broadly divided into red muscle and white muscle, dark meat and light meat, long before the basis for the difference was understood. The red or dark color is now known to result from the presence of the instruments for oxidative metabolism: myoglobin, mitochondria, and a vascular network for delivery of oxygen to the metabolizing muscle cells. Histochemical stains help separate the different types of muscle fibers and often allow the appreciation of structural detail and abnormalities not seen with routine hematoxylin and eosin stains. The myosin ATPase (adenosine triphosphatase) histochemical stain identifies two distinct populations of muscle fibers, referred to as type 1 and type 2, which correspond to type 1 and 2 motor units. Further adjustment of pH allows separation of type 2 muscle fibers into types 2A and 2B (Box 23.1). An average muscle contains about 40% type 1 fibers and 60% type 2 fibers. However, this ratio varies with the anatomical location and function of the muscle,

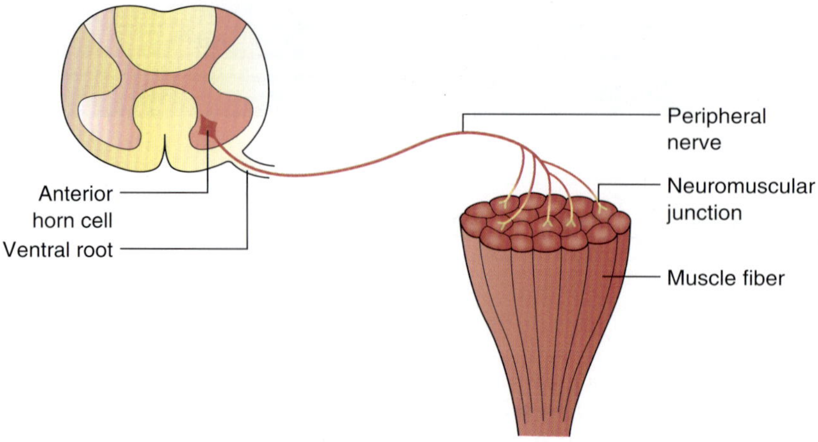

FIGURE 23.1 The motor unit. An alpha motor neuron in the anterior horn gives rise to an axon, which branches and arborizes in the periphery to innervate scattered muscle fibers within a muscle fascicle.

and similar muscles may vary among individuals. All fibers in a particular motor unit are of the same type, and there is good correlation between the mechanical properties and other attributes of a motor unit and the histochemical reactions of its muscle fibers. The fiber type mix of a muscle is determined by its innervation and ultimately by its function. In needle electromyography, the summated electrical activity of all the muscle fibers of a motor unit—a motor unit action potential—is recorded by a needle electrode inserted into the muscle.

Type 1 muscle fibers are rich in oxidative enzymes and mitochondria but sparse in glycogen; they are designed for sustained, long-duration contraction under aerobic conditions. Red, or dark, meat is high in type 1 fibers. Type 2 fibers are rich in glycogen and glycolytic enzymes but sparse in oxidative enzymes, mitochondria, and lipid. They are designed for brief, intense bursts of activity under anaerobic conditions. White meat is high in type 2 fibers. The mnemonic "one, slow, red ox" helps recall the essentials: type 1 fibers, slow muscle, red meat, oxidative metabolism.

In another functional and physiologic scheme, motor units are classified into three different types: fast twitch, fatigue sensitive, or fast fatigable (FF);

BOX 23.1

Type 1 and Type 2 Muscle Fibers

The myosin ATPase (adenosine triphosphatase) stain identifies the two distinct populations of type 1 and type 2 muscle fibers; the differences are summarized in Table 23.1. Cross sections reveal a random admixture of the two fiber types creating a checkerboard pattern. The type 2 fibers stain darkly and the type 1 fibers lightly at pH 9.4; the staining characteristics reverse at pH 4.3. Preincubation at pH 4.6 identifies two kinds of type 2 fibers: type 2A and type 2B. The 2B fibers are the classic fast twitch, fatigue-sensitive glycolytic fibers, whereas 2A fibers have characteristics intermediate between type 1 and type 2B, with some oxidative capability, slower twitch, and more fatigue resistance than the 2B fibers. Pathologic processes may cause characteristic abnormalities of fiber type distribution or proportion or produce changes primarily in one particular fiber type.

TABLE 23.1 Attributes and Characteristics of Type 1 and Type 2 Muscle Fibers

Attribute	Type 1	Type 2
ATPase stain at pH 4.6	Dark	Light
ATPase stain at pH 9.4	Light	Dark
Oxidative enzymes	High	Low
Lipid	High	Low
Mitochondria	High	Low
Glycogen	Low	High
Glycolytic enzymes	Low	High
Function	Sustained contraction	Brief contraction
Twitch speed	Slow	Fast
Metabolism	Aerobic	Anaerobic
Fatigue	Resistant	Sensitive

ATPase, adenosine triphosphatase.

slow twitch, fatigue resistant (S); and intermediate or fast fatigue resistant (FR). Type FF units are fast twitch and fatigue sensitive, type 2B histochemically, rich in glycogen but poor in oxidative enzymes, and designed for brief, phasic activity. Type S units are slow twitch, fatigue resistant, type 1 histochemically, low in glycolytic but high in oxidative enzymes, and designed for sustained, tonic activity. Type FR is intermediate, fast twitch but more fatigue resistant than type FF, type 2A histochemically, high in glycolytic, and intermediate in oxidative enzyme activity.

Myotomes

A myotome consists of all the muscles innervated by a specific nerve root. Most skeletal muscles receive innervation from two or more roots, and there is inherent variability in the myotomal patterns among individuals. Early anatomists reported myotome innervation from detailed dissections, and some errors have been perpetuated through the years. Many different innervation charts are available, and most vary in some details. Some misinformation remains, such as the inclusion of C6-C7 innervation to the thenar muscles, which does not fit clinical reality. The issue has been compounded by observations during intraoperative recordings that indicate contributions from unexpected sources to leg muscles and anomalous innervation so frequent as to be the rule rather than the exception. Liveson and Ma present charts derived from seven different sources, separating "new myotomes" derived from electromyographic data.

Microanatomy of the Peripheral Nerve

Peripheral nerves are composed of myriad axons, ensheathed by myelin of varying thickness and supported by Schwann cells, all imbedded in a matrix of connective tissue. Nerves are divided into discrete internal fascicular compartments by perineurium. The blood-nerve barrier is a physiologic partition, created by the perineurium and the endothelium of intrafascicular capillaries. It regulates the nerve microenvironment and acts as a diffusion barrier. The extreme terminal ends of nerve fibers are not protected by perineurium and have no effective blood-nerve barrier, a detail of probable importance in the pathogenesis of some peripheral neuropathies. Within each fascicle, endoneurium separates individual axons and their Schwann cells (Figure 23.2). Fascicles are bound together into nerve trunks by the epineurium, loose areolar connective tissue that also contains blood vessels, lymphatics, and the nervi nervorum. The epineurium also serves an important cushioning role. The interfascicular (internal) epineurium lies between fascicles; the epifascicular (external) epineurium circumferentially envelops the entire nerve.

Fascicles bifurcate, join with adjacent fascicles, redivide, and recombine to create a complex internal fascicular network (Figure 23.3). Yoon et al. have imaged the individual fascicles beautifully with 7T MRI (Figure 23.4). Nerves can be classified into monofascicular, oligofascicular, and polyfascicular types. A polyfascicular pattern is common in regions subject to mechanical stress and where there is heavy

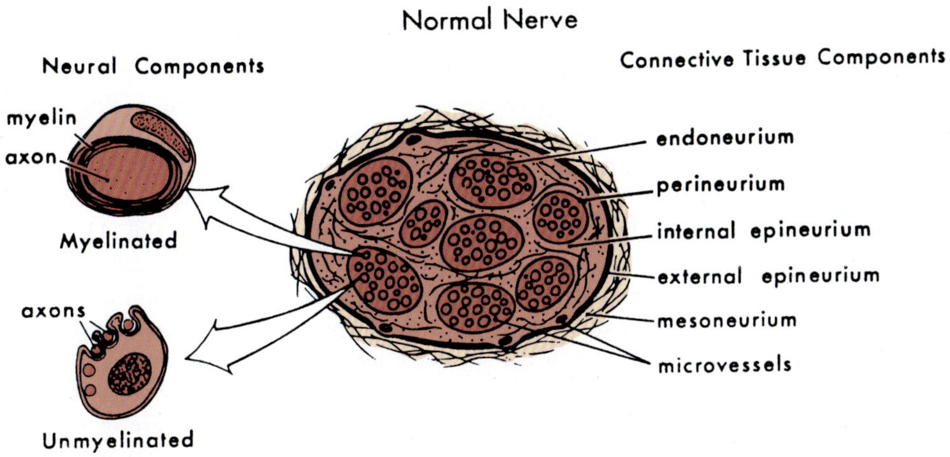

FIGURE 23.2 The normal peripheral nerve is composed of connective tissue and neural tissue components. The nerve fibers may be myelinated or unmyelinated. (Modified with permission of Georg Thieme Verlag KG from Mackinnon SE, Dellon AL. *Surgery of the Peripheral Nerve.* 1st ed. New York: Thieme, 1988; permission conveyed through Copyright Clearance Center, Inc.)

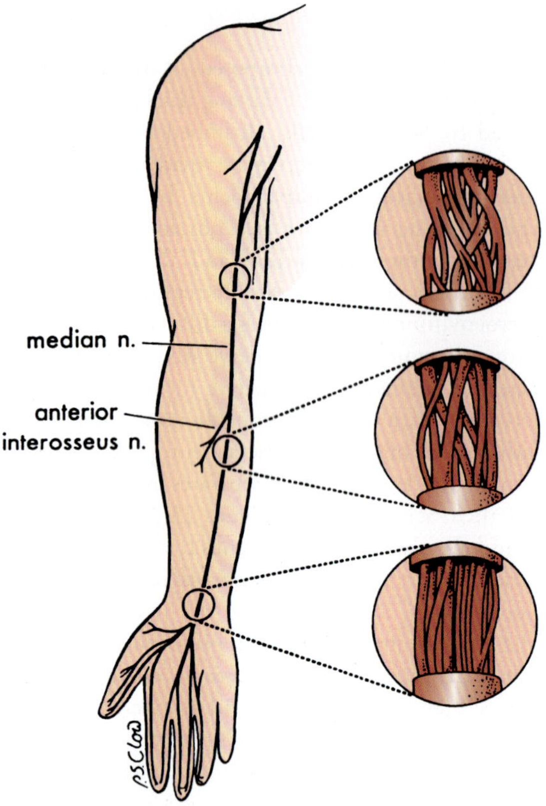

FIGURE 23.3 An illustration of the internal topography of the median nerve at different levels. The complexity of the internal fascicular anatomy is apparent. The degree of plexus formation between fascicles decreases in the distal portion of the nerve as the bundles approach their target muscles. (Modified with permission of Georg Thieme Verlag KG from Mackinnon SE, Dellon AL. *Surgery of the Peripheral Nerve.* 1st ed. New York: Thieme, 1988; permission conveyed through Copyright Clearance Center, Inc.)

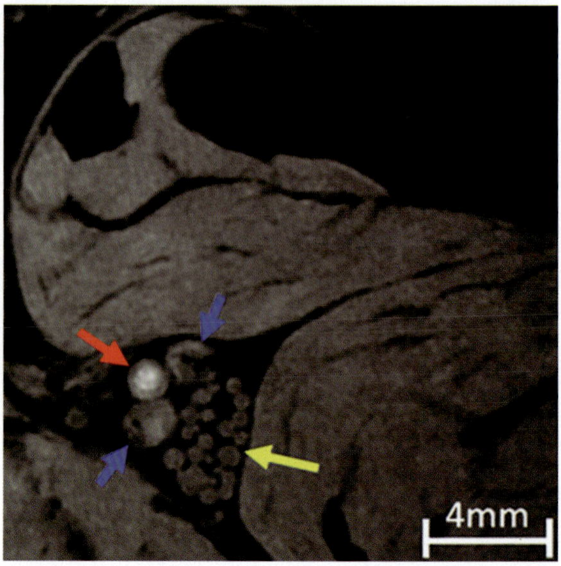

FIGURE 23.4 Individual fascicles of the tibial nerve are clearly identified at high resolution on 7T MRI, marked by the *yellow arrow*. Posterior tibial artery is marked by the *red arrow* and posterior tibial veins are marked by the *blue arrows*. (Modified from Yoon D, Biswal S, Rutt B, et al. Feasibility of 7T MRI for imaging fascicular structures of peripheral nerves. *Muscle Nerve.* 2018;57(3):494-498. Copyright © 2017 Wiley Periodicals, Inc. Reprinted by permission of John Wiley & Sons, Inc.)

fiber exchange, such as the brachial plexus. Plexiform fascicular exchange is most prominent proximally, and a constant fascicular pattern is present for only a short distance in proximal regions of a nerve. Fascicles innervating a particular muscle or sensory zone become more discrete and constant in position as they approach the target organ. This complex intraneural topography has important clinical, surgical, and electrophysiologic implications.

Axons are divided into three major size groups: large myelinated, small myelinated, and unmyelinated. Large myelinated axons have diameters in the 6- to 12-μm range, small myelinated axons are 2 to 6 μm, and unmyelinated axons are 0.2 to 2.0 μm. Small myelinated fibers are about three times more numerous than large myelinated axons. The myelin sheath adds additional thickness. Conduction is most efficient when the ratio of the axon diameter to total fiber diameter is 0.5 to 0.7.

Ultrastructurally, axons contain cytoskeletal elements, neurofilaments, and neurotubules, which are synthesized in the cell body and move slowly down the axon at a rate of 3 mm/d. Neurotubules consist of polymerized dimers of tubulin protein forming longitudinally oriented hollow tubes about 20 nm in diameter and 1 mm long, linked by crossbridges to the neurofilaments. Neurofilaments are smaller organelles that maintain axonal structure. Neurotubules are responsible for fast antegrade and retrograde axonal transport (see Physiology of the Peripheral Nerve below).

In myelinated axons, a single Schwann cell wraps a single internodal segment in concentric layers of myelin (Figure 23.5). Schmidt-Lanterman incisures are bits of Schwann cell cytoplasm sequestered between layers of myelin. The external plasma membrane of the Schwann cell is continuous with the outermost layer of myelin; the inner membrane of the Schwann cell is immediately adjacent to the outer surface of the axolemma. The external lamina is a condensation of extracellular matrix surrounding the entire external surface of the Schwann cell. The nodes of Ranvier are gaps in the myelin coverage between the territories of adjacent Schwann cells. Internodal length varies with fiber size; it is about 1 mm for large-diameter fibers. For unmyelinated axons, a single Schwann cell, sometimes referred to as

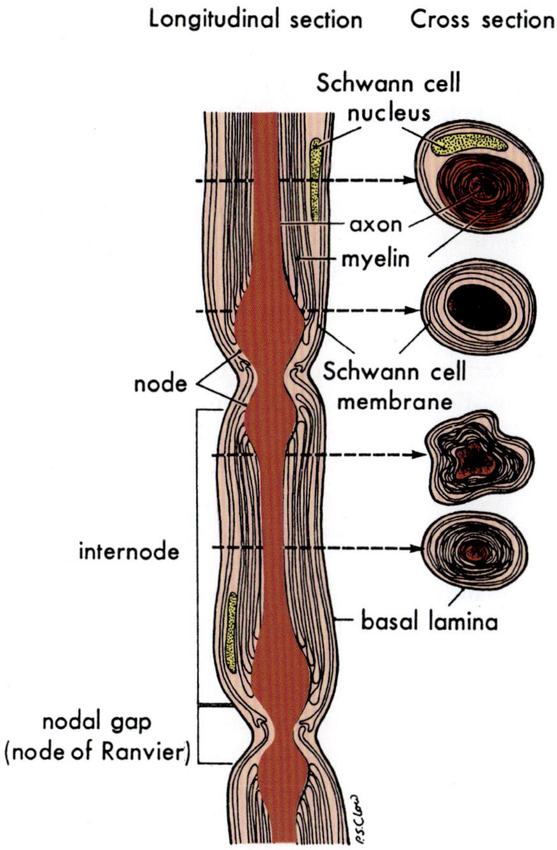

FIGURE 23.5 Illustration of a single myelinated nerve fiber demonstrates the relationships between the axon, the Schwann cell, and the myelin sheath at different points. (Modified with permission of Georg Thieme Verlag KG from Mackinnon SE, Dellon AL. *Surgery of the Peripheral Nerve.* 1st ed. New York: Thieme, 1988; permission conveyed through Copyright Clearance Center, Inc.)

a Remak cell, sends out processes to support several adjacent axons, lending to each primarily a cytoplasmic coat and only a minimal investment of myelin. A complex of several unmyelinated axons and their supporting Remak cell is encased by an external lamina.

Peripheral nerves receive blood supply from penetrating segmental arteries usually derived from adjacent vessels. Penetrating arterioles then form an extensive longitudinal anastomotic network that runs within the nerve. Watershed zones of precarious perfusion within the nerve may explain some of the clinical manifestations seen in ischemic neuropathies, especially in vasculitis.

Physiology of the Peripheral Nerve

Peripheral nerve fibers are classified according to two schemes: the ABC and the I/II/III/IV systems (Chapter 31), both ranging from largest (A, I) to smallest (C, IV). The conduction velocity (CV) of a fiber depends on its diameter and degree of myelination; it ranges from less than 1 m/s for small, unmyelinated fibers to greater than 100 m/s for large, myelinated fibers. The compound nerve action potential—recorded in vitro from a mixed peripheral nerve—separates fibers into groups based on their CV. Aa and Ag fibers are efferent fibers from alpha and gamma motoneurons, respectively. Ab and Ad fibers are primarily cutaneous afferents. Group B fibers are preganglionic autonomics. Group C fibers are postganglionic autonomics, visceral afferents, and pain and temperature fibers. The Roman numeral system applies only to afferent fibers. The Ia fibers arise from nuclear bag muscle spindle fibers and joint receptors, the Ib fibers from Golgi tendon organs, and the II fibers from nuclear chain muscle spindle fibers. Class III fibers are cutaneous axons that correspond more or less to Ad fibers, and type IV fibers correspond to C fibers. Some neuropathies have a predilection for certain types and sizes of fibers. Large-fiber neuropathies affect strength, reflexes, and proprioception with relative sparing of pain and temperature sensation, whereas small-fiber neuropathies primarily affect pain, temperature, and autonomic function. Differential involvement of large versus small sensory fibers can sometimes be discerned clinically. The immunologic and biochemical differences between fibers, which might explain differential involvement, are just beginning to be understood. For example, the L2 membrane protein is expressed only on motor axon Schwann cells, and the nerves to the extraocular muscles are especially rich in ganglioside GQ1b, which may relate to their involvement in Miller-Fisher syndrome.

The axoplasm is in constant flux, containing elements that flow to and fro along its length between the cell body and the periphery. Antegrade axoplasmic flow moves from the cell body distally; retrograde flow moves centripetally. Antegrade flow has multiple components. Slow axonal transport, 1 to 3 mm/d, conveys cytoskeletal proteins to the periphery for maintenance and renewal of axoplasm, along with neurotransmitters, enzymes, and other components. Fast axonal transport, 400 mm/d, largely transports membrane-bound vesicles that are propelled by kinesin, a microtubule-associated ATPase. Abnormalities of axonal transport are likely important in the mechanism of dying back or length-dependent neuropathies. Several substances produce neuropathy by disrupting the cytoskeletal elements: vinca alkaloids, taxoids, and hexacarbons, for example. Retrograde flow moves materials from the periphery back to the cell body; it is the mechanism through which some neurotrophic viruses reach the central nervous system.

Anatomy and Physiology of the Neuromuscular Junction

In the nervous system, presynaptic electrical events are converted to chemical events at the synapse and are converted again into electrical events postsynaptically. The NMJ is a specialized synapse through which electrical events in the peripheral nerve are transduced into chemical events that then induce depolarization of the postsynaptic muscle membrane, which in turn induces muscle contraction. Disturbed neuromuscular transmission (NMT) results in several different clinical disorders, which are characterized primarily by weakness and fatigability.

An intramuscular nerve branch ends by forming a bulbous swelling—the terminal bouton. The primary synaptic cleft separates the terminal bouton from the postsynaptic muscle membrane, which is in turn divided into a number of secondary synaptic clefts, or junctional folds. The postsynaptic muscle membrane is blanketed by a dense array of nicotinic acetylcholine receptor (AChR) molecules. Freeze-fracture techniques show the AChR as large particles concentrated on the tips of junctional folds, extending about halfway down into the secondary synaptic clefts. The AChR is a complex structure, consisting of two alpha subunits and beta, gamma, and delta subunits, plus an ion channel. The main immunogenic region of the AChR is the site that is attacked by autoantibodies in the majority of cases of myasthenia gravis. In addition, there are acetylcholine esterase molecules on both presynaptic and postsynaptic membranes (Figure 23.6).

The terminal bouton is a beehive of metabolic activity. It is packed with cytoskeletal proteins, mitochondria, and numerous chemicals. Most importantly, it contains vesicles, which are membrane-bound collections of acetylcholine (ACh). In the cytoplasm of the terminal bouton, ACh is packaged into vesicles, which then migrate to and collect at primary release sites, or active zones. The active zones of the presynaptic membrane tend to line up opposite the secondary synaptic clefts of the postsyn-

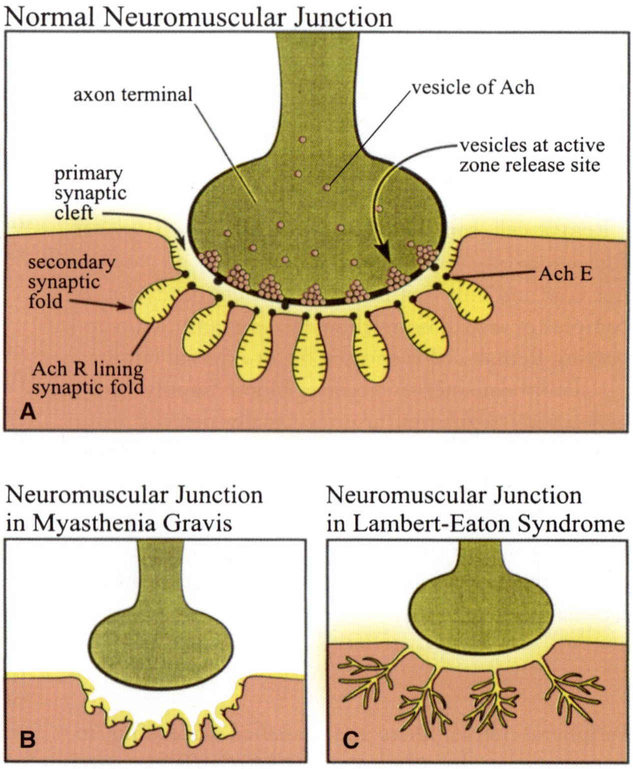

FIGURE 23.6 **A.** A normal neuromuscular junction (NMJ). **B.** An NMJ in myasthenia, degraded by immunologic attack, simplified, and depopulated of acetylcholine receptor. **C.** An NMJ in Lambert-Eaton's syndrome, highly complex and convoluted with increased surface area. (From Campbell WW. *Essentials of Electrodiagnostic Medicine.* Philadelphia: Lippincott Williams & Wilkins, 1999. Modified with permission of Dr. William W. Campbell.)

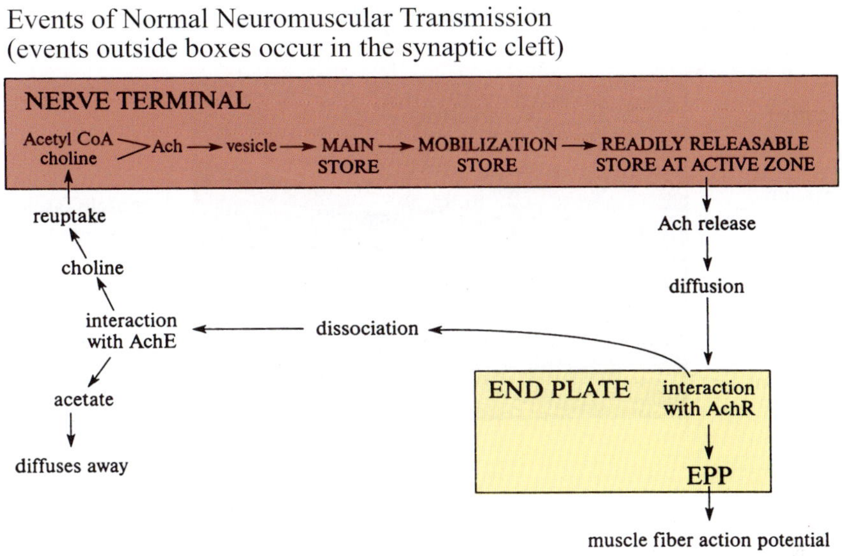

FIGURE 23.7 Schematic of the events of normal neuromuscular transmission. Ach, acetylcholine; AchE, acetylcholinesterase; AchR, acetylcholine receptor; EPP, end plate potential. (From Campbell WW. *Essentials of Electrodiagnostic Medicine*. Philadelphia: Lippincott Williams & Wilkins, 1999. Modified with permission of Dr. William W. Campbell.)

aptic membrane. The active zones are the sites of both exocytosis of ACh vesicles and ingress of calcium.

The presynaptic membrane contains voltage-gated calcium channels. In response to nerve depolarization, these channels permit the influx of calcium into the presynaptic terminal, which greatly facilitates the release of neurotransmitter with the next nerve impulse. Magnesium has the opposite effect and inhibits the release of transmitter. After a nerve impulse, calcium diffuses out of the nerve terminal and is largely gone within 100 to 200 ms. Repetitive nerve impulses also increase the mobilization of ACh vesicles toward the active zones. As a result, sustained voluntary muscle contraction has a transient facilitatory effect on transmitter release. Repetitive nerve stimulation (RNS) is a clinical neurophysiologic technique used to investigate NMT disorders. The timing of the calcium fluxes is extremely important in determining the response to different rates of RNS.

Vesicles of ACh are released sporadically and irregularly while the membrane is at rest and in flurries after nerve depolarization. Each vesicle contains about 5,000 to 10,000 molecules of ACh. Upon activation, the vesicles fuse with the presynaptic membrane and pour their ACh contents into the primary synaptic cleft. The molecules of ACh diffuse rapidly across the primary synaptic cleft and into the secondary clefts. Anywhere two molecules of ACh encounter an AChR, a chemical interaction takes place. This causes opening of sodium channels in the postsynaptic membrane, producing a brief nonpropagated localized depolarization. The depolarization produced by the contents of one vesicle is referred to as a miniature end-plate potential (MEPP). The summation of many MEPPs produces a localized, nonpropagated depolarization in the region of the end plate, referred to as an end-plate potential (EPP). The EPPs in turn summate, and if above threshold spawn a propagated, all-or-none muscle fiber action potential. The summated electrical activity of hundreds to thousands of muscle fiber action potentials produces the motor unit action potential, which can be recorded by needle electromyography.

The events of normal NMT are summarized in Figure 23.7. Defects in NMT may develop at a number of points in the process.

Anatomy and Physiology of Muscle

A muscle is composed of hundreds to thousands of individual muscle fibers (Figure 23.8). Each fiber is a multinucleated syncytium, roughly cylindrical in shape and encased in a connective tissue covering of endomysium, which extends over a long

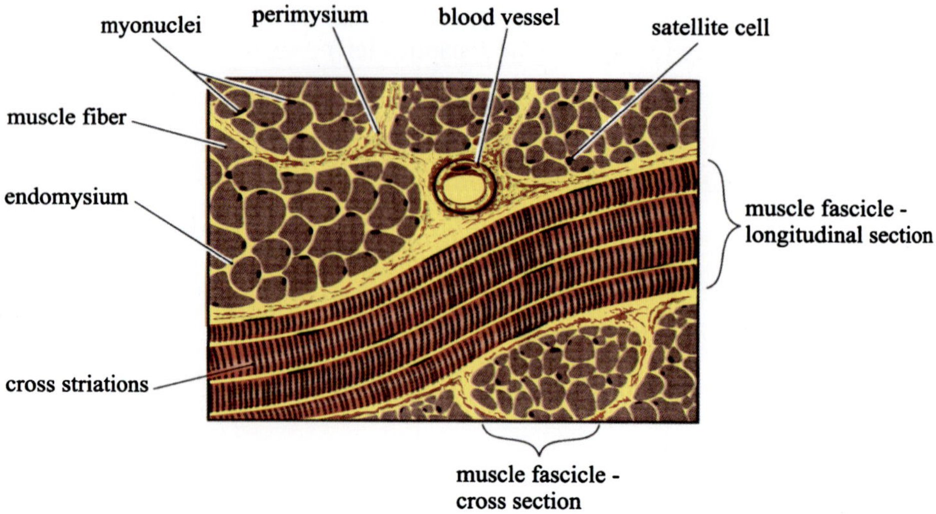

FIGURE 23.8 Cross section of muscle showing several fascicles, with muscle fibers, connective tissue septa, and blood vessels. Note the endomysium surrounding individual muscle fibers, the perimysium surrounding and separating fascicles, and the epimysium surrounding the entire muscle. Myonuclei and satellite cells lie peripherally and cannot be distinguished histologically. Longitudinal fibers demonstrate cross striations. (From Campbell WW. *Essentials of Electrodiagnostic Medicine.* Philadelphia: Lippincott Williams & Wilkins, 1999. Modified with permission of Dr. William W. Campbell.)

distance within a muscle fascicle. Fibers are polygonal in cross section; the diameter may vary depending on a number of factors but is relatively constant within a given muscle. A muscle fascicle is a group of fibers lying together within a sheath of perimysium. Intramuscular nerve twigs, capillaries, and muscle spindles also occupy the perimysium.

Epimysium separates groups of fascicles and also provides a covering for the entire muscle. The surface epimysium, which encases the muscle proper, is continuous with the fascia, which covers the muscle, and in turn with the tendons, which anchor it at the origin and insertion. The nuclei supporting a fiber lie peripherally just under the sarcolemmal membrane. Just external to the sarcolemma is the dense basement membrane. Satellite cells lie between the basement membrane and the sarcolemma. These dormant, omnipotential stem cells, whose nuclei resemble the sarcolemmal nuclei, can serve as the source of regeneration of muscle fibers following injury. Cellular organelles, glycogen granules, and lipids lie interspersed between the myofibrils and near the sarcolemmal nuclei.

Each muscle fiber is composed of thousands of myofibrils, which are in turn made up of myriad myofilaments, the contractile elements (Figure 23.8). The myofibril is composed of repeating identical segments called sarcomeres. A sarcomere is anchored at each end by a condensation of protein referred to as a Z disk. From each Z disk arise thin filaments, made up of a long double helix of two chains of actin, which project toward the center of the sarcomere. From a condensation in the center of the sarcomere—the M line—thick filaments of myosin project outward toward the Z lines. Where the myosin and actin filaments overlap, the sarcomere appears denser and transmits less light—the anisotropic or A band. At the sarcomere's ends, where thin actin filaments exist alone, the appearance is lighter—the isotropic or I band. In the paramedian zone, where myosin filaments exist alone, the appearance is intermediate—the H zone. There are twice as many actin filaments as myosin filaments. During muscle contraction, the filaments slide past each other as side arms on the myosin molecule ratchet the actin molecule and draw it past. At maximal shortening, the Z disks are drawn together and the I bands are obliterated as the overall length of the sarcomere decreases (Figure 23.9).

Myosin is composed of two fragments: heavy meromyosin, which has ATPase activity, and light meromyosin, which does not. Actin is composed of three fragments: actin, troponin, and tropomyosin. Lying in the groove between the two chains in the actin are long filaments of tropomyosin molecules. Troponin molecules are small globular units located at intervals along the tropomyosin molecules. Troponin is made up of three subunits: troponin T, troponin I, and troponin C. Troponin T binds the troponin components to tropomyosin, troponin I

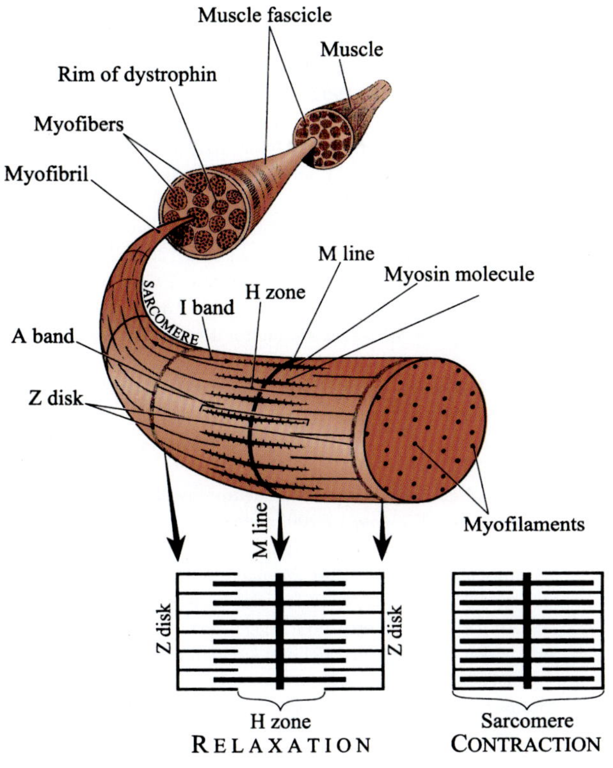

FIGURE 23.9 Myofibrils are composed of repeating sarcomeres. The sarcomere extends from Z line to Z line and consists of the I band (actin filaments only), the A band (actin and myosin filaments overlapping), the H zone (myosin filaments only), and the M line (a central condensation of the myosin filaments). The myosin molecules have cross bridges that interact with the actin molecules. When the muscle shortens, the overlapping of the myosin and actin molecules increases as the filaments slide, drawing the Z lines together and obliterating the I band. Dystrophin lies beneath the sarcolemma and helps reinforce it against stretching and buckling. (From Campbell WW. *Essentials of Electrodiagnostic Medicine*. Philadelphia: Lippincott Williams & Wilkins, 1999. Modified with permission of Dr. William W. Campbell.)

inhibits the interaction of myosin with actin, and troponin C contains the binding sites for the Ca^{2+} that helps to initiate contraction. Troponin can reversibly bind with calcium. A troponin-tropomyosin complex inhibits the interaction of myosin and actin while the muscle is at rest. The binding of calcium to troponin disinhibits the interaction and allows reactions to occur between the cross bridges on the myosin molecule and active sites on the actin molecule. Other important skeletal muscle proteins are actinin, titin, and desmin. Actinin binds actin to the Z lines. Titin connects the Z lines to the M lines and provides a scaffold for the sarcomere. Desmin adds structure to the Z lines.

At the junction of the A and I bands, the transverse (T) tubular systems arise as invaginations of the plasmalemma and ramify as an intricate network within the sarcomere. The T tubules allow communication between the muscle interior and the extracellular space and are the conduits along which the action potential is transmitted to the depths of the sarcomere. The sarcoplasmic reticulum (SR) is a closed internal labyrinth of vesicles that surrounds the myofibrils. The SR ends as focal dilatations, the terminal cisterns, which contain calcium. A pair of terminal cisterns abuts a T tubule to form a triad. The action potential conducted into the fiber along the T tubule causes calcium release from the terminal cisterns, which in turn activates myosin ATPase and initiates sliding of the filaments. This sequence is referred to as excitation contraction coupling. Following contraction, calcium ions are sequestered back into the terminal cisterns of the SR.

In addition to the contractile elements, skeletal muscle contains important cytoskeletal proteins, which help provide it structure. Elastic elements are vital to allow for contraction and relaxation. One of the key cytoskeletal proteins is dystrophin, a large molecule that forms a reinforcing meshwork just beneath the sarcolemma, and links the sarcomere to the sarcolemma and the extracellular matrix. Dystrophin is not directly connected to the membrane, but anchored to it at each end by a glycoprotein complex (dystrophin-associated glycoprotein), which spans the membrane and binds externally to laminin in the extracellular matrix. Dystrophin appears to lend mechanical support to the sarcolemma to help stabilize and brace it against the forces of muscle contraction. Genetic derangements of these cytoskeletal proteins underlie many of the muscular dystrophies.

BIBLIOGRAPHY

Anthony DC, Vogel FS. Peripheral nervous system. In: Damjanov I, Linder J, eds. *Anderson's Pathology*. 10th ed. St. Louis: Mosby, 1996:2799–2831.

Barrett KE, Barman SM, Boitano S, et al. *Ganong's Review of Medical Physiology*. 23rd ed. Los Altos: Lange, 2010.

Brown RH, Al-Chalabi A. Amyotrophic lateral sclerosis. *N Engl J Med* 2017;377:162–172.

Campbell WW. Diagnosis and management of common compression and entrapment neuropathies. *Neurol Clin* 1997;15: 549–567.

Campbell WW. *Essentials of Electrodiagnostic Medicine*. 2nd ed. New York: Demos Medical, 2014.

Campbell WW, Pridgeon RP. *Practical Primer of Clinical Neurology*. Philadelphia: Lippincott Williams & Wilkins, 2002.

Donofrio PD, Albers JW. AAEM minimonograph #34: polyneuropathy: classification by nerve conduction studies and electromyography. *Muscle Nerve* 1990;13:889–903.

Drachman DB. Myasthenia gravis. *N Engl J Med* 1994;330: 1797–1810.

Eisen A. Amyotrophic lateral sclerosis. *Intern Med* 1995;34: 824–832.

Ernste FC, Reed AM. Idiopathic inflammatory myopathies: current trends in pathogenesis, clinical features, and up-to-date treatment recommendations. *Mayo Clin Proc* 2013;88:83–105.

Gath I, Stalberg E. In situ measurement of the innervation ratio of motor units in human muscles. *Exp Brain Res* 1981;43: 377–382.

Gilhus NE. Myasthenia gravis. *N Engl J Med* 2016;375:2570–2581.

Jabaley ME, Wallace WH, Heckler FR. Internal topography of major nerves of the forearm and hand: a current view. *J Hand Surg [Am]* 1980;5:1–18.

Keesey J. Myasthenia gravis. *Arch Neurol* 1998;55:745–746.

Levin KH. Common focal mononeuropathies and their electrodiagnosis. *J Clin Neurophysiol* 1993;10:181–189.

Liveson JA, Ma DM. *Laboratory Reference for Clinical Neurophysiology*. Philadelphia: FA Davis Co., 1992:408–414.

Matloub HS, Yousif NJ. Peripheral nerve anatomy and innervation pattern. *Hand Clin* 1992;8:201–214.

McComas AJ. Invited review: motor unit estimation: methods, results, and present status. *Muscle Nerve* 1991;14:585–597.

Myers RR. Anatomy and microanatomy of peripheral nerve. *Neurol Clin* 1991;2:1–20.

Nicolle MW. Myasthenia gravis and Lambert-Eaton myasthenic syndrome. *Continuum (Minneap Minn)* 2016;22(6, Muscle and Neuromuscular Junction Disorders):1978–2005.

Pham M, Bäumer P, Meinck HM, et al. Anterior interosseous nerve syndrome: fascicular motor lesions of median nerve trunk. *Neurology* 2014;82:598–606.

Plotz PH, Dalakas M, Leff RL, et al. Current concepts in the idiopathic inflammatory myopathies: polymyositis, dermatomyositis, and related disorders. *Ann Intern Med* 1989;111(2):143–157.

Ruff RL. Neurophysiology of the neuromuscular junction: overview. *Ann N Y Acad Sci* 2003;998:1–10.

Sanders DB. Clinical neurophysiology of disorders of the neuromuscular junction. *J Clin Neurophysiol* 1993;10:167–180.

Stewart JD. Peripheral nerve fascicles: anatomy and clinical relevance. *Muscle Nerve* 2003;28:525–541.

Stewart JD. Magnificent MRI and fascinating selective nerve fascicle damage. *Neurology* 2014;82:554–555.

Tzartos SJ, Cung MT, Demange P, et al. The main immunogenic region (MIR) of the nicotinic acetylcholine receptor and the anti-MIR antibodies. *Mol Neurobiol* 1991;5:1–29.

Verschuuren J, Strijbos E, Vincent A. Neuromuscular junction disorders. *Handb Clin Neurol* 2016;133:447–466.

Vincent A, Palace J, Hilton-Jones D. Myasthenia gravis. *Lancet* 2001;357:2122–2128.

Wertsch JJ, Oswald TA, Roberts MM. Role of intraneural topography in diagnosis and localization in electrodiagnostic medicine. *PMR Clinics North Am* 1994;5:465–475.

CHAPTER 24

The Spinal Cord Level

Above the motor unit, the next level of motor system integration is the spinal cord. The spinal cord begins at the cervicomedullary junction and ends at the conus medullaris. It is slightly flattened in an anteroposterior direction. Fissures and sulci mark the external surface of the spinal cord; most are of little clinical importance. A deep anterior median fissure and a posterior median sulcus partially divide it into two symmetrical halves. The anterior and posterior roots form the spinal nerves, which are segmentally arranged in 31 pairs. There are 8 pairs of cervical nerves, 12 thoracic, 5 lumbar, 5 sacral, and 1 coccygeal (Figure 24.1). Situated on each dorsal root is a dorsal root ganglion (DRG).

In newborns, the spinal cord may extend as far caudally as L3. During maturation, the vertebral column elongates more than the spinal cord, and the adult spinal cord is about 25 cm shorter than the vertebral column. The variability of the lower level has some correlation with the length of the trunk, especially in females. Radiographically, the conus is usually seen at the L1-L2 interspace in adults; if the level of the tip of the conus is below the mid-L2 vertebral body, the conus is considered low-lying. Because the spinal cord normally ends at the level of the L1-L2 interspace, lumbar punctures are done well below this level.

The length discrepancy between the spine and the spinal cord creates a difference between the segments of the spinal cord and the vertebral level that progressively increases from rostral to caudal. In the upper cervical area, the numerical cord level is about one segment greater than the corresponding vertebral spinous process (e.g., the C5 spinous process lies at the C6 segment of the spinal cord). In the lower cervical and thoracic areas, there is a difference of about two segments; in the lumbar region, there is a difference of almost three segments (Figure 24.1). Because of the offset, the spinal nerves below the cervical region course downward before exiting through the intervertebral foramina. Nerve roots exit through the foramen above the vertebra of like number from C1 to C7. The C8 root exits below C7 and sets the pattern of root exit below like-numbered vertebra followed down the rest of the vertebral column. The lumbar and sacral roots descend almost vertically to reach their points of exit. These long trailing roots from the lower cord segments make up the cauda equina.

The spinal cord is greater in width and diameter in the cervical and lumbosacral regions, forming the cervical and lumbar enlargements, the site of nuclear centers that supply the extremities. The cervical enlargement extends from the C3-T2 spinal cord segments; it innervates muscles of the upper limb (Figure 24.2). The lumbar enlargement extends from the L1-S3 spinal cord segments; it innervates muscles of the lower limb. The segments of the cervical enlargement match fairly well with the corresponding vertebral levels. The lumbar enlargement extends over vertebral levels T9-T12. Below T12, the spinal cord tapers to form the conus medullaris.

Each segment of the spinal cord gives rise to a mixed spinal nerve that contains motor, sensory, and autonomic fibers (Figure 24.3). Motor axons arising from the anterior horn cells of the spinal cord travel in the converging filaments of the anterior spinal root. On each posterior root, within the intervertebral foramen and just proximal to the junction with the anterior root, lies a DRG. The DRG is made up of unipolar neurons, and the posterior roots are made up of the central processes of these neurons. Acetylcholine is the only neurotransmitter in the anterior roots; the posterior roots contain several, including substance P, glutamate, calcitonin gene–related peptide, vasoactive intestinal polypeptide, cholecystokinin, somatostatin, and dynorphin. The anterior roots convey motor and autonomic fibers

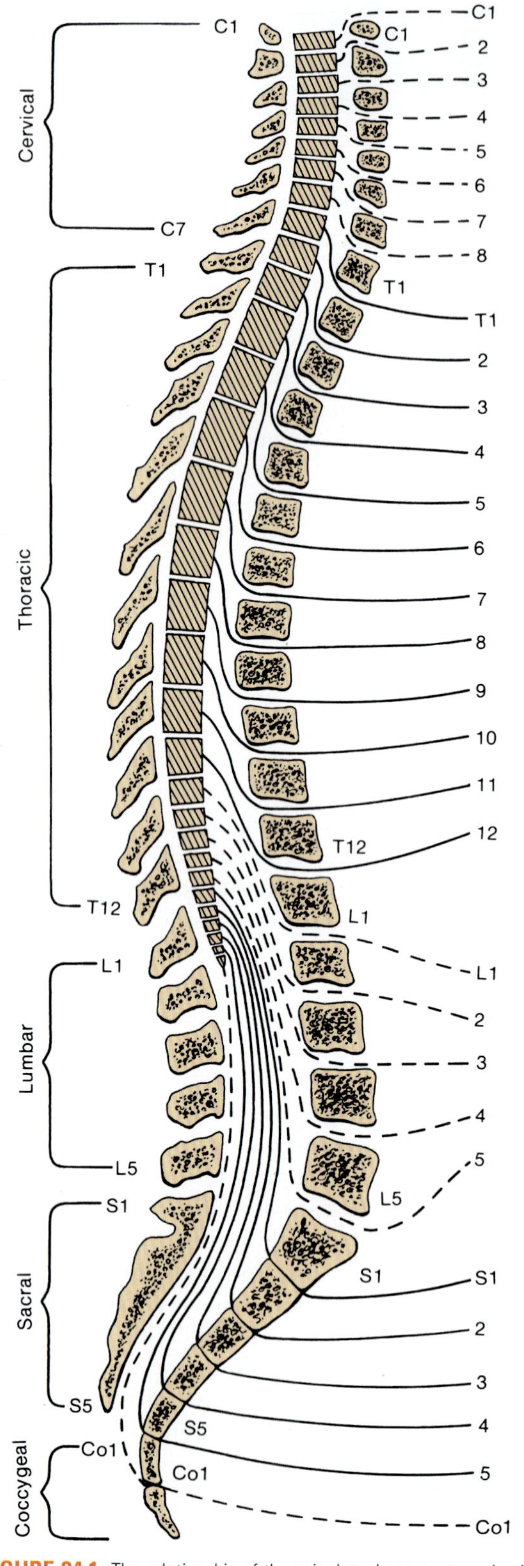

FIGURE 24.1 The relationship of the spinal cord segments and spinal nerves to the vertebral bodies and spinous processes.

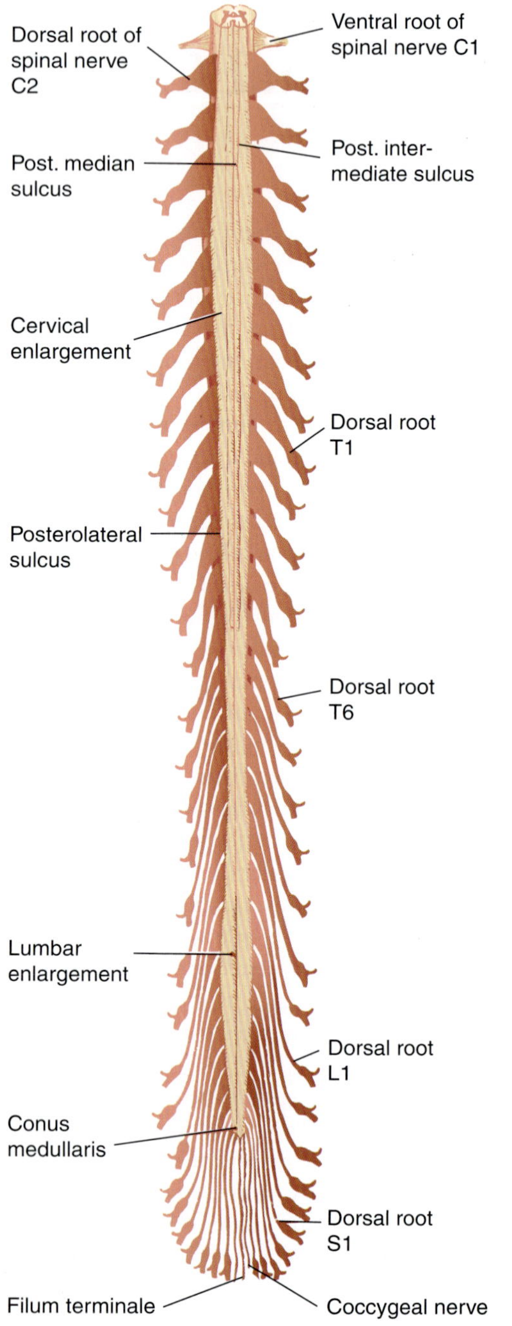

FIGURE 24.2 Posterior view of the spinal cord showing attached dorsal root filaments and spinal ganglia. Letters and numbers indicate corresponding spinal nerves. (Modified from Carpenter MB, Sutin J. *Human Neuroanatomy*. 8th ed. Baltimore: Williams & Wilkins, 1983, with permission.)

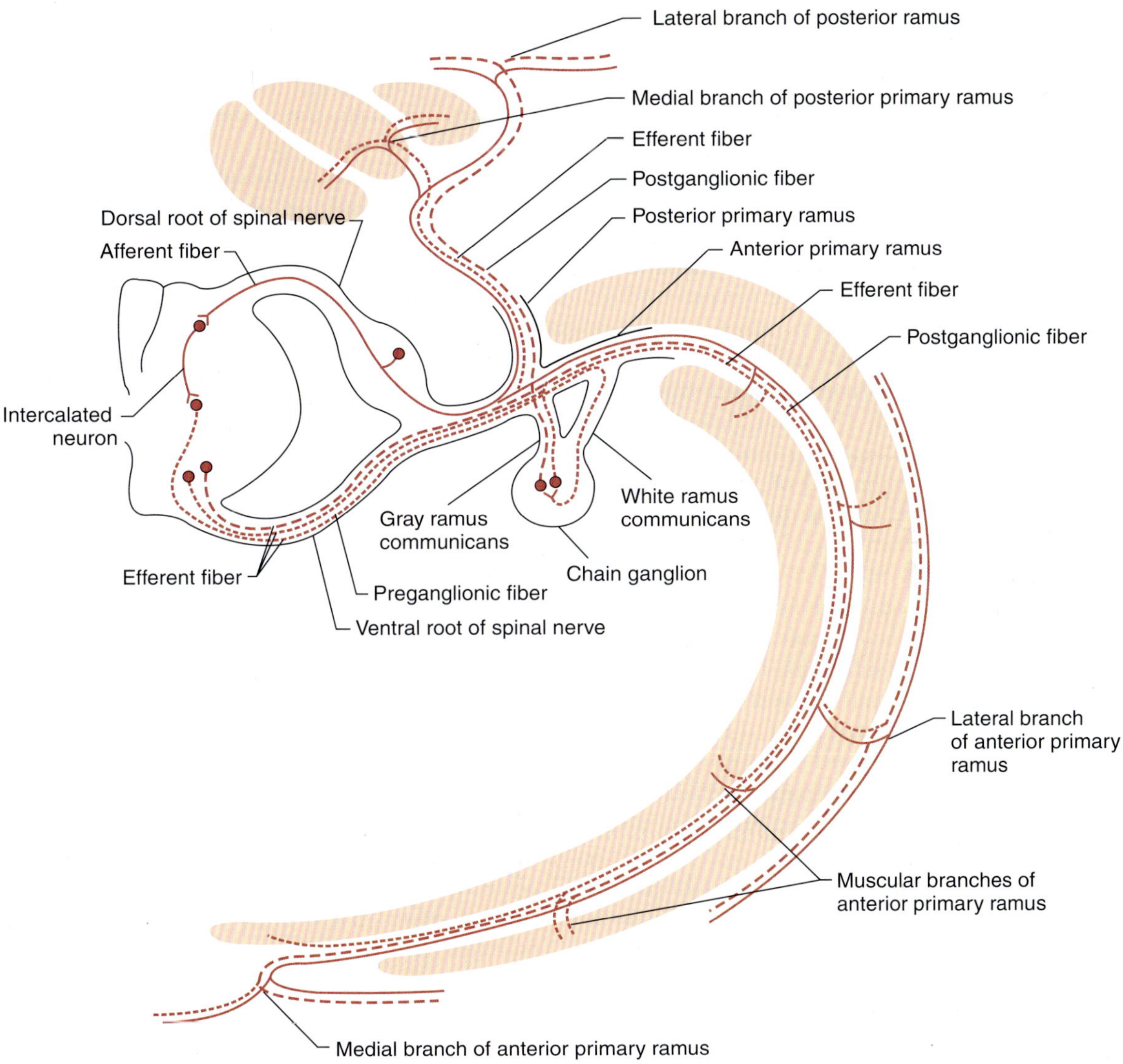

FIGURE 24.3 Segmental spinal nerve showing the course of motor, sensory, and preganglionic and postganglionic sympathetic fibers.

into the peripheral nerve; they join the posterior root to form the mixed spinal nerve. In the thoracolumbar region, white and gray rami communicantes connect the spinal nerve to the paravertebral sympathetic chain (Figure 24.3).

The Bell-Magendie law (for Sir Charles Bell and Francois Magendie) states that the anterior roots are motor and the posterior roots sensory; this discovery was one of the seminal developments in early neurobiology. However, it now appears there may be some afferent nerve fibers in the anterior roots, and up to 3% of the fibers in the posterior root may be efferent. The roots pass through the dura separately and then unite in the intervertebral foramina just distal to the DRG to form the mixed spinal nerve. After the mixed spinal nerve exits the intervertebral foramen, it divides into anterior and posterior primary rami. The smaller posterior primary rami supply the skin of the back and the paraspinal muscles. The anterior primary rami are continuations of the mixed spinal nerves and supply motor and sensory innervation to all other structures of the body. The anterior primary rami from the cervical and lumbar enlargements form the brachial and lumbosacral plexuses that innervate the limbs. The anterior primary rami of the thoracic segments of the spinal cord continue as the intercostal nerves. The anterior primary ramus of the mixed spinal nerve is sometimes referred to as a root, especially by surgeons and especially regarding the brachial plexus. When anatomy sources say that the C5 and C6 roots join to form the upper trunk, they are actually referring to the anterior primary rami of the spinal nerve. Similarly, when the dorsal scapular nerve is said to arise from the C5 root.

The delicate pia-arachnoid closely invests the spinal cord. The tough, fibrous membrane of the dura mater forms a firm, tubular sheath around the exiting nerve roots. The spinal cord is separated from the walls of the vertebral canal by the epidural space, which contains areolar tissue and a plexus of veins. The subdural space is a potential space containing a small amount of fluid. The subarachnoid space is a well-defined cavity containing cerebrospinal fluid that extends to about the level of the second sacral vertebra, forming the lumbar thecal sac. Systemic malignancies frequently metastasize to the capacious spinal epidural space. Spinal hematomas may accumulate in the epidural, subdural, or subarachnoid space. Subarachnoid hematomas can extend along the entire length of the subarachnoid space. Epidural and subdural spinal hematoma present with intense, knifelike pain at the location of the hemorrhage ("coup de poignard") followed by progressive paralysis below the affected level. Spinal epidural abscess classically causes a triad of fever, back pain, and a neurologic deficit.

A section of spinal cord where the rootlets of a pair of spinal nerves attach is referred to as a segment, although there is no internal demarcation to separate one segment from another. Each spinal cord segment can function as an independent entity for purposes of some very basic functions, such as the segmental muscle stretch reflex. Each segment controls the resting muscle tone of the muscles it innervates. The motor units supplying the myotomal muscles innervated by a segment carry out voluntary activity. The motor function of a spinal cord segment is modulated and influenced by suprasegmental impulses from several descending motor tracts.

The spinal cord parenchyma consists of an H- or butterfly-shaped core of gray matter that contains nerve cells, surrounded by white matter made up of longitudinally arranged ascending and descending nerve fibers, mainly myelinated. The relative proportion of white to gray matter varies depending on the cord level. In the center of the gray matter, running throughout the entire length of the cord and for a short distance into the filum terminale, is a minute central canal consisting of a single layer of ependymal cells. The two halves of the spinal cord are joined by a commissure made up of a core of gray matter surrounded by anterior and posterior white commissures. Internally, the white matter of the spinal cord is divided into posterior, lateral, and anterior funiculi. The posterior funiculus extends from the posterior median sulcus to the attachment of the posterior rootlets at the posterolateral sulcus. Rostral to the upper thoracic segments, a posterior intermediate sulcus separates the medial fasciculus gracilis from the lateral fasciculus cuneatus. The lateral funiculus lies between the attachments of the posterior and anterior spinal rootlets. The anterior funiculus extends from the anterior rootlets to the anterior median fissure.

The spinal cord gray matter consists of anterior and posterior horns with a lateral concavity. In the thoracic and upper lumbar regions, an intermediolateral column of autonomic neurons forms a small projecting lateral horn between the anterior and posterior horns. The sympathetic axons project through the anterior horn and anterior root and then through the gray rami communicantes to enter the sympathetic chain ganglia. The gray matter contains neurons, nerve fibers, supporting neuroglia, and blood vessels. Neurons are not distributed uniformly but are collected into functional groups that consist of columns of cells extending over many segments (Figure 24.4). The most elementary division is into posterior horns that contain sensory neurons and anterior horns that contain motor neurons. The posterior horn is relatively narrow and capped by a thin crescent of tissue, the substantia gelatinosa (of Rolando). The tip of the posterior horn is separated from the surface by a thin white matter tract, the dorsolateral tract (of Lissauer).

Within the anterior horn, there are alpha motor (skeletomotor) neurons, gamma motor (fusimotor) neurons, beta motor neurons, and interneurons. The alpha motoneurons innervate common, extrafusal striated skeletal muscle; the gamma motoneurons innervate intrafusal, muscle spindle fibers (L. fusus "spindle"). Beta motor neurons innervate both intrafusal and extrafusal fibers. All of these fibers are classified as general somatic efferent. At any given level, there is a somatotopic arrangement of motor neurons. A medial cell group that extends throughout the length of the spinal cord innervates the trunk and proximal muscles. A lateral cell group found only in the cervical and lumbar enlargements innervates limb muscles. The expansion of the anterior horns in the cervical and lumbar enlargements reflects the presence

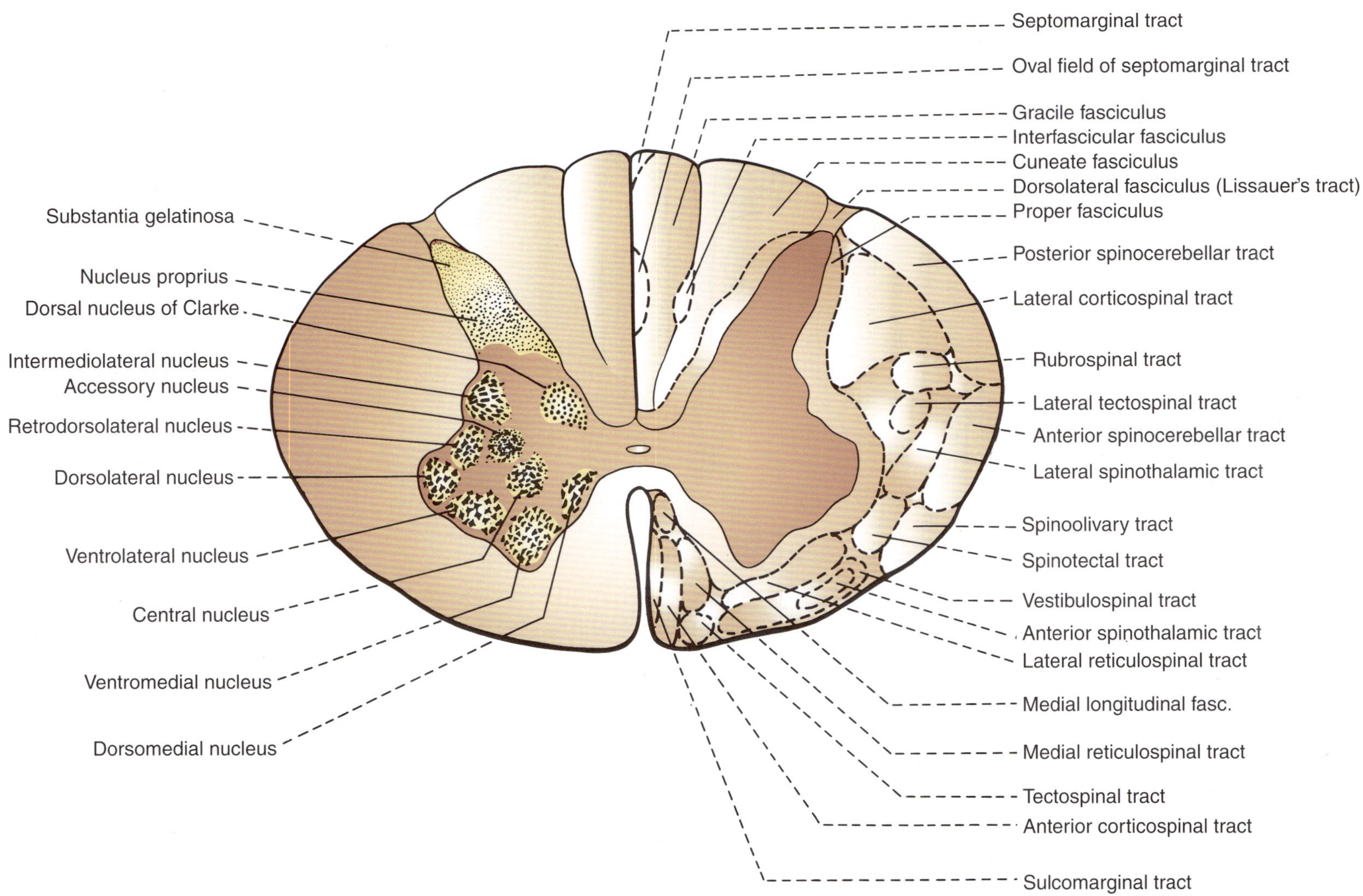

FIGURE 24.4 Cross section of the spinal cord showing the arrangement of cellular groups in the gray matter and fiber pathways in the white matter.

of this lateral cell column that supplies limb muscles. In both the cervical and lumbar enlargements, neurons innervating proximal muscles are located more rostrally and those innervating distal muscles more caudally; cells supplying extensors are more ventral than cells innervating flexors. Some motor neurons are aggregated into well-defined nuclear groups. The phrenic nucleus is a central collection of cells from C3 to C7 that innervates the diaphragm. Onuf's nucleus is a ventrolateral cell group at S1 and S2 that supplies the striated muscles of the perineum. For unknown reasons, the cells of Onuf's nucleus are relatively spared in motor neuron disease but disproportionately involved in multiple system atrophy.

The collections of neurons in the gray matter of the spinal cord are not as well defined as nuclei in other parts of the nervous system. In experimental animals, Rexed identified 10 regions, or laminae, of the spinal cord gray matter. Rexed laminae are more commonly used in the study of spinal cord neurons than the named nuclei (Figure 24.5, Box 24.1). There is evidence supporting the laminar scheme in humans as well. Laminae I to IV make up most of the posterior horn and receive cutaneous primary afferents. Lamina IX contains the motor neurons that supply striated muscles. Small motor neurons tend to innervate type S (slow twitch, fatigue resistant) motor units, and larger neurons type FF (fast twitch, fatigue sensitive) and FR (intermediate, fast twitch but more fatigue resistant than FF) motor units.

The white matter of the spinal cord consists of ascending and descending long fiber tracts and short intersegmental and intrasegmental tracts (Figure 24.4). The ascending pathways carry sensory impulses of various types from the extremities, trunk, or neck to higher centers. The major ascending tracts are the posterior columns, the spinothalamic/anterolateral system, and the spinocerebellar tracts.

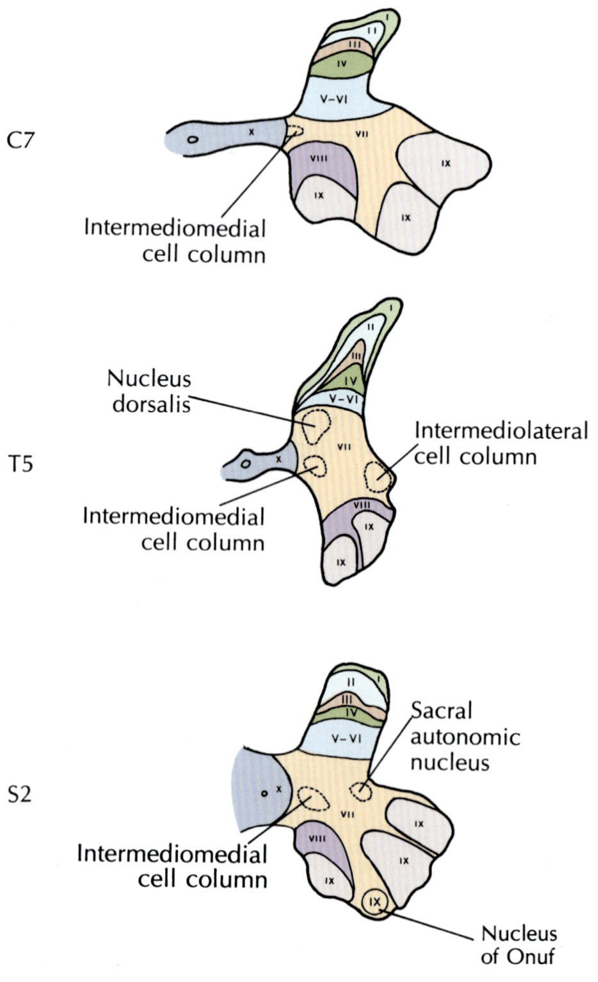

FIGURE 24.5 Positions of the Rexed cytoarchitectonic laminae at three levels of the spinal cord gray matter. (Modified from Kiernan JA. *Barr's The Human Nervous System: An Anatomical Viewpoint.* 9th ed. Philadelphia: Wolters Kluwer Health/Lippincott Williams & Wilkins, 2009, with permission.)

BOX 24.1

The Rexed Laminae

Lamina I consists of scattered large neurons in the superficial region of the posterior horn that receive afferents from Lissauer's tract; these neurons are primarily involved with pain impulses. Lamina II, with overlap into lamina III, is approximately coterminous with the substantia gelatinosa. These regions contain interneurons that receive pain and temperature afferents from Lissauer's tract but make no contribution to the long ascending sensory pathways. Lamina IV contains polymodal, or wide dynamic range, sensory neurons that are activated by many different stimuli. Cells in lamina IV give rise to the contralateral spinothalamic tract. Laminae V and VI are indistinguishable in humans. Cells in laminae IV and V to VI make up the nucleus proprius. Laminae V to VI receive many descending fibers, particularly those of the corticospinal tract. Lamina VII is the most extensive cytoarchitectonic layer. Between C8 and L3, the medial portion of lamina VII contains the nucleus dorsalis (of Clarke), which is the origin of the posterior spinocerebellar tract. Laterally in lamina VII is the intermediolateral gray column that contains preganglionic sympathetic neurons between T1 and L2 and preganglionic parasympathetic neurons between S2 and S4. Lamina VIII contains interneurons involved in motor control, including Renshaw cells that receive collaterals from nearby lamina IX motor neurons. Lamina IX contains the motor neurons. There is a medial nuclear group at all levels that innervates axial and proximal muscles and a lateral nuclear group in the cervical and lumbar enlargements that innervates distal extremity muscles. Lamina X surrounds the central canal and contains small neurons that receive dorsal root afferents involved with pain, temperature, and visceral sensation.

The descending pathways carry impulses from higher centers; these terminate in spinal cord nuclei on which they have regulatory and inhibitory functions. The major descending pathway is the pyramidal tract, which includes the lateral corticospinal (crossed pyramidal) and ventral corticospinal (uncrossed pyramidal) tracts. The lateral corticospinal tract is a massive bundle taking up most of the lateral funiculus of the cord. It contains descending pyramidal tract fibers from the giant pyramidal Betz cells in the motor cortex, but these comprise only 3% of the bundle; fibers making up the bulk of the tract come from other cortical areas. Lateral corticospinal axons drop off to innervate segmental motor neurons all along the cord, so the tract becomes progressively smaller as it descends.

In humans, corticospinal tract fibers originating in areas 4 and 6 synapse not only with interneurons but directly with the large, multipolar, spinal motor neurons in lamina IX. The direct synapse with anterior horn motor neurons is one of the defining characteristics of the corticospinal system. The direct projections from the precentral gyrus to spinal motor neurons are concerned with discrete, fractionated limb movements and fine motor control, and the distribution of precentral corticospinal fibers is primarily to motor neurons that supply distal extremity muscles. Other descending tracts that influence segmental spinal cord motor activity include the rubrospinal, vestibulospinal, medial and lateral reticulospinal, olivospinal, and the tectospinal tract. Fractionated, fine movements of distal extremity muscles are controlled primarily by the corticospinal and rubrospinal tracts; control of proximal and postural muscles is primarily by extrapyramidal pathways, particularly the reticulospinal and vestibulospinal tracts. There are other less well-defined tracts, as well as intersegmental, intrasegmental, and association pathways. There is some intermingling of fibers within the various tracts, and individual pathways are not as distinctly delineated as diagrams would indicate.

BLOOD SUPPLY

There is some individual variation in the blood supply of the spinal cord (Figure 24.6). The anterior spinal artery is formed by the union of the arterial branches that pass caudally from each vertebral artery and unite in the midline near the foramen magnum. It descends the entire length of the spinal cord, taking a somewhat undulating course, and lies in or near the anterior median fissure. Below the fourth or fifth cervical segment, the anterior spinal artery is fed

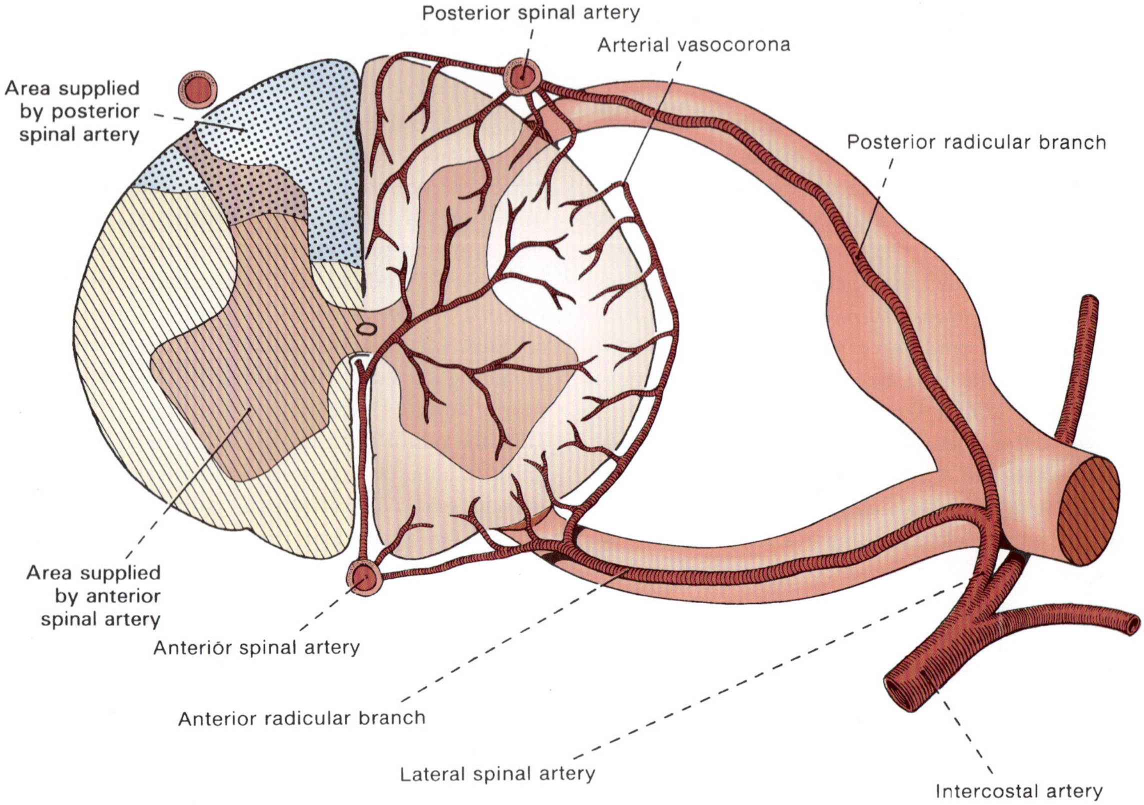

FIGURE 24.6 Arterial supply of the spinal cord.

or reinforced by unpaired anterior medullary arteries that arise from the lateral spinal arteries. These latter vessels enter the vertebral canal through the intervertebral foramina, and in the cervical region are branches of the ascending cervical artery; in the thorax, of the intercostals; and in the abdomen, of the lumbar, iliolumbar, and lateral sacral arteries. They pierce the dural sheaths of the spinal roots and split into anterior and posterior radicular branches. The radicular arteries are asymmetric and sometimes absent. The largest medullary artery, the great anterior radicular artery of Adamkiewicz, arises between T9 and L2, usually on the left side, and supplies the lumbar enlargement. The blood supply to any given level of the spinal cord is proportional to its cross-sectional area of gray matter, and the caliber of the anterior spinal artery is largest at the level of the lumbar and cervical enlargements.

The posterior spinal arteries are really plexiform channels rather than distinct single vessels that lie near the posterolateral sulci and the entrance of the rootlets of the posterior spinal nerves. They also arise from the vertebral arteries, and posterior medullary arteries join them at irregular intervals. Central arteries, branches of the anterior spinal, are given off alternately to the right and left halves of the spinal cord at different levels to supply the anterior and central portions of the cord. Branches of the anterior and posterior spinal arteries form a peripheral anastomosis, the arterial vasocorona, which supplies the periphery of the cord, including the lateral and ventral funiculi. This anastomosis is least efficient in the region of the lateral columns. Within the substance of the cord, the posterior spinal arteries supply the posterior horns and most of the dorsal funiculi; the anterior spinal artery supplies most of the remainder of the cord. Certain boundary zones between ascending and descending sources of the blood supply are sites of least adequate circulation in the spinal cord. The cervical and lumbosacral spinal cord are more richly vascularized than the thoracic cord. The upper thoracic segments near T4 have been traditionally thought particularly vulnerable to ischemia. More recent evidence finds the lower thoracic or upper lumbar cord more vulnerable. Patients with myelopathy after cardiac arrest or severe hypotension were found to have predominant involvement of the lumbosacral level with relative sparing of the thoracic region; none of the patients had damage isolated to the thoracic region. In a series of 44 cases of spinal cord infarction, the mean level of deficit in cases of global ischemia was at T9.

The venous drainage of the spinal cord courses from the capillary plexuses to peripheral venous plexuses that correspond somewhat to the arterial supply. The major portion of the venous drainage takes place through the intervertebral foramina into veins in the thoracic, abdominal, and pelvic cavities, but the valveless spinovertebral venous plexus (Batson's plexus) also continues upward into the intracranial cavity and venous sinuses and may be a means of transport of tumor cells. Abnormalities of the cerebrospinal venous system have been implicated in the pathogenesis of multiple sclerosis (MS).

PHYSIOLOGY AND PATHOPHYSIOLOGY

Spinal reflexes are responses to stimuli that are mediated at the spinal cord level. A spinal reflex may be monosynaptic, with an afferent and efferent limb mediated by only two neurons joined by a single synapse, or polysynaptic when one or more interneurons are involved. A spinal reflex may be segmental (intrasegmental), mediated at only one level, or intersegmental, with several levels participating. Long-loop reflexes involve circuits that reach as far as the cerebral cortex, allowing modulation of spinal reflexes by suprasegmental mechanisms.

The motor unit consists of an alpha motor neuron and all its subject muscle fibers (Chapter 23). A parallel system of innervation arises from gamma motor neurons that innervate muscle spindles. Muscle spindles, or neuromuscular spindles, are small structures (1 to 3 mm long in small muscles, 7 to 10 mm long in large muscles), composed of specialized muscle fibers. Spindles lie widely interspersed in the muscle, affixed with connective tissue parallel to the larger, extrafusal muscle fibers. Muscles that require finely graded contractile control, such as small hand muscles, have a greater density of spindles. The extrafusal fibers provide the force for muscle contraction; the muscle spindles provide modulation and control of that force. They also help regulate the underlying tone in the muscle. Muscle contraction always occurs against some setting of background tone. When the underlying, background level of muscle tone is either too high or too low, voluntary activity cannot occur with normal effectiveness. Thus, the gamma efferent system is a critical component of motor control. The descending extrapyramidal motor pathways, such as the reticulospinal and vestibulospinal tracts, have an important influence on the gamma efferent system. Pathways from the motor cortex and cerebellum tend to influence both the alpha and gamma motor neurons simultaneously, an effect referred to as alpha-gamma coactivation.

Muscle spindles consist of a small group of intrafusal muscle fibers surrounded by a connective tissue capsule. Tonic firing of the gamma motor neuron produces slight contraction of the intrafusal fibers, leaving them under tension. The spindles send information regarding the level of tension to the spinal cord. There are two primary types of intrafusal fibers, nuclear chain and nuclear bag, in a ratio of 3 to 4:1. In nuclear bag fibers, a collection of myonuclei creates a bulge in the fiber's center; in nuclear chain fibers, the myonuclei are linear. There are two types of nuclear bag fibers: bag 1 and bag 2. The bag 2 fibers are smaller than the bag1 fibers, intermediate in size between the bag 1 fibers and the nuclear chain fibers. Muscle spindles supply the nervous system with information about the length of a muscle and, if the length is changing, about the rate of change. The bag 1 fibers convey dynamic information about changes in length; the bag 2 fibers relay data about static muscle length. Nuclear chain fibers respond only to static muscle length.

The efferent nerve supply to the muscle spindles arises from gamma or beta motor neurons. There are two types of efferent nerve ending configurations: plate endings occur primarily on nuclear bag fibers; trail endings are common on both bag and chain fibers. Afferent nerve fibers from the muscle spindles are group Ia (primary spindle afferents) and group II (secondary spindle afferents). The group Ia afferents arise from primary annulospiral endings that form spirals around the equatorial region of nuclear bag fibers; the group II afferents arise from both annulospiral and flower spray endings, primarily on nuclear chain fibers. Primary spindle afferents are large, heavily myelinated, rapidly conducting fibers; they are the fastest conducting fibers in the peripheral nervous system. Centrally, they make monosynaptic contact with alpha motor neurons innervating agonist and synergist muscles. They also send collaterals to the gamma motor neurons innervating the same muscle, as well as inhibitory collaterals to alpha motor neurons innervating antagonist muscles (reciprocal inhibition). Secondary spindle afferents make monosynaptic contact only with agonist muscle motor neurons. Spindle afferents are classified as general somatic afferent type fibers.

Renshaw described the effect of the discharge of motoneurons on neighboring motoneurons. Alpha motor neurons give off collateral fibers that synapse on nearby inhibitory interneurons, which then modulate the discharge of the alpha motor neuron (recurrent inhibitory Renshaw loop, lateral inhibition). Renshaw cells are present in laminae VII and VIII, immediately medial to the motor neurons in lamina IX. The synapse of the alpha motor neuron on the Renshaw cell is cholinergic. Both glycine and gamma-amino butyric acid (GABA)—inhibitory amino acids—appear to play a role in the recurrent inhibition mechanism of Renshaw cells on motor neurons. Autoantibodies to glutamic acid decarboxylase—a key enzyme in GABA synthesis—cause stiff-person syndrome, a condition of generalized stiffness and increased tone because of impaired inhibitory mechanisms.

Another important component in this system is the Golgi tendon organ (GTO). The GTO, from its position in the tendon, further helps to regulate muscle tone. In contrast to the parallel arrangement of the muscle spindles, GTOs are connected in series with the muscle. The GTO is a mechanism for force feedback to the contracting muscle. It may also serve as a protective mechanism against overstretch of the muscle tendon, either from active contraction of the muscle or from passive stretch. When tension in the tendon increases beyond a certain level, afferent traffic travels centrally via group Ib fibers from the GTO to inhibit contraction of the agonist and to cause contraction of the antagonist. The inhibition of the agonist (autogenic inhibition) is mediated by glycinergic interneurons. For force generated by active muscle contraction, autogenic inhibition helps to unload the tension on the tendon by causing the muscle to relax. The effects of the GTO/Ib fiber system are opposite (inhibition of the agonist) those of the muscle spindle/Ia fiber system (facilitation of the agonist). Further modulation of the motor system at the local segmental level is provided by afferents coming from the skin and joints that help to convey additional information regarding the position of the limb in space.

The simplest example of spinal cord segmental modulation of motor unit activity is the monosynaptic stretch reflex. If a muscle is suddenly stretched, as by percussion of its tendon with a reflex hammer, the passive stretch of the tendon stretches the muscle belly, which in turn leads to passive stretch of the muscle spindles. This lengthening of the intrafusal fibers triggers a volley of impulses in the primary spindle afferents. These synapse with alpha motor neurons innervating the muscle. The alpha motor neurons fire, producing a contraction of the muscle, which then, because of the parallel configuration of intrafusal and extrafusal fibers, unloads or takes the stretch off the muscle spindles. The muscle then returns to a state of relaxation. The sequence of percussion, contraction, and then relaxation is a muscle stretch or myotatic reflex (myo + Gr. teinein "to stretch"). Because the muscle stretch is produced by percussion of the tendon, the terms tendon reflex and deep tendon reflex are also commonly used. The contraction of the agonist may be accompanied by relaxation of the antagonist mediated by inhibitory interneurons (inverse myotatic reflex). If the resting tone of the muscle spindles is increased, and the tension of the intrafusal fibers at a higher than normal level, then the additional passive stretch due to percussion of the tendon produces a markedly exaggerated response. This is hyperreflexia, which is seen with upper motor neuron lesions.

In addition to the monosynaptic reflex arc, there are complex polysynaptic spinal reflexes that involve excitation or inhibition of agonists, synergists, and antagonist muscles and even contralateral muscles. The withdrawal reflex consists of a movement to escape from a cutaneous stimulus, usually noxious (e.g., flexion of the lower extremity in response to a painful stimulus on the sole of the foot). Afferent cutaneous nociceptive fibers synapse on both excitatory and inhibitory interneurons, which cause flexion of the hip and thigh, and dorsiflexion of the foot, with appropriate inhibition of their antagonists. The reflex activity is intersegmental, spread over several cord segments. More complex yet is the crossed extensor (Phillipson) reflex, in which withdrawal of the ipsilateral limb is accompanied by extension of the contralateral limb to provide body support whereas the stimulated limb escapes the provoking trigger. The crossed extensor reflex is not merely polysynaptic and intersegmental; the contralateral side of the spinal cord also participates. The crossed flexor reflex is when the contralateral leg flexes rather than extends.

CLINICAL MANIFESTATIONS OF DISINHIBITED SPINAL CORD SEGMENTS

The activity of the motor neurons in the spinal cord is regulated and modulated by the descending motor pathways. When the influence of the descending motor pathways is removed, as in a spinal cord injury, the result is a disinhibition of the segmental motor neuron pools below the level of the lesion, resulting in a higher level of gamma efferent resting traffic. This increases the gain on the muscle spindles, leaving them under an increased level of resting tone, which leads to spasticity and hyperreflexia.

Segmental spinal cord reflexes can be responsible for fairly elaborate motor phenomena. A dog making vigorous kicking movements with one leg in response to being scratched is exhibiting a complex, polysynaptic, intersegmental spinal reflex. The descending motor pathways—particularly the pyramidal tract—in general inhibit segmental reflexes and act to suppress excess activity. Because descending motor pathways normally suppress segmental activity, the eloquence of spinal reflexes is seen to best advantage when suprasegmental control is defective. In the immature nervous system of the neonate, suprasegmental pathways are not fully developed; a variety of spinal reflexes occur normally, such as stepping and placing reactions, crossed extensor reflex, and the tonic neck reflex. In the normal neonate, the crossed extensor and placing/stepping reactions disappear by 1 to 2 months of age, the tonic neck reflex by 3 months, and the extensor plantar response by 12 months. In patients with severe myelopathy that has interrupted the suprasegmental pathways rostrally, spinal reflex activity may be prominent, including withdrawal and crossed extensor reflexes. The Babinski's sign and related extensor plantar responses are fragments of the withdrawal reflex that occur with damage to the descending motor pathways. A more fully developed variation is the triple flexion response, in which extension of the great toe is accompanied by dorsiflexion of the foot and flexion of the knee and hip, essentially a withdrawal reflex. Brain-dead patients can display impressive spinal reflex movements, including the dramatic "Lazarus sign" (bilateral arm flexion, shoulder adduction, raising of the arms, and crossing of the hands). These are all ostensibly due to local spinal cord reflexes, which have become autonomous and are under no suprasegmental control.

SPINAL CORD SYNDROMES AND DISORDERS

Common or classic spinal cord syndromes include transverse myelopathy, Brown-Séquard syndrome, central cord syndrome, syringomyelic syndrome, anterior cord syndrome, posterior column syndrome, posterolateral column syndrome, anterior horn syndrome, and anterior horn-corticospinal tract syndrome.

Complete transverse myelopathy causes total loss of function below the level of the lesion; with incomplete myelopathy, there is some preservation of function (see Chapter 53). Common etiologies include trauma, cord compression, and myelitis, due to MS, neuromyelitis optica, a parainfectious event, or an isolated clinical syndrome. Patients present with acute transverse myelopathy if compression involves the spinal cord proper. If compression involves the cauda equina, the patient presents with a cauda equina syndrome rather than a transverse myelopathy (see Chapter 47). Longitudinally extensive transverse myelitis refers to florid and widespread inflammation of the spinal cord causing T2 hyperintensity on spinal magnetic resonance imaging that is seen to extend over three or more vertebral segments. It is classically associated with neuromyelitis optica, but there are many other causes, including other inflammatory etiologies, infection, malignancy, and metabolic disturbances.

Brown-Séquard described the clinical picture that follows functional hemisection of the spinal cord. It is actually more often seen with extramedullary tumor compression than with trauma. Patients with Brown-Séquard syndrome have corticospinal tract and posterior column dysfunction ipsilateral to the lesion and spinothalamic tract–mediated pain and temperature loss contralateral to the lesion. There may be evidence of root dysfunction at the level of the lesion. Brown-Séquard-plus syndrome is associated with additional neurologic findings involving the eyes, bowel, or bladder.

Central cord syndrome is one of the regularly recurrent variants seen with incomplete cervical spinal cord injury; it involves necrosis with softening of the central aspect of the spinal cord, with relative sparing of the periphery. Patients have segmental weakness at the involved level because of anterior horn gray matter necrosis, with only minor long tract findings, that is, they are not paraplegic or quadriplegic. The segmental weakness typically involves the

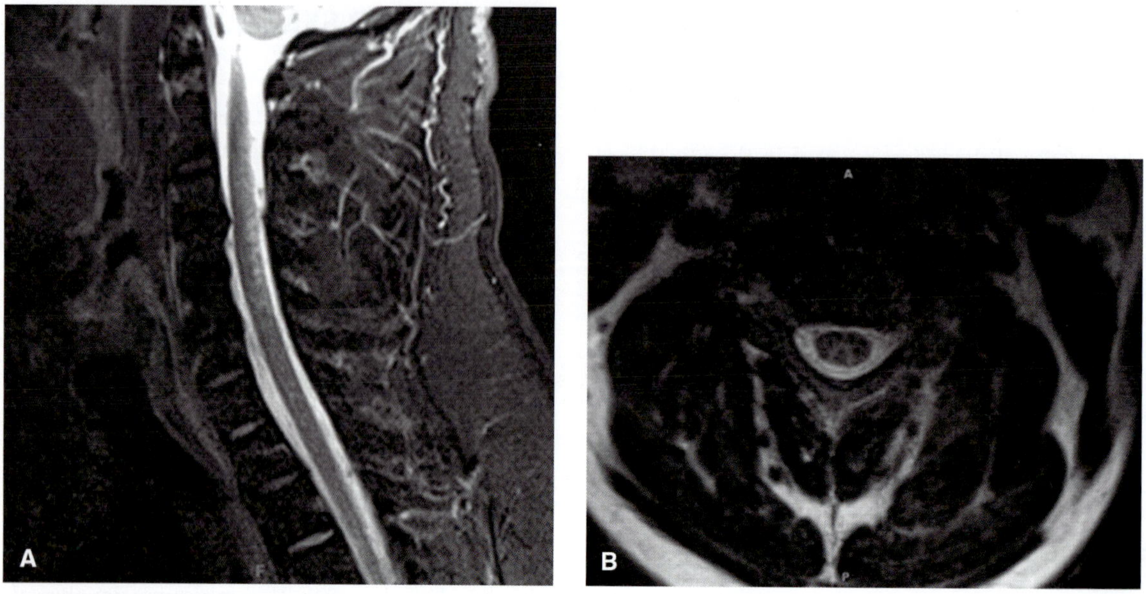

FIGURE 24.7 Nitrous oxide abuse myelopathy. Sagittal short T1 inversion recovery MRI showing hyperintensity in the posterior cervical and thoracic spinal cord **(A)**; axial T2 hyperintensity **(B)**. (Reprinted from Probasco JC, Felling RJ, Carson JT, et al. Teaching NeuroImages: myelopathy due to B_{12} deficiency in long-term colchicine treatment and nitrous oxide misuse. *Neurology*. 2011;77[9]:e51, with permission.)

hands and distal upper extremities. Hand weakness may also occur with a lesion several segments higher.

Anterior cord syndrome is due to ischemia in the distribution of the anterior spinal artery (anterior spinal artery syndrome). There is dysfunction of the entire spinal cord, except for the posterior columns. Patients are typically paraplegic or quadriplegic with loss of pain and temperature sensation below the level of the lesion but with retained sensation to light touch, position, and vibration. In the posterolateral column syndrome (subacute combined degeneration), most often because of vitamin B_{12} deficiency, there is demyelination and gliosis of the posterior and lateral columns. Clinically, affected patients have weakness, spasticity, and prominent loss of vibratory and position sense with relative preservation of pain and temperature. A similar syndrome may occur in nitrous oxide exposure, HIV myelopathy, copper deficiency, or zinc toxicity (Figure 24.7). Syringomyelia, often associated with Chiari malformations, produces suspended, dissociated sensory loss (see Chapter 36).

In the posterior column syndrome, dysfunction is limited to the posterior columns. The primary cause is syphilitic myelopathy, now rarely seen (tabes dorsalis; tabes, L. consumption). Isolated degeneration of the posterior column, without demonstrable etiology, occurs as a clinically benign rare condition, without progression to other systems. The etiology is most likely a sporadic degenerative disease of the cord. The anterior horn syndrome is characterized by loss of anterior horn cells and occurs in such conditions as spinal muscular atrophy (hereditary or acquired) and poliomyelitis. The anterior horn-corticospinal tract syndrome causes a combination of spasticity and anterior horn cell dysfunction and occurs in amyotrophic lateral sclerosis.

BIBLIOGRAPHY

Brown RH, Al-Chalabi A. Amyotrophic lateral sclerosis. *N Engl J Med* 2017;377:162–172.

Bueri JA, Saposnik G, Maurino J, et al. Lazarus' sign in brain death. *Mov Disord* 2000;15:583–586.

Byrne TN. Metastatic epidural cord compression. *Curr Neurol Neurosci Rep* 2004;4:191–195.

Byrne TN, Borges LF, Loeffler JS. Metastatic epidural spinal cord compression: update on management. *Semin Oncol* 2006;33:307–311.

Cikes N, Bosnic D, Sentic M. Non-MS autoimmune demyelination. *Clin Neurol Neurosurg* 2008;110:905–912.

Duggal N, Lach B. Selective vulnerability of the lumbosacral spinal cord after cardiac arrest and hypotension. *Stroke* 2002;33:116–121.

Fox RJ, Diaconu C, Baus L, et al. No association of chronic cerebrospinal venous insufficiency with multiple sclerosis. *Can J Neurol Sci* 2016;43:195–197.

Frohman EM, Wingerchuk DM. Clinical practice. Transverse myelitis. *N Engl J Med* 2010;363:564–572.

Geiman EJ, Zheng W, Fritschy JM, et al. Glycine and GABA(A) receptor subunits on Renshaw cells: relationship with presynaptic neurotransmitters and postsynaptic gephyrin clusters. *J Comp Neurol* 2002;444:275–289.

Gilman S, Newman SW. *Manter and Gatz's Essentials of Clinical Neuroanatomy and Neurophysiology*. 10th ed. Philadelphia: FA Davis, 2003.

Gould DJ, Fix JD. *Neuroanatomy*. 5th ed. Philadelphia: Wolters Kluwer Health/Lippincott Williams & Wilkins, 2014.

Gruener G, Biller J. Spinal cord anatomy, localization, and overview of spinal cord syndromes. CONTINUUM Lifelong Learning in Neurology. *Spinal Cord Root Plexus Disord* 2008;14:11–35.

Hohl JB, Lee JY, Horton JA, et al. A novel classification system for traumatic central cord syndrome: the central cord injury scale (CCIS). *Spine (Phila Pa 1976)* 2010;35:E238–E243.

Issaivanan M, Nhlane NM, Rizvi F, et al. Brown-Sequard-plus syndrome because of penetrating trauma in children. *Pediatr Neurol* 2010;43:57–60.

Jaiser SR, Winston GP. Copper deficiency myelopathy. *J Neurol* 2010;257:869–881.

Jeffery DR, Mandler RN, Davis LE. Transverse myelitis. Retrospective analysis of 33 cases, with differentiation of cases associated with multiple sclerosis and parainfectious events. *Arch Neurol* 1993;50:532–535.

Kastrup O, Timman D, Diener HC. Isolated degeneration of the posterior column as a distinct entity—a clinical and electrophysiologic follow-up study. *Clin Neurol Neurosurg* 2010; 112:209–212.

Kiernan JA, Rajakumar N. *Barr's The Human Nervous System: An Anatomical Viewpoint*. 10th ed. Philadelphia: Wolters Kluwer Health/Lippincott Williams & Wilkins, 2014.

Kitley J, Leite M, George J, et al. The differential diagnosis of longitudinally extensive transverse myelitis. *Mult Scler* 2012; 18:271–285.

Kreppel D, Antoniadis G, Seeling W. Spinal hematoma: a literature survey with meta-analysis of 613 patients. *Neurosurg Rev* 2003;26:1–49.

Kumar N. Pearls: myelopathy. *Semin Neurol* 2010;30:38–43.

Lin RJ, Chen HF, Chang YC, et al. Subacute combined degeneration caused by nitrous oxide intoxication: case reports. *Acta Neurol Taiwan* 2011;20:129–137.

Mannen T. Neuropathological findings of Onuf's nucleus and its significance. *Neuropathology* 2000;20(Suppl):S30–S33.

Marignier R, Cobo Calvo A, Vukusic S. Neuromyelitis optica and neuromyelitis optica spectrum disorders. *Curr Opin Neurol* 2017;30:208–215.

Meinck HM, Thompson PD. Stiff man syndrome and related conditions. *Mov Disord* 2002;17:853–866.

Parent A. *Carpenter's Human Neuroanatomy*. 9th ed. Baltimore: Lippincott Williams & Wilkins, 1996.

Pawate S, Sriram S. Isolated longitudinal myelitis: a report of six cases. *Spinal Cord* 2009;47:257–261.

Pearce JM. The craniospinal venous system. *Eur Neurol* 2006; 56:136–138.

Pittock SJ, Payne TA, Harper CM. Reversible myelopathy in a 34-year-old man with vitamin B_{12} deficiency. *Mayo Clin Proc* 2002;77:291–294.

Pouw MH, van Middendorp JJ, van Kampen A, et al. Diagnostic criteria of traumatic central cord syndrome. Part 3: descriptive analyses of neurological and functional outcomes in a prospective cohort of traumatic motor incomplete tetraplegics. *Spinal Cord* 2011;49:614–622.

Probasco JC, Felling RJ, Carson JT, et al. Teaching NeuroImages: myelopathy due to B_{12} deficiency in long-term colchicine treatment and nitrous oxide misuse. *Neurology* 2011;77:e51.

Prodan CI, Holland NR, Wisdom PJ, et al. Myelopathy due to copper deficiency. *Neurology* 2004;62:1655–1656.

Pryse-Phillips W. *Companion to Clinical Neurology*. 3rd ed. Oxford: Oxford University Press, 2009.

Renard D, Dutray A, Remy A, et al. Subacute combined degeneration of the spinal cord caused by nitrous oxide anaesthesia. *Neurol Sci* 2009;30:75–76.

Ropper AH, Samuels MA, Klein J. *Adams and Victor's Principles of Neurology*. 10th ed. New York: McGraw-Hill Education Medical, 2014.

Ruet A, Deloire MS, Ouallet JC, et al. Predictive factors for multiple sclerosis in patients with clinically isolated spinal cord syndrome. *Mult Scler* 2011;17:312–318.

Saposnik G, Bueri JA, Maurino J, et al. Spontaneous and reflex movements in brain death. *Neurology* 2000;54:221–223.

Schneider SP, Fyffe RE. Involvement of GABA and glycine in recurrent inhibition of spinal motoneurons. *J Neurophysiol* 1992;68:397–406.

Sonstein WJ, LaSala PA, Michelsen WJ, et al. False localizing signs in upper cervical spinal cord compression. *Neurosurgery* 1996;38:445–448.

Standring S, ed. *Gray's Anatomy: The Anatomical Basis of Clinical Practice*. 41st ed. New York: Elsevier Limited, 2016.

Traynor BJ, Codd MB, Corr B, et al. Clinical features of amyotrophic lateral sclerosis according to the El Escorial and Airlie House diagnostic criteria: a population-based study. *Arch Neurol* 2000;57:1171–1176.

Weidauer S, Nichtweiss M, Lanfermann H, et al. Spinal cord infarction: MR imaging and clinical features in 16 cases. *Neuroradiology* 2002;44:851–857.

Yazbeck PG, Al Rouhban RB, Slaba SG, et al. Anterior spinal artery syndrome after percutaneous vertebroplasty. *Spine J* 2011;11:e5–e8.

Young J, Quinn S, Hurrell M, et al. Clinically isolated acute transverse myelitis: prognostic features and incidence. *Mult Scler* 2009;15:1295–1302.

Zhao B, He L, Lai XH. A case of neuro-Behcet's disease presenting with lumbar spinal cord involvement. *Spinal Cord* 2010;48:172–173.

CHAPTER 25

The Corticospinal (Pyramidal) Level

In common parlance, the corticospinal level of motor integration is also referred to as the pyramidal level, cortical level, or upper motor neuron level. From a strict anatomical perspective, these terms are not synonymous. Objections can be raised to the terminology because neither corticospinal, pyramidal, nor upper motor neuron precisely and unambiguously describes the voluntary, direct descending motor pathway, but a better term has not come into use. The pyramidal tract is only one of the descending motor systems that converge on the anterior horn cell, so there are other "upper motor neurons." The corticobulbar tract supplies brainstem structures in the same way the corticospinal tract (CST) innervates the spinal cord but does not pass through the medullary pyramids and is not therefore "pyramidal." Neurons that are not part of the pyramidal system project from the cortex to the spinal cord. The terms pyramidal and extrapyramidal have become blurred anatomically; some anatomists suggest that they be abandoned. Clinicians, however, continue to find them useful because the clinical manifestations of lesions of the direct (pyramidal) motor pathways differ from those of the indirect (extrapyramidal) system.

ANATOMY AND PHYSIOLOGY

For clinical purposes, the CST is the principal efferent system through which purposive movements are initiated and performed. The CST is by no means the sole cortical mechanism for movement; it acts primarily to integrate highly skilled, fine, discrete movements of the distal extremities. It is responsible for the contraction of agonist muscles as well as the inhibition, or graded relaxation, of antagonist muscles necessary to perform skilled acts. By its integration and control, individual muscle contractions are coalesced into complex motor acts. The corticospinal level does not function independently. Normally, and in the presence of disease, it is closely integrated with other levels of motor activity, as well as with a constant stream of incoming sensory impulses. The CST, along with other cortical and brainstem pathways, constantly supplies lower centers with impulses that have a generally inhibitory effect. Disease involving the pyramidal pathways results in a release of this inhibiting effect, resulting in hyperactive and autonomous function of the affected spinal cord segmental levels. This results in excessive activity of the lower centers that are normally suppressed by cortical control mechanisms.

Area 4 (area gigantopyramidalis) of the precentral gyrus is the primary motor cortex (M-I); it is the region having the lowest threshold for stimulation to cause contraction of muscles of the opposite side of the body. The cortex of M-I is agranular and heterotypical; its most characteristic feature is the presence of giant pyramidal neurons (Betz cells) in lamina V. The localization of function within the precentral gyrus is depicted by the motor homunculus (Figure 6.5). The corticospinal system is phylogenetically relatively new. It is fully developed only in mammals and reaches its highest development in apes and man. The phylogenetic acquisition of speech and complex hand function resulted in expansion of cortical areas representing the tongue, mouth, lips, thumb, and fingers, displacing the cortical representation for the lower extremities and sacral regions upward and onto the medial surface of the hemisphere. Areas for the tongue, face, and digits are exceptionally large and out of proportion to those of the proximal musculature. The extension of the precentral gyrus onto the medial aspect of the frontal lobe forms the anterior portion of the paracentral lobule. Neurons controlling the lower extremities and perineal musculature are in the paracentral lobule, which plays an important role in bowel and bladder sphincter control.

There are reciprocal connections between the primary motor cortex and the primary somatosensory cortex in the postcentral gyrus. M-I receives association fibers from the premotor and supplementary motor areas and from the insula. These connections are involved in the preparation and planning for voluntary movements that are then executed by the primary motor cortex. There are also connections between the primary motor cortices in the two hemispheres. The posterior division of the ventral lateral nucleus of the thalamus receives input from the cerebellum and projects to area 4.

The term pyramidal tract arose because these fibers make up most of the medullary pyramids. It was once thought that the pyramidal tract consisted mainly of the axons of the Betz cells in the primary motor cortex. However, of the approximately 1 million fibers in the CST at the level of the pyramids, only 20% to 30% arise from M-I and only 3% arise from the Betz cells. These fibers are large, heavily myelinated and conduct rapidly. In addition to the contribution from M-I, the CST contains fibers from the premotor cortex (area 6), the supplementary motor area and adjacent regions, and the postcentral gyrus (areas 3, 1, and 2). The majority of the CST arises in approximately equal thirds from area 4, area 6, and the postcentral gyrus, with an additional contribution from the adjoining parietal cortex (area 5) and other portions of the brain, including the temporal and occipital lobes, cingulate gyrus, and certain subcortical centers (Figures 25.1 and 25.2).

The premotor region (area 6), located just rostral to area 4, is closely related to the motor cortex, both anatomically and functionally. The premotor cortex is similar histologically to the motor cortex but lacks the giant pyramidal cells. Some fibers from area 6 pass to area 4 and then downward with the CST; others descend with the pyramidal fibers. There is probably less complete crossing of the fibers from the premotor cortex than of those from the motor cortex. In addition, the premotor region communicates with the basal ganglia and other portions of the extrapyramidal system, including the subthalamic nucleus, red nucleus, superior colliculus, vestibular nuclei, inferior olive, and brainstem reticular formation (Figure 25.3).

The CST is important in controlling discrete, isolated motor responses, especially fine voluntary movement of individual digits. The CST provides speed and agility of distal extremity movements. The

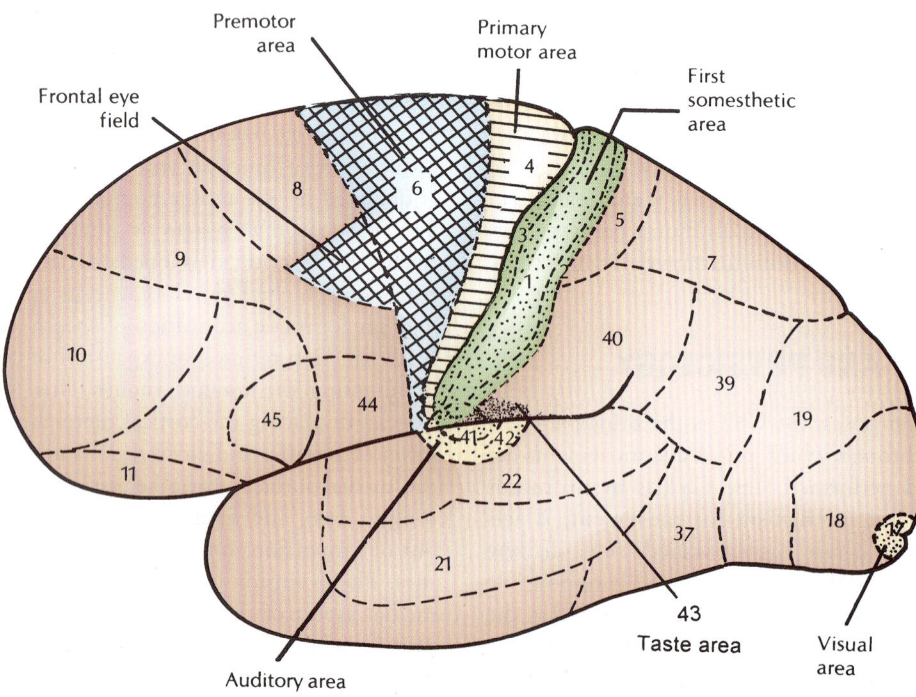

FIGURE 25.1 A lateral view of some of the clinically relevant cortical areas from the Brodmann cytoarchitectonic map. (Modified from Kiernan JA. *Barr's The Human Nervous System: An Anatomical Viewpoint.* 7th ed. Philadelphia: Lippincott-Raven, 1998, with permission.)

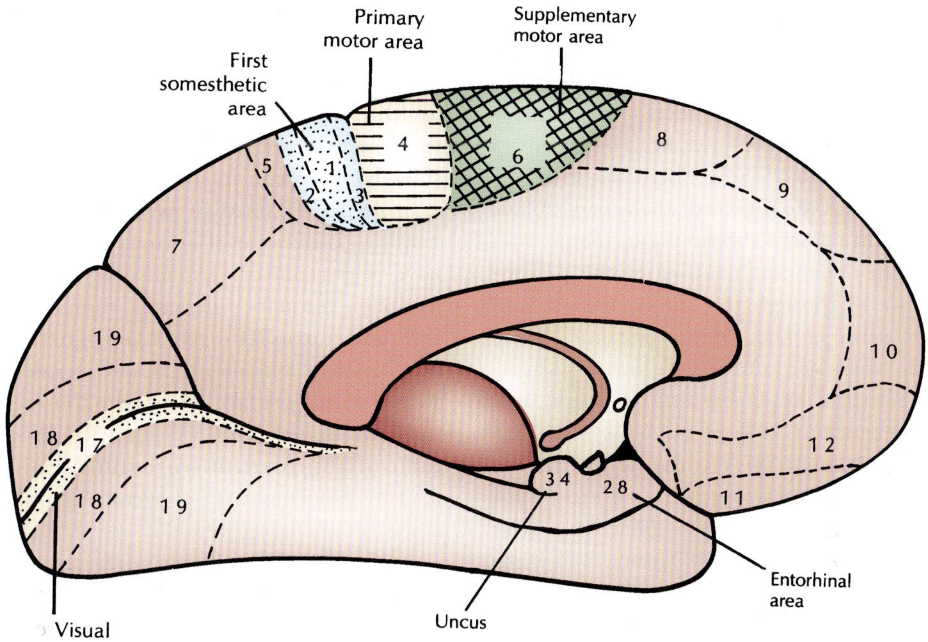

FIGURE 25.2 A medial view of some of the clinically relevant cortical areas from the Brodmann cytoarchitectonic map. (Modified from Kiernan JA. *Barr's The Human Nervous System: An Anatomical Viewpoint.* 7th ed. Philadelphia: Lippincott-Raven, 1998, with permission.)

premotor cortex and its pathways are concerned with larger coordinated responses, with more stereotyped movements that are partly automatic and involve the trunk and the proximal limbs, and with postural mechanisms. It is the principal cortical component of the extrapyramidal system. Stimulation of area 6 causes contraversive movements of the head and trunk. The premotor region is involved in movements guided by visual, auditory, and somatosensory stimuli. The supplementary motor area (M-II) is part of area 6 that lies on the medial aspect of the frontal lobe just anterior to the paracentral lobule (area 6ab). It communicates with the primary motor cortex as well as with the supplementary motor cortex in the opposite hemisphere. M-II seems to be involved particularly in planning and integrating bilateral body

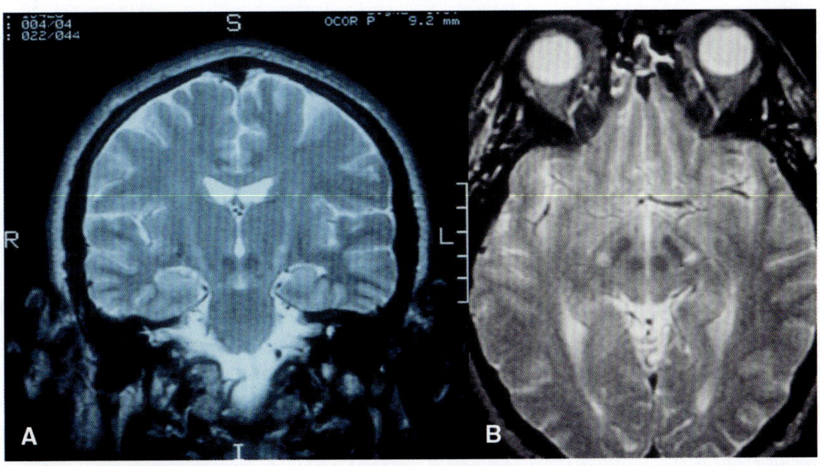

FIGURE 25.3 Degeneration of the corticospinal tracts in primary lateral sclerosis. In **(A)**, there are streaks of high signal on the coronal view. In **(B)**, the transverse view demonstrates ovoid areas of high signal intensity in the posterior portions of the internal capsules.

movements. M-II is also somatotopically organized, but the homunculus is cruder and less detailed than the one in M-I. The cingulate motor area in the anterior half of the cingulate gyrus projects to the primary motor cortex and also contributes descending fibers to the corticobulbar and CSTs. There is also a secondary motor area in the depths of the central sulcus where the precentral and postcentral gyri merge.

Axons from the motor neurons of the precentral gyrus descend through the corona radiata and the posterior limb of the internal capsule where corticobulbar fibers are anterior, followed posteriorly by those to the upper extremity, trunk, and lower extremity. About 90% of the CST fibers are small myelinated axons with a diameter of 1 to 4 μm, and most of the remaining fibers are 5 to 10 μm in diameter. The small numbers of fibers that arise from Betz cells are very large, with diameters of 10 to 22 μm. The posterior limb of the internal capsule is that portion of the capsule between the lenticular nucleus and the thalamus. The retrolenticular part lies posterior to the lenticular nucleus. In the rostral part of the internal capsule, the corticospinal fibers lie in the anterior portion of the posterior limb. As the capsules descend, the corticospinal fibers move posteriorly and come to occupy a position in the posterior third to posterior quarter of the posterior limb. In normal individuals, the CST can often be visualized as a subtle hyperintensity in the posterior portion of the posterior limb of the internal capsule on T2-weighted axial magnetic resonance images. These areas of hyperintensity are found near the junction of the posterior limb and the retrolenticular portion of the capsule. The signal change is thought to mark the very large heavily myelinated, rapidly conducting fibers that constitute the Betz cell component of the pyramidal tract. Degeneration of the CST, as occurs in amyotrophic lateral sclerosis or primary lateral sclerosis, accentuates this signal change and may be useful diagnostically (Figure 25.4).

At the midbrain level, pyramidal fibers traverse the middle three-fifths of the cerebral peduncle, with corticobulbar fibers most medial (Figure 25.5). The majority of corticobulbar fibers decussate before synapsing with the specific cranial nerve nuclei, but most of the cortical innervation of brainstem centers is both crossed and uncrossed. The descending fibers then pass through the basilar portion of the pons as disjointed fascicles and enter the medulla. In the caudal medulla, the CSTs gather into the discrete twin columns of the medullary pyramids that make up the base of the medulla (Figure 11.11). Approximately 85% to 90% of the fibers cross in the decussation of the pyramids, with those destined for the upper extremity decussating more rostrally than those for the lower extremity (Figure 11.12). There is considerable variation in the proportion of crossed and uncrossed CST fibers in man. Instances of ipsilateral hemiplegia because of an uncrossed pyramidal tract have been reported. Terakama et al. used functional magnetic resonance imaging, motor-evoked potentials, and somatosensory-evoked potentials to investigate a patient with an ipsilateral hemiplegia following a cerebral hemorrhage. They were able to demonstrate that the affected limbs were controlled by the ipsilateral cerebral cortex. In some instances, an uncrossed CST is associated with congenital anomalies of various sorts.

The fibers that decussate descend in the lateral funiculus of the spinal cord in the lateral CST, lying anterolateral to the posterior gray horn, medial to the posterior spinocerebellar tract, and posterior to the plane of the denticulate ligaments, to supply the muscles of the opposite side of the body. In the lumbosacral cord, where there is no posterior spinocerebellar tract, the lateral CST abuts the surface of the cord. The lateral CSTs may also contain other corticofugal fibers as well as some ascending ones. About 50% of the fibers of the lateral CST terminate in the cervical region, 20% in the thoracic area, and 30% in the lumbosacral portion of the cord. The tract ends at about the S4 level. The smaller anterior CST usually contains about 10% to 15% of the corticospinal fibers; it descends uncrossed in the ipsilateral anterior funiculus and usually does not extend below the midthoracic region. These fibers cross in the anterior white commissure at the segmental spinal cord level before terminating; they primarily supply axial muscles.

The axons of the corticobulbar and CSTs terminate on motor nuclei of the cranial nerves and the anterior horn cells of the spinal cord. Those traveling to the cord terminate primarily in laminae IV to VI, lamina VII, lamina VIII, and lamina IX on the side opposite the hemisphere of origin. Fibers from areas 4 and 6 end more ventrally, mainly in laminae VII and VIII, and are concentrated in the cervical and lumbosacral enlargements. The majority of CST fibers synapse on an interneuron, but about 10% end directly on alpha motor neurons in lamina IX. Those fibers that project directly from the cortex to anterior horn cells mediate discrete, skilled, fine motor movements of the distal extremities. Impulses then travel from

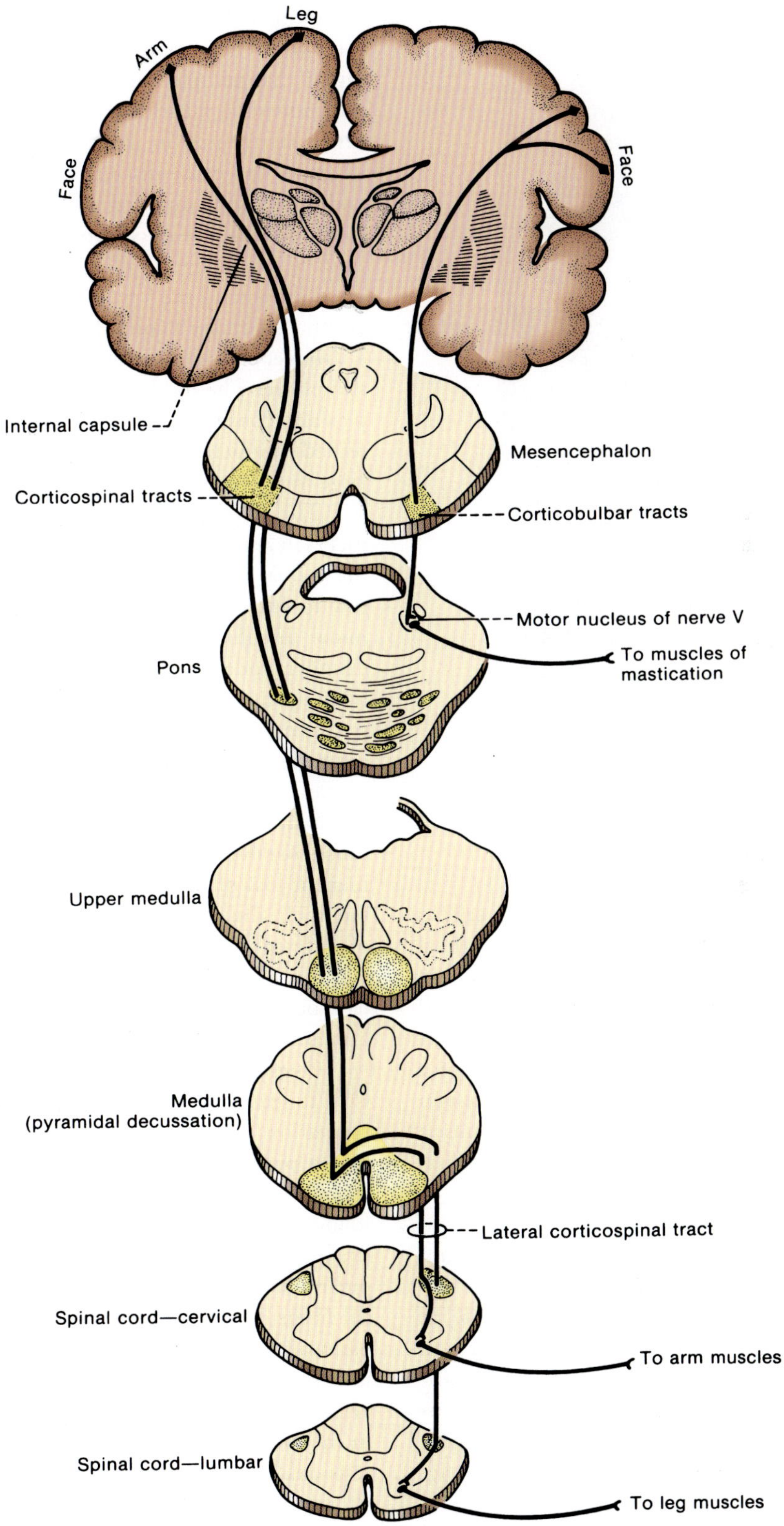

FIGURE 25.4 The corticobulbar and corticospinal pathways.

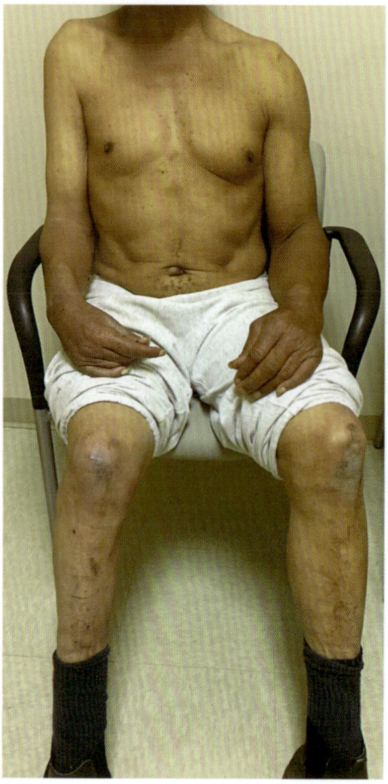

FIGURE 25.5 This patient suffered a major intracranial injury at age 3 and was left with refractory seizures and a spastic right hemiplegia with hemiatrophy.

the brainstem motor nuclei and anterior horn cells to the neuromuscular junctions of striated muscles (final common pathway). A single corticospinal fiber innervates more than one neuron in the spinal cord, and some probably innervate many. The pyramidal tract affects the activity of both alpha and gamma motor neurons. Alpha gamma coactivation serves to maintain a consistent level of stretch on the intrafusal muscle fibers during contraction and relaxation of the extrafusal fibers.

The CST preferentially innervates certain muscles, and this "pyramidal distribution" is important clinically. Lateral vestibulospinal tract effects are largely the opposite of CST effects. Glutamate or aspartate may be the excitatory neurotransmitters in some corticospinal neurons. The fibers from the parietal lobe that descend in the pyramidal tract terminate on sensory neurons in the dorsal horn and play a role in modulating sensory impulses in the long, ascending sensory pathways.

Neuronal discharge of the primary motor cortex, as from electrical stimulation or seizure activity, causes muscular contractions on the opposite side of the body. The response is one of groups of muscles rather than simple contraction of isolated muscles, but individual muscles as well as movements may be finely represented in the motor cortex. Stimulation of area 4 can cause discrete movements of the digits and the muscles supplied by the cranial nerves. With some overlap, areas controlling movements of the thumb, index finger, hallux, and face have the widest distribution and the lowest threshold. Stimulation of area 6 also causes a contralateral motor response, but a stronger stimulus is necessary than when area 4 is stimulated. The resulting movements are more complex and consist of slow, synergistic, postural, or patterned contractions of a generalized type that involve large muscle groups.

The CST lesions induced by ablation experiments in animals cause various deficits, depending on the animal and the area ablated. From a phylogenetic standpoint, voluntary motor control is extrapyramidal in submammalian species, mixed pyramidal/extrapyramidal in nonhuman mammals, and essentially pyramidal in humans. The effects of medullary pyramid transection (pyramidotomy) illustrate the differences in the function of the CST in different species. In the chimpanzee, it causes paralysis of the whole limb. In the rhesus monkey, the same lesion causes paralysis of distal extremity muscles with permanent loss of independent hand and finger movements. In the cat, it causes minimal deficits. Because of differences between the effects of lesions in man and those in experimental animals, such experiments have been of only limited usefulness in understanding human CST pathophysiology.

Questions remain about the relationship of the CST to spasticity. Primarily because of animal experimentation, it has been thought that lesions restricted to the pyramidal tract may cause weakness but not spasticity or hyperreflexia. The increase in tone that follows CST lesions may be related more closely to dysfunction of the extrapyramidal rather than the pyramidal system or to interruption of corticofugal fibers other than pyramidal in the corticospinal pathway. Although experimental pyramidotomies in animals may not lead to spasticity, in humans the evidence is that spasticity does eventually develop in the majority of cases. This is true even after very restricted lesions involving the medullary pyramids, although after a longer interval than is typical of other pyramidal lesions. It is likely that early flaccidity followed by the development of spasticity occurs with infarction of the CST at any level. More slowly developing lesions are likely to manifest spasticity at the time of initial presentation. Spasticity probably results from imbalance of the facilitatory and inhibitory centers in the midbrain and brainstem reticular formations, as well as altered balance between the alpha and gamma motor systems in the spinal cord. The reduction in the threshold and exaggeration of the stretch reflexes, an essential aspect of spasticity, may be mediated by the reticulospinal and vestibulospinal rather than the CSTs.

Hemiplegia in man is often produced by combined lesions of the motor and premotor components of the upper motor neuron. Various pathologic responses—such as the Babinski, Chaddock, and Hoffmann signs—appear. The affected extremities may at first be flaccid with depressed reflexes, but spasticity and reflex exaggeration typically develop within a few days. The pathologic reflexes may remain permanently.

CLINICAL MANIFESTATIONS OF DISEASE OF THE CORTICOSPINAL LEVEL

The corticospinal pathways may be involved in diverse disease processes, including vascular disease, neoplasm, degeneration, trauma, and others. The essential manifestations of a CST lesion consist of loss of skilled voluntary movements, or impairment of integration of movements, along with an overactivity of lower segmental centers because of disinhibition. The loss of voluntary movement is accompanied by increased tone in the involved muscles. The paresis from a lesion involving the pyramidal tract tends to involve entire extremities or certain muscle groups. Pyramidal lesions disrupt movements; any muscle that participates in the movement will be weakened, regardless of its specific lower motor neuron innervation. In contrast, lower motor neuron lesions involve muscles innervated by a specific structure, such as a nerve root or peripheral nerve. For instance, a CST lesion causes weakness of external rotation of the shoulder. This movement is carried out by both the infraspinatus and teres minor muscles. The teres minor is innervated by the axillary nerve and the infraspinatus by the suprascapular nerve; both are weakened despite their different segmental innervations.

Pyramidal tract lesions do not cause the sort of severe, early focal muscle atrophy seen in lower motor neuron lesions, but there may be some mild, late atrophy of the involved part because of disuse (see Chapter 29). With lesions that are congenital or occur early in life, the involved limbs may fail to grow normally, resulting in hemiatrophy to varying degrees in adulthood (Figure 25.5). Such hemiatrophy may be difficult to detect; comparing the size of the thumbnails is a traditional technique for detecting subtle hemiatrophy. When atrophy does occur with CST disorders, it usually affects the small muscles of the hand. There are no fasciculations.

Deep tendon (muscle stretch) reflexes—rather than being lost as is the usual case with neurogenic atrophy because of a lower motor neuron lesion—are increased, and clonus may be elicited (see Chapter 38). The superficial reflexes are diminished or absent (see Chapter 39). Various pathologic reflexes, such as the Babinski sign, often termed pyramidal reflexes or upper motor neuron signs, often appear (see Chapter 40). Normal associated movements may be lost, and abnormal associated movements may appear (see Chapter 42). Trophic changes are uncommon, but occasionally, there is edema, desquamation, pigmentary changes, or glossy skin.

A pyramidal tract lesion causes weakness in a characteristic distribution. Facial weakness is limited to the lower face, although occasionally eyelid closure may be slightly weak. Voluntary facial movements are affected more than emotional ones, and movement in response to emotional stimuli may be normal (dissociated facial palsy; Chapter 16). There is slight, if any, detectable involvement of the muscles innervated by the spinal accessory nerve. There may be slight weakness of the affected side of the tongue, but the throat and jaw muscles function normally. Deglutition, articulation, movements of the trunk, and other functions with bilateral supranuclear innervation are little affected. Voluntary, skilled, and learned actions are most impaired, and there is loss of the ability to carry out fine, independent, fractionated movements, especially with the distal portions of the extremities, with precision and delicacy. Gross movements and those that are habitual or have little voluntary control are relatively spared.

The extremity weakness reflects the preferential CST innervation of certain muscle groups and has a characteristic pattern: the pyramidal or corticospinal distribution. When weakness is mild, it may be detectable only in the corticospinal distribution. Distal muscles, especially hand muscles, receive more pyramidal innervation than proximal muscles and are particularly affected. In the upper extremity, weakness preferentially involves the wrist, finger and elbow extensors, supinators, and external rotators and abductors of the shoulder; there is relative sparing of the flexor, pronator, and internal rotation muscles. In the lower extremity, weakness is most marked in the foot and toe dorsiflexors, knee flexors, and flexors and internal rotators of the hip, with relative sparing of the extensors, external rotators, and plantar flexors. When weakness is severe, the stronger, non–CST-innervated muscles overcome the weak muscles, producing the characteristic posture of a spastic hemiplegia. The arm is held in adduction, with internal rotation at the shoulder, flexion and pronation at the elbow, and flexion of the wrist and fingers. Additional flexion may still be carried out, but there is marked weakness of extension. There is loss of isolated movements of the wrist and fingers; movements at the elbow and shoulder are less affected. In the lower extremity, there is weakness of flexion at the hip and knee; the hip is extended, adducted, and often externally rotated, and the knee is extended. There is weakness of the dorsiflexors and everters of the foot, often with a pes equinovarus deformity causing plantar flexion and inversion of the foot and toes.

The spasticity, or increase in tone, is most marked in the flexor and pronator muscles of the upper limb and the extensors of the lower, more apparent with an attempt to extend or supinate the muscles of the upper extremity or flex those of the lower. Passive motion may be carried out with little difficulty if done through a small range of movement, but resistance increases if an attempt is made to move the extremities through a greater range. Slow, passive movement may be carried out with relative ease, but on rapid movement, there is a "blocking" or "catching," often with a waxing followed by a sudden waning of tone at the extremes of the range of motion (clasp-knife phenomenon). Abnormalities of muscle tone are discussed further in Chapter 28.

The paralysis that follows a vascular lesion of the internal capsule provides a common example of the effects of a CST lesion. Examination soon after the event typically reveals flaccid paralysis and areflexia on the opposite side of the body ("cerebral shock") but is soon followed by spasticity and hyperreflexia. When the corticospinal pathways are affected by a spinal cord lesion of sudden onset, especially if bilateral, there may also be a period of flaccidity and areflexia accompanying the paralysis below the level of the lesion. This is the period of "spinal shock," which sooner or later gives way, in most instances, to the corticospinal syndrome. During the neural shock phase, the plantar responses may be mute and the superficial reflexes absent. The pyramidal, or upper motor neuron, syndrome gradually emerges over hours to weeks with spasticity, hyperactive tendon reflexes, extensor plantar responses, and continued absence of superficial reflexes. With spinal cord lesions, there is also impairment of bowel, bladder, and sexual function.

The motor deficit with CST lesions is only occasionally complete. This may be the result of the same, largely unknown, factors and mechanisms responsible for the recovery of function that follows many such lesions. Some muscles may have bilateral innervation, or there may be incomplete decussation in the medulla. The CST receives fibers from regions of the cortex other than the motor strip, and many of the motor centers in the cortex occupy a large area with overlap of the foci of localization. The primary motor cortex is only one portion of the motor system; other cortical and subcortical centers, such as the supplementary and secondary motor cortices, may assume function in the face of disease of the corticospinal system. Sensory factors influence the type and degree of paralysis and the degree of motor recovery; the prognosis for return of function is less optimistic if there is significant sensory loss. In patients with infantile hemiplegia, hemispherectomy done for seizure control may not increase the motor deficit. Removal of normally developed cortex in an adult (e.g., surgical extirpation of a neoplasm) causes a spastic hemiplegia. Yet similar removal in patients who have had a spastic hemiparesis since birth or early childhood causes a transient flaccid deficit that later becomes spastic, and the residual weakness after surgery is no more than before, sometimes less. In such patients, it is likely that either the other hemisphere or some subcortical or cortical structures have previously assumed a portion of the function of the diseased cortex.

With cerebral neoplasms or other pathologic processes affecting the motor cortex, there may be a corticospinal type of paresis, together with recurrent jacksonian convulsions of the involved extremities. A lesion of the pyramidal pathway after it has left the cortex, however, produces only paresis, and convulsions do not occur.

BIBLIOGRAPHY

Davidoff RA. The pyramidal tract. *Neurology* 1990;40:332–339.

Dol JA, Louwerse ES. Images in clinical medicine. Wallerian degeneration of the pyramidal tract on magnetic resonance imaging. *N Engl J Med* 1994;331:88.

Hardy TA, Wang C, Beadnall HN, et al. Wallerian degeneration in the corticospinal tract following tumefactive demyelination: conventional and advanced magnetic resonance imaging. *Can J Neurol Sci* 2016;43:726–727.

Hosokawa S, Tsuji S, Uozumi T, et al. Ipsilateral hemiplegia caused by right internal capsule and thalamic hemorrhage: demonstration of predominant ipsilateral innervation of motor and sensory systems by MRI, MEP, and SEP. *Neurology* 1996;46:1146–1149.

Jagiella WM, Sung JH. Bilateral infarction of the medullary pyramids in humans. *Neurology* 1989;39:21–24.

Kiernan JA, Rajakumar N. *Barr's The Human Nervous System: An Anatomical Viewpoint*. 10th ed. Philadelphia: Wolters Kluwer Health/Lippincott Williams & Wilkins, 2014.

Marti-Fabregas J, Pujol J. Selective involvement of the pyramidal tract on magnetic resonance imaging in primary lateral sclerosis. *Neurology* 1990;40:1799–1800.

Paulson GW, Yates AJ, Paltan-Ortiz JD. Does infarction of the medullary pyramid lead to spasticity? *Arch Neurol* 1986;43:93–95.

Penfield W, Rasmussen T. *The Cerebral Cortex of Man: A Clinical Study of Localization of Function*. New York: Macmillan, 1950.

Powers RK, Marder-Meyer J, Rymer WZ. Quantitative relations between hypertonia and stretch reflex threshold in spastic quadriparesis. *Ann Neurol* 1988;23:115–124.

Pryse-Phillips W. *Companion to Clinical Neurology*. 3rd ed. Oxford: Oxford University Press, 2009.

Ropper AH, Fisher CM, Kleinman GM. Pyramidal infarction in the medulla: a cause of pure motor hemiplegia sparing the face. *Neurology* 1979;26:91–95.

Standring S, ed. *Gray's Anatomy: The Anatomical Basis of Clinical Practice*. 41st ed. New York: Elsevier Limited, 2016.

Terakawa H, Abe K, Nakamura M, et al. Ipsilateral hemiparesis after putaminal hemorrhage due to uncrossed pyramidal tract. *Neurology* 2000;54:1801–1805.

Welniarz Q, Dusart I, Roze E. The corticospinal tract: evolution, development, and human disorders. *Dev Neurobiol* 2017;77:810–829.

Wiesendanger M. Pyramidal tract function and the clinical "pyramidal syndrome." *Human Neurobiol* 1984;2:227.

Yagishita A, Nakano I, Oda M. Location of the corticospinal tract in the internal capsule at MR imaging. *Radiology* 1994;191:455–460.

CHAPTER 26

The Extrapyramidal Level

The extrapyramidal system is more of a functional concept—derived primarily from the study of patients with neurologic disease—than an anatomic or physiologic entity. Patients with disease of the extrapyramidal system have disorders that involve the motor system, but the clinical phenomenology is distinctly different from the weakness, spasticity, and hyperreflexia that mark the pyramidal syndrome. The term extrapyramidal was first used by Wilson in describing hepatolenticular degeneration (Wilson's disease). Wilson's patients had a type of motor disturbance with different clinical characteristics than seen with pyramidal system disease, which was associated with lesions in the basal ganglia (BG). Because the principal component of the extrapyramidal motor system is the BG, the term extrapyramidal came to be used to refer to the BG and their connections. Extrapyramidal disorders cause a category of neurologic illness now more often referred to as movement disorders. Such conditions may produce excessive movement (e.g., Huntington's chorea), a poverty of movement (e.g., Parkinson's disease), or a disturbance of posture, tone, righting reflexes, or other manifestations.

The extrapyramidal system is phylogenetically old. Much of its function arises through modulation of the pyramidal system rather than by direct projections to the spinal cord. The extrapyramidal system can be looked at as a neural network that influences motor control. It is not directly concerned with the production of voluntary movement but is closely integrated with other levels of the motor system to modulate and regulate the motor activity that is carried out by way of the pyramidal system.

ANATOMY AND PHYSIOLOGY

Anatomists disagree as to what should be properly included in the extrapyramidal system and even whether it should be recognized as an entity. They speak of "nonpyramidal corticofugal systems" but are loath to discuss the "extrapyramidal system." Many decry the continued use of the expression, and the term does not even appear in many major neuroanatomy textbooks. There are other important nonpyramidal motor systems that are not related to the BG. Other nonpyramidal, nonbasal ganglia pathways include the rubrospinal, vestibulospinal, olivospinal, and reticulospinal tracts. The pyramidal system is the final effector because the extrapyramidal system serves to modulate the activity of the pyramidal system and does not itself project to the spinal cord. Despite these limitations, the concept of an extrapyramidal level continues to be clinically useful. Although the cerebellum is a nonpyramidal motor system, it is not considered part of the extrapyramidal system.

As mentioned in Chapter 2, BG nomenclature is not used consistently. The BG that contribute most extensively to the extrapyramidal system and are most important for clinical purposes include the caudate, putamen, globus pallidus (GP), substantia nigra (SN), and subthalamic nucleus (STN). In addition to the motor circuits controlling voluntary movement, the BG have limbic connections involved with the emotional aspects of movement, as well as connections with the oculomotor system. They also play a role in cognition.

The caudate and putamen are frequently referred to as the striatum, in contrast to the GP, or pallidum. Sometimes, all three are included as parts of the striatum, with the caudate- and putamen-labeled neostriatum and the GP-labeled paleo- (less often archi-) striatum. The terms striatum and corpus striatum are sometimes used synonymously; at other times, a distinction is drawn between the striatum as caudate and putamen (or caudatoputamen) and the corpus striatum as caudate, putamen, and GP. For purposes of this discussion, striatum refers to the neostriatum, the caudate and putamen. Some authorities include other gray matter masses that lie at the base of the brain as part of the BG, including the substantia innominata, nucleus accumbens, claustrum, amygdala, anterior perforated substance, and olfactory tubercle. Most of these are not functionally related to the BG motor system and are usually not considered parts of the extrapyramidal system for clinical purposes. There is a dorsal striatum, or dorsal division of the striatum, and a smaller ventral striatum, or ventral division. The dorsal striatum is the caudate and putamen; the ventral striatum consists of the nucleus accumbens and the anterior portion of the anterior perforated substance and olfactory tubercle. The connections of the ventral striatum are predominantly with the limbic system. Similarly, there is a dorsal pallidum (the GP proper) and a ventral pallidum (the posterior portion of the anterior perforated substance). For clinical purposes, neither the ventral striatum nor the ventral pallidum plays a significant role in voluntary motor function.

The caudate nucleus lies deep in the substance of the cerebral hemisphere between the lateral ventricle and the insula (Figure 26.1). The head of the caudate nucleus is a pear-shaped mass of gray matter that bulges into the lateral aspect of the frontal horn of the lateral ventricle; its tail runs backward in the floor of the ventricle and then downward and forward in the roof of the temporal horn. The tail of the caudate abuts but remains separate from the amygdala. The sulcus terminalis is a groove that separates the caudate nucleus from the thalamus; it contains the stria terminalis and the thalamostriate vein. The lenticular, or lentiform, nucleus is composed of the putamen and GP, with the putamen forming the most lateral

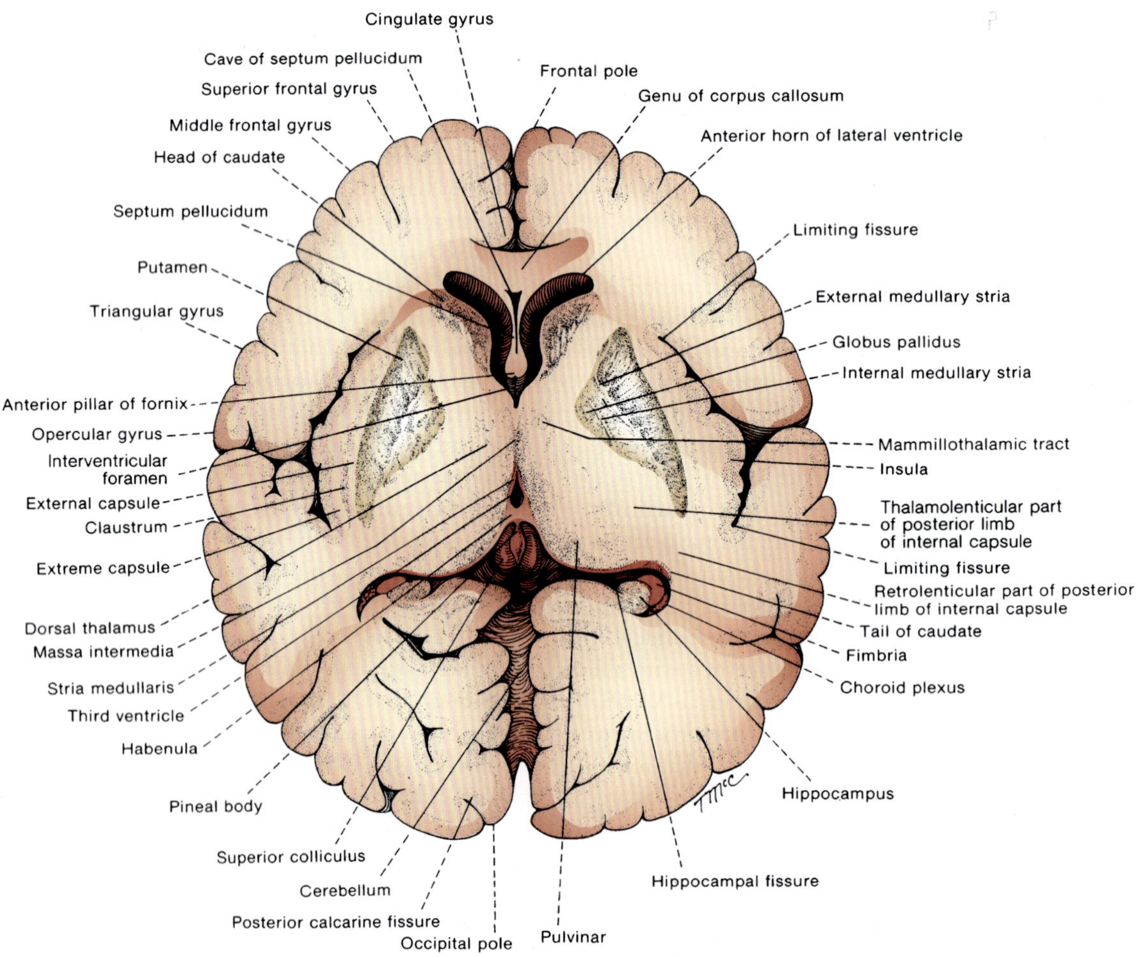

FIGURE 26.1 Drawing of the superior surface of an unstained horizontal section of the adult human brain, through the internal capsule, basal ganglia (BG), and thalamus.

part of the lentiform complex and the GP the medial part. The claustrum is an island of gray matter in the subcortical white matter of the insula. The putamen is separated from the insula by, in order, the external capsule, claustrum, and extreme capsule.

The internal capsule thrusts itself squarely through the region of the BG, vastly complicating its anatomy and connections. Important components of the BG and extrapyramidal system lie separated on opposite sides of the capsule. The putamen and GP are lateral to it; the caudate, thalamus, STN, and SN lie medial. All efferent and many afferent connections of the BG are made with the diencephalon and midbrain, which are separated from the BG by the internal capsule and crus cerebri. The caudate and putamen are cytologically and functionally nearly identical, but the anterior limb of the internal capsule separates one from the other. Fibers of the internal capsule and crus cerebri also separate the SN from the GP, which are functionally closely related.

The caudate nucleus and putamen are semicontinuous, separated by the streaming fibers of the anterior limb of the internal capsule (Figure 26.1). The alternating gray and white strands led to the name striatum (striped). Bundles of finely myelinated, small-diameter fibers ("Wilson's pencils") crossing the striatum toward the GP also contribute to the marbled appearance. Inferiorly, just above the anterior perforated substance, the head of the caudate fuses with the inferior part of the putamen and is continuous medially with the nucleus accumbens. Histologically, the caudate and putamen are identical; they have a common embryologic origin. They contain a few large and many small neurons, with the small cells predominating by 20:1. Dendrites may be spiny or aspiny. The most common cell type in the striatum is small and spiny and contains gamma-amino butyric acid (GABA), plus enkephalin (ENK), dynorphin, or substance P (SP). The small, spiny neurons are the primary source of striatal efferents. The small, aspiny neurons are cholinergic.

The microstructure of the striatum consists of a matrix of cells that stain histochemically for acetylcholine (ACh), with patches or islands of cells that contain other neurotransmitters. The islands are referred to as striosomes, and the striatum is a mosaic arrangement of islands or patches of striosomes lying in the matrix of cholinergic cells. The striosomes primarily contain SP and ENK. The ENKergic neurons have D2 dopamine receptors; SP neurons have D1 receptors. In the caudate, striosomes have a higher concentration of dopamine compared to the matrix. The striosome-matrix pattern is not as evident in the putamen, which consists mostly of matrix, or in the ventral striatum, which consists mostly of striosomes. The cholinergic neurons of the matrix are facilitatory to the projection neurons and are inhibited by dopamine.

The GP is medial to the putamen, just lateral to the third ventricle. An external medullary lamina separates the GP from the putamen. Internally, the GP is divided by an internal medullary lamina into a lateral, or external, zone (the globus pallidus externa, GPe); and a medial, or internal, zone (the globus pallidus interna, GPi). The GP contains only about 5% as many cells as the striatum, and all are large neurons. Neurons throughout the GP use primarily GABA as a neurotransmitter, less often ACh. The associated neuropeptide is SP in the GPi and ENK in the GPe.

The SN is a gray mass that lies in the cerebral peduncle between the crus cerebri and the tegmentum of the midbrain at the level of the superior colliculi. The SN is composed of two parts: the deep pars or zona compacta (SNc), which contains the large, melanin-containing, dopaminergic neurons that give the structure its name; and the more superficial zona reticulata (SNr), which contains large, multipolar, nonpigmented, GABAergic neurons similar to those in the GP. The SNr is closely related functionally to—essentially a midbrain extension of—the GPi; they are separated only by fibers of the internal capsule and crus cerebri, and both are involved in BG efferent functions. The SNr receives afferents through the striatonigral comb system or comb bundle, which crosses through the crus cerebri obliquely. The STN (corpus Luysii) is a small, lens-shaped gray mass situated in the ventral thalamic region just dorsal and medial to the cerebral peduncle (Figure 26.2).

Other important structures involved in the extrapyramidal motor control system include the thalamus, red nucleus (RN), the brainstem reticular formation (RF), the inferior olivary nucleus in the medulla, the zona incerta (ZI), the vestibular nuclei, the pedunculopontine nucleus (PPN), and the gray matter of the quadrigeminal plate. Several thalamic nuclei are involved, and these are sometimes referred to as the motor thalamus, including the nucleus ventralis lateralis (VL), pars oralis (VLo); ventralis lateralis, pars caudalis (VLc); ventralis posterior lateralis, pars oralis (VPLo); and portions of ventralis anterior

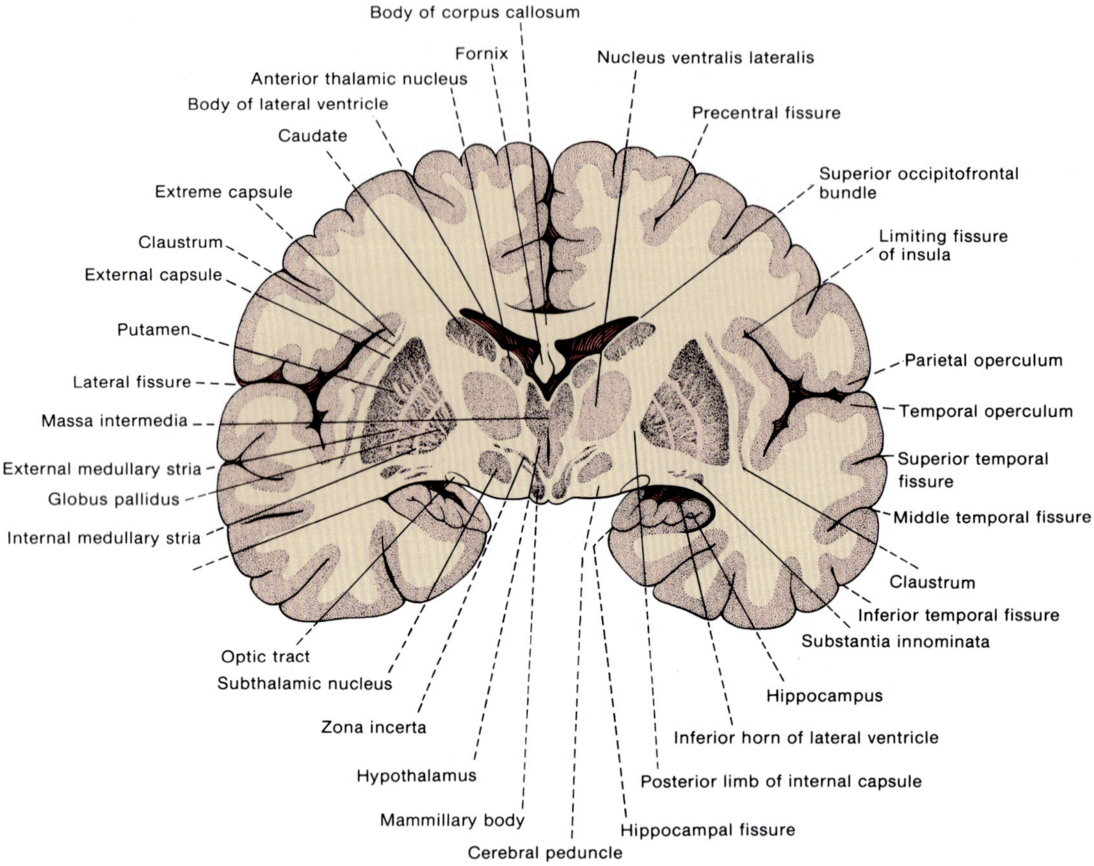

FIGURE 26.2 Drawing of the posterior surface of an unstained coronal section of the adult human brain, through the posterior limb of the internal capsule, BG, and mammillary bodies.

(VA). The RN is located in the tegmentum of the midbrain at the level of the superior colliculi. It has magnocellular (large-celled) and parvocellular (small-celled) portions. The caudal magnocellular part gives rise to the rubrospinal tract and the parvocellular part to the central tegmental tract. The lateral and medial nuclear groups of the RF are situated in the tegmentum of the midbrain, and other constituents of the RF that either inhibit or facilitate motor responses are placed caudally in the brainstem. The PPN is a cholinergic nucleus that lies caudal to the SN in the brainstem tegmentum, partially buried in the superior cerebellar peduncle. It receives afferents primarily from GPi/SNr and sends cholinergic projections to the dopaminergic neurons in the SNc. It may be involved in locomotion. Patients with Parkinson's disease have significant loss of PPN neurons, and dysfunction of the PPN may be important in the pathophysiology of the locomotor and postural disturbances of parkinsonism.

The BG have rich connections with one another and with brainstem structures, as well as with the cerebral cortex and with lower centers (Figure 26.3). The area of the cortex involved is the motor cortex, which includes the precentral motor regions including the supplementary and premotor areas. In essence, the cerebral cortex projects to the striatum, which in turn projects to the GP and SNr; efferents go to the thalamus, which then projects back to cerebral cortex, primarily to the motor areas. Table 26.1 summarizes some of the major connections.

Striatal Afferents

The striatum receives topographically organized glutaminergic axons that originate from small pyramidal cells in layers V and VI of the entire ipsilateral neocortex. The striatum also receives afferents from the thalamus. These connections provide the striatum with sensory and cognitive inputs. The head of the caudate

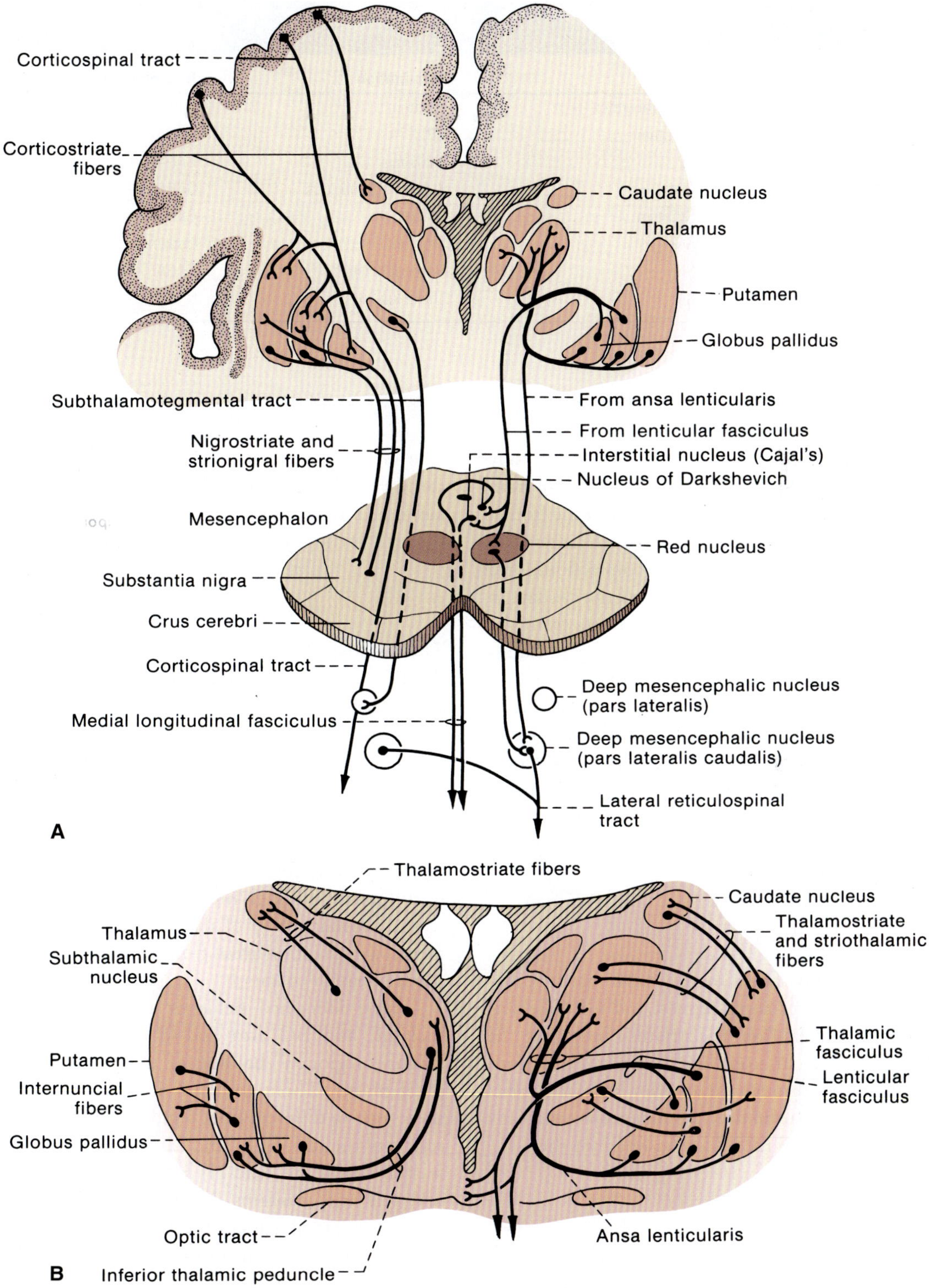

FIGURE 26.3 **A.** Principal connections of the BG. The thalamocortical portions of the loops (cortex-BG-thalamus-cortex) are omitted. **B.** Detail giving connections between the BG and thalamus.

TABLE 26.1 Major Basal Ganglia Pathways

Tract	Origin	Termination	Neurotransmitter
Corticostriate	Cerebral cortex	Striatum*	Glutamate
Striatopallidal	Striatum	GP	GABA
Pallidothalamic†	GP	Thalamus	GABA
Pallidosubthalamic‡	GPe	Subthalamic nucleus	GABA
Striatonigral	Striatum	SN	GABA
Nigrostriatal	SNc	Striatum	Dopamine
Nigrotectal	SNr	Superior colliculus	GABA
Nigrothalamic	SNr	Thalamus	GABA

*The dorsal striatum, the caudate, and putamen.
†Via the fasciculus and ansa lenticularis.
‡Via the subthalamic fasciculus.
GABA, gamma-amino butyric acid; GP, globus pallidus; SN, substantia nigra; SNc, pars compacta; SNr, pars reticulata.

receives projections from the frontal lobe, the body from the parietal and occipital lobes, and the tail from the temporal lobe. The massive input from the frontal lobe to the head is the reason it is so much larger than the remainder of the nucleus. These connections form the anatomical substrate for the role of the caudate in cognition. The caudate also receives fibers from the dorsomedial (DM) and VA nuclei of the thalamus (thalamostriate fibers) and from the putamen.

The connections of the putamen are more focused; it receives fibers from cortical areas 4 and 6 and from the parietal lobe, the perirolandic motor centers, which are essentially the same areas that give rise to the corticospinal tract. It has a large connection with the caudate. It also receives fibers from the SN by the comb bundle.

Striatal Efferents

The caudate sends fibers to the thalamus (striothalamic fibers) and to the putamen and GP. The primary efferent fibers from the striatum project to the GP and SN. The striatopallidal fibers from the caudate run directly through the anterior limb of internal capsule, and those from the putamen project medially through the external medullary lamina into the GP.

Pallidal Afferents

The principal afferents to the GP are from the caudate and putamen. The STN also sends fibers to the GP in the subthalamic fasciculus; some pass through the internal capsule into the medial segment of the GP; some cross in the supraoptic commissure (of Gudden). There are also fibers from the SNc to the GP. The GP also receives impulses from DM and VA, through thalamostriate fibers in the inferior thalamic peduncle, and from area 6 and possibly area 4 through corticospinal collaterals.

Pallidal Efferents

The pallidal efferents are the principal outflow of the BG. There are four major bundles: (a) the fasciculus lenticularis; (b) the ansa lenticularis; (c) pallidotegmental fibers, which arise from GPi; and (d) pallidosubthalamic fibers, which arise from GPe. Pallidofugal fibers are often discussed in terms of their relationships to the “fields of Forel.” August Forel performed some of the early anatomical studies of the BG and subthalamic region using degeneration techniques. (Although his name is inextricably linked to the neuroanatomy of the subthalamic region, his principal reputation arises from seminal studies of the social behavior of ants.)

Forel identified fields or regions in the subthalamic and BG area and labeled them “H” for “Haubenregionen” because of their resemblance to a hat plume. There are Forel fields H, H_1, and H_2; these refer to different fiber bundles that course in the region of the RN, STN, and ZI. The prerubral or tegmental field (Forel field H) lies just rostral to the RN and primarily contains dentatothalamic fibers from the contralateral superior cerebellar peduncle and rubrothalamic fibers from the ipsilateral RN ascending toward the thalamus through the subthalamic region. The dentatothalamic and rubrothalamic fibers form a capsule around the RN; the portion of this capsule just rostral to the RN is the prerubral field. Pallidofugal fibers stream into the prerubral field and then turn upward. As these fibers ascend toward the thalamus, the prerubral field divides into dorsal and ventral lamina; the dorsal division consists of the lenticular fasciculus (Forel field H_2), and the ventral division is the thalamic fasciculus (Forel field H_1).

Both the ansa and fasciculus lenticularis have the same origin, GPi, and the same destination, the thalamus; the difference is that the fasciculus penetrates through, and the ansa curves around, the internal capsule. Both pass through field H, and both join with the thalamic fasciculus. The fasciculus lenticularis emerges from the dorsal surface of GPi and then pierces the internal capsule to lie just above the STN and below the ZI. The ansa lenticularis emerges from the ventral surface of GPi, runs ventromedially to loop around the posterior limb of the internal capsule, and then enters the prerubral field. After traversing the internal capsule, the fasciculus lenticularis joins the ansa lenticularis at the medial border of the ZI; both then enter the thalamic fasciculus just above the ZI.

The thalamic fasciculus (Forel field H_1) is a complex bundle that lies just dorsal to the ZI. It carries pallidofugal fibers as well as rubrothalamic and dentatothalamic fibers. The thalamic fasciculus enters the rostral ventral tier of thalamic nuclei, primarily VL and VA. Some pallidofugal fibers separate from the thalamic fasciculus and enter the centromedian thalamic nucleus. The dentatothalamic fibers in the thalamic fasciculus are destined primarily for VL, but some enter the intralaminar nuclei. The VL is involved in integration and coordination of BG and cerebellar function. The VL in turn projects to area 4 of the motor cortex. The point where the thalamic fasciculus converges on VL is of singular strategic importance in the function of the motor system.

Subthalamic Nucleus

The STN is reciprocally connected with the GP via the subthalamic fasciculus, a bundle that runs directly through the internal capsule. The connection to the STN is the only pallidal efferent to arise from GPe; all others come from GPi. The STN sends fibers back to GPe, as well as to GPi, through the subthalamic fasciculus.

Substantia Nigra

The SN extends from the pons to the subthalamic region and makes up the primary dopaminergic cell population of the midbrain; cholinergic cells are also present. The SNc of one side is continuous across the midline with the SNc of the opposite side. Cells of the SNc contain neuromelanin, a by-product of dopamine synthesis. The striatonigral afferents from the striatum use GABA and either SP or ENK as transmitters. The SNr receives strionigral fibers from the striatum, GP, and STN. The primary efferents from the SN are to the striatum, midbrain tectum, and thalamus (Table 26.1). The SNr is functionally related to the GPi; its efferents are GABAergic. Dopaminergic nigrostriatal fibers from SNc project to the striatum. The nigrothalamic tract runs to VA and DM. The nigrotectal tract connects the SN with the ipsilateral superior colliculus and may be involved in the control of eye movements. There are also connections between the SN and the PPN and RF.

BASAL GANGLIA PHYSIOLOGY

The connections of the motor system are complex (Figure 22.2). There are two major loops: the BG and the cerebellar. The essential connections in the BG loop are cortex → striatum → globus pallidus → thalamus → cortex. The projections of the thalamus, cortex, and STN are excitatory; the outputs of the striatum and pallidum are primarily inhibitory. The projections from the cortex to the striatum and from the thalamus to the cortex are both excitatory (glutaminergic). The pathway from the striatum to the thalamus may be either excitatory or inhibitory depending on the route. Current models of BG function include a direct and an indirect loop or pathway for the connection between the striatum and thalamus (Box 26.1). In brief, the direct loop is excitatory and the indirect loop is inhibitory. The indirect loop brings in GPe and STN, which are not involved in the direct pathway (Figure 26.4). The caudate, putamen, and STN make up the BG input nuclei; the GPi and SNr are the output nuclei. The input and output nuclei are connected by the direct and indirect loops. In essence, the output nuclei, GPi and SNr, tonically inhibit the motor thalamus; the input nuclei either facilitate cortical motor activity by disinhibiting the thalamus or inhibit motor activity by increasing thalamic inhibition. The direct pathway serves to facilitate cortical excitation and carry out voluntary movement. The indirect pathway serves to inhibit cortical excitation and prevent unwanted movement. Disease of the direct pathway produces hypokinesia, for example, parkinsonism; disease of the indirect

BOX 26.1

Direct and Indirect Pathways

As an overview, the direct pathway is mediated by D1 dopamine receptors and results in a facilitation of movement; the indirect pathway is mediated by D2 receptors and results in an inhibition of movement. In the direct pathway, the motor cortex sends glutaminergic-activating signals to the caudate and putamen and excites D1 receptors. Striopallidal fibers to the globus pallidus interna (GPi) and superficial zona reticulata (SNr) are inhibitory (GABAergic); fibers from the GPi to the thalamus are also inhibitory (GABAergic). At rest, GPi/SNr exert in inhibitory influence on the thalamus, which decreases the excitatory influence of the thalamus on the cortex. Activation of the direct pathway inhibits the activity of GPi/SNr. The direct loop projections from the striatum to GPi inhibit the inhibitory pallidothalamic pathway and result in net cortical excitation and facilitation. The direct loop excites the thalamic projections to the cortex by inhibiting the pallidothalamic pathway.

In the indirect pathway, the motor cortex sends glutaminergic-activating signals to the caudate and putamen and excites D2 receptors. Striopallidal fibers then project to the globus pallidus externa (GPe), causing inhibition (GABAergic). The resting activity of GPe decreases. The GPe projects inhibitory GABAergic fibers to the subthalamic nucleus (STN) by the subthalamic fasciculus. The STN then projects to the GPi, but its fibers are excitatory (glutaminergic). Indirect pathway activity reduces the inhibition of the STN. The STN then facilitates the inhibitory projection of the GPi to the thalamus, resulting in a net decrease in activity in the thalamocortical pathways. The indirect loop inhibits the thalamic projections to the cortex by increasing the inhibition mediated by the pallidothalamic projection. Activity in the indirect loop prevents activation of motor cortical areas that might interfere with the voluntary movement executed by the direct pathway.

Activity in the direct loop results in a net increase in cortical excitation; activity in the indirect loop results in a net decrease. When cortical excitation is at a normal level, voluntary movements are normal. When there is a pathologic net decrease in cortical activation because of disease involving the direct pathway, voluntary movements are inhibited; this causes hypokinetic movement disorders, such as Parkinson's disease. When there is a pathologic net increase in cortical activation because of disease involving the indirect pathway, movements are augmented; this causes hyperkinetic movement disorders, such as chorea. The final common result in Parkinson's disease is an increase in the firing rate of the GPi, resulting in a suppression of activity in the thalamocortical circuits (the GPi rate theory).

The direct and indirect pathway model and GPi rate theory fail to explain some features of movement disorders, for example, the hyperkinetic component, tremor, in a disease primarily producing hypokinesia. It fails to explain some of the effects of deep brain stimulation in Parkinson's disease or the efficacy of anticholinergic agents. Various authors have proposed refinements, modifications, and alternatives, including the bursting neurons theory, synchronization theory, prokinetic/antikinetic oscillators theory, and the systems oscillators theory. Changes in GPi firing patterns rather than simply the overall firing rate as emphasized in traditional wiring diagrams of the basal ganglia may explain many disease features not well accounted for by the GPi rate theory.

pathway produces hyperkinesias, for example, chorea or hemiballismus.

The SNc projects dopaminergic fibers to the striatum, causing excitation or inhibition depending on the receptor. There are five subtypes of dopamine receptor, D1 through D5. The D1 and D2 receptors are the primary ones involved in regulating movement. The dopamine effect on the D1 family of receptors is excitatory; the effect on D2 receptors is inhibitory. The direct loop is routed through the D1 receptors and the indirect loop through the D2 receptors. Dopamine excitation of D1 receptors increases the inhibitory effect of the striatum on the GPi/SNr through the direct pathway, which results in a decrease of the inhibitory effect of GPi/SNr on the thalamus and a net increase in thalamocortical excitation. The net effect of dopamine on the D1 receptor is to facilitate the direct loop and increase

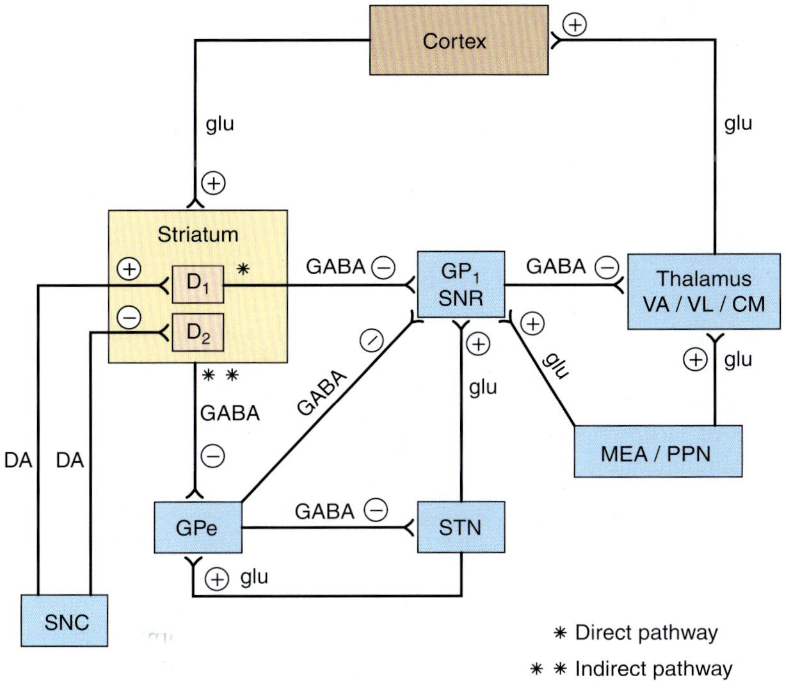

FIGURE 26.4 The direct and indirect BG loops. The indirect loop includes the GPe and subthalamic nucleus. The direct loop results in excitation of the thalamus and cortex, the indirect loop in inhibition. +, excitatory; –, inhibitory; CM, centromedian thalamic nucleus; D1, D1 dopamine receptor; D2, D2 dopamine receptor; DA, dopamine; GABA, gamma-amino butyric acid; glu, glutamic acid; GPe, globus pallidus externa; GPi, globus pallidus interna; MEA, midbrain extrapyramidal area; PPN, pedunculopontine nucleus; SNc, substantia nigra, compacta; SNr, substantia nigra, reticulata; STN, subthalamic nucleus; VA, ventral anterior thalamic nucleus; VL, ventral-lateral thalamic nucleus.

thalamocortical excitation. Dopamine inhibition of D2 receptors decreases the inhibitory effect of the striatum on the GPe through the indirect pathway, which results in a decrease of the inhibitory effect of GPe on STN. The disinhibition of STN causes an increase in its ability to excite GPi/SNr, increasing the inhibitory output of GPi/SNr and causing a net decrease in thalamocortical excitation. The net result is that the nigrostriatal system facilitates activity in the direct loop, which increases thalamocortical excitation and inhibits activity in the inhibitory indirect loop, which also increases thalamocortical excitation. When there is dopamine deficiency, cortical activation is decreased both because of decreased facilitation through the excitatory direct loop and lack of inhibition of the inhibitory indirect loop.

The inhibitory effect of the BG output neurons affects not only the motor thalamus but the midbrain extrapyramidal areas as well. The effects have been likened to a brake. Increased braking through increased activity from GPi/SNr inhibits motor pattern generators in the cerebral cortex and brainstem; decreased GPi/SNr activity decreases the braking and results in a net facilitation of cortical and brainstem motor activity. The STN increases the braking, whereas the striatum decreases it. The striatal input to GPi/SNr is organized to provide a specific, focused inhibition (unbraking) in order to selectively facilitate desired movements, whereas the input from the STN causes a more global excitation of GPi/SNr (braking), perhaps to inhibit potentially competing movements.

BASAL GANGLIA PATHOPHYSIOLOGY

Hypokinetic movement disorders, such as parkinsonism, are thought to result from an increase of the normal inhibitory effects of the BG output neurons. Hyperkinetic movement disorders—such as chorea, hemiballismus, and dystonia—presumably result from a reduction in the normal inhibition.

The most common hypokinetic movement disorder is Parkinson's disease. Pathologically, there is loss of the pigmented cells in the SNc, as well as loss of other pigmented cells in the central nervous system, such as the locus coeruleus. The SNc cells are the origin of the nigrostriatal dopaminergic pathway. Loss of dopamine input to the striatum decreases thalamocortical activation by effects mediated by both D1 and D2 receptors. There is decreased activity in the direct loop, mediated by the D1 receptor, causing loss of striatal inhibition of GPi/SNr and increased inhibition of the motor thalamus, resulting in decreased cortical activation. There is also decreased inhibition of the indirect loop, mediated by the D2 receptor. The STN is released from the inhibitory control of

GPe, which causes increased activity of the STN; this in turn increases the inhibitory effects of GPi/SNr. Both of these effects decrease the thalamic drive to the motor cortex, causing hypokinesia and bradykinesia. There is a net increase in activity through the indirect over the direct pathway, resulting in a net hyperactivity of GPi/SNr and subsequent inhibition or braking of the thalamocortical circuits.

In hyperkinetic movement disorders, the inhibition of the motor thalamus by the GPi/SNr is impaired. Hemiballismus results from a lesion of the contralateral STN, usually infarction. The damage to the STN removes its normal facilitation of the inhibitory effects of GPi/SNr. The loss of facilitation of GPi/SNr output (less braking) disinhibits the motor thalamus and the cortex, resulting in hyperkinetic movements of the involved extremities. In Huntington's disease, there is loss of ENKergic spiny neurons in the striatum, which project primarily to GPe. Loss of these neurons removes inhibition from GPe, the effect of which is to profoundly inhibit STN, incapacitating it. As with hemiballismus, without STN input, GPi/SNr inhibition of the motor thalamus decreases, releasing the brake, disinhibiting VL, and causing increased thalamocortical activity and hyperkinesis. Experimentally, chorea can be produced by lesioning STN, disinhibition of GPe, or the administration of dopaminergic agents.

OTHER BASAL GANGLIA FUNCTIONS

In addition to its functions in the regulation of voluntary movement, the BG also have connections involved in cognition, emotion, and oculomotor control. The BG have links to parts of the brain involved in behavior, memory, attention, and reward processes. In the motor loop, cortical projections are to the putamen; in the other loops, cortical projections are to the caudate. In the cognitive loop, projections from the frontal lobe to the caudate travel via the GP to the VA and DM thalamic nuclei, which then send fibers back to the frontal lobe. The cognitive connections of the BG are important in learning new motor tasks. The limbic loop originates in the orbitofrontal and anterior cingulate cortex and travels via the ventral striatum, particularly the nucleus accumbens, to the ventral pallidum, and then to DM, which projects back to the cortex. The limbic loop may be involved in the motor expressions of emotion. The oculomotor loop originates in the cortical eye movement control areas, including the frontal eye fields and posterior parietal cortex, and projects to the caudate and then to both the SNr and the superior colliculus. Impulses from SNr are routed via VA and DM back to the cortex. The oculomotor loop is involved in the control of saccadic eye movements.

BIBLIOGRAPHY

Afifi AK. Basal ganglia: functional anatomy and physiology. Part 1. *J Child Neurol* 1994a;9:249–260.

Afifi AK. Basal ganglia: functional anatomy and physiology. Part 2. *J Child Neurol* 1994b;9:352–361.

Afifi AK. The basal ganglia: a neural network with more than motor function. *Semin Pediatr Neurol* 2003;10:3–10.

Albin RL, Young AB, Penney JB. The functional anatomy of basal ganglia disorders. *Trends Neurosci* 1989;12:366–375.

Bronstein JM, Tagliati M, Alterman RL, et al. Deep brain stimulation for Parkinson disease: an expert consensus and review of key issues. *Arch Neurol* 2011;68:165.

DeLong MR, Wichmann T. Circuits and circuit disorders of the basal ganglia. *Arch Neurol* 2007;64:20–24.

DeLong M, Wichmann T. Update on models of basal ganglia function and dysfunction. *Parkinsonism Relat Disord* 2009; 15(Suppl 3):S237–S240.

FitzGerald MJT, Folan-Curran J. *Clinical Neuroanatomy and Related Neuroscience*. 4th ed. Edinburgh: W. B. Saunders, 2002.

Gilman S, Newman SW. *Manter and Gatz's Essentials of Clinical Neuroanatomy and Neurophysiology*. 10th ed. Philadelphia: FA Davis, 2003.

Gould DJ, Fix JD. *Neuroanatomy*. 5th ed. Philadelphia: Wolters Kluwer Health/Lippincott Williams & Wilkins, 2014.

Herrero MT, Barcia C, Navarro JM. Functional anatomy of thalamus and basal ganglia. *Childs Nerv Syst* 2002;18:386–404.

Holt DJ, Graybiel AM, Saper CB. Neurochemical architecture of the human striatum. *J Comp Neurol* 1997;384:1–25.

Kiernan JA, Rajakumar N. *Barr's The Human Nervous System: An Anatomical Viewpoint*. 10th ed. Philadelphia: Wolters Kluwer Health/Lippincott Williams & Wilkins, 2014.

Kingsley RE. *Concise Text of Neuroscience*. 2nd ed. Philadelphia: Lippincott Williams & Wilkins, 2000.

Kopell BH, Rezai AR, Chang JW, et al. Anatomy and physiology of the basal ganglia: implications for deep brain stimulation for Parkinson's disease. *Mov Disord* 2006;21(Suppl 14):S238–S246.

Koprich JB, Johnston TH, Huot P, et al. New insights into the organization of the basal ganglia. *Curr Neurol Neurosci Rep* 2009;9:298–304.

Lozano AM, Snyder BJ, Hamani C, et al. Basal ganglia physiology and deep brain stimulation. *Mov Disord* 2010;25 Suppl 1:S71–S75.

Mink JW. The basal ganglia and involuntary movements: impaired inhibition of competing motor patterns. *Arch Neurol* 2003;60: 1365–1368.

Montgomery EB Jr. Basal ganglia physiology and pathophysiology: a reappraisal. *Parkinsonism Relat Disord* 2007;13:455–465.

Obeso JA, Rodriguez-Oroz MC, Benitez-Temino B, et al. Functional organization of the basal ganglia: therapeutic implications for Parkinson's disease. *Mov Disord* 2008;23(Suppl 3): S548–S559.

Pahapill PA, Lozano AM. The pedunculopontine nucleus and Parkinson's disease. *Brain* 2000;123(Pt 9):1767–1783.

Parent A, Hazrati LN. Functional anatomy of the basal ganglia. I. The cortico-basal ganglia-thalamo-cortical loop. *Brain Res Brain Res Rev* 1995a;20:91–127.

Parent A, Hazrati LN. Functional anatomy of the basal ganglia. II. The place of subthalamic nucleus and external pallidum in basal ganglia circuitry. *Brain Res Brain Res Rev* 1995b;20:128–154.

Pollack AE. Anatomy, physiology, and pharmacology of the basal ganglia. *Neurol Clin* 2001;19:523–534.

Postuma RB, Land AE. Hemiballism: revisiting a classic disorder. *Lancet Neurol* 2003;2:661–668.

Pryse-Phillips W. *Companion to Clinical Neurology*. 3rd ed. Oxford: Oxford University Press, 2009.

Ring HA, Serra-Mestres J. Neuropsychiatry of the basal ganglia. *J Neurol Neurosurg Psychiatry* 2002;72:12–21.

Ropper AH, Samuels MA, Klein J. *Adams and Victor's Principles of Neurology*. 10th ed. New York: McGraw-Hill Education Medical, 2014.

Standring S, ed. *Gray's Anatomy: The Anatomical Basis of Clinical Practice*. 41st ed. New York: Elsevier Limited, 2016.

Welniarz Q, Dusart I, Roze E. The corticospinal tract: evolution, development, and human disorders. *Dev Neurobiol* 2017;77:810–829.

Wilson SAK. Progressive lenticular degeneration. A familial nervous disease associated with cirrhosis of the liver. *Brain* 1912; 34:295.

CHAPTER 27

Motor Strength and Power

Motor strength and power indicate the capacity of muscles to exert force and expend energy. Decreased strength is weakness, or paresis; absence of muscle contraction is paralysis, or plegia. Weakness may cause loss of the speed, rapidity, or agility of movement and a decrease in the range, or amplitude, of movement before there is loss of power to formal strength testing. Other manifestations of impaired motor function include fatigability, variation in strength on repeated tests, diminished range and rate of movement, loss of coordination, irregularity and clumsiness of motion, tremulousness, loss of associated movements, and lack of ability to carry out skilled acts.

Although judgment of the force exerted in either initiating or resisting movement is the major criterion in the evaluation of strength, observation and palpation of either the contraction of the muscle belly or its movement of its tendon may be helpful adjuncts. The contraction of an extremely weak muscle may sometimes be felt when it cannot be seen. In nonorganic weakness, contraction of the apparently weak muscle may be felt when the patient is asked to carry out movements with synergistic muscles (cocontraction sign), or the antagonists may be felt to contract when the patient is asked to contract the weak muscle. Weakness may be masked when attempts to contract individual weak muscles are accompanied by activation of other muscles to compensate for the loss of power. In these substitution, or "trick," movements, the patient exploits a strong muscle with similar function to compensate for the loss of action of a weak muscle. Careful observation for alterations in normal movement patterns and substitution movements may indicate loss of function. Endurance is the ability to perform the same act repeatedly. Loss of endurance, or abnormal fatigability, may occur in myasthenia gravis. Conversely, a patient with Lambert-Eaton myasthenic syndrome may grow transiently stronger with successive contractions.

For clinical purposes, it is usually possible to evaluate muscle strength adequately without resorting to special equipment. Although the subjective impression of the examiner is usually adequate, it is at best semiquantitative and varies with the experience and ability of the examiner. There is a subjective element, with significant interexaminer and intraexaminer variability. When more quantitative determinations are necessary, various dynamometers, myometers, and ergometers are available.

The strength examination assesses primarily voluntary, or active, muscle contraction rather than reflex contraction. Strength may be classified as kinetic (the force exerted in changing position) and static (the force exerted in resisting movement from a fixed position). Strength may be tested in two ways. The patient may place a joint in a certain position, and then the examiner tries to move it. Alternately, the patient may try to move a joint or contract a muscle against the fixed resistance of the examiner. In most disease processes, both are equally affected, and the two methods can be used interchangeably. Some patients may comprehend and cooperate better with the first method, but having the patient initiate movement may better detect mild weakness. There is disagreement about how the examiner should apply force. Some authorities recommend a slow application of resistance in which the patient and examiner match effort; others contend that a rapid movement by the examiner will better detect mild weakness. With very weak muscles, strength may have to be judged without resistance or only against the resistance offered by gravity.

Many factors may complicate the strength examination and make assessment more difficult. The experience gained from examining many patients helps in buttressing an examiner's impression of loss of strength, especially when the impairment is mild. Fatigue, systemic illness, failure to understand or cooperate with strength testing, and many other factors may result in a false or distorted impression of weakness. In extrapyramidal disease, rigidity may interfere with apparent muscle power, and bradykinesia delays the onset of muscle contraction and causes retardation of movement. Hyperkinesias of various types and ataxia may make motor activity difficult. Loss or impairment of motion may also occur with pain, swelling, spasm, fractures, dislocations, adhesions or ankylosis of joints, contractures of either agonists or antagonists, loss of position sense, hysteria, malingering, and catatonia.

There is wide individual variation in the speed of voluntary movement. It may be increased in hyperthyroidism and mania and decreased in hypothyroidism, depression, parkinsonism, fatigue, and various myopathies. Slowness of movement (bradykinesia) may be the first manifestation of extrapyramidal disease. Abnormalities in the smoothness and regularity of movement may be due to ataxia, tremor, or chorea, but incoordination may also be caused by weakness. Motor impersistence is the inability to sustain voluntary motor acts that have been initiated on verbal command. The patient is unable to sustain an activity, such as keeping the eyes closed or the hand raised. It may be a form of apraxia and has been said to occur most often with left hemisphere lesions.

Weakness of a muscle must be distinguished from loss of range of motion for other reasons and from contracture of antagonists. Passive movements to assess range of motion are sometimes necessary to help distinguish whether limitation of movement is due to weakness, pain, muscle spasm, or fibrous or bony changes. Limitation of movement due to severe weakness may ultimately result in contracture and deformity. With contracture, a muscle cannot be stretched to its normal limits without considerable resistance and the production of pain. Patients with spasticity are at particular risk for contractures, especially if the muscles are not passively stretched at regular intervals. Contractures are particularly common in the calf muscles, drawing the foot downward. There is lack of full range of motion on attempted passive dorsiflexion ("tight heel cords"). Contractures may ultimately result in periarthritic changes, joint ankylosis, and fixed deformities.

In evaluating contractures and deformities, it is important to differentiate between those of neurogenic origin and those due to orthopedic disease, congenital abnormalities, habitual postures, occupational factors, or other factors that cause mechanical difficulty with movement. An equinus or equinovarus deformity of the foot may result from any of the following: footdrop due to peroneal (fibular) nerve palsy; spasm of the calf muscles in foot dystonia; spasticity due to a corticospinal tract (CST) lesion; a developmental anomaly, such as a congenital clubfoot; or trauma or arthritis of the ankle joints. The limitation of movement in the shoulder that often complicates hemiplegia must be differentiated from shoulder joint or rotator cuff disease. Flexion contracture of the wrist joint associated with a long-standing wrist drop due to a radial nerve palsy, and the claw hand due to ulnar neuropathy, must be differentiated from the deformities seen in such conditions as arthritis, Volkmann's contracture, and Dupuytren's contracture.

The motor examination may have to be modified, often with only a rough estimation of function, in various disease states, in confused or stuporous patients, and in infants and young children. Detection of weakness in the patient with altered consciousness or coma requires special techniques. In coma, assessment of motor function depends on spontaneous movements, the position of an extremity, or withdrawal of an extremity in response to painful stimulation, noting particularly any asymmetry of spontaneous or reflex movements on the two sides. The only manifestations of hemiplegia in the comatose patient may be the absence of contraction of the facial muscles on one side following pressure on the supraorbital ridge, the flail dropping of the wrist and forearm when released while the flexed elbow is resting on the bed, and extension and external rotation of the thigh and leg when released after having been placed in flexion with the heel resting on the bed. These are discussed in Chapter 51. In infants and young children, the motor examination may be largely limited to observing spontaneous activity and noting the general posture and the positions of the extremities when the patient is prone, supine, seated, and upright. Resistance to passive movement, reflex motor responses, and palpation may provide indirect evidence of muscle strength.

Strength may be assessed in absolute terms (e.g., the examiner comparing the patient's power to a belief of what normal should be), or it may be assessed in comparison with the patient's other muscles. The comparison is most often to a homologous muscle on the other side, as in comparing the two biceps muscles. But proximal strength should be commensurate with distal strength in the same patient. A patient with polymyositis may have weakness of the deltoids on both sides, so one deltoid cannot be judged against the other. But the deltoids may be obviously weaker than the wrist extensors, so there is a proximal to distal gradient of increasing strength that is clearly abnormal. The muscles on the dominant side are usually slightly stronger.

STRENGTH SCALES

Quantitative measurements and permanent records help in diagnosis and in evaluating disease progression or recovery. In manual muscle testing, the strength of individual muscles is tested and graded quantitatively using some scale. Strength is most commonly graded using the five-level MRC (Medical Research Council) scale, which was developed in Britain in World War II to evaluate patients with peripheral nerve injuries (Table 27.1). The MRC scale has been widely applied to the evaluation of strength in general. However, the scale is heavily weighted toward the evaluation of very weak muscles **(Video 27.1)**. In a severe peripheral nerve injury, improvement from grade 0 (no contraction) to grade 1 (a flicker) is highly significant, as it signals the beginning of reinnervation. A patient with a nerve injury who eventually recovers to grade 4 has had an excellent outcome. In contrast, a patient with polymyositis who is diffusely grade 4 has severe disease and is doing poorly. So, the most commonly used strength grading scale has significant limitations when dealing with many patients.

The levels of the MRC scale are precisely defined, but not linear. It is a common error to believe the MRC grades are evenly spaced and that grade 5 is normal, grade 4 is minimal or mild weakness, grade 3 is moderate weakness, grade 2 is severe, and so forth. In fact, anything less than grade 5 denotes significant weakness. Grade 4 is moderate weakness, and anything less is severe weakness. A patient who is diffusely 4/5 does not have mild or equivocal weakness but major and serious involvement. One must not confuse poor effort with weakness. A muscle is graded by the maximal power demonstrated, even if it is only briefly.

TABLE 27.1 The Medical Research Council Scale of Muscle Strength

0	No contraction
1	A flicker or trace of contraction
2	Active movement with gravity eliminated
3	Active movement against gravity
4–	Active movement against gravity and slight resistance
4	Active movement against gravity and moderate resistance
4+	Active movement against gravity and strong resistance
5	Normal power

The muscle strength scale used by physical therapists grades muscles on a 6-point scale from 0 (no motion) through trace, poor, fair, and good to normal. The scale used at the Mayo Clinic grades muscle strength on a 5-point scale that is more linear. Normal is designated as 0, mild weakness is –1, and total paralysis is –4.

The different levels of the MRC scale are so precisely defined that there is good interexaminer consistency once the fine points of proper positioning and other details are mastered. In clinical practice, the MRC scale is often expanded to include subgrades (e.g., 5–, 4+). The MRC eventually saw the need to include grades 4– and 4+. Mendell and Florence developed a formal modified MRC scale. In general use, the subgrades are not so precisely defined, and there is much less inter- and even intraexaminer consistency. Approximate guidelines are all that is possible. Before attempting to describe these guidelines, the important issue of examiner-patient mismatch should be recognized.

There is obviously considerable individual variation in muscle power, dependent in part upon size, gender, body build, age, and activity level. This variability affects examiners as well as patients. Patients come large and small, young and old, male and female, and physically strong and relatively weak. So do physicians. A large, young, powerful, physician examining a small, old, sick, patient has an unfair advantage. The physician may tend to think the patient is weak when they are in fact normal for his or her age, sex, and circumstances. Conversely, a small, relatively weak physician examining a large, powerful patient may miss significant weakness because of strength mismatch.

As a general principle, reliable strength testing should attempt to break a given muscle. Muscles are most powerful when maximally shortened. Another consideration is the lever effect. Attempting to overpower a muscle, such as a deltoid, using a very short lever (examiner's hand at the mid-upper arm) is much less likely to meet with success than using a long lever (patient's elbow extended and examiner pressing down on the wrist). A small, weak examiner can overcome the deltoid of the most powerful person by keeping the patient's elbow extended and using both hands to pull down the wrist. Technique matters.

By varying the length of lever and the shortening of the muscle permitted, the examiner may give or take mechanical advantage as necessary to compensate for strength mismatch. Many patients of different ages, sizes, and strength levels must be examined in this fashion in order to develop an appreciation of the expected strength of a muscle for a given set of circumstances.

So, for an examiner of average size and strength examining a patient of average size and presumed normal strength, the following is a useful guideline for assessing power in the major muscle groups. If it requires the whole hand and a firm push to break the muscle, the power is grade 4+. If the muscle can be broken using three fingers, it is grade 4. If it can be broken using one finger, it is grade 4–. Some clinicians use the grades of 3– and 2– to describe muscles that can move against gravity or with gravity eliminated, but not through a full range, and the grade of 5– to indicate borderline or equivocal weakness.

Some muscles are "special cases." The small hand muscles are best examined by matching them against the examiner's like muscle (e.g., abductor pollicis brevis [APB] to abductor pollicis brevis). This method is beautifully described and illustrated in *Segmental Neurology* by John K. Wolf. The gastrocnemius muscles are normally so powerful it is virtually useless to examine them using hand and arm strength, unless they are very weak. Having the patient walk on tiptoe, hop, support the entire body weight on one tiptoe, or do one-legged toe raises are usually better methods.

PATTERNS OF WEAKNESS

There are common patterns of weakness. Recognition of a pattern may help greatly in lesion localization and differential diagnosis. Identification of the process causing weakness is further aided by accompanying signs, such as reflex alterations and sensory loss. Table 27.2 reviews the features of upper motor neuron versus lower motor neuron weakness. Table 27.3 summarizes some common patterns of weakness and their localization.

Weakness may be focal or generalized. When focal, it may follow the distribution of some structure in the peripheral nervous system, such as a peripheral nerve or spinal root. It may affect one side of the body in a "hemi" distribution. A hemi distribution may affect the arm, leg, and face equally on one side of the body, or one or more areas may be more involved than others. The CST preferentially innervates certain muscle groups, and these are often selectively impaired (see Chapter 25). When weakness is nonfocal, it may be generalized, predominantly proximal, or predominantly distal.

Generalized Weakness

The term *generalized weakness* implies that the weakness involves both sides of the body, more or less symmetrically. When a patient has truly generalized weakness, bulbar motor functions—such as facial movements, speech, chewing, and swallowing—are involved as well. Weakness of both arms and both legs with normal bulbar function is quadriparesis or tetraparesis. Weakness of both legs is paraparesis. When weakness affects all four extremities, the likely causes

TABLE 27.2 Features of Upper Motor Neuron versus Lower Motor Neuron Weakness

Feature	Upper Motor Neuron	Lower Motor Neuron
Weakness distribution	Corticospinal distribution; hemiparesis, quadriparesis, paraparesis, monoparesis, faciobrachial	Generalized, predominantly proximal, predominantly distal or focal. No preferential involvement of corticospinal innervated muscles
Sensory loss distribution	Central pattern	None, stocking glove or peripheral nerve or root distribution
Deep tendon reflexes	Increased unless very acute	Normal or decreased
Superficial reflexes	Decreased	Normal
Pathologic reflexes	Yes	No
Sphincter function	Sometimes impaired	Normal (except for cauda equina lesion)
Muscle tone	Increased	Normal or decreased
Pain	No	Sometimes
Other CNS signs	Possibly	No

CNS, central nervous system.

TABLE 27.3 Common Patterns of Weakness with Lesions at Different Locations in the Neuraxis

Location of Lesion	Distribution of Weakness	Sensory Loss	DTRs*	Possible Accompanying Signs
Middle cerebral artery	Contralateral arm and face > leg†	Y	Incr	Aphasia, apraxia, visual field deficit, gaze palsy
Anterior cerebral artery	Contralateral leg > arm and face†	Y	Incr	Cortical sensory loss in contralateral leg, frontal lobe signs, sometimes incontinence
Internal capsule	Contralateral face = arm = leg†	N	Incr	None ("pure motor stroke")
Brainstem	Ipsilateral cranial nerve and contralateral body†	Y	Incr	Variable, depending on level
Cervical cord (transverse)	Both arms and both legs†	Y	Incr	Bowel, bladder, or sexual dysfunction common
Thoracic cord (transverse)	Both legs†	Y	Incr	Bowel, bladder, or sexual dysfunction common
Cauda equina	Both legs, asymmetric, multiple root pattern	Y	Decr	Occasional bowel, bladder, or sexual dysfunction; sometimes pain
Anterior horn cell	Focal early, generalized late	N	Incr	Atrophy, fasciculations, bulbar weakness
Single nerve root	Muscles of the affected myotome	Y	Decr	Pain
Plexus	Plexus pattern, complete or partial	Usually	Decr	Pain is common, especially with brachial "plexitis"
Mononeuropathy	Muscles of the affected nerve	Usually	Decr	Variable atrophy, variable pain
Polyneuropathy	Distal > proximal	Usually	Decr	Variable pain, atrophy late
Neuromuscular junction	Bulbar, proximal extremities	N	Normal	Ptosis, ophthalmoparesis, fatigable weakness, fluctuating weakness
Muscle	Proximal > distal	N	Normal	Pain uncommon, many potential patterns (limb girdle, facioscapulohumeral, etc.), pseudohypertrophy, myotonia

*With corticospinal lesions, DTRs acutely may be normal or decreased (neural shock).
†Extremity weakness in a corticospinal tract distribution.
Decr, decreased; DTR, deep tendon reflex; Incr, increased; N, no; Y, yes.

include spinal cord disease, peripheral neuropathy, a neuromuscular junction disorder, or a myopathy.

When spinal cord disease is the culprit and the deficit is incomplete, more severe involvement of those muscles preferentially innervated by the CST can frequently be discerned. Reflexes are usually increased (though in the acute stages they may be decreased or absent); there is usually some alteration of sensation, sometimes a discrete spinal "level"; superficial reflexes disappear; and there is often bowel and bladder dysfunction. Generalized peripheral nerve disease tends to predominantly involve distal muscles, although there are exceptions. There is no preferential involvement of CST innervated muscles; reflexes are usually decreased; sensory loss is frequently present; and bowel and bladder functions are not disturbed. With a neuromuscular junction disorder, the weakness is likely to be worse proximally; sensation is spared; reflexes are normal; and there is usually involvement of bulbar muscles, especially with ptosis and ophthalmoplegia. When the problem is a primary muscle disorder, weakness is usually more severe proximally; reflexes are normal; sensation is normal; and with only a few exceptions, bulbar function is spared except for occasional dysphagia.

Amyotrophic lateral sclerosis (ALS) causes a characteristic pattern of weakness. The weakness and wasting due to lower motor neuron involvement are accompanied by weakness and hyperreflexia due to upper motor neuron involvement.

Focal Weakness

Weakness of the arm and leg on one side of the body is hemiparesis. Monoparesis is weakness limited to one extremity. Diplegia is weakness of like parts on the two sides of the body; the term spastic diplegia refers to weakness of both legs that occurs in cerebral palsy; and facial diplegia is weakness of both sides of the face. Spastic weakness of one arm and the opposite leg is referred to as cruciate or crossed paralysis, or hemiplegia alternans.

Certain patterns of muscle weakness point to a peripheral nerve, plexus, or root lesion. With a peripheral nerve lesion, all muscles below the level of the lesion are at risk. It is increasingly recognized, however, that not all muscles distal to a peripheral nerve lesion are necessarily equally affected. When multiple muscles of an extremity are weak, localization depends on recognizing the common innervating structure. In cervical radiculopathy, the muscles involved are innervated by different peripheral nerves and different brachial plexus components, but all by the same root. For instance, lesions of the middle trunk of the brachial plexus are exceedingly rare, so weakness of the triceps (radial nerve) and the pronator teres (PT) (median nerve) usually means a lesion of the C7 root.

A focal neuropathy, such as a radial nerve palsy, or a spinal root lesion, such as from a herniated disc, causes weakness limited to the distribution of the involved nerve or root. A complete plexopathy, such as a traumatic brachial plexopathy, may cause weakness of the entire limb. Partial lesions may cause weakness only in the distribution of certain plexus components. With such lower motor neuron pathology, reflexes are typically decreased, and there is often accompanying sensory loss. Localization of focal weakness due to root, plexus, and peripheral nerve pathology requires intimate familiarity with peripheral neuroanatomy. Anterior horn cell disease often begins with focal weakness that may simulate mononeuropathy, but it evolves into a more widespread pattern as the disease progresses, culminating in generalized weakness. Except for extraocular muscle involvement in myasthenia gravis, it is rare for a myopathy or neuromuscular junction disorder to cause focal weakness.

NONORGANIC (FUNCTIONAL) WEAKNESS

Nonorganic weakness due to psychiatric disorders—such as conversion disorder, malingering, or somatization by patients with underlying depression or anxiety—is common. The first step in evaluating weakness is often deciding whether it is organic or nonorganic. This distinction is not always easy. Patients with nonorganic weakness are commonly thought to have neurologic disease, but it seems nearly as often patients with real weakness are thought to have psychogenic weakness or malingering. Organic and functional deficits may coexist—the problem of functional or psychogenic overlay. Some patients embellish by nature; others may exaggerate a real deficit for fear the physician may not take them seriously. A patient may have real weakness in one area and functional weakness in another area. Some patients with organic weakness may allow resistance to collapse when the examiner begins to defeat a muscle so that real weakness may appear to be related to poor effort. When a movement causes pain, resistance may be less than full and the effort may be erratic.

Coaching is often helpful. The examiner exhorts the patient not to give up, to keep pushing or pulling no matter what. Simple encouragement to keep trying even if the patient is losing may suffice to improve effort. Some patients, in spite of all, will simply not give full effort. Their efforts are erratic and variable. Some things are often useful in distinguishing organic from psychogenic weakness. Patients with bona fide organic muscle weakness will yield smoothly as the examiner defeats the weak muscle. The patient gives uniform resistance throughout the movement. If the examiner decreases his resistance, the patient will begin to win the battle. If the examiner drops the resistance level, the patient with nonorganic weakness will not continue to push or pull. Instead, the patient will also stop resisting so that no matter how little force the examiner applies, there is an absence of follow-through and the patient never overcomes the examiner. When there is nonorganic weakness, resistance is erratic and often collapses abruptly. The muscular contractions are poorly sustained and may give way suddenly, rather than gradually, as the patient resists the force exerted by the examiner. Some patients will give up entirely and allow the muscle or limb to flop; others will provide variable resistance throughout the range of motion with alternating moments of effort and no effort. At the peaks of contraction, strength is normal; in the valleys, there is little or no resistance. This pattern of variable strength is referred to as "collapsing," "ratchety," "give way," "breakaway," or "catch and give." It is characteristic of nonorganic weakness. With nonorganic weakness, there may be an increase or a decrease in strength with repeated testing. Contraction of the apparently weak muscle may be felt when the patient is asked to carry out movements with synergistic muscles, or the antagonists may be felt to contract when the patient is asked to contract the agonist (e.g., the triceps muscle twitches when the patient is told to flex the elbow). Functional testing may fail to confirm weakness suspected during strength testing. For example, there may be apparent foot dorsiflexion weakness, yet the patient is able to stand on the heel without difficulty.

The patient with nonorganic weakness may make little effort to contract the muscles necessary to execute a particular movement. He may be calm and indifferent while demonstrating the lack of strength, showing little sign of alarm at the presence of complete paralysis, and smile cheerfully during the examination. If the examiner raises and drops an extremity, a limb with psychogenic paralysis may drop slowly to avoid injury, whereas an extremity with real weakness would drop rapidly, especially if the paralysis is flaccid. In psychogenic paralysis of the arm, the latissimus dorsi may appear paretic when tested by having the patient adduct the arm but contract normally on coughing. In simulated hemiplegia, the patient may be unable to adduct either the affected arm or leg against resistance, yet if asked to keep both arms against the body or both legs close together, the adductors contract strongly on both sides because it is difficult to adduct one extremity without adducting its apparently paralyzed fellow. In testing paralysis of the finger muscles, the patient may be asked to pronate the forearms and interlock the fingers so that the left fingers are on the right and vice versa (Figure 36.6); the examiner then points to the individual fingers and tells the patient to move them. It is difficult for one to determine immediately whether the indicated finger is on the right side or on the left; if the patient attempts to respond promptly, he or she makes many mistakes. Similar tests may be carried out by asking the patient to perform individual movements with the hands behind the back.

The patient with functional weakness cannot control associated movements, which forms the basis of the Hoover and abductor signs. The Hoover (automatic walking) sign is useful for evaluating suspected nonorganic leg weakness. When a normal supine patient flexes the hip to lift one leg, there is an involuntary downward movement of the other leg. The extension countermovement of the opposite leg is a normal associated movement (see Chapter 42). An extension movement of one leg normally accompanies flexion of the other leg, as in walking. In organic leg weakness, the downward pressure of the contralateral heel occurs when the patient tries to raise the weak leg, and the examiner can feel the extension pressure by placing a hand beneath the heel that remains on the bed. In nonorganic leg weakness, there is no downward pressure of the contralateral heel as the patient tries to raise the weak leg, but an extension movement of the "paralyzed" leg may be felt as the good leg is raised. Hoover's sign is the absence of the expected extension movement of the good leg on attempting to raise the bad leg and normal involuntary extension of the bad leg on raising the good leg.

In the quest for ways to distinguish real from psychogenic weakness at the turn of the 20th century, Hoover thought this maneuver was more useful than the Babinski sign (Chapter 40). The abductor sign is similar and seeks to elicit synergistic movement of the nonparetic leg when the patient is asked to abduct the paretic leg. In nonorganic paresis, the paretic leg demonstrates synergistic abduction when the sound leg is tested, and the sound leg does not exert normal abduction power and can be moved into a hyperadducted position when the paretic limb is tested. It may be useful when relatively preserved hip extensor strength limits the utility of Hoover's test. In the Spinal Injuries Center (SIC) test, patients unable to raise their knees spontaneously have a positive test, indicating nonorganic weakness, when their knees remain up after being lifted by the examiner. See LaFrance for video of the Hoover, abduction, and SIC tests. Dynamometers have been used in various ways in an attempt to prove weakness is nonorganic, and investigators have developed computerized, quantitative methods for detecting functional weakness based on these principles.

Patients with nonorganic hemiparesis are more likely to have weakness of the sternomastoid, usually ipsilateral, but this muscle is rarely involved in bona fide hemiparesis because of its bilateral innervation (Chapter 19). With the arm-dropping test, transient voluntary contraction in functional weakness may cause a brief hang-up before the arm collapses. On the Babinski trunk-thigh test, a leg with nonorganic weakness fails to flex as expected. Looking for the presence or absence of other associated movements may sometimes help in the differentiation between organic and psychogenic weakness (Chapter 42). The patient with functional weakness may have a dramatic display of effort, grimacing and grunting when trying to contract the weak muscle. A movement such as a squat may be executed in a slow and laborious manner that actually requires greater than normal strength. The onset of functional weakness is often sudden.

In psychogenic weakness, muscle tone may be normal, decreased, or variable, but it is often increased with pseudorigidity or pseudospasticity. Rigidity, if present, resembles voluntary resistance. The part may be held firmly in a bizarre position. Abnormalities in tone usually vary from time to time, especially under the influence of suggestion.

Normal tone, normal deep tendon reflexes (DTRs), normal facial movements in the face of hemiparesis, an absence of trophic changes, normal sphincter function despite paraparesis or quadriparesis, aphonia, and a monoplegic dragging gait all may suggest that weakness is nonorganic. It is very unusual for functional weakness to present in a peripheral nerve, plexus, or root distribution or to display a proximal/distal gradient. Evidence does not support the notion that functional weakness is more common on the left.

DSM-V emphasizes the importance of "positive signs" of nonorganicity to support a diagnosis of conversion disorder. Many such positive signs have been reported, but only a minority have been validated. The positive signs that have been carefully studied generally have low sensitivity but high specificity. In a carefully done pilot study, Daum et al. concluded that four positive signs were highly reliable in the diagnosis of functional weakness: Hoover's sign, giveaway weakness, cocontraction, and drift without pronation.

EXAMINATION OF MOTOR STRENGTH AND POWER

Evaluation of the strength of various muscle groups and movements can become complex, depending upon the degree of detail necessary. Isolated contraction of a single muscle is rarely possible because muscles with similar functions participate in almost every movement. Normal contraction of synergists and fixating muscles and relaxation of antagonists are also necessary. Still, the predominant action of a single muscle can usually be determined and tested. Some functions are carried out by many muscles acting synergistically (e.g., flexion and extension of the trunk), and the muscles must be tested as a group by assessing the movement rather than individual muscles. It is helpful to be fluent with the primary actions of the major muscles and their peripheral nerve, plexus, and root innervations. The strength of each major pertinent muscle group should be determined individually and its strength grade recorded.

Reliable strength testing requires proper patient positioning and avoidance of unwanted movements. Testing may be done in various positions, depending on the muscle to be tested and its power. Testing in the seated position suffices under most circumstances. It is important to fix the proximal portion of a limb when the movements of the distal portion are being tested. For instance, when testing forearm pronation strength, the patient must not be allowed to internally rotate the shoulder to compensate for lack of pronation power. When evaluating very weak muscles, gravity must be eliminated to detect residual power. A very weak biceps muscle (MRC grade 2/5), even when it cannot succeed against gravity, may be able to flex the elbow if the arm is raised to shoulder height so that the forearm can be moved horizontally. The wrist and finger drop of radial nerve palsy creates such a mechanical disadvantage for contraction that the patient may appear to have weakness of grip and finger abduction, but these functions are intact when the wrist and fingers are passively extended.

EXAMINATION OF SPECIFIC MOVEMENTS AND MUSCLES

The motor examination of the muscles supplied by those cranial nerves that have motor functions is discussed separately. For the trunk and extremities, the strength and power of the individual muscles and of movements are assessed as appropriate for the clinical circumstances. Many reference sources are available to assist in learning muscle examination techniques. There is some difference regarding the exact innervation of individual muscles among different reference sources, and occasionally, there is variable or anomalous innervation. Tables 27.4 to 27.7 give the most generally accepted spinal cord segment and peripheral nerve innervation of the more important muscles. Tables 27.8 and 27.9 give the innervation by root.

The action of a muscle about a joint may vary depending on the part of the muscle activated and the position of the joint. Parts of some large muscles, such as the gluteus maximus, may have secondary actions that are different from other parts. For instance, the upper part of the gluteus maximus abducts the hip, whereas the lower part adducts it. Still, each muscle has a primary action in which all parts participate, and in this instance, it is hip extension. The angle of the joint about which a muscle acts may influence its leverage and angle of pull. In extreme cases, a muscle may move to the opposite side of the axis of rotation and have an action in one joint position that

TABLE 27.4 Innervation of Muscles Responsible for Movements of the Head and Neck

Parentheses signify minor contribution

Muscle	Segmental Innervation	Peripheral Nerve
Sternocleidomastoid	Cranial XI; C(1)2-C3	Spinal accessory nerve
Trapezius	Cranial XI; C(2)3-C4	Spinal accessory nerve
Scalenus anterior	C4-C7	
Scalenus medius	C4-C8	
Scalenus posterior	C6-C8	
Longus capitis	C1-C4	
Longus colli	C2-C6	
Rectus capitis anterior	C1-C2	Suboccipital nerve
Rectus capitis lateralis	C1	Suboccipital nerve
Rectus capitis posterior	C1	Suboccipital nerve
Obliquus capitis inferior	C1	Suboccipital nerve
Obliquus capitis superior	C1	Suboccipital nerve
Splenius capitis	C2-C4 (C1-C6)	
Splenius cervicis	C2-C4 (C1-C6)	
Semispinalis capitis	C1-C4	
Semispinalis cervicis	C3-C6	
Spinalis cervicis	C5-C8	
Sacrospinalis	C1-C8	
Iliocostalis cervicis	C1-C8	
Longissimus capitis	C1-C8	
Longissimus cervicis	C1-C8	
Intertransversarii	C1-C8	
Rotatores	C1-C8	
Multifidi	C1-C8	

is different from its action in another joint position (inversion of action). For instance, the hip adductors act secondarily as hip flexors when the hip is extended but as extensors when the hip is flexed; the piriformis externally rotates the extended hip but internally rotates the flexed hip.

Examination of Movements and Muscles of the Neck

The principal neck movements are flexion, extension (retraction), rotation (turning), and lateral bending (tilting, abduction). Many different muscle groups contribute to the various neck movements. Except for the sternocleidomastoid (SCM) and trapezius, it is not possible to examine them individually, and the assessment is made of movement (e.g., neck flexion) rather than particular muscles. The spinal accessory nerve, along with the second, third, and fourth cervical segments, supplies the SCM and trapezius muscles. The SCM is a flexor and rotator of the head and neck; the trapezius retracts the neck and draws it to one side. Other muscles that contribute to neck flexion include the platysma, suprahyoid, infrahyoid, scalenes, and prevertebral group of muscles (longus colli and capitis, rectus capitis).

Many muscles contribute to neck extension, including the trapezius and the paravertebral muscles. Many of these muscles when contracting unilaterally rotate the spine. The paravertebral musculature is a massive, complex amalgam of individual muscle groups that primarily serve to extend and rotate the neck and trunk. Four principal muscle subgroups combine to form the paravertebral muscles: the splenii, erector spinae, transversospinalis, and interspinal-intertransverse. All of these muscles lie deep and medial in the groove formed between the transverse and spinous processes of the vertebral bodies. They are further named for the vertebral segment in which they lie (e.g., transversospinalis cervicis). The splenius capitis is a powerful ipsilateral rotator of the head; the splenii contracting bilaterally extend the neck. Muscles commonly injected with botulinum toxin to treat cervical dystonia include the SCM, trapezius, splenius capitis, scalenes, longissimus, and levator scapula. The paraspinal muscle complex generally receives its innervation from multiple levels. These muscles arise from a common embryologic precursor muscle mass, and their innervation shows extensive longitudinal overlap (Table 27.4).

Neck flexors are tested by having the patient try to place the chin on the chest as the examiner applies extension force to the forehead (Figure 27.1). Extensors are tested by having the patient extend against the examiner's resistance applied to the occiput (Figure 27.2). Neck rotation is accomplished by the contralateral SCM and ipsilateral splenius capitis and trapezius; examination of the SCM and trapezius muscles is discussed in Chapter 19. Neck flexor strength may be tested with the patient sitting or supine and neck extension sitting or prone. The neck flexion test consists of measuring the time the supine patient can keep the head raised with the chin on the chest; most patients can keep their

TABLE 27.5 Innervation of Muscles Responsible for Movements of the Shoulder Girdle and Upper Extremity

Parentheses signify minor contribution

Muscle	Segmental Innervation	Peripheral Nerve
Trapezius	Cranial XI; C(2)3-C4	Spinal accessory nerve
Levator scapulae	C3-C4	Nerves to levator scapulae
	C5	Dorsal scapular nerve
Rhomboideus major	C4-C5	Dorsal scapular nerve
Rhomboideus minor	C4-C5	Dorsal scapular nerve
Serratus anterior	C5-C7	Long thoracic nerve
Deltoid	C5-C6	Axillary nerve
Teres minor	C5-C6	Axillary nerve
Supraspinatus	C(4)5-C6	Suprascapular nerve
Infraspinatus	C(4)5-C6	Suprascapular nerve
Latissimus dorsi	C6-C8	Thoracodorsal nerve
Pectoralis major	C5-T1	Lateral and medial anterior thoracic nerves
Pectoralis minor	C7-T1	Medial anterior thoracic nerve
Subscapularis	C5-C7	Subscapular nerves
Teres major	C5-C7	Lower subscapular nerve
Subclavius	C5-C6	Nerve to subclavius
Coracobrachialis	C6-C7	Musculocutaneous nerve
Biceps brachii	C5-C6	Musculocutaneous nerve
Brachialis	C5-C6	Musculocutaneous nerve
Brachioradialis	C5-C6	Radial nerve
Triceps brachii	C6-C8	Radial nerve
Anconeus	C7-C8	Radial nerve
Supinator	C6-C7	Radial nerve
Extensor carpi radialis longus	C(5)6-C7	Radial nerve
Extensor carpi radialis brevis	C7-C8	Radial nerve
Extensor carpi ulnaris	C7-C8	Radial nerve
Extensor digitorum communis	C7-C8	Radial nerve
Extensor indicis proprius	C7-C8	Radial nerve
Extensor digiti minimi	C7-C8	Radial nerve
Extensor pollicis longus	C7-C8	Radial nerve
Extensor pollicis brevis	C7-C8	Radial nerve
Abductor pollicis longus	C7-C8	Radial nerve
Pronator teres	C6-C7	Median nerve
Flexor carpi radialis	C6-C7	Median nerve
Pronator quadratus	C7-C8	Median nerve
Palmaris longus	C7-C8	Median nerve
Flexor digitorum sublimis	C7-T1	Median nerve
Flexor digitorum profundus (radial half)	C8-T1	Median nerve
Lumbricales 1 and 2	C8-T1	Median nerve
Flexor pollicis longus	C7-T1	Median nerve
Flexor pollicis brevis (FPB) (lateral head)	C8-T1	Median nerve
Abductor pollicis brevis	C8-T1	Median nerve
Opponens pollicis	C8-T1	Median nerve
Flexor carpi ulnaris	C7-T1	Ulnar nerve
Flexor digitorum profundus (ulnar half)	C8-T1	Ulnar nerve
Interossei	C8-T1	Ulnar nerve
Lumbricales 3 and 4	C8-T1	Ulnar nerve
FPB (medial head)	C8-T1	Ulnar nerve
Flexor digiti minimi brevis	C8-T1	Ulnar nerve
Abductor digiti minimi (ADM)	C8-T1	Ulnar nerve
Opponens digiti minimi	C8-T1	Ulnar nerve
Palmaris brevis	C8-T1	Ulnar nerve
Adductor pollicis	C8-T1	Ulnar nerve

head in this position for at least 1 minute. This test is sometimes useful in the evaluation of myopathies and neuromuscular junction disorders, the principal conditions that cause neck flexor or extensor weakness. Abnormalities of neck position may occur in conditions in which there is no muscle weakness, and these can sometimes be confused with the effects of a weak muscle. The patient with meningismus may have the head retracted, whereas the patient with Parkinson disease may have it flexed. Cervical

TABLE 27.6 Innervation of Muscles Responsible for Movements of the Thorax and Abdomen

Parentheses signify minor contribution

Muscle	Segmental Innervation	Peripheral Nerve
Diaphragm	C3-C5	Phrenic nerve
Intercostal muscles (internal and external)	T1-T12	Intercostal nerves
Levatores costarum	C8-T11	Intercostal nerves
Transversus thoracis	T2-T7	Intercostal nerves
Serratus posterior superior	T1-T4	Intercostal nerves
Serratus posterior inferior	T9-T12	Intercostal nerves
Rectus abdominis	T5-T12	Intercostal nerves
Pyramidalis	T11-T12	Intercostal nerves
Transversus abdominis	T7-L1	Intercostal, ilioinguinal, and iliohypogastric nerves
Obliquus internus abdominis	T7-L1	Intercostal, ilioinguinal, and iliohypogastric nerves
Obliquus externus abdominis	T7-L1	Intercostal, ilioinguinal, and iliohypogastric nerves

dystonia can cause an almost infinite number of abnormal head positions, including torticollis (head turned or tilted), anterocollis (head flexed), and retrocollis (head extended). Examination of the neck muscles must be done carefully in any patient at risk for cervical spine disease.

Examination of Movements and Muscles of the Upper Extremities

The responsible muscles and their innervation are given in Table 27.5.

The Shoulder

Movements of the shoulder take place at the sternoclavicular, acromioclavicular, and glenohumeral joints. Because the scapula is firmly connected to the clavicle at the acromioclavicular joint, the two bones tend to move as a unit with the motion taking place primarily at the sternoclavicular joint. Movements of the scapula are elevation, depression, retraction (movement away from the chest wall), protraction (movement toward the chest wall), and rotation. The ventral surface of the scapula is a concavity known as the subscapular fossa that is filled mostly with the subscapularis muscle. The serratus anterior lies between the subscapularis and the chest wall and inserts into a thin rim of the scapula along the vertebral border and slightly expanded triangular areas at the superior and inferior angles (Figure 27.3). The serratus runs obliquely from its origination from the upper eight ribs along the lateral chest wall to its attachment to the scapula. The trapezius is a diamond-shaped muscle that attaches widely to the shoulder girdle. The superior fibers insert along the posterior border of the clavicle and scapular spine, the middle and lower fibers along the scapular spine. The upper and middle fibers insert laterally along the scapular spine and the lower fibers more medially. The rhomboids (major and minor) arise from the spinous process of the upper thoracic vertebrae and insert along the medial border of the scapula. The levator scapulae originates from the upper cervical vertebra and drops diagonally to insert along the upper medial border of the scapula.

The upper fibers of the trapezius, assisted by the levator scapulae, elevate the scapula and the point of the shoulder and rotate the scapula upward. The middle fibers rotate the scapula upward and assist the rhomboids in retraction. The lower fibers rotate and depress the scapula and draw it toward the midline. The rhomboids act primarily to retract the scapula, bracing the shoulder backward. The levator scapulae acts with the trapezius to elevate the scapula. The serratus anterior, assisted by the pectoralis minor, protracts the scapula, pulling it anteriorly. It is critical in all functions that involve reaching or pushing forward. The expanded insertion at the inferior angle helps to pull the inferior scapular angle forward around the chest wall. It also, along with the trapezius, rotates the scapula and raises the point of the shoulder to abduct the arm above horizontal. It helps to fix the scapula while other muscles abduct or flex the arm.

Elevation of the scapula, as in shrugging the shoulder, is carried out by the upper trapezius and levator scapulae muscles, assisted by the SCM. The levator scapulae is innervated by direct branches from C3 and C4 with a contribution from C5 via the dorsal scapular nerve. The levator scapulae draws the scapula upward and rotates it so that the inferior angle approaches the spinal column. Depression of

TABLE 27.7 Innervation of Muscles Responsible for Movements of the Lower Extremities

Parentheses signify minor contribution

Muscle	Segmental Innervation	Peripheral Nerve
Psoas major	L(1)2-L3(4)	Nerve to psoas major
Psoas minor	L1-L2	Nerve to psoas minor
Iliacus	L2-L3(4)	Femoral nerve
Quadriceps femoris	L2-L4	Femoral nerve
Sartorius	L2-L3	Femoral nerve
Pectineus	L2-L3	Femoral nerve
Gluteus maximus	L5-S2	Inferior gluteal nerve
Gluteus medius	L4-S1	Superior gluteal nerve
Gluteus minimus	L4-S1	Superior gluteal nerve
Tensor fasciae latae	L4-S1	Superior gluteal nerve
Piriformis	(L5)S1-S2	Nerve to piriformis
Adductor longus	L2-L4	Obturator nerve
Adductor brevis	L2-L4	Obturator nerve
Adductor magnus	L2-L4	Obturator nerve
Adductor magnus	L4-L5	Sciatic nerve
Gracilis	L2-L4	Obturator nerve
Obturator externus	L2-L4	Obturator nerve
Obturator internus	L5-S1	Nerve to obturator internus
Gemellus superior	L5-S1	Nerve to obturator internus
Gemellus inferior	L5-S1	Nerve to quadratus femoris
Quadratus femoris	L5-S1	Nerve to quadratus femoris
Biceps femoris (long head)	L5-S1	Tibial nerve
Semimembranosus	L5-S1	Tibial nerve
Semitendinosus	L5-S2	Tibial nerve
Popliteus	L5-S1	Tibial nerve
Gastrocnemius	S1-S2	Tibial nerve
Soleus	S1-S2	Tibial nerve
Plantaris	S1-S2	Tibial nerve
Tibialis posterior	L5-S1	Tibial nerve
Flexor digitorum longus	L5-S1	Tibial nerve
Flexor hallucis longus	L5-S1	Tibial nerve
Biceps femoris (short head)	L5-S2	Common peroneal nerve
Tibialis anterior	L4-L5	Deep peroneal nerve
Peroneus tertius	L5-S1	Deep peroneal nerve
Extensor digitorum longus	L5-S1	Deep peroneal nerve
Extensor hallucis longus	L5	Deep peroneal nerve
Extensor digitorum brevis	L5-S1	Deep peroneal nerve
Extensor hallucis brevis	L5-S1	Deep peroneal nerve
Peroneus longus	L5-S1	Superficial peroneal nerve
Peroneus brevis	L5-S1	Superficial peroneal nerve
Flexor digitorum brevis	S1-S2	Medial plantar nerve
Flexor hallucis brevis	S1-S2	Medial plantar nerve
Abductor hallucis	S1-S2	Medial plantar nerve
Lumbricales (medial 1 or 2)	S1-S3	Medial plantar nerve
Quadratus plantae	S1-S2	Lateral plantar nerve
Adductor hallucis	S2-S3	Lateral plantar nerve
ADM pedis	S1-S3	Lateral plantar nerve
Flexor digiti minimi brevis	S2-S3	Lateral plantar nerve
Lumbricales (lateral 2 or 3)	S1-S3	Lateral plantar nerve
Interossei	S2-S3	Lateral plantar nerve

the scapula is carried out primarily by the lower trapezius, pectoralis minor, and subclavius muscles.

Retraction of the scapula is carried out primarily by the rhomboids and the middle trapezius. The rhomboids also draw the scapulae together, as in standing at attention. The rhomboids are innervated by a twig directly from the C5 nerve root, and not via the brachial plexus. Examination of the rhomboids is important in the differentiation of C5 radiculopathy from upper trunk brachial plexopathy.

In protraction of the scapula, the scapula moves forward as in throwing a punch. This movement is carried out primarily by the serratus anterior (long thoracic nerve, C5-C7). The serratus keeps the vertebral border of the scapula applied to the thorax and pulls the scapula forward and laterally. Rotation of the scapula is accomplished by the trapezius, serratus anterior, pectorals, rhomboids, and latissimus dorsi. Normal scapular rotation is essential to efficient shoulder abduction.

TABLE 27.8 Major Upper-Extremity Muscles Innervated by Different Roots

Parentheses signify minor contribution

Root	Muscles Supplied
C4	Levator scapulae, rhomboids
C5	Levator scapulae, rhomboids, supraspinatus, infraspinatus, teres major and minor, deltoid, biceps, brachialis, BR, serratus anterior, pectoralis
C6	Supraspinatus, infraspinatus, teres major and minor, deltoid, biceps, brachialis, BR, supinator, serratus anterior, pectoralis, FCR, pronator teres, latissimus dorsi, ECRL (triceps)
C7	Serratus anterior, pectoralis, teres major, latissimus dorsi, triceps, anconeus, pronator teres, FCR, ECRL, EDC, ECU, supinator (EIP, FCU, FDS, FPL, extensor pollicis longus/brevis)
C8	Latissimus dorsi, pectoralis, triceps, anconeus, EDC, ECU, EIP, extensor pollicis longus/brevis, FCU, FDS, FDP, FPL, PQ, APB, APL, OP, AP, ADM, lumbricals, interossei
T1	T1 Pectoralis, FCU, FDS, FDP, FPL, APB, OP, AP, ADM, lumbricals, interossei

ADM, abductor digiti minimi; AP, adductor pollicis; APB, abductor pollicis brevis; APL, abductor pollicis longus; BR, brachioradialis; ECRL, extensor carpi radialis longus; ECU, extensor carpi ulnaris; EDC, extensor digitorum communis; EIP, extensor indicis proprius; FCR, flexor carpi radialis; FCU, flexor carpi ulnaris; FDP, flexor digitorum profundus; FDS, flexor digitorum superficialis; FPL, flexor pollicis longus; OP, opponens pollicis; PQ, pronator quadratus.

Scapulohumeral Rhythm

There are two motions involved in abducting the arm: scapulothoracic and glenohumeral. The scapulothoracic motion is the movement of the scapula in relation to the chest wall; the glenohumeral is the movement at the shoulder joint. These two motions normally occur in harmony to effect smooth arm movements. When the scapula does not move normally, the arm cannot raise normally. As abduction begins, the scapular muscles—especially serratus anterior—fix the scapula, so the pull of the deltoid is on the humerus and not the scapula. As the deltoid abducts the shoulder toward 90 degrees, the serratus anterior and trapezius rotate the scapula. The serratus pulls forward and laterally on the inferior angle, holding the scapula close to the chest wall, while the upper fibers of the trapezius pull up on the lateral end of the clavicle and the lower fibers pull down on the medial part of the scapular spine (Figure 27.4). The smooth interaction of scapula and shoulder joint movements is referred to as the scapulohumeral rhythm. For every 2 degrees of motion at the glenohumeral joint, there is 1 degree of scapular rotation. After the deltoid abducts the arm to the horizontal, further action by the upper trapezius elevates and rotates the scapula further to allow the arm to be raised overhead.

TABLE 27.9 Major Lower-Extremity Muscles Innervated by Different Roots

Parentheses signify minor contribution

Root	Muscles Supplied
L2	Iliopsoas, sartorius, quadriceps (adductors, gracilis)
L3	Iliopsoas, sartorius, adductors, gracilis, quadriceps
L4	Gracilis, gluteus medius, TFL, quadriceps, adductor magnus, TA (iliopsoas, adductor longus)
L5	Gluteus maximus, internal hamstring, biceps femoris, gluteus medius, TFL, peronei, TA, EHL, EDL, EDB, TP, FDL, FHL (adductor magnus)
S1	Internal hamstring, biceps femoris, gluteus maximus, gastrocnemius, soleus, FDL, FHL, ADMP, AH, EDB, lumbricals (gluteus medius, TFL, peronei, EDL, TP)
S2	Gluteus maximus, gastrocnemius, soleus, AH, ADMP, interossei, lumbricals (internal hamstring, short head of biceps femoris)
S3	Interossei, lumbricals, ADMP

ADMP, abductor digiti minimi pedis; AH, abductor hallucis; EDB, extensor digitorum brevis; EDL, extensor digitorum longus; EHL, extensor hallucis longus; FDL, flexor digitorum longus; FHL, flexor hallucis longus; TA, tibialis anterior; TFL, tensor fascia lata; TP, tibialis posterior.

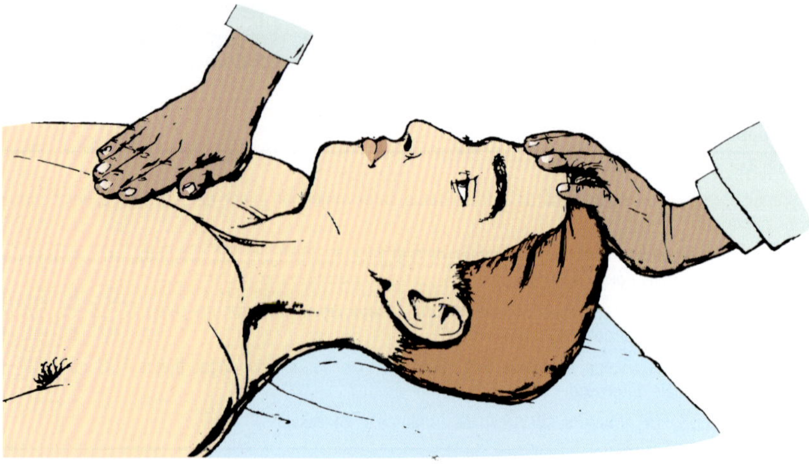

FIGURE 27.1 Examination of flexion of the neck. The patient attempts to flex his neck against resistance; the sternocleidomastoid, platysma, and other flexor muscles can be seen and palpated.

The Scapular Muscles

The rhomboids can be tested by having the patient, with hand on hip, retract the shoulder against the examiner's attempt to push the elbow forward (Figure 27.5). If the patient braces the shoulders backward as if standing at attention, the bulge of the rhomboids can be seen and palpated along the medial border of the scapula. Another test of rhomboid function is to have the patient place the back of the hand against the small of the back and to push backward with the palm against the examiner's resistance. The rhomboid major contracts vigorously as a downward rotator of the scapula. Lifting the hand off the small of the back is also used to test the subscapularis. The levator scapulae is tested by observing elevation of the scapula; it is rarely possible to detect weakness of the levator scapulae on clinical examination.

The different parts of the trapezius must be tested separately. One test of the upper fibers is to have the patient shrug the shoulders against resistance (Figure 19.4). A better test is resisting the patient's

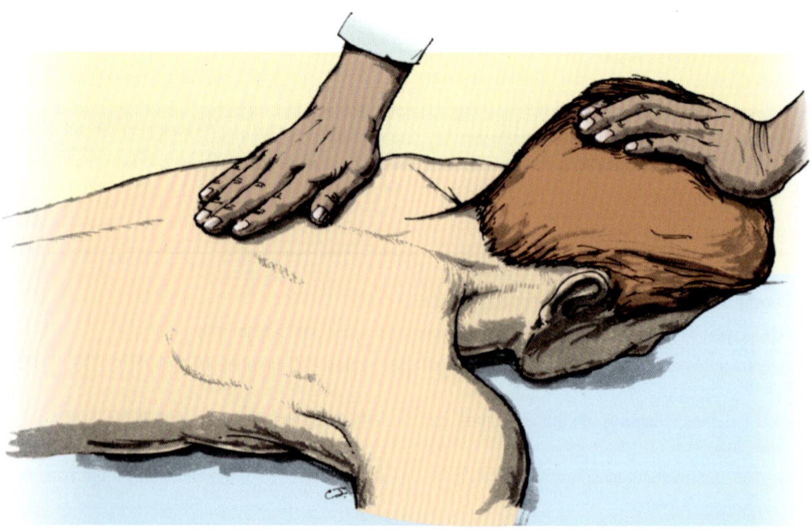

FIGURE 27.2 Examination of extension of the neck. The patient attempts to extend his neck against resistance; contraction of the trapezius and other extensor muscles can be seen and felt, and strength of movement can be judged.

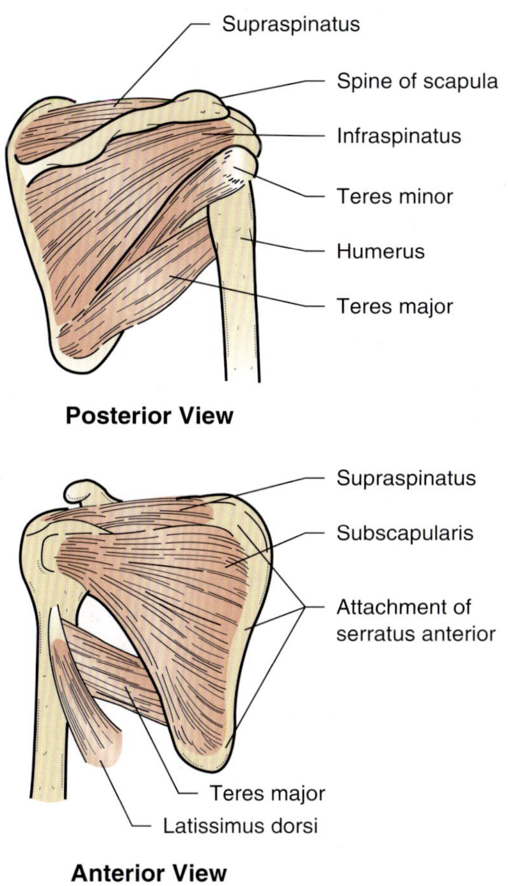

FIGURE 27.3 The muscles of the scapula.

attempt to touch the occiput to the acromion. The middle fibers may be tested by having the patient retract the scapula against resistance (Figure 27.6) or having the patient hold the arm horizontally abducted, palm up, and attempting to push the elbow forward.

With unilateral trapezius paralysis, the patient cannot retract the shoulder or abduct the arm above horizontal. Because of the weight of the arm, the upper portion of the scapula falls laterally, the inferior angle moves medially, and the vertebral border is flared. The sagging of the shoulder causes a drooping of the entire arm, and the fingertips on the involved side are at a lower level than on the normal side. With trapezius atrophy, the superior angle of the scapula may bulge beneath the skin. There is little loss of shoulder-shrug ability because the levator scapulae and rhomboids are able to elevate the scapula, but the normal slant from the base of the neck to the shoulder becomes squared off because of loss of trapezius bulk.

The patient may be able to elevate the arms forward with little or no difficulty because the serratus anterior is primarily responsible for scapular fixation and rotation in that plane.

The serratus anterior can be tested by having the patient make movements that involve forward reaching or pushing and observing for evidence of scapular winging (see next section). When there is significant weakness, abnormalities may appear when the patient simply tries to raise the arm overhead. More subtle degrees of weakness may be brought out by having the patient push forward against resistance. The classical test is to have the patient push against a wall, comparing how well the scapulae remain against the chest wall on the two sides (Figure 27.7).

Winging of the Scapula

Normally, the medial border of the scapula remains close to the chest wall when the arms are raised. However, with weakness of either the serratus anterior or the trapezius, the vertebral border or the entire scapula protrudes posteriorly, away from the thoracic wall. This causes the deformity known as "winging" (Figure 27.8). The trapezius is a rotator and retractor of the scapula and functions primarily during abduction of the arm to the side in the coronal plane of the body. When the trapezius is weak, scapular winging is more apparent on attempted abduction of the arm than on forward elevation. Trapezius winging may be made more conspicuous by having the patient bend forward at the waist so the upper body is parallel to the ground and then raise the arms to the sides, as if beginning a swan dive. This requires strong action by the trapezius to retract the scapula and accentuates the posterior displacement of the shoulder girdle.

The serratus anterior is primarily a protractor of the scapula and functions during forward arm elevation. When the serratus is weak, the inferior angle is shifted medially and the entire vertebral border rides up from the chest wall. Serratus anterior weakness causes winging that is more obvious when trying to elevate the arm in front, in the sagittal plane of the body; it is less obvious when the arms are abducted to the sides. This difference aids in differentiating serratus anterior winging (as from a long thoracic nerve palsy) from the flaring of the scapula that occurs with trapezius weakness (as from a spinal accessory nerve palsy). Serratus winging may be accentuated by having the patient

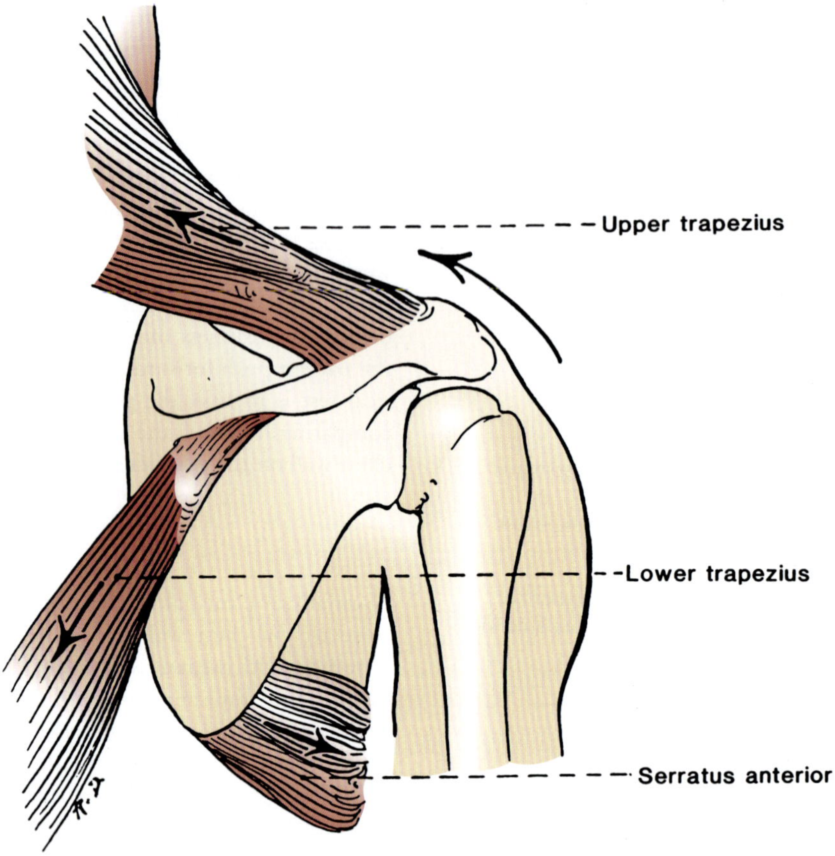

FIGURE 27.4 Upward rotators of the scapula. (Modified from Weibers DO, Dale AJD, Kokmen E, et al., eds. *Mayo Clinic Examinations in Neurology*. 7th ed. St. Louis: Mosby, 1998. Copyright © 1998 Elsevier. With permission.)

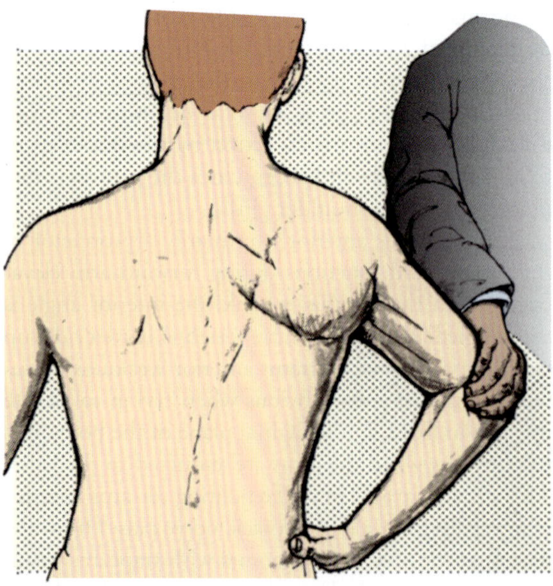

FIGURE 27.5 Examination of the rhomboids. With hand on hip, the patient retracts the shoulder against the examiner's effort to push the elbow forward; the contracting muscles can be seen and palpated.

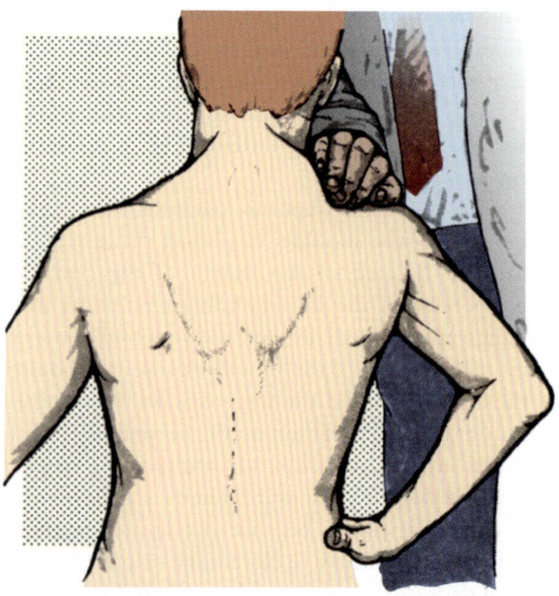

FIGURE 27.6 Examination of the trapezius. On retraction of the shoulder against resistance, the middle fibers of the muscle can be seen and palpated.

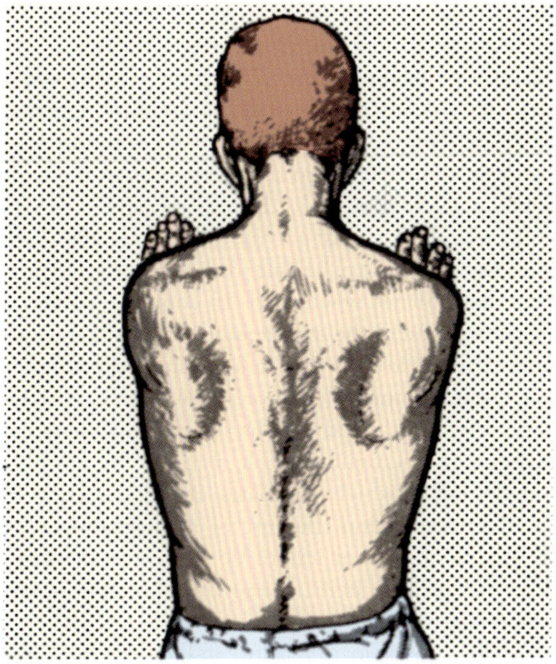

FIGURE 27.7 Examination of the serratus anterior. The patient pushes against a wall with his arms extended horizontally in front of him; normally, the medial border of the scapula remains close to the thoracic wall.

protract the scapula against resistance (Figure 27.7). Another method to bring out mild serratus winging is to have the patient slowly lower the outstretched arms. This downward movement may exacerbate the winging, and at a certain point as the arms descend the scapula will suddenly snap backward. Scapular winging is also discussed in Chapter 19. For a video of scapular winging, see **Video Link 27.1**.

In the muscular dystrophies, particularly facioscapulohumeral (FSH) dystrophy, there is often weakness of all the shoulder girdle muscles, with prominent scapular winging, typically bilateral (Figures 27.8 and 29.6). Another manifestation of shoulder girdle weakness, seen most often in patients with myopathy, is a change in the position of the arms. Normally, as the arms hang at the sides, the thumb faces to the front. With shoulder girdle weakness, the scapula tends to slip laterally so that even at rest the shoulders tend to turn slightly anteriorly. This causes the entire arm to rotate internally, making the back of the hand rather than the thumb face anteriorly. Another effect, especially if there is also pectoral muscle atrophy, may be to produce a crease running diagonally from the anterior axillary fold toward the neck **(Video Link 27.2)**.

The Glenohumeral Joint

The principal movements at the glenohumeral joint are abduction, adduction, external and internal rotation, flexion, extension, and elevation of the arm. These movements are best appreciated as taking place in the plane of the body of the scapula rather than in the body as a whole.

The deltoid is the most prominent muscle in the shoulder region. It is supplied by C5 and C6 through the axillary nerve, a branch of the posterior cord of

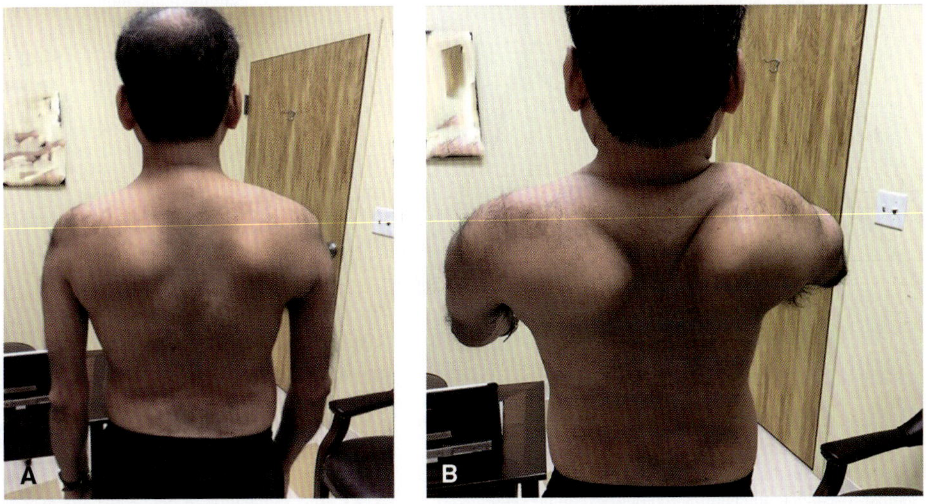

FIGURE 27.8 Scapular winging in a patient with facioscapulohumeral muscular dystrophy. **A.** With the arms at rest. **B.** With the arms raised.

the brachial plexus. The deltoid has three portions: anterior, middle, and posterior. The middle deltoid and supraspinatus muscles, aided by the subscapularis and the upper part of the infraspinatus, abduct the shoulder. With deltoid contraction, the arm is abducted (raised laterally) to the horizontal plane. Further abduction, or elevation above the horizontal plane, is carried out by the associated action of the trapezius and the serratus anterior, which rotate the scapula and tilt the angle of the glenoid fossa upward. In the first 15 degrees, the abduction motion by the deltoid is aided by the supraspinatus, and the synergistic actions of the subscapularis, infraspinatus, and teres minor prevent the humeral head from translating upward. The posterior fibers of the deltoid also assist in extension and external rotation of the arm and the anterior fibers in flexion and internal rotation; but electromyography shows the deltoid is not very active in these movements.

The major function of the deltoid is tested by noting the ability of the patient either to abduct the arm through the range up to 90 degrees against resistance (Figure 27.9) or to hold the arm in abduction to the horizontal level, either laterally or forward (the elbow may be either flexed or extended) and to resist the examiner's attempt to push it down. Testing both sides simultaneously helps the patient maintain balance and also helps in the comparison of strength on the two sides. With MRC grade 3/5 weakness, the patient can abduct the arm against gravity but not against significant resistance. With more severe weakness, the patient may lean in the opposite direction and raise the tip of the shoulder to aid in the attempt (trick movement). When active elevation to the horizontal plane is impossible, the passively abducted arm may be held up against gravity. With grade 2/5 weakness, the patient may be able to abduct the arm when lying flat but not when erect. In complete paralysis, no contraction of the muscle is possible. When weakness of the deltoid is due to a lesion of the anterior horn cells, brachial plexus, or axillary nerve, atrophy appears promptly and may be severe. This leaves the bulge of the acromion visible through the atrophic muscle belly, which simulates the appearance of shoulder dislocation. Because of myotomal overlap, isolated cervical root lesions do not cause the same degree of atrophy. In ALS or cervical spondylosis, fasciculations are often noted.

The supraspinatus helps abduct the shoulder through the first 15 degrees. The muscle belly lies in the supraspinous fossa of the scapula; its contraction can be palpated and sometimes seen when the arm is abducted less than 15 degrees against resistance (Figure 27.10). The supraspinatus is innervated primarily by C5 and C6 and by the suprascapular

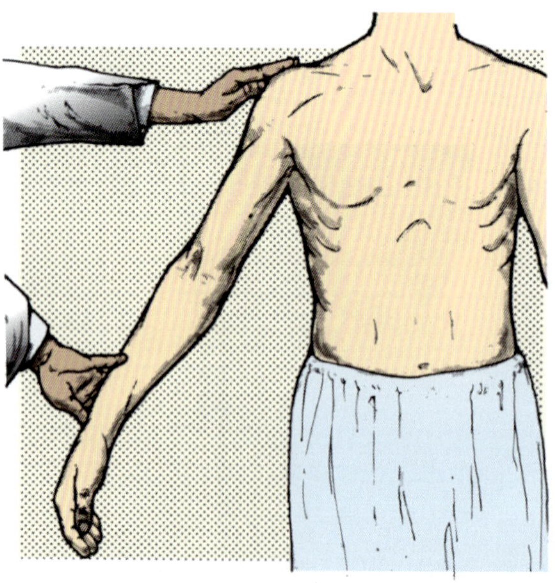

FIGURE 27.9 Examination of the deltoid. The patient attempts to abduct his arm against resistance; the contracting deltoid can be seen and palpated.

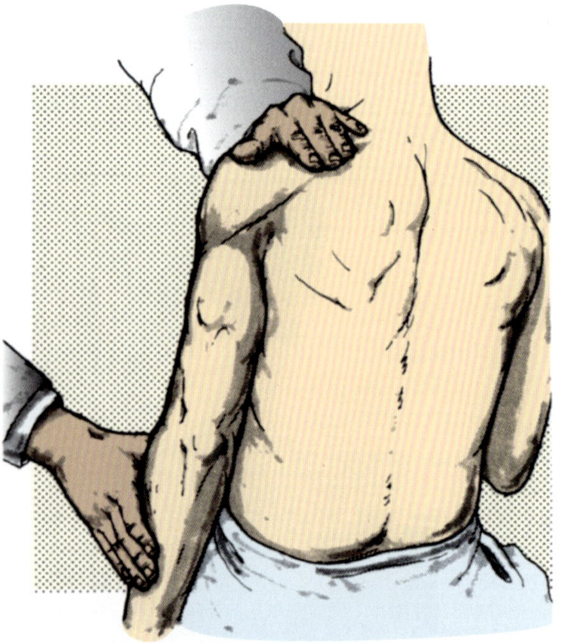

FIGURE 27.10 Examination of the supraspinatus. Contraction of the muscle fibers can be felt during early stages of abduction of the arm.

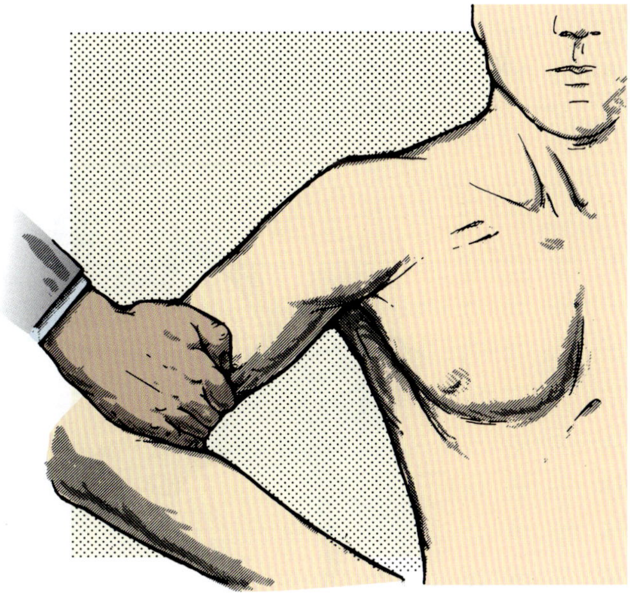

FIGURE 27.11 Examination of the pectoralis major. Contraction of the muscle can be seen and felt during attempts to adduct the arm against resistance.

nerve, which arises directly from the upper trunk of the brachial plexus. Its tendon crosses over the shoulder joint to attach to the greater tuberosity of the humerus, forming one component of the rotator cuff (Chapter 47).

The primary adductors of the shoulder are the pectoralis major and latissimus dorsi. Their adduction actions are difficult to separate. The pectoralis major receives innervation from all levels of the brachial plexus, C5-T1, through the medial and lateral pectoral nerves. It is the principal shoulder adductor and is also a flexor and internal rotator. When the arm is fixed, the muscle draws the chest upward, as in climbing. On attempts to adduct the horizontally abducted arm against resistance, the contraction of the sternocostal and clavicular portions of the muscle can be seen and felt (Figure 27.11). The muscle can also be tested and palpated by having the patient move the horizontally abducted arm forward, try to press the hands together with the arms in front, or try to internally rotate the forearms with the elbows at the side and flexed, in a position as if holding a book.

The latissimus dorsi is supplied by C6-C8 through the thoracodorsal nerve off the posterior cord of the brachial plexus. It adducts, extends, and medially rotates the shoulder and may be tested in various ways. The muscle acts when the patient tries to adduct the raised arm against resistance (Figure 27.12). Along with the teres major, the latissimus forms the posterior axillary fold. The fold becomes prominent when the arm is adducted against resistance and the muscle belly can be easily seen and palpated. The muscle belly can also be felt when the patient coughs or pushes the arm downward and backward. When the humerus is fixed, the latissimus draws the pelvis and the lower part of the trunk forward and upward. When the arm is hanging by the side, it depresses, retracts, and rotates the scapula.

External rotation of the shoulder is carried out principally by the infraspinatus with a minor contribution by the teres minor (axillary nerve, C5-C6). The infraspinatus is innervated by the suprascapular nerve, C5 and C6, which also innervates the supraspinatus. To test these muscles, the patient attempts to externally rotate the shoulder by turning the forearm laterally and backward against resistance while the elbow is flexed at an angle of 90 degrees and held at the side (Figure 27.13).

Internal rotation at the shoulder chiefly results from contraction of the subscapularis and teres major muscles. These muscles are tested by having the patient move the forearm medially against resistance with the elbow flexed and at the side—the opposite motion from external rotation. Internal rotation can also be tested by having the patient lift the back of the hand off the small of the back against resistance, as is done when testing the rhomboids (see "The Scapular Muscles" above).

Flexion of the shoulder (forward elevation of the arm in the sagittal plane of the body) is carried out by the anterior fibers of the deltoid and the pectoralis

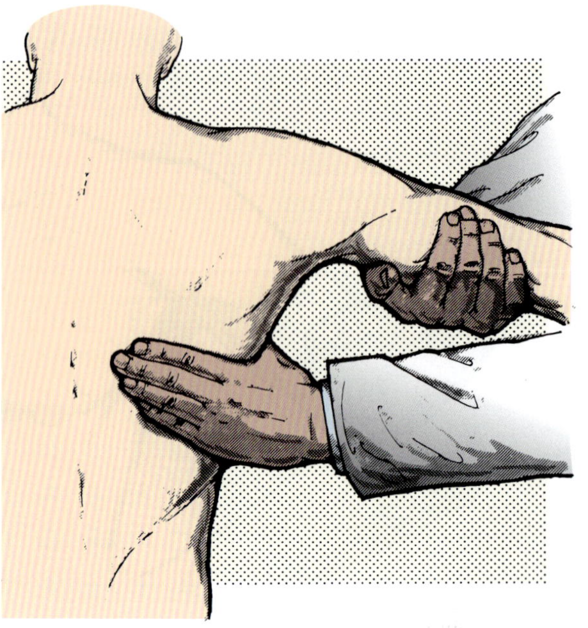

FIGURE 27.12 Examination of the latissimus dorsi. On adduction of the horizontally and laterally abducted arm against resistance, the contracting muscle fibers can be seen and palpated. An effective way to compare the latissimus contraction strength on the two sides is to firmly grasp the muscle bellies from behind and have the patient cough.

major, subscapularis, coracobrachialis, and biceps muscles. The muscles, especially the deltoid and pectoralis, may be palpated when raising the arm forward against resistance. Extension of the shoulder (backward elevation of the arm) is carried out by the posterior fibers of the deltoid together with the latissimus dorsi, triceps, subscapularis, and teres major muscles. This action can be tested by having the patient attempt to extend the arm against resistance. The individual muscles concerned are better examined by the tests discussed in the preceding paragraphs.

The Rotator Cuff

The subscapularis, supraspinatus, infraspinatus, and teres minor form the rotator cuff. The infraspinatus and teres minor rotate the humerus externally and the

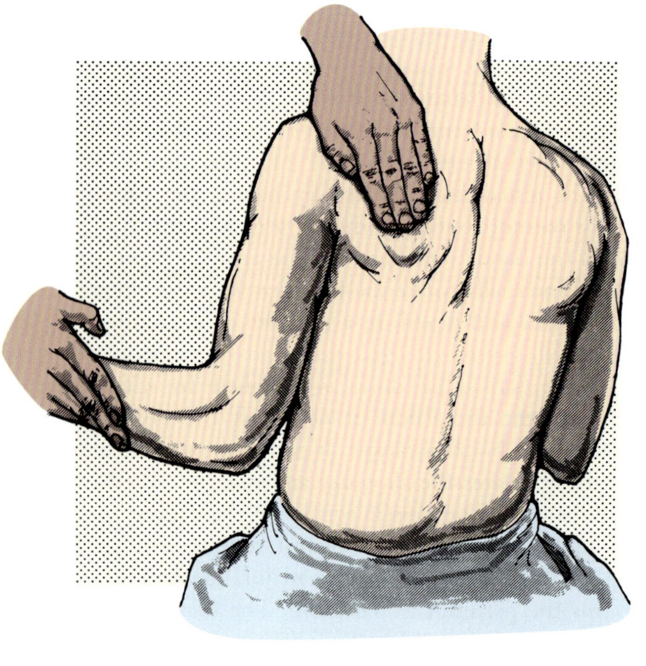

FIGURE 27.13 Examination of the external rotators of the arm. On external rotation of the arm while the elbow is flexed and kept close to the body, the contracting infraspinatus muscle can be seen and palpated.

subscapularis internally. The subscapularis, infraspinatus, and teres minor help keep the humeral head from sliding upward when the deltoid contracts during the initial stages of abduction. The supraspinatus, more than the deltoid, keeps the humeral head from migrating downward when the arm is hanging down. Rotator cuff tears are a common clinical problem. Rotator cuff pathology often enters the differential diagnosis in patients with arm pain and weakness. A torn rotator cuff, especially impaired arm abduction due to a ruptured supraspinatus muscle or tendon (the most common component of the rotator cuff to suffer a tear), can be confused with a neurologic process (Chapter 47).

The Elbow

The principal movements at the elbow are flexion and extension of the forearm at the elbow joint and pronation and supination at the radioulnar joint.

Many muscles contribute to elbow flexion; the primary ones are the biceps brachii, brachialis, and brachioradialis. Which muscle is the prime mover depends on the position of the forearm. The biceps muscle is innervated by C5-C6 through the musculocutaneous nerve, a branch of the lateral cord of the brachial plexus. It is an elbow flexor and also a strong supinator of the forearm. Its supination power is greatest when the forearm is flexed and pronated. Its flexion power is greatest when the forearm is supinated. The brachialis has the same innervation; it flexes the elbow regardless of forearm position. The musculocutaneous nerve passes through the coracobrachialis and may be compressed there, causing weakness of the biceps and brachialis muscles. The brachioradialis is innervated by C5-C6 through the radial nerve. It acts as an elbow flexor when the forearm is held midway between pronation and supination (thumb up). The brachioradialis acts as a supinator when the forearm is extended and pronated but as a pronator when the forearm is flexed and supinated.

Biceps and brachialis functions are tested by having the patient attempt to flex the elbow against resistance. The biceps contraction can be seen and felt, but the brachialis is buried (Figure 27.14). The brachioradialis is tested by attempts to flex the semipronated forearm (Figure 27.15). Even when the biceps and brachialis are completely paralyzed, the brachioradialis is still capable of flexing the elbow to some degree. When the biceps muscle is weak, the patient may employ trick movements by putting the forearm into midpronation and bringing in the brachioradialis or pulling the elbow backwards. The latter resembles the movement bartenders make when drawing a draft beer and has been called the "bartender's sign."

The triceps brachii is the principal elbow extensor. It is innervated by C6, C7, and C8 through the radial nerve, a branch of the posterior cord of the

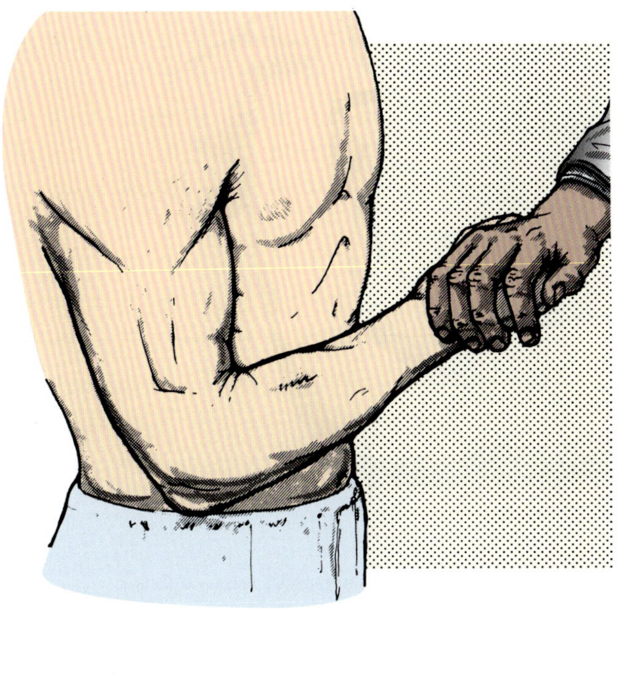

FIGURE 27.14 Examination of the biceps brachii. On attempts to flex the forearm against resistance, the contracting biceps muscle can be seen and palpated.

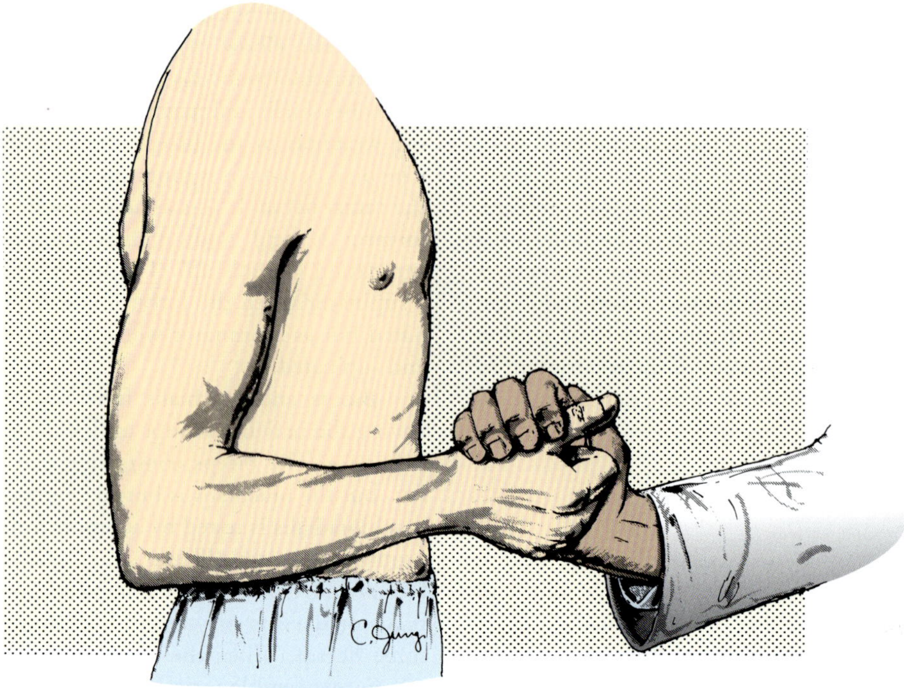

FIGURE 27.15 Examination of the brachioradialis. On flexion of the semipronated forearm (thumb up) against resistance, the contracting muscle can be seen and palpated.

brachial plexus. The branches to the triceps come off before the nerve enters the spiral groove. The anconeus aids the triceps in extension. To test these muscles, place the elbow in a position midway between flexion and extension and have the patient attempt to either extend the elbow or to hold position against the examiner's resistance (Figure 27.16). The triceps muscle is less powerful when the elbow is fully flexed,

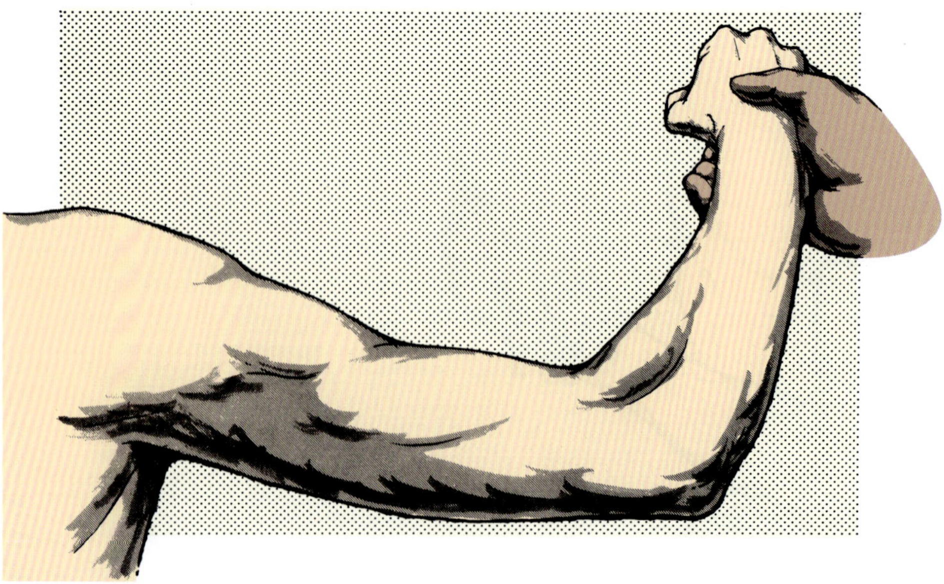

FIGURE 27.16 Extension of the forearm. On attempts to extend the partially flexed forearm against resistance, contraction of the triceps can be seen and palpated.

and slight weakness may be more easily detected with testing in this position. With mild triceps weakness, the examiner may be able to pin the triceps in extreme flexion on the involved but not the normal side.

Supination of the forearm is done primarily by the supinator muscle, assisted by stronger muscles, especially the biceps, for movements requiring power.

The supinator has superficial and deep layers; the proximal edge of the superficial head is the arcade of Frohse. The posterior interosseous nerve passes beneath the arcade and may be compressed there. The supinator is innervated by C6 and C7, either by the posterior interosseous nerve or the radial in different individuals. The biceps muscle is the most powerful forearm supinator; its action is strongest when the forearm is flexed and pronated. The supinator is less powerful, but it acts through all degrees of flexion and supination. Supination is tested by having the patient supinate against the examiner's resistance. With the forearm in extension, the brachioradialis also participates; with the forearm in flexion, the biceps also participates (Figure 27.17).

Pronation is brought about primarily by the pronator quadratus (PQ), which is assisted by the much stronger PT for movements requiring power. Other muscles may play a minor role. The PT originates from the common flexor tendon (CFT) that arises from the medial epicondyle. Like the other muscles that arise from the CFT (flexor carpi radialis [FCR], palmaris longus, flexor carpi ulnaris [FCU], and flexor digitorum superficialis [FDS]), the PT is also an elbow flexor. To test the PT and PQ, the patient attempts to pronate against resistance (Figure 27.18). The PT has a humeral and an ulnar head. The median nerve usually enters the forearm between the two heads and supplies the muscle (C6 and C7). The PQ is innervated by the anterior interosseous branch of the median nerve (C7-C8). The anterior interosseous nerve comes off the median nerve between the two heads of the PT. The anterior interosseous nerve, less often the main trunk of the median nerve, may be compressed between the two heads of the PT (pronator syndrome). To isolate the action of the PQ, pronation should be tested with the elbow extended, when the PT is maximally lengthened and exerts its weakest pull. Flexion of the elbow would signal that the patient is trying to bring the PT into play.

The Wrist

The principal movements at the wrist are flexion and extension; adduction (ulnar flexion) and abduction (radial flexion) are minor movements.

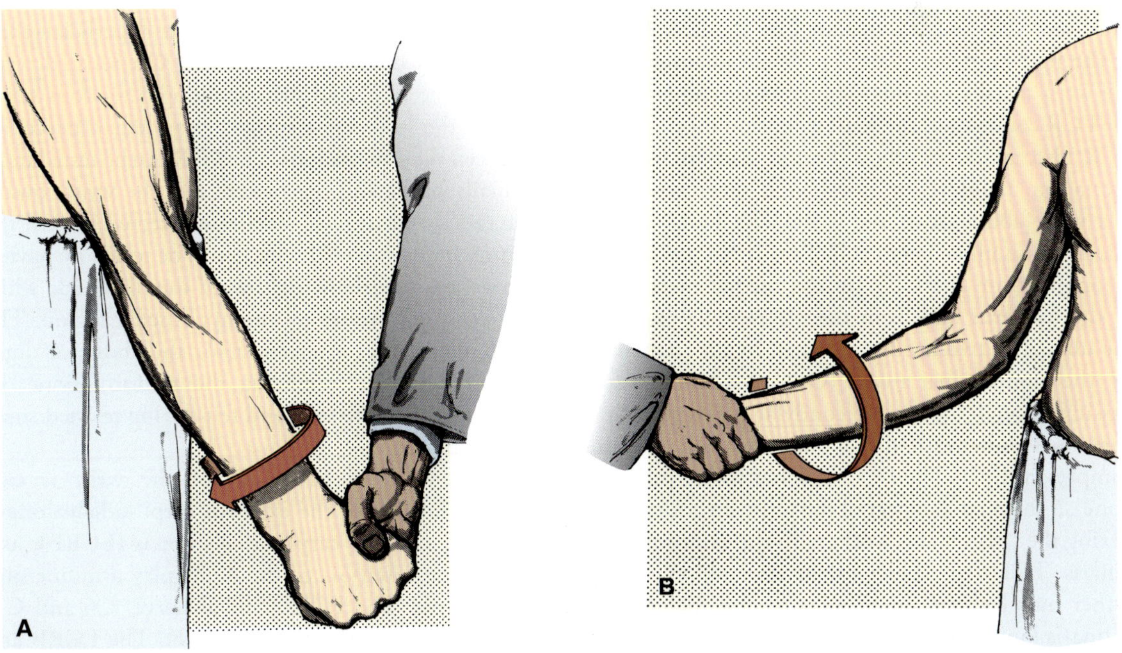

FIGURE 27.17 Supination of the forearm. **A.** On attempts to supinate the extended forearm against resistance, the contracting brachioradialis can be seen and palpated. **B.** On attempts to supinate the flexed forearm against resistance, the contracting biceps can be seen and palpated.

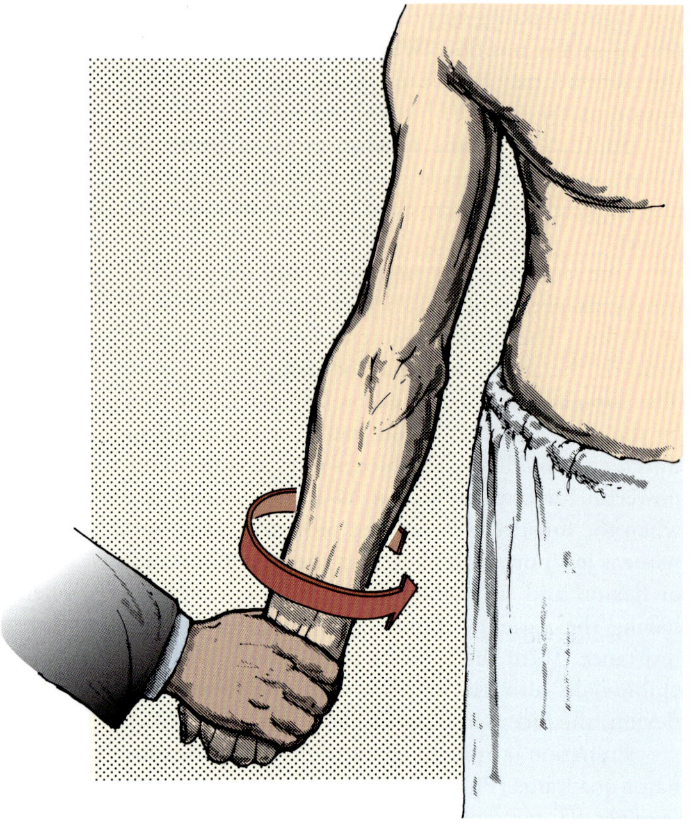

FIGURE 27.18 Pronation of the forearm. On pronation of the forearm against resistance, contraction of the pronator teres can be seen and palpated.

Flexion of the wrist is carried out principally by the FCR and FCU muscles. The FCR originates from the CFT and is innervated by the lateral head of the median nerve (C6-C7). When making a fist, the wrist usually extends slightly as the fingers flex; the FCR counteracts the wrist extension motion. The FCR also assists in elbow flexion and in forearm pronation. It inserts on the second metacarpal and is a weak abductor of the wrist. The FCU is supplied by the ulnar nerve (C7-T1). It has two heads of origin: from the CFT on the medial epicondyle of the humerus and from the olecranon process of the ulna. The two heads are joined by an aponeurosis, the humeroulnar arcade (Osborne's band). After passing through the retroepicondylar grove, the ulnar nerve passes beneath the aponeurosis and may be compressed by it. The FCU attaches to the pisiform bone on the medial aspect of the wrist. In addition to flexing the wrist, it also works with the extensor carpi ulnaris (ECU) to adduct (ulnar deviate) the hand. Other muscles that aid in wrist flexion include the palmaris longus, flexor digitorum profundus (FDP), FDS, flexor pollicis longus (FPL), and abductor pollicis longus (APL).

Wrist flexion is tested by having the patient resist the examiner's attempts to extend the wrist (Figure 27.19). Both the FCR and FCU are superficial; their contraction can be seen and felt. On resisted wrist flexion, the FCR and palmaris longus tendons stand out on the volar wrist surface; the median nerve lies between the two tendons. The FCR can be tested individually by having the patient flex the wrist toward the radial side against resistance directed toward the thumb. Function of the FCU can be tested by having the patient flex the wrist toward the ulnar side while the examiner presses on the hypothenar region. The FCU also acts as a synergist for the abductor digiti minimi (ADM), stabilizing the pisiform bone; its contraction can be seen and felt during resisted small finger abduction.

Extension (dorsiflexion) of the wrist is executed primarily by the extensor carpi radialis longus (ECRL), extensor carpi radialis brevis (ECRB), and ECU. The extensors of the digits play a minor supportive role. The ECRL (radial nerve, C6 and C7) is the most powerful wrist extensor. The ECRB and ECU are innervated by the posterior interosseous branch of the radial nerve (C7-C8). In a posterior

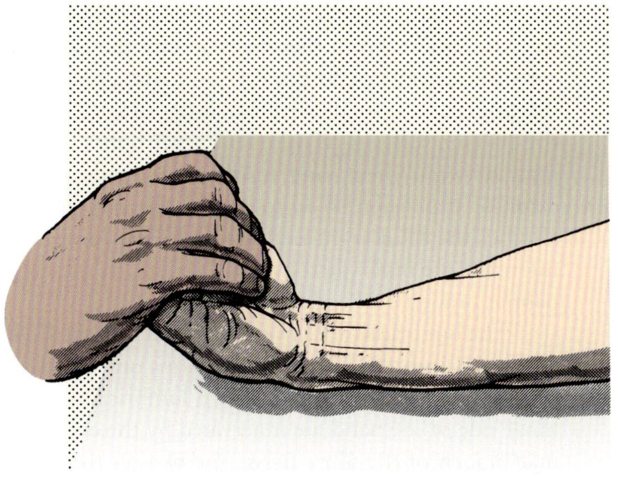

FIGURE 27.19 Flexion at the wrist. On flexion of the hand at the wrist against resistance, the tendon of the flexor carpi radialis can be seen and palpated on the radial side of the wrist and that of the flexor carpi ulnaris on the ulnar side; the tendon of the palmaris longus can also be seen and palpated.

interosseous neuropathy, the wrist deviates radially on extension because of the unbalanced pull of the ECRL.

To test the wrist extensors, the forearm is held in pronation with the wrist partially extended. The patient then resists the examiner's attempts to pull the wrist into flexion (Figure 27.20). With mild weakness, the examiner may be able to hold the wrist in extreme flexion using one or two fingers against the patient's efforts to extend it on the involved but not the normal side. Moderate weakness of the extensors results in involuntary flexion at the wrist when the patient attempts to make a fist; marked weakness causes a wrist drop, the major finding in a radial nerve palsy.

Adduction, or ulnar deviation or flexion, of the wrist is carried out principally by the FCU and ECU; abduction, or radial deviation or flexion, is carried out by the FCR, ECRL, and ECRB. Other muscles may make minor contributions. These movements, too, may be tested by carrying them out against resistance.

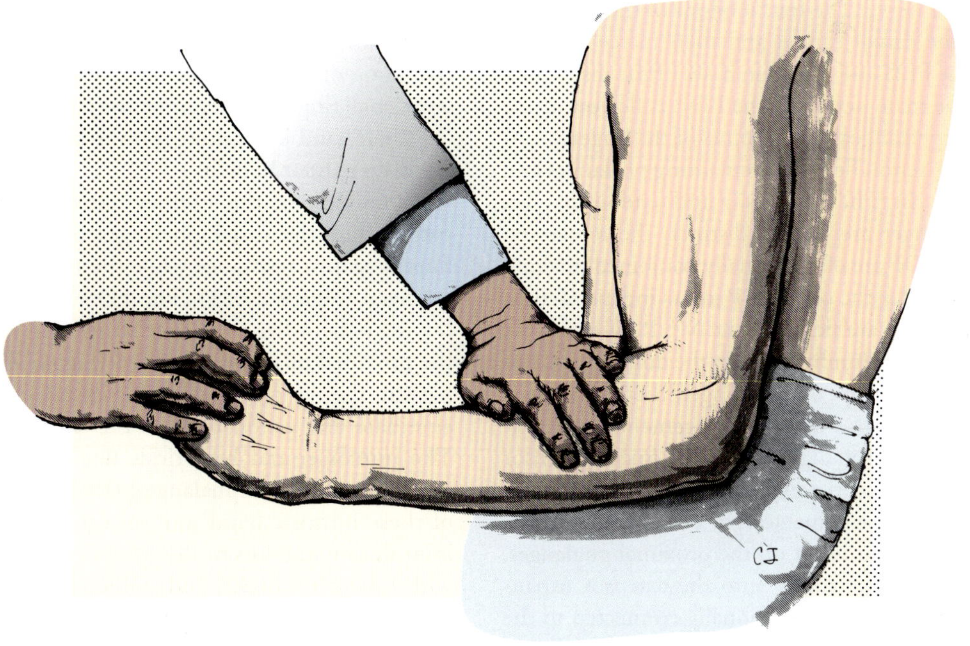

FIGURE 27.20 Extension at the wrist. On attempts to extend the hand at the wrist against resistance, the bellies of the extensors carpi radialis longus, carpi ulnaris, and digitorum communis can be seen and palpated.

The Hands and Fingers

Examination of the hand and finger muscles is difficult. Innervation is complex, and the numerous possible substitution movements can lead to misinterpretation. Possible movements include flexion, extension, adduction, abduction, and opposition. The muscles that power the hand can be divided into extrinsics and intrinsics. The extrinsic muscles originate in the forearm and insert on hand structures; the intrinsics originate and insert within the hand.

Flexion of the Fingers

The primary finger flexors are the FDS and the FDP. The FDS and FDP are both innervated by C8 and T1. The FDS is supplied by the main trunk of the median nerve. Its tendons pass through the carpal tunnel and then diverge to insert on the palmar surfaces of the middle phalanges. The FDS primarily flexes the proximal interphalangeal (PIP) joints of the four fingers; a continuation of its action flexes the metacarpophalangeal (MCP) joints and ultimately the wrist. There are separate muscle slips for each finger, so the PIP joints can be flexed independently. The FDP has two parts: (a) The lateral or radial head is innervated by the anterior interosseous branch of the median nerve and (b) the medial or ulnar head by the ulnar nerve. The four tendons of the FDP pass through the carpal tunnel and then pierce the tendons of the FDS and insert on bases of the distal phalanges. The main action of the FDP is flexion of the distal interphalangeal (DIP) joints of the fingers; continuing this action flexes the remaining phalanges and finally the wrist. The muscle slip and tendon that flex the index finger are usually distinct; the remaining slips of the FDP are often partially conjoined, making it difficult to flex the other DIP joints independently.

The fingers are flexed at the MCP joints by the interossei and the lumbricals. On the dorsal surface of the proximal phalanx of each finger, there is a dorsal extensor expansion, a fibrous enlargement of the tendon of the extensor digitorum. The finger extensor tendons blend into the expansion. The dorsal interossei lie between the metacarpal bones, from which they originate, and insert on the proximal phalanges. They also insert separately into the extensor expansions and are therefore functionally connected to the finger extensor tendons. Finger adduction and abduction are judged in relation to an imaginary line down the center of the middle finger. From the insertion on the proximal phalanx, the dorsal interossei flex the MCP joint. From their insertion on the extensor expansion, they extend the PIP joint and also abduct the fingers. The smaller palmar interossei arise from the palmar surfaces of the metacarpal bones, rather than between them, and insert on the side of the extensor expansion so as to adduct the finger; they also flex the MCP joint and extend the PIP joint. The interossei are innervated by C8-T1 through the deep palmar branch of the ulnar nerve.

The lumbricals arise from the tendons of the FDP and insert into the extensor expansions on the dorsal surfaces of the phalanges. The two lumbricals on the ulnar side of the hand are innervated by the deep palmar branch of the ulnar nerve, the two on the radial side of the hand by the median nerve, all C8-T1. The lumbricals are weak flexors of the MCP joints. Their more important function is to extend the PIP joints.

The flexor digiti minimi brevis flexes and slightly abducts the proximal phalanx of the little finger. Two other muscles acting on the little finger are the ADM, which abducts the little finger, flexes its proximal phalanx, and extends the middle phalanx, and the opponens digiti minimi, which flexes, adducts, and slightly rotates the fifth metacarpal. All three muscles are supplied by C8-T1 through the ulnar nerve proximal to the origin of the deep palmar branch. The palmaris brevis has the same innervation; it wrinkles the skin over the hypothenar eminence and deepens the hollow of the hand. The palmaris brevis sign is wrinkling of the skin over the hypothenar eminence with small finger abduction in the face of weakness of the ulnar hand intrinsics; it proves the lesion involves the deep palmar branch.

Function of the FDP is tested by having the patient flex the distal phalanges of the individual fingers against resistance while the middle phalanges are fixed (Figure 27.21). The FDS is tested by having the patient flex the fingers at the PIP joints while the proximal phalanges are fixed (Figure 27.22). The patient should try to relax the distal phalanges to eliminate any action of the FDP on the PIP joint. The interossei and lumbricals flex the MCP joints and extend the interphalangeal (IP) joints. Weakness of these intrinsic hand muscles causes loss of MCP joint flexion and loss of PIP joint extension, together with loss of adduction and abduction of the fingers. The hand assumes a position of rest in which the MCP joints are held in extension and the PIP and DIP joints are flexed (claw hand). Ulnar neuropathy is the most common cause of claw hand (ulnar griffe).

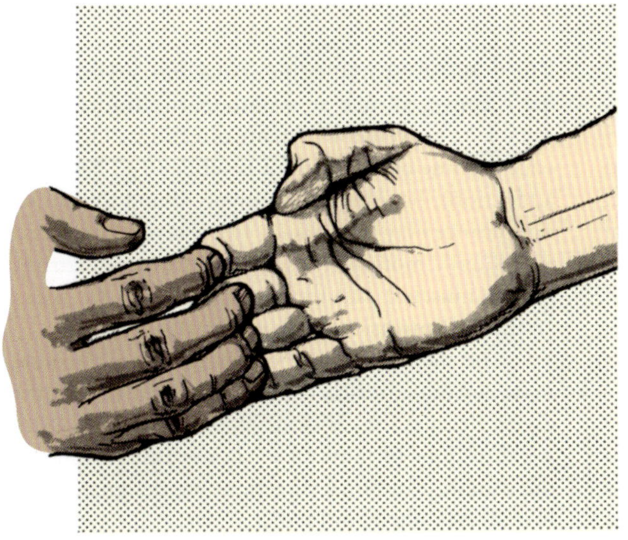

FIGURE 27.21 Examination of the flexor digitorum profundus. The patient resists attempts to extend the distal phalanges while the middle phalanges are fixed.

Ulnar clawing primarily affects the ring and small fingers because both lumbrical and interosseous functions are lost.

Making a fist requires flexion of the fingers at all joints. The strength of the grip depends on the degree of flexion at the MCP and IP joints, on the position of the thumb and its ability to flex and to brace the fingers, and on the synergistic actions of the wrist extensors in fixation of the wrist. A firm fist can be made only with the wrist in extension. Grip is commonly used in the assessment of upper-extremity strength. An examiner cannot easily extricate his fingers from the clenched hand of a person with normal grip strength. For quantitative testing, a dynamometer may be used. In fact, although commonly done, grip power is not very useful in assessing upper-extremity motor function in neurologic patients for the following reasons. The finger and wrist flexors are not corticospinal innervated and are not likely to be weak with a mild CST lesion. Grip strength is so unaffected by CST pathology that many patients with a severe, spastic hemiparesis have a tightly fisted hand—enough that palmar hygiene may become a problem. In addition, grip is a complex movement with many different muscles involved, so it is insensitive to peripheral pathology as well. A good rule is that one can use grip as a strength test only if prepared to name all the muscles involved along with their peripheral nerve, brachial plexus, and root innervations. An examiner sophisticated enough to know this information will be testing individual hand muscles, not grip strength.

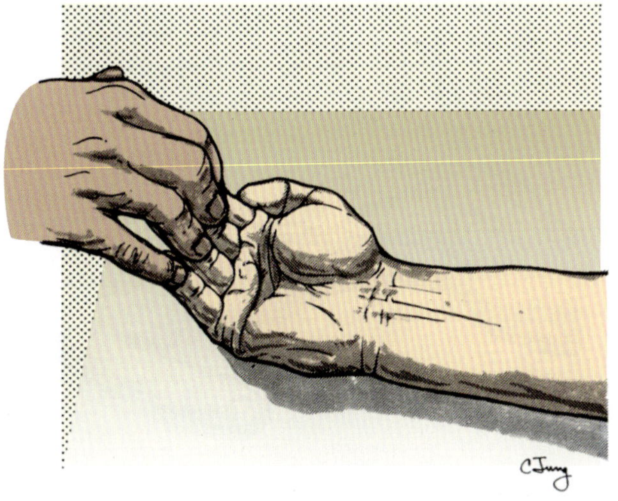

FIGURE 27.22 Examination of the flexor digitorum superficialis. The patient resists attempts to straighten the fingers at the first interphalangeal (IP) joint.

Extension of the Fingers

The long extensors of the fingers include the extensor digitorum communis (EDC), extensor indicis proprius (EIP, aka extensor indicis), and the extensor digiti minimi (EDM). All the finger extensors are innervated by C7-C8 through the posterior interosseous branch of the radial nerve. The tendons insert on the dorsal extensor expansions of the first phalanges of the fingers. The primary action of the EDC is extension of the MCP joints. However, the EDC can exert some force to extend each joint it crosses, including the wrist and—through the extensor expansion complexes—the PIP and DIP joints. Its action on the MCP joints causes some spreading of the fingers, and patients with weakness of the interossei may use this as a trick movement to abduct the fingers. The EIP extends the index finger and adducts it slightly. The EDM extends the little finger. The interossei and lumbricals also extend the PIP and DIP joints of the fingers.

To test the action of the EDC, EIP, and EDM, the patient resists attempts to push the fingers down at the MCP joints with the forearm pronated and the wrist stabilized (Figure 27.23). A useful technique is for the examiner to try to overcome the patient's finger extensors with his own. Because they have separate muscles, the index and little fingers can extend independently, but it is very difficult to extend either the middle or ring finger without moving the other. The extensor function of the lumbricals and interossei is tested by having the patient try to extend the PIP and DIP joints against resistance while the MCP joints are hyperextended and fixed (Figure 27.24).

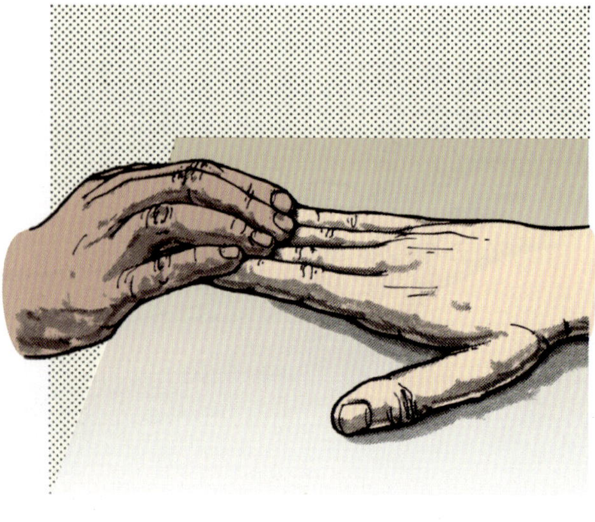

FIGURE 27.23 Examination of the extensor digitorum communis. With hand outstretched and IP joints held in extension, the patient resists the examiner's attempt to flex the fingers at the metacarpophalangeal (MCP) joints.

The Thumb and Its Muscles

The thumb is a complex bit of machinery; small wonder it conveyed such an evolutionary advantage. It is capable of movement in many directions. The difference in some of the motions is subtle (e.g., flexion vs. adduction), but the muscle involved and the clinical significance may be marked. Two sets of muscles control thumb motion: those in the forearm (extrinsic thumb muscles) and those that make up the thenar eminence (intrinsic thumb muscles).

The mobility of the opposable thumb requires more elaborate muscle control compared to the other digits. Because the classical anatomical terms describing directions of movement are not easily applied to the thumb, additional directions are designated: palmar, dorsal, ulnar, and radial.

The IP and MCP joints can flex and extend. The carpometacarpal joint can move in many directions. In palmar abduction, the thumb moves upward at right angles to the plane of the palm; in radial abduction, the thumb moves away in the plane of the palm. Ulnar and palmar adductions are movements that touch the first and second metacarpals together. Opposition (anteposition) is the motion of circumduction of the thumb with extended MCP and IP joints; this turns the thumb into semipronation and touches the palmar surface of the tip of the thumb to the palmar surface of the tip of the small finger.

The forearm muscles involved in controlling the thumb are the APL, extensor pollicis longus (EPL), extensor pollicis brevis (EPB), and FPL. The APL abducts the thumb and extends it to a slight degree. The EPL extends the terminal phalanx; the

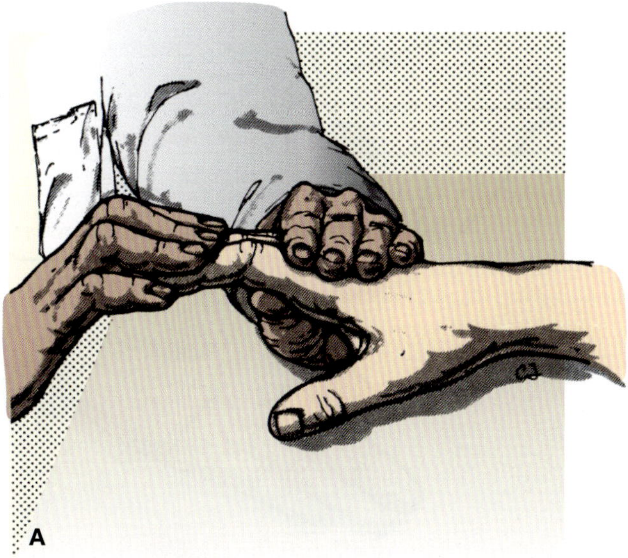

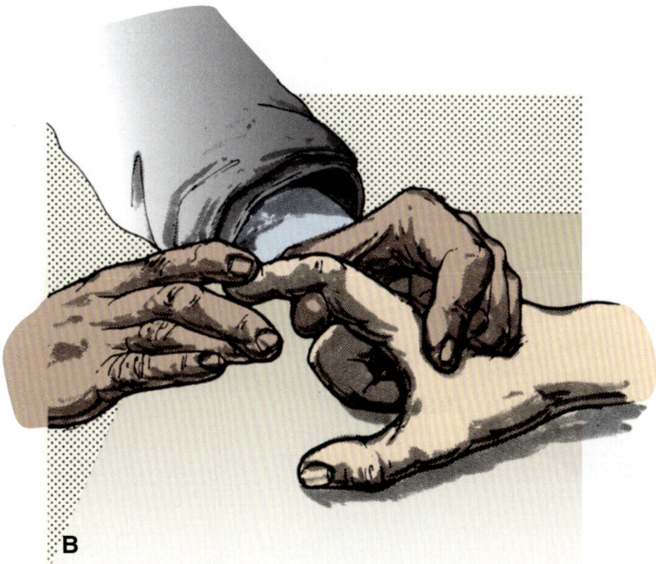

FIGURE 27.24 A and B. Extension of the middle and distal phalanges. The patient attempts to extend the fingers against resistance while the MCP joints are fixed.

EPB extends the proximal phalanx. These three muscles are supplied by the C7-C8 cervical segments through the posterior interosseous branch of the radial nerve. The APL is the only muscle in the flexor pronator compartment of the forearm supplied by the radial nerve. The FPL (anterior interosseous branch of the median nerve, C8-T1) flexes the distal phalanx of the thumb. To test the FPL, the patient flexes the distal phalanx of the thumb while the proximal phalanx is flexed and immobilized (Figure 27.25). The EPL is tested by having the patient extend the thumb at the IP joint while the proximal phalanx is immobilized (Figure 27.26). The EPB is tested by having the patient extend the thumb at the MCP joint while the metacarpal bone is immobilized (Figure 27.27). Hyperextending the thumb, especially at both joints, causes the tendons of the EPL, EPB, and APL to stand out, forming the "anatomic snuff box."

The thenar eminence is the mass of muscles on the palmar surface overlying the first metacarpal. The muscles that make up the thenar eminence are the APB, opponens pollicis (OP), and flexor pollicis brevis (FPB). The APL and APB muscles produce palmar abduction. The OP pronates the thumb, turning the volar thumb surface down, to touch the tip of the

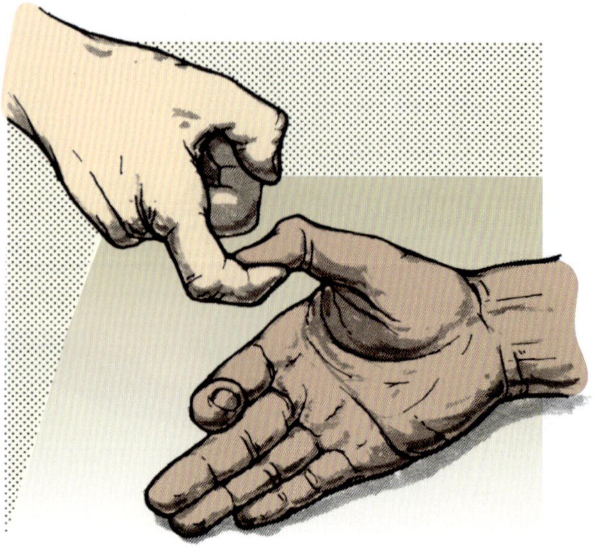

FIGURE 27.25 Examination of the flexor pollicis longus. The patient resists attempts to extend the distal phalanx of the thumb while the proximal phalanx is fixed.

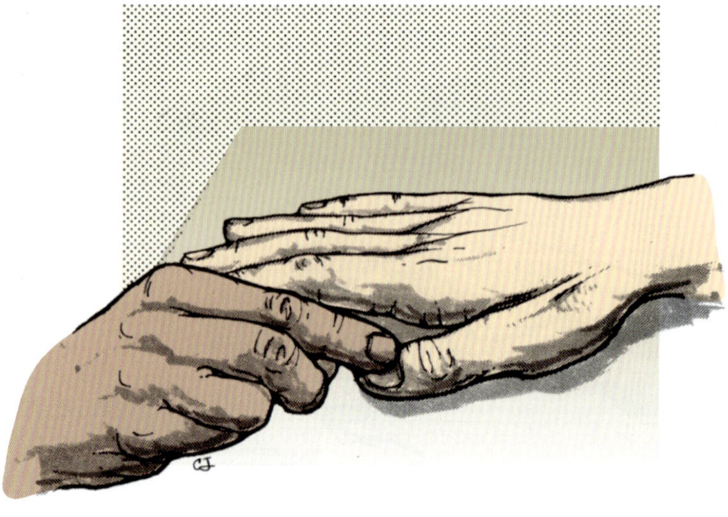

FIGURE 27.26 Examination of the extensor pollicis longus. The patient attempts to resist passive flexion of the thumb at the IP joint; the tendon can be seen and palpated.

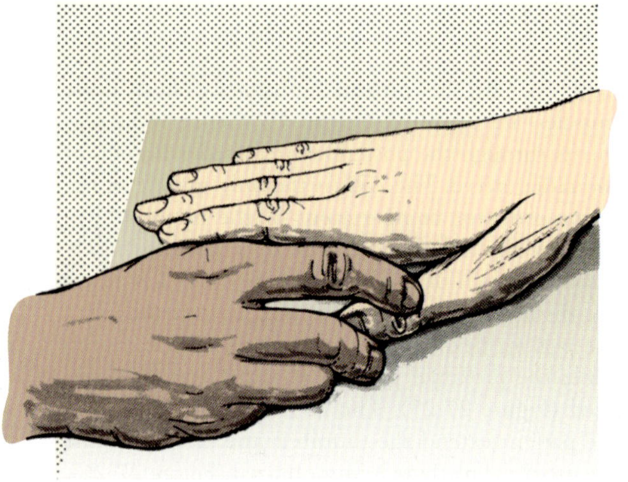

FIGURE 27.27 Examination of the extensor pollicis brevis. The patient attempts to resist passive flexion of the thumb at the MCP joint; the tendon can be seen and palpated.

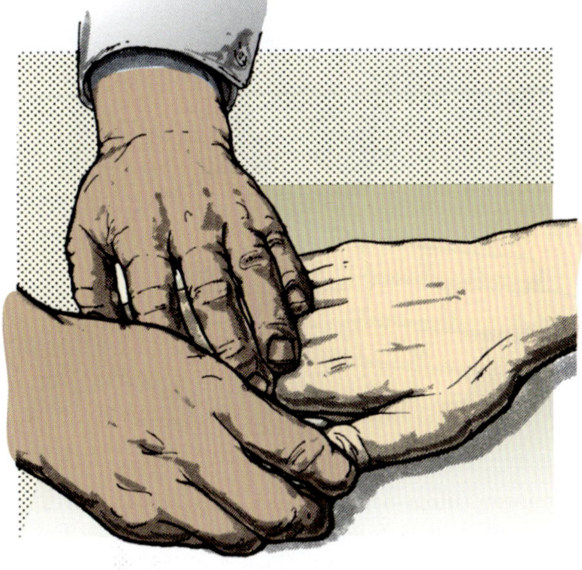

FIGURE 27.28 Radial abduction of the thumb. The patient attempts to abduct the thumb in the same plane as that of the palm; the tendon of the abductor pollicis longus can be seen and palpated.

thumb to the small finger. The FPB flexes the MCP joint of the thumb. In testing the FPB, the patient is asked to flex the MCP joint of the thumb while keeping the IP joint extended. The FPB has a superficial head supplied by the median nerve and a deep head by the deep palmar branch of the ulnar nerve, all C8-T1. The rest of the thenar muscles are supplied by C8-T1 through the median nerve.

Abduction of the thumb is carried out in two planes: in the same plane as the palm (radial abduction) and at right angles to the plane of the palm (palmar abduction). To test radial abduction, the thumb is moved outward if the hand is horizontal, and upward if the hand is vertical, against resistance. This movement is executed by the APL and EPB (Figure 27.28). The APB is a thin sheet of muscle lying just medial to the first metacarpal that performs palmar abduction. To test palmar abduction, the thumb is moved upward at right angles to the palm, inside the radial margin of the hand, against resistance. It is very easy for both patient and physician to confuse abduction with extension. One trick is to place a pencil or similar object between the thumb and the palm, or radial to the thumb, perpendicular to the palm. The patient then raises the thumb to a point vertically above its original position, keeping it parallel to the pencil with the thumbnail at right angles to the palm (Figure 27.29). In paralysis of abduction, the thumb is adducted and rotated, thumbnail parallel rather than perpendicular to the fingernails, falling into the plane of the palm (simian or ape hand, Figure 46.6).

The APB is most often tested by having the patient place the thumb in full palmar abduction and hold it there as the examiner tries to force the thumb down toward the palm. The examiner may do this in several ways. A commonly used technique is for the examiner to hold the back of the patient's hand in his palm, touch the radial side of the patient's thumb with the palmar aspect of his own (usually right hand against right hand), and then make a compound motion with the long and short flexors and opponens to pull the patient's thumb down. The patient, using only his thumb abductors, is outnumbered and outgunned and will usually lose. A better technique is to use APB against APB. The examiner holds the patient's hand as above. The examiner and patient both hold their thumbs in full abduction, radial aspect to radial aspect, IP joint to IP joint; then, the examiner, using only his thumb abductors, tries to press the patient's thumb down. This is normally a match. If the patient's APB yields, the degree of weakness may be semiquantitated if the examiner then uses progressively weaker muscles against the patient's APB. This is sometimes useful for follow-up. Suppose the patient's APB could be overcome by the examiner's APB, first dorsal interosseous (first DI), and ADM on the first visit, but after treatment, the patient's APB can stand up to the examiner's ADM. This means that there has been improvement. If the patient's APB could stand up to the examiner's ADM initially but fails later, then there has been worsening.

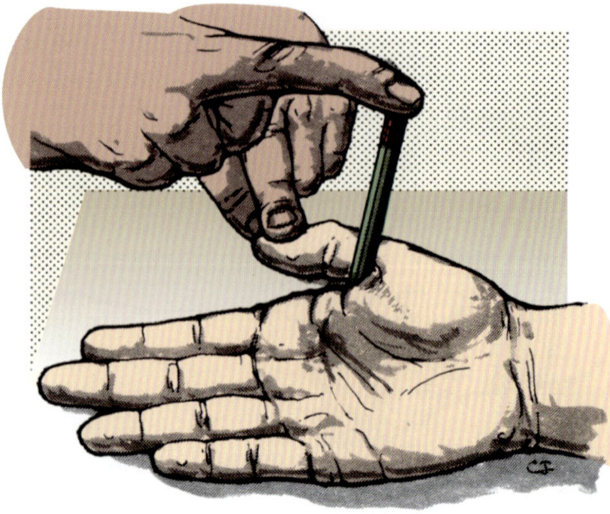

FIGURE 27.29 Palmar abduction of the thumb. The patient attempts, against resistance, to bring the thumb to a point vertically above its original position.

Side-to-side "confrontational testing" is a similar like-muscle-against-like-muscle method for testing hand intrinsic strength. The patient pushes his own abducted small fingers or index fingers together. If one side is weak, the finger on the strong side will force the finger on the weak side into adduction. See Dr. John K. Wolf's *Segmental Neurology* for further elaboration on these elegant muscle-to-muscle techniques.

Opposition of the thumb is tested by having the patient touch the little finger with the thumb (Figure 27.30). With the thumbnail on a plane approximately parallel to the palm, the palmar surface of the tip of the thumb should contact the palmar surface of the tip of the little finger. When the OP is weak, the patient may be able to oppose the thumb to the index or middle finger, but not the little finger. In testing opposition of the little finger by the opponens digiti minimi (ulnar nerve, C8-T1), the patient moves the extended little finger in front of the other fingers and toward the thumb (Figure 27.31). Opposition of the thumb and little finger may be tested in one maneuver. When both are opposed, their extended tips meet and form an arch over the cupped palm (Figure 27.32). The strength of the combined movement may be gauged by the patient's ability to hold onto a piece of paper held between finger and thumb as the examiner tries to pull it free, or the examiner may attempt to pull his finger between the touching tips of the thumb and little finger. The flexors of the thumb and little finger and the short abductor of the thumb probably enter into these movements.

The adductor pollicis is the final muscle innervated by the deep palmar branch of the ulnar nerve (C8-T1). It adducts the thumb and flexes the first

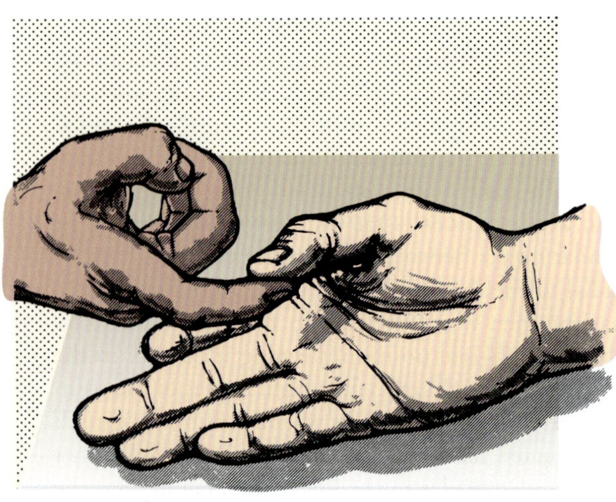

FIGURE 27.30 Examination of the opponens pollicis. The patient attempts, against resistance, to touch the tip of the little finger with the thumb.

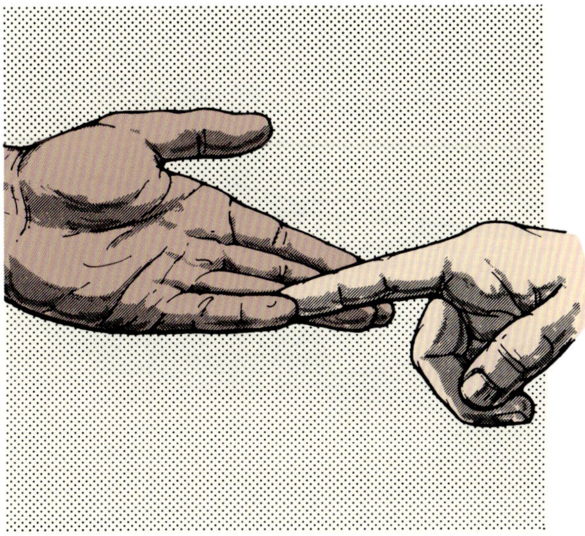

FIGURE 27.31 Examination of the opponens digiti minimi. The patient attempts to move the extended little finger in front of the other fingers and toward the thumb.

metacarpal. Adduction of the thumb is also carried out in two planes: in the plane of the palm (ulnar adduction) and in a plane at right angles to the palm (palmar adduction). Ulnar adduction is touching the ulnar aspect of the thumb to the radial aspect of the second metacarpal, the thumb in the same plane as the palm and the thumbnail as nearly as possible parallel with the other fingernails, as if to put the hand into salute position. In palmar adduction, the ulnar aspect of the thumb touches the palmar aspect of the second metacarpal so that the thumb and index finger lie perpendicular to each other, with the thumbnail at right angles to the other fingernails (Figure 27.33). A commonly used test of adduction power in either of these positions is to have the patient try to hold a piece of paper tightly between thumb and hand as the examiner tries to extract it (Figure 27.34). When thumb adduction is weak, the patient may make a substitution movement, flexing the IP joint with the FPL and trying to secure the paper with the tip of the thumb (Froment's sign), a common finding in ulnar neuropathy.

Adduction of the fingers is the movement that brings the fingers tightly together; abduction spreads the fingers apart. Adduction is a function of the volar

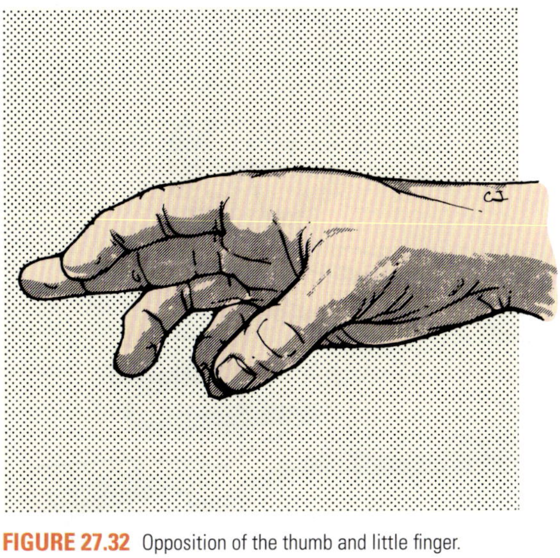

FIGURE 27.32 Opposition of the thumb and little finger.

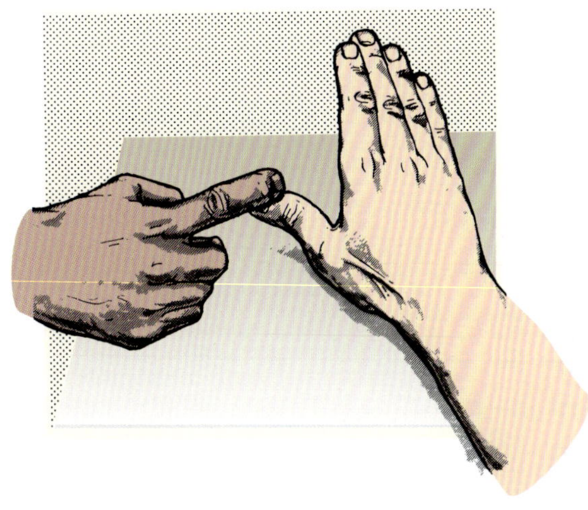

FIGURE 27.33 Palmar adduction of the thumb. The patient, against resistance, attempts to approximate the thumb to the palmar aspect of the index finger; the thumbnail is kept at a right angle to the nails of the other fingers.

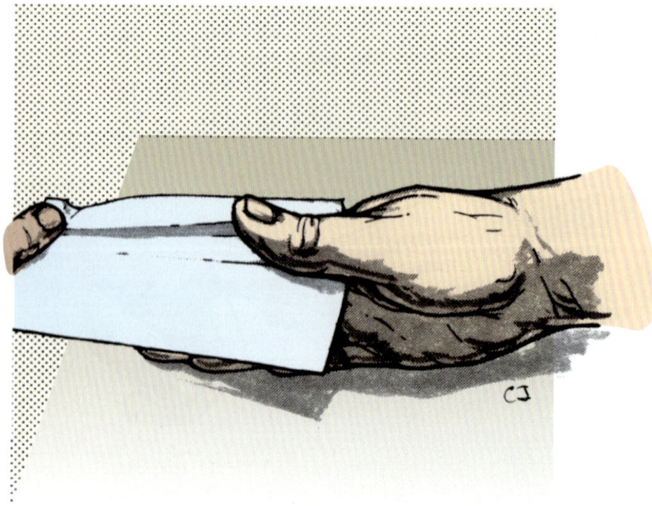

FIGURE 27.34 Ulnar adduction of the thumb. The patient attempts to grasp a piece of paper between the thumb and the radial border of the index finger while the thumbnail is parallel to the nails of the other fingers. In ulnar neuropathy, the IP joint flexes to compensate for weakness of the adductor pollicis (Froment's sign, Chapter 46).

interossei, whereas abduction is a function of the dorsal interossei. Abduction of the little finger is done by the ADM. Adduction may be tested in several ways. With the fingers abducted and extended, the patient may try to adduct the fingers against resistance (Figure 27.35). The patient may try to clutch a piece of paper between two fingers and resist the examiner's attempts to withdraw it. The examiner may interdigitate his fingers between the patient's and have the patient squeeze as tightly as possible. Another test is to have the patient make a "finger cone," by holding the hand palm up, touching the index and ring fingers together above the middle finger, and then laying the small finger atop the ring finger. This movement requires good adduction power. If the patient then opposes the thumb to the small finger, all major muscle groups of the hand have been tested in one quick maneuver. Yet another adduction test is to have the patient, palm down, lay the middle finger across the index finger as far as possible, trying to touch the ulnar aspect of the middle finger to the radial aspect of the index finger.

The usual test of abduction is to have the patient keep the fingers fully extended and spread apart and resist the examiner's attempt to bring them together

FIGURE 27.35 Adduction of the fingers. The patient attempts to adduct the fingers against resistance.

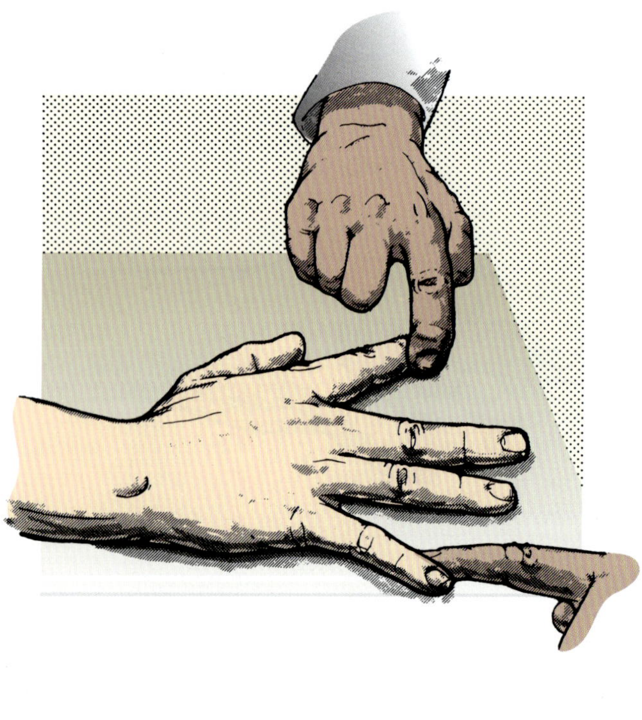

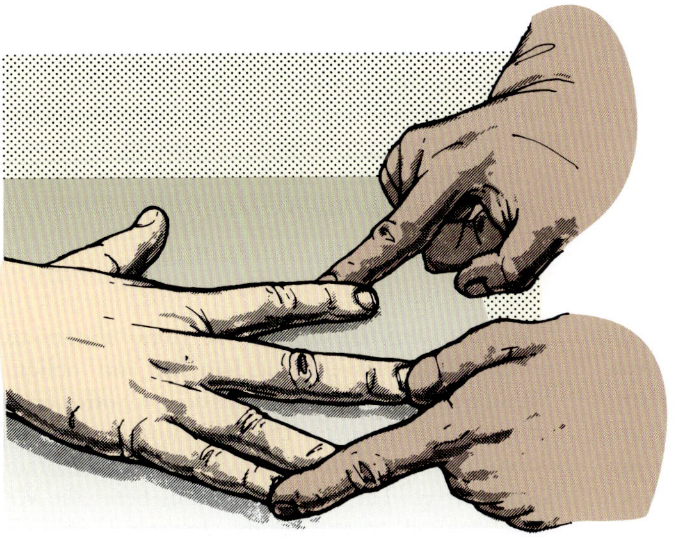

FIGURE 27.36 Examination of the abduction of the fingers. The patient resists the examiner's attempt to bring the fingers together.

(Figure 27.36). In most circumstances, the examination concentrates on the first DI and the ADM. A commonly used technique is for the examiner to use a claw-like grip with his palm against the back of the patient's fingers, patient and examiner both palm down, examiner's small finger hooked around the patient's small finger, and thumb around the patient's index finger; then, the examiner pulls the thumb and small finger together to overpower the patient's finger abductors. This is a mismatch in that the muscles the examiner is using are more powerful than the muscles the patient is using, so the examiner always overcomes the finger abductors and must develop a feel for how much resistance is normal. A better technique is for the patient and examiner to match muscles. The patient and examiner both have their hands palms down, fingers extended and abducted. With the radial aspect of his right index finger against the radial aspect of the patient's right index finger, the fingertip of each about at the level of the PIP joint of the other, the examiner tries to overcome the patient's first DI with his own first DI, like muscle against like muscle (as described for the APB above). Similarly for the ADM, but patient and examiner are both palms up. If the patient and examiner are both right handed or both left handed, this method has the advantage of pitting dominant hand against dominant hand and nondominant against nondominant. A more efficient if less ideal technique for testing finger abduction of the patient's right hand is as follows. The patient holds his right hand palm down, fingers fully abducted. The examiner holds his right hand palm down, his left palm up, right index finger against the patient's right index finger, and left small finger against the patient's right small finger. Using these like muscles, the examiner then tries to force the patient's fingers together.

Examination of Movements and Muscles of the Thorax, Abdomen, and Trunk

The actions of the large muscles of the trunk, chest, and abdomen are often combined, and it is difficult to evaluate them individually (Table 27.6). Except for the respiratory muscles, most of these muscles have scant neurologic significance.

The Muscles of the Thorax

The major thoracic muscles consist of the internal and external intercostals and diaphragm. Muscles attached to the sternum, clavicles, and scapulae act as accessory muscles of respiration. The intercostal muscles are innervated by the intercostal nerves, which are the anterior divisions of the 12 thoracic spinal nerves. The diaphragm is innervated by C3-C5 through the phrenic nerves, which arise directly from the nerve roots. The diaphragm is the principal muscle of respiration. During quiet inspiration, intercostal contraction expands the anteroposterior and transverse diameters of the thorax, and the vertical diameter is increased by the descent of the diaphragm. In deep inspiration, additional muscles are brought into action, including the scaleni, SCMs, and other muscles that act on the shoulders, clavicles, and scapulae. The diaphragm also contracts during various expulsive acts such as coughing, sneezing, laughing, vomiting, hiccuping, urination, defecation, and parturition.

Weakness of the intercostal muscles causes adduction of the costal margins and abdominal respiration, with alternate bulging and retraction of the epigastrium as increased diaphragmatic contraction compensates for the intercostal weakness (abdominal breathing). The intercostal spaces may retract during inspiration, and the ribs do not rise and separate. When bilateral paralysis of the diaphragm is present, the excursion of the costal margins is increased and the epigastrium does not bulge during inspiration. The moving shadow caused by retraction of the lower intercostal spaces during inspiration (Litten's sign) is absent. The expulsive acts, primarily coughing, are carried out with difficulty. Quick, forceful diaphragmatic contractions are impaired; one manifestation of this may be the inability to sniff. Unilateral diaphragmatic weakness is difficult to detect, but the excursion of the costal margin on the affected side during quiet inspiration may be slightly increased, and Litten's sign is absent. Fluoroscopy, ultrasonography, and phrenic nerve conduction studies, not to mention pulmonary function tests, are far superior to physical examination in detecting diaphragmatic impairment. Diaphragm function should be particularly assessed in patients with spinal cord lesions that involve the C3-C5 segments. If there is diaphragmatic or intercostal weakness, the accessory muscles that act in deep inspiration are brought into play, and breathing recruits the scaleni, SCMs, serrati, and pectorals.

The Muscles of the Abdomen

The abdominal muscles are the rectus abdominis, pyramidalis, transversus abdominis, and obliqui. Weakness of these muscle groups does not often occur in neurologic patients. The abdominal muscles are innervated by the anterior divisions of the thoracic spinal nerves. The rectus abdominis flexes the vertebral column, compresses the abdominal viscera in such acts as defecation and parturition, and aids in forced expiration.

When performing a sit-up, the abdominal muscles contract strongly during the initial phase of the movement, when raising the head and shoulders. After the shoulders have been raised about 8 in, the hip flexors contract strongly and bring the trunk to an upright position. The abdominal muscles may be tested by having the patient raise the head against resistance (Figure 27.37), cough, or do a sit-up. If the

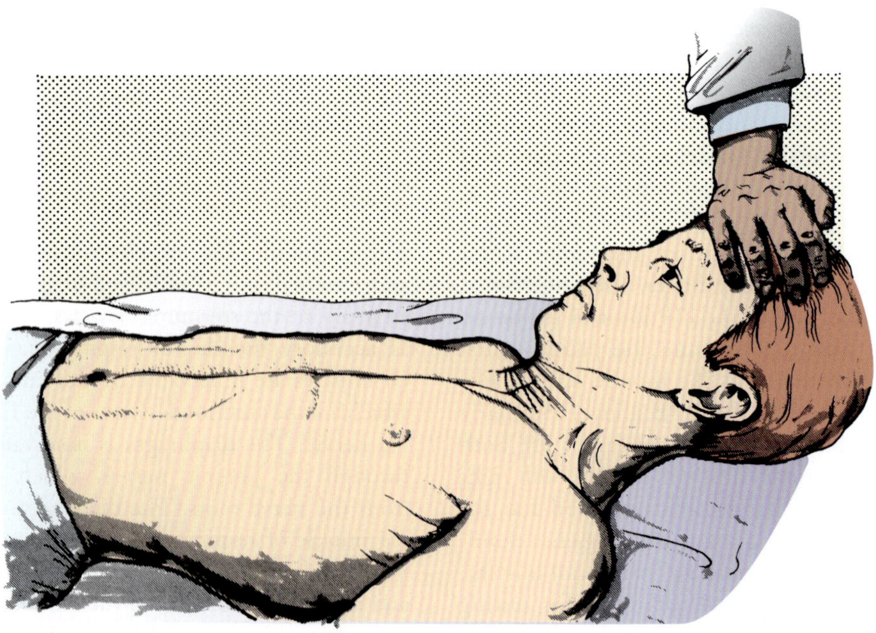

FIGURE 27.37 Examination of the abdominal muscles. The recumbent patient attempts to raise his head against resistance.

abdominal muscles are weak but the hip flexors normal, hyperextension of the spine will occur during an attempted sit-up. If the abdominal muscles contract equally in all four quadrants, the umbilicus will not move. If the lower abdominal muscles are paralyzed, as in a T10 myelopathy, the upper abdominal muscles will pull the umbilicus cephalad when the patient raises the head or attempts a sit-up (Beevor's sign, see **Video Link 27.3**). More rarely, abnormal movement of the umbilicus may occur with weakness of the upper abdominals or if the weakness is unilateral.

The Muscles of the Pelvis

The pelvic muscles, including the urinary bladder and the perineal and external genital muscles, are not accessible for the usual clinical testing. A crude assessment can be obtained by reflex activation, for example, cremasteric, bulbocavernosus, and anal wink. These are discussed in Chapter 39. The bladder and some of the functions of the genitalia are discussed in Chapter 45.

The Muscles of the Spine

The muscles that extend and rotate the spine were introduced above in the discussion of neck muscles. Most of these muscle groups extend down the entire spine, and for general clinical purposes, they are considered as a group: the erector spinae, paravertebral, or paraspinal muscles. Paraspinal examination is an important part of needle electromyography. Abnormalities in the paraspinal muscles help differentiate nerve root disease from plexus and peripheral nerve disease. The paraspinals are also often abnormal electromyographically in myopathies. The movements of the spine are flexion, extension, rotation, and lateral bending. The muscles that produce these movements are examined en masse by examining the movements rather than individual muscles. All the paraspinal muscles are innervated by the posterior primary rami of the spinal nerves.

The extensors of the spine are tested by having the prone patient raise the head and shoulders without the assistance of the hands (Figure 27.38); in a continuation of this, the young and supple may be able to raise the legs and balance on the belly. The ability to perform these maneuvers indicates normality, but further assessment may be done by pressing downward against the patient's extension motion. The most common cause of paraspinal weakness is primary muscle disease, particularly muscular dystrophies, especially FSH dystrophy. Patients with weak spine extensors often adopt a lordotic, sometimes hyperlordotic, posture. This is because the paraspinals normally function like guy-wires on a tower antenna, helping to balance the spine above the pelvis. With forward bending,

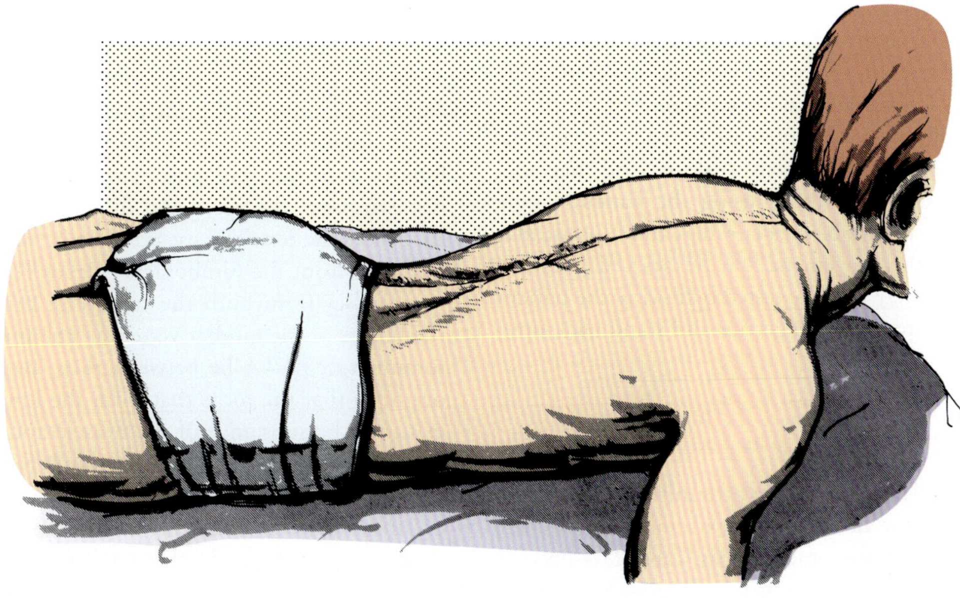

FIGURE 27.38 Examination of the extensors of the spine. The patient, lying prone, attempts to raise the head and upper part of the trunk.

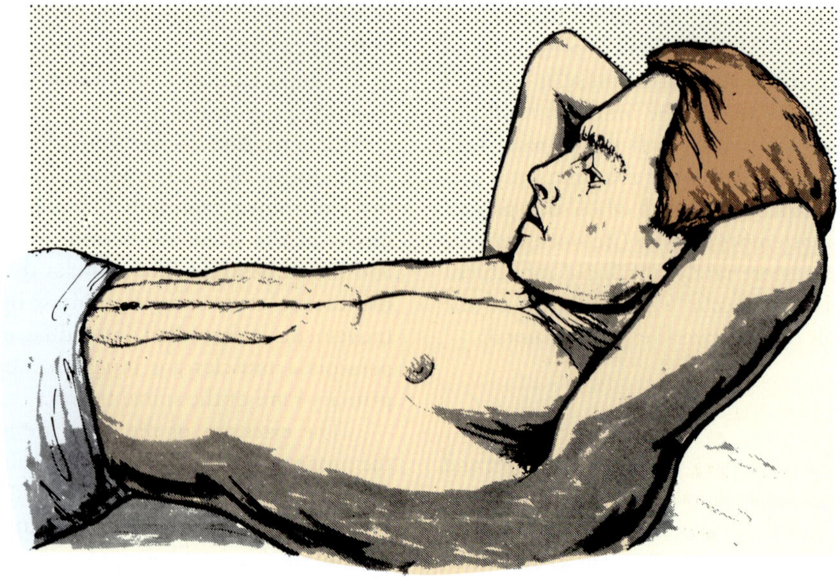

FIGURE 27.39 Examination of the abdominal muscles and flexor muscles of the spine. The patient attempts to rise from a recumbent to a sitting position without the use of the hands.

contraction of the paraspinals prevents tipping over. Patients with paraspinal weakness cannot rely on their spine extensors to keep them from falling forward, so they lean backward to compensate and maintain balance. The result is the lordotic posture. In FSH, the hyperlordosis may reach bizarre proportions, with the patient leaning so far backward the spine approaches horizontal. The lordosis disappears when the patient lies down. When patients with some dystrophies, particularly Duchenne's, become wheelchair bound, the paraspinal weakness may lead to scoliosis, often severe enough to require surgical intervention.

The flexors of the spine are tested by having the patient rise from recumbent to seated and then to a standing position without using the hands (Figure 27.39). The flexors of the abdomen and hips are also involved in this movement. The flexors and extensors of the spine may both be tested by having the patient try to touch toes with fingertips and stand back up.

Examination of the Movements and Muscles of the Lower Extremities

The movements of the lower extremities are less complex than those of the upper extremities, and there are fewer substitution movements. Table 27.7 lists the pertinent muscles and their innervation. Some muscles of the lower extremity have complicated actions that seem discordant (e.g., the hamstrings flex the knee but extend the hip). This is largely due to the rotation of the lower extremity into a new functional position that occurred during the evolution to land vertebrates. The ventral surface of the thigh came to lie posterior so that the knee flexes backward even though the hip flexes forward.

The Hip Joint

The movements that take place at the hip are flexion, extension, abduction, adduction, and internal and external rotation. The principal hip flexor is the iliopsoas. Important accessory hip flexors are the rectus femoris, sartorius, and tensor fascia lata. The iliopsoas has two parts, the psoas and the iliacus, which have the same function. The psoas portion is innervated by branches from the lumbosacral plexus (L1-L4). The psoas arises from both the transverse processes and the bodies of the lumbar vertebra. The intervertebral foramina of L1-L4 lie between these two points of origin so that the roots that form the lumbar plexus exit into the substance of the muscle and the plexus lies within it. This anatomy accounts for the severe damage to the lumbosacral plexus that commonly occurs with hemorrhage into the psoas muscle. The iliacus portion arises in the iliac fossa and is innervated by the femoral nerve (L2-L4).

The two iliopsoas muscles acting together from each side help to maintain an erect posture by

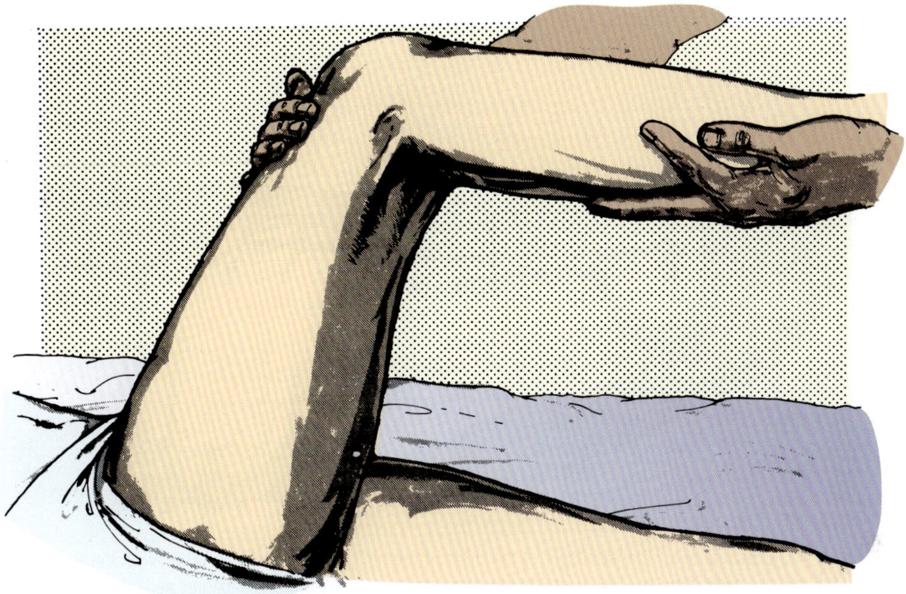

FIGURE 27.40 Examination of the flexors of the thigh. The patient attempts to flex the thigh against resistance; the knee is flexed and the leg rests on the examiner's arm.

balancing the spine and pelvis over the femurs, preventing a backward tilt. When the legs are fixed, they flex the trunk and pelvis forward, as in doing a sit-up. Hip flexor strength is tested by having the patient flex the hip against resistance (Figure 27.40). This may be done in the sitting or supine position. If sitting, the patient should not be permitted to lean backward. When testing in the sitting position, normal hip flexors cannot be overcome by an examiner using hand and arm strength from an arm's length away. If the examiner stands close and uses his body weight, the hip flexors can usually be defeated. When testing supine, a patient with mild hip flexor weakness may still be able to raise the leg with the knee extended; with more severe weakness, the hip can only be flexed with the knee flexed. Another hip flexor test is to have the supine patient attempt to maintain both lower extremities flexed at the hip and extended at the knee, the legs at about a 45-degree angle off the bed, feet apart. This is a difficult callisthenic maneuver that not all patients can perform. If the hip flexors are mildly weak unilaterally, as in a CST lesion, the involved lower extremity will drift downward more rapidly than its fellow (leg drift). Another version of this test can be used to look for subtle hamstring weakness (see "The Knee Joint").

The major hip extensor is the gluteus maximus (inferior gluteal nerve, L5-S2). The gluteus maximus is the most powerful extensor and external rotator of the thigh. Accessory hip extensors are the glutei medius and minimus, hamstrings, and hip adductors. The gluteus maximus is important in climbing steps, jumping, and rising from a chair. Hip extensor function is best tested with the patient prone, raising the flexed knee up from the table against downward pressure from the examiner (Figure 27.41). Having the knee flexed minimizes any contribution from the hamstrings. The gluteus maximus can also be tested with the patient lying on the side and extending the hip, or seated and trying to press the raised knee back down as the examiner holds it up, or by testing the ability to stand upright from a stooped position. With hip girdle weakness, particularly in the muscular dystrophies, there is marked weakness of the hip extensors, and the patient arises from a stooped position by using his hands to "climb up the legs" (Gowers' sign or maneuver, see **Video Link 27.4**).

The primary abductors of the hip are the gluteus medius, gluteus minimus, and tensor fasciae lata (TFL). These muscles are supplied by L4-S1 through the superior gluteal nerve. They also function as internal rotators of the hip. The TFL also tightens the fascia lata and flexes the hip. The hip abductors may be tested either supine or sitting by having the patient attempt to hold the lower extremities outward with ankles spread far apart as the examiner tries to force the ankles together (Figure 27.42). Weakness of hip abduction is often present in myopathies affecting the hip girdle musculature.

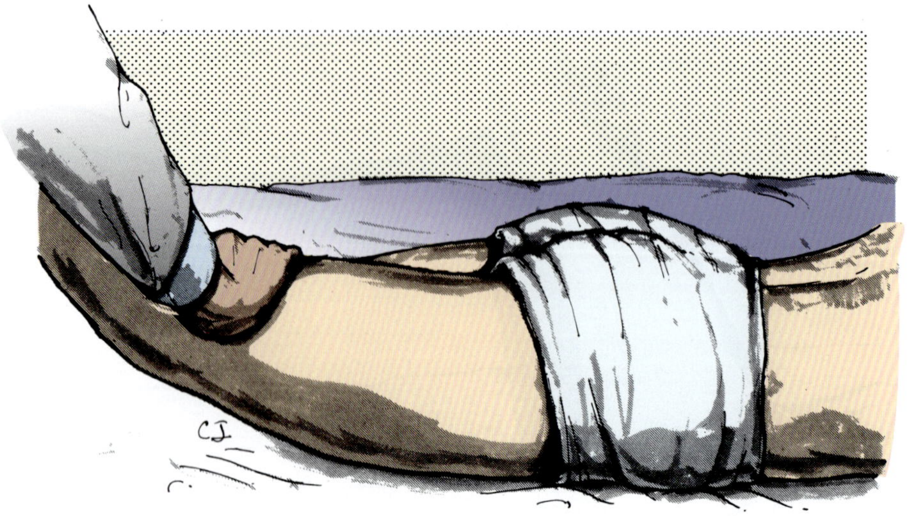

FIGURE 27.41 Examination of the extensors of the thigh at the hip. The patient, lying prone with the leg flexed at the knee, attempts to extend the thigh against resistance; contraction of the gluteus maximus and other extensors can be seen and palpated.

The hip abductors are very important in walking. With each step, the abductors of the stance leg must generate enough force to balance all the weight of the rest of the body in order to keep the pelvis level. Without contraction of the hip abductors, the hip would slide laterally toward the stance leg as the pelvis tilted and the stance leg adducted. When the hip abductors are weak, there is an exaggerated pelvic swing during the stance phase as the pelvis on the side of the swing leg drops downward (Trendelenburg's sign). When bilateral, the result is a gait pattern referred to as a pelvic waddle, which resembles the exaggerated hip swing of a fashion model. The waddling gait is particularly common in myopathies that weaken the pelvic girdle musculature. A unilateral Trendelenburg sign can occur with processes that weaken the hip abductors unilaterally, such as lumbosacral radiculopathy (Chapters 44 and 47).

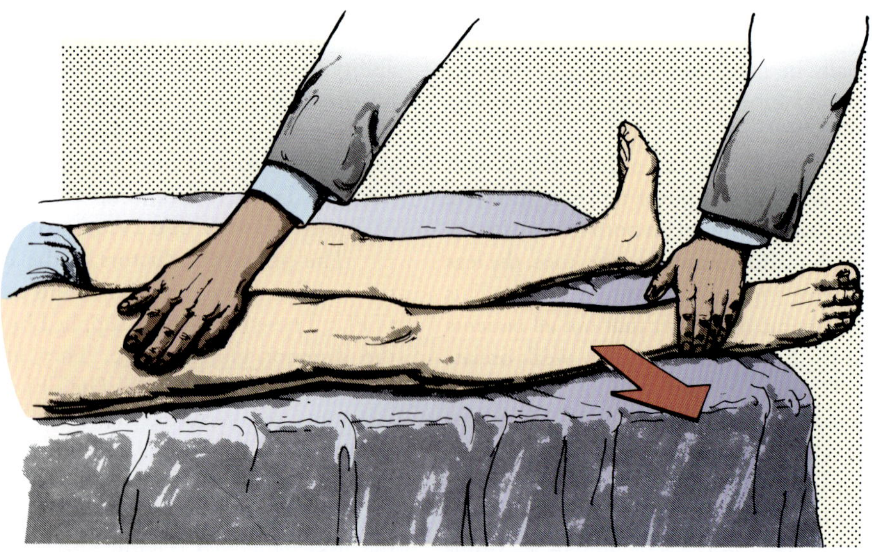

FIGURE 27.42 Abduction of the thigh at the hip. The recumbent patient attempts to move the extended leg outward against resistance; contraction of the gluteus medius and tensor fasciae latae can be palpated.

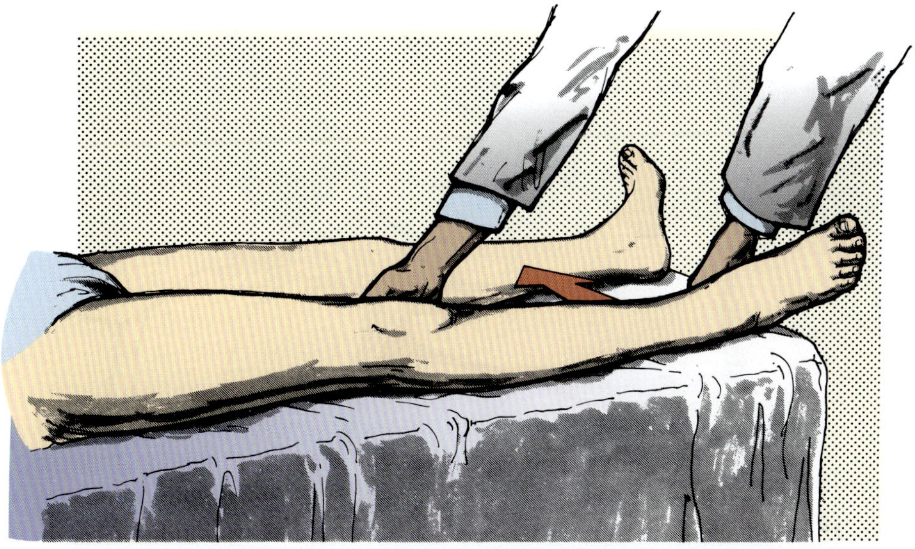

FIGURE 27.43 Examination of adduction of the thigh at the hip. The recumbent patient attempts to adduct the extended leg against resistance; contraction of the adductor muscles can be seen and palpated.

Adduction of the hip is principally a function of the three adductors: longus, brevis, and magnus. The adductor magnus is the longest and strongest hip adductor. Other muscles may play a minor role. The three adductors are supplied by L2-L4 through the obturator nerve. The adductor magnus also receives a twig from the sciatic nerve carrying innervation from L4 to L5. The adductors can be tested with the patient supine, sitting, or lying on one side. The patient attempts to bring the legs together as the examiner tries to keep them apart (Figure 27.43). As with the abductors, the adductors are so powerful it is helpful to keep the patient's knees extended to give the examiner the advantage of a longer lever. When testing with the patient in the decubitus position, the examiner raises the uppermost leg with the patient trying to keep the legs together; this should raise the entire body, with the lowermost leg remaining apposed and following the upward movement. When the uppermost adductors are weak, the leg will passively abduct and the torso will not move upward; when the lowermost adductors are weak, the lower leg will not follow the upward motion, remaining behind on the bed.

Internal, or medial, rotation of the hip is carried out principally by the hip abductor muscles (glutei medius and minimus, and TFL), with some contribution from the adductors. To test internal rotation, the patient lies supine with the hip and knee flexed or prone with the knee flexed. He then attempts to move the foot laterally against resistance, thus rotating the hip medially (Figure 27.44). Internal rotation can also be tested with the patient supine and the leg extended, rotating the foot medially as if to touch the big toe to the bed. Rotating the foot medially with the knee extended produces the same hip motion as carrying the foot laterally with the knee flexed. With a unilateral CST lesion (e.g., acute stroke), the internal rotators are weak. When the patient lies supine, the involved leg lies externally rotated compared to its fellow. This asymmetry of leg position may be a clue to the presence of a hemiparesis in an obtunded patient.

External, or lateral, rotation of the thigh at the hip is carried out primarily by the gluteus maximus. The piriformis externally rotates the extended thigh but abducts the flexed thigh. External rotation is tested by maneuvers similar to those for testing internal rotation, but the patient rotates the hip externally by attempting to carry the foot medially against resistance with the knee flexed. If these muscles are paralyzed, the entire leg is turned inward.

An array of short muscles around the hip (obturators, gemelli, quadratus femoris, piriformis, and pectineus) probably play a more important role as postural muscles maintaining hip stability than as prime movers. The sartorius (femoral nerve, L2-L3), the longest muscle in the body, has a complex set of actions. It is an abductor, flexor, and lateral rotator of the hip and a flexor and medial rotator of the knee. The sartorius would be active when trying to look at the bottom of one's foot.

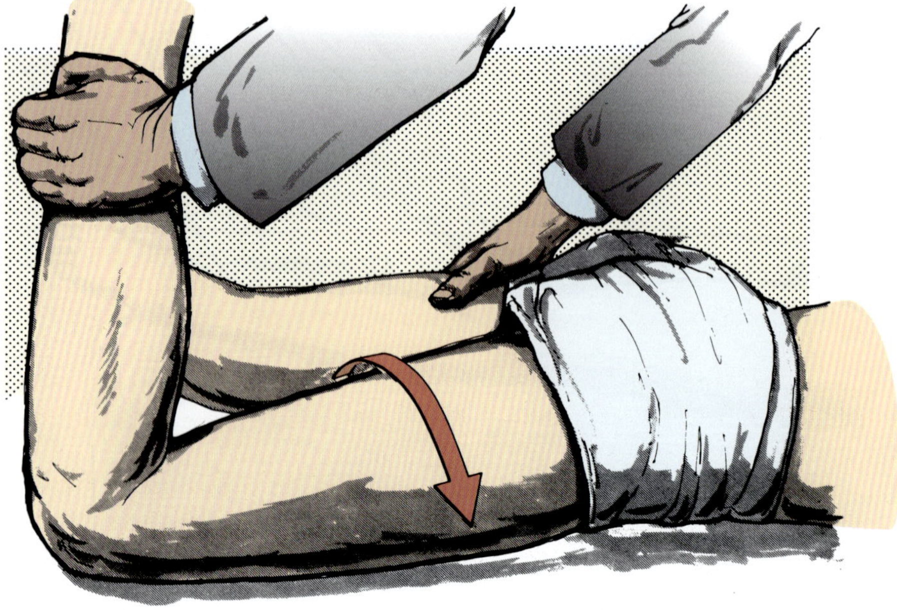

FIGURE 27.44 Examination of internal rotation of the thigh. The patient, lying prone with the leg flexed at the knee, attempts to carry the foot laterally against resistance, thus rotating the thigh medially.

The Knee Joint

The major movements that take place at the knee joint are flexion and extension. Flexion of the knee is carried out primarily by the hamstring muscles (biceps femoris, semimembranosus, and semitendinosus). Other muscles may play a contributory role. The hamstrings also act as powerful hip extensors. The biceps femoris (external or lateral hamstring) has two heads, long and short. The belly of the long head overlies the short head except just above the popliteal fossa. Both heads are innervated by the sciatic nerve (L5, S1-S2), but the long head is supplied by the tibial division and the short head by the peroneal division. The innervation of the short head by the peroneal division is important in distinguishing lesions involving the peroneal (fibular) nerve at the knee from those involving the peroneal division of the sciatic, which may be otherwise inseparable. Involvement of the short head is not detectable by physical examination but can be detected electromyographically. The common peroneal nerve at the knee lies just medial to the biceps femoris tendon. The semimembranosus and semitendinosus muscles (internal or medial hamstrings) are supplied by branches of the sciatic nerve (L5, S1-S2).

The knee flexors may be tested with the patient prone (Figure 27.45), supine, or sitting. With the knee in partial flexion, the patient resists the examiner's attempts to straighten the knee. The knee flexors are powerful and cannot normally be overcome. Another test is to have the prone patient attempt to maintain both knees flexed at about 45 degrees from horizontal with the feet slightly apart. When the knee flexors are weak on one side, as in a CST lesion, the involved leg will sink, gradually or rapidly (leg drift, leg sign of Barré). Examination of knee flexion with the patient prone makes it easier to see and palpate the muscle contractions and lessens the likelihood of misinterpretation because of simultaneous action of the hip flexors. The sartorius may be examined by having the patient attempt to flex the knee against resistance with the hip flexed and rotated laterally (Figure 27.46).

The quadriceps femoris (femoral nerve, L2-L4) is the primary knee extensor. It is composed of four large muscles, rectus femoris, vastus lateralis, vastus medialis, and vastus intermedius, which are united into a common tendon inserted into the upper border of the patella. The quadriceps is very powerful. It is capable of generating as much as 1,000 lb of force—three times more than the hamstrings. The rectus femoris originates from the ilium and runs straight down the middle of the thigh. The other three muscles originate from the shaft of the femur and only cross the knee joint. Because the rectus femoris also crosses the hip, it serves as a hip flexor as well as a knee extensor. The vastus medialis is sometimes divided into two

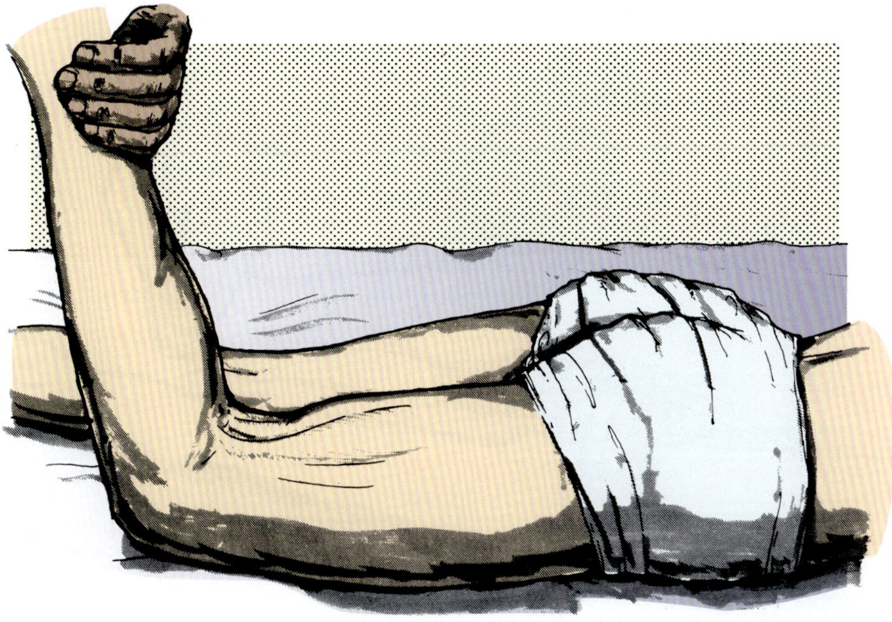

FIGURE 27.45 Examination of flexion at the knee. The prone patient attempts to maintain flexion of the leg while the examiner attempts to extend it; the tendon of the biceps femoris can be palpated laterally and the tendons of the semimembranosus and semitendinosus medially.

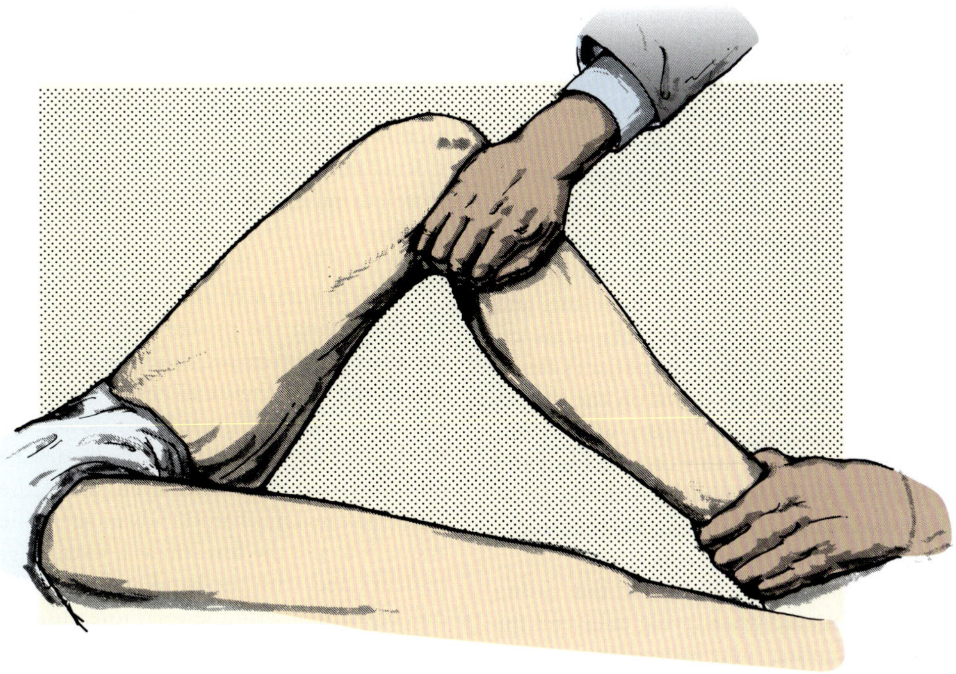

FIGURE 27.46 Examination of the sartorius. With the thigh flexed and rotated laterally and the knee moderately flexed, the patient attempts further flexion of the knee against resistance.

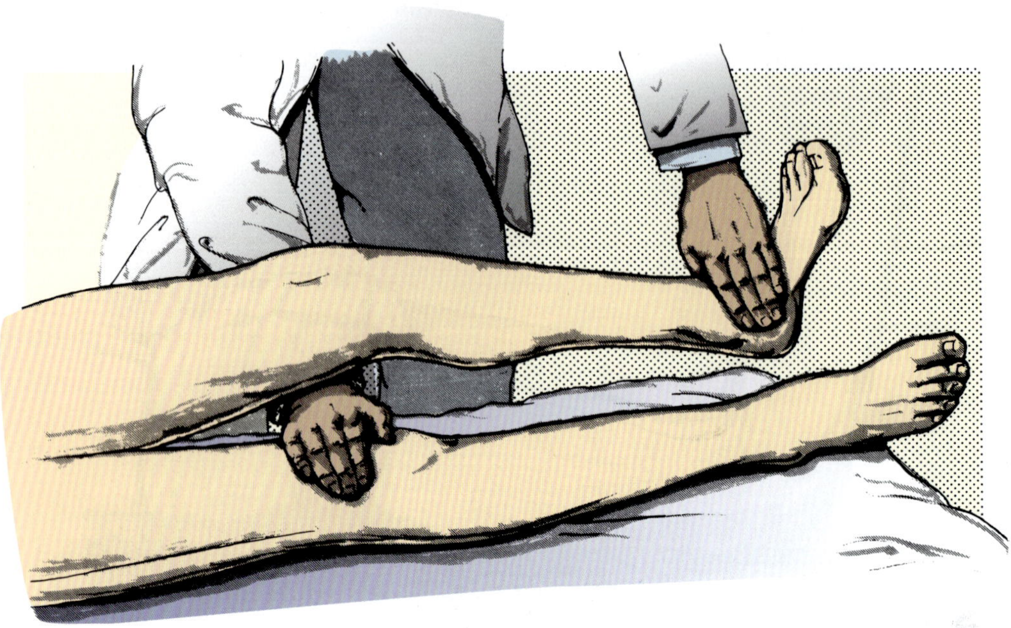

FIGURE 27.47 Examination of extension of the leg at the knee. The supine patient attempts to extend the leg at the knee against resistance; contraction of the quadriceps femoris can be seen and palpated.

parts: vastus medialis longus and vastus medialis oblique. Although the oblique head is often examined electromyographically, it in fact is the only portion of the quadriceps that is incapable of extending the knee.

The quadriceps may be tested when the patient, sitting or supine, attempts to extend the knee against the examiner's resistance (Figure 27.47). The quadriceps is so powerful it is nearly impossible to overcome in the normal adolescent or adult except by taking extreme mechanical advantage. A sometimes useful technique for testing knee extension is the "barkeeper's hold," a hold usually applied to the elbow to control unruly patrons. To examine the right quadriceps, the examiner, standing on the outer aspect of the knee and reaching around from the inner aspect, places his left elbow, forearm pronated, beneath the patient's flexed knee, puts his right hand as far down on the shin as possible, and then grips his right forearm with his left hand, locking the patient's leg in a vice from front and back. The examiner then pulls upward with the elbow while pushing downward with the hand as the patient tries to extend his knee (Figure 27.48).

With severe quadriceps weakness, the sitting patient may lean backward when trying to extend the knee, attempting to muster some knee extension force by allowing the rectus femoris to contract across the hip. The patient will have marked difficulty in rising from a kneeling position and in climbing stairs; he can walk backward but has difficulty walking forward.

The Ankle Joint

Movements about the ankle joint are plantar flexion, dorsiflexion, eversion, and inversion. Plantar flexion (flexion) of the foot is carried out principally by the gastrocnemius and soleus muscles (gastrosoleus, triceps surae). Other muscles cross posterior to the axis of rotation of the ankle but because of mechanical factors are not very effective plantar flexors. The gastrocnemius also assists in flexing the knee. The gastrosoleus raises the heel, as in walking, and inverts the foot. The calf muscles are innervated by the tibial nerve (S1-S2).

The function of these muscles is tested manually by having the patient plantar flex the ankle as the examiner offers resistance by pressure against the sole of the foot (Figure 27.49). The plantar flexors of the ankle are among the most powerful muscles in the body. They cannot normally be defeated by hand and arm strength alone, even when the examiner takes maximal mechanical advantage. A helpful technique is to use the forearm as a lever by grasping the patient's heel with the hand and pushing against the ball of the foot with the volar forearm. Normal plantar flexors will hold fast even against this power move. A better test of plantar flexor strength is to have the patient stand on tiptoe. Normally, a patient can easily support the entire body weight on one tiptoe, hop on one foot, and even do multiple toe raises on one foot.

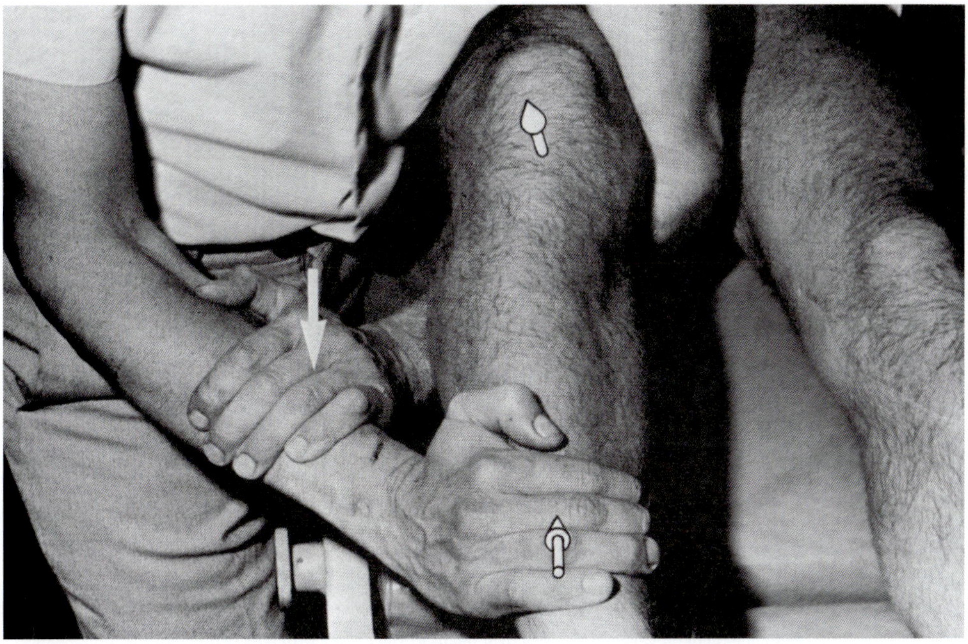

FIGURE 27.48 The "barkeeper's hold," a powerful move against the quadriceps. (From Wolf JK. *Segmental Neurology.* Baltimore: University Park Press, 1981. Reprinted with permission from Dr. John K. Wolf.)

The number and ease of toe raise repetitions on the two sides may be compared to detect subtle weakness, as in S1 radiculopathy.

Dorsiflexion (extension) of the ankle is carried out primarily by the tibialis anterior muscle, assisted by the extensor digitorum longus (EDL) and extensor hallucis longus (EHL). The tibialis anterior is supplied by the deep peroneal nerve (L4-L5). It also functions as an invertor, more so when the ankle is dorsiflexed. When the foot is planted on the ground, the tibialis anterior tilts the lower leg forward, as in walking. The foot dorsiflexors are tested by having the patient pull

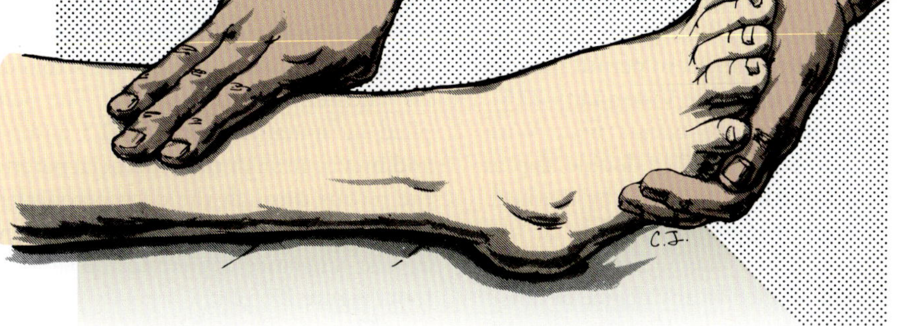

FIGURE 27.49 Examination of plantar flexion of the foot. The patient attempts to plantar flex the foot at the ankle joint against resistance; contraction of the gastrocnemius and associated muscles can be seen and palpated.

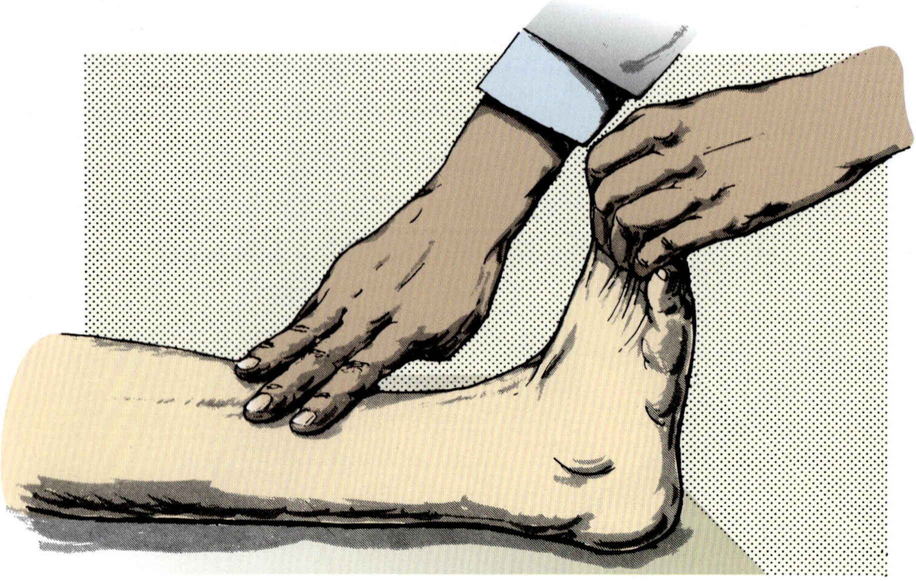

FIGURE 27.50 Examination of dorsiflexion (extension) of the foot. The patient attempts to dorsiflex the foot against resistance; contraction of the tibialis anterior can be seen and palpated.

the foot up against the examiner's resistance (Figure 27.50). The dorsiflexors are powerful and cannot normally be overcome, even with maximal effort from the examiner. Subtle weakness can sometimes be detected by placing the patient at maximal mechanical disadvantage with the foot plantar flexed and trying to hold the foot in that position as the patient tries to dorsiflex it. This technique is most useful with unilateral weakness when the two sides can be compared. Dorsiflexion may also be tested by having the patient stand on the heels, raising the toes as high as possible. The toes on the weak side cannot be lifted as far. The tibialis anterior is the major muscle innervated by the L5 myotome; L5 radiculopathy and peroneal neuropathy are the most common causes of weakness.

With severe weakness of dorsiflexion, there is a footdrop. The patient walks with a "steppage gait," raising the affected leg higher off the ground by exaggerated flexion at the hip and knee, to permit the toes to clear during the stride phase (see **Video Link 27.5**). In normal walking, heel strike occurs first. With a footdrop, there may be an audible double slap as the toes contact the floor first, followed by the heel. There may be inability to raise the forefoot off the ground while trying to stand on the heel. The term footdrop is sometimes applied to any degree of dorsiflexion weakness, even when too mild to cause a steppage gait. The term steppage gait is also used to refer to the high-stepping, drum-major gait of a patient with sensory ataxia as he slams the feet to the ground to reinforce proprioception (Chapter 44).

Inversion at the ankle is elevation of the inner border of the foot to turn the sole medially. Several muscles can perform this action with different degrees of efficiency, determined in part by whether the ankle is dorsi- or plantar flexed. The tibialis posterior (tibial nerve, L5-S1), the strongest invertor, is also a plantar flexor and is strongest as an invertor when the ankle is plantar flexed. The tibialis anterior functions as an invertor when the ankle is dorsiflexed. Inversion is tested by having the patient attempt to invert the ankle against resistance (Figure 27.51). Weakness of ankle inversion is a key clinical sign indicating that a footdrop is due to L5 radiculopathy and not peroneal neuropathy at the knee.

Eversion, or lateral deviation, is elevation of the outer border of the foot to turn the sole laterally. This movement is carried out by the peroneus longus, brevis, and tertius and the EDL. The peronei are supplied by spinal segments L4-L5 and S1, the longus and brevis through the superficial peroneal nerve, and the tertius through the deep peroneal nerve. To test these muscles, the patient attempts to evert the ankle against resistance applied to the lateral border of the foot (Figure 27.52).

The evertors and invertors of the ankle are very important in ankle stability. When these muscles are weak, the patient is susceptible to ankle sprains; an

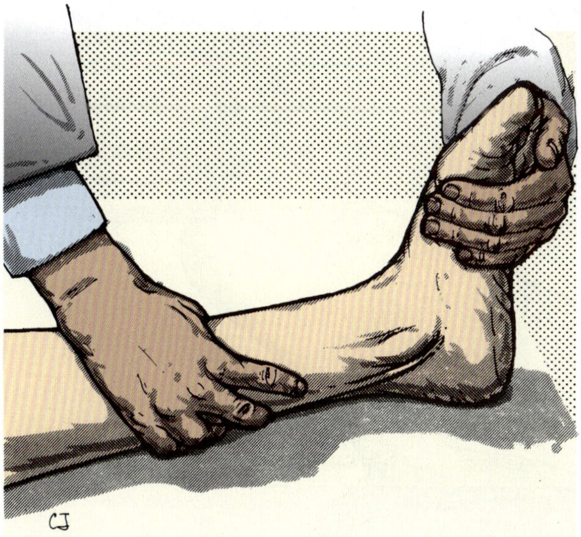

FIGURE 27.51 Examination of inversion of the foot. The patient attempts to raise the inner border of the foot against resistance; the tendon of the tibialis posterior can be seen and palpated just behind the medial malleolus.

early symptom of ankle instability is difficulty walking over rough or uneven terrain.

Muscles of the Foot and Toes

The function of individual foot and toe muscles is not as clearly defined as in the hand, and muscle testing cannot be carried out with as much detail. The principal movements are extension (dorsiflexion) and flexion (plantar flexion) of the toes. With plantar flexion, there is cupping of the sole. Abduction and adduction of the toes are minimal.

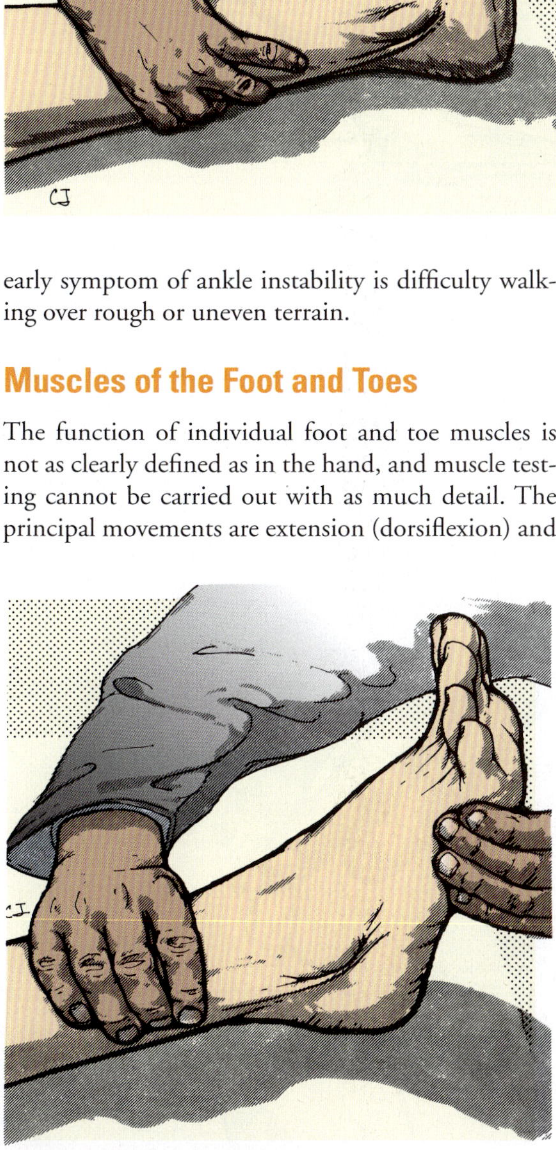

FIGURE 27.52 Examination of eversion of the foot. The patient attempts to raise the outer border of the foot against resistance; the tendons of the peronei longus and brevis can be seen and palpated just above and behind the lateral malleolus.

The toe extensors are the extensor digitorum longus (EDL) and extensor digitorum brevis (EDB) and the extensor hallucis longus (EHL) and extensor hallucis brevis (EHB). These muscles are all supplied by the deep peroneal nerve (EHL, L5; EDL and EDB, L5-S1).

The long toe extensors extend the metatarsophalangeal (MTP) and IP joints and dorsiflex the ankle joint. The EDL is also an evertor. The EDB aids the EDL in extending the four medial toes. Dorsiflexion of the toes against resistance may be used as a test for the function of these muscles. The tendons of the long extensors and the belly of the EDB can be palpated during this maneuver (Figure 27.53). The EDB normally forms a prominent bulge on the dorsolateral aspect of the foot. Its most medial and largest belly is the EHB. The EDB is the muscle used for recording the compound muscle action potential when performing peroneal nerve conduction studies. The EDB atrophies easily in neurogenic processes, and its bulge may disappear in patients with radiculopathy or peripheral neuropathy. Preservation of EDB bulk in the face of foot dorsiflexion weakness suggests a myopathic process (e.g., distal myopathy, scapuloperoneal dystrophy, FSH dystrophy). Weakness of the EHL is a key clinical sign of L5 radiculopathy; it is sometimes the only weak muscle. In testing for subtle weakness between the two sides, a useful technique is for the examiner to test the muscle using a relatively weak hand muscle, such as the first DI or the

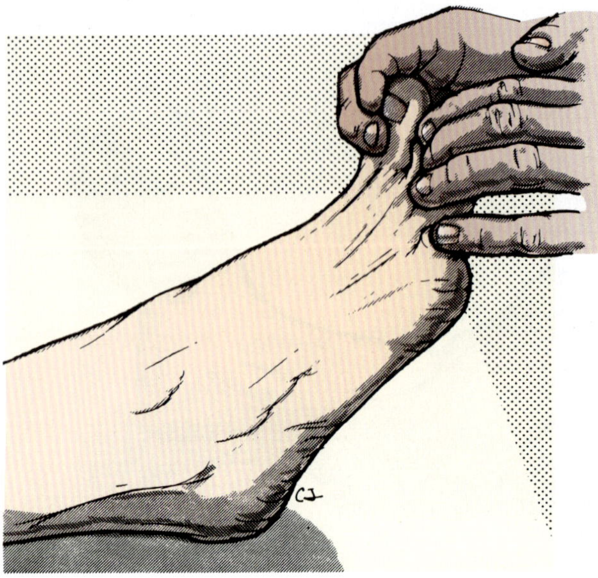

FIGURE 27.53 Examination of dorsiflexion (extension) of the toes. On attempts to dorsiflex the toes against resistance, the tendons of the extensors digitorum and hallucis longus and the belly of the extensor digitorum brevis can be seen and palpated.

ADM. Either of these muscles may be able to overcome the EHL on the weak side but not the normal side. When the EHL is severely weak in the absence of severe weakness of the other foot and toe extensors, the patient may have a "toe drop" rather than a "footdrop."

Flexion of the toes is carried out by the flexors digitorum and hallucis longus, flexors digitorum and hallucis brevis, and some of the intrinsic muscles of the sole of the foot. These muscles are tested by having the patient flex the toes against resistance (Figure 27.54). The long toe flexors are calf muscles, innervated by the tibial nerve (L5, S1-S2). These muscles flex the phalanges of all five toes, acting chiefly at the distal IP joints. They also plantar flex the ankle joint and invert the foot. The short toe flexors (medial

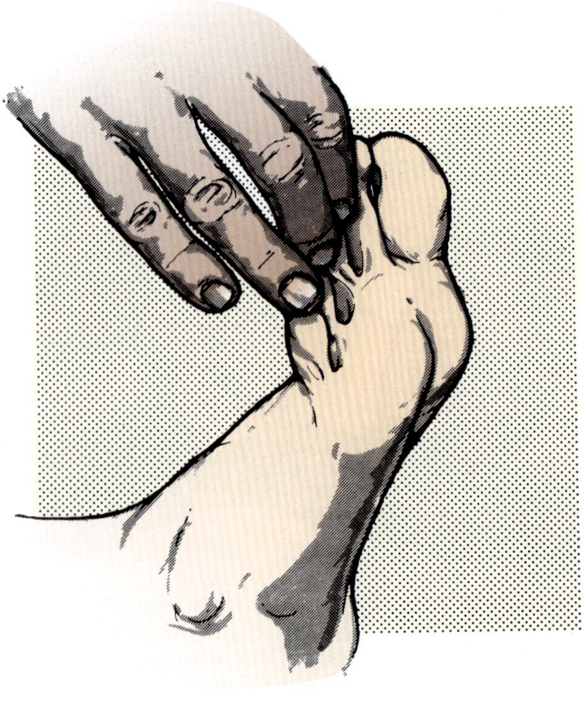

FIGURE 27.54 Examination of flexion of the toes. The patient attempts to flex the toes against resistance.

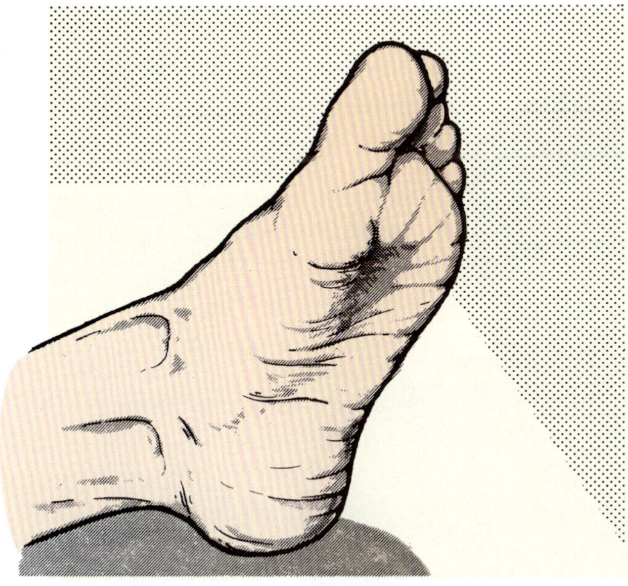

FIGURE 27.55 Cupping of the sole of the foot.

plantar nerve, S1-S2) act at the proximal IP and MTP joints. Testing of the intrinsic muscles of the sole of the foot is difficult and not clinically useful. Abduction and adduction are extremely weak movements, and the short toe flexors are more powerful than the other intrinsic muscles. These muscles may be tested together by asking the patient to cup the sole of the foot (Figure 27.55). Most of the intrinsic foot muscles are more important in maintaining the longitudinal arches of the foot than in moving the toes.

EXAMINATION FOR SUBTLE HEMIPARESIS

The motor examination is not concluded just with the formal strength assessment. Patients with mild CST lesions may have normal strength to routine testing, but the neurologic deficit may be brought out using ancillary maneuvers. The most important of these is the examination for pronator drift (Barré's sign). With the patient's upper extremities outstretched to the front, palms up and with the eyes closed, observe the position of each extremity (Figure 27.56). The patient should hold this position for at least 20 to 30 seconds. In normals, the palms will remain flat, the elbows straight, and the limbs horizontal. Any deviation from this position will be similar on the two sides. One exception to the usual symmetry is that the dominant hand occasionally may pronate slightly more than the nondominant, perhaps because the nondominant extremities tend to be more flexible than the dominant extremities, making it more difficult to stretch the dominant hand to a horizontal position. Slight pronation, without downward drift, of the dominant arm (pseudodrift) due to decreased flexibility is not necessarily abnormal and must be interpreted in clinical context. However, greater pronation of the nondominant arm is sometimes an indication of subtle hemiparesis. Except for pseudodrift and for coincidental orthopedic or musculoskeletal problems, there should be no difference between the positions of the two limbs.

The patient with a mild CST deficit may demonstrate "pronator drift" to varying degrees **(Video 27.2)**. With mild drift, there is slight pronation of the hand and slight flexion of the elbow on the abnormal side. With more severe drift, there is more prominent pronation and obvious flexion of the elbow, and there may be downward drift of the entire arm (Figure 27.57). Because of the innervation pattern of the CST, the minimally weak CST innervated muscles are overcome by the non-CST muscles. With a mild CST lesion, the minimally weak muscles in the upper extremity are the extensors, supinators, and abductors. These are overcome by the uninvolved and therefore stronger muscles: the pronators, biceps, and internal rotators of the shoulder. As these overcome the slightly weakened CST innervated muscles, the hand pronates, the elbow flexes, and the arm drifts downward. The tendency to pronation and

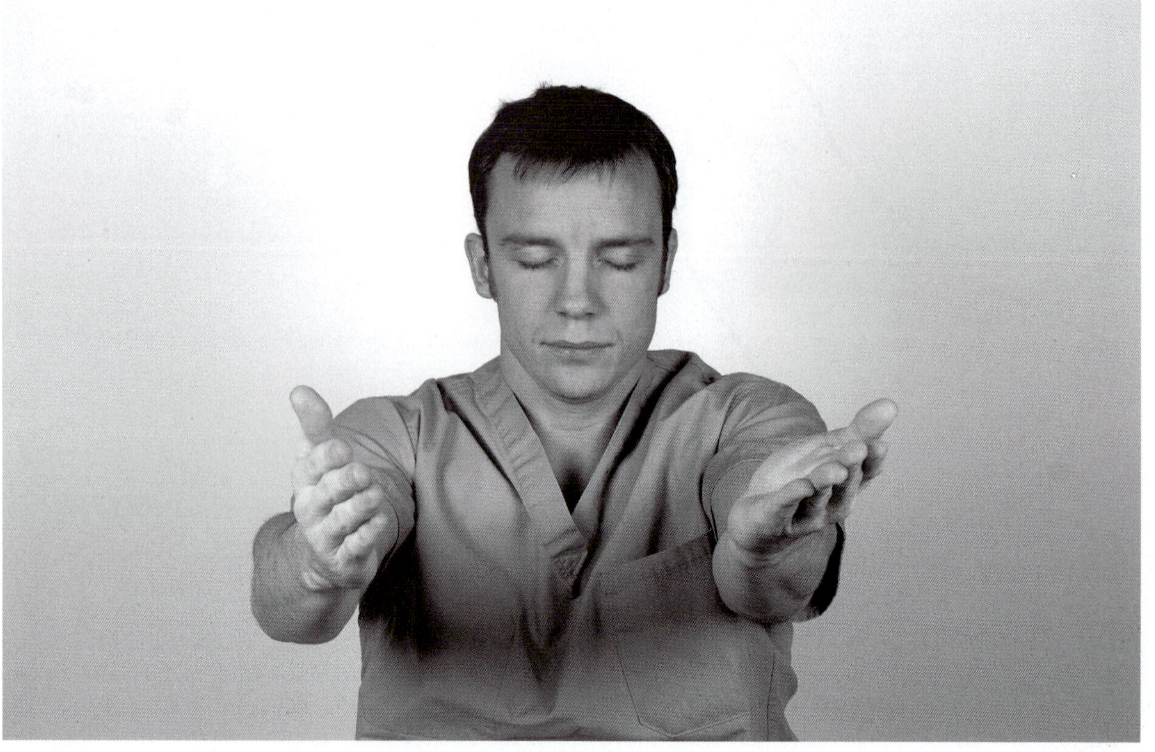

FIGURE 27.56 Technique for testing for pronator drift. In the presence of a corticospinal tract (CST) lesion, the selectively weakened muscles are the shoulder abductors and external rotators, the supinators, and the elbow extensors. These muscles are overcome by their antagonists to cause pronation, elbow flexion, and downward drift. This is an illustration of mild pronator drift of the right upper extremity. Patients with mild CST lesions may demonstrate a pronator drift or have an abnormal arm or finger roll test in the absence of clinically detectable weakness to formal strength testing.

flexion in mild hemiparesis has also been attributed to subtle hypertonicity in the pronator and flexor muscle groups. Imagine what would occur if this motion continued to the extreme: the hand would become hyperpronated, the elbow fully flexed, and the shoulder internally rotated, that is, the position of spastic hemiparesis (Figure 27.58). The abnormal upper limb positions in minimal pronator drift and in severe spastic hemiparesis are due to the same underlying phenomenon: strong non-CST muscles overcome variably weak CST muscles involved by the disease process. Another sign occasionally useful is the digiti quinti sign (see **Video Link 27.6**). With the hands outstretched in drift position, the small finger on the hemiparetic side may be abducted more than on the normal side.

Hachinski recently described the upgoing thumb sign as a subtle clinical finding in minor stroke. The thumb is extended (radially abducted) but with the palms facing it is upgoing. Souques described the "interosseous phenomenon" in 1907, in which elevation of a paretic arm caused abduction of all the fingers. The interosseous phenomenon, or finger sign, is usually classified as an associated movement (Chapter 42). Several subtle upper motor neuron signs that involve finger abduction are probably all related to the interosseous phenomenon originally described by Souques, including the digiti quinti sign; the upgoing thumb sign; myelopathy hand, a hand posture seen in patients with cervical spondylotic myelopathy; and the finger escape sign, widely cited in Orthopedic and Neurosurgery textbooks as a sign of cervical spondylotic myelopathy.

The examination for pronator drift is a very important part of the neurologic examination. If only one motor test could be done on a patient, the best single test to use would probably be examining for drift. While waiting for drift to occur, because it is not instantaneous, the examiner may simply wait or hasten the development of drift by tapping on the palms or having the patient turn the head back and forth or both. The examination for drift is often combined with the Romberg test because both require the patient to have the eyes closed.

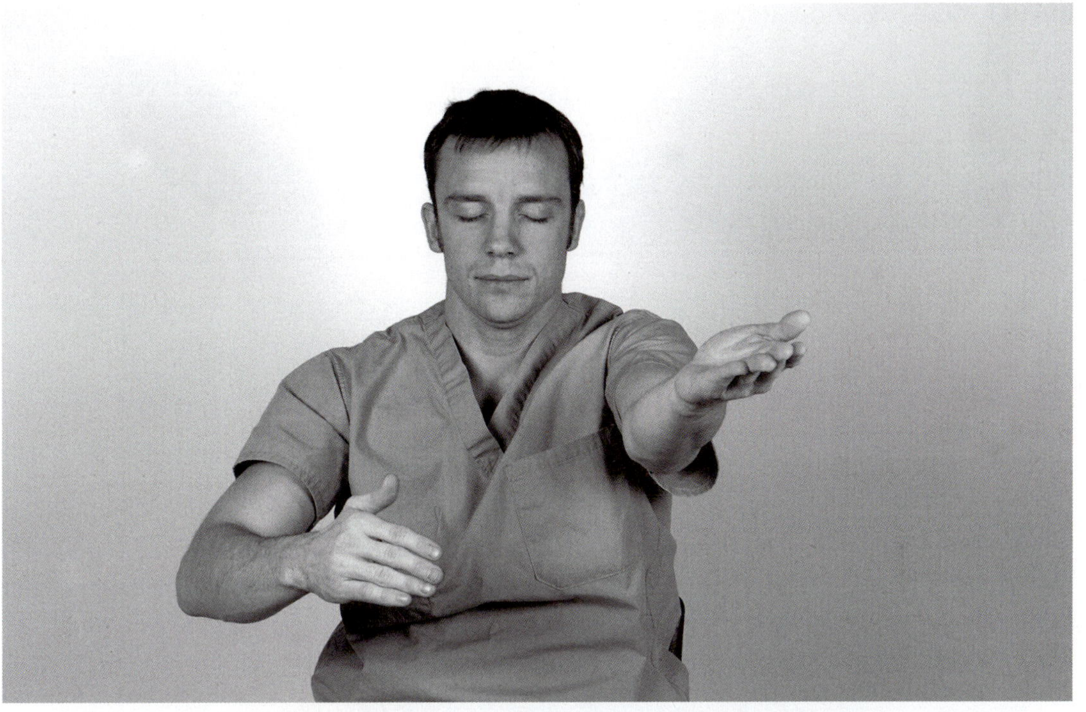

FIGURE 27.57 Moderate drift with further development of the posture.

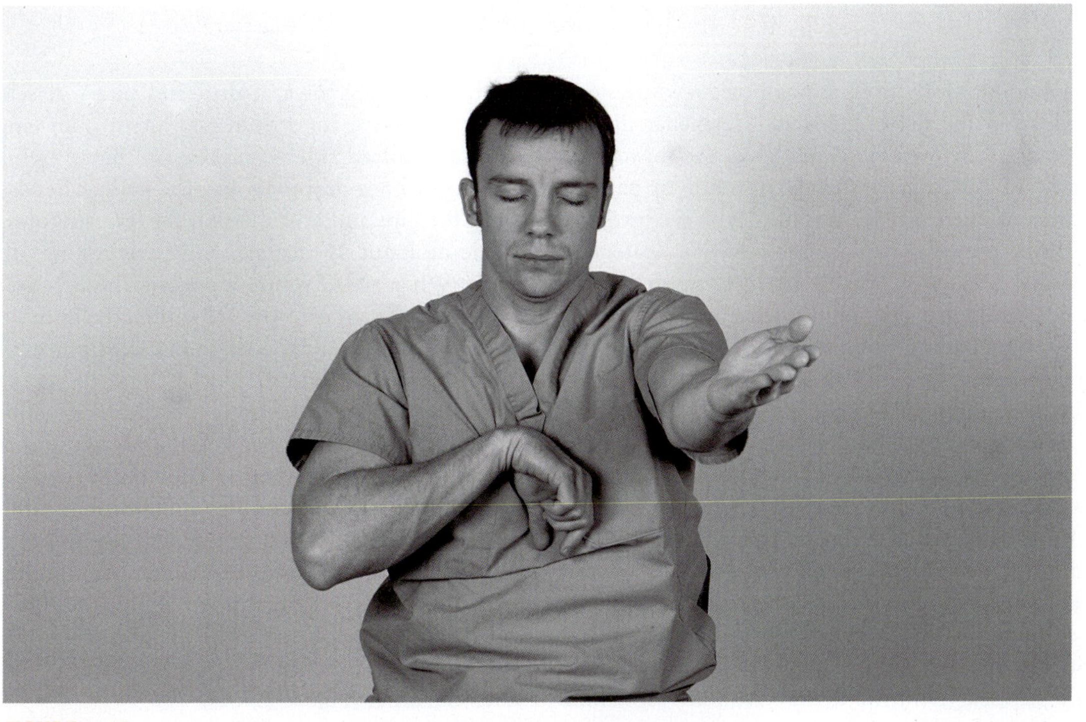

FIGURE 27.58 Further development of pronator drift, with the evolution of severe drift to show how marked weakness of the corticospinal innervated muscles produces the posture of spastic hemiparesis. The pathophysiologic basis for pronator drift and for the upper-extremity posture of fully developed spastic hemiparesis and for the upper-extremity posture of decorticate rigidity is the same; it is only a matter of degree. A mild CST lesion results in mild pronator drift; a severe lesion results in spastic hemiparesis.

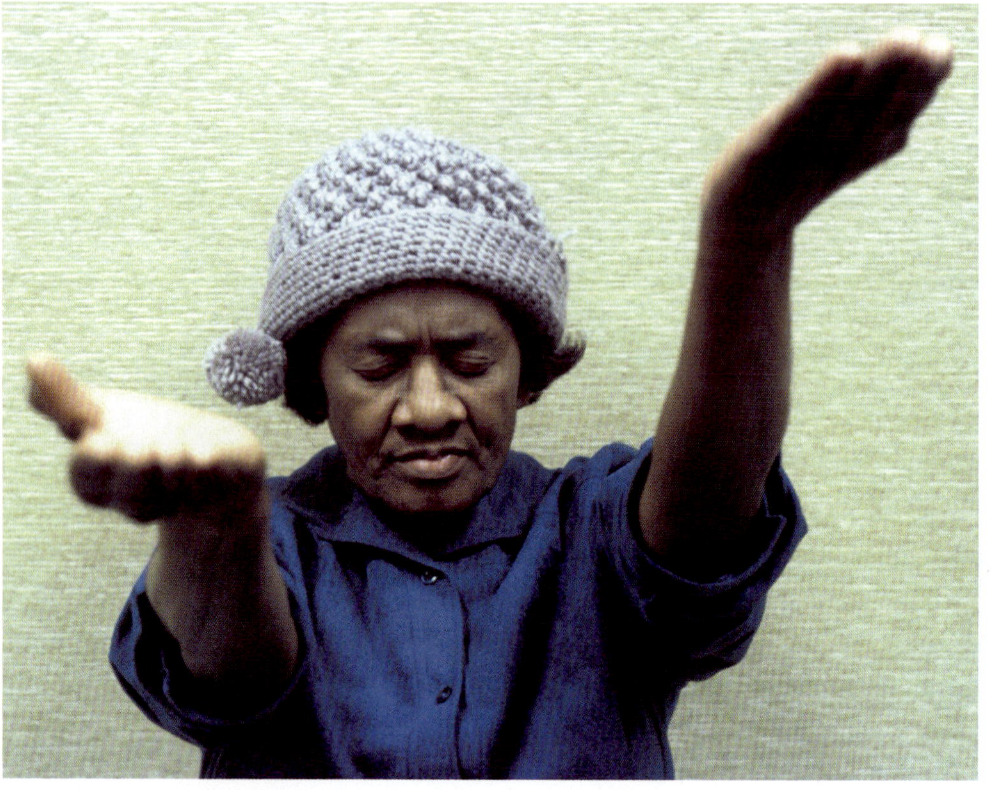

FIGURE 27.59 Updrift due to a parietal lobe lesion with loss of position sense.

Abnormal drift can occasionally occur with lesions elsewhere in the nervous system. Cerebellar disease may cause drift to some degree, but the movement is outward and usually slightly upward. In parietal lobe lesions, there may be "updrift," with the involved arm rising overhead without the patient's awareness, ostensibly because of loss of position sense (Figure 27.59). Additional pronation phenomena have been described by Babinski and Wilson. In the former, the palmar aspects of the hands are held in approximation with the thumbs up and are then jarred or shaken; the paretic hand falls into a position of pronation. In the latter, there is pronation of the forearm along with internal rotation at the shoulder when the arms are held overhead, palms facing; as a result, the affected palm turns outward. Pronation may also occur on the paretic side when the arms are actively abducted with the forearm supinated or when the arms are passively abducted with the forearm supinated and then suddenly released. Downward drift without pronation has been reported as a sign of nonorganic weakness.

Similar procedures can be used to detect lower-extremity weakness. Examination for leg drift is possible (see "The Hip Joint") but is not nearly as useful as testing for arm drift and therefore seldom done. Checking for a decreased rate of foot tapping on the involved side is simpler and more useful. In the leg or knee-dropping test, the patient lies supine with the hips and knees flexed, the knees forming an angle of about 45 degrees, and heels resting on the table. When a CST lesion is present, the affected heel will gradually slide downward so that the knee slowly extends, and the hip goes into extension, external rotation, and abduction.

Other useful maneuvers include examination of forearm roll, finger roll, thumb roll, and rapid alternating movements **(Video 27.3)**. Abnormal forearm rolling is a sensitive indicator of neurologic pathology. To test it, the patient is instructed to make fists, to hold the forearms horizontally so that the fists and distal forearms overlap with the palms pointed more or less toward the umbilicus, and then to rotate the fists around each other, first in one direction and then the other (Figure 27.60).

Normal patients will have about an equal excursion of both forearms so that the fists and forearms roll about each other symmetrically. With a unilateral corticospinal lesion, the involved side does not move as

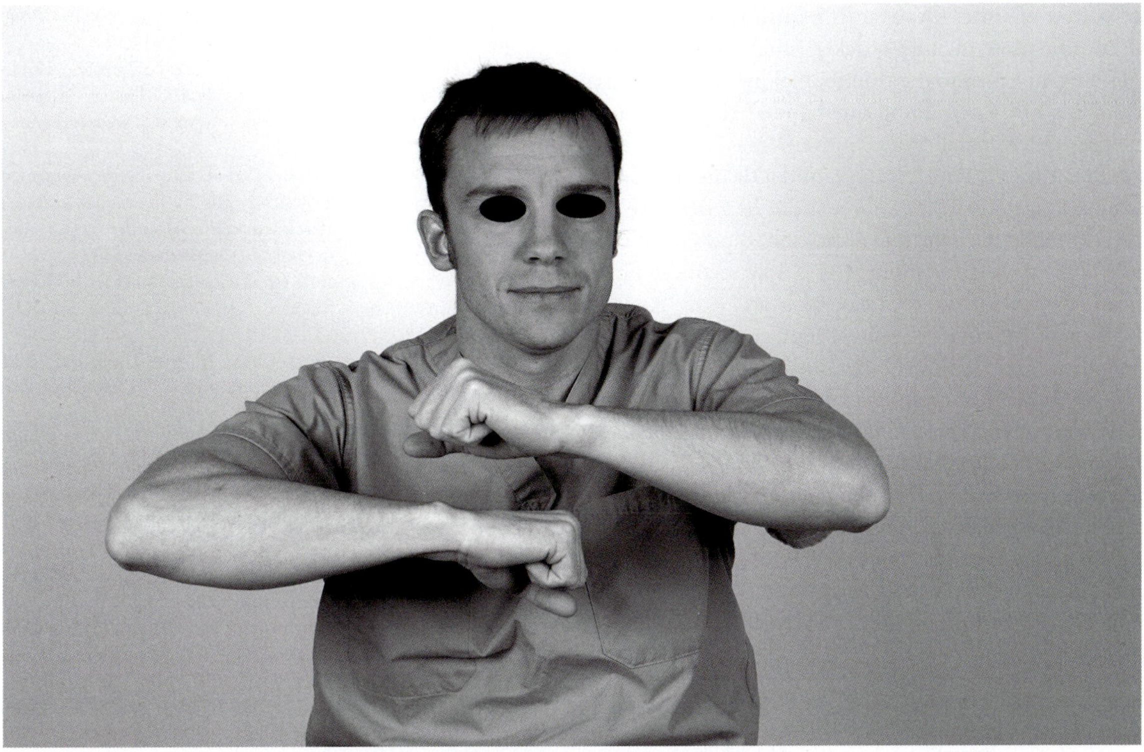

FIGURE 27.60 Testing for a CST lesion using arm roll. The involved extremity tends to have a lesser excursion as the forearms roll about each other so that the normal extremity tends to rotate around the abnormal extremity, which tends to remain relatively fixed ("posted"). Patients with mild CST lesions may have an abnormal arm roll test in the absence of clinically detectable weakness to formal strength testing.

much as the normal side, so the patient will appear to plant, fix, or "post" one forearm and to rotate the opposite forearm around it **(Video 27.4)**. Finger roll is an even more sensitive version of the same test. The patient is asked to rotate the extended forefingers around each other, moving just the fingers. Again, the finger on the abnormal side will move less than its fellow. In the thumb rolling test, the patient rotates each thumb around its fellow. Forearm rolling has a sensitivity of 17% to 87%, specificity of 97% to 98%, positive LR of 15.6, and negative LR of 0.6 in the detection of contralateral hemispheric disease. Index finger rolling has a sensitivity of 33% to 42%, a specificity of 92% to 98%, positive LR of 6.0, and negative LR of 0.7 in the detection of contralateral hemispheric disease. In a series of patients with mild hemiparesis, thumb rolling was more sensitive (88%) than pronator drift (47%), forearm rolling (65%), or index finger rolling (65%). Patients with bradykinesia or rigidity from extrapyramidal disease may also show decreased excursion of the affected limbs.

Normal fine motor control requires functional integrity of both the CST and the cerebellum. Testing for rapid alternating movements is part of the cerebellar examination, but the primary function of the CST is to provide discrete, fractionated movements to the distal extremities. Either CST or cerebellar disease may interfere with fine motor control of distal muscles. Normal fine motor control also requires intact proprioceptive pathways. Traditionally, different tests have been done to look for CST signs than for cerebellar signs, but both involve rapid alternating movements. This test is also referred to as assessment of alternate motion rate, but in fact more than the rate of motion provides useful information. Fine motor control can be tested in numerous ways, most advantageously by comparing the dexterity and precision of the two hands while performing rapid, repetitive movements, making allowance of course for hand dominance. The patient may be asked to repetitively, and as quickly as possible, touch the tip of the index finger to the tip of the thumb, as in making the OK sign. Any finger can be used, but the index and small fingers are favorites. The movements will be slower and less agile on the abnormal side. This test is often done by having the patient touch the IP joint rather than the tip of the thumb. Rough quantitation can be done by counting the number of touches in a set period of time. Other tests requiring a high level of coordination include quickly touching the tip of each finger in turn to the thumb, flicking the fingers as if flicking off water, doing one-handed clapping, and making quick, small finger movements as if playing a piano. Patients with extrapyramidal disorders, especially parkinsonism, may show more of a decrease in the amplitude than the rate of motion, especially if the task is continued for more than a few seconds. Fine motor control of the foot can be assessed by having the patient do rapid, repetitive foot taps on the floor if standing and against the examiner's palm if supine.

Abnormalities of associated movements may also occur relatively early in a CST lesion. These may include the absence of a normal associated movement, such as a decreased arm swing while walking, or the presence of an abnormal associated movement, such as Wartenberg's thumb adduction sign, the Babinski trunk-thigh sign, or the anterior tibial sign (Chapter 42).

Video Links

Video Link 27.1. Scapular winging. http://www.youtube.com/watch?v=dfTe0nPclDE
Video Link 27.2. Pectoral crease in shoulder girdle weakness. http://neurosigns.org/wiki/Pectoral_crease
Video Link 27.3. Beevor's sign. http://neurosigns.org/wiki/Beevor%27s_sign
Video Link 27.4. Gowers' sign. http://neurosigns.org/wiki/Gower%27s_sign
Video Link 27.5. Steppage gait. http://neurosigns.org/wiki/Steppage_Gait
Video Link 27.6. Digiti quinti sign. http://neurosigns.org/wiki/Digiti_quinti_sign

BIBLIOGRAPHY

Anderson NE. The forearm and finger rolling tests. *Pract Neurol* 2010;10:39–42.

Brendler SJ. The human cervical myotomes: functional anatomy studied at operation. *J Neurosurg* 1968;28:105–111.

Brooke MH. *A Clinician's View of Neuromuscular Disease*. 2nd ed. Baltimore: Williams & Wilkins, 1986.

Buschbacher R. Side-to-side confrontational strength-testing for weakness of the intrinsic muscles of the hand. *J Bone Joint Surg Am* 1997;79:401–405.

Campbell WW. *Clinical Signs in Neurology: A Compendium*. Philadelphia: Wolters Kluwer Health, 2016.

Campbell WW, Pridgeon RP. *Practical Primer of Clinical Neurology*. Philadelphia: Lippincott Williams & Wilkins, 2002.

Carter AB. The functional overlay. *Lancet* 1967;2:1196–1200.

Chabrol H, Peresson G, Clanet M. Lack of specificity of the traditional criteria for conversion disorders. *Eur Psychiatry* 1995;10:317–319.

Crimlisk HL, Bhatia K, Cope H, et al. Slater revisited: 6 year follow up study of patients with medically unexplained motor symptoms. *BMJ* 1998;316:582–586.

Daum C, Aybek S. Validity of the "Drift without pronation" sign in conversion disorder. *BMC Neurol* 2013;13:31.

Daum C, Hubschmid M, Aybek S. The value of 'positive' clinical signs for weakness, sensory and gait disorders in conversion disorder: a systematic and narrative review. *J Neurol Neurosurg Psychiatry* 2014;85:180–190.

Daum C, Gheorghita F, Spatola M, et al. Interobserver agreement and validity of bedside 'positive signs' for functional weakness, sensory and gait disorders in conversion disorder: a pilot study. *J Neurol Neurosurg Psychiatry* 2015;86425–86430.

Espay AJ, Aybek S, Carson A, et al. Current concepts in diagnosis and treatment of functional neurological disorders. *JAMA Neurol* 2018;75(9):1132–1141.

Gerscovich EO, Cronan M, McGahan JP, et al. Ultrasonographic evaluation of diaphragmatic motion. *J Ultrasound Med* 2001;20:597–604.

Gould R, Miller BL, Goldberg MA, et al. The validity of hysterical signs and symptoms. *J Nerv Ment Dis* 1986;174:593–597.

Hachinski V, Alsubaie R, Azarpazhooh MR. Upgoing thumb sign: a sensitive indicator of brain involvement? *Neurology* 2017; 89:370–375.

Koehler PJ, Okun MS. Important observations prior to the description of the Hoover sign. *Neurology* 2004;63:1693–1697.

LaFrance WC Jr. Video NeuroImage: diagnosing conversion weakness with the Spinal Injuries Center test: when Hoover doesn't help. *Neurology* 2008;71:e57.

Lanska DJ. Functional weakness and sensory loss. *Semin Neurol* 2006;26:297–309.

Lehmkuhl LD, Smith LK. *Brunnstrom's Clinical Kinesiology*. 4th ed. Philadelphia: F.A. Davis Company, 1983.

Lempert T, Dieterich M, Huppert D, et al. Psychogenic disorders in neurology: frequency and clinical spectrum. *Acta Neurol Scand* 1990;82:335–340.

Lemyze M, Bart F. Hoover sign. *CMAJ* 2011;183:E133.

Liguori R, Krarup C, Trojaborg W. Determination of the segmental sensory and motor innervation of the lumbosacral spinal nerves. An electrophysiological study. *Brain* 1992;115:915–934.

Mace CJ, Trimble MR. Ten-year prognosis of conversion disorder. *Br J Psychiatry* 1996;169:282–288.

Massey EW, Pleet AB, Scherokman BJ. *Diagnostic Tests in Neurology: A Photographic Guide to Bedside Techniques*. Chicago: Year Book Medical Publishers, Inc., 1985.

McGee S. *Evidence Based Physical Diagnosis*. 3rd ed. Philadelphia: Elsevier/Saunders, 2012.

McWhirter L, Stone J, Sandercock P, et al. Hoover's sign for the diagnosis of functional weakness: a prospective unblinded cohort study in patients with suspected stroke. *J Psychosom Res* 2011; 71:384–386.

Mendell JR, Florence J. Manual muscle testing. *Muscle Nerve* 1990;13:S16–S20.

Nowak DA. The thumb rolling test: a novel variant of the forearm rolling test. *Can J Neurol Sci* 2011;38:129–132.

Ono K, Ebara S, Fuji T, et al. Myelopathy hand. New clinical signs of cervical cord damage. *J Bone Joint Surg Br* 1987;69: 215–219.

Phillips LH II, Park TS. Electrophysiologic mapping of the segmental anatomy of the muscles of the lower extremity. *Muscle Nerve* 2011;43:1–2.

Pleet AB, Massey EW. Palmaris brevis sign in neuropathy of the deep palmar branch of the ulnar nerve. *Ann Neurol* 1978;3: 468–469.

Reuber M, Mitchell AJ, Howlett SJ, et al. Functional symptoms in neurology: questions and answers. *J Neurol Neurosurg Psychiatry* 2005;76:307–314.

Sawyer RN Jr, Hanna JP, Ruff RL, et al. Asymmetry of forearm rolling as a sign of unilateral cerebral dysfunction. *Neurology* 1993;43:1596–1598.

Slater E. Diagnosis of "hysteria". *Br Med J* 1965;1:1395–1399.

Slater ET, Glithero E. A follow-up of patients diagnosed as suffering from "hysteria". *J Psychosom Res* 1965;9:9–13.

Sonoo M. Abductor sign: a reliable new sign to detect unilateral non-organic paresis of the lower limb. *J Neurol Neurosurg Psychiatry* 2004;75:121–125.

Standring S, ed. *Gray's Anatomy: The Anatomical Basis of Clinical Practice*. 41st ed. New York: Elsevier Limited, 2016.

Stone J, Zeman A, Sharpe M. Functional weakness and sensory disturbance. *J Neurol Neurosurg Psychiatry* 2002a;73:241–245.

Stone J, Sharpe M, Carson A, et al. Are functional motor and sensory symptoms really more frequent on the left? A systematic review. *J Neurol Neurosurg Psychiatry* 2002b;73:578–581.

Stone J, Sharpe M, Rothwell PM, et al. The 12 year prognosis of unilateral functional weakness and sensory disturbance. *J Neurol Neurosurg Psychiatry* 2003;74:591–596.

Stone J, Smyth R, Carson A, et al. La belle indifference in conversion symptoms and hysteria: systematic review. *Br J Psychiatry* 2006;188:204–209.

Stone J, Warlow C, Sharpe M. The symptom of functional weakness: a controlled study of 107 patients. *Brain* 2010;133(Pt 5): 1537–1551.

Stone J, Warlow C, Sharpe M. Functional weakness: clues to mechanism from the nature of onset. *J Neurol Neurosurg Psychiatry* 2012;83:67–69.

Tinazzi M, Simonetto S, Franco L, et al. Abduction finger sign: a new sign to detect unilateral functional paralysis of the upper limb. *Mov Disord* 2008;23:2415–2419.

Tremolizzo L, Susani E, Riva MA, et al. Positive signs of functional weakness. *J Neurol Sci* 2014;340:13–18.

Weibers DO, Dale AJD, Kokmen E, et al., eds. *Mayo Clinic Examinations in Neurology*. 7th ed. St. Louis: Mosby, 1998.

Wolf JK. *Segmental Neurology*. Baltimore: University Park Press, 1981.

Yamamoto T. Forearm-rolling test. *Neurology* 1995;45:2299.

Young A, Getty J, Jackson A, et al. Variations in the pattern of muscle innervation by the L5 and S1 nerve roots. *Spine* 1983; 8:616–624.

Yugué I, Shiba K, Ueta T, et al. A new clinical evaluation for hysterical paralysis. *Spine (Phila Pa 1976)* 2004;29:1910–1913.

Ziv I, Djaldetti R, Zoldan Y, et al. Diagnosis of "non-organic" limb paresis by a novel objective motor assessment: the quantitative Hoover's test. *J Neurol* 1998;245:797–802.

CHAPTER 28

Muscle Tone

Muscle tone has been defined as the tension in the relaxed muscle or the resistance to passive movement when voluntary contraction is absent. Because of resting tone, normal muscles have slight resistance to passive movement even in the relaxed state. The inherent attributes of muscle tissue—such as viscosity, elasticity, and extensibility—contribute to resting tone. Even apparently relaxed muscle fibers have a constant slight fixed tension by which they hold their resting position, resist changes in length, prevent undue mobility at joints, and are in position to contract when necessary. Resting muscle tone is greatest in the antigravity muscles that maintain the body in an erect position.

The resting level of tone in a muscle is dependent on activity in the spinal cord segment that innervates it, primarily the gamma motor neuron. Efferent impulses from the gamma motor neuron set the level of contraction of the intrafusal fibers of the muscle spindles. Spindle afferents in turn convey impulses to the spinal cord segment to complete the gamma loop. Descending influences from higher motor centers regulate and modulate the activity at the local spinal cord segment. All of these factors interact to determine the level of resting tone. When a muscle with normal segmental innervation is passively stretched, reflex shortening may occur; this is the stretch reflex.

The background level of muscle tone maintains normal resting limb positions and attitudes. Active muscle contraction takes place on the background of the resting level of muscle tone, and normal background tone is important for proper coordination of movement. Activity mediated by the reticular formation, the otolith organs, the vestibular apparatus, and other higher centers is important in maintaining the steady contraction of the antigravity muscles that is necessary to the standing position, as well as to other postural and righting reflexes.

Tone may be affected by disease at different levels of the nervous system. Interruption of the local spinal reflex arc abolishes resting muscle tone. Most types of hypertonicity can be abolished by interrupting either the gamma efferent impulses to the intrafusal fibers or the afferent impulses from the muscle spindles. Denervated muscle is flaccid and behaves as noncontractile tissue. Loss of impulses from the supraspinal pathways that normally inhibit lower reflex centers usually causes an increase in tone. Loss of the normal balance between higher facilitatory and inhibitory centers may either decrease or increase tone.

EXAMINATION OF TONE

Tone is difficult to assess. The determination of tone is subjective and prone to interexaminer variability. There are no methods that can measure tone quantitatively. The determination is based solely on the clinical judgment of the examiner; accurate assessment of tone requires clinical experience. It is difficult to separate slightly increased tone from poor relaxation in a tense or apprehensive patient. Tone is especially difficult to evaluate in infants, where there may be wide variations in apparent tone on different examinations, in either health or disease.

The examination of tone requires a relaxed and cooperative patient. Small talk may help the patient relax. Simple observation may reveal an abnormality of posture or resting position that indicates an underlying change in tone. Muscle palpation is sometimes useful, but well-muscled individuals may have firm muscles despite normal resting tone, whereas in other individuals, the muscles may feel flabby despite an underlying hypertonicity. Muscles may have a firm consistency to palpation because of edema, inflammation, spasm due to pain, or pseudohypertrophy.

The most important part of the examination of tone is determination of the resistance of relaxed muscles to passive manipulation as well as the extensibility, flexibility, and range of motion. Abnormalities of tone are more easily detected in extremity than in trunk muscles. The limb is moved passively, first slowly and through a complete range of motion and then at varying speeds. The examiner may shake the forearm to and fro and note the excursions of the patient's hand, brace a limb and then suddenly remove the support, or note the range of movement of a part in response to a slight blow. Bilateral examination of homologous parts helps compare for differences in tone on the two sides of the body.

Tone should be assessed by both slow and rapid motion and through partial and full range of motion, documenting the distribution, type, and severity of any abnormality. Certain specific maneuvers may be helpful in evaluation of abnormal tone.

The Babinski Tonus Test

The arms are abducted at the shoulders, and the forearms are passively flexed at the elbows. With hypotonicity, there is increased flexibility and mobility, and the elbows can be bent to an angle more acute than normal. With hypertonicity, there is reduced flexibility, and passive flexion cannot be carried out beyond an obtuse angle.

The Head-Dropping Test

The patient lies supine without a pillow, completely relaxed, eyes closed, and attention diverted. The examiner places one hand under the patient's occiput and with the other hand briskly raises the head and then allows it to drop. Normally, the head drops rapidly into the examiner's protecting hand, but in patients with extrapyramidal rigidity, there is delayed, slow, gentle dropping of the head because of rigidity affecting the flexor muscles of the neck. When meningismus is present, there is resistance to and pain on flexion of the neck.

Pendulousness of the Legs

The patient sits on the edge of a table, relaxed with legs hanging freely. The examiner either extends both legs to the same horizontal level and then releases them (Wartenberg pendulum test, see **Video Link 28.1**) or gives both legs a brisk, equal backward push. If the patient is completely relaxed and cooperative, there will normally be a swinging of the legs that progressively diminishes in range and usually disappears after six or seven oscillations. In extrapyramidal rigidity, there is a decrease in swing time but usually no qualitative change in the response. In spasticity, there may be little or no decrease in swing time, but the movements are jerky and irregular, the forward movement may be greater and more brisk than the backward, and the movement may assume a zigzag pattern. In hypotonia, the response is increased in range and prolonged beyond the normal. In all of these maneuvers, a unilateral abnormality will be more apparent.

The Shoulder-Shaking Test

The examiner places her hands on the patient's shoulders and shakes them briskly back and forth, observing the reciprocal motion of the arms. With extrapyramidal disease, there will be a decreased range of arm swing on the affected side. With hypotonia, especially that associated with cerebellar disease, the excursions of the arm swing will be greater than normal.

The Arm-Dropping Test

The patient's arms are briskly raised to shoulder level and then dropped. In spasticity, there is a delay in the downward movement of the affected arm, causing it to hang up briefly on the affected side (Bechterew's or Bekhterew's sign); with hypotonicity, the dropping is more abrupt than normal. A similar maneuver may be carried out by lifting and then dropping the extended legs of the recumbent patient.

Hand Position

Hypotonicity, especially that associated with cerebellar disease or Sydenham's chorea, may cause the hands to assume a characteristic posture. With the arms and hands outstretched, there is flexion at the wrists and hyperextension of the fingers ("spooning") accompanied by moderate overpronation. With the arms raised overhead, the overpronation is exaggerated with the palms turned outward. This overpronation phenomenon differs from the pronator drift sign, in which the overpronation is due to weakness of corticospinal innervated muscles or increased tone in the pronator muscles.

MYOTATIC IRRITABILITY, MYOEDEMA, AND TENDERNESS

In addition to the inspection, palpation, and resistance to passive motion used in the assessment of tone, it is sometimes useful to observe the reaction to direct percussion of the muscle belly. The idiomuscular contraction is the brief and feeble contraction of a muscle belly after it is tapped with a percussion hammer, causing a slight depression even when the deep tendon reflex (DTR) is absent. Myotactic irritability has been defined as both the response to direct percussion as well as the ability of a muscle to contract in response to sudden stretch.

The response to direct muscle percussion in normal muscle is very slight and, in most muscles, is seen or felt with difficulty. The reaction may be more pronounced in wasting diseases, such as cachexia and emaciation, and in some diseases of the lower motor neuron. Hyperexcitability to such stimulation occurs in tetanus, tetany, and certain electrolyte disturbances. Occasionally, after a muscle is percussed with a reflex hammer, a wave of contraction radiates along the muscle away from the point of percussion. A small ridge or temporary swelling may persist for several seconds at the point of stimulation. This stationary muscle mounding is known as myoedema. There is no accompanying electrical muscle activity. The idiomuscular contraction causes a slight depression, myoedema a rounding up. The mechanism of myoedema is poorly understood, but it is probably a normal physiologic phenomenon. Its presence alone does not indicate a neuromuscular disorder, but the response may be exaggerated in some circumstances, most notably hypothyroid myopathy and cachexia. Myoedema is electrically silent on electromyography. Hypothyroidism may also cause an electrically active muscle mounding and spreading contraction, manifest by a burst of normal motor unit action potentials upon percussion (for video, see Loomis et al.). Myotonia is a persisting contraction following mechanical stimulation of muscle that is quite different from myoedema (see below). In rippling muscle disease, there are wave-like muscle contractions evoked by muscle stretch that move laterally along the muscle over 5 to 20 seconds. The phenomenon is especially prominent in large proximal muscles (see **Video Link 28.2**).

During muscle palpation, muscle tenderness may sometimes be elicited. Muscle tenderness on squeezing the muscle belly, or even with very slight pressure, may cause exquisite pain. Widespread muscle tenderness to palpation may occur with inflammatory myopathy, especially polymyositis and dermatomyositis, in some neuropathies, and in acute poliomyelitis. Focal muscle tenderness occurs with trauma or overexertion of muscles.

ABNORMALITIES OF TONE

Pathologic conditions may cause an increase or decrease in tone. In addition, there are different varieties of hypotonicity and hypertonicity. Hypotonicity may develop from disease of the motor unit, the proprioceptive pathways, cerebellar lesions and in the choreas. The muscle may be flaccid, flabby, and soft to palpation. The involved joints offer decreased resistance to passive movement. The excursion of the joint may be increased with an absence of the normal "checking" action on extreme passive motion. If the involved extremity is lifted and allowed to drop, it falls abruptly. A slight blow causes it to sway through an excessive excursion. The DTRs are usually decreased or absent when hypotonia is due to a lesion involving the motor unit or proprioceptive pathways.

Hypotonia

When hypotonia is due to disease of the motor unit, there is invariably some degree of accompanying weakness. The hypotonia that results from central processes (e.g., cerebellar disease) does not cause weakness; muscle power is preserved even though hypotonia is demonstrable on examination. Infantile hypotonia (floppy baby syndrome) is a common clinical condition in which there is a generalized decrease in muscle tone, typically affecting a neonate. There are numerous causes, both central and peripheral.

Tone may also be decreased when disease affects the muscle spindle afferent system. Tabes dorsalis affects proprioceptive fibers in the posterior root and may cause muscle hypotonia with joint hyperextensibility. Hypotonia may occur with some lesions of the parietal lobe, probably because of disturbances of sensation. Hypotonicity may occur with various types of cerebellar disease but is never as severe as that which occurs with diseases of the lower motor neuron. Cerebellar hypotonia is not associated with weakness and the reflexes are not lost, although they may be pendular; there are no pathologic reflexes. Muscle tone is, of course, decreased in deep sleep, coma, and other states of impaired consciousness.

Sudden attacks of impaired muscle tone in an awake patient occur in akinetic epilepsy and in cataplexy. With atonic (akinetic) seizures, the attacks of sudden loss of muscle tone occur spontaneously, and the patient may fall to the ground (drop attack or drop seizure). Less severe attacks may cause only a head drop. In cataplexy, there are attacks of decreased tone after strong emotion, such as laughter or anger. With severe attacks, the patient falls to the ground but without loss of consciousness. With incomplete attacks, there may be slackening of facial muscles, jaw drop, head drop, slumping of the shoulders, or knee buckling without a fall. Cataplexy is usually a component of narcolepsy. Sleep paralysis is a state common in narcolepsy, in which a patient has diffusely decreased tone and is unable to move immediately after awakening from sleep. The hemiparesis that is present acutely following hemispheric stroke may be associated with hypotonia (cerebral or neural "shock"), which gradually evolves into hypertonia with the passage of time. Some conditions may cause abnormal joint laxity, which may be confused with muscle hypotonia (e.g., Ehlers-Danlos syndrome).

Hypertonia

Hypertonia occurs under many circumstances. It is a routine feature of lesions that involve the corticospinal tract after the acute stage. It can occur with diffuse cerebral disorders, with disease involving the extrapyramidal system, with disease of spinal cord interneurons (e.g., stiff-person syndrome), and even with muscle disorders in continuous muscle fiber activity syndromes. The most common causes of hypertonia are spasticity and rigidity. For a discussion and demonstration of spasticity versus rigidity from the 2015 Stanford Medicine 25 Skills Symposium, see **Video Link 28.3**.

Extrapyramidal Rigidity

Extrapyramidal rigidity is a diffuse increase in muscle tone to passive movement that occurs primarily with lesions that involve the basal ganglia. There is a fairly constant level of increased tone that affects both agonist and antagonist and is equally present throughout the range of motion at a given joint. Both flexor and extensor muscles are involved, with resistance to passive movement in all directions. The increased tone is equally present from the beginning to the end of the movement and does not vary with the speed of the movement. This type of rigidity is referred to as "lead-pipe." The involved muscles may be firm and tense to palpation. After being placed in a new position, the part may remain there, causing the limbs to assume awkward postures. Both neural-mediated excitation of shortening muscles (the shortening reaction) and inhibition of stretched muscles contribute to the rigidity; which mechanism predominates is associated with the direction of movement. An increase in spinal interneuron excitability mediated through specific descending motor pathways may underlie parkinsonian rigidity.

In cogwheel rigidity, there is a jerky quality to the hypertonicity. As the part is manipulated, it seems to give way in a series of small steps as if the limb were attached to a heavy cogwheel or ratchet. The jerky quality of the resistance may be due to tremor superimposed on lead-pipe rigidity. Cogwheel rigidity is most commonly encountered in Parkinson's disease and other parkinsonian syndromes. It appears first in proximal muscles and then spreads distally. Any muscle may be affected, but there is predominant involvement of neck and trunk muscles and the flexor muscles of the extremities. The rigidity of extrapyramidal disease may be brought out by the head-dropping, shoulder-shaking, and similar tests. The rigidity on one side may be exaggerated by active movements of the contralateral limbs (see Chapter 30).

In extrapyramidal disease, there is usually associated hypokinesia and bradykinesia, but no real paralysis. With repeated active movements, there is a gradual decrease in speed and amplitude. This may be brought out by having the patient rapidly open and close the eyes or mouth, open and close the hand, or oppose finger and thumb. Patients may also show slowness of starting and limitation of the amplitude of movement, loss of pendulousness of the arms and legs, inability to carry out rapid repeated movements or to maintain two simultaneous voluntary movements, and impairment of associated movements, such as swinging of the arms when walking.

Paratonia is an alteration in tone to passive motion that is often a manifestation of diffuse frontal lobe disease. It has been divided into inhibitory paratonia and facilitatory paratonia. Gegenhalten (inhibitory paratonia, paratonic rigidity) is a form of rigidity in which the resistance to passive movement seems proportional to the vigor with which the movement is attempted. The resistance of the patient increases in proportion to the examiner's efforts to move the part; the harder the examiner pushes, the harder the patient seems to push back. It seems as though the patient is actively fighting, but the response is involuntary. It is said that the severity of gegenhalten can be judged by the loudness of the examiner's exhortations to relax.

In the limb placement test, the examiner passively lifts the patient's arm, instructs the patient to relax, releases the arm, and notes whether or not it remains elevated. The arm remaining aloft, in the absence of parkinsonism or spasticity, indicates paratonia. In facilatory paratonia (mitgehen), the patient cooperates too much. The patient actively assists the examiner's passive movements, and the limb may continue to move even after the examiner has released it. In the modified Kral procedure, the examiner instructs the seated patient to relax and then passively flexes and extends the elbow several times through a full range of motion, releasing the arm with the patient's hand at the level of the thigh. Further movement is scored on a scale of 0 (no movement) to 4 (elbow flexes fully or cycles of flexion and extension continue).

Using a Delphi procedure, experts agreed on the following definition of paratonia: paratonia is a form of hypertonia with an involuntary variable resistance during passive movement; the nature of paratonia may vary from active assistance to active resistance; the degree of resistance depends on the speed of movement (e.g., slow → low resistance, fast → high resistance); the degree of paratonia is proportional to the amount of force applied; and the resistance to passive movement is in any direction and there is no clasp-knife phenomenon. The Paratonia Assessment Instrument is an assessment tool for paratonia. For a training video on paratonia from the Geriatric Medicine Research Unit at Dalhousie University, see **Video Link 28.4**.

Spasticity

Spasticity is due to lesions involving the corticospinal pathways. The hypertonicity to passive movements differs from that of rigidity because it is not uniform throughout the range of movement, and it varies with the speed of movement. In addition, rigidity tends to affect all muscles to about the same degree, whereas the hypertonia of spasticity varies greatly from muscle to muscle. In spasticity, if the passive movement is made slowly, there may be little resistance. But if the movement is made quickly, there will be a sudden increase in tone partway through the arc, causing a catch or a block as though the muscle had impacted a stop. The relationship of the hypertonus to the speed of movement is a key feature distinguishing spasticity from rigidity. In the upper extremity, it is useful to look for spasticity involving the pronator muscles. With the patient's elbow flexed to about 90 degrees and the forearm fully pronated, the examiner slowly supinates the patient's hand. Unless spasticity is severe, there will be little or no resistance to this slow movement. If, after several slow repetitions, the examiner supinates the patient's hand very quickly, there will be sudden resistance at about the midrange of movement, referred to as a "pronator catch." The catch will then relax, and the supination movement can be completed. When hypertonus is severe, this maneuver may elicit pronator clonus.

A similar slow then rapid motion technique can be used to detect lower-extremity spasticity. With hands behind the knee, the examiner slowly flexes and extends the knee of the supine and relaxed patient. With adequate relaxation, the foot remains on the bed. After several slow repetitions, from the position of full extension, the examiner abruptly and forcefully pulls the knee upward. When tone is normal, the foot will scoot back, remaining in contact with the bed. When there is spasticity, the foot flies upward in a kicking motion (spastic kick). In the heel- or foot-dropping test, the examiner holds the patient's leg flexed at the knee and hip, one hand behind the knee and the other supporting the foot. The foot is suddenly released. Normally, its descent is smooth, but when there is spasticity in the quadriceps muscle, the foot may hang up and drop in a succession of choppy movements.

Spastic muscles may or may not feel firm and tense to palpation. The range of movement of spastic extremities, and the degree of hypertonicity, often varies between examinations. No devices for quantitating spasticity exist, and clinical evaluation remains the most useful tool. The Ashworth scale is commonly used to quantitate spasticity on a scale from 1 (no increase in muscle tone) to 5 (affected part rigid in flexion or extension). Its validity and reliability have been questioned. In the presence of spasticity, the DTRs are exaggerated, and pathologic reflexes such as the Babinski and Chaddock signs can often be elicited. Clonus is often present. There may be abnormal associated movements.

Upper motor neuron weakness is often accompanied by sustained contraction of specific groups of muscles. With hemiparesis or hemiplegia, spasticity is most marked in the flexor and pronator muscles of the upper and the extensor muscles of the lower extremity; this causes a posture of flexion of the arm and extension of the leg, the characteristic distribution in cerebral hemiplegia (Figure 25.6). The arm is adducted, flexed at the elbow, and the wrist and fingers are flexed; there may be forced grasping. The lower extremity is extended at the hip, knee, and ankle, with inversion and plantar flexion of the foot; there may be marked spasm of the hip adductors. There is more passive resistance to extension than to flexion in the upper extremities and to flexion than to extension in the lower extremities. With bilateral lesions, the increased tone of the hip adductors causes a scissors gait, in which one leg is pulled toward the other as each step is taken (see Chapter 44). Although spasticity in the lower extremities usually affects the extensors most severely, in some patients with severe myelopathy or extensive cerebral lesions, there is marked hypertonicity in the flexor muscles, drawing the legs into a position referred to as paraplegia in flexion.

Catatonic Rigidity

The abnormal muscle tone in catatonia is in many respects similar to extrapyramidal rigidity and may be physiologically related. There is a waxy or lead-pipe type of resistance to passive movement that may be accompanied by posturing, bizarre mannerisms, and evidence of psychosis. It may be possible to mold the extremities into any position, in which they remain indefinitely. Catatonia may be induced by neuroleptics and may progress to neuroleptic malignant syndrome.

Decerebrate and Decorticate Rigidity

Decerebrate rigidity is characterized by marked rigidity and sustained contraction of the extensor muscles of all four extremities; in decorticate rigidity, there is flexion of the elbows and wrists with extension of the legs and feet. These are discussed further in Chapter 41.

Similar generalized rigidity with neck extension can occur with severe meningismus (opisthotonos), as well as in the tonic phase of a generalized seizure. Cerebellar or posterior fossa fits are probably attacks of decerebrate rigidity due to brainstem dysfunction related to mass effect in the posterior fossa.

Voluntary Rigidity

Various muscle groups may be consciously tensed or braced to protect against injury or in response to pain. It is often difficult to differentiate between tension that is truly volitional and that which is unconscious or involuntary, especially when related to excitement, alarm, pain, or fatigue. Tense, apprehensive individuals may show increased muscular tension at all times and may have exaggerated tendon reflexes. The reflex exaggeration is one of range of response, and the latent period is not shortened. Conversely, the reflexes may be suppressed because the semivoluntary contraction prevents normal movement.

Involuntary Rigidity

Rigidity that is involuntary, reflex, or nonorganic may resemble voluntary rigidity. Rigidity of psychogenic origin may be bizarre and may simulate any type of hypertonicity. Hysterical rigidity may simulate decerebration or catatonia. It may be extreme, with neck retraction and opisthotonos, the body resting with only the head and heels upon the bed (arc de cercle, Chapter 52).

Reflex Rigidity

Muscles may develop reflex rigidity, or spasm, in response to afferent impulses, particularly pain. Muscle spasm is a state of sustained involuntary contraction accompanied by muscle shortening. The abnormal contraction is visible and palpable. Common examples of reflex muscle spasm are the board-like abdomen of acute abdominal disorders, rigidity of the neck and back in meningitis, and the localized spasm in the extremities following trauma. Reflex rigidity may follow other sensory stimuli, such as cold. Muscle contracture may follow prolonged spasm. In some metabolic myopathies (e.g., McArdle's disease), painful muscle cramps and spasms are brought on by exercise; the muscle cramp is a physiologic form of contracture due to abnormal metabolism and is not accompanied by electrical activity.

Myotonia

Myotonia is a disorder of the muscle membrane that can occur in many different conditions. Tone is usually normal when the muscles are relaxed, but contraction produces a temporary involuntary tonic perseveration of muscle contraction with slow relaxation **(Video 28.1)**. Sudden movements may cause marked spasm and inability to relax. In grip myotonia, the patient has difficulty letting go of an object after gripping it strongly. The myotonia usually decreases with repetition of the movement. In rare instances, the myotonia increases with repetitive movement (paradoxical myotonia). Percussion myotonia is elicited by tapping on the muscle. Percussion over the thenar eminence produces a prolonged tonic abduction and opposition movement lasting several seconds, over which the patient has no control. Tapping over the extensor digitorum communis to the middle finger causes the finger to snap into extension, after which it slowly falls over a much longer period of time than normal. Percussion myotonia can also be elicited over other muscles. Oblique elimination with a penlight may help to make the slowly disappearing depression or dimple more visible. Percussion of a tongue blade placed transversely on edge across the tongue may produce a segmental myotonic contraction that constricts the tongue circumferentially (napkin-ring sign, Chapter 20).

Other Types of Rigidity

Muscular rigidity may also occur in epilepsy, tetany, and tetanus. In epilepsy, there may be generalized rigidity during the tonic phase of the fit. Occasionally, there are tonic seizures with no clonic phase (tonic fits). In tetany, there is generalized irritability of the peripheral and central nervous systems, with tonic muscle spasms leading to localized or generalized hypertonicity, hypersensitivity to stimuli, cramps, and muscle twitching (see Chapter 52).

In tetanus, there is usually generalized rigidity with increased muscle tone in the entire body. In most instances, it begins in the face and jaw muscles and then spreads to affect the abdominal muscles, extremities, and spinal muscles, causing abdominal rigidity, extensor rigidity, and opisthotonos. In cephalic tetanus, disease manifestations occur primarily in head and neck muscles (for video, see You et al.). Both agonist and antagonist muscles are simultaneously hypertonic. Spasm of the muscles of mastication causes trismus (lockjaw). Retraction of the angles of the mouth causes the facial dystonia referred to as risus sardonicus. Paroxysms of muscle spasm progressively increase in intensity and propagate to other muscles. Spasms may occur spontaneously, after voluntary contraction or after mechanical, tactile, auditory, visual, or other stimuli. Between spasms, there is usually some persisting muscular rigidity. The reflexes are grossly exaggerated, and a light tap on a tendon may throw the limb into violent spasms. The clinical manifestations of tetanus are due to the action of the exotoxin of *Clostridium tetani* on the inhibitory internuncial neurons of the brainstem and spinal cord. In the stiff-person (stiff-man) syndrome, there are painful tonic muscular spasms and progressive rigidity of the muscles of the trunk, neck, abdomen, back, and proximal parts of the extremities. Other disorders causing increased muscle tone are discussed in Chapter 30.

Video Links

Video Link 28.1. Wartenberg pendulum test. https://www.youtube.com/watch?v=yYtGjvCcA7o

Video Link 28.2. Rippling muscle disease. https://www.youtube.com/watch?v=bdiwylu3Oro

Video Link 28.3. Discussion and demonstration of spasticity versus rigidity from the 2015 Stanford Medicine 25 Skills Symposium. https://www.youtube.com/watch?v=gLZoYLxdXCQ&index=5&list=PL5o6KWShAMajcL3piv2wiiVm0BIDyE9rL

Video Link 28.4. Training video on paratonia. https://www.youtube.com/watch?v=Z-NjgIPbuEU&t=89s

BIBLIOGRAPHY

Andersson PB, Rando TA. Neuromuscular disorders of childhood. *Curr Opin Pediatr* 1999;11:497–503.

Ashby P, Mailis A, Hunter J. The evaluation of "spasticity". *Can J Neurol Sci* 1987;14(3 Suppl):497–500.

Beversdorf DQ, Heilman KM. Facilitory paratonia and frontal lobe functioning. *Neurology* 1998;51:968–971.

Brown RA, Lawson DA, Leslie GC, et al. Observations on the applicability of the Wartenberg pendulum test to healthy, elderly subjects. *J Neurol Neurosurg Psychiatry* 1988;51:1171–1177.

Brown RA, Lawson DA, Leslie GC, et al. Does the Wartenberg pendulum test differentiate quantitatively between spasticity and rigidity? A study in elderly stroke and Parkinsonian patients. *J Neurol Neurosurg Psychiatry* 1988;51:1178–1186.

Campbell WW. *Clinical Signs in Neurology: A Compendium.* Philadelphia: Wolters Kluwer Health, 2016.

Chatterjee A. Feeling frontal dysfunction: facilitory paratonia and the regulation of motor behavior. *Neurology* 1998;51:937–939.

Fowler EG, Nwigwe AI, Ho TW. Sensitivity of the pendulum test for assessing spasticity in persons with cerebral palsy. *Dev Med Child Neurol* 2000;42:182–189.

Ghiglione P, Mutani R, Chiò A. Cogwheel rigidity. *Arch Neurol* 2005;62:828–830.

Harris SR. Congenital hypotonia: clinical and developmental assessment. *Dev Med Child Neurol* 2008;50:889–892.

Hobbelen JS, Koopmans RT, Verhey FR, et al. Paratonia: a Delphi procedure for consensus definition. *J Geriatr Phys Ther* 2006;29:50–56.

Hobbelen JS, Koopmans RT, Verhey FR, et al. Diagnosing paratonia in the demented elderly: reliability and validity of the Paratonia Assessment Instrument (PAI). *Int Psychogeriatr* 2008;20:840–852.

Hornung K, Nix WA. Myoedema. A clinical and electrophysiological evaluation. *Eur Neurol* 1992;32:130–133.

Hughes BN, Hogue JS, Hsieh DT. Grip and percussion myotonia in myotonic dystrophy type 1. *J Pediatr* 2014;164:1234–1234.e1.

Ivanhoe CB, Reistetter TA. Spasticity: the misunderstood part of the upper motor neuron syndrome. *Am J Phys Med Rehabil* 2004;83(10 Suppl):S3–S9.

Johnston HM. The floppy weak infant revisited. *Brain Dev* 2003;25:155–158.

Lance JW. The control of muscle tone, reflexes, and movement: Robert Wartenberg Lecture. *Neurology* 1980;30:1303.

Lee HM, Huang YZ, Chen JJ, et al. Quantitative analysis of the velocity related pathophysiology of spasticity and rigidity in the elbow flexors. *J Neurol Neurosurg Psychiatry* 2002;72:621–629.

Lin CC, Ju MS, Lin CW. The pendulum test for evaluating spasticity of the elbow joint. *Arch Phys Med Rehabil* 2003;84: 69–74.

Loomis C, Bird SJ, Levine JM. Teaching video neuroimages: involuntary muscle contractions in Hoffman syndrome. *Neurology* 2010;75:836.

Mayer NH. Clinicophysiologic concepts of spasticity and motor dysfunction in adults with an upper motoneuron lesion. *Muscle Nerve Suppl* 1997;6:S1–S13.

Messina C. Pathophysiology of muscle tone. *Funct Neurol* 1990;5:217–223.

Pandyan AD, Johnson GR, Price CI, et al. A review of the properties and limitations of the Ashworth and modified Ashworth Scales as measures of spasticity. *Clin Rehabil* 1999;13: 373–383.

Perlmutter JS. Assessment of Parkinson disease manifestations. *Curr Protoc Neurosci* 2009;Chapter 10:Unit10.1.

Pickett JB, Tatum EJ. Pendular knee reflexes: a reliable sign of hypotonia? *Lancet* 1984;2:236–237.

Powers RK, Marder-Meyer J, Rymer WZ. Quantitative relations between hypertonia and stretch reflex threshold in spastic hemiparesis. *Ann Neurol* 1988;23:115.

Rekand T. Clinical assessment and management of spasticity: a review. *Acta Neurol Scand Suppl* 2010;(190):62–66.

Sadeh M, Berg M, Sandbank U. Familial myoedema, muscular hypertrophy and stiffness. *Acta Neurol Scand* 1990;81:201–204.

Sehgal N, McGuire JR. Beyond Ashworth. Electrophysiologic quantification of spasticity. *Phys Med Rehabil Clin N Am* 1998;9:949–979.

Tucci V, Plazzi G. Cataplexy: an affair of pleasure or an unpleasant affair? *Neurosci Lett* 2009;450:90–91.

Tyrrell P, Rossor M. The association of gegenhalten in the upper limbs with dyspraxia. *J Neurol Neurosurg Psychiatry* 1988;51:995–997.

van der Meché FG, van Gijn J. Hypotonia: an erroneous clinical concept? *Brain* 1986;109(Pt 6):1169–1178.

Vendrame M, Zarowski M, Alexopoulos AV, et al. Localization of pediatric seizure semiology. *Clin Neurophysiol* 2011;122:1924–1928.

Wartenberg R. Some useful neurological tests. *JAMA* 1951;147: 1645.

White DA. Catatonia and the neuroleptic malignant syndrome—a single entity? *Br J Psychiatry* 1992;161:558–560.

Woodbury MM, Woodbury MA. Neuroleptic-induced catatonia as a stage in the progression toward neuroleptic malignant syndrome. *J Am Acad Child Adolesc Psychiatry* 1992;31:1161–1164.

Xia R, Powell D, Rymer WZ, et al. Differentiation between the contributions of shortening reaction and stretch-induced inhibition to rigidity in Parkinson's disease. *Exp Brain Res* 2011;209:609–618.

Xia R, Rymer WZ. The role of shortening reaction in mediating rigidity in Parkinson's disease. *Exp Brain Res* 2004;156: 524–528.

You S, Kim MJ, Jang EH, et al. Teaching Video NeuroImages: Cephalic tetanus as a pseudodystonic emergency. *Neurology* 2011;77:e77–e78.

Zhao J, Afra P, Adamolekun B. Partial epilepsy presenting as focal atonic seizure: a case report. *Seizure* 2010;19:326–329.

CHAPTER 29

Muscle Volume and Contour

A search for evidence of muscle atrophy or hypertrophy is an important part of the motor examination. There is normally an appreciable individual variation in muscular development, but noteworthy changes in the size or shape of individual muscles or muscle groups, especially when focal or asymmetric, may be significant.

Muscle atrophy (amyotrophy) causes a decrease in muscle volume or bulk and is usually accompanied by changes in shape or contour. Neurologic conditions likely to cause muscle atrophy are primarily those that affect the following components of the motor unit: the anterior horn cell, the nerve root(s), the peripheral nerve, or the muscle. Neuromuscular junction disorders do not cause muscle atrophy. Atrophy may also result from such things as disuse or inactivity, immobilization, tendonotomy, muscle ischemia, malnutrition, endocrine disorders, and normal aging.

Muscle hypertrophy is an increase in the bulk, or volume, of muscle tissues. It may result from excessive use of the muscles (physiologic hypertrophy) or occur on a pathologic basis. Hypertrophied muscle is not necessarily stronger than normal. Persistent abnormal muscle contraction may cause hypertrophy. Patients with myotonia congenita have a diffuse muscularity without significant increase in strength. Patients with dystonia may develop hypertrophy of the abnormally active muscle. In cervical dystonia (spasmodic torticollis), it is common to see hypertrophy of one sternomastoid muscle. Muscular dystrophies, especially Duchenne's dystrophy, often cause pseudohypertrophy of muscle, with enlargement because of infiltration of the muscle with fat and connective tissue without an actual increase in muscle fiber size or number.

EXAMINATION OF MUSCLE VOLUME AND CONTOUR

There is a great deal of individual variation in muscular development, in part constitutional and in part because of training, activity, and occupation. Certain individuals have small or poorly developed muscles, whereas others show outstanding muscular development. The sedentary, the elderly, and those with chronic disease may have small muscles without evidence of wasting or atrophy. Athletes may develop physiologically hypertrophic muscles. In normal individuals, the dominant side may exhibit an increase in the size of the muscles, even of the hand and foot. The appraisal of bulk and contour should be correlated with the other parts of the motor examination, especially with the evaluation of strength and tone.

Muscle volume and contour may be appraised by inspection, palpation, and measurement. Inspection generally compares symmetric parts on the two sides of the body, noting any flattening, hollowing, or bulging of the muscle masses. The muscles of the face, shoulder, and pelvic girdles, and distal parts of the extremities—especially the palmar surfaces of the hands, the thenar and hypothenar eminences, and the interosseous muscles—should be examined specifically. A useful technique for comparing extremities is to look down the long axis. Hold the patient's arms outstretched and close together, comparing "down the barrel" from fingertips to shoulders for any asymmetry.

Palpation assesses muscle bulk, contour, and consistency. Normal muscles are semielastic and regain their shape at once when compressed. When hypertrophy is present, the muscles are firm and hard; in pseudohypertrophy, they appear enlarged but may feel doughy or rubbery on palpation. The feel of pseudohypertrophy has been likened to that of a plastic, gelatinous toy such as an imitation snake. Atrophic muscles are often soft and pulpy in consistency. When degenerated muscles have undergone fibrotic changes, they may feel hard and firm. Those infiltrated or replaced by fat may feel pliant and flabby.

Measurements may be very useful in assessing atrophy or hypertrophy. A pronounced difference in muscle size may be recognized at a glance, especially when confined to one side of the body, one extremity, or one segment of a limb. Slight differences are more difficult to detect, and measurements with a tape measure or calipers may be necessary. Measurements should be made from fixed points or landmarks and the sites—such as the distance above or below the olecranon, anterior superior iliac spine, or patella—recorded. The extremities should be in the same position and in comparable states of relaxation. It may also be valuable to measure the length of the limbs.

Atrophy or hypertrophy may be limited to an individual muscle, to muscles supplied by a specific structure (e.g., a nerve or root), to those muscles supplied by certain spinal cord segments, or to one-half of the body; or it may be multifocal or generalized. In atrophy related to arthritis and disuse, there may be a pronounced decrease in volume with little change in strength. In myopathies, on the other hand, there is often little atrophy in spite of a striking loss of power. Examination of the skin and subcutaneous tissues may also be relevant, especially in such conditions as dermatomyositis.

ABNORMALITIES OF VOLUME AND CONTOUR

Muscular Atrophy

Many processes may cause muscular atrophy. Neurogenic atrophy follows disease of the anterior horn cell, root, or peripheral nerve. Atrophy because of other neurologic processes, such as the hemiatrophy associated with congenital hemiplegia, is not typically considered neurogenic atrophy even though it is related to nervous system disease. The term neurogenic atrophy as commonly used implies disease affecting some part of the lower motor neuron. Myogenic atrophy is that due to muscle disease, such as muscular dystrophy. As a generalization, when weakness and wasting are comparable, the process is more likely to be neurogenic; when the weakness is disproportionately greater than the wasting, the process is more likely to be myopathic. When a muscle appears wasted but is not weak, the cause is likely to be nonneurologic, such as disuse.

Neurogenic Atrophy

The anterior horn cell and its processes exert a trophic effect on skeletal muscle. The nature of the trophic effect remains poorly understood, but it is not as simple as the effect of nerve impulses. Electrical stimulation of the peripheral nerve, sometimes done after peripheral nerve injury or Bell's palsy, does not help prevent or reverse neurogenic atrophy. Nerves may be involved in regulating the trophic actions of insulin-like growth factor, calcitonin gene–related peptide, and other neurotrophic factors that have an influence on skeletal muscle. When a lesion completely disrupts the lower motor neuron or its peripheral processes, the affected muscle lies inert and flaccid and no longer contracts voluntarily or reflexively. Muscle fibers decrease in size, causing wasting or atrophy of the entire muscle mass. Without timely reinnervation, the muscle may become fibrotic, with an increase in connective tissue and fatty infiltration.

The more abrupt or extreme the interruption of nerve supply, the more rapid the wasting. The atrophy may either precede or follow other signs, such as weakness. In rapidly progressing diseases, weakness precedes atrophy, but in slowly progressive diseases, the atrophy may precede appreciation of weakness. If the pathologic process is confined to the anterior horn cells or the spinal cord, the neurogenic atrophy is segmental in distribution. Some conditions cause rapid destruction of the anterior horn cells and atrophy in the distribution of the affected spinal cord segments that develops within a short period of time (e.g., poliomyelitis).

In more slowly progressive disorders of the motor neuron (e.g., amyotrophic lateral sclerosis [ALS]), there is a gradual but widespread degeneration of the brainstem motor nuclei and anterior horn cells, causing progressive muscular atrophy that may appear before paralysis is evident (Figure 29.1). The distribution of the atrophy is important. To make a diagnosis of motor neuron disease, it is necessary to demonstrate widespread denervation in a multiple nerve, multiple root distribution. Eventually, the disease becomes widespread, but it often begins segmentally in one limb. Rarely, it may remain confined to one limb (monomelic motor neuron disease, Hirayama

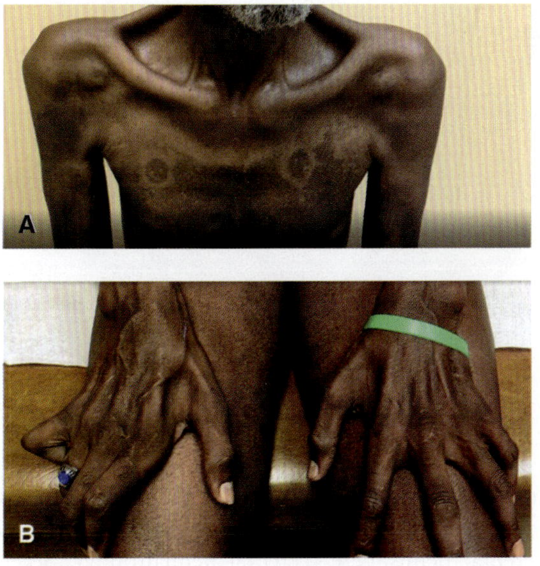

FIGURE 29.1 A patient with amyotrophic lateral sclerosis showing advanced atrophy of the muscles of the shoulder girdle and upper arms **(A)** and intrinsic hand muscles **(B)**.

disease, O'Sullivan-McLeod syndrome). Particular groups of muscles are often affected. In classical ALS and in progressive spinal muscular atrophy (SMA) of the Aran-Duchenne type, atrophy is usually first seen in the distal musculature—the thenar, hypothenar, and interosseous muscles of the hand and the small muscles of the foot—and then spreads up the limbs to the proximal parts. In some patients, ALS seems to have a tendency to preferentially involve the muscles of the lateral half of the hand, median-innervated thenar, and ulnar-innervated first dorsal interosseous muscles while sparing the hypothenar muscles (split hand syndrome). Although not common, this pattern seems to be relatively specific for anterior horn cell disorders. In progressive bulbar palsy, the atrophy is first noted in the muscles supplied by the 12th, 10th, and 7th cranial nerves. In hereditary motor neuron syndromes, the involvement is often proximal. In SMA type 1 (infantile progressive SMA, Werdnig-Hoffmann disease), the atrophy first involves the trunk, pelvic, and shoulder muscles and then spreads toward the periphery. The proximal distribution and slow progression in SMA type 3 (juvenile proximal SMA, Kugelberg-Welander disease) may simulate muscular dystrophy. Segmental atrophy may also follow focal spinal cord lesions involving the anterior horn cells (e.g., syringomyelia). The rapidity of the progress depends upon the type of pathologic change.

Involvement of nerve roots, plexus elements, or peripheral nerves leads to atrophy of the muscles supplied by the diseased or injured component (Figure 29.2). With severe lesions involving a peripheral nerve or nerve plexus, atrophy may develop within a short period of time. Within 1 month after denervation, there may be a 30% loss of weight in the affected muscle and a 50% loss within 2 months; thereafter, the atrophy progresses more slowly and replacement by connective tissue and infiltration by fat follows. Lesions involving single nerve roots usually do not cause much atrophy, because most muscles are innervated from more than one level. Marked wasting in a disease that appears consistent with radiculopathy suggests multiple root involvement. In generalized peripheral neuropathy, weakness and wasting are usually greatest in the distal portions of the extremities. The amount of atrophy depends on the severity and chronicity of the neuropathy. The hereditary peripheral neuropathy, Charcot-Marie-Tooth disease (peroneal muscular atrophy), typically causes marked atrophy in a characteristic distribution involving the lower legs (inverted champagne bottle deformity; Figure 29.3).

The complete syndrome of peripheral nerve dysfunction, with paralysis, atrophy, sensory impairment, areflexia, and trophic changes in the skin and other tissues, is the result of interruption of motor, sensory, and autonomic fibers. Interruption of sensory nerve fibers alone does not lead to muscular atrophy except as related to disuse, but loss of pain sensation may predispose one to painless injuries, including ulcerations following minor trauma and burns. The autonomic system is involved in trophic function by regulating the nutrition and metabolism of muscle and other tissues. Because of interruption of autonomic pathways, diseases of the lower motor neuron may be associated with trophic changes in the skin and subcutaneous tissues: edema, cyanosis or pallor, coldness, sweating, changes in the hair and nails, alterations in the texture of the skin, osteoporosis, and even ulcerations and decubiti. Autonomic fibers may be a factor in muscle atrophy because of "trophic dysfunction" and loss of vasomotor control.

Upper motor neuron lesions in adults are usually not followed by atrophy of the paralyzed muscles except for some generalized loss of muscle volume and secondary wasting because of disuse, which is seldom severe. With lesions dating from birth or early childhood, there may be a failure of growth of the contralateral body (Figure 25.5). Such congenital hemiatrophy

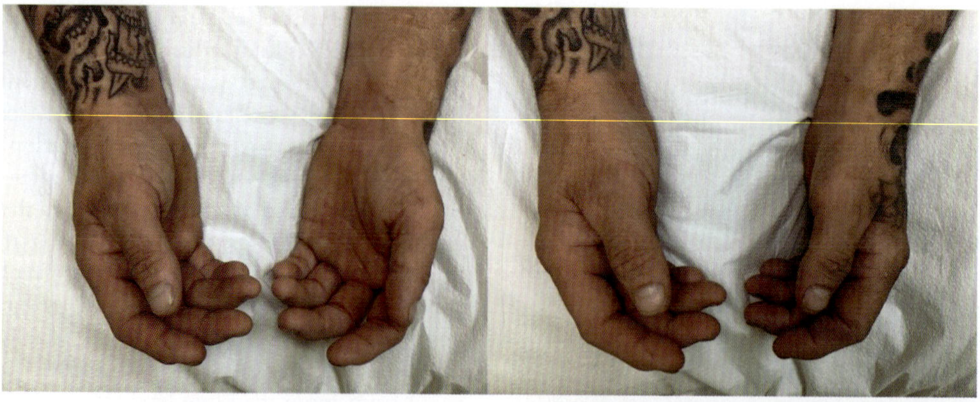

FIGURE 29.2 Atrophy of the left abductor pollicis brevis in a plumber with carpal tunnel syndrome.

may involve one side of the face or the face and corresponding half of the body; it is characterized by underdevelopment not only of the muscles but also of the skin, hair, subcutaneous tissues, connective tissue, cartilage, and bone. Congenital hemihypertrophy is rarer than the corresponding hemiatrophy, and there are usually other anomalies. There may be underdevelopment of one-half of the body because of either lack of development or atrophy of the opposite cerebral hemisphere (cerebral hemiatrophy). Severe cerebral insults in early life may lead to hemiplegia, hemiatrophy, partial or hemiseizures, and the development of delayed hemidystonia ("4-hemi" syndrome). Experimentally, lesions of the motor cortex and the descending corticospinal pathways may be followed by muscular atrophy, and on occasion, severe wasting appears with cerebral hemiplegias. Usually, there are associated trophic and sensory changes, and the wasting may in part be secondary to involvement of the postcentral gyrus or parietal lobe, lesions of which are known to be followed by contralateral atrophy. The loss of muscle bulk associated with lesions of the parietal lobe may appear promptly; the degree of atrophy depends upon the size and character of the lesion and the extent of the hypotonia and sensory change. The distribution is determined by the localization of the process within the parietal lobe. It is most severe if the motor cortex or pathways are involved along with the sensory areas of the brain. Hemiatrophy may also complicate hemiparkinsonism. Rarely, hemiatrophy is idiopathic.

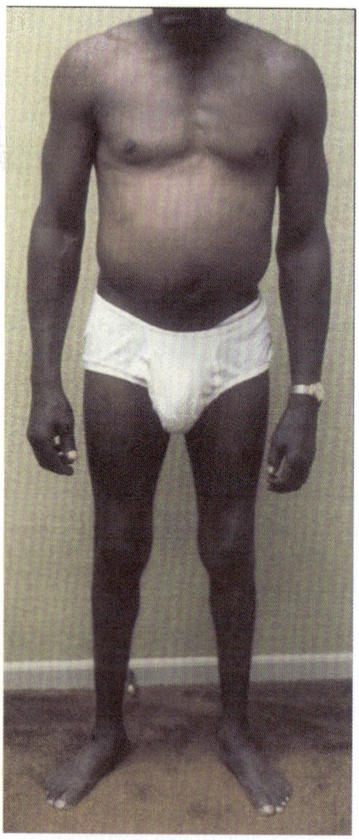

FIGURE 29.3 A patient with type 1 Charcot-Marie-Tooth disease. Despite a muscular upper body, there is marked atrophy of the lower extremities below the knees.

Other Varieties of Muscular Atrophy

Myogenic, or myopathic, atrophy occurs as a result of primary muscle disease. In some conditions, there may be prominent wasting without much weakness. In most of these, the primary pathologic change is type 2 fiber atrophy. Wasting with little weakness occurs in disuse, aging, cachexia, and some endocrine myopathies. Weakness out of proportion to wasting occurs in inflammatory myopathy, myasthenia gravis, and periodic paralysis.

Muscle wasting is common in muscular dystrophy, and the distribution of the wasting parallels the weakness. In dystrophinopathies, the weakness and atrophy primarily involve the pelvic and shoulder girdle muscles (Figure 29.4). Weakness of the hip and spine extensors causes difficulty in assuming the erect position, and the patient "climbs up his thighs" (Gowers' sign or maneuver) in order to stand **(Video Link 29.1)**. As the disease progresses, there is increasing wasting of all muscles of the shoulders,

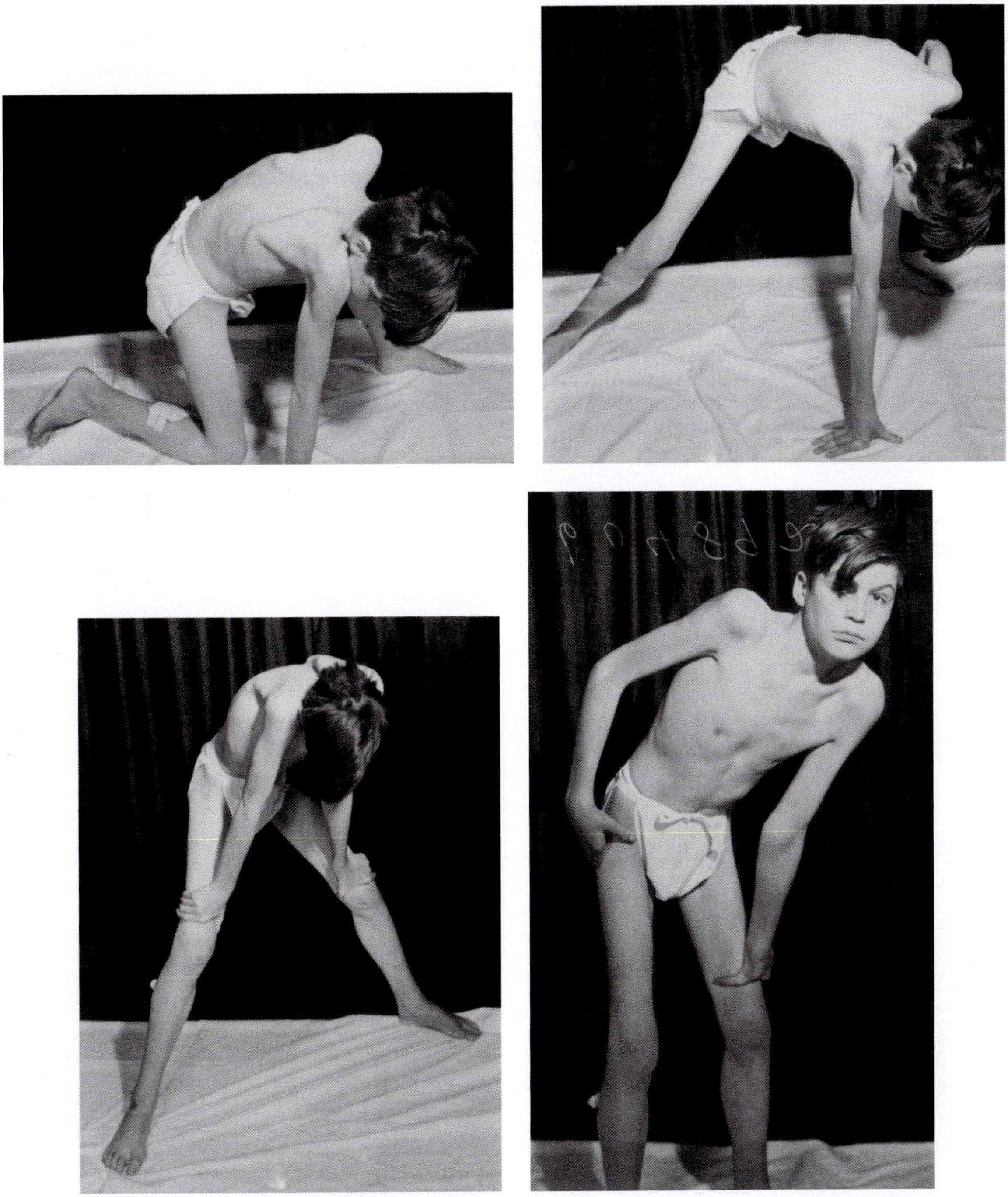

FIGURE 29.4 A boy with Duchenne's muscular dystrophy, showing wasting of the musculature in the shoulders and thighs; weakness and atrophy of the glutei cause difficulty in assuming the erect position, and the patient "climbs up on his thighs" (Gowers' maneuver) in order to stand erect.

upper arms, pelvis, and thighs. In the face of all of the atrophy, certain muscles—particularly the calf muscles—are paradoxically enlarged because of pseudohypertrophy (see below). The limb-girdle syndromes also primarily involve the pelvic and shoulder girdles. In facioscapulohumeral (FSH) (Landouzy-Dejerine) dystrophy, the atrophy predominates in the muscles of the face, shoulder girdles (especially the trapezius and periscapular muscles), and upper arms, especially the biceps (Figure 29.5). Involvement is often asymmetric, and occasionally, there is pseudohypertrophy of the deltoid and other shoulder muscles.

Distal myopathies, affecting the muscles of the hands and feet, are occasionally seen. Wasting involving the distal extremities, with relative sparing of the hands and feet, is likely to be myopathic. In contrast, denervation atrophy involves the entire distal extremity, including the hand or foot. Some myopathies cause striking weakness and atrophy involving certain muscles or muscle groups. In myotonic dystrophy, there is prominent atrophy of the sternocleidomastoid muscles. Scapuloperoneal syndromes involve the periscapular and peroneal muscles. Selective involvement of the quadriceps occurs in inclusion body myositis and type 2B limb-girdle muscular dystrophy (dysferlin deficiency). Some myopathies have a curious tendency to affect certain muscles while sparing nearby muscle groups. FSH characteristically causes wasting of the biceps and triceps with sparing of the deltoid and forearm musculature creating the "Popeye" arm appearance (Figure 29.6). The diamond on quadriceps sign refers to asymmetric diamond-shaped bulges seen in the anterolateral thighs of patients with dysferlinopathy (LGMD 2B and Miyoshi myopathy) when standing with the knees slightly bent. Proximal and distal atrophy causes the curious island of sparing to stand out. Other unusual muscle shapes have been described as a manifestation of dysferlinopathy, such as selective biceps atrophy causing a "bowl-shaped biceps."

Disuse atrophy follows prolonged immobilization of a part of the body. It may be rapid in onset and can sometimes simulate neurogenic atrophy. Disuse atrophy may occur in an extremity after immobilization, such as casting, one that cannot be moved normally because of joint disease, such as arthritis, paresis following a cerebral lesion, or after prolonged bed rest. The quadriceps femoris is particularly susceptible to

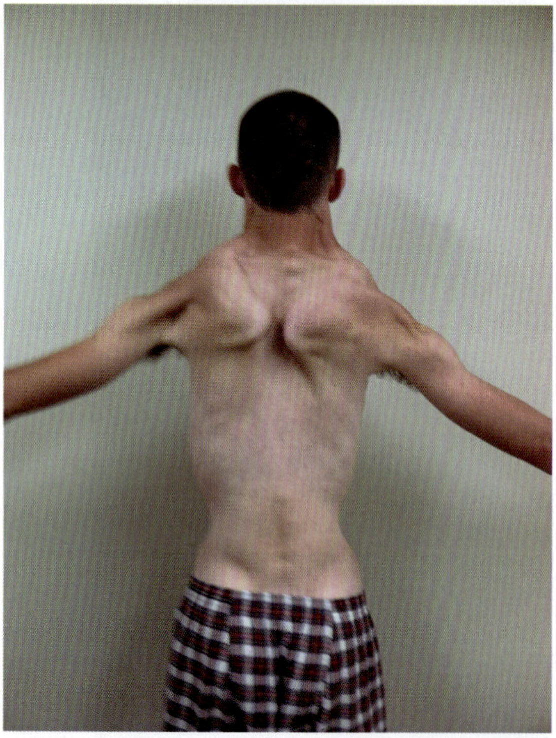

FIGURE 29.5 A patient with facioscapulohumeral muscular dystrophy showing atrophy of the muscles of the shoulders and upper arms and pronounced scapular winging.

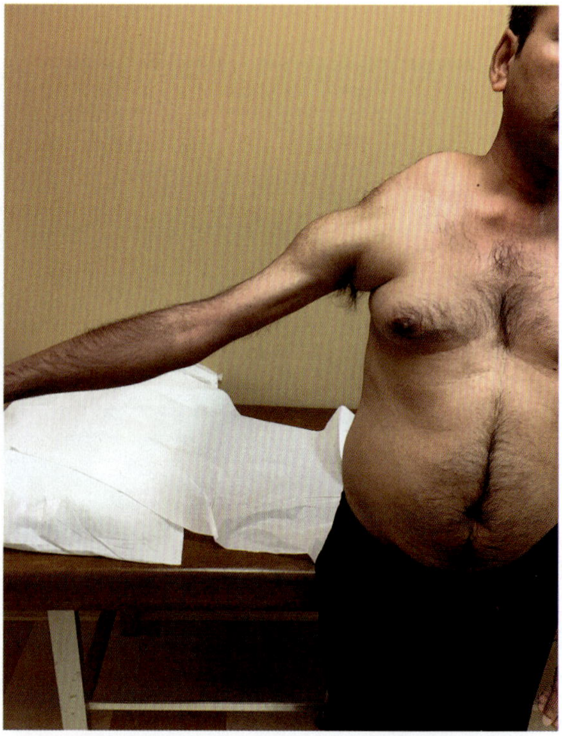

FIGURE 29.6 The Popeye arm appearance in FSH dystrophy.

disuse atrophy because of bed rest or because of pain in the knee or hip. The degree of muscle wasting is greater than the degree of weakness, which may be minimal or absent. Muscle biopsy shows atrophy of type 2 fibers, with the earliest changes in the type 2B fibers. Disuse atrophy can occasionally occur in extremities that are not used because of nonorganic paralysis.

Arthrogenic atrophy may appear in association with joint disease. It is more severe and develops more rapidly in acute arthritis. Both rheumatoid arthritis and osteoarthritis may cause periarticular atrophy, with loss of muscle bulk around involved joints. Periarticular muscle atrophy may be particularly prominent in patients with HIV-associated arthritis. Atrophy of this type may in part be the result of inactivity or disuse, but other factors are likely involved.

Muscle atrophy may accompany malnutrition, weight loss, cachexia, and other wasting diseases. The loss of muscle mass is typically greater than the degree of accompanying weakness. A normal blood supply is essential to the nutrition and oxygenation of muscles, and ischemia may lead to muscle atrophy as well as to alterations in the skin and other trophic changes. In Volkmann ischemic contracture, atrophy accompanies the muscle shortening.

Endocrine dysfunction of various types may lead to atrophy and other changes in muscle. In thyrotoxic myopathy, atrophy is particularly prone to involve the shoulder girdle and may lead to scapular winging. Coarse fasciculations are often seen in the affected areas. With primary hyperparathyroidism, weakness may be associated with atrophy, hyperreflexia, and fasciculations simulating ALS (Vical's syndrome). Myopathy because of excess corticosteroids, exogenous or endogenous, may be associated with muscle wasting. Muscular weakness and atrophy are also frequent findings in hypopituitarism because of loss of thyroid and adrenal cortical hormones. Muscle wasting also occurs with diabetes. Distal weakness and atrophy are common in diabetic distal axonopathy. Diabetic amyotrophy (or radiculoplexus neuropathy) is a common syndrome of bilateral but asymmetric weakness and atrophy that involves the pelvic and thigh muscles because of involvement of the lumbosacral plexus and nerve roots. It is usually associated with severe pain. Patients with diabetes may also develop either localized lipoatrophy or areas of focal muscular atrophy because of repeated injections of insulin in the same area. The loss of subcutaneous tissue may simulate muscle atrophy. In adiposis dolorosa (Dercum's disease), the muscles may be replaced with fat.

Congenital hypoplasia or absence of a muscle may be mistaken for atrophy. Almost any muscle may be congenitally absent, but some are particularly prone, including the depressor anguli oris, palmaris longus, trapezius, peroneus tertius, and anterior abdominal muscles (prune-belly syndrome). In the Holt-Oram syndrome, there are absent or hypoplastic thenar muscles. Poland syndrome is a rare anomaly characterized by unilateral absence of the pectoral muscles and ipsilateral hand abnormalities; it may be associated with a variety of other congenital anomalies. Other syndromes of congenital muscle abnormality include Duane retraction syndrome, Möbius' syndrome, and congenital ptosis.

Muscular Hypertrophy and Pseudohypertrophy

Enlarged muscles are encountered less frequently than atrophy. In true muscle hypertrophy, the muscle is enlarged; in pseudohypertrophy, the muscle appears enlarged because it is replaced by fat and fibrous tissue. Extremely muscular individuals may show pronounced development of certain groups of muscles because of functional or physiologic hypertrophy, often found in athletes and heavy manual laborers. Microscopic examination shows an increase in the diameter of muscle fibers, primarily the type 2 fibers, without any increase in the number of fibers. Except for physiologic hypertrophy because of exercise, pseudohypertrophy is encountered more commonly than true hypertrophy.

Pseudohypertrophy is common in some forms of muscular dystrophy. Muscle biopsy reveals severe myopathy, with fatty and connective tissue infiltrations. Pseudohypertrophy is common in Duchenne's and Becker's dystrophy; an alternate term for Duchenne's dystrophy is pseudohypertrophic muscular dystrophy. Certain muscles, particularly the calf muscles and the infraspinatus, are often strikingly enlarged because of pseudohypertrophy (Figure 29.7). Comparing the circumference of the calf to the knee is most informative. In the early stages of the disease, the enlarged muscles may feel firm and hard and remain strong, and there may actually be an element of true hypertrophy. With progression, they develop a soft doughy or rubbery feeling.

Muscle hypertrophy is common in myotonia congenita, especially the dominant form (Thomsen's disease), because of the excessive contraction. These patients may have the impressive muscularity of a

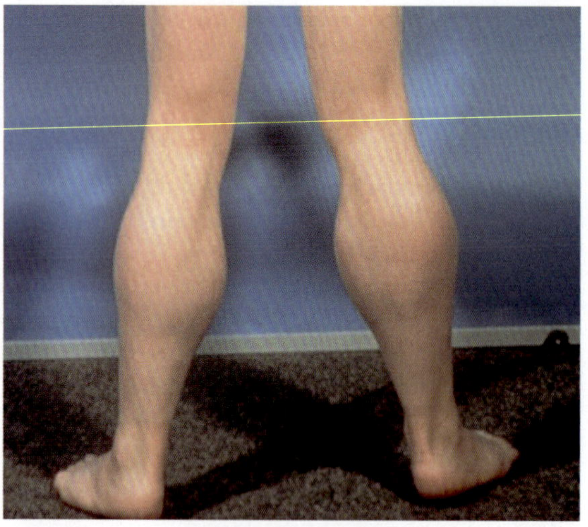

FIGURE 29.7 Pseudohypertrophy of the calves in Duchenne's muscular dystrophy. (Reprinted from Schaaf CP, Zschocke J, Potocki L. *Basiswissen Humangenetik*. Heidelberg: Springer Midizin; 2008. Figure 31.11. Reproduced with permission of Springer in the format Book via Copyright Clearance Center.)

bodybuilder; although they may appear strong and muscular, strength is normal, or there is even slight weakness. Hypertrophia musculorum vera is a hereditary syndrome causing enlargement of the muscles, usually those of the limbs, but any area may be affected. Mutations in the myostatin gene may cause muscle hypertrophy.

Muscle enlargement, either true hypertrophy or pseudohypertrophy, occurs as an occasional feature in other neuromuscular disorders, including Kugelberg-Welander disease, central core disease, centronuclear myopathy, autosomal recessive limb-girdle muscular dystrophy, acid maltase deficiency, polymyositis, FSH muscular dystrophy, inclusion body myositis, hyperkalemic periodic paralysis, paramyotonia congenita, proximal myotonic myopathy, Isaac's syndrome, focal myositis, and in manifesting dystrophinopathy carriers. Chronic partial denervation of muscle occasionally leads to focal muscle hypertrophy, presumably because of compensatory physiologic hypertrophy of unaffected fibers or parts of the muscle. Muscle hypertrophy has been reported as a manifestation of radiculopathy and rarely in other neurogenic processes. Use or abuse of androgenic steroids or beta-2 adrenergic agonists may lead to muscle hypertrophy.

Muscle enlargement may occur in hypothyroidism. The enlarged muscles have reduced strength, fatigability, and slowness of contraction and relaxation. The Kocher-Debré-Semelaigne (infant Hercules) syndrome is diffuse muscular hypertrophy because of hypothyroidism, particularly early in life. Hoffman syndrome refers to a hypertrophic myopathy because of hypothyroidism in adults. Early acromegaly may cause generalized muscular hypertrophy with increased strength, but in later stages, there is weakness and amyotrophy. Edema and inflammation of muscles may simulate hypertrophy. Muscle enlargement may also occur due to interstitial infiltrates, as occurs in cysticercosis, trichinosis, sarcoidosis, and amyloidosis. Focal muscle enlargement may occur with benign or malignant neoplasms. The masseters may become enlarged because of bruxism or as a familial condition.

Loss of body fat may lend the appearance of muscle enlargement. In the lipodystrophies, which may be familial and acquired, there is loss of adipose tissue that may be focal or generalized, often associated with metabolic complications, such as diabetes mellitus and hypertriglyceridemia. Köbberling-Dunnigan syndrome is a familial partial lipodystrophy that may result in an appearance of excessive muscularity, particularly in females.

Video Links

Video Link 29.1. Gowers' sign. http://neurosigns.org/wiki/Gower%27s_sign

BIBLIOGRAPHY

Appell HJ. Muscular atrophy following immobilisation. A review. *Sports Med* 1990;10:42–58.

Brooke MH. *A Clinician's View of Neuromuscular Disease*. 2nd ed. Baltimore: Williams & Wilkins, 1986.

Buchman AS, Goetz CG, Klawans HL. Hemiparkinsonism with hemiatrophy. *Neurology* 1988;38:527–530.

De Beuckeleer L, Vanhoenacker F, De SA Jr, et al. Hypertrophy and pseudohypertrophy of the lower leg following chronic radiculopathy and neuropathy: imaging findings in two patients. *Skeletal Radiol* 1999;28:229–232.

Delmont E, Roth S, Heudier P, et al. Primary hyperparathyroidism, a differential diagnosis of motor neuron diseases. *Rev Med Interne* 2001;22:1253–1255.

Edgerton VR, Roy RR, Allen DL, et al. Adaptations in skeletal muscle disuse or decreased-use atrophy. *Am J Phys Med Rehabil* 2002;81(11 Suppl):S127–S147.

Fokin AA, Robicsek F. Poland's syndrome revisited. *Ann Thorac Surg* 2002;74:2218–2225.

Garg A. Lipodystrophies. *Am J Med* 2000;108:143–152.

Harwood SC, Honet JC. Calf enlargement associated with neurologic disease: two uncommon cases. *Arch Phys Med Rehabil* 1988;69:48–50.

Kim DG, Hong YH, Shin JY, et al. Split-hand phenomenon in amyotrophic lateral sclerosis: a motor unit number index study. *Muscle Nerve* 2016;53:885–888.

Kugelberg E, Welander L. Heredofamilial juvenile muscular atrophy simulating muscular dystrophy. *Arch Neurol Psychiatry* 1956;75:500.

Lang AE. Hemiatrophy, juvenile-onset exertional alternating leg paresis, hypotonia, and hemidystonia and adult-onset hemiparkinsonism: the spectrum of hemiparkinsonism-hemiatrophy syndrome. *Mov Disord* 1995;10:489–495.

Mastropasqua M, Spagna G, Baldini V, et al. Hoffman's syndrome: muscle stiffness, pseudohypertrophy and hypothyroidism. *Horm Res* 2003;59:105–108.

Mehrotra P, Chandra M, Mitra MK. Kocher Debre Semelaigne syndrome: regression of pseudohypertrophy of muscles on thyroxine. *Arch Dis Child* 2002;86:224.

Menon P, Kiernan MC, Vucic S. ALS pathophysiology: insights from the split-hand phenomenon. *Clin Neurophysiol* 2014;125:186–193.

Nair KS. Age-related changes in muscle. *Mayo Clin Proc* 2000;75(Suppl):S14–S18.

O'Donnell PP, Leshner RT, Campbell WW Jr. Hypertrophia musculorum vera in familial ataxia. *Arch Neurol* 1986;43:146–147.

Pestronk A. http://www.neuro.wustl.edu/neuromuscular/

Pradhan S, Mittal B. Infraspinatus muscle hypertrophy and wasting of axillary folds as the important signs in Duchenne muscular dystrophy. *Clin Neurol Neurosurg* 1995;97:134–138.

Pryse-Phillips W. *Companion to Clinical Neurology*. 3rd ed. Oxford: Oxford University Press, 2009.

Reimers CD, Schlotter B, Eicke BM, et al. Calf enlargement in neuromuscular diseases: a quantitative ultrasound study in 350 patients and review of the literature. *J Neurol Sci* 1996;143:46–56.

Ruff RL, Weissmann J. Endocrine myopathies. *Neurol Clin* 1988;6:575–592.

Soraru' G, Negrin P, Angelini C. Unilateral calf hypertrophy due to S1-radiculopathy. *Neuromuscul Disord* 2000;10:514.

Thajeb P. The syndrome of delayed posthemiplegic hemidystonia, hemiatrophy, and partial seizure: clinical, neuroimaging, and motor-evoked potential studies. *Clin Neurol Neurosurg* 1996;98:207–212.

Walton JN, Karpati G, Hilton-Jones D, eds. *Disorders of Voluntary Muscle*. 6th ed. Edinburgh: Churchill Livingstone, 1994.

Wilbourn AJ. The "split hand syndrome". *Muscle Nerve* 2000;23:138.

Wildermuth S, Spranger S, Spranger M, et al. Kobberling-Dunnigan syndrome: a rare cause of generalized muscular hypertrophy. *Muscle Nerve* 1996;19:843–847.

CHAPTER 30

Abnormalities of Movement

Movement disorders may involve any portion of the body. They usually result from disease involving various parts of the motor system, and the etiologies are many. The character of the movement depends on both the site of the lesion and the underlying pathology. Lesions in different sites sometimes cause identical movements, but different etiologic processes involving the same part of the motor system may cause different movement abnormalities.

Movement disorders disrupt motor function not by causing weakness but by producing either abnormal, involuntary, unwanted movements (hyperkinetic movement disorders) or by curtailing the amount of normal free-flowing, fluid movement (hypokinetic movement disorders). The hypokinetic movement disorders are usually accompanied by abnormal states of increased muscle tone. Pathology in movement disorders primarily involves the basal ganglia: caudate, putamen, globus pallidus, substantia nigra, or subthalamic nucleus. The rich connections between the subcomponents of the basal ganglia and between the basal ganglia and other motor systems, as well as the numerous neurotransmitters involved, make the clinical manifestations of basal ganglia disease complex and varied. Depending on the precise location of the abnormality, the particular cell type involved, and the neurotransmitter affected, the clinical picture may range from abnormally decreased movement (the akinesia/bradykinesia of Parkinson's disease [PD]) to abnormally increased movement (chorea, hemiballismus, dystonia).

HYPOKINETIC MOVEMENT DISORDERS

The archetype of hypokinetic movement disorders is PD. Other disease processes may produce a similar clinical picture, characterized by decreased movement and rigidity; these have been grouped together as the akinetic-rigid syndromes. About 80% of the instances of akinetic-rigid syndrome are due to PD (Table 30.1). The terms Parkinson syndrome and Parkinson plus are sometimes used to designate such other disorders, and the features that resemble PD are referred to as parkinsonism, or parkinsonian. Parkinsonism is a clinical diagnosis appropriate in the presence of resting tremor, bradykinesia, rigidity, and impaired postural reflexes. PD is but one cause of parkinsonism, and it must be differentiated from other conditions that may have some of its typical features as a component of another disorder.

Parkinson's Disease

PD is due to a degeneration of neurons in the dopaminergic nigrostriatal pathway. It is the second most common movement disorder behind essential tremor (ET), affecting about 1% of the population over the age of 50. The prevalence increases exponentially between the ages of 65 and 90 and reaches 3% of the population over 65. Cardinal manifestations include bradykinesia, rigidity, tremor, an expressionless face, and postural instability. Asymmetry is characteristic. The disease often begins asymmetrically; the signs may be so lateralized as to warrant the designation of hemi-PD, and some asymmetry usually persists even when the disease is well established. The major manifestations vary from case to case. In some, tremor is the outstanding symptom and in others the rigidity, the bradykinesia, or the loss of associated movements. Akinetic, tremor, and postural instability subtypes have been recognized. Asymmetric rest tremor is the most common presentation of PD, occurring in about 75% of patients.

PD causes marked hypertonia, or rigidity, which principally affects the axial muscles and the proximal and flexor groups of the extremities, causing an

TABLE 30.1 The Differential Diagnosis of Parkinson's Disease (PD)

- PD
- Parkinsonian syndromes
  - Progressive supranuclear palsy
  - Multisystem atrophy (MSA)
    - MSA-parkinsonian (striatonigral degeneration)
    - MSA-cerebellar (olivopontocerebellar degeneration, sporadic form)
    - MSA-autonomic (Shy-Drager syndrome)
  - Diffuse Lewy body disease
  - Corticobasal degeneration
  - Drug-induced parkinsonism
  - Dopa-responsive dystonia
- Other non-Parkinson's akinetic-rigid syndromes
- Huntington's disease (rigid or juvenile form)
- Wilson's disease
- Essential tremor
- Depression
- Arthritis, polymyalgia, and fibromyalgia

increased tone to passive movement. The rigidity has a rhythmic quality referred to as cogwheel rigidity (Negro's sign), presumably because of the superimposition of the tremor. Cogwheeling may be brought out as the examiner passively moves an elbow or wrist by having the patient grit the teeth, look at the ceiling, use the opposite hand to make a fist, trace circles in the air, or imitate throwing a ball. The rigidity is present evenly throughout the range of movement, without the ebb at the extremes of the range that occurs in spasticity.

In PD, there is a paucity of movement and a slowing of movements. Strictly speaking, akinesia means an absence of movement; bradykinesia, a slowness of movement; and hypokinesia, a decreased amount or amplitude of movement, but the term bradykinesia is often used to encompass all three. Bradykinesia is not due simply to the rigidity and may have an independent pathophysiologic basis. There is loss of associated and automatic movements, with masking of the face, infrequent smiling and blinking, and loss of swinging of the arms in walking (Figure 30.1). Normal fidgeting and adventitial movements are decreased or absent. Because of the rigidity and bradykinesia, strength may seem to be decreased, but (although an alternate name for PD is paralysis agitans and Parkinson referred to the disorder as "shaking palsy") there is no true loss of power such as is seen in corticospinal lesions. The rigidity and bradykinesia involve movements and not muscles or muscle groups and do make locomotion and

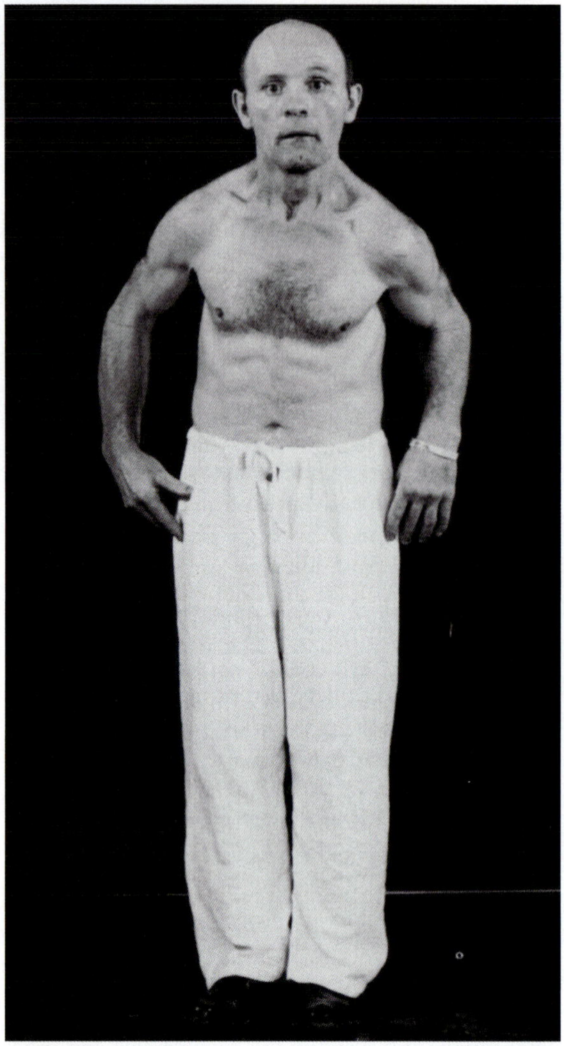

FIGURE 30.1 A patient with Parkinson's disease, showing rigidity, masked facies, and typical posture.

motor activity slow and difficult. Under acute emotional stress, the extremities can often be used rapidly and effectively, as when an otherwise immobile patient escapes from a fire (kinesia paradoxica).

The tremor of PD is a coarse "pill-rolling" movement, so named because of its resemblance to the motion pharmacists of a bygone era used to make pills **(Video 30.1)**. The tremor is fairly rhythmic and gross, from 2 to 6 Hz, and may involve the hands, feet, jaw, tongue, lips, and pharynx, but not the head. It is typically a resting tremor that lessens during voluntary movement and disappears in sleep. Parkinson said the tremor was present "whilst the limb is at rest and unemployed." The tremor fluctuates, increasing in amplitude but not rate when the patient becomes excited. The tremor often is more apparent when the patient is walking. Some patients may also have a low-amplitude 7- to 8-Hz tremor during voluntary movement that is suppressed by relaxation.

Patients with PD have poor balance, a tendency to fall, and difficulty walking. Gait and balance are not prominently affected in most patients with early PD, and significant postural instability early in the course suggests an alternate diagnosis, such as progressive supranuclear palsy (PSP) (see below). The gait abnormality is stereotypical: slow and shuffling with a reduced stride length, sometimes markedly so; a stooped flexed posture of the body and extremities (simian posture); a tendency to turn "en bloc;" and reduced arm swing **(Video 30.2)**. Head drop and camptocormia may occur. Lower-half (lower-body, arteriosclerotic) parkinsonism causes gait difficulty out of proportion to other manifestations (Chapter 44). Impaired postural reflexes lead to a tendency to fall forward (propulsion), which the patient tries to avoid by walking with increasing speed but with very short steps, the festinating gait. Falls are common. If a patient, standing upright, is gently pushed either backward or forward, she cannot maintain balance and will fall in the direction pushed. When a patient, seated in a chair, is suddenly tilted backward, there is absence of the normal reflex leg extension to counteract the loss of balance (Souques' leg sign).

Facial immobility and lack of expressiveness are common features of PD (hypomimia, masked face; **Video 30.3**). A decreased rate of blinking (5 to 10 per minute rather than the normal 12 to 20), accompanied by slight eyelid retraction (Stellwag's sign, also seen in thyroid eye disease), causes patients to have a staring expression (reptilian stare). Hanes describes the whistle-smile sign as efficient way to bring out the masked facies in PD. When the normal individual is asked to whistle, he does so and then smiles, probably as a response to the apparent absurdity of the request. The patient suffering from parkinsonism does not smile after whistling because of bradykinesia affecting the facial muscles.

Abnormalities of phonation and articulation are common (bradylalia). The voice is typically soft, breathy, monotonous, and tremulous. Lack of movement of the lips and tongue causes articulatory imprecision. Temporarily overcoming vocal bradykinesia, words pour out in a short rush of rapid speech. Patients with PD tend to be soft, fast, mumbly talkers. They are often unable to speak loudly or shout. There is also slowness of chewing and swallowing, and the decreased swallowing is largely responsible for the drooling that sometimes occurs.

The freezing phenomenon is common in PD. In the midst of a motor act, the patient will suddenly freeze in place, unable to move for a short time because of simultaneous activation of agonists and antagonists **(Video 30.2)**. Freezing may occur when first starting to walk (start hesitation), when turning (turn hesitation), when approaching an obstacle, and even when talking or eating. Associated involvement of midbrain structures may cause changes in ocular movements, including fixation instability, hypometric saccades, convergence insufficiency, and impaired upgaze. Oculogyric crisis, forced involuntary eye deviation, usually upward, is a feature of postencephalitic PD and can occur in drug-induced parkinsonism, but it does not happen in idiopathic PD.

In PD, there is no atrophy, fasciculations, reflex changes, or pathologic reflexes of the type seen in corticospinal tract disorders (see Table 22.1). Reflex changes may occur if there is associated corticospinal tract involvement, but this does not occur in idiopathic PD. Even when the extrapyramidal signs are asymmetric, the reflexes remain normal and equal. Fragments of dystonia sometimes occur. A "striatal toe" (dystonic toe) is an apparent extensor plantar response, without fanning of the toes that occurs in isolation, without other signs suggesting corticospinal tract dysfunction, in patients with extrapyramidal disorders such as PD (Figure 30.2). The extended toe may occur as part of a foot dystonia that includes ankle inversion, arching of the sole, and flexion of the other toes (striatal foot). The parkinsonian hand is slightly extended at the wrist and flexed at the metacarpophalangeal joints with the fingers extended and adducted. There is often exaggeration of the orbicularis oculi and orbicularis oris reflexes. Myerson's sign (glabellar tap reflex) is blinking of the eyes on tapping over the glabella. In PD, the patient is unable to inhibit the response and will continue to blink over and over; normals do not continue to blink with repetitive tapping (see Chapter 16). Patients with PD may exhibit a variety of nonmotor manifestations, such as anosmia, hyperhidrosis, greasy seborrhea, constipation, somnolence, REM sleep behavior disorder, difficulty turning over in bed, blepharospasm, apraxia of eyelid opening, depression, and dementia. Nonmotor manifestations may occur before motor symptoms develop.

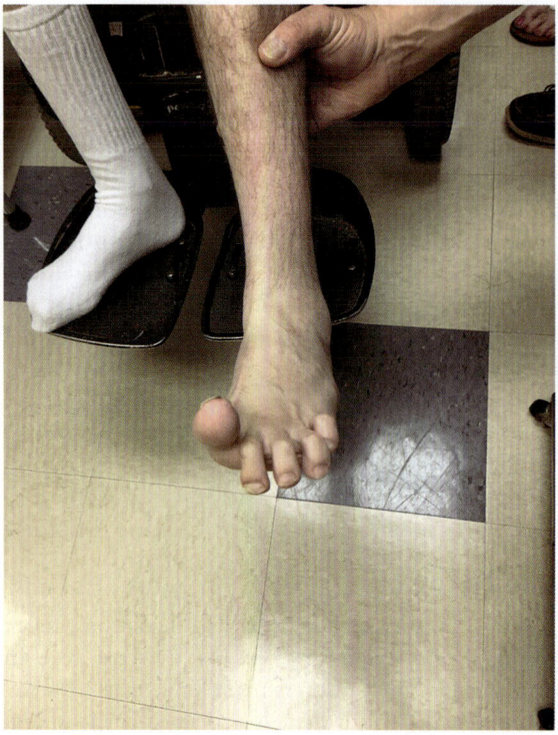

FIGURE 30.2 A "striatal toe" (dystonic toe) resembles the great toe extension of Babinski's plantar sign but is tonic and sustained, not accompanied by fanning of the toes, and occurs without plantar stimulation; it occurs in extrapyramidal disease, in this case Wilson's disease.

In the early stages of PD, typical signs are often subtle, and patients may present complaining only of stiffness, impaired handwriting (especially micrographia), or difficulty getting about. Stiffness and myalgic pains may suggest a diagnosis of arthritis, polymyalgia, or fibromyalgia. The facial masking and bradykinesia often lead to a misdiagnosis of depression. Early PD may also be mistaken for the effects of aging. Rest tremor, a flexed posture, and mild cogwheel rigidity provide important clues to the possibility of early parkinsonism in such patients. The clinical diagnosis of PD at the time of initial presentation is occasionally wrong. The pattern of disease progression and the response to medication are important additional factors in determining whether the patient suffers from PD or one of the other akinetic-rigid syndromes.

Advancing disease is characterized by increasing gait difficulty, worsening of tremor and bradykinesia, motor fluctuations related to levodopa therapy, behavioral changes, dysphagia, speech difficulty, intractable drooling, and sleep impairment **(Video 30.3)**. Some degree of cognitive blunting may occur in 20% to 40% of patients. Severe dementia is rare; when present, especially early in the course, the possibility of dementia with Lewy bodies should be considered. Depression occurs in approximately one-third of patients, and psychosis and hallucinations occur in about one-fourth of patients. Early, prominent, and nonvisual hallucinations raise the possibility of dementia with Lewy bodies. The absence of tremor in the early stages may suggest a possible Parkinson-plus syndrome. Advanced age at onset, severe depression, dementia, and an akinetic-rigid presentation are risk factors for rapid disease progression. The tremor may begin to abate in the very late stages.

PD usually affects older patients, the mean age at onset is around 60 years, but some cases began relatively early in life. The nosology describing these patients is inconsistent. Juvenile Parkinson's disease (JPD) has its onset before 20 and young-onset Parkinson's disease (YOPD) between 20 and 50, but the terms are sometimes used interchangeably. JPD was first described by Ramsay Hunt and is one of the several "Ramsay Hunt syndromes" (Box 16.2). YOPD is probably the same entity as idiopathic PD, with a younger age of onset. In a series of 953 individuals with YOPD, 17% were found to have a genetic etiology. In contrast, JPD is a heterogeneous group of disorders. Many patients with JPD have a genetic disorder due to a parkin gene mutation. Patients with parkin mutations may have atypical clinical features such as dystonia at onset and marked diurnal symptom fluctuation. YOPD tends to have more gradual progression of parkinsonian signs and symptoms and earlier treatment-related complications. Susceptibility to developing late-onset PD has been associated with polymorphisms or mutations in several genes.

The diagnosis of PD is predominantly clinical, and differential diagnosis essentially is between other conditions causing tremor, of which ET is the commonest, and other akinetic-rigid syndromes. Clinical features that favor PD include prominent rest tremor, asymmetric signs, preservation of balance and postural reflexes in the early stages of the disease, and a good response to levodopa replacement therapy. The other degenerative disorders with parkinsonian features typically produce other neurologic signs, such as gaze limitation, cerebellar signs, pyramidal signs, severe dementia, apraxia and other parietal lobe signs, or dysautonomia, although these other manifestations may not be apparent early in the course. In the past, a diagnosis of PD required two of three parkinsonian features (tremor, rigidity, bradykinesia). Using these criteria resulted in a 24% error rate based on pathologic studies. Using revised criteria (the UK Brain Bank criteria) of rest tremor, asymmetry, and a good response to levodopa improved accuracy and resulted in pathologic confirmation of the diagnosis in 99% of cases determined by clinicopathologic correlation studies. The most common condition confused with PD is PSP (see below).

Certain drugs can induce a reversible condition that mimics PD. The most common agents that cause drug-induced parkinsonism are antipsychotics, especially the high-potency piperazine compounds such as haloperidol. The atypical neuroleptics are as potent in their antipsychotic effects as traditional compounds but less likely to induce parkinsonism. Drug-induced parkinsonism can mimic PD closely, even to the point of causing asymmetric signs. Although dopamine receptor–blocking agents, especially those that block the D2 receptor, are the most common offenders, other agents can induce parkinsonism. Some patients are much more prone to develop extrapyramidal side effects than others, but most individuals will eventually develop parkinsonism if treated with high doses. Metoclopramide is a dopamine blocker most often used for gastrointestinal disease; it may have extrapyramidal side effects.

In the presence of typical clinical signs and symptoms and the typical age of onset, extensive workup is not required. Imaging studies are usually normal. A thorough medication history, complete neurologic examination to look for nonextrapyramidal abnormalities, and screening for orthostatic hypotension are useful. Certain features suggest an alternative diagnosis, such as prominent dementia and hallucinations in the patient suffering from dementia with Lewy bodies, prominent dysautonomia in the patient with multisystem atrophy (MSA), dysarthria, and early age of onset in Wilson's disease. Single-photon emission computed tomography (SPECT) imaging of the dopamine transporter system can confirm or exclude loss of nigrostriatal dopaminergic neurons and help distinguish PD from some of the conditions that may mimic it, such as ET. These scans cannot distinguish between PD and conditions such as MSA and PSP.

Pathologically, the disease is characterized by depigmentation and cystic degeneration of the pars compacta of the substantia nigra with cell loss and the presence of intracytoplasmic Lewy bodies in surviving neurons. A major chemical constituent of the Lewy body is alpha-synuclein, a synaptic protein. Abnormal aggregation of alpha-synuclein has been advocated in the pathogenesis of PD, dementia with Lewy bodies, and multisystem atrophy, and these conditions have been grouped together as synucleinopathies. In PD, there is depletion of dopamine; replacement by its precursor, levodopa, has been well recognized as effective therapy since the landmark studies of the 1960s. The etiology of PD remains unknown, but the basis is likely multifactorial, possibly involving hereditary factors, environmental influences that may selectively affect dopaminergic nigral cells, and free radical toxicity.

The pathophysiology of parkinsonism is complex. Dopamine deficiency ultimately results in an increased output from the internal segment of the globus pallidus and subthalamic nuclei, which results in excessive inhibition of the thalamus and suppression of the cortical motor system (see Chapter 26). Pharmacologic treatment modalities include anticholinergic drugs, dopamine-releasing agents, dopamine agonists that directly stimulate the dopamine receptor in the striatum, catechol-*O*-methyl transferase inhibitors, and levodopa. Dopamine and acetylcholine are in balance in the striatum, and anticholinergics increase the effect of dopamine by influencing this balance. These agents were the earliest treatment available for PD. The discovery of L-dopa as a treatment for PD was a major medical advance. The story of that discovery is told in British neurologist Oliver Sacks' book, *Awakenings*, and its motion picture adaptation. Over 90% of patients with PD respond very well to the initiation of levodopa replacement. The absence of a good initial response suggests the possibility of another diagnosis, although some of the mimickers of PD, especially MSA, may also have a good initial response.

Some of the other conditions important in the differential diagnosis of PD include multisystem atrophy, PSP, corticobasal degeneration (CBD), and diffuse Lewy body disease.

Multisystem Atrophy

MSA produces degeneration involving the basal ganglia, cerebellum, anterior horn cells, cerebral cortex, and brainstem in varying combinations and usually includes parkinsonian features. Patients with MSA may have elements of cerebellar ataxia, dementia, amyotrophy, parkinsonism, corticospinal tract dysfunction, dysautonomia, and urinary dysfunction.

There are three subtypes: MSA-P (parkinsonian), MSA-C (cerebellar), and MSA-A (autonomic). In MSA-P (formerly striatonigral degeneration), the primary manifestation is parkinsonism; it accounts for about 80% of the cases of MSA. About 10% of patients presenting with parkinsonism will evolve into MSA-P. In MSA-C (formerly the sporadic form of olivopontocerebellar atrophy), the primary manifestations are cerebellar. In MSA-A (formerly Shy-Drager syndrome), the primary manifestation is dysautonomia, particularly postural hypotension. Suspicion of MSA should arise in the patient with atypical parkinsonism in conjunction with cerebellar signs and/or early and prominent autonomic dysfunction, usually orthostatic hypotension. There is some overlap of pathologic findings in the different forms of MSA. Recently discovered glial cytoplasmic inclusions containing alpha-synuclein confirm these three disorders are different forms of the same disease. The dysautonomia is due to degeneration of the neurons in the intermediolateral gray column of the thoracic and lumbar spinal cord. Impaired peripheral vasomotor control in MSA may cause cold, dusky, purplish discoloration of the digits (cold hands sign; Figure 30.3).

Parkinsonism is the most frequent motor manifestation of MSA. MSA-P has been associated with relative symmetry of findings, urinary incontinence, frequent falls, an absence of tremor, and the frequent presence of pyramidal or cerebellar signs. MSA-A consists of a combination of parkinsonian signs and symptoms coupled with severe dysautonomia, most often manifest as orthostatic hypotension. The primary manifestations of MSA-C are ataxia and brainstem dysfunction. Approximately one-quarter of patients with MSA-C will develop parkinsonian features within 5 years; such evolution carries a poor prognosis for survival.

Progressive Supranuclear Palsy

In PSP (Steele-Richardson-Olszewski syndrome, Richardson's syndrome), degenerative changes in the rostral brainstem and thalamus result in impairment first of downgaze, then of upgaze, and eventually in global gaze paresis. Three subtypes are currently recognized: classic Richardson's syndrome (PSP-RS), PSP parkinsonism (PSP-P), and pure akinesia with gait freezing. In PSP-P, the clinical picture resembles PD early in the course. In PSP-RS, the gaze abnormalities are accompanied by parkinsonian signs, frontal lobe–type dementia, postural instability, pseudobulbar palsy, and a pronounced tendency to extensor axial rigidity, especially involving the neck muscles, and sometimes causing frank retrocollis. Gait difficulty is prominent, and a tendency to fall is an early and conspicuous feature. Some have likened the hypererect gait with abducted arms seen in PSP to that of a gunslinger. The falls are often backward because of the increased extensor tone and postural instability. There is particular difficulty walking downstairs because of the combination of retrocollis and impaired downgaze. Tremor is not usually pronounced, and the disease does not respond

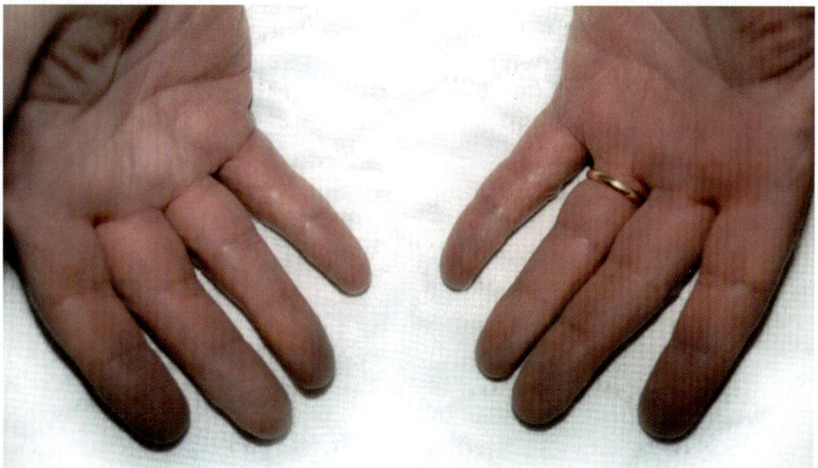

FIGURE 30.3 Dusky, violaceous fingers typical of multisystem atrophy. (Reprinted from Reich SG. The cold hands sign in MSA. *Neurology* 2003;60[4]:719, with permission.)

significantly to levodopa. The gaze abnormalities at first involve voluntary, vertical, saccadic gaze, sparing reflex eye movements; the name of the disease refers to this supranuclear ocular motility disturbance. The disordered motility may progress to complete ophthalmoplegia terminally.

Facial dystonia may contort the face, particularly the forehead muscles, into a characteristic expression of "perpetual surprise" or astonishment with raised eyebrows, lid retraction, and reduced blinking (procerus sign; Figure 16.4). The facial expression is markedly different from the hypomimia and masking of PD. The characteristic ocular motility disturbance may not be present early in the course and, in rare instances, never appears. The "applause sign" is an inability to stop clapping after being asked to clap three times. It was initially touted as a way to distinguish PSP from PD and frontotemporal dementia. Later studies found the applause sign in cortical dementia and suggested that it is a nonspecific sign of frontal lobe dysfunction. On magnetic resonance imaging (MRI), a characteristic atrophy of the midbrain with relative preservation of the pons (the "hummingbird sign" on midsagittal images) may be seen. MRI measurement of the midbrain/pons ratio and combined measurements, such as midbrain area/pons area and especially the magnetic resonance parkinsonism index, are very useful in distinguishing PSP from other parkinsonian syndromes.

Corticobasal Syndrome

In CBD (corticobasal degeneration), abnormalities involve both the basal ganglia and the cerebral cortex. Pathologically, there is asymmetric frontoparietal neuronal loss and gliosis, with swollen, achromatic neurons, tau-immunoreactive neuronal and glial inclusions, and nigral degeneration. Clinically, the corticobasal syndrome (CBS) is characteristically very asymmetric initially, with rigidity, bradykinesia, and occasionally tremor, accompanied by evidence of higher cortical dysfunction such as apraxia, agnosia, cortical sensory loss, focal myoclonus, or pyramidal signs. It has been increasingly recognized that not all patients with CBS have CBD pathologically. Many have other pathology, most commonly PSP or Alzheimer's disease. Conversely, some patients with a clinical picture of PSP, frontotemporal dementia, or Alzheimer's disease may have CBD pathologically.

CBS typically begins with clumsiness, stiffness, or jerking of an arm. The alien limb phenomenon is common. There may be dystonic posturing as well as spontaneous and reflex myoclonus of the involved limbs. The involved limbs become stiff, jerky, and eventually useless. The combination of unilateral parkinsonism unresponsive to levodopa, accompanied by ideomotor apraxia of the involved extremities, is very suggestive. MRI frequently shows asymmetric cortical atrophy. Cognitive impairment may emerge as the disease progresses and becomes generalized. The disorder progresses slowly and does not respond to levodopa. Tau protein is a microtubule-associated protein, which when aggregated causes neurofibrillary tangles. Other conditions are associated with abnormalities of tau protein, especially PSP and frontotemporal dementia, collectively referred to as tauopathies.

Diffuse Lewy Body Disease

In diffuse Lewy body disease, the usual clinical picture is progressive dementia with added parkinsonian features in an elderly patient. It is the second most common degenerative dementia after Alzheimer's disease (Chapter 8). Parkinsonism may occur early or late and varies in severity. The parkinsonian features are typically more symmetric and milder than in PD. Tremor occurs but is less common and less severe than in PD. Another characteristic feature is psychotic behavior with visual hallucinations, delirium, and paranoia. Other common clinical features include cognitive fluctuations; dysautonomia; sleep disorders, especially REM sleep behavior disorder; and neuroleptic sensitivity.

Wilson's Disease

Wilson's disease (hepatolenticular degeneration) is a rare, autosomal recessive disorder due to abnormal copper deposition in the brain, especially the basal ganglia, liver, eye, and other tissues because of a genetic defect in an ATPase involved in copper transport (ATP7B), usually accompanied by a defect in the copper transport protein ceruloplasmin. The genetic defect leads to impaired copper excretion and systemic copper accumulation. A low ceruloplasmin level is found in the serum in 95% of patients. Ceruloplasmin is involved in the transfer of copper to copper-containing enzymes such as cytochrome oxidase, and the dysfunction of these enzymes may underlie the clinical manifestations.

The usual age of onset is between the ages of 10 and 20, and major manifestations include tremor, rigidity, dystonia, abnormal involuntary movements of various types, dysarthria, dementia, parkinsonian features, spasticity, cerebellar signs, and psychiatric abnormalities (anxiety, depression, psychosis). The tremor may be present at rest and increased by voluntary movement. Most characteristic is a "wing-beating" tremor of the proximal upper extremities, consisting of a slow, high-amplitude, up-and-down movement of the elbow when the arm is held with the shoulder abducted and the elbow flexed (see **Video Link 30.1**). Pathologically, there is symmetric degeneration of the lenticular nuclei, with widespread neuronal loss and proliferation of Alzheimer-type II astrocytes.

Kayser-Fleischer rings are crescents of green-brown discoloration of the cornea because of copper deposits in Descemet's membrane (Figure 30.4); these are essentially always present in patients with neurologic involvement but may not be visible without a slit lamp. Rarely, the disease may present without the rings. Slit lamp examination may also detect sunflower cataracts because of copper deposition in the lens.

Risus sardonicus refers to an unusual forced "smile" because of facial dystonia and may be seen in Wilson's disease and other disorders (Figure 30.5). Other manifestations of the disease include cirrhosis, atypical hepatitis, hemolytic anemia, and renal disease. Patients may present with liver disease alone, brain disease alone, or evidence of both. In a series of 282 patients seen over three decades, the mean age at diagnosis was 16, and the predominant features were neurologic (in 69%); the predominant neurologic manifestations were parkinsonism (62%) and dystonia (35%).

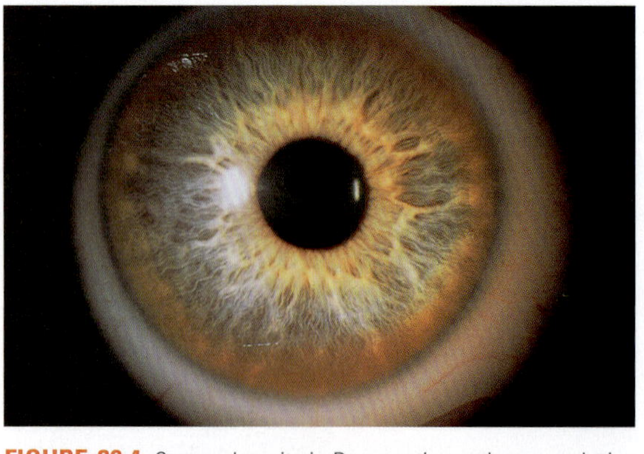

FIGURE 30.4 Copper deposits in Descemet's membrane producing the brownish Kayser-Fleischer ring in Wilson's disease. (Reprinted from Chern KC, Saidel MA. *Ophthalmology Review Manual*. 2nd ed. Philadelphia: Wolters Kluwer Health/Lippincott Williams & Wilkins, 2012, with permission.)

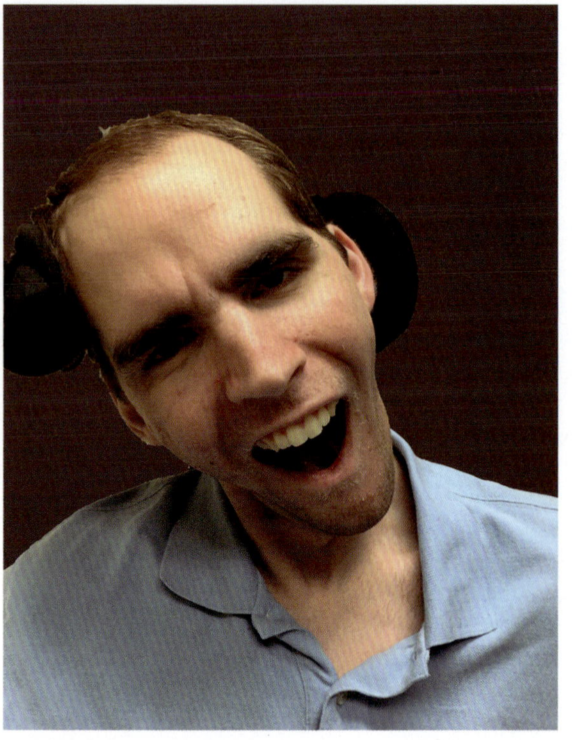

FIGURE 30.5 Risus sardonicus in a patient with Wilson's disease.

Pantothenate Kinase–Associated Neurodegeneration

Pantothenate kinase–associated neurodegeneration (PKAN, neurodegeneration with brain iron accumulation type 1, Hallervorden-Spatz syndrome) is a rare autosomal recessive disorder associated with macroscopic rust-brown discoloration of the globus pallidus and substantia nigra because of iron deposition. The clinical phenotype is variable. The disease usually begins in the first to the fourth decade of life, with rigidity, involuntary movements, ataxia, and dystonia, followed by pyramidal signs and progressive dementia. MRI findings are characteristic. T2-weighted sequences show bilaterally symmetric low signal intensity in the globus pallidus, because of iron deposition, surrounding a focus of high signal intensity, because of gliosis. This "eye of the tiger" image pattern is virtually diagnostic for PKAN.

Dentatorubropallidoluysian Atrophy

Dentatorubropallidoluysian atrophy is a heredofamilial degeneration, because of CAG repeats, in which the pathologic changes involve primarily the dentate, globus pallidus externa, red nucleus, and subthalamic nucleus. Clinical manifestations include choreoathetosis, dystonia, dementia, myoclonus, and ataxia; the disease is often included as one of the hereditary ataxia syndromes. Most reported cases have been from Japan. A cluster of cases occurred in the United States around the Haw River in North Carolina (Haw River syndrome).

HYPERKINETIC MOVEMENT DISORDERS

Hyperkinesia refers to increased movement. Hyperkinesias are abnormal involuntary movements that occur in a host of neurologic conditions. Hyperkinesias come in many forms, ranging from tremor to chorea to muscle fasciculations to myoclonic jerks. Any level of the motor system, from the motor cortex to the muscle itself, may be involved in their production. The only common characteristic is that the movements are spontaneous and, for the most part, not under volitional control. They may be rhythmic or random, fleeting or sustained, and predictable or unpredictable and may occur in isolation or accompanied by other neurologic signs. Table 30.2 summarizes some of these features.

In the examination of abnormal movements, the following should be noted: (a) the part of the body involved or the exact location of the movements; (b) the extent of the movement, or its distribution as it regards to part of a muscle, an entire muscle, movement involving joints, or more complex or composite patterns consisting of a sequence of different movements; (c) the pattern, rhythmicity, uniformity, multiformity, and regularity of recurrence—there may be a regular or rhythmic recurrence of activity involving the same muscle or groups, or there may be an irregular pattern of constantly changing motion of different parts; (d) the course, speed, and frequency of each particular movement; (e) the amplitude and force of the movement; (f) the relationship to posture, rest, voluntary activity or exertion, involuntary activity, various stimuli, fatigue, and time of day; (g) the response to heat and cold; (h) the relationship to emotional tension and excitement; (i) the degree that movements are suppressible by attention or the use of sensory tricks; and (j) the presence or absence of the movements during sleep. In general, involuntary movements are increased by stress and anxiety and decrease or disappear with sleep. Truly involuntary movements must be separated from complex or bizarre voluntary movements, such as mannerisms or compulsions.

It may be possible to name movements that fit a well-defined clinical pattern, but it is often better to describe the abnormality. Palpation may sometimes be useful, especially if the movements are very fine and limited to individual muscles. Videos are often very useful in the diagnosis and management of movement disorders.

TABLE 30.2 Abnormal Involuntary Movements as a Spectrum of Movements

Regular/ Predictable	Intermediate	Fleeting/ Unpredictable
Tremor	Most dystonias	Fasciculations
Hemiballism	Myokymia	Myoclonus
Palatal myoclonus	Athetosis	Chorea
	Tic	Dyskinesias
	Stereotypy	
	Myorhythmia	

TREMOR

A tremor is a series of involuntary, relatively rhythmic, purposeless, oscillatory movements. The excursion may be small or large and may involve one or more parts of the body. A simple tremor involves only a single muscle group; a compound tremor involves several muscle groups and may have several elements in combination, resulting in a series of complex movements (e.g., alternating flexion and extension together with alternate pronation and supination). Not only the agonist and antagonist, but muscles of fixation and synergists may play a part in the movements. A tremor may be present at rest or with activity. Some tremors are accentuated by having the patient hold the fingers extended and separated with the arms outstretched. Slow movements, writing, and drawing circles or spirals may bring tremor out.

Tremors may be classified in various ways: by location, rate, amplitude, rhythmicity, relationship to rest and movement, etiology, and underlying pathology. Other important factors may include the relationship to fatigue, emotion, self-consciousness, heat, cold, and the use of medications, alcohol, or street drugs. Tremor may be unilateral or bilateral and most commonly involves distal parts of the extremities—the fingers or hands—but may also affect the arms, feet, legs, tongue, eyelids, jaw, and head and may occasionally seem to involve the entire body. The rate may be slow, medium, or fast. Oscillations of 3 to 5 Hz are considered slow and 10 to 20 Hz rapid. Amplitude may be fine, coarse, or medium. Tremor may be constant or intermittent, rhythmic or relatively nonrhythmic, although a certain amount of rhythmicity is implied in the term tremor. Irregular "tremor" may be due to myoclonus.

The relationship to rest or activity is the basis for classification into two primary tremor types: rest and action. Resting (static) tremors are present mainly during relaxation (e.g., with the hands in the lap) and attenuate when the part is used. Rest tremor is seen primarily in PD and other parkinsonian syndromes.

Action tremors appear when performing some activity. Action tremors are divided into subtypes: postural, kinetic, task-specific, and isometric. Only when they are very severe are action tremors present at rest. Postural tremors become evident when the limbs are maintained in an antigravity position (e.g., arms outstretched). Common types of postural tremor are enhanced physiologic tremor and ET. Kinetic tremor appears when making a voluntary movement and may occur at the beginning, during, or at the end of the movement. The most common example is an intention (terminal) tremor. Intention tremor is a form of action tremor seen primarily in cerebellar disease (see Chapter 43). The tremor appears when precision is required to touch a target, as in the finger-nose-finger or toe-to-finger test. It progressively worsens during the movement. Approaching the target causes the limb to shake, usually side-to-side perpendicular to the line of travel, and the amplitude of the oscillation increases toward the end of the movement. Some tremors fall into more than one potential classification. Most tremors are accentuated by emotional excitement, and many normal individuals develop tremor with anxiety, apprehension, and fatigue. A shivering type of tremor (rigors) may be brought on by cold, but identical movements can be psychogenic.

Physiologic tremor is present in normal individuals. The frequency varies from 8 to 12 Hz, averaging about 10 Hz in the young adult, somewhat slower in children and older persons. The frequency for an individual is the same at different sites in the body. The visible tremor brought out in normal persons by anxiety, fright, fatigue (rock climber's tremor, Elvis leg), and other conditions with increased adrenergic activity is accentuated or enhanced physiologic tremor. A typical example of enhanced physiologic tremor is that seen in hyperthyroidism. The tremor involves principally the fingers and hands and may be fine and difficult to see. It may be brought out by placing a limb in a position of postural tension, by performing voluntary movements at the slowest possible rate, or holding the index fingertips as close together as possible without touching. The tremor may be better appreciated by placing a sheet of paper on the outstretched fingers; shaking of the paper may be obvious even though tremor is not grossly visible. Physiologic tremor may be present both at rest and on activity, but it is accentuated by activity as well as by anxiety and emotional stress. Similar tremor occurs due to the effects of alcohol, nicotine, caffeine, amphetamines, ephedrine, and other stimulants (Table 30.3). A fine tremor of the closed eyelids is seen in hyperthyroidism (Rosenbach's sign).

TABLE 30.3 Some Drugs That Cause Tremor

Sympathomimetics (epinephrine, pseudoephedrine, isoproterenol, metaproterenol, albuterol, terbutaline, ritodrine)
Aminoglycoside antibiotics (amikacin, kanamycin, tobramycin)
Methylxanthines (aminophylline, theophylline)
Amphetamines
Anticholinergics
Antihistamines
Bupropion
Carisoprodol, orphenadrine (centrally acting muscle relaxants)
Antipsychotics
Cyclosporine
Benzodiazepines (diazepam, oxazepam)
Selective serotonin reuptake inhibitors
Other antidepressants (mirtazapine, amoxapine, trazodone, clomipramine)
Lithium
Thyroid supplements
Antiarrhythmics (mexiletine, amiodarone, quinidine)
Opioid antagonists (naloxone)
Phenytoin
Tramadol
Valproic acid
Vasopressin
Yohimbine

Tremor of medium amplitude and rate is often evident in anxiety. Such tremor may occur in the absence of neurologic disease. The tremor is usually postural, most evident with the hands outstretched, made worse by movement, and may interfere with motor activity. ET is often of medium amplitude and rate but may be coarse when severe. The intention tremor of multiple sclerosis (MS) and cerebellar disease is usually of medium amplitude and may vary in degree from mild to severe; it may be coarse and irregular, especially when associated with ataxia. Coarse tremors occur in a variety of disease states and are usually slow. Parkinsonian tremor is one of the most characteristic. Coarse tremor also occurs in Wilson's disease and other extrapyramidal syndromes. The tremor of general paresis and alcoholism may also be coarse, especially if the movements are diffuse, as in delirium tremens. Psychogenic tremor and the tremor associated with midbrain and cerebellar disease may also be coarse and slow.

Parkinsonian Tremor

Resting, static, or nonintention tremor occurs most frequently in diseases of the basal ganglia and extrapyramidal pathways **(Video 30.1)**. The most characteristic tremor of this type is seen in PD and the various parkinsonian syndromes (see PD above). The tremor is slow, coarse, and compound in type. The rate may vary from 2 to 6 Hz, averaging 4 to 5 Hz. The movement in the hand characteristically consists of alternate contractions of agonist and antagonist, involving the flexors, extensors, abductors, and adductors of the fingers and thumb, together with motion of the wrist and arm, including flexion, extension, pronation, and supination. As a result, there is a repetitive movement of the thumb on the first two fingers, together with the motion of the wrist, producing the classical pill-rolling. The tremor is relatively rhythmic, present at rest, and may be temporarily suppressed by movement. It may disappear temporarily, whereas the limb is engaged in a voluntary effort. Because of the uniformly alternating movements at regular intervals, it is sometimes called an alternating tremor. The tremor may be unilateral at onset; it may even begin in a single digit but, in most cases, eventually becomes bilateral. It disappears during sleep and is aggravated by emotional stimulation, fatigue, and anxiety. Tremor resembling that of parkinsonism may also occur in other extrapyramidal syndromes.

Essential Tremor

ET is the most common of all movement disorders **(Video 30.1)**. It is higher in frequency and lower in amplitude than the tremor of PD. The etiology and pathophysiology remain obscure, but recent evidence suggests a cerebellar abnormality.

ET is often familial. The prevalence of ET increases with age, may first appear anywhere between the second and sixth decades of life, and tends to be slowly progressive. ET is a postural and action tremor that tends to affect the hands, head, and voice. It is made worse by anxiety. The movement of the head may be in an anteroposterior (affirmative, yes-yes) or a lateral (negative, no-no) direction. Senile tremor is ET occurring during senescence with a negative family history.

A common problem is differentiating the tremor of early PD from ET. The tremor of PD is most prominent at rest, whereas that of ET occurs with a sustained posture, such as with the hands outstretched, or on action. Parkinsonian tremor may persist with hands outstretched but usually damps, at least momentarily, when making a deliberate movement, whereas ET usually worsens with any attempt at a precise action. The ET patient may have great difficulty sipping water from a cup, but the PD patient may do so without spilling a drop. The head and voice are often involved with ET, only rarely with PD, although the tremor in PD may involve the lips and jaw. Alcohol and beta-blockers often improve ET but have no effect on parkinsonian tremor. Some patients thought to have ET go on to develop PD.

Other Forms of Tremor

Cerebellar tremor is a low-frequency tremor that occurs primarily as the finger approaches a target (intention tremor); it may have a postural component (see Chapter 43). Rubral (Holmes, cerebellar outflow, midbrain) tremor refers to a severe, large-amplitude, relatively slow (2 to 5 Hz) tremor, involving both proximal and distal muscles, present at rest but made worse with action. The clinical picture resembles a combination of parkinsonian and cerebellar tremors. It may be unilateral and is usually due to stroke or trauma. Formerly thought to result from an abnormality of the red nucleus, it is now believed to be due to a lesion involving cerebellar efferent and nigrostriatal fibers coursing through the midbrain.

Orthostatic tremor (shaky legs syndrome) is a variant of ET that involves the legs. It is an isometric tremor most apparent when standing, and it abates when walking. Neuropathic tremor is a coarse postural and action tremor seen in patients with peripheral neuropathy. Dystonic tremor is typically a localized, irregular postural tremor that resembles ET but is more irregular and asymmetric. It usually but not invariably occurs with evidence of dystonia. Head tremor in a patient with cervical dystonia and hand tremor in a patient with writer's cramp are examples. Task-specific tremors appear during performance of a particular activity (e.g., primary writing tremor). Nonorganic or psychogenic tremor is typically complex and does not fit well into the classification scheme. The patient may have action as well as resting tremor, with rapidly changing clinical features and disability out of proportion to the tremor. Typical features include abrupt onset with maximal disability immediately, onset in one limb with rapid generalization, spontaneous resolution and recurrence, easy distractibility, entrainment, and refractoriness to conventional antitremor treatment.

CHOREA

Chorea (Gr. "dance") is characterized by involuntary, irregular, purposeless, random, and nonrhythmic hyperkinesias **(Video 30.4)**. The movements are spontaneous, abrupt, brief, rapid, jerky, and unsustained. Individual movements are discrete, but they are variable in type and location, causing an irregular pattern of chaotic, multiform, constantly changing movements that seem to flow from one body part to another. The movements may at times appear purposeful to a casual observer, but they are actually random and aimless. They are present at rest but are increased by activity, tension, emotional stress, and self-consciousness. The patient may be able to temporarily and partially suppress the movements, and they disappear in sleep.

The distribution of the choreic movements is variable. They may involve one extremity, one-half of the body (hemichorea), or be generalized. They occur most characteristically in the distal parts of the upper extremities but may also involve the proximal parts, lower extremities, trunk, face, tongue, lips, and pharynx. There may be repeated twitching and grimacing movements of the face that change constantly in character and location. Involvement of the vocal tract may cause abnormal vocalizations, difficulty in maintaining phonation, or aphonia.

The abnormal movements interrupt the harmonious coordination of prime movers, synergists, and antagonists. They interfere with and distort voluntary movements, and the latter may be short, jerky, and unsustained. Difficulty with rapid, repetitive movements and problems performing a sequence of hand movements indicate the disturbed motor function. Constant unwanted movements of the hands may interfere with activities of daily living. When asked to hold the hands outstretched, there may be constant random movements of individual fingers (piano-playing movements). If the patient holds the examiner's finger in her fist, there are constant twitches of individual fingers (milkmaid grip). Choreic movements may often be brought out by having the patient carry out two simultaneous acts. She may touch finger to nose or protrude the tongue in isolation, but when attempting to do both at the same time, the jerky movements become noticeable. The patient may also have difficulty chewing and swallowing.

The patient may try to incorporate a spontaneous, involuntary movement into a semipurposeful movement in order to mask the chorea (parakinesia). If a choreic movement suddenly makes a hand fly upward, the patient may continue the movement and reach up and scratch her nose. When chorea is generalized, the patient is in a constant state of motion with continual adventitial movements randomly scattered.

In addition to the abnormal movements, there is hypotonia of the skeletal muscles, with decreased resistance to passive movement. The outstretched hands are held with hyperextension of the fingers with flexion and dorsal arching of the wrist (spooning). The fingers are separated and the thumb is abducted and droops downward. When the arms are raised overhead, the hands may turn into a position of hyperpronation. Motor impersistence—the inability to sustain a contraction—frequently accompanies chorea. The patient is frequently unable to hold the tongue out for any length of time; when asked to do so, the tongue shoots out and then jerks back quickly (snake, darting, flycatcher, or trombone tongue). The blink rate is increased.

There is no paralysis, but the hypotonia and constantly repeated hyperkinesias may interfere with voluntary movement enough to cause significant impairment of motor function. The hypotonia may result in pendular deep tendon reflexes.

Many disorders may cause chorea, among them Huntington's disease (HD) and Sydenham's chorea.

Huntington's Disease

HD (Huntington's chorea) is a progressive, fatal, AD, neurodegenerative condition with variable penetrance, because of an unstable CAG trinucleotide repeat expansion on chromosome 4. The gene produces a protein called huntingtin. The mutant protein results in an expanded polyglutamine tract and a buildup of deleterious β-amyloid–like aggregates, which primarily affect the caudate and putamen. The onset is usually between the ages of 35 and 50, but the disease may begin in childhood or senescence. Onset is often earlier when the disease is inherited from the father. Age of onset correlates inversely with the length of trinucleotide repeats. Repeats tend to lengthen in succeeding generations, causing earlier onset (anticipation), particularly with paternal transmission. DNA diagnostic testing can confirm the diagnosis, even in presymptomatic individuals.

Huntington described three cardinal features: dementia, emotional disturbance, and the familial nature of the disorder. The condition is inexorably progressive and ultimately fatal. The typical course is from 15 to 20 years. Some symptomatic treatments are available, but nothing which will arrest the progression. The choreic movements may cause the patient to complain of clumsiness or tremor. The movements are similar to those of Sydenham's chorea but are often somewhat slower, less jerky, and more bizarre, widespread, and violent. They may be seemingly purposeful, and the same pattern may be repeated over and over. Frequently, the larger muscle groups and the proximal extremities are affected; there may be repeated shrugging of the shoulder or flail-like movements of the arm and twisting and lashing movements that lie between those of chorea and athetosis. Facial grimacing may be marked. Movements of the fingers and hands are often accentuated as the patient walks. Pronounced chorea of the arms and legs when walking may lead to a bizarre, prancing gait (see **Video Link 30.2**). In the later stages of the disease, the chorea may progress to athetosis or dystonia. Rigidity may become a conspicuous feature in the later stages of choreic disease. In juvenile HD, with onset prior to age 20, rigidity is often more prominent than chorea (Westphal, rigid, or pseudoparkinsonian variant).

HD is accompanied by progressive intellectual deterioration. Cognitive impairment usually begins at about the same time as the abnormal movements but may precede it and progresses in tandem. Most patients also develop psychiatric abnormalities, particularly personality changes and mood disorders. The degree of dementia is out of proportion to the cortical pathology and may reflect impairment related to the role of the caudate in cognition. Patients are typically reduced to a vegetative state about 10 to 15 years after onset.

Neuropathologically, there is atrophy most prominent in the caudate, putamen, and cerebral cortex. The neuron loss initially affects the enkephalinergic (ENKergic) spiny neurons of the striatum. Loss of ENKergic striatal neurons lessens the inhibitory influence of the striatum on the external segment of the globus pallidus, allowing it to increase its inhibition of the subthalamic nucleus. This results in a decrease in the facilitatory influence of the subthalamic nucleus on the internal segment of the globus pallidus, decreasing the inhibition of the motor thalamus (releasing the brake), increasing thalamocortical activity, and resulting in hyperkinesis (see Chapter 26). Imaging studies may show atrophy of the caudate, producing a square-shaped lateral ventricle (Figure 30.6). The cortical atrophy primarily affects the frontal and temporal regions. HD-like 1 and 2 are hereditary disorders clinically and pathologically very similar to HD.

Other Forms of Chorea

Sydenham's chorea (chorea minor, rheumatic chorea, St. Vitus' dance) occurs in childhood and adolescence in relationship to streptococcal infection. Like rheumatic fever, it has become a rarity in developed countries. After recovery, a patient may retain minimal choreic movements or have minor tic-like movements that are difficult to differentiate from chorea. Some of the other conditions associated with chorea include chorea gravidarum (occurs during pregnancy), systemic lupus erythematosus, antiphospholipid syndrome, neurosyphilis (usually with concomitant HIV infection), hyperthyroidism, polycythemia vera, nonketotic hyperglycemia, adult polyglucosan body disease, Behçet's disease, and neuroacanthocytosis. In children, chorea may occur after cardiac surgery (postpump chorea). Sydenham's chorea may recur, at times, as chorea gravidarum. There is also a form of

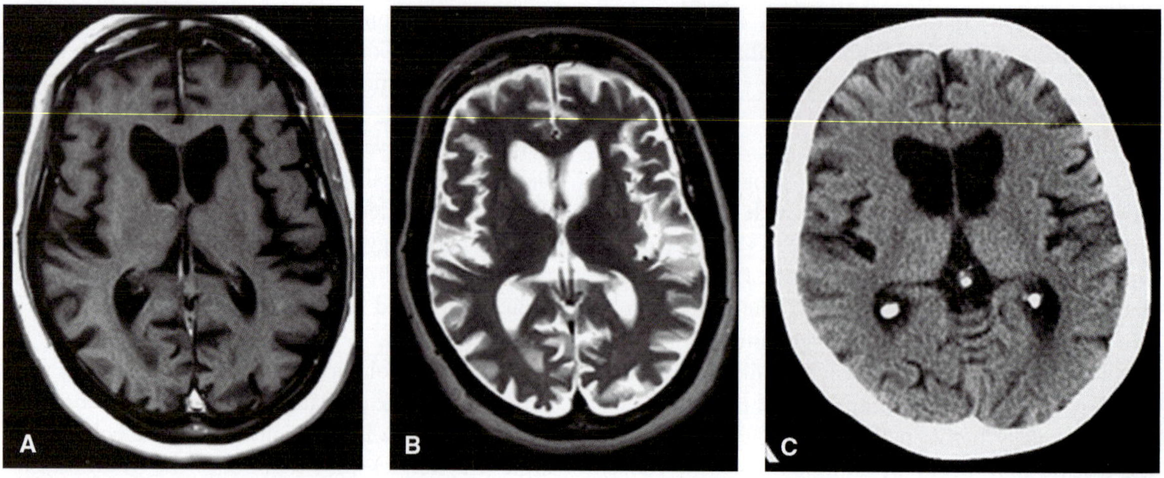

FIGURE 30.6 T1-weighted MRI **(A)**, T2-weighted MRI **(B)** and axial CT **(C)** images show atrophy of the caudate and frontal horn enlargement. (From Sethi KD. Magnetic resonance imaging in Huntington's disease. *Mov Disord* 1991;6[2]:186. Copyright © 1991 Movement Disorder Society. Reprinted by permission of John Wiley & Sons, Inc.)

nonprogressive chorea that is inherited as a recessive trait (benign hereditary chorea).

Structural lesions of the basal ganglia, such as infarct, neoplasm, or trauma, may occasionally cause chorea. It may occur with inborn errors of metabolism, such as Lesch-Nyhan syndrome, Niemann-Pick disease, and gangliosidosis. Chorea is nearly universal in the neuroacanthocytosis syndromes, in which various neurologic abnormalities are associated with the presence of acanthocytes on peripheral smear. Some patients have a genetic abnormality involving the protein chorein. Others may have decreased or absent (Bassen-Kornzweig disease) beta-lipoproteins. Neuroferritinopathy is an AD disorder in which various extrapyramidal features, including chorea, develop in the third to fifth decade. It is often mistaken for HD. Low serum ferritin is common but not invariable.

Chorea may be a transient side effect of many medications, such as psychotropic agents, phenytoin, antihistamines, levodopa, methylphenidate, lithium, oral contraceptives, estrogen, tricyclic antidepressants, isoniazid, and others. Drugs of abuse may cause chorea, including cocaine ("crack dancing") and amphetamines. Cocaine abuse is also associated with other movement disorders, including dystonia, exacerbation of Tourette's syndrome, multifocal tics, opsoclonus-myoclonus, and stereotyped behavior. Chorea may be a persisting feature of past or present exposure to psychoactive drugs as part of the syndrome of tardive dyskinesia. It may be a remote effect of carcinoma or be part of multisystem familial degenerative disorders. Hemichorea may follow structural lesions of the contralateral basal ganglia (see Hemiballism).

ATHETOSIS

In athetosis (Hammond's disease), the hyperkinesias are slower, more sustained, and larger in amplitude than those in chorea. They are involuntary, irregular, coarse, somewhat rhythmic, and writhing or squirming in character. They may involve the extremities, face, neck, and trunk. In the extremities, they affect mainly the distal portions, the fingers, hands, and toes. The movements are characterized by any combination of flexion, extension, abduction, pronation, and supination, often alternating and in varying degrees (Figure 30.7). They flow randomly from one body part to another, and the direction of movement changes randomly. The affected limbs are in constant motion (athetosis means "without fixed position"). Hyperextension of the fingers and wrist and pronation of the forearm may alternate with full flexion of the fingers and wrist and supination of the forearm. Facial grimacing, slower and more sustained than in chorea, often accompanies the movements of the extremities, and there may be synkinesias affecting other parts of the body. The hyperkinesias may not be constant or continuous. The movements can often be brought out or intensified by voluntary activity of another body part (overflow phenomenon). They disappear

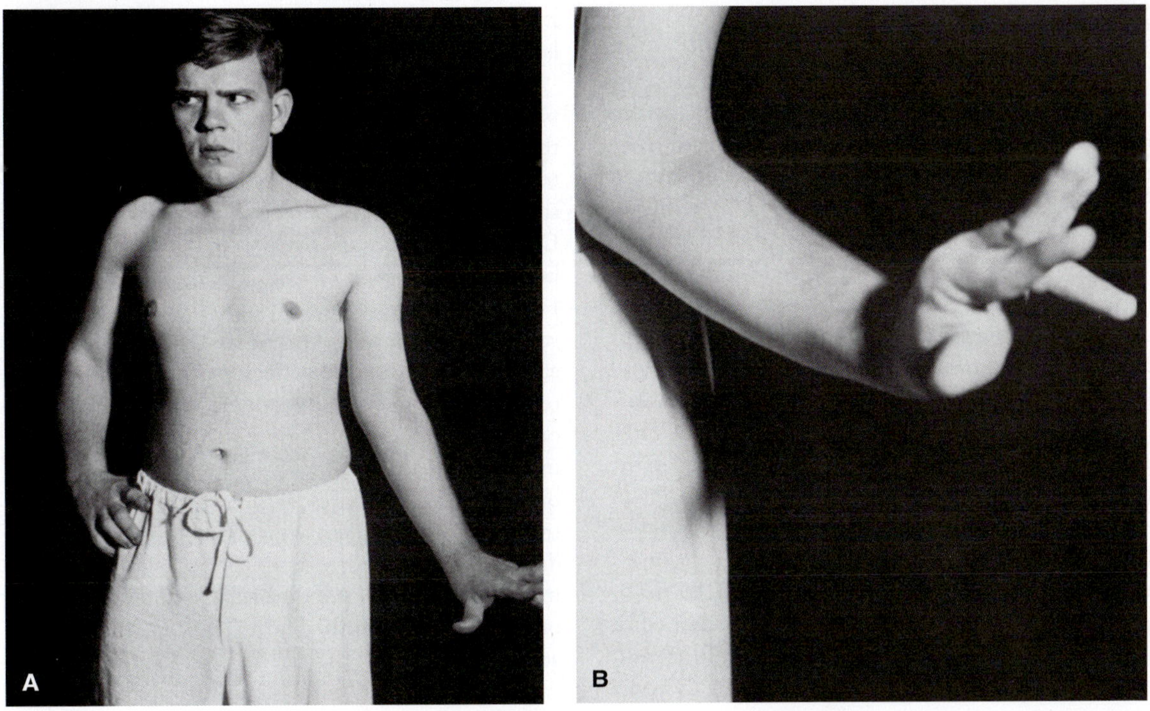

FIGURE 30.7 **A and B:** A patient with congenital unilateral athetosis.

in sleep. Voluntary movements are impaired and coordinated action may be difficult or impossible. Athetosis is usually unilateral; bilateral involvement is called double athetosis.

Athetosis is usually congenital, the result of perinatal injury to the basal ganglia, and may be present in association with other neurologic deficits (athetotic cerebral palsy). It may be either unilateral or bilateral. The predominant pathologic changes are in the caudate and putamen, although there may also be cortical involvement. Double athetosis may be associated with status marmoratus of the basal ganglia, which is usually due to anoxic birth injury. Acquired athetosis may follow disease or trauma in later life. Many of its causes overlap with those of chorea, and in fact, many patients have features of athetosis plus chorea. Choreoathetosis refers to movements that lie between chorea and athetosis in rate and rhythmicity and may represent a transitional form. Slow athetoid movements begin to blend with dystonia. Pseudoathetosis (sensory athetosis) is a term used to describe similar undulating and writhing movements of the extremities because of loss of position sense as a result of a parietal lobe lesion or peripheral deafferentation because of such conditions as tabes dorsalis, posterolateral sclerosis, and peripheral nerve disease (Figure 30.8). The movements are more marked when the eyes are closed and are usually unassociated with an increase in muscle tone.

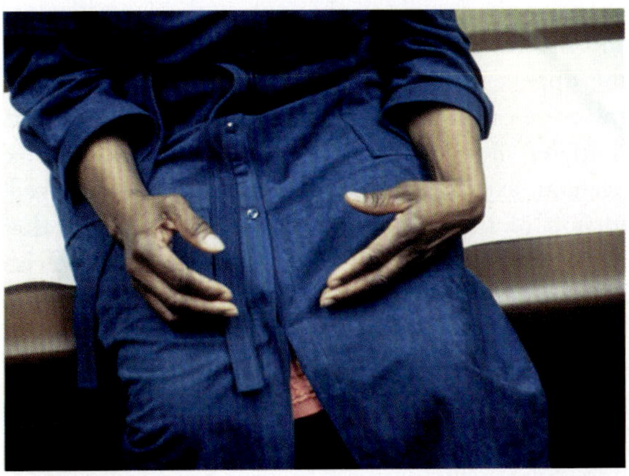

FIGURE 30.8 Pseudoathetosis of the hand in a patient with a parietal lobe lesion.

DYSTONIA

Dystonia refers to spontaneous, involuntary, sustained muscle contractions that force the affected parts of the body into abnormal movements or postures, sometimes with cocontraction of agonists and antagonists. Dystonia often affects the extremities, neck, trunk, eyelids, face, or vocal cords. It may be either constant or intermittent and generalized, segmental, focal, multifocal, or in a hemidistribution. Dystonic movements are patterned, tending to recur in the same location, in contrast to the random and fleeting nature of chorea. The speed of dystonia varies widely, from slow, sustained, and cramp-like (athetotic dystonia) to quick and flicking (myoclonic dystonia). When the duration is very brief (less than 1 second), the movement may be referred to as a dystonic spasm, when more sustained (several seconds) as a dystonic movement, and when prolonged (minutes to hours) as a dystonic posture. Occasionally, dystonia is associated with rapid rhythmic tremulous movements (dystonic tremor). Action dystonia occurs when carrying out a voluntary movement. As in athetosis, overflow may occur, with the dystonia brought out by use of another part of the body.

Generalized dystonia causes involuntary movements similar in many respects to athetosis but involving larger portions of the body, often producing distorted postures of the limbs and trunk. The movements are slow, bizarre, and sometimes grotesque, with an undulating, writhing, twisting, turning character, and a tendency for the contraction to be sustained at the peak of the movement (torsion dystonia, torsion spasm). Generalized dystonia may start distally, usually in the foot, with plantarflexion and inversion, and then spread to the opposite side, the upper extremities, the trunk, face, and tongue. In severe cases, there are writhing movements of the shoulder muscles, hip girdles, and trunk. There is peculiar, axial twisting of the spine, causing marked torsion of the entire vertebral column with lordosis, scoliosis, and tilting of the shoulders and pelvis. Dysarthria, facial grimacing, and torticollis may also be present. The muscles are often in a constant state of hypertonicity, and the muscular contractions may cause severe pain. The movements are involuntary but are increased by voluntary activity and emotion. Eventually, postures become fixed by contractures, and deformities develop. The term dystonia is sometimes used to describe the postures or positions assumed by the patient, as well as for the hyperkinesia itself. Dystonia may be intermittent or paroxysmal, lasting minutes.

Dystonia musculorum deformans (DMD, idiopathic torsion dystonia) is a rare progressive disease that usually begins in childhood. DMD-1 (DYT1 dystonia) is AD, and DMD-2 (DYT2 dystonia) is recessive; numerous other genetic forms of dystonia exist. Dystonia also occurs in Wilson's disease, acquired hepatocerebral degeneration, PKAN, kernicterus, in HD as it progresses, in PD, and occasionally with structural lesions affecting the basal ganglia. Dystonia can occur as a drug side effect, particularly as a dose-related manifestation of treatment with levodopa and other dopaminergic drugs. Other offending agents include cimetidine, anticonvulsants, calcium channel blockers, and anxiolytics. Tardive dystonia is related to treatment with phenothiazines and other psychotropic drugs. Dopa-responsive dystonia (Segawa's disease and many other names) is a distinctive and common type of generalized dystonia that presents in childhood or adolescence and is characterized by marked diurnal variation in severity and exquisite responsiveness to small doses of levodopa. It is a consideration in the differential diagnosis of diplegic cerebral palsy, sporadic spastic paraplegia, hereditary spastic paraplegia, and JPD. Misdiagnosis is frequent. Hemidystonia is along the spectrum of hemichorea and hemiballismus but because of a lesion of the contralateral striatum.

The focal dystonias are disorders causing involuntary contractions in a limited distribution. A relatively common form of focal dystonia is cervical dystonia (spasmodic torticollis; Chapter 19), which affects the neck, and sometimes the shoulder, muscles, producing either a sustained or jerky turning of the head to one side, often with some element of head tilt. "Torti" implies a twisting or turning movement; less common variants of cervical dystonia include retrocollis (extension movement) and anterocollis (flexion movement). In the beginning, the twisting and turning may be intermittent or present only in paroxysms (spasmodic), but later in the course of the syndrome, there is persistent contraction of the involved muscles with resulting deviation of the head. Many if not most patients with cervical dystonia learn they can straighten their head by placing a hand or finger somewhere on the face or performing some other maneuver to provide sensory stimulation or light counterpressure (geste antagoniste, sensory trick, counterpressure sign; Figure 30.9). Notoriously refractory to medical therapy, cervical dystonia is now often treated by the injection of infinitesimally small

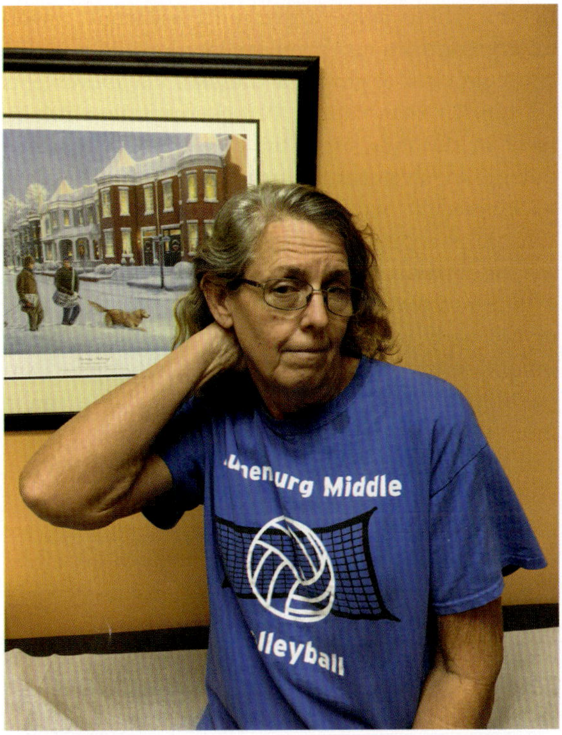

FIGURE 30.9 Sensory trick in cervical dystonia. The patient found that keeping her right hand behind the neck helped keep her head straight. She kept the right elbow flexed so constantly she developed a right ulnar neuropathy at the elbow.

amounts of botulinum toxin to weaken the abnormally contracting muscles.

Writer's cramp (graphospasm) is a focal dystonia of the hand or forearm muscles brought on by use of the part, most frequently by writing. There are a number of other focal, occupational, or task-specific dystonias related to specific activities. Musicians may develop hand or embouchure dystonia. The *yips* in golfers may be a task-specific dystonia. Blepharospasm (upper facial dystonia) causes involuntary closure of both eyes. The spasms may be brief or sustained. Patients with sustained spasms become functionally blind during the paroxysms. Involuntary closure of one eye is usually due to early hemifacial spasm. Oromandibular dystonia involves the mouth, lips, and jaw. The combination of blepharospasm and oromandibular dystonia constitutes Meige's (Brueghel's) syndrome **(Video 30.5)**. Auctioneer's jaw is a task-specific oromandibular dystonia. Spasmodic dysphonia is dystonia of the vocal cords (see Chapter 9). Belly dancer's dystonia refers to involuntary movements affecting the abdominal musculature. Focal dystonias of peripheral origin have been described in relation to nerve, plexus, or nerve root lesions. A segmental dystonia is more extensive than a focal dystonia and involves contiguous body regions (e.g., cervical dystonia accompanied by oromandibular dystonia).

HEMIBALLISMUS

Hemiballismus (hemiballism) refers to a dramatic neurologic syndrome of wild, flinging, incessant movements that occur on one side of the body **(Video 30.6)**. It is classically due to infarction or hemorrhage in the region of the contralateral subthalamic nucleus; the lesion results in disinhibition of the motor thalamus and the cortex, resulting in contralateral hyperkinetic movements. Case series with modern neuroimaging have shown that only a minority of cases have lesions in the subthalamic nucleus. Nonketotic hyperglycemia is also a common etiology. The ballistic movements of hemiballismus resemble those of chorea but are more pronounced. The clinical distinction between severe hemichorea and hemiballismus becomes arbitrary. Like chorea, hemiballistic movements are involuntary and purposeless movements, but they are much more rapid and forceful and involve the proximal portions of the extremities. When fully developed, there are continuous, violent, swinging, flinging, rolling, throwing, and flailing movements of the involved extremities. The movements are ceaseless during the waking state and disappear only with deep sleep. They are usually unilateral and involve one entire half of the body; their intensity may cause movement of the entire body. Rarely, they are bilateral (biballismus or paraballismus) or involve a single extremity (monoballismus). The movements may spare the face and trunk. Hemiballismus is difficult to treat, incredibly disabling, and sometimes fatal because of exhaustion and inanition.

DYSKINESIAS

All hyperkinetic movements are technically dyskinesias, but the term is often used to encompass complex involuntary movements that do not neatly fit into another category. Dyskinesia is used most often to refer to abnormal involuntary movements related to drugs. Dyskinesias are a common dose-related complication of the treatment of PD with levodopa and dopamine agonists. In some disorders, the dyskinesias occur paroxysmally. Paroxysmal dyskinesias strike suddenly and unexpectedly when the patient is engaged in otherwise normal motor behavior. The dyskinesias may be precipitated by movement (paroxysmal kinesigenic dyskinesia) or by other factors, such as stress, heat, or fatigue (paroxysmal nonkinesigenic dyskinesia). Paroxysmal hypnogenic dyskinesias occur during sleep.

OROFACIAL DYSKINESIAS

Orofacial dyskinesias are involuntary movements of the mouth, face, jaw, or tongue that may consist of grimacing, pursing of the mouth and lips, "fish-gaping" movements, and writhing movements of the tongue. These often develop as tardive dyskinesias (TD) after the use of phenothiazines and other psychotropic drugs.

TD are involuntary movements that usually develop in patients who have received phenothiazines or related compounds, usually as treatment for major psychosis, for prolonged periods. Dyskinesias may also occur shortly after initiation of psychotropic therapy and may be associated with the use of other drugs. The movements typically involve primarily the mouth, tongue, and jaw with incessant chewing, smacking, licking, and tongue-thrusting movements that are difficult to eradicate. Some patients are unaware they have these movements. It seems likely that long-term dopamine receptor blockade leads to denervation hypersensitivity of the receptor. The movements not infrequently first appear when the dose of dopamine-blocking agent is reduced and can often be controlled, at least temporarily, by reinstituting or increasing the dose of the drug. TD are more prone to develop in older patients, especially women. Unfortunately, the term TD is often used for all involuntary orofacial movements, which may develop with no drug exposure, especially in older or edentulous patients. Other abnormal movements may arise as a tardive phenomenon, including tremor, dystonia, akathisia, tics, and chorea. Rabbit syndrome refers to a rhythmic perioral tremor, generally associated with the use of psychotropics. The movements are more rapid and regular and do not involve the tongue, helping distinguish them from TD.

MYOCLONUS

The term myoclonus has been used for several differing motor phenomena. In general, myoclonus may be defined as single or repetitive, abrupt, brief, rapid, lightning-like, jerky, arrhythmic, asynergic, involuntary contractions, involving portions of muscles, entire muscles, or groups of muscles. The movements are quicker than chorea. Myoclonus is seen principally in the muscles of the extremities and trunk, but the involvement is often multifocal, diffuse, or widespread. It may involve the facial muscles, jaws, tongue, pharynx, and larynx. There may be successive or simultaneous involvement of many muscles. Myoclonus may appear symmetrically on both sides of the body; such synchrony may be an attribute unique to myoclonus. The sudden, shock-like contractions usually appear in paroxysms at irregular intervals, during either the resting or active state, and may be activated by emotional, mental, tactile, visual, and auditory stimuli. Myoclonic movements, like fasciculations and myokymia, occasionally are too weak to cause joint movement. More often, they affect entire muscles or muscle groups, producing clonic movements of the extremities. They may be so violent as to cause an entire limb to be suddenly flung out and may even throw the patient to the ground. An excessive startle response causing a massive whole-body myoclonic jerk occurs in some conditions, especially Creutzfeldt-Jakob disease (see "Hyperekplexia"). Myoclonus may also be subtle, a quick flick of a finger or foot.

Myoclonus has been classified in numerous ways, including the following: positive versus negative, epileptic versus nonepileptic, stimulus sensitive (reflex) versus spontaneous, rhythmic versus arrhythmic, anatomically (peripheral, spinal, segmental, brainstem, or cortical), and by etiology (physiologic, essential, epileptic, and symptomatic). Asterixis may be viewed as negative myoclonus, the transient, unwanted, abnormal relaxation of a muscle group. As typically used, the term myoclonus refers to positive myoclonus: abnormal jerks. Cortical reflex myoclonus is focal myoclonus triggered by stimulation or movement of the affected part.

Myoclonic movements may occur in a variety of conditions, and their significance varies. Physiologic myoclonus occurs in normals. Sleep starts (hypnic jerks) are myoclonic jerks that appear during the process of falling asleep but disappear during sleep. Hiccups are another form of physiologic myoclonus. In essential myoclonus, there are no accompanying abnormalities; it may be sporadic or familial. Paramyoclonus multiplex is a disorder of adult life causing paroxysmal contractions of the limb and trunk muscles. The etiology is not known, and the existence of the entity has been questioned.

Myoclonus is frequently encountered in epilepsy. Many epileptic patients have occasional random myoclonic jerks of the axial or proximal limb musculature, which may appear or increase in frequency immediately prior to a seizure. Beginning around puberty, patients with juvenile myoclonic epilepsy (Janz syndrome) have generalized tonic-clonic seizures that are associated with frequent myoclonic jerks predominantly affecting the arms, especially on awakening. Massive myoclonic spasms of infancy are characterized by frequent, sudden, violent jerking attacks with flexion of the neck and trunk and adduction or abduction and extension of the arms and legs (infantile spasms, West syndrome). The body may bend forward (salaam or jackknife attacks).

The progressive myoclonic epilepsies are a group of disorders that include Unverricht-Lundborg syndrome and Lafora body disease. Progressive myoclonic epilepsy can also occur without Lafora bodies and in type 3 Gaucher's disease, sialidosis, gangliosidoses, ceroid lipofuscinoses, and myoclonic epilepsy with ragged red fibers. In dyssynergia cerebellaris myoclonica, one of the several Ramsay Hunt syndromes, myoclonus is accompanied by progressive cerebellar degeneration and seizures.

Myoclonus occurs without prominent seizures in a number of other conditions, including metabolic disorders (especially uremic and anoxic encephalopathy), subacute sclerosing panencephalitis, PKAN, Creutzfeldt-Jakob disease, Alzheimer's disease, Wilson's disease, HD, CBD, viral encephalitis, general paresis, Hashimoto's encephalopathy, and the lipidoses. Opsoclonus refers to random, chaotic, lightning-fast eye movements (see Chapter 14). Opsoclonus accompanied by myoclonus (opsoclonus-myoclonus syndrome, dancing eyes-dancing feet, Kinsbourne's syndrome) may occur as a postinfectious encephalopathy or as a paraneoplastic syndrome, especially because of occult neuroblastoma. Action myoclonus occurs with use of the involved limb. A syndrome of action or intention myoclonus may develop as a sequel to cerebral anoxia (Lance-Adams syndrome).

Myoclonus may sometimes be benign and without serious significance and even have a psychogenic basis. Movements difficult to differentiate from myoclonus may be nonorganic. Benign nocturnal myoclonus may occur in healthy persons. Paroxysmal kinesigenic myoclonus has also been described.

Myoclonus is typically arrhythmic and diffuse, but the term has also been applied to rhythmic and localized motor phenomena. Palatal myoclonus is characterized by involuntary, rhythmic movements of the soft palate and pharynx, sometimes of the larynx, eye muscles, and diaphragm, and occasionally of other muscles. The movements are generally not influenced by drugs or sleep. The palate may bounce up and down or twitch rhythmically to one side **(Video 30.7)**. The posterior pharyngeal wall moves laterally, and the larynx moves in an upward and downward direction. Movements involving the diaphragm or larynx may cause a grunting respiratory noise. Opening and closing of the eustachian tube sometimes causes a clicking sound accompanying the movements, audible to the patient and sometimes the examiner.

Palatal myoclonus occurs in essential and symptomatic forms. Symptomatic palatal myoclonus occurs with lesions involving the connections between the inferior olivary, dentate, and red nuclei. The Guillain-Mollaret (myoclonic) triangle is a loop: inferior olive → inferior cerebellar peduncle → dentate nucleus → superior cerebellar peduncle → red nucleus → central tegmental tract → inferior olive. A lesion anywhere in this loop, most often brainstem infarction, may cause palatal myoclonus and its variants. Lesions of the central tegmental tract may cause hypertrophy (pseudohypertrophy) of the olive. There is gliosis of the amiculum of the olive, increasing the size of the olive grossly, which may be visualized by MRI.

Palatal myoclonus is also referred to as palatal microtremor. Tremors are due to alternating agonist-antagonist contractions, rhythmic myoclonus to contraction-relaxation cycles of an agonist. In addition, tremors usually disappear in sleep and these palatal movements do not. Whether palatal myoclonus is best characterized as rhythmic myoclonus or a tremor remains unclear.

ASTERIXIS

Seen primarily in metabolic encephalopathy, particularly hepatic encephalopathy, asterixis is an inability to sustain normal muscle tone **(Video 30.8)**. With the arms outstretched and wrists extended, "like stopping traffic," the lapse in postural tone may cause the hands to suddenly flop downward, then quickly recover, causing a slow and irregular flapping motion that led to the term "liver flap." When severe, the entire arm may drop. Other body parts may exhibit the phenomenon (e.g., inability to keep the foot dorsiflexed [foot flap]). Unilateral asterixis may occur with focal brain lesions, particularly involving the contralateral thalamus. In metabolic encephalopathy, there may be a high-frequency postural tremor that begins after a latent period of 2 to 30 seconds and attenuates on movement (mini-asterixis, metabolic tremor). In unresponsive patients, asterixis at the hip joints can sometimes be brought out by passively flexing and abducting to hips so that the thighs form a "V." In this position, the knees may flap up and down.

MYORHYTHMIA

The term myorhythmia refers to slow (typically 2 to 3 Hz), rhythmic alternating movements that resemble tremor. The primary distinguishing characteristics are the slow rate and the often widespread involvement. It may be intermittent or continuous, synchronous, or asynchronous when involving multiple body parts and is absent during sleep. The movements may involve one or several limbs, the head, the eyes, or various combinations. Myorhythmia has been described in cerebrovascular disease, anti-NMDA receptor encephalitis, Hashimoto's encephalopathy, and other disorders. Oculomasticatory myorhythmia refers to pendular vergence movements of the eyes synchronous with contractions of the masticatory muscles. It is a distinctive movement disorder that appears to be specific for central nervous system (CNS) Whipple's disease (see **Video Link 30.3**).

TICS

The hyperkinesias discussed to this point have been involuntary movements. In another type of abnormal movement, the patient has some degree of awareness of the movement but must make a movement in response to the urge of some compelling inner force. The patient experiences tension and restlessness, which are temporarily relieved by making a particular movement. Such movements have been called "unvoluntary." Examples include tics, akathisia, stereotypies, compulsions, and restless legs.

Tics (habit spasms) are quick, irregular but repetitive movements that are more often seen in children than adults. A tiqueur is a person who is subject to one or multiple tics. A tic may be defined as a coordinated, repetitive, seemingly purposeful act involving a group of muscles in their normal synergistic relationships. Tics are stereotyped, recurrent movements that may seem purposeful but are relatively involuntary, consisting of brief contractions of whole muscles or groups of muscles, always accompanied by motion of the affected part. Patients are able to suppress the movements temporarily with concentration, but they quickly return when attention is diverted to some other task. Voluntary suppression causes a sense of intolerable mounting tension and an urge to move that is temporarily relieved by indulgence in a tic. Tics are exaggerated by emotional strain and tension; they cease during sleep.

Tics may involve any portion of the body. Common examples of simple motor tics include repetitive blinking, facial contortions, or shoulder shrugging. More complicated tics can occur, and tics can also involve the vocal tract (phonic or vocal tic), producing throat-clearing as well as bizarre vocalizations, such as barking and grunting or sounds resembling a hiccup.

Patients affected with Gilles de la Tourette syndrome (maladie des tics) have multifocal tics, compulsive behavior, imitative gestures, stereotyped movements, grunts and groans, and evidence of regressive behavior. There are explosive vocalizations, and the patient may utter profanity and obscenities over which they have no control (coprolalia). The condition has its onset in childhood and occurs most frequently in boys, usually in the preadolescent period. Tics are very common and usually benign; patients with Tourette's syndrome have exaggerated, complex tics, which together with the other features of the disease can be very disabling (see **Video Link 30.4**). The large repertoire of tics and the combination of motor and vocal tics distinguish Tourette's syndrome from ordinary tics. The disease is hereditary, probably AD with variable expressivity, and related to some dysfunction of dopamine receptors. It is likely that the noted historical literary figure, Dr. Samuel Johnson, the famously eccentric author of the first English language dictionary, suffered from Tourette's syndrome.

AKATHISIA

Patients suffering from akathisia experience an inner restlessness and urge to move that causes them to remain in almost constant motion. It occurs most often as a result of treatment with dopamine-blocking agents. Patients with PD may experience akathisia but are not able to move in response to it.

STEREOTYPY

A stereotypy is a repetitive, purposeless but often seemingly purposeful, involuntary, patterned motor activity. Common foot shaking and other mannerisms are examples of simple stereotypies. More complex stereotypies may involve ritualistic behavior, such as the compulsions of obsessive-compulsive disorder. Stereotypies most commonly occur in psychiatric disorders: anxiety, obsessive-compulsive disorder, schizophrenia, autism, and intellectual disability. They may also be a part of neurologic disorders, such as tardive dyskinesia and Tourette's syndrome. The hand-wringing in Rett's syndrome is a stereotypy. "Punding" refers to complex, purposeless, stereotyped behavior seen in cocaine and amphetamine abuse and in patients with PD disease treated with dopaminergic agents. Stereotypies may resemble motor tics but do not share the suppressibility, variability, or mounting-tension compulsion to make the movement. Mannerisms are somewhat more complicated and stereotyped and are usually carried out in a more leisurely manner. They may appear only under emotional stress or when the patient is engaged in some particular activity.

HYPEREKPLEXIA

Hyperekplexia (startle disease, pathologic startle) refers to disorders characterized by an excessive startle response in the absence of other evidence of neurologic disease, sometimes accompanied by echolalia, automatic behavior, or automatic obedience (see **Video Link 30.5**). It may be sporadic or hereditary. Colorful names have been used for variants of the condition described in different geographic regions (jumping Frenchmen of Maine, latah, myriachit). An exaggerated startle response may also occur in Creutzfeldt-Jakob disease, Tay-Sachs disease, stiff-person syndrome, and lipidoses.

SLEEP-RELATED DYSKINESIAS

Except for palatal myoclonus, involuntary movements generally do not occur during sleep. There are some disorders, however, that occur primarily during sleep. Restless legs syndrome (RLS, Ekbom's syndrome, fidgety feet, jimmy legs) is a common disorder causing unpleasant and difficult-to-describe sensations in the legs that are temporarily relieved by movement. The symptoms commonly occur at night as the patient is drifting off to sleep. Many affected individuals get up and walk around to obtain respite. The patient support newsletter is NightWalkers. In many patients, RLS is accompanied by spontaneous movements of the legs during sleep (periodic movements in sleep, nocturnal myoclonus), best documented by polysomnography. The disorder is likely due to a central disturbance of dopamine metabolism. The restless red legs syndrome is RLS associated with telangiectasias of the legs. Patients with spinal stenosis may have leg pain in recumbency with similarities to RLS (vespers curse; Chapter 47). Restless arms and restless abdomen may also occur.

FASCICULATIONS

Fasciculations are fine, rapid, flickering or vermicular twitching movements due to contraction of a bundle, or fasciculus, of muscle fibers. They are usually not extensive enough to cause movement of joints, except occasionally the digits. They vary in size and intensity, from so faint and small as to only slightly ripple the surface of the overlying skin to coarse and impossible to overlook. They are random, irregular, fleeting, and inconstant. At times, they are abundant; at other times, they require a careful search. Fasciculations often seem to strike where the examiner is not looking and are usually seen from the corner of the eye.

Fasciculations are brought out by fatigue and cold. When assessing fasciculations, the patient should be warm, comfortable, and completely relaxed. It is written that fasciculations may be brought out by mechanical stimulation of the muscle (e.g., light tapping), and neurologists frequently engage in a ritual of tapping a muscle with a reflex hammer and peering intently for a resultant fasciculation. Whether this really occurs is debatable. Good light is necessary in order to visualize fasciculations; oblique lighting is best. They may be more difficult to see in women than men because of the overlying subcutaneous fat. When not visible, they can occasionally be palpated or heard with a stethoscope. Many patients are unaware of fasciculations; others may see or feel them, or both. Needle electromyography can detect their presence even when they cannot be seen. High-resolution sonography may reveal fasciculations not visible from the surface.

Fasciculations continue in sleep. They are exaggerated by the administration of cholinergic drugs (e.g., pyridostigmine). Hypercaffeinism is a common cause of fasciculations in normal individuals. At one time, the terms fibrillation and fasciculation were used synonymously. But fibrillation potentials are the contractions of single muscle fibers too small to be visible through the skin; they can only be detected by needle electromyography. Fasciculations are contractions of a large group of fibers, all or part of a single motor unit. Fasciculations are much more gross than fibrillations and can be seen through intact skin.

Fasciculations are a characteristic feature of motor neuron disease **(Video 30.9)**. They serve as a very useful marker for the disease, and the diagnosis should remain circumspect when fasciculations are not present. Their exact mechanism remains debatable. Fasciculations were once thought to represent the dying gasps of sick motor neurons, but current evidence indicates they more likely arise much more distally in the neuron, perhaps in immature, unstable peripheral sprouts. In amyotrophic lateral sclerosis (ALS), abundant fasciculations may be an indication that disease progression will be rapid. Fasciculations of small hand muscles in chronic anterior horn cell disease, particularly spinal muscular atrophy, may cause small amplitude, subtle finger twitches called minipolymyoclonus, which are of course not real myoclonus.

Although fasciculations are most characteristic of motor neuronopathies, they can occur in any chronic denervating process, including radiculopathy and peripheral neuropathy. Fasciculations can also occur when anterior horn cells are involved in intrinsic spinal cord disease, such as syringomyelia or tumor. Except for thyrotoxicosis, myopathies generally do not cause fasciculations. In chronic denervating disease resulting in an enlarged motor unit territory, slight muscle contraction may activate a larger than normal number of muscle fibers causing a visible twitch referred to as a contraction fasciculation. These do not have the same significance as spontaneous fasciculations. In Kennedy's disease (bulbospinal muscular atrophy), contraction fasciculations occur in the chin with slight pursing of the lips. Contraction fasciculations may be seen occasionally in normal individuals, especially in the small hand muscles.

Fasciculations unaccompanied by atrophy or weakness do not necessarily indicate the presence of a serious disease process. About 70% of the population, especially health care workers, have occasional benign fasciculations. Some patients, most often older men, have prominent fasciculations without other abnormality. These most often occur in the calves, and the patients are quite aware of the movements, whereas most patients with ALS seem surprisingly oblivious to their fasciculations. The clinical examination is otherwise normal, and needle electromyography is normal except for the fasciculations. There is no infallible way to distinguish benign from malignant fasciculations from the fasciculations alone; judgment is made by the company they keep. A nonprogressive course over time is more reassuring than a single normal electrodiagnostic evaluation. Of 121 patients with benign fasciculations followed up to 32 years, none developed ALS. In another report, 6.7% of ALS patients had fasciculations as an isolated, initial manifestation of the disease. Cramp-fasciculation syndrome is a syndrome of cramps and fasciculations because of hyperexcitability of the peripheral nerve.

MYOKYMIA

Myokymia (Gr. kyma, "wave") refers to involuntary, spontaneous, localized, transient or persistent quivering movements that affect a few muscle bundles within a single muscle but usually are not extensive enough to cause movement at a joint. The movements are somewhat coarser, slower, and undulating ("wormlike"), usually more prolonged, and involve a wider local area than fasciculations. They usually are not affected by motion or position, and they persist during sleep. On needle electromyography, clinical myokymia is accompanied by electrical discharges, either myokymic discharges or, less often, neuromyotonic discharges. Myokymic discharges, the electrical phenomenon, may or may not be accompanied by clinical myokymia, the visible, vermicular undulations on the skin surface.

Myokymia often occurs in normal individuals, causing persistent, focal twitching of a muscle, most commonly the orbicularis oculi. Myokymia usually occurs in isolation, without evidence of an accompanying neurologic disease; it is exacerbated by fatigue, anxiety, and caffeine. Myokymia in normal individuals and benign fasciculations may represent similar alterations in muscle physiology. Myokymia occurs in a variety of disease states; it is thought to arise because of biochemical perturbations in the nerve microenvironment because of demyelination, a toxin (such as rattlesnake venom or gold salts), edema, a decrease in ionized Ca^{++} concentration, or other factors (see **Video Link 30.6**). The generator lies somewhere along the motor axon.

Myokymia may be generalized or focal/segmental. Focal myokymia is much more common than generalized myokymia. The superior oblique muscle may develop episodic twitching producing a low-amplitude monocular intorsional movement (microtremor) that may cause annoying monocular oscillopsia and diplopia. It may be a microvascular compression syndrome with contact between the trochlear nerve and a vascular structure that may be seen by high-resolution thin slice magnetic resonance images. Myokymia sometimes occurs in the facial muscles in patients with MS or other lesions of the brainstem or cranial nerves, such as pontine glioma, syrinx, or Guillain-Barré syndrome. Facial myokymia is usually transient but may persist for long periods when due to channelopathy or a structural lesion, such as pontine glioma or syringobulbia. Other abnormal facial movements, including synkinesias because of aberrant facial nerve regeneration and hemifacial spasm, are discussed in Chapter 16. Focal limb myokymia is particularly characteristic of radiation damage to a nerve or plexus. Myokymia is only rarely associated with nerve compression syndromes. Myokymia may be seen, along with fasciculations, in motor neuronopathies. The pacemaker site varies with the condition. The response pattern of myokymic discharges to sleep, anesthesia, nerve blocks, and curare suggests a distal origin in many instances.

Generalized myokymia (Isaacs' syndrome, syndrome of continuous muscle fiber activity, neuromyotonia) causes generalized muscle stiffness and persistent contraction because of underlying continuous muscle fiber activity. Needle electromyography discloses spontaneous repetitive firing of motor unit potentials, creating myokymic and neuromyotonic discharges. Morvan's syndrome (Morvan's fibrillary chorea) is a dubious entity also associated with clinical myokymia. Generalized myokymia also occurs in episodic ataxia with myokymia.

STIFF-PERSON SYNDROME

Stiff-person (stiff-man, Moersch-Woltman) syndrome is due to hyperexcitability of anterior horn cells related to interference with gamma-aminobutyric acid–mediated spinal cord inhibitory mechanisms. There is progressive, often painful rigidity, punctuated by intense muscle spasms, particularly affecting the axial and paraspinal muscles. The axial rigidity causes hyperlordosis and prominent paraspinal muscle contractions. Superimposed on the stiffness are spasms provoked by movement or external stimuli. Most patients have antibodies to glutamic acid decarboxylase. In stiff-limb syndrome, symptoms are limited to one extremity. Jerking stiff-person syndrome is characterized by muscles stiffness and spasms affecting the legs. Progressive encephalomyelitis with rigidity and myoclonus causes a clinical picture similar to classic stiff-person syndrome but is more rapidly progressive.

SPASMS

Spasms are involuntary contractions of a muscle or group of muscles. The tonic contraction may cause either alteration of position or limitation of movement. They may occur in almost any muscle. A painful, tonic, spasmodic muscular contraction is often spoken of as a cramp. Spasms that limit movement may be defensive or protective. Prolonged spasm may cause reflex rigidity or be followed by muscle contracture. Spasms are often of reflex origin because of peripheral irritation affecting either muscles or nerves. Pain is a common cause of defensive spasm and reflex rigidity. Muscle spasm may also be voluntary or occur in response to fear or excitement. Carpopedal spasm is a common manifestation of tetany and hyperventilation (Chapter 52). Muscle spasms may also result from central processes. Prolonged and severe muscle spasms occur in tetany and tetanus. Characteristic painful tonic spasms occur in MS and stiff-person syndrome.

OTHER HYPERKINESIAS

In the painful legs and moving toes syndrome, there are continuous, involuntary movements of the toes associated with pain in the legs (see **Video Link 30.7**). The condition is sometimes a manifestation of peripheral neuropathy, but the responsible lesion in many is not clear. Variants are painful arms and moving fingers and painless legs and moving toes. Jumpy stump is involuntary movements of an amputated limb.

FUNCTIONAL MOVEMENT DISORDERS

Functional (psychogenic, nonorganic) movement disorders can simulate virtually any type of movement disorder. Functional disorders do not correspond to any of the organic types of abnormal involuntary movement; they are bizarre, change in type from time to time, and are influenced by emotional state and suggestion. Onset is often sudden. If a movement disorder is bizarre and defies classification, the possibility that it may be psychogenic should be borne in mind. Peculiar motor behaviors occur frequently in major psychiatric illnesses such as schizophrenia. However, being bizarre and difficult to characterize does not necessarily mean a movement disorder is psychogenic.

Psychogenic tremor is typically complex and does not fit well into the tremor classification scheme. The patient may have rapidly changing clinical features including variable resting, postural and kinetic components, and disability out of proportion to the tremor. Typical features include abrupt onset with severe involvement and maximal disability immediately, onset in one limb with rapid generalization, spontaneous resolution and recurrence, a decrease in the tremor with distraction, refractoriness to conventional antitremor treatment, and entrainment. Entrainment is a change in the frequency of the tremor to match that of a task performed by another body part. The patient with a psychogenic 10-Hz right-hand tremor asked to pat on the left thigh with the left hand at 3 Hz soon has a 3-Hz right-hand tremor. Normally, tremor amplitude and frequency have an inverse relationship, but a psychogenic tremor may be paradoxically both high amplitude and high frequency, especially when attention is focused on the tremor.

Video Links

Video Link 30.1. "Wingbeating" tremor in Wilson's disease. https://www.youtube.com/watch?v=_LJXgDQV2Vo

Video Link 30.2. Choreic gait. http://neurosigns.org/wiki/Hyperkinetic_gait_disorders

Video Link 30.3. Oculomasticatory myorhythmia in CNS Whipple's disease. http://neurosigns.org/wiki/Oculomasticatory_myorhythmia

Video Link 30.4. Multiple tics and coprolalia in Tourette's syndrome. http://neurosigns.org/wiki/Tics

Video Link 30.5. Hyperekplexia. https://www.youtube.com/watch?v=c0IYpOLWdSU

Video Link 30.6. Facial myokymia after rattlesnake bite. https://www.youtube.com/watch?v=KaM3-qy8uqU

Video Link 30.7. Painful legs and moving toes. http://neurosigns.org/wiki/Painful_legs_and_moving_toes

BIBLIOGRAPHY

Adler CH, Crews D, Kahol K, et al. Are the yips a task-specific dystonia or "golfer's cramp"? *Mov Disord* 2011;26:1993–1996.

Alvarez MV, Driver-Dunckley EE, Caviness JN, et al. Case series of painful legs and moving toes: clinical and electrophysiologic observations. *Mov Disord* 2008;23:2062–2066.

Armstrong MJ. Progressive supranuclear palsy: an update. *Curr Neurol Neurosci Rep* 2018;18:12.

Asmus F, Horber V, Pohlenz J, et al. A novel TITF-1 mutation causes benign hereditary chorea with response to levodopa. *Neurology* 2005;64:1952–1954.

Azher SN, Jankovic J. Camptocormia: pathogenesis, classification, and response to therapy. *Neurology* 2005;65:355–359.

Azher SN, Jankovic J. Clinical aspects of progressive supranuclear palsy. *Handb Clin Neurol* 2008;89:461–473.

Bader B, Walker RH, Vogel M, et al. Tongue protrusion and feeding dystonia: a hallmark of chorea-acanthocytosis. *Mov Disord* 2010;25:127–129.

Baizabal-Carvallo JF, Cardoso F, Jankovic J. Myorhythmia: phenomenology, etiology, and treatment. *Mov Disord* 2015;30:171–179.

Bajaj N, Hauser RA, Grachev ID. Clinical utility of dopamine transporter single photon emission CT (DaT-SPECT) with (123I) ioflupane in diagnosis of parkinsonian syndromes. *J Neurol Neurosurg Psychiatry* 2013;84:1288–1295.

Barclay CL, Bergeron C, Lang AE. Arm levitation in progressive supranuclear palsy. *Neurology* 1999;52:879–882.

Barker RA, Revesz T, Thom M, et al. Review of 23 patients affected by the stiff man syndrome: clinical subdivision into stiff trunk (man) syndrome, stiff limb syndrome, and progressive encephalomyelitis with rigidity. *J Neurol Neurosurg Psychiatry* 1998;65:633–640.

Batla A, Nehru R, Vijay T. Vertical wrinkling of the forehead or procerus sign in progressive supranuclear palsy. *J Neurol Sci* 2010;298:148–149.

Berkovic SF, Bladin PF. Rubral tremor: clinical features and treatment of three cases. *Clin Exp Neurol* 1984;20:119–128.

Bhatia KP. Paroxysmal dyskinesias. *Mov Disord* 2011;26:1157–1165.

Blexrud MD, Windebank AJ, Daube JR. Long-term follow-up of 121 patients with benign fasciculations. *Ann Neurol* 1993;34:622–625.

Bokhari MR, Bokhari SRA. Hallervorden Spatz Disease (Pantothenate Kinase-Associated Neurodegeneration, PKAN). *StatPearls [Internet]*. Treasure Island: StatPearls Publishing, 2018. Available at: http://www.ncbi.nlm.nih.gov/books/NBK430689/

Borchert A, Moddel G, Schilling M. Teaching video NeuroImages: paroxysmal kinesigenic dyskinesia. *Neurology* 2009;72:e118.

Boxer AL, Geschwind MD, Belfor N, et al. Patterns of brain atrophy that differentiate corticobasal degeneration syndrome from progressive supranuclear palsy. *Arch Neurol* 2006;63:81–86.

Brinar VV, Barun B, Zadro I, et al. Progressive ataxia and palatal tremor. *Arch Neurol* 2008;65:1248–1249.

Brown P, Marsden CD. The stiff man and stiff man plus syndromes. *J Neurol* 1999;246:648–652.

Burke JR, Wingfield MS, Lewis KE, et al. The Haw River syndrome: dentatorubropallidoluysian atrophy (DRPLA) in an African-American family. *Nat Genet* 1994;7:521–524.

Burkhard PR, Delavelle J, Du PR, et al. Chronic parkinsonism associated with cirrhosis: a distinct subset of acquired hepatocerebral degeneration. *Arch Neurol* 2003;60:521–528.

Catena M, Fagiolini A, Consoli G, et al. The rabbit syndrome: state of the art. *Curr Clin Pharmacol* 2007;2:212–216.

Caterino M, Squillaro T, Montesarchio D, et al. Huntingtin protein: a new option for fixing the Huntington's disease countdown clock. *Neuropharmacology* 2018;135:126–138.

Caviness JN, Truong DD. Myoclonus. *Handb Clin Neurol* 2011;100:399–420.

Cetlin RS, Rodrigues GR, Pena-Pereira MA, et al. Teaching video NeuroImages: excessive grinning in Wilson disease. *Neurology* 2009;73:e73.

Chhibber S, Greenberg SA. Teaching video NeuroImages: widespread clinical myokymia in chronic inflammatory demyelinating polyradiculoneuropathy. *Neurology* 2011;77:e33.

Collins SJ, Ahlskog JE, Parisi JE, et al. Progressive supranuclear palsy: neuropathologically based diagnostic clinical criteria. *J Neurol Neurosurg Psychiatry* 1995;58:167–173.

da Silva-Junior FP, Machado AA, Lucato LT, et al. Copper deficiency myeloneuropathy in a patient with Wilson disease. *Neurology* 2011;76:1673–1674.

Dale RC. Tics and Tourette: a clinical, pathophysiological and etiological review. *Curr Opin Pediatr* 2017;29:665–673.

Dawson TM, Dawson VL. Molecular pathways of neurodegeneration in Parkinson's disease. *Science* 2003;302:819–822.

Delmaire C, Vidailhet M, Elbaz A, et al. Structural abnormalities in the cerebellum and sensorimotor circuit in writer's cramp. *Neurology* 2007;69:376–380.

Demirkiran M, Jankovic J, Lewis RA, et al. Neurologic presentation of Wilson disease without Kayser-Fleischer rings. *Neurology* 1996;46:1040–1043.

Deuschl G, Bergman H. Pathophysiology of nonparkinsonian tremors. *Mov Disord* 2002;17(Suppl 3):S41–S48.

Deuschl G, Krack P, Lauk M, et al. Clinical neurophysiology of tremor. *J Clin Neurophysiol* 1996;13:110–121.

Dickson DW, Lin W, Liu WK, et al. Multiple system atrophy: a sporadic synucleinopathy. *Brain Pathol* 1999;9:721–732.

Dobyns WB, Goldstein NP, Gordon H. Clinical spectrum of Wilson's disease (hepatolenticular degeneration). *Mayo Clin Proc* 1979;54:35–42.

Dubinsky RM, Gray CS, Koller WC. Essential tremor and dystonia. *Neurology* 1993;43:2382–2384.

Dubois B, Slachevsky A, Pillon B, et al. "Applause sign" helps to discriminate PSP from FTD and PD. *Neurology* 2005;64:2132–2133.

Edwards MJ, Deuschl G. Tremor syndromes. *Continuum (Minneap Minn)* 2013;19(5 Movement Disorders):1213–1224.

Eisen A, Stewart H. Not-so-benign fasciculation. *Ann Neurol* 1994;35:375–376.

Ellul MA, Cross TJ, Larner AJ. Asterixis. *Pract Neurol* 2017;17:60–62.

El-Youssef M. Wilson disease. *Mayo Clin Proc* 2003;78:1126–1136.

Espay AJ, Aybek S, Carson A, et al. Current concepts in diagnosis and treatment of functional neurological disorders. *JAMA Neurol* 2018;75(9):1132–1141.

Fanciulli A, Wenning GK. Multiple-system atrophy. *N Engl J Med* 2015;372:249–263.

Ferenci P. Diagnosis of Wilson disease. *Handb Clin Neurol* 2017;142:171–180.

Findley LJ. Classification of tremors. *J Clin Neurophysiol* 1996;13:122–132.

Findley LJ. Expanding clinical dimensions of essential tremor. *J Neurol Neurosurg Psychiatry* 2004;75:948–949.

Finke C, Jumah MD, Jons T, et al. Teaching video NeuroImages: an endoscopic view of symptomatic palatal tremor. *Neurology* 2010;74:e16.

Fishman PS, Oyler GA. Significance of the parkin gene and protein in understanding Parkinson's disease. *Curr Neurol Neurosci Rep* 2002;2:296–302.

Galvin JE, Price JL, Yan Z, et al. Resting bold fMRI differentiates dementia with Lewy bodies vs Alzheimer disease. *Neurology* 2011;76:1797–1803.

Gilman S, Low PA, Quinn N, et al. Consensus statement on the diagnosis of multiple system atrophy. *J Neurol Sci* 1999;163:94–98.

Gilman S, Little R, Johanns J, et al. Evolution of sporadic olivopontocerebellar atrophy into multiple system atrophy. *Neurology* 2000;55:527–532.

Golbe LI. Young-onset Parkinson's disease: a clinical review. *Neurology* 1991;41(2 Pt 1):168–173.

Hanes FM. Two clinically useful signs. *J Am Med Assoc* 1943;121:1152–1153.

Hardie RJ, Pullon HW, Harding AE, et al. Neuroacanthocytosis. A clinical, haematological and pathological study of 19 cases. *Brain* 1991;114(Pt 1A):13–49.

Hawley JS, Weiner WJ. Hemiballismus: current concepts and review. *Parkinsonism Relat Disord* 2012;18:125–129.

Hayat GR, Kulkantrakorn K, Campbell WW, et al. Neuromyotonia: autoimmune pathogenesis and response to immune modulating therapy. *J Neurol Sci* 2000;181:38–43.

Heckmann JG, Lang CJ, Neundörfer B, et al. Neuro/Images. Kayser-Fleischer corneal ring. *Neurology* 2000;54:1839.

Hobson DE. Clinical manifestations of Parkinson's disease and parkinsonism. *Can J Neurol Sci* 2003;30(Suppl 1):S2–S9.

Houlden H, Baker M, Morris HR, et al. Corticobasal degeneration and progressive supranuclear palsy share a common tau haplotype. *Neurology* 2001;56(12):1702–1706.

Isaacson SH, Fisher S, Gupta F, et al. Clinical utility of DaTscan™ imaging in the evaluation of patients with parkinsonism: a US perspective. *Expert Rev Neurother* 2017;17:219–225.

Jan MM. Misdiagnoses in children with dopa-responsive dystonia. *Pediatr Neurol* 2004;31:298–303.

Jankovic J, Ashoori A. Movement disorders in musicians. *Mov Disord* 2008;23:1957–1965.

Jellinger KA. Recent developments in the pathology of Parkinson's disease. *J Neural Transm Suppl* 2002;62:347–376.

Josephs KA. Current understanding of neurodegenerative diseases associated with the protein tau. *Mayo Clin Proc* 2017;92:1291–1303.

Kamath S, Bajaj N. Crack dancing in the United Kingdom: apropos a video case presentation. *Mov Disord* 2007;22:1190–1191.

Kelly DM, Kelleher EM, O'Shea A, et al. Teaching video NeuroImages: primary writing tremor: lessons from a patient with multiple sclerosis. *Neurology* 2016;87:e131.

Kim YJ, Pakiam AS, Lang AE. Historical and clinical features of psychogenic tremor: a review of 70 cases. *Can J Neurol Sci* 1999;26:190–195.

Koutsis G, Karadima G, Kladi A, et al. The challenge of juvenile Huntington disease: to test or not to test. *Neurology* 2013;80:990–996.

LaBan MM. "Vespers Curse" night pain—the bane of Hypnos. *Arch Phys Med Rehabil* 1984;65:501–504.

Lang AE. Corticobasal degeneration: selected developments. *Mov Disord* 2003;18(Suppl 6):S51–S56.

Langston JW, Tan LC. Juvenile parkinsonism: a term in search of an identity. *Eur J Neurol* 2000;7:465–466.

Lanska DJ. Early controversies over athetosis: I. Clinical features, differentiation from other movement disorders, associated conditions, and pathology. *Tremor Other Hyperkinet Mov (NY)* 2013;3. pii: tre-03-132-2918-1.

Lees AJ, Hardy J, Revesz T. Parkinson's disease. *Lancet* 2009;373:2055–2066.

Litvan I, Grimes DA, Lang AE, et al. Clinical features differentiating patients with postmortem confirmed progressive supranuclear palsy and corticobasal degeneration. *J Neurol* 1999;246(Suppl 2):II1–II5.

Longoni G, Agosta F, Kosti VS, et al. MRI measurements of brainstem structures in patients with Richardson's syndrome, progressive supranuclear palsy-parkinsonism, and Parkinson's disease. *Mov Disord* 2011;26:247–255.

Louis ED. Samuel Adams' tremor. *Neurology* 2001;56:1201–1205.

Louis ED. Linking essential tremor to the cerebellum: neuropathological evidence. *Cerebellum* 2016;15:235–242.

Louis ED, Faust PL, Vonsattel JP, et al. Neuropathological changes in essential tremor: 33 cases compared with 21 controls. *Brain* 2007;130(Pt 12):3297–3307.

Luzzi S, Fabi K, Pesallaccia M, et al. Applause sign: is it really specific for Parkinsonian disorders? Evidence from cortical dementias. *J Neurol Neurosurg Psychiatry* 2011;82:830–833.

Margolis RL, Ross CA. Diagnosis of Huntington disease. *Clin Chem* 2003;49:1726–1732.

McKeith IG, Dickson DW, Lowe J, et al. Diagnosis and management of dementia with Lewy bodies: third report of the DLB Consortium. *Neurology* 2005;65:1863.

Mhoon JT, Nandigam K, Juel VC. Teaching video NeuroImages: painful legs and moving toes syndrome. *Neurology* 2010;75(2):e6.

Michaud M, Chabli A, Lavigne G, et al. Arm restlessness in patients with restless legs syndrome. *Mov Disord* 2000;15:289–293.

Mink JW. The basal ganglia and involuntary movements: impaired inhibition of competing motor patterns. *Arch Neurol* 2003;60:1365–1368.

Morelli M, Arabia G, Novellino F, et al. MRI measurements predict PSP in unclassifiable parkinsonisms: a cohort study. *Neurology* 2011a;77:1042–1047.

Morelli M, Arabia G, Salsone M, et al. Accuracy of magnetic resonance parkinsonism index for differentiation of progressive supranuclear palsy from probable or possible Parkinson disease. *Mov Disord* 2011b;26:527–533.

Mori F, Piao YS, Hayashi S, et al. Alpha-synuclein accumulates in Purkinje cells in Lewy body disease but not in multiple system atrophy. *J Neuropathol Exp Neurol* 2003;62:812–819.

Morimatsu M. Procerus sign in progressive supranuclear palsy and corticobasal degeneration. *Intern Med* 2002;41:1101–1102.

Muller J, Wissel J, Masuhr F, et al. Clinical characteristics of the geste antagoniste in cervical dystonia. *J Neurol* 2001;248:478–482.

Noda S, Ito H, Umezaki H, et al. Hip flexion-abduction to elicit asterixis in unresponsive patients. *Ann Neurol* 1985;18:96–97.

Pahwa R, Lyons KE. Essential tremor: differential diagnosis and current therapy. *Am J Med* 2003;115:134–142.

Pal G, Lin MM, Laureno R. Asterixis: a study of 103 patients. *Metab Brain Dis* 2014;29:813–824.

Pankratz ND, Wojcieszek J, Foroud T. Parkinson disease overview. In: Pagon RA, Bird TD, Dolan CR, et al., eds. *GeneReviews [Internet]*. Seattle: University of Washington, 1993.

Pharr V, Uttl B, Stark M, et al. Comparison of apraxia in corticobasal degeneration and progressive supranuclear palsy. *Neurology* 2001;56:957–963.

Quinn N, Schrag A. Huntington's disease and other choreas. *J Neurol* 1998;245:709–716.

Rajagopalan S, Andersen JK. Alpha synuclein aggregation: is it the toxic gain of function responsible for neurodegeneration in Parkinson's disease? *Mech Ageing Dev* 2001;122:1499–1510.

Ramsden DB, Parsons RB, Ho SL, et al. The aetiology of idiopathic Parkinson's disease. *Mol Pathol* 2001;54:369–380.

Rana AQ, Vaid HM. A review of primary writing tremor. *Int J Neurosci* 2012;122:114–118.

Reich SG. The cold hands sign in MSA. *Neurology* 2003;60:719.

Reich SG. Psychogenic movement disorders. *Semin Neurol* 2006;26:289–296.

Renard D, Taieb G, Castelnovo G, et al. Teaching video NeuroImages: painful legs, moving toes associated with partial transverse myelitis. *Neurology* 2010;75:e74.

Respondek G, Höglinger GU. The phenotypic spectrum of progressive supranuclear palsy. *Parkinsonism Relat Disord* 2016;22(Suppl 1):S34–S36.

Rice JE, Thompson PD. Movement disorders I: parkinsonism and the akinetic-rigid syndromes. *Med J Aust* 2001;174: 357–363.

Riley DE, Lang AE. Non-Parkinson akinetic-rigid syndromes. *Curr Opin Neurol* 1996;9:321–326.

Rio J, Montalban J, Pujadas F, et al. Asterixis associated with anatomic cerebral lesions: a study of 45 cases. *Acta Neurol Scand* 1995;91:377–381.

Rizek P, Kumar N, Jog MS. An update on the diagnosis and treatment of Parkinson disease. *CMAJ* 2016;188:1157–1165.

Rowin J, Lewis SL. Copper deficiency myeloneuropathy and pancytopenia secondary to overuse of zinc supplementation. *J Neurol Neurosurg Psychiatry* 2005;76:750–751.

Sarva H, Deik A, Ullah A, et al. Clinical spectrum of stiff person syndrome: a review of recent reports. *Tremor Other Hyperkinet Mov (N Y)* 2016;6:340.

Satoh M, Narita M, Tomimoto H. Three cases of focal embouchure dystonia: classifications and successful therapy using a dental splint. *Eur Neurol* 2011;66:85–90.

Schneider SA, Bhatia KP. Huntington's disease look-alikes. *Handb Clin Neurol* 2011;100:101–112.

Schwartz MA, Selhorst JB, Ochs AL, et al. Oculomasticatory myorhythmia: a unique movement disorder occurring in Whipple's disease. *Ann Neurol* 1986;20:677–683.

Scolding NJ, Smith SM, Sturman S, et al. Auctioneer's jaw: a case of occupational oromandibular hemidystonia. *Mov Disord* 1995;10:508–509.

Sharma P, Eesa M. Teaching NeuroImage: posttraumatic palatal tremor. *Neurology* 2008;71:e30.

Shimizu N, Asakawa S, Minoshima S, et al. PARKIN as a pathogenic gene for autosomal recessive juvenile parkinsonism. *J Neural Transm Suppl* 2000;58:19–30.

Stoessl AJ, Rivest J. Differential diagnosis of parkinsonism. *Can J Neurol Sci* 1999;26(Suppl 2):S1–S4.

Stover NP, Watts RL. Corticobasal degeneration. *Semin Neurol* 2001;21:49–58.

Stremmel W, Meyerrose KW, Niederau C, et al. Wilson disease: clinical presentation, treatment, and survival. *Ann Intern Med* 1991;115:720–726.

Subramanian I, Vanek ZF, Bronstein JM. Diagnosis and treatment of Wilson's disease. *Curr Neurol Neurosci Rep* 2002;2:317–323.

Tadic V, Kasten M, Brüggemann N, et al. Dopa-responsive dystonia revisited: diagnostic delay, residual signs, and nonmotor signs. *Arch Neurol* 2012;69:1558–1562.

Tagawa A, Ono S, Shibata M, et al. A new neurological entity manifesting as involuntary movements and dysarthria with possible abnormal copper metabolism. *J Neurol Neurosurg Psychiatry* 2001;71:780–783.

Taly AB, Meenakshi-Sundaram S, Sinha S. Wilson disease: description of 282 patients evaluated over 3 decades. *Medicine (Baltimore)* 2007;86:112.

Tani T, Piao Y, Mori S, et al. Chorea resulting from paraneoplastic striatal encephalitis. *J Neurol Neurosurg Psychiatry* 2000;69:512–515.

Tarsy D, Simon DK. Dystonia. *N Engl J Med* 2006;355:818–829.

Thenganatt MA, Jankovic J. Parkinson disease subtypes. *JAMA Neurol* 2014;71:499–504.

Timmermann L, Gross J, Kircheis G, et al. Cortical origin of mini-asterixis in hepatic encephalopathy. *Neurology* 2002;58:295–298.

Topper R, Schwarz M, Lange HW, et al. Neurophysiological abnormalities in the Westphal variant of Huntington's disease. *Mov Disord* 1998;13:920–928.

Tsuji S. Dentatorubral-pallidoluysian atrophy. *Handb Clin Neurol* 2012;103:587–594.

van Dijk JG, van der Velde EA, Roos RA, et al. Juvenile Huntington disease. *Hum Genet* 1986;73:235–239.

Volles MJ, Lansbury PT Jr. Zeroing in on the pathogenic form of alpha-synuclein and its mechanism of neurotoxicity in Parkinson's disease. *Biochemistry* 2003;42:7871–7878.

Wadia PM, Lang AE. The many faces of corticobasal degeneration. *Parkinsonism Relat Disord* 2007;13(Suppl 3):S336–S340.

Walker RH, Jung HH, Dobson-Stone C, et al. Neurologic phenotypes associated with acanthocytosis. *Neurology* 2007;68: 92–98.

Walker RH, Jung HH, Danek A. Neuroacanthocytosis. *Handb Clin Neurol* 2011;100:141–151.

Whitwell JL, Jack CR Jr, Boeve BF, et al. Imaging correlates of pathology in corticobasal syndrome. *Neurology* 2010;75:1879–1887.

Williams DR, Holton JL, Strand C, et al. Pathological tau burden and distribution distinguishes progressive supranuclear palsy-parkinsonism from Richardson's syndrome. *Brain* 2007;130(Pt 6):1566–1576.

Winkler AS, Reuter I, Harwood G, et al. The frequency and significance of 'striatal toe' in parkinsonism. *Parkinsonism Relat Disord* 2002;9:97–101.

Xia C, Dubeau F. Teaching video NeuroImages: dystonic posturing in anti-NMDA receptor encephalitis. *Neurology* 2011;76: e80.

Yokochi M. Development of the nosological analysis of juvenile parkinsonism. *Brain Dev* 2000;22(Suppl 1):S81–S86.

Zhang YQ. Teaching video NeuroImages: regional myokymia. *Neurology* 2010;74(23):e103–e104.

SECTION F The Sensory System

CHAPTER 31

Overview of the Sensory System

The sensory system places the individual in relationship to the environment. Every sensation depends on impulses that arise by stimulation of receptors or end organs. These impulses are carried to the central nervous system (CNS) by sensory nerves and then conveyed through fiber tracts to higher centers for conscious recognition, reflex action, or other consequences of sensory stimulation. Somatic sensation is all senses other than the special senses. In this section, only general somatic sensory modalities are considered; the special senses—smell, vision, taste, hearing, and vestibular sensation—are discussed with the cranial nerves that mediate them.

The sensory system can be classified in several different ways. Sherrington divided sensation into exteroceptive, interoceptive, and proprioceptive. Exteroceptive sensation provides information about the external environment, including somatosensory functions and special senses. The interoceptive system conveys information about internal functions, blood pressure, or the concentration of chemical constituents in bodily fluids. Proprioception senses the orientation of the limbs and body in space. Anatomists differentiate between somatic and visceral sensation, with general and special varieties of each. General somatic afferent fibers carry exteroceptive and proprioceptive information; general visceral afferent fibers carry impulses from visceral structures. Special somatic afferent fibers subserve the special senses; special visceral afferent fibers mediate smell and taste. Other terms used to categorize types of sensation, such as epicritic, protopathic, vital, and gnostic, are of historical interest but have fallen into disuse.

Sensory systems may function on a conscious or unconscious level. Unconscious visceral sensory systems help regulate the internal environment. The monitoring of limb position in space has both a conscious component—the posterior column pathways—and an unconscious component—the spinocerebellar pathways. The conscious somatosensory system has two components: the position/vibration/fine discriminatory touch system and the pain/temperature/crude touch system. The different sensory modalities are carried over nerve fibers that vary in size, diameter, and myelination. Sensory impulses are carried to the dorsal (posterior) root ganglia and then into the CNS. After one or more synapses, the impulses ascend specific fiber tracts and reach the central sensory areas of the brain. Fine touch, position, and vibration from the body are carried over the posterior column/medial lemniscus system. These sensations from the head and face are processed by the trigeminal principal sensory nucleus in the pons. Pain and temperature from the body is carried over the spinothalamic tracts and from the head and face over the spinal tract and nucleus of the trigeminal. The major sensory pathways are depicted in Figure 31.1.

SENSORY RECEPTORS

The interface between the sensory nervous system and the environment is the receptor. There are many different types of receptors in the skin, subcutaneous tissues, muscles, tendons, periosteum, and visceral

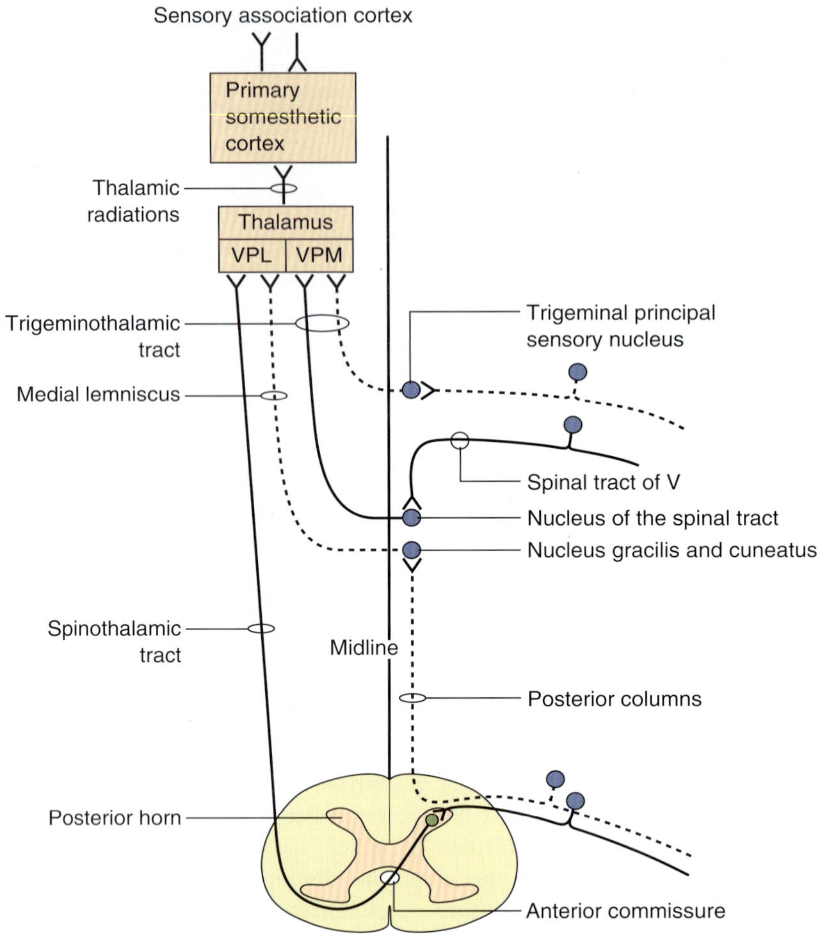

FIGURE 31.1 The light touch, pressure, position, and vibration pathways from the body and face are indicated by the *dashed line*; the pain and temperature fibers from the body and face are indicated by the *solid line*. Fibers from these various sources ultimately converge on the ventral posterior nuclei of the thalamus, which projects via the thalamic radiations to the primary sensory cortex in the postcentral gyrus. V, trigeminal; VPL, ventral posterior lateral; VPM, ventral posterior medial.

structures to subserve the transduction of various types of sensory information into nerve impulses. Sensory end organs are found in the skin and mucous membranes throughout the body. They are denser on the tongue, lips, genitalia, and fingertips and farther apart on the upper arms, buttocks, and trunk. One nerve fiber may innervate more than one receptor, and each end organ may receive filaments from more than one nerve fiber. Receptors may respond to more than one type of stimulus but have "specificity" because their threshold is lowest for a particular type of stimulus. Polymodal receptors respond efficiently to more than one modality, especially stimuli that cause tissue damage and pain. An "adequate" stimulus for a receptor is the type of stimulus that has the lowest threshold for receptor activation.

Receptor stimulation causes a change in the permeability of its membrane that gives rise to a receptor or generator potential—a local, nonpropagated potential whose intensity is proportional to the intensity of the stimulus. Receptors may adapt to a stimulus to varying degrees. Some receptors are rapidly adapting, or phasic, and most sensitive to on-and-off stimuli. Others are slowly adapting, or tonic, and function to constantly monitor a stimulus. Receptors are the terminal part of, and are continuous with, a sensory nerve. Receptor potentials induce action potentials in the nerve, with the frequency of the action potential discharge usually in proportion to the amplitude of the receptor potential, which is in turn proportional to the intensity of the applied stimulus. Each neuron has a specific receptive field, which consists of all the receptors it can respond to. The receptive fields form more or less discrete maps in the nervous system in which specific regions of the body are represented in specific regions of the brain. Some systems have a highly organized map (e.g., the somatosensory homunculus in the postcentral gyrus). In other systems, the maps are crude. In the cortex, neurons subserving the same modality and with similar receptive fields are organized into vertical rows, which extend from the cortical surface to the white matter and are referred to as cortical columns.

Receptors may be free nerve endings (FNE), or they may be encapsulated or connected to specialized nonneural components to form the sense organ. The nonneural elements are not excitable, but they help to form a structure that efficiently stimulates and excites the sensory nerve fiber. Exteroceptors respond to external stimuli and lie at or near the interfaces between the body and the environment. Special sensory exteroceptors subserve vision, hearing, smell, taste, and vestibular function. General or cutaneous sensory organs include the free and encapsulated receptor terminals in the skin. Proprioceptors respond to stimulation of deeper tissues, such as muscles and tendons, and are designed particularly to detect movement and the position of body parts. Receptors around hair follicles are activated by distortion of the hairs.

Receptors may be classified by the specific modality to which they are more responsive, such as mechanoreceptors, thermoreceptors, chemoreceptors, photoreceptors, and osmoreceptors. Mechanoreceptors respond to deformation, such as touch or pressure. Stimulation of mechanoreceptors causes a physical deformation of the receptor that results in the opening of ion channels. There is a great deal of variation in the density of sensory receptors between different body surface regions. Also, receptor density decreases with advancing age.

Receptors may also be classified morphologically, but the correlation between function and morphology is not nearly as close as was once believed. There are FNE, epidermal endings, and encapsulated endings. The FNE are fine, unmyelinated terminal fibers that arborize in the skin, fascia, ligaments, tendons, and other connective tissues throughout the body. They mediate several sensory modalities; some are exclusively nociceptors. The FNE are the terminals of sensory C fibers or A-delta fibers (see Nerve Fiber Classification below) and are located in both glabrous and hairy skin. The FNE terminals of unmyelinated nerve fibers are mainly nociceptive, but they may also be thermoreceptors or mechanoreceptors. Merkel cell endings (tactile discs or menisci) are specialized nerve endings lying just below the epidermis, especially in glabrous skin, and around hair follicles that function as mechanoreceptors. In encapsulated nerve endings, nonneural cells form a capsule around the terminal axon. Examples include Golgi tendon organs, muscle spindles, Ruffini endings, peritrichial endings, and Meissner's and Pacinian corpuscles.

There is evidence that abnormalities may be limited to sensory receptors in some neuropathies previously thought to selectively affect small nerve fibers.

NERVE FIBER CLASSIFICATION

In the peripheral nervous system, axons are divided into three major size groups: large myelinated, small myelinated, and unmyelinated. The largest fibers are the spindle afferents and the motor fibers arising from alpha motor neurons. The smallest, unmyelinated fibers are pain and postganglionic autonomic fibers. Large myelinated axons have diameters in the 6 to 12 μm range, small myelinated axons 2 to 6 μm, and unmyelinated axons 0.2 to 2 μm. Small myelinated fibers are about three times more numerous than large myelinated axons. The conduction velocity (CV) of a fiber depends on its diameter and degree of myelination. Large fibers conduct more rapidly than small ones, and myelinated fibers, more rapidly than unmyelinated ones. The CV ranges from less than 1 m/s for small, unmyelinated fibers to greater than 100 m/s for large, myelinated fibers. In large, myelinated fibers, the fiber diameter (in μm) × 6 approximates the CV (in m/s).

Peripheral nerve fibers are classified by size and CV according to two schemes: the ABC and the I/II/III/IV systems (see Chapter 23). The ABC scheme includes both motor and sensory fibers. The A-alpha and A-gamma fibers are motor. The A-alpha group also includes afferents from encapsulated receptors in the skin, joints, and muscles, including the primary spindle afferents. The A-beta and A-delta fibers are primarily cutaneous afferents. Group B fibers are preganglionic autonomics. Group C fibers include postganglionic autonomics, general visceral afferents, and pain and temperature fibers. The I/II/III/IV system applies only to afferent fibers. Groups I to III are myelinated; group IV is unmyelinated. The Ia fibers are spindle afferents from nuclear bag fibers; the Ib fibers arise from Golgi tendon organs; and the II fibers are spindle afferents from nuclear chain fibers. Group III fibers are cutaneous axons approximately the same as A-delta fibers. Group IV fibers correspond to C fibers and are primarily nociceptive. Sympathetic fibers do not carry sensation but may modulate the activity of central pain processing neurons.

In addition to the relationships between nerve fiber diameter, CV and sensory modality, the vulnerability to various types of injury varies with size and type of fiber. Cocaine, which blocks the conduction of the smaller fibers first, causes loss of sensation in the order of slow pain, cold, warmth, fast pain, touch, and position. Pressure, which blocks the conduction of the larger fibers first, causes loss of sensation in the order of position, vibration, pressure, touch, fast pain, cold, warmth, and slow pain. Most peripheral neuropathies affect both large and small fibers, but in some conditions, the involvement primarily affects either the large or the small fibers.

DERMATOMES

Sensory nerve roots supply cutaneous innervation to specific dermatomes. The dermatome innervation of the extremities is complex, in part because of the migration of the limb buds during embryonic development. As a result, the C4-C5 dermatomes abut T1-T2 on the upper chest, and the L1-L2 dermatomes are close to the sacral dermatomes on the inner aspect of the thigh near the genitalia. The generally available dermatomal charts are primarily derived from three sources: Head and Campbell, Foerster, and Keegan and Garrett, who all used very different approaches. Head and Campbell were primarily interested in herpes zoster and mapped dermatomes according to the distribution of herpetic eruptions. Foerster performed posterior rhizotomies in patients with chronic pain. He mapped the distribution of an intact root when one or more of those above and below had been severed or by electrically stimulating the stump of a severed root and observing the area of cutaneous vasodilation. The observation of dermatomal overlap originated partly from this work, and for a time, many believed a lesion of a single root would produce no detectable deficit. Keegan and Garrett examined a large series of patients with clinical involvement of various roots and mapped the sensory deficits due to single root lesions; there was surgical correlation in 53% of the patients. The loss of sensation because of isolated involvement of a single root, as occurs clinically, produces a different dermatomal map than the preserved sensation in a zone of anesthesia as found by Foerster. It is clear that the dermatomal overlap is such that the clinical deficit from an isolated root lesion is typically much more restricted than that expected from the anatomical geography of the dermatome. Deficits to pin prick are smaller than those to light touch. Figure 36.5 shows the dermatome distributions as depicted by Keegan and Garrett.

ANATOMY OF THE POSTERIOR ROOT

The oval-shaped dorsal root ganglia (DRG) lie on the posterior root in the intervertebral foramen, just lateral to the point where the posterior root penetrates the dura. The connective tissue capsule around each DRG is continuous with the epineurium of the spinal root. The DRG is composed of neurons, satellite cells, and a highly vascular supporting stroma. The DRG neurons are unipolar. A single nonmyelinated "dendroaxonal" process leaves the cell and then bifurcates into peripheral and central branches. The peripheral processes conduct afferent impulses toward the cell body; they are functionally elongated dendrites but more closely resemble axons from a structural standpoint and by convention are referred to as axons. Large sensory neurons may be found singly or in small groups proximal or distal to the DRG.

Sometimes, the entire DRG lies in an ectopic intraspinal location, well proximal to its usual position, making it vulnerable to involvement by herniated nucleus pulposus or osteophytic spur. Such ectopic DRGs have been mistaken for tumors, with unfortunate results. The DRG for the C1 posterior root is often missing.

The dorsal root is divided into a medial zone, conveying large fiber proprioceptive traffic and a lateral zone conveying small fiber pain and temperature traffic. As the posterior root exits the DRG to enter the spinal cord, two discrete fascicles may be visible; these correspond to the medial and lateral divisions. After the posterior root joins the spinal cord, the pathways serving different sensory modalities diverge and follow very different central courses through the spinal cord and lower brainstem, only to draw closer together as they ascend through the upper brainstem to ultimately reconverge as they enter the thalamus.

The major central somatosensory pathways are diagrammed in Figure 31.1 and discussed in more detail in subsequent chapters.

CLINICAL EXAMINATION

Sensory function is divided clinically into primary modalities and secondary or cortical modalities. The primary modalities for clinical purposes include light touch, pain, temperature, joint position sense (proprioception), and vibration. The cortical or secondary modalities are those that require synthesis and interpretation of primary modalities by the sensory association area in the parietal lobe. These include two-point discrimination, stereognosis, graphesthesia, tactile localization, and others. When the primary modalities are normal in a particular body region, but the cortical modalities are impaired, a parietal lobe lesion may be responsible. Itch and tickle sensations are closely allied to pain; they are probably perceived by the same nerve endings and are absent following procedures used for the relief of pain.

Many terms have been used, not always consistently, to describe sensory abnormalities. The definition of esthesia is perception, feeling, or sensation (Gr. *aesthesis* "sensation"). Algesia refers to the sense of pain (Gr. *algos* "pain"). Hypalgesia is a decrease, and analgesia an absence, of pain sensation. The combining form "algia" refers to any painful condition. Hypesthesia is a decrease, and anesthesia an absence, of all sensation. Hyperesthesia refers to an increase in sensation. The terms hyperalgesia, hyperpathia, and allodynia refer to pain felt following a stimulus that is not normally painful, or an exaggerated response to a stimulus that should be only minimally painful. Allodynia often occurs after a peripheral nerve injury in the setting of a complex regional pain syndrome in which there is sensory loss, but once the sensory threshold is exceeded, the response is excessive. Such patients may also have a painful response to any stimulus, even a puff of air. Paresthesia is an abnormal sensation; dysesthesia is an abnormal, unpleasant, or painful sensation. Table 31.1 summarizes some of the definitions. Seldom-used terms and those of primarily historical interest have been omitted. When describing sensory examination findings, it is preferable to simply refer to an increase or a decrease in sensation to a particular modality. Avoiding the Greek-derived terms can eliminate fusion.

Sensory abnormalities may be characterized by an increase, decrease, absence, or a perversion or distortion of sensation. An example of increased sensation is pain—an unpleasant or disagreeable feeling that results from excessive stimulation of certain sense organs, fibers, or tracts. Perversions of sensation take

TABLE 31.1 Generally Accepted Definitions of Commonly Used Terms Regarding the Sensory System and Abnormalities of Sensation

Term	Definition
Allodynia	Increase in sensibility to pain; pain in response to a stimulus not normally painful
Alloesthesia (allesthesia)	Perception of a sensory stimulus at a site other than where it was delivered; tactile allesthesia is feeling something other than at the site of the stimulus; visual allesthesia is seeing something other than where it actually is. *Mitempfindung* refers to distant referral of cutaneous sensation
Analgesia	Absence of sensibility to pain
Astereognosis	Absence of spatial tactile sensibility; inability to identify objects by feel
Anesthesia	Absence of all sensation
Dysesthesias	Unpleasant or painful abnormal perverted sensations, either spontaneous or after a normally nonpainful stimulus (e.g., burning in response to touch); often accompany paresthesias
Hypalgesia	Decrease in sensibility to pain
Hypesthesia	Decrease in sensibility to sensory stimuli
Hyperalgesia	Increase in sensibility to pain; pain in response to a stimulus not normally painful
Hyperpathia	Increase in sensibility to pain; pain in response to a stimulus not normally painful
Hyperesthesia	Increased sensitivity to sensory stimuli, often with added unpleasant quality
Kinesthesia	The sense of movement
Pallesthesia	Vibratory sensation
Paresthesias	Abnormal spontaneous sensations experienced in the absence of specific stimulation (feelings of cold, warmth, numbness, tingling, burning, prickling, crawling, heaviness, compression, or itching)

the form of paresthesias, dysesthesias, and phantom sensations. Impairment and loss of sensation result from decreased acuity of the sensory organs or receptors, impaired conduction in sensory fibers or tracts, or dysfunction of higher centers causing impairment in the powers of perception or recognition.

The sensory examination is performed to discover whether areas of absent, decreased, exaggerated, or distorted sensation are present and to determine the type of sensation affected, the degree of abnormality, and the distribution of the abnormality. Findings may include loss, decrease, or increase of one or more types of sensation; dissociation of sensation with loss of one modality type but not of others; loss of ability to recognize differences in degrees of sensation; misinterpretations (perversions or distortions) of sensation; or areas of localized hyperesthesia. More than one of these may occur simultaneously.

The sensory examination is arguably the most difficult and tedious part of the neurologic examination. Useful information is more likely to be obtained if the examiner performs a practical, goal-directed examination. Some examiners prefer to assess sensory functions early in the course of the examination, when the patient is most likely to be alert and attentive. Fatigue causes faulty attention and slowing of the reaction time, and the findings are less reliable when the patient has become weary during the examination. Others argue that the routine sensory examination is the most subjective and least useful part of the neurologic examination and prefer to leave it until the end. If one of the patient's complaints involves sensation, it is preferable to perform the sensory examination early rather than later. Because the results depend largely on subjective responses, the full cooperation of the patient is necessary if conclusions are to be accurate. Occasionally, objective evidence, such as withdrawal of the part stimulated, wincing, blinking, and changes in countenance, may aid in the delineation of areas of sensory change. Keenness of perception and interpretation of stimuli differ in individuals, in various parts of the body, and in the same individual under different circumstances.

For a reliable sensory examination, the patient must understand the procedure and be ready and willing to cooperate. Accurate communication is vital. The purpose and method of testing should be explained in simple terms, so that the patient understands the expected responses. During the examination, the patient should be warm, comfortable, and relaxed. The best results are obtained when the patient is lying comfortably in a warm, quiet room. Obtaining patient confidence is important. Satisfactory results cannot be obtained when the patient is suspicious, in pain, uncomfortable, fearful, confused, or distracted by sensations such as noise or hunger. If the patient is in pain or discomfort, or if he has recently been sedated, the examination should be postponed. The areas under examination should be uncovered, but it is best to expose the various parts of the body as little as possible. In general, the patient's eyes should be closed or the areas under examination shielded to eliminate distractions and to avoid misinterpretation of stimuli. However, it is sometimes helpful when performing a sensory examination for suspected peripheral neuropathy to have the patient watch as the stimuli are moved distal to proximal to more accurately report an area of change. Proprioception and vibration are always best tested with the eyes closed. Homologous areas of the body should be compared whenever possible.

The detail and technique used for the sensory examination depend on the history. For example, a patient with no sensory complaints referred for evaluation of headache or vertigo requires only a screening examination. A patient who is seen for possible carpal tunnel syndrome, radiculopathy, peripheral neuropathy, or a suspected parietal lobe lesion requires a very different approach. Too much time can be spent on the sensory examination when there are no sensory complaints, but investing too little time can lead to errors when certain information is essential to an accurate diagnosis.

The examiner should first determine whether the patient is aware of subjective changes in sensation or is experiencing abnormal spontaneous sensations. Sensory symptoms may be divided into negative symptoms, lack of sensation, and positive symptoms, abnormal sensory discharges such as paresthesias and dysesthesias. Positive and negative symptoms may occur together. Inquire whether the patient has noticed pain, paresthesias, or loss of feeling; whether any part of the body feels numb, dead, hot, or cold; whether he has perceived sensations such as tingling, burning, itching, "pins and needles," pressure, distention, formication, or feelings of weight or constriction. If such symptoms are present, determine their type and character, intensity, distribution, duration, and periodicity, as well as exacerbating and relieving factors. Spontaneous pain must be differentiated from tenderness. Pain and numbness may exist together, as in thalamic pain and peripheral neuropathy. The patient's manner of describing the pain or sensory disturbance and the associated affective responses, the nature of the terms used, the localization, and the precipitating and relieving factors may aid in differentiating between organic and nonorganic disturbances. Nonorganic abnormalities are often associated with inappropriate affect (either excessive emotionality or indifference), are often vague in character or location, and reactions to them are not consistent with the degree of disability.

If the patient has no sensory symptoms, testing can be done rapidly, bearing in mind the major sensory nerve and segmental supply to the face, trunk, and extremities. In certain situations, more careful sensory testing is required. If there are specific sensory symptoms; if there are motor symptoms such as atrophy, weakness, or ataxia; or if any areas of sensory abnormality are detected on the survey examination, or if the clinical situation suggests the likelihood of sensory abnormalities, then detailed sensory examination should be performed. The presence of trophic changes, especially painless ulcers and blisters, is also an indication for careful sensory testing because these may be the first manifestations of a sensory disorder of which the patient is unaware. In patients with limited cooperation, it may be desirable to examine the areas of sensory complaint first and then survey the rest of the body. It is difficult to perform an adequate sensory examination of the lower extremities unless the shoes and socks are removed.

The simpler the method of examination, the more satisfactory the conclusions. Explain to the patient what is to be done and demonstrate in an area expected to be normal what the stimulus feels like. Then, have the patient close the eyes and begin the testing. The subject should be asked to tell the type of stimulus perceived and its location, with the examiner taking care not to suggest responses. Responses are normally prompt, and a consistent delay in answering may indicate an abnormal delay in perception. There are two general screening patterns: side to side and distal to proximal. The side-to-side screening should usually compare the major dermatomes and peripheral nerve distributions, although more abbreviated screening may be appropriate in certain clinical circumstances. Distal to proximal testing is appropriate when peripheral neuropathy is part of the differential diagnosis. If the patient is complaining of a discrete area of abnormal sensation, such as an area on an arm or leg, it can be helpful to begin testing in a distant location, or in a homologous area of the opposite limb, so that the patient understands what the stimulus feels like in the normal region. Then proceed to the area in question and define the extent of the abnormality. The distribution of abnormalities can be drawn on the skin with a marker and recorded on a chart (Figure 36.5), indicating areas of change in the various modalities by horizontal, vertical, or diagonal lines, stippling or different colors. A key helps to explain the meaning of the various symbols and colors, as does a note regarding the cooperation and insight of the patient and an estimate of the reliability of the examination. Sensory charts are helpful for comparison with the results of subsequent examinations in following the course of the patient's illness and for comparison with the results of other examiners.

Accuracy in localization of pain, temperature, and tactile stimuli is also informative. Tactile localization is a sensitive test of sensory function; there may be loss of localization before there is a detectable change in sensory threshold. Tactile localization is most accurate on the palmar surfaces of the fingers, especially the thumb and index finger. The patient should name or point to the area stimulated, comparing responses on the two sides of the body.

The results of the sensory examination may at times seem unreliable and confusing. The process can become tedious, and the findings can be difficult to interpret. Sensory changes because of suggestion are notoriously frequent in emotionally labile individuals, but suggestion can produce nonorganic findings in patients with organic disease. Care must be taken in drawing conclusions. To obtain reliable results, it may be necessary to postpone the sensory examination if the patient has become fatigued or to repeat the testing at a later time. The sensory examination should always be repeated at least once to confirm the findings. Sensory testing, more than any other part of the neurologic examination, requires patience and detailed observation for reliable interpretation.

The following are some of the difficulties that may be encountered in performing the sensory examination. The uncooperative patient may be indifferent to the sensory examination or object to the use of painful stimuli. The overly cooperative patient, on the other hand, may make too much of small differences and report changes that are not present. Some areas of the body, such as the antecubital fossae, the supraclavicular fossae, the breast region, and the neck, are more sensitive than others; apparent sensory changes in these regions may lead to fallacious conclusions, including false sensory levels on the upper chest. A normal individual may report an increased sensitivity to pin when a sharp stimulus moves from the dorsum of the foot to the distal leg. This is not an abnormal sensory gradient but rather because of the decrease in density of sensory receptors in the skin of the dorsal foot just distal to the ankle. The last in a series of identical stimuli may be interpreted as the strongest. Even though pain sensibility is absent, a patient may still be able to identify a sharp stimulus with a pin. Occasionally in syringomyelia, with lost pain but preserved tactile sensibility, the patient may recognize the pin point in an analgesic area and give confusing and inconsistent responses. Sensory findings are difficult to evaluate in individuals with intellectual disability, language difficulties, or a clouded sensorium, but it may be necessary to carry out the examination despite these obstacles. In patients with altered mental status or a decreased sensorium, pain may be tested grossly by pricking or pinching the skin, comparing responses on the two sides of the body. In such patients, it may only be possible to determine whether or not the patient reacts to painful stimuli in various parts of the body. A child may be fearful of testing, requiring assurance at the outset that the examination will be brief and not actually painful. In young children, it is often best to delay sensory testing until the end of the examination, particularly when even mildly uncomfortable, yet threatening, stimuli are applied. This may also hold true for some apprehensive adults.

BIBLIOGRAPHY

Bell J, Bolanowski S, Holmes MH. The structure and function of Pacinian corpuscles: a review. *Prog Neurobiol* 1994;42:79–128.

Bell-Krotoski J, Weinstein S, Weinstein C. Testing sensibility, including touch-pressure, two-point discrimination, point localization, and vibration. *J Hand Ther* 1993;6:114–123.

Birder LA, Perl ER. Cutaneous sensory receptors. *J Clin Neurophysiol* 1994;11:534–552.

Campbell WW, Pridgeon RP. *Practical Primer of Clinical Neurology*. Philadelphia: Lippincott Williams & Wilkins, 2002.

Davidoff RA. The dorsal columns. *Neurology* 1989;39(10): 1377–1385.

DeMyer W. Pointers and pitfalls in the neurologic examination. *Semin Neurol* 1998;18:161–168.

Foerster O. The dermatomes in man. *Brain* 1933;56:1–39.

Freeman C, Okun MS. Origins of the sensory examination in neurology. *Semin Neurol* 2002;22:399–408.

Gilman S. Joint position sense and vibration sense: anatomical organization and assessment. *J Neurol Neurosurg Psychiatry* 2002;73:473–477.

Gilman S, Newman SW. *Manter and Gatz's Essentials of Clinical Neuroanatomy and Neurophysiology*. 10th ed. Philadelphia: FA Davis, 2003.

Head H, Campbell AW. The pathology of herpes zoster and its bearing on sensory localization. *Brain* 1900;23:353–523.

Head H, Campbell AW, Kennedy PG. The pathology of Herpes Zoster and its bearing on sensory localisation. *Rev Med Virol* 1997;7:131–143.

Kandel ER. *Principles of Neural Science*. 5th ed. New York: McGraw-Hill Medical, 2013.

Keegan J. Dermatome hypalgesia associated with herniation of intervertebral disk. *Arch NeurPsych* 1943;50:67–83.

Keegan JJ, Garrett FD. The segmental distribution of the cutaneous nerves in the limbs of man. *Anat Rec* 1948;102:409–437.

Mochizuki H, Kakigi R. Central mechanisms of itch. *Clin Neurophysiol* 2015;126:1650–1660.

Pryse-Phillips W. *Companion to Clinical Neurology*. 3rd ed. Oxford: Oxford University Press, 2009.

Saade NE, Baliki M, El Khoury C, et al. The role of the dorsal columns in neuropathic behavior: evidence for plasticity and non-specificity. *Neuroscience* 2002;115:403–413.

Shibasaki H. Central mechanisms of pain perception. *Suppl Clin Neurophysiol* 2004;57:39–49.

Stone J, Vermeulen M. Functional sensory symptoms. *Handb Clin Neurol* 2016;139:271–281.

Standring S, ed. *Gray's Anatomy: The Anatomical Basis of Clinical Practice*. 41st ed. New York: Elsevier Limited, 2016.

Vierck CJ Jr, Cooper BY. Cutaneous texture discrimination following transection of the dorsal spinal column in monkeys. *Somatosens Mot Res* 1998;15:309–315.

Williams D, Conn J, Talley N, et al. Reviewing the evidence base for the peripheral sensory examination. *Int J Clin Pract* 2014;68:756–760.

Wolf JK. *Segmental Neurology*. Baltimore: University Park Press, 1981.

CHAPTER 32

The Exteroceptive Sensations

Exteroceptive sensations originate in peripheral receptors in response to external stimuli and changes in the environment. There are four main types of general somatic sensation: pain, thermal or temperature sense, light touch or touch-pressure, and position sense or proprioception. Some include pruritic (itch) as a separate modality, and there is growing evidence for a modality that conveys the positive affective (pleasant) properties of touch.

PAIN AND TEMPERATURE SENSATION

Anatomy and Physiology

Impulses carrying superficial pain sensation arise in nociceptors—free or branched nerve endings in the skin and mucous membranes. Some nociceptors respond to specific types of stimuli, whereas others are polymodal. Thermoreceptors for heat and cold sensation are free nerve endings in the dermis. Warm and cold stimuli activate different fibers. Pain and thermal sensation are carried along small myelinated A-delta and unmyelinated C nerve fibers to the dorsal root ganglion (DRG), where the first cell body is situated (Figure 32.1). The impulses in response to moderate heat or cold travel primarily over A-delta and some C fibers. The response to the pain associated with the extremes of temperature is conveyed along C fibers. Axons from small and intermediate size neurons in the DRG traverse the lateral division of the dorsal root to enter the dorsolateral fasciculus of the spinal cord (Lissauer's tract), where they ramify longitudinally for one or two segments. The axons leave Lissauer's tract, enter the posterior gray horn, and synapse in laminae I to V. Second-order neurons for the spinothalamic system lie primarily in laminae I, II, and V (see Chapter 24). The other related posterior horn cells are interneurons in the pain pathway. The posterior horn contains a variety of neurotransmitters; pain impulses are thought to be mediated primarily by substance P and glutamate. Activity in the spinothalamic tract (ST) neurons of the posterior horn is modulated by descending pathways. Stimulation of certain brain regions inhibits the response of ST cells to noxious stimuli. Descending influences are known to arise from the nucleus raphe magnus, periaqueductal gray, brainstem reticular formation, periventricular gray, ventral posterior lateral (VPL) thalamic nucleus, and parietal cortex and travel primarily in the corticospinal tract and dorsolateral funiculus. These pathways are important in pain control mechanisms.

The majority of axons originating from second-order spinothalamic neurons cross the midline in the anterior white commissure and gather into the anterior and lateral STs; a small proportion of fibers ascend ipsilaterally. Fibers crossing in the anterior white commissure are affected early in syringomyelia. In the past, anatomists thought the anterior ST carried crude touch and the lateral ST pain and temperature; current evidence suggests all these modalities are carried in both tracts, so the lateral and anterior STs are now sometimes lumped together as the anterolateral or ventrolateral system (ALS) or simply the spinothalamic tract or system. For clinical purposes, it remains useful to consider the pain and temperature pathways in the ST as a distinct system. The ST ascends in an anterolateral position, just medial to the anterior spinocerebellar tract (Figure 32.2). Intermingled with the fibers of the ST are ascending spinoreticulothalamic fibers, which contribute to the ALS. The ST is somatotopically organized, and the distribution of fibers is clinically relevant. Lowermost, sacral and lumbar, fibers entering first are displaced progressively more laterally by subsequently entering fibers. As the tract ascends, the sacral fibers come to lie most lateral and superficial,

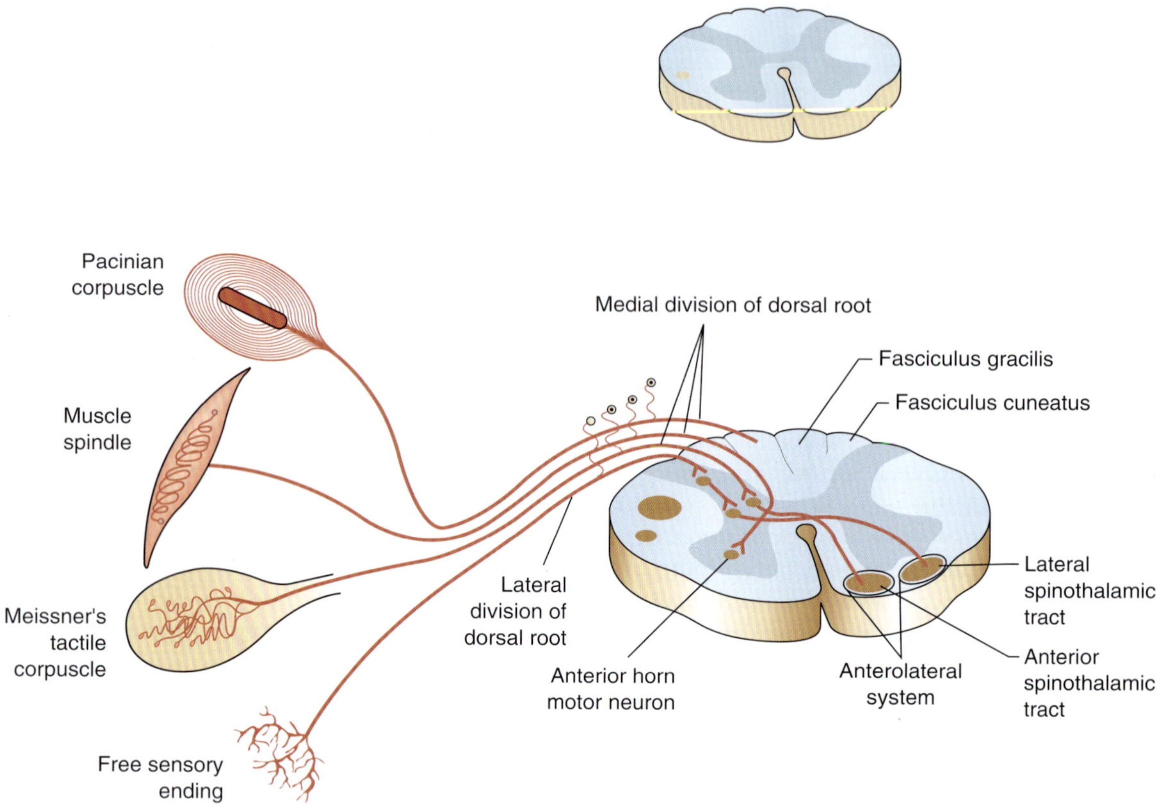

FIGURE 32.1 Diagram of the spinal cord and dorsal root showing the peripheral receptors and terminations of fibers within the spinal cord.

nearer to the surface of the cord (Figure 32.3), with cervical fibers most medial. There is also a slight rotation so that the sacral fibers also come to lie somewhat more posterior as the tract ascends. At midbrain levels, lower extremity and sacral fibers are posterior, and those from the upper limb and trunk are more anterior. Because the sacral fibers lie most laterally, an intramedullary spinal cord lesion, such as a neoplasm, may produce "sacral sparing," preservation of sensation in a saddle distribution in the face of sensory loss otherwise present below a certain spinal level. Conversely, a compressive lesion pressing on the upper spinal cord may preferentially involve the sacral spinothalamic fibers, causing sacral dysfunction first. Fibers carrying deep pain are in general thought to lie nearer the midline than those carrying superficial pain. The spinoreticulothalamic fibers in the ALS subserve diffuse, poorly localized pain from deep and visceral structures. They may also be involved in the affective aspects of pain.

In the medulla, the ST lies peripherally, dorsolateral to the inferior olivary nuclei; in the pons, it is lateral to the medial lemniscus (ML) and medial to the middle cerebellar peduncle; in the mesencephalon, it is peripheral, dorsal to the ML and just dorsolateral to the red nucleus. It passes near the colliculi and enters the diencephalon just medial to the brachium of the inferior colliculus.

Pain and temperature fibers from the face enter the pons through the gasserian ganglion and then descend in the spinal tract of the trigeminal nerve to varying levels, where they synapse on neurons in the adjacent nucleus of the spinal tract (see Chapter 15). These second-order neurons decussate and form the trigeminothalamic tract, which runs near the ascending spinothalamic and lemniscal fibers (Figure 15.2). The other cranial nerves carrying exteroceptive pain sensation have ganglia comparable to the DRG and pathways corresponding to the trigeminothalamic tract. These are discussed in the chapters on the individual cranial nerves.

In the upper lateral midbrain, all the somatosensory fibers begin to converge. The ST fibers are joined in the rostral brainstem by the laterally migrating fibers from the ML and by ascending trigeminothalamic fibers so that ultimately all the fibers subserving somatosensory function run together as they approach the thalamus. The tracts enter the ventrobasal and

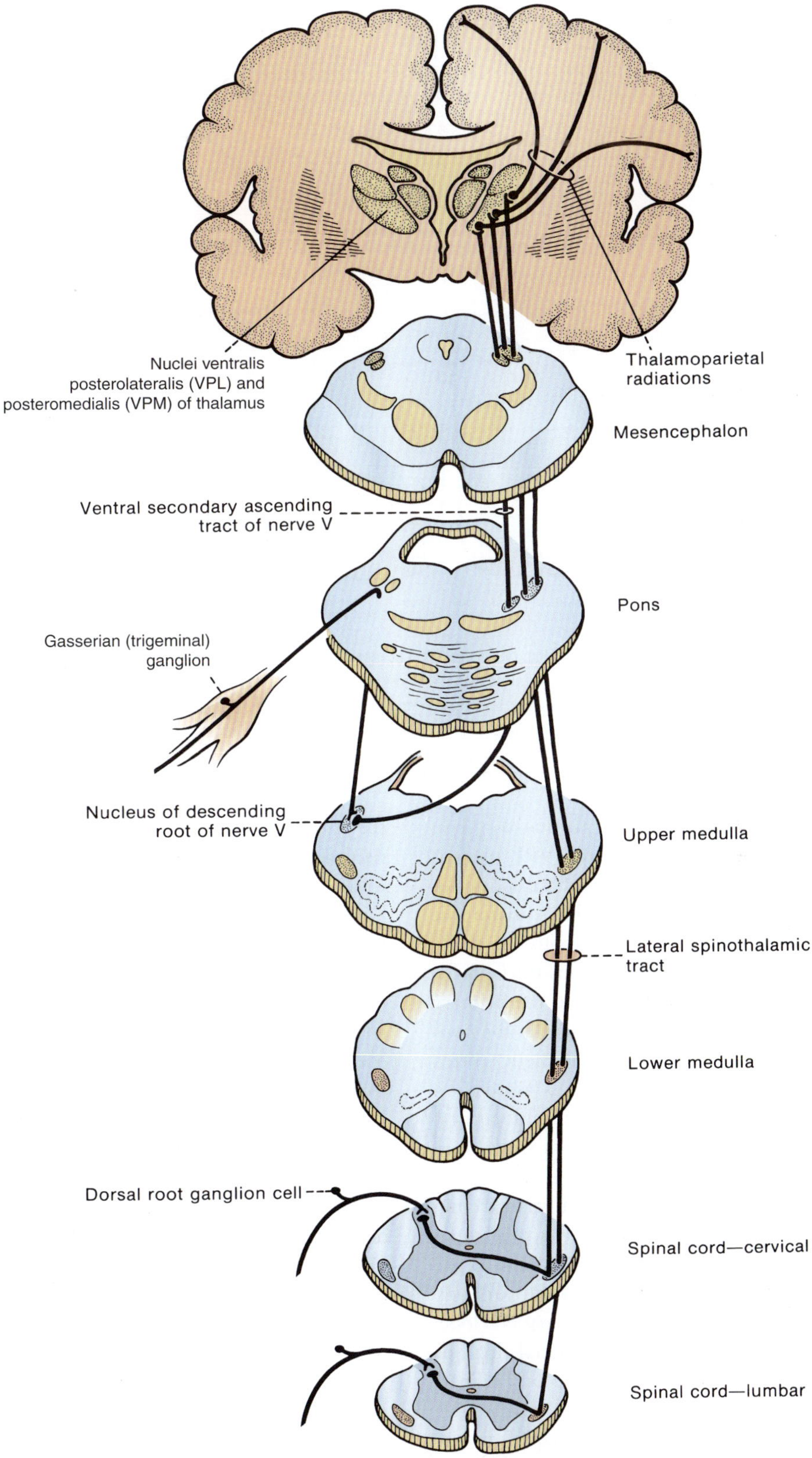

FIGURE 32.2 The lateral spinothalamic tract.

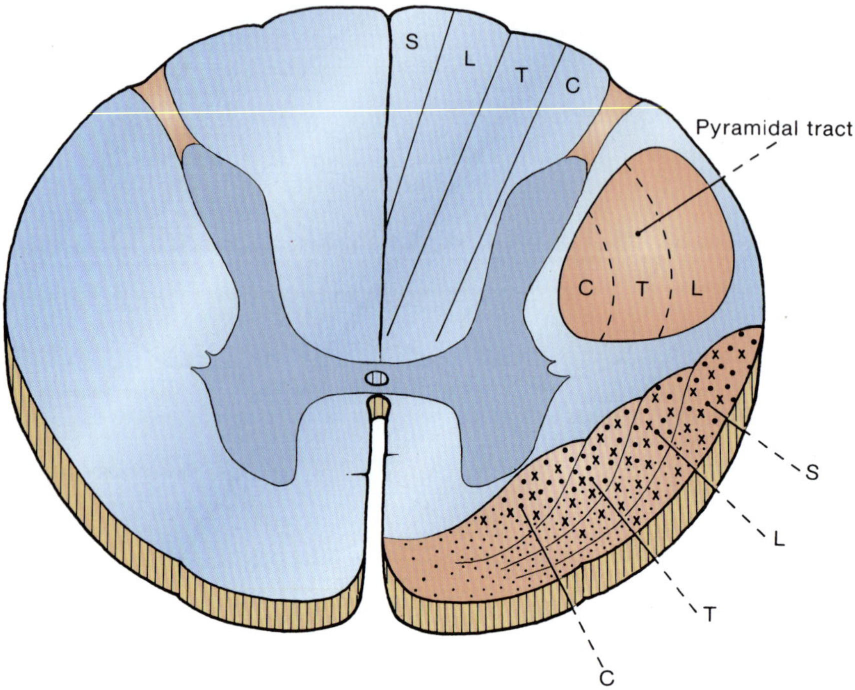

FIGURE 32.3 Diagram of cross section of the cervical region of the spinal cord showing the arrangement of fibers in the spinothalamic and pyramidal tracts and dorsal columns. *Heavy dots* indicate fibers carrying temperature sensation, *crosses* indicate fibers carrying pain sensation, and *fine dots* indicate fibers carrying tactile impulses. *C, T, L,* and *S* indicate fibers from or destined for cervical, thoracic, lumbar, and sacral levels of the spinal cord.

ventral posterior nucleus of the thalamus together; body sensation fibers terminate in the VPL nucleus and facial sensation fibers in the ventral posterior medial (VPM) nucleus. There is detailed somatotopic organization within VPL and VPM. From the thalamus, fibers run in the thalamic radiations through the posterior limb of the internal capsule to the primary somesthetic cortex in the postcentral gyrus for conscious recognition. The primary somesthetic cortex communicates with the parietal sensory association cortex and with other cortical areas. Thalamocortical fibers also project to the superior bank of the sylvian fissure.

In the thalamoparietal radiations, fibers carrying lower-extremity sensation curve medially to the superior medial surface of the hemisphere adjacent to the medial longitudinal fissure; those from the upper body go to the midportion of the surface of the parietal lobe; those from the face terminate on the lateral, inferior portion of the postcentral gyrus (Figure 6.7). Fibers of the spinoreticulothalamic tract carry nociceptive information in the ALS. There are synapses in the brainstem reticular formation and medial part of the thalamus. Spinoreticulothalamic fibers terminate in the intralaminar thalamic nuclei. The thalamic neurons that mediate pain project both to the parietal lobe and to the limbic cortex. Projections from the intralaminar nuclei terminate in the hypothalamus and limbic system and probably mediate the affective and autonomic responses to pain. Evidence from both humans and nonhuman primates suggests that the posterior insula and medial operculum is an important cortical target of the spinothalamic system, and that operculo-insular (parasylvian) pain may exist as a distinct entity.

Descending pathways serve to modulate pain. Fibers from the frontal cortex and hypothalamus project to the midbrain periaqueductal gray. The descending pain modulation pathway then descends in the dorsal part of the lateral funiculus to the posterior horn. Descending fibers from the locus caeruleus, the raphe nuclei, and other brainstem areas also modulate the pain response. These descending pathways are important in endogenous pain control and opiate analgesia.

Clinical Examination

There are many methods for testing superficial pain sensation. A simple and commonly used method, as reliable as any, is to use a common safety pin bent at right angles so its clasp may serve as a handle. The instrument should be sharp enough to create a mildly painful sensation, but not so sharp as to draw blood. A hypodermic needle is far too sharp unless its point has been well blunted against some hard surface. A broken wooden applicator stick is often used and is usually satisfactory provided the shards are sharp. Adequately sharp ends can be obtained by holding the stick at the very ends while breaking it. Disposable sterile devices, sharp on one end and dull on the other, are commercially available. Although it is not necessary for the stimulating instrument to be sterile, whatever is used must be discarded after use on a single patient to avoid the risk of transmitting disease from accidental skin puncture. There is no place in modern neurology for reusable sharp instruments such as the Wartenberg wheel, but disposable pinwheels are available. Various sensory testing devices have been used experimentally. Instruments for evaluating sensation quantitatively are available commercially **(Video 32.1)**.

A helpful trick is to hold the pin or shaft of the applicator stick lightly between thumb and fingertip and let the shaft slide between fingertip and thumb tip with each stimulation. This helps insure more consistent stimulus intensity than putting a fingertip on the end of the instrument and trying to control the force with the hand or wrist. Experience teaches how to gauge the intensity of the applied stimulus and the expected reaction to it. The clinical evaluation of superficial pain, temperature, and touch sensation shows a reasonably good correlation with quantitative assessment.

It is best to do the examination with the patient's eyes closed. The patient should be asked to judge whether the stimulus feels as sharp on one side as on the other, and whether it is as sharp distally as proximally. Always suggest that the stimuli should be the same, as by language such as, "Does this feel about the same as that?" Avoid such language as "Does this feel any different?" or "Which feels sharper?" Suggesting there should be a difference encourages some patients to overanalyze and predisposes them to spurious findings and a tedious, often unreliable examination. A commonly used technique is asking the patient to compare one side to the other in monetary or percentage terms, for example, "If this (stimulating the apparently normal side) side is a dollar's worth (or 100%), how much is this (stimulating the apparently abnormal side) worth?" The overanalytical but neurologically normal patient often responds with an estimate on the order of "95 cents," whereas the patient with real, clinically significant sensory loss is more apt to respond with "5 cents" or "25 cents." Delivering alternately sharp and dull stimuli, as with the sharp and blunt ends of a safety pin and instructing the patient to reply "sharp" or "dull" may not elicit subtle sensory loss only detectable in comparison with an uninvolved area. Slight changes can sometimes be demonstrated in a cooperative patient by asking her to indicate the alterations in sensation when a pinpoint is drawn lightly over the skin. A cooperative patient with a discrete distribution of sensory loss may be able to map out the involved area quite nicely if instructed how to proceed and left alone for a short time with tools and a marking instrument. The affected area can then be compared with a figure showing sensory distributions (see **Web Link 32.1**). As noted in Chapter 31, if the presenting complaint is a discrete area of altered sensation, begin testing in a presumably normal area, then proceed to the involved area, and map out the extent of the abnormality.

The latent time in the response to stimulation is eliminated and the delineation more accurate if the examination proceeds from areas of lesser sensitivity to those of greater sensitivity rather than the reverse. If there is subjective hypalgesia, move from areas of decreased sensation to those of normal sensation; if there is hyperalgesia, proceed from the normal to the hyperalgesic area. There may be a definite line of demarcation between the areas of normal and abnormal sensation, a gradual change, or at times a zone of hyperesthesia between them. It is occasionally useful to move from the normal to the numb area. In myelopathy, a spinal sensory level that is the same going from rostral to caudal as from caudal to rostral suggests a very focal and destructive lesion; when the two levels are far apart, the lesion is usually less severe.

If testing is done too rapidly, the area of sensory change may be misjudged. Applying the stimuli too close together may produce spatial summation; stimulating too rapidly may produce temporal summation. Either of these may lead to spurious findings. If stimulation is too rapid, or if conduction is delayed, a given response may refer to a previous stimulation. Stimuli should be applied at irregular intervals to avoid patient anticipation. If the patient knows when to expect a stimulus, a seemingly normal response can occur even from an anesthetic area. Include control stimuli from time to time, especially if the patient is comparing sharp and dull (e.g., using the dull end of the pin while asking if it is sharp), to be sure the patient has understood the instructions and is paying attention.

Temperature testing is difficult. Temperature sensation may be tested with test tubes containing warm and cool water, or by using various objects with different thermal conductivity. Ideally, for testing cold, the stimuli should be 5°C to 10°C (41°F to 50°F), and for warmth, 40°C to 45°C (104°F to 113°F). The extremes of free-flowing tap water are usually about 10°C and 40°C. Temperatures much lower or higher than these elicit pain rather than temperature sensations. Normally, it is possible to detect a difference of about 1°C in the range around 30°C. The tubes must be dry, as dampness may be interpreted as cold. The tines of a tuning fork are naturally cool and work well for giving a quick impression of the ability to appreciate coolness. The tines quickly warm with repeated skin contact; applying the tines alternately and waving the fork in the air between stimuli helps prevent this warming. Holding the tines under cold running tap water may also be helpful. Some examiners warm one tine deliberately by rubbing and then test the ability to discriminate between the warm side and the cool side of the fork. This technique has limited practicality because the cool side warms so rapidly with skin contact. The latency for detecting temperature is longer than for other sensory modalities, and the application of the stimulus may need to be extended.

In temperature testing, it is usually sufficient to determine whether the patient can distinguish hot and cold stimuli. In peripheral neuropathy, a gradient sometimes occurs where the patient begins sensing cold or hot sensation more normally. To detect more subtle impairment in temperature sensibility, the Mayo Clinic developed disks of variable temperature conductance (steel, copper, glass, plastic) to determine if patients could discern subtle temperature variations.

In most instances, heat and cold sensibility are equally impaired. Rarely, one modality may be involved more than the other; the area of impaired heat sensibility is usually the larger. Pain and temperature sensibility are usually involved equally with lesions of the sensory system, and it is rarely necessary to test both. Temperature testing is more difficult and less often done. Testing temperature may be useful when the patient does not tolerate pinprick stimuli, has confusing or inconsistent responses to pain testing, or to help map an area of sensory loss. In some instances, the deficit is more consistent with temperature testing than with pinprick. Temperature testing may not be very reliable in patients with circulatory insufficiency or vasoconstriction causing acral coolness.

Quantitative sensory testing (QST) uses computerized neurophysiologic methods to examine sensation. It provides very accurately measured stimuli of various types and uses strict paradigms for recording responses. Temperature sensation is tested by delivering pulses of hot and cold and determining the threshold for detection. Extremes of temperature assess pain. Testing is expensive, is time consuming, and must be administered by trained technicians. There is good correlation between QST and clinical methods. QST is very useful for longitudinal research studies but of little clinical utility.

TACTILE SENSATION

Anatomy and Physiology

Cutaneous receptors that mediate light touch or general tactile sensibility include free nerve endings, Merkel cell endings, and encapsulated endings such as Meissner's and Pacinian corpuscles and Ruffini endings. All the encapsulated receptors function as mechanoreceptors with afferent nerve fibers in the group II and III range. Pacinian corpuscles are large, lamellated structures located subcutaneously in the palmar, plantar and digital skin, genitalia, and other sensitive areas; they function as rapidly adapting mechanoreceptors. They are especially responsive to vibration, most notably in the 40 to 1,000 Hz frequency range. Meissner tactile corpuscles are found primarily in thick hairless skin, such as the hand, foot, and lips, and are most highly developed in the finger pads. They also respond to vibration in the low-frequency range (10 to 400 Hz) and are maximally sensitive at 100 to 200 Hz. Merkel cell receptors are also slowly adapting mechanoreceptors that respond to low-frequency vibration. Ruffini endings are slowly adapting mechanoreceptors located in hairy as well as glabrous skin, in joint capsules, tendon insertions, and elsewhere. They are particularly responsive to stretching or indentation of the skin.

Light touch sensation is conveyed over large and small myelinated peripheral nerve fibers to unipolar DRG cells. The neurons subserving fine discriminative touch are the largest cells in the DRG. Tactile sensation follows several different pathways within the central nervous system. The central processes enter the spinal cord via the medial division of the posterior roots and bifurcate into ascending and descending fibers (Figure 32.4). Fibers carrying fine

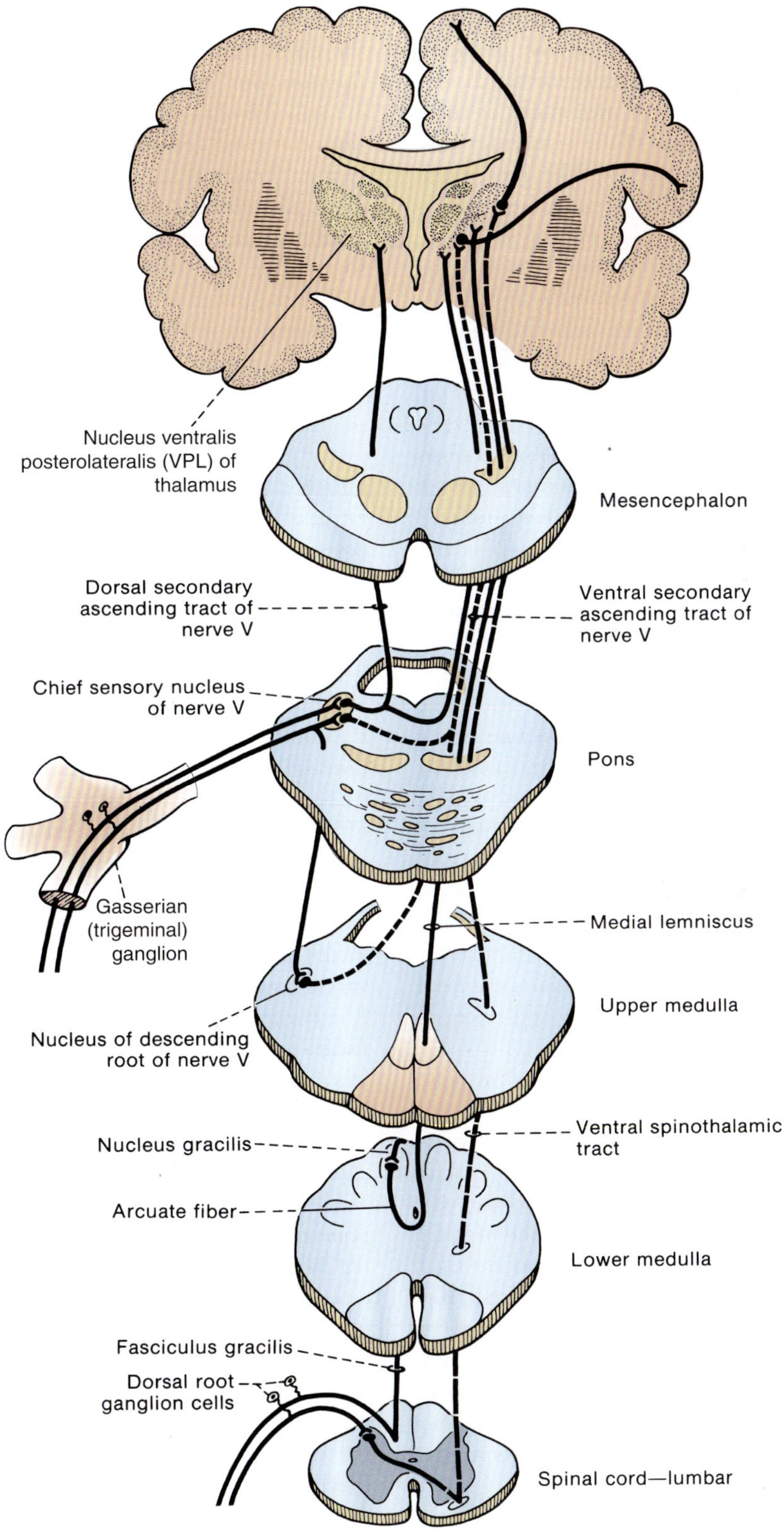

FIGURE 32.4 The tactile pathways.

discriminatory and localized tactile sensibility then, without synapsing, turn upward in the ipsilateral posterior column. Fibers carrying crude touch synapse within several segments of their point of entry, and the axons of the neurons of the next order cross to the opposite ALS. Other tactile fibers have a synapse in the posterior horn and ascend in the dorsolateral funiculus to the lateral cervical nucleus at C1-C2, where axons of the next order neurons decussate and join the ML. In the posterior columns, fibers from the lumbosacral region aggregate near the midline, and fibers from successively more rostral regions aggregate in a progressively more lateral position, producing somatotopic lamination that is the reverse of the STs (Figure 32.3). In the STs, the sacral fibers are most lateral; in the posterior columns, the lowest fibers are most medial. All the fibers below about T8 are grouped together in the fasciculus gracilis; analogous fibers above T8 form the fasciculus cuneatus.

ALS fibers transmit light touch and light pressure sensations, without accurate localization. The posterior column fibers are concerned with highly discriminatory and accurately localized sensibility, including spatial and two-point discrimination. Because of the overlap and duplication of function, and because of the multisynaptic pathways for general tactile sensation, tactile sensibility is the sensory modality least likely to be completely abolished with lesions of the spinal cord, and disturbances of it may fail to give localizing information. A myelopathy severe enough to abolish light touch will often render the patient nonambulatory. However, loss of light touch is common in peripheral neuropathy, and identifying the severity and extent of loss of touch sensation is extremely useful.

Axons in the gracile and cuneate fasciculi synapse with second-order neurons in the gracile and cuneate nuclei at the cervicomedullary junction. The second-order neurons sweep anteriorly as internal arcuate fibers, cross the midline, and accumulate in the ML. Within the medulla, the ML is a vertical band of fibers situated along the median raphe; in the pons, the tract becomes more horizontal and shifts to a ventral position; and in the mesencephalon, the tract migrates to lie far laterally in an oblique position. Somatotopic organization is maintained in the ML. In the medulla, the fibers from the nucleus gracilis lie ventrally and those from the nucleus cuneatus dorsally (homunculus erect). As the ML ascends the brainstem, it moves from a vertical, paramidline position gradually to a horizontal position (homunculus sits, then lies down). In the pons, fibers from the nucleus gracilis lie laterally and those from cuneatus medially. In the midbrain, the fibers from the nucleus gracilis lie dorsolaterally (homunculus in Trendelenburg). The lemniscal fibers are joined by analogous fibers subserving facial sensation that have decussated after synapsing in the trigeminal principal sensory nucleus in the pons. These fibers all terminate in the thalamus, from which the thalamocortical radiations project to the somatosensory cortex. The distribution of the tactile impulses within the thalamic nuclei and their radiation to the parietal cortex in general follow that for pain and temperature impulses.

Clinical Examination

Chapters 32 to 35 discuss sensory examination techniques. Interpretation and sensory localization are covered in Chapter 36.

There are many methods available for evaluating tactile sensation. Light touch can be tested with a wisp of cotton, tissue paper, a feather, a soft brush, light stroking of the hairs, or even using a very light touch of the fingertip. Creating a wisp of cotton on the end of a cotton-tipped applicator stick serves the purpose well. Some appreciation of light touch may be obtained by noting the responses to the blunt end of the stimulus used to test pinprick. More detailed and quantitative evaluation can be accomplished using Semmes-Weinstein filaments, an aesthesiometer, or von Frey hairs. These methods employ filaments of different thicknesses to deliver stimuli of varying, graded intensity.

For routine testing, simple methods using cotton, tissue, or fingertip suffice. It is enough to determine whether the patient recognizes and roughly localizes light touch stimuli and differentiates intensities. The stimulus should not be heavy enough to produce pressure on subcutaneous tissues. Ask the patient to say "now" or "yes" on feeling the stimulus or to name or point to the area stimulated. Allowance must be made for the thicker skin on the palms and soles and the especially sensitive skin in the fossae. Similar stimuli are used for evaluating discriminatory sensory functions such as tactile localization and two-point discrimination. It is best to avoid hairy skin because the sensory stimulation due to hair motion may be confused with the test stimulus; hairy skin is exceptionally sensitive to touch. Two-point discrimination is considered both a delicate tactile modality and a more complex sensation requiring cortical interpretation; it can be reduced in both peripheral and cortical lesions.

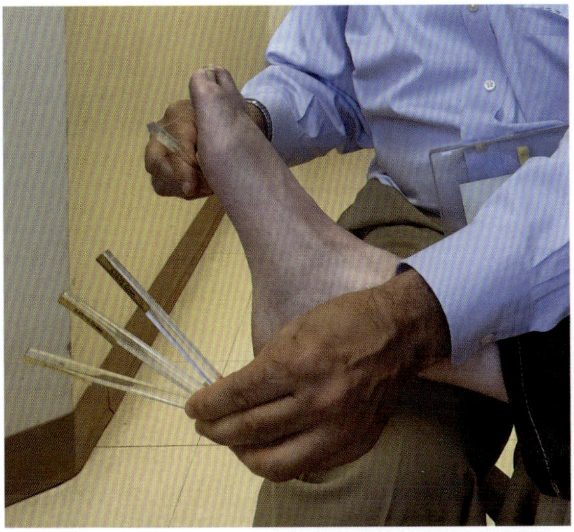

FIGURE 32.5 Examination of protective foot sensation using Semmes-Weinstein monofilaments.

Semmes-Weinstein monofilaments are now used rather than von Frey hairs, after use in leprosy clinics showed that patients who could not detect the 10-g filament on the plantar foot surface were likely to develop ulcers (Figure 32.5). This concept was then used in diabetic neuropathy. Detailed bedside QST is tedious.

Using painless and noninvasive reflectance in vivo confocal microscopy of skin, investigators are able to visualize and quantitate Meissner's corpuscles (MC) in dermal papillae. Comparing the density of MC may prove very useful for noninvasive detection and monitoring of patients with sensory neuropathy. Epidermal nerve fiber layer assessment on skin biopsy has been used to evaluate patients with small fiber neuropathies and is rapidly becoming a useful clinical tool to assess the degree of small fiber loss in patients with normal electrophysiologic studies and the suggestion of predominant small fiber involvement on the neurologic examination. Other detectable changes in neuropathy include distortion of MC structure, focal thinning, or loss of myelin and short myelin internodes.

Web Links

Web Link 32.1. Peripheral nerve sensory distributions. http://www.neuroguide.com/nerveindex.html

BIBLIOGRAPHY

Bourne S, Machado AG, Nagel SJ. Basic anatomy and physiology of pain pathways. *Neurosurg Clin N Am* 2014;25:629–638.

Cohen MS, Wall EJ, Brown RA, et al. 1990 AcroMed Award in basic science. Cauda equina anatomy. II: Extrathecal nerve roots and dorsal root ganglia. *Spine* 1990;15:1248–1251.

Defrin R, Ohry A, Blumen N, et al. Sensory determinants of thermal pain. *Brain* 2002;125:501–510.

Dyck PJ. Enumerating Meissner corpuscles: future gold standard of large fiber sensorimotor polyneuropathy? *Neurology* 2007;69:2116–2118.

Friehs GM, Schrottner O, Pendl G. Evidence for segregated pain and temperature conduction within the spinothalamic tract. *J Neurosurg* 1995;83:8–12.

Fuller G. *Neurological Examination Made Easy*. 5th ed. New York: Churchill Livingstone–Elsevier, 2013.

Garcia-Larrea L. Insights gained into pain processing from patients with focal brain lesions. *Neurosci Lett* 2012;520:188–191.

Garcia-Larrea L. The posterior insular-opercular region and the search of a primary cortex for pain. *Neurophysiol Clin* 2012; 42:299–313.

Gilman S. *Clinical Examination of the Nervous System*. New York: McGraw-Hill, 2000.

Gilman S, Newman SW. *Manter and Gatz's Essentials of Clinical Neuroanatomy and Neurophysiology*. 10th ed. Philadelphia: FA Davis, 2003.

Herrmann DN, Boger JN, Jansen C, et al. In vivo confocal microscopy of Meissner corpuscles as a measure of sensory neuropathy. *Neurology* 2007;69:2121–2127.

Ikoma A, Rukwied R, Stander S, et al. Neurophysiology of pruritus: interaction of itch and pain. *Arch Dermatol* 2003;139:1475–1478.

Kandel ER. *Principles of Neural Science*. 5th ed. New York: McGraw-Hill, 2013.

Kennedy WR, Selim MM, Brink TS, et al. A new device to quantify tactile sensation in neuropathy. *Neurology* 2011;76:1642–1649.

Kiernan JA, Rajakumar N. *Barr's The Human Nervous System: An Anatomical Viewpoint*. 10th ed. Philadelphia: Wolters Kluwer/ Lippincott Williams & Wilkins, 2014.

Kikuchi S, Sato K, Konno S, et al. Anatomic and radiographic study of dorsal root ganglia. *Spine* 1994;19:6–11.

Krumova EK, Geber C, Westermann A, et al. Neuropathic pain: is quantitative sensory testing helpful? *Curr Diab Rep* 2012;12:393–402.

Massey EW, Pleet AB, Scherokman BJ. *Diagnostic Tests in Neurology: A Photographic Guide to Bedside Techniques*. Chicago: Year Book Medical Publishers, Inc., 1985.

McGlone F, Reilly D. The cutaneous sensory system. *Neurosci Biobehav Rev* 2010;34:148–159.

Nathan PW, Smith MC, Cook AW. Sensory effects in man of lesions of the posterior columns and of some other afferent pathways. *Brain* 1986;109:1003–1041.

Nathan PW, Smith M, Deacon P. The crossing of the spinothalamic tract. *Brain* 2001;124:793–803.

Nolano M, Provitera V, Crisci C, et al. Quantification of myelinated endings and mechanoreceptors in human digital skin. *Ann Neurol* 2003;54(2):197–205.

Noseworthy JH, Murray TJ, Lee SHA. Risks of the neurologist's pin. *N Engl J Med* 1979;301:1288.

Posnick JC, Zimbler AG, Grossman JA. Normal cutaneous sensibility of the face. *Plast Reconstr Surg* 1990;86:429–433.

Ropper A, Samuels M, Klein J. *Adams and Victor's Principles of Neurology*. 10th ed. New York: McGraw-Hill Medical, 2014.

Ross RT. *How to Examine the Nervous System*. 4th ed. Totowa: Humana Press, 2006.

Shy ME, Frohman EM, So YT, et al. Quantitative sensory testing: report of the Therapeutics and Technology Assessment Subcommittee of the American Academy of Neurology. *Neurology* 2003;60:898–904.

Siao P, Cros DP. Quantitative sensory testing. *Phys Med Rehabil Clin N Am* 2003;14:261–286.

Standring S, ed. *Gray's Anatomy: The Anatomical Basis of Clinical Practice*. 41st ed. New York: Elsevier Limited, 2016.

Weibers DO, Dale AJD, Kokmen E, et al., eds. *Mayo Clinic Examinations in Neurology*. 7th ed. St. Louis: Mosby, 1998.

Wolf JK. *Segmental Neurology*. Baltimore: University Park Press, 1981.

CHAPTER 33

The Proprioceptive Sensations

The proprioceptive sensations arise from the deeper tissues of the body, principally from the muscles, ligaments, bones, tendons, and joints. Proprioception, or kinesthesia, refers to either the sense of position of a body part or motion of a body part. Proprioception has both a conscious and an unconscious component. The conscious component travels with the fibers subserving fine, discriminative touch; the unconscious component forms the spinocerebellar pathways. The conscious proprioceptive sensations that can be tested clinically are motion, position, vibration, and pressure.

ANATOMY

The primary receptors for proprioception are the muscle spindles. Other peripheral sense organs dealing with proprioception are located in the muscles, tendons, and joints, particularly Pacinian corpuscles. These respond to pressure, tension, stretching or contraction of muscles fibers, joint movement, changes in the position of the body or its parts, and related stimuli. Cutaneous afferents play a contributory role. Proprioceptors are essential for the normal coordination and grading of muscle contraction and the maintenance of equilibrium. Conscious proprioceptive impulses travel along large, myelinated fibers from the periphery to the first-order neuron in the dorsal root ganglion (DRG) and then via the medial division of the posterior root (Figure 32.1). These fibers then enter, without a synapse, the ipsilateral fasciculi gracilis and cuneatus and ascend to the nuclei gracilis and cuneatus in the lower medulla, where a synapse occurs. The spinocervical and dorsal spinocerebellar tracts also convey proprioceptive impulses.

Axons of the second-order neuron decussate as internal arcuate fibers and then ascend in the medial lemniscus (ML) to the thalamus (Figure 33.1). The somatotopic organization in the posterior columns and lemniscal pathways is the same as for light touch (Figure 32.3). Other DRG fibers subserving kinesthesia synapse in the dorsal horn and then ascend in the dorsolateral funiculus to the lateral cervical nucleus, where they join the ML. The thalamoparietal radiations then go through the posterior limb of the internal capsule, and the fibers are distributed to the cortex.

Proprioceptive impulses from the head and neck enter the central nervous system with the cranial nerves. Many terminate on the mesencephalic root of the trigeminal nerve; others accompany motor nerves from the muscles they supply. Impulses probably reach the thalamus through the ML. Recently, the higher cognitive neurophysiology for position sense was described by researchers who were awarded the Nobel prize in Medicine for their work. Grid cells in the medial entorhinal cortex create a neural representation of space, which was popularly referred to as the brain's internal GPS.

SENSES OF MOTION AND POSITION

The sense of motion, also known as the kinetic or kinesthetic sense, or the sensation of active or passive movement, consists of an awareness of motion of various parts of the body. The sense of position, or posture, is awareness of the position of the body or its parts in space. These sensations depend on impulses arising as a result of motion of the joint and of lengthening and shortening of the muscles. Motion and position sense are usually tested together by passively moving a part and noting the patient's appreciation of the movement and recognition of the direction, force, and range of movement; the minimum angle of movement the patient can detect; and the ability to judge the position of the part in space.

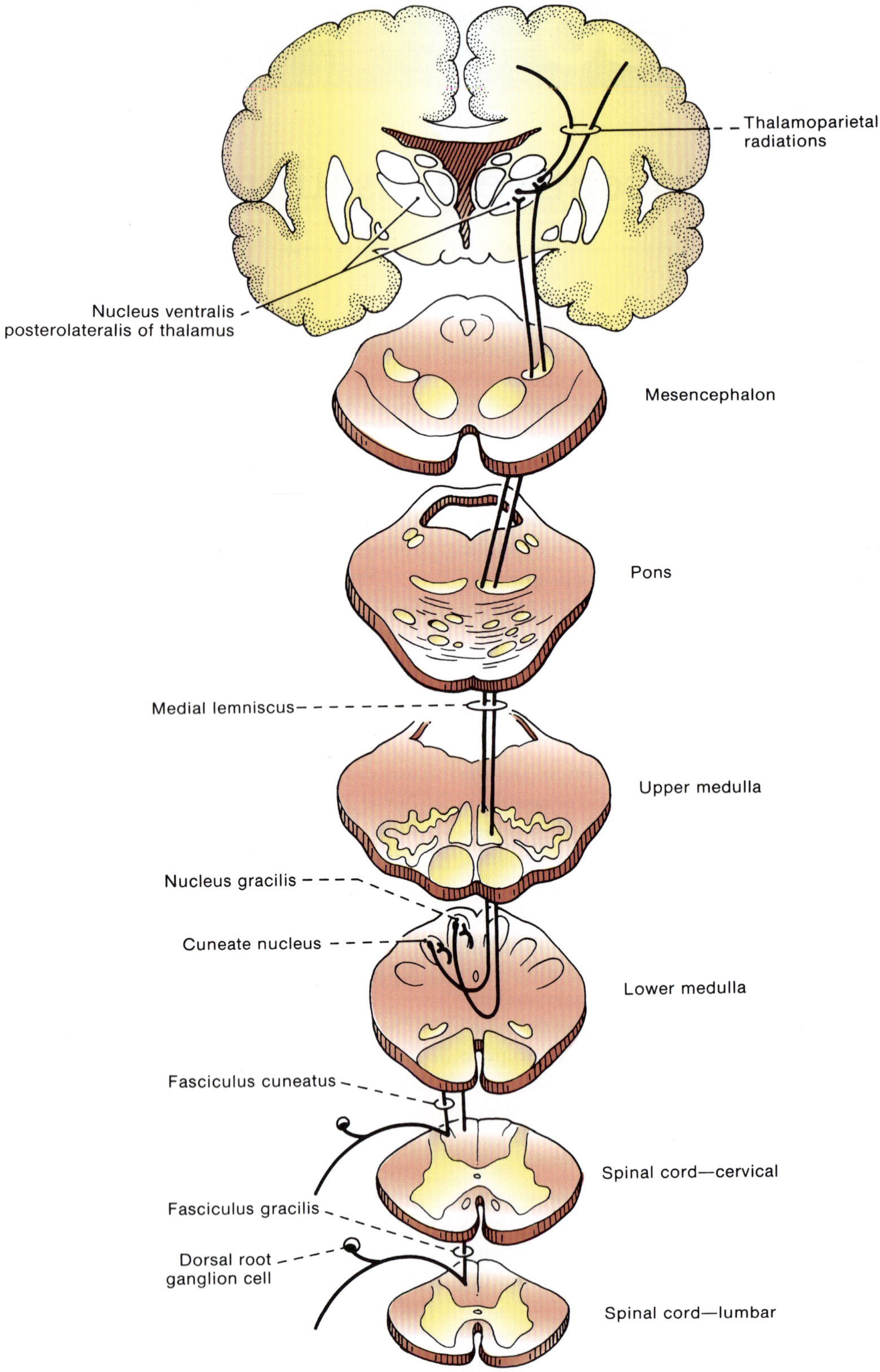

FIGURE 33.1 The pathways for position sense and fine discriminative touch through the posterior columns and medial lemniscus.

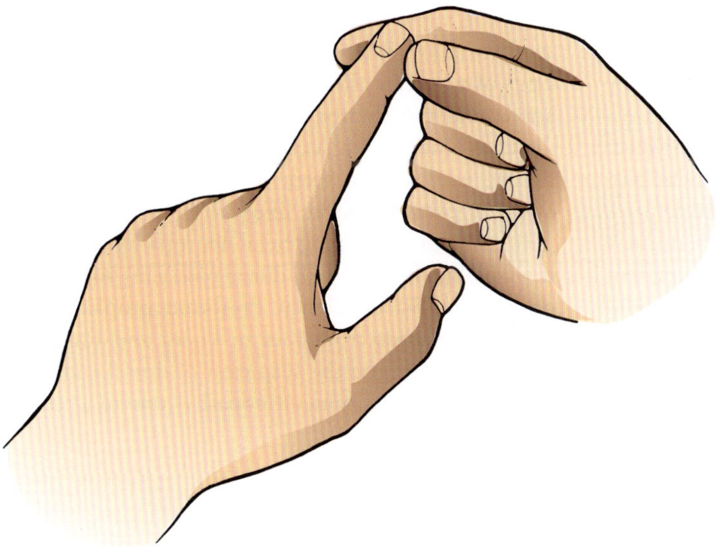

FIGURE 33.2 Method of testing position sense, done similarly with toe.

In the lower extremity, testing usually begins at the metatarsophalangeal joint of the great toe, in the upper extremity at one of the distal interphalangeal joints. If these distal joints are normal, there is no need to test more proximally. Testing is done with the patient's eyes closed. It is extremely helpful to instruct the patient, eyes open, about the responses expected before beginning the testing. No matter the effort, nonsensical replies are frequent. The examiner should hold the patient's completely relaxed digit on the sides, away from the neighboring digits, parallel to the plane of movement, exerting as little pressure as possible to eliminate clues from variations in pressure. If the digit is held dorsoventrally, the grip must be firm and unwavering so that the pressure differential to produce movement provides no directional clue. The patient must relax and not attempt any active movement of the digit that may help to judge its position. The part is then passively moved up or down, and the patient is instructed to indicate the direction of movement from the last position (Figure 33.2). Even when instructed that the response is two alternative, forced choice, up or down, some patients cannot be dissuaded from reporting the absolute position (e.g., down), even if the movement was up from a down position; a surprising number insist on telling the examiner the digit is "straight" when it is moved into that position. It is often useful simply to ask the patient to report when he first detects movement and then move the digit up and down in tiny increments, gradually increasing the excursion until the patient is aware of the motion. Quick movements are more easily detected than very slow ones; attempt to make the excursions over about 1 to 2 seconds. Healthy young individuals can detect great toe movements of about 1 mm, or 2 to 3 degrees; in the fingers, virtually invisible movements, 1 degree or less, at the distal interphalangeal joint are accurately detected. There is some rise in the threshold for movement and position sense with advancing age. To quantitate proprioception at the bedside, move the joint (toe, finger, ankle, etc.) four times and record the proportion of correct responses.

Minimal impairment of position sense causes first loss of the sense of position of the digits, then of motion. In the foot, these sensations are lost in the small toes before they disappear in the great toe; in the hand, involvement of the small finger may precede involvement of the ring, middle, or index finger or thumb. Loss of small movements in the midrange is of dubious significance, especially in an older person. Loss of ability to detect the extremes of motion of the great toe is abnormal at any age. Errors between these two extremes require clinical correlation. If the senses of motion and position are lost in the digits, one should examine more proximal joints, such as ankle, wrist, knee, or elbow. Abnormality at such large joints is invariably accompanied by significant sensory ataxia and other neurologic abnormalities.

Position sense may also be tested by placing the fingers of one of the patient's hands in a certain position (e.g., the "OK" sign) while his eyes are closed and then asking him to describe the position or to imitate it with the other hand. This is sometimes referred to as parietal copy because both parietal lobes (and their connections) must be intact: one side to register the position and the other side to copy it. The foot may be passively moved while the eyes are closed, and the patient asked to point to the great toe or heel. With the hands outstretched and eyes closed, loss of position sense may cause one hand to waver or droop. One of the outstretched hands may be passively raised or lowered, and the patient asked to place the other extremity at the same level. One hand may be passively moved, with eyes closed, and the patient asked to grasp the thumb or forefinger of that hand with the opposite hand. Abnormal performance on these latter tests does not indicate the side of involvement when a unilateral lesion is present.

Loss of position sense may cause involuntary, spontaneous movements (pseudoathetosis, Figure 30.8). Pseudoathetosis can occur because of severe proprioceptive loss in juvenile vitamin E deficiency. Reduction in the ability to perceive the direction of passive skin movement may indicate impairment of position sense superficial to the joint. Such impairment is usually associated with joint-sense deficit as well. The methods available for evaluating the senses of motion and position are all relatively crude, and there may be functional impairment not adequately brought out by the testing procedures.

Normal coordination requires intact proprioceptive sensory function in order to keep the nervous system informed about the moment-to-moment position of the limbs and body in space. Patients with severe proprioceptive deficits (akinesthesia) may have ataxia and incoordination, which closely resembles that seen in cerebellar disease, except that it is much worse when the eyes are closed. The incoordination due to proprioceptive loss is referred to as sensory ataxia. The ataxia and incoordination are significantly influenced by vision. Visual input allows for conscious correction of errors and permits the patient to compensate to some degree for the proprioceptive loss. There may be some degree of incoordination with eyes open, but performance is significantly degraded with eyes closed. The incoordination may be apparent on the tests usually employed for cerebellar function, such as finger to nose and heel to shin. When trying to stand and walk, the patient with sensory ataxia may not be aware of the position of his feet or the posture of his body. He may walk fairly well with eyes open, but with eyes closed, he staggers and may fall. Although the standing posture with eyes open is stable, with eyes closed, there is a tendency to sway and fall. The Romberg test explores for imbalance due to proprioceptive sensory loss. The patient is able to stand with feet together and eyes open but sways or falls with eyes closed; it is one of the earliest signs of posterior column disease. The gait of sensory ataxia and the Romberg sign are discussed in more detail in Chapter 44. A classic disease causing sensory ataxia, now seldom seen, is tabes dorsalis. Sensory ataxia is currently more likely to be encountered in patients with severe peripheral neuropathy (especially if it involves large fibers), dorsal root ganglionopathy, or vitamin B_{12} deficiency. Profound proprioceptive loss that extends from toes to knees and fingers to elbows should raise the suspicion of dorsal root ganglionopathy (sensory neuronopathy) due to a remote effect of cancer.

SENSE OF VIBRATION (PALLESTHESIA)

Vibratory sensation is the ability to perceive the presence of vibration when an oscillating tuning fork is placed over certain bony prominences. For clinical purposes, it can be considered a specific type of sensation, but more probably results from a combination of other sensations. Bone may act largely as a resonator. The receptors for vibratory stimuli are primarily the very rapidly adapting mechanoreceptors such as Pacinian corpuscles, located deep in the skin, subcutaneous tissues, muscles, periosteum, and other deeper structures of the body; and Merkel disk receptors and Meissner corpuscles in the more superficial skin layers. The Merkel disk receptors and Meissner corpuscles respond best to relatively low frequencies and Pacinian corpuscles to higher frequencies. The oscillations of the tuning fork invoke impulses that are coded so that one cycle of the sinusoidal wave produces one action potential. The frequency of action potentials in the afferent nerve fiber signals the vibration frequency. The intensity of vibration is related to the total number of sensory nerve fibers activated.

Impulses are relayed with the proprioceptive and tactile sensations through large, myelinated nerve fibers and enter the spinal cord through the medial division of the posterior root. Vibration had been traditionally considered to ascend the spinal cord with other proprioceptive impulses in the dorsal columns, but likely other pathways are involved, particularly the posterior portion of the lateral funiculus. On entering the spinal cord, some fibers turn upward in the posterior columns. Others bifurcate, sending one branch into the deeper layers of the posterior horn and another into the posterior columns. Axons of the second-order neurons in the posterior horn ascend in the spinocervical tract in the ipsilateral dorsolateral funiculus and terminate in the lateral cervical nucleus. Axons from neurons in the lateral cervical nucleus cross in the anterior commissure and ascend to the medulla where they join the ML. The fibers in the dorsolateral funiculus may be the most important pathway subserving vibratory sensation in man. This divergence of the position sense and vibration sense pathways may partially explain the dissociation occasionally encountered clinically between changes in position sense and vibration sense. In subacute combined degeneration, it is not uncommon for vibration loss to be much worse than position sense loss, conversely for tabes dorsalis. With a parietal lobe lesion, position sense is often impaired and vibration preserved. Thalamocortical fibers from the ventral posterior lateral and the ventral posterior medial nuclei project to the primary somatosensory areas in the postcentral gyrus and terminate on vibration-responsive neurons.

A tuning fork of 128 Hz, with weighted ends, is most frequently used. Sensation may be tested on the great toes, the metatarsal heads, the malleoli, the tibia, anterior superior iliac spine, sacrum, spinous processes of the vertebrae, sternum, clavicle, styloid processes of the radius and ulna, and the finger joints. It is possible to test vibration perceived from the skin by testing on the pads of the fingertips or even on the skin overlying muscle and other tissues. Both the intensity and duration of the vibration perceived depend to a great extent on the force with which the fork is struck and the interval between the time it is set in motion and the time of application. Devices for measuring vibratory sensation quantitatively are commercially available; the primary applicability is in the evaluation and management of patients with peripheral neuropathy. Because of time and expense, quantitative vibratory testing (QVT) is reserved for special situations and routine clinical testing is most often employed.

For clinical testing, the tuning fork is struck and placed on a bony prominence, usually the dorsum of the interphalangeal joint of the great toe initially and held there until the patient no longer feels the vibration. Testing should compare side to side and distal to proximal sensation. If vibration is absent distally, the stimulus is moved proximally to the metatarsophalangeal joints, then the ankle, then the knee, then the iliac spines, and so forth. Upper extremity areas frequently tested include the distal joints of the fingers, the radial and ulnar styloids, the olecranon, and the clavicles. Gradual loss of sensation, such as from toe to ankle to knee, favors a peripheral nerve problem. Uniform loss of vibration beyond a certain point, for example, the iliac crests, favors myelopathy. In some patients with myelopathy, a "vibration level" can be detected by placing the fork on successively more rostral spinous processes.

A frequent problem is failure to adequately instruct the patient in the desired response. The novice examiner strikes the tuning fork, touches it to the patient's great toe, and says, "Do you feel that?" A deceptive problem lies in the definition of "that." A patient with absent vibratory sensation may feel the touch of the handle of the tuning fork, misinterpret it as the "that" inquired about, and respond affirmatively. Thus, very gross defects in vibratory sensibility may be completely missed. Always set the fork in motion, touch it to some presumably normal body part, and tell the patient "this is vibrating or buzzing"; then dampen the tines, reapply the stimulus, and tell the patient "this is just touching," or something similar that clearly differentiates the nature of the two stimuli; and then proceed with the testing with the patient's eyes closed.

With normal vibratory sensation, the patient can feel the fork over the great toe until it has almost stopped vibrating. If vibration is impaired, when the fork is no longer perceptible distally, it is moved to progressively more proximal locations until a level is found that is normal. It is also important to compare pallesthesia at homologous sites on the two sides. Sensing the vibration briefly when moving to one side after vibration has ceased on the other side is not abnormal; it probably has to do with sensory adaptation. Consistent asymmetry of vibratory sensation is abnormal; feeling the vibration for more than 3 to 5 seconds on one side compared to the other is probably abnormal. The most subtle abnormality would be to fail to feel the vibration briefly when moving from the normal to the abnormal side but not vice versa. It is important to include occasional control applications, striking the fork so the patient hears the hum, and then quickly grabbing and damping the tines before applying the handle. The patient who then claims to feel the vibration has not understood the instructions. Occasional peripheral neuropathy patients with constant tingling in the feet may think they feel a vibration even when the fork is silent.

The threshold for vibratory perception is normally somewhat higher in the lower than in the upper extremities. There is progressive loss of vibratory sensibility with advancing age, and the sensation may be entirely absent at the great toes in the elderly. The best control is an approximately age-matched normal, such as the patient's spouse. If patient and examiner are about the same age, the examiner can compare the patient's perception of vibration with his own.

Vibration is a sensitive modality because the nervous system must accurately perceive, transmit, and interpret a rapidly changing stimulus. An early physiologic change due to demyelination is prolongation of the nerve refractory period, which causes an inability of the involved fiber to follow a train of impulses. The ability to follow a train of stimuli is one of the first functions impaired when there is demyelination in the nervous system, either peripheral or central. Testing vibratory sensibility measures this functional ability, and loss of vibratory sensation is a sensitive indicator of dysfunction of the peripheral nervous system or the posterior columns, especially when there is any degree of demyelination.

Vibratory sensation can be quantitated fairly simply by noting where the patient can perceive it and for how long (e.g., "absent at the great toes and first metatarsal heads, present for 5 seconds over the medial malleoli [128 Hz fork]"). If the patient returns having lost vibration over the malleoli, then the condition is progressing. If on follow-up, vibration is present for 12 seconds over the malleoli and can now be perceived for 3 seconds over the metatarsal heads, then the patient is improving.

In a large series of patients, routine clinical testing was compared to QVT. Neuromuscular physicians more often overestimated than underestimated vibratory loss when compared to QVT. The graduated Rydel-Seiffer tuning fork provides a more quantitative assessment of vibratory sensation (Figure 33.3). This method is no more time consuming than routine qualitative vibratory testing, and

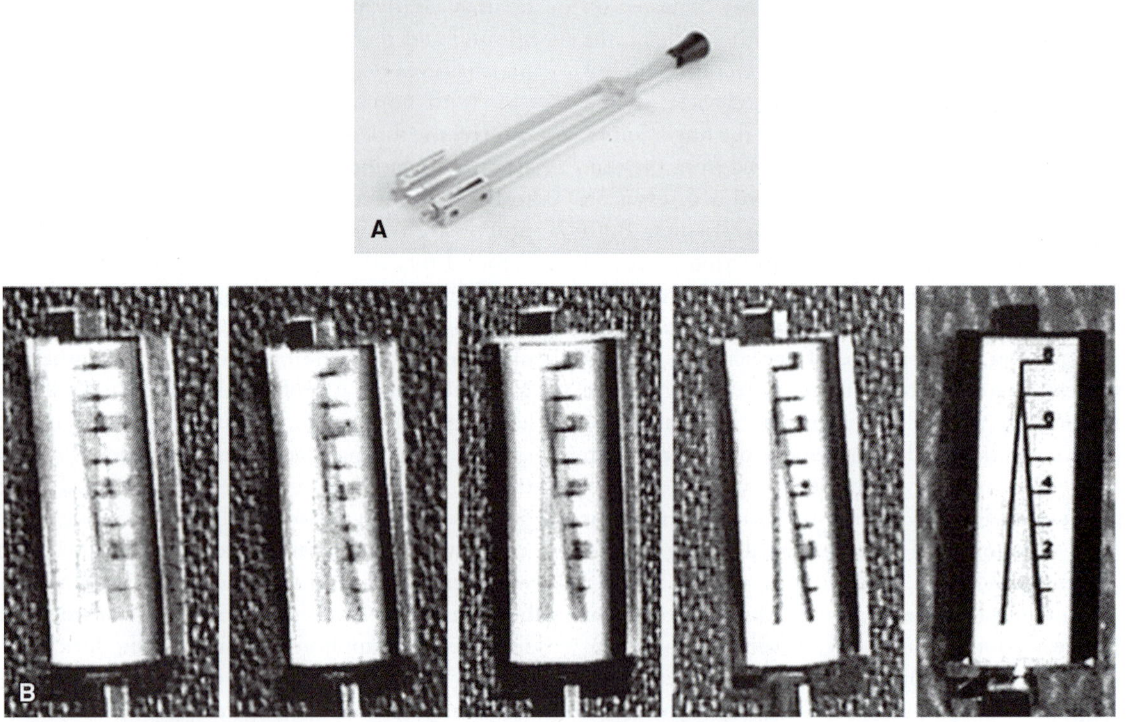

FIGURE 33.3 **A.** Rydel-Seiffer tuning fork. **B.** Fork in motion; arbitrary scale from 0 to 8 at rest (*right*). The intersection of the two virtual *white triangles* moves up from 0 to 8 with decreasing vibration amplitude of the arms (*left* to *right*). (Reprinted from Pestronk A, Florence J, Levine T, et al. Sensory exam with a quantitative tuning fork: rapid, sensitive and predictive of SNAP amplitude. *Neurology* 2004;62[3]:461–464, with permission.)

some have suggested it replace traditional testing (see **Video Link 33.1**). The results correlate with more expensive and time-consuming QVT. In a series of 184 subjects, quantitative vibration testing with the Rydel-Seiffer fork correlated with the amplitude of the sural sensory nerve action potential recorded electrophysiologically.

Vibratory sensation may be impaired or lost in lesions of the peripheral nerves, nerve roots, DRG, posterior columns, and lesions involving the ML and other central connections. In patients with posterior column or peripheral nerve disease, vibratory sensation is lost in the lower extremities much earlier than in the upper. The finding of a normal vibratory threshold in the distal lower extremities usually obviates the need for testing proximally or in the upper extremities, absent specific symptoms involving these areas. A moderate decrease in vibratory perception in the lower extremities or a difference between the lower and the upper extremities may be clinically significant. Marked vibratory loss distally (e.g., the toe), with a transition to normal more proximally (e.g., the knee), is more consistent with peripheral neuropathy. Impaired vibration from posterior column disease is more likely to be uniform at all sites in the involved extremities. Occasionally, in localized spinal cord lesions, a "level" of vibration sensory loss may be found on testing over the spinous processes. Loss of position sense and vibration sense does not always parallel one another, and in some clinical conditions, one is affected much more and much earlier than the other. Because bone is such an efficient resonator, occasional patients with severe deficits to vibration in the distal lower extremities may feel transmitted vibrations in the hip and pelvis. When vibration seems more intact than it should, ask the patient where he feels the sensation.

PRESSURE SENSATION

Pressure or touch-pressure sensation is closely related to tactile sense but involves the perception of pressure from the subcutaneous structures rather than light touch from the skin. It is also closely related to position sense and is mediated via the posterior columns. Pressure sense is tested by a firm touch on the skin or by pressure on deep structures (muscle masses, tendons, nerves), using finger pressure or a blunt object. The patient should both detect and localize the pressure. Strong pressure over muscles, tendons, and nerves tests deep pain sensibility.

DEEP PAIN SENSE OR PRESSURE PAIN

Pain originating from the deeper tissues of the body is more diffuse and less well localized than superficial pain. The pathways for deep pain are the same as for superficial pain. Deep pain may be tested by squeezing muscles, tendons, or the testicles; by pressing on superficial nerves or on the eyeballs; or by pushing a finger interphalangeal joint into extreme, forced hyperflexion. Firm pressure on the base of a nail with a hammer or tuning fork handle also hurts a great deal. Loss of deep pain sensibility is a classic finding in tabes dorsalis, because of involvement of the DRG. The response to superficial or deep pain stimulation may be simply delayed before it is lost. Abadie's sign is the absence of pain on squeezing the Achilles tendon, which is normally quite uncomfortable, Biernacki's sign is the absence of pain on pressure on the ulnar nerve, and Pitres' sign is loss of pain squeezing the testicles; all these are classic signs of tabes dorsalis.

Video Links

Video Link 33.1. The Rydel-Seiffer quantitative tuning fork. http://neurosigns.org/wiki/Vibration_testing_with_the_Rydel-Seiffer_tuning_fork

BIBLIOGRAPHY

Alanazy MH, Alfurayh NA, Almweisheer SN, et al. The conventional tuning fork as a quantitative tool for vibration threshold. *Muscle Nerve* 2017;57(1):49–53.

Allen C. Testing joint-position sense: does it matter how you hold the toe? *Pract Neurol* 2017;17(6):497–498.

Bosco G, Poppele RE. Proprioception from a spinocerebellar perspective. *Physiol Rev* 2001;81:539–568.

Botez SA, Liu G, Logigian E, et al. Is the bedside timed vibration test reliable? *Muscle Nerve* 2009;39:221–223.

Burns TM, Taly A, O'Brien PC, et al. Clinical versus quantitative vibration assessment: improving clinical performance. *J Peripher Nerv Syst* 2002;7:112–117.

Davidoff RA. The dorsal columns. *Neurology* 1989;39:1377.

Dyck PJ. Enumerating Meissner corpuscles: future gold standard of large fiber sensorimotor polyneuropathy? *Neurology* 2007;69:2116–2118.

Findlater SE, Desai JA, Semrau JA, et al. Central perception of position sense involves a distributed neural network—evidence from lesion-behavior analyses. *Cortex* 2016;79:42–56.

Fuller G. *Neurological Examination Made Easy*. 5th ed. Edinburgh: Churchill Livingstone, 2013.

Gilman S. *Clinical Examination of the Nervous System*. New York: McGraw-Hill, 2000.

Gilman S. Joint position sense and vibration sense: anatomical organisation and assessment. *J Neurol Neurosurg Psychiatry* 2002;73:473–477.

Gilman S, Newman SW. *Manter and Gatz's Essentials of Clinical Neuroanatomy and Neurophysiology*. 10th ed. Philadelphia: FA Davis, 2003.

Hilz M, Axelrod FB, Hermann K, et al. Normative values of vibratory perception in 530 children, juveniles and adults aged 3–79 years. *J Neurol Sci* 1998;159:219–225.

Jackson CE, Amato AA, Barohn RJ. Case of the month: isolated vitamin E deficiency. *Muscle Nerve* 1996;19:1161–1165.

Johnson EO, Babis GC, Soultanis KC, et al. Functional neuroanatomy of proprioception. *J Surg Orthop Adv* 2008;17: 159–164.

Kandel ER. *Principles of Neural Science*. 5th ed. New York: McGraw-Hill, 2013.

Kaplan FS, Nixon JE, Reitz M, et al. Age-related changes in proprioception and sensation of joint position. *Acta Orthop Scand* 1985;56:72.

Liniger C, Albeanu A, Bloise D, et al. The tuning fork revisited. *Diabet Med* 1990;7:859–864.

Lockard BI, Kempe LG. Position sense in the lateral funiculus? *Neurol Res* 1988;10:81–86.

Massey EW, Pleet AB, Scherokman BJ. *Diagnostic Tests in Neurology: A Photographic Guide to Bedside Techniques*. Chicago: Year Book Medical Publishers, Inc., 1985.

Moser EI, Moser MB, McNaughton BL. Spatial representation in the hippocampal formation: a history. *Nat Neurosci* 2017;20:1448–1464.

Nathan PW, Smith MC, Cook AW. Sensory effects in man of lesions of the posterior columns and of some other afferent pathways. *Brain* 1986;109:1003.

Panosyan FB, Mountain JM, Reilly MM, et al. Rydel-Seiffer fork revisited: beyond a simple case of black and white. *Neurology* 2016;87:738–740.

Pestronk A, Florence J, Levine T, et al. Sensory exam with a quantitative tuning fork: rapid, sensitive and predictive of SNAP amplitude. *Neurology* 2004;62:461–464.

Peters EW, Bienfait HM, de Visser M, et al. The reliability of assessment of vibration sense. *Acta Neurol Scand* 2003;107: 293–298.

Ross RT. *How to Examine the Nervous System*. 4th ed. Totowa: Humana Press, 2006.

Ross ED, Kirkpatrick JB, Lastimosa AC. Position and vibration sensations: functions of the dorsal spinocerebellar tracts? *Ann Neurol* 1979;5:171–176.

Rowland DC, Roudi Y, Moser MB, et al. Ten years of grid cells. *Annu Rev Neurosci* 2016;39:19–40.

Schwartzman RJ. *Neurologic Examination*. 1st ed. Malden: Blackwell Publishing, 2006.

Standring S, ed. *Gray's Anatomy: The Anatomical Basis of Clinical Practice*. 41st ed. New York: Elsevier Limited, 2016.

Weibers DO, Dale AJD, Kokmen E, et al., eds. *Mayo Clinic Examinations in Neurology*. 7th ed. St. Louis: Mosby, 1998.

Wolf JK. *Segmental Neurology*. Baltimore: University Park Press, 1981.

CHAPTER 34

The Interoceptive, or Visceral, Sensations

Interoceptive sensations are general visceral sensations that arise from the internal organs. The special visceral sensations (smell and taste) are discussed with the cranial nerves. General visceral afferent fibers are found in cranial nerves VII, IX, and X and in the thoracolumbar and sacral autonomic nerves. Visceral afferent fibers run with autonomic efferent fibers to the viscera. Cell bodies are in the dorsal root and associated cranial ganglia; impulses enter the central nervous system through the posterior roots and ascend to higher centers through pathways close to those that carry general somatic afferent impulses.

Visceral afferent fibers are involved with unconscious visceral and autonomic reflexes and also likely convey visceral sensations such as hunger, nausea, sexual excitement, vesical distention, and visceral pain. Afferent impulses from the viscera may reach consciousness by a variety of routes. Some travel in somatic nerves and some with efferent autonomic nerves. Some synapse in the dorsal horn, and axons of the next-order neurons cross to the opposite spinothalamic tract, where the fibers that carry visceral pain lie medial to those that carry superficial pain and temperature sensations. Others may travel in the ipsilateral spinothalamic tract. Many ascend for a great distance in Lissauer's tract before synapsing, and some ascend by long intersegmental fibers in the white matter at the border of the dorsal horn, reaching the hypothalamus and thalamus without decussating. As a consequence of the multiple pathways and redundancy, localization of visceral pain is not precise. The gyms rectus, rather than the parietal cortex, may be the end station for visceral afferent sensation.

In the history, symptoms related to visceral function and conveyed by visceral afferent fibers include such things as gastric fullness and early satiety, gastric discomfort, intestinal spasm, a pressure sensation in the chest, a sensation of fullness in the bladder or rectum, a desire for micturition, a sense of engorgement from the genitalia, or pain in the internal organs.

The viscera are generally insensitive to the usual stimuli that cause pain, but spasm, inflammation, trauma, pressure, distention, or tension on the viscera may produce severe pain, some of which results from involvement of the surrounding tissues. Pain endings are found in the parietal pleura over the thoracic wall and the diaphragm, although probably none are present in the visceral pleura or the lungs. The parietal peritoneum is sensitive, especially to distention, but the visceral peritoneum is probably not sensitive.

Visceral pain is often vaguely localized or diffuse and likely to be described by the patient as deep seated. In addition to the pain experienced in the viscus itself, there may be pain referred to other areas, and the area where the referred pain is felt may be hyperalgesic to stimulation. At times, there may also be tenderness and muscle spasm in the same area. Wide dynamic range (WDR) neurons in the dorsal horn respond both to ordinary somatic sensory input and to noxious stimuli. They respond progressively as stimulus intensity increases. Nociceptive visceral afferents activate the same WDR neurons that respond to somatic sensation.

The convergence of somatic and visceral sensation on the same neuronal population may be one explanation for referred pain. The zones of referred pain and hyperalgesia found in disease of the various viscera are rather poorly localized and vary widely. Referred pain may be felt in the dermatome or skin segment directly over the involved organ as a result of corresponding segmental innervation in the area of cutaneous distribution of the spinal nerves that correspond to the segmental spinal cord level that supplies the viscus, or the pain may be quite distant from the diseased area, as a result of shifting of the viscus during embryonic development. Appendiceal pain is felt directly over the appendix; the pain of angina pectoris may radiate down the left arm; and renal pain is referred to the groin. The phrenic nerve (C3-C5) is sensory as well as motor to the diaphragm and to the contiguous structures—the extrapleural and extraperitoneal connective tissues in the vicinity of the gallbladder and liver. As a consequence, in disease of the gallbladder, liver, or central portion of the diaphragm, there may be pain and hyperesthesia not only in the viscus involved but also on the side of the neck and shoulder in the C3-C5 cutaneous distribution, the area supplied by the posterior roots of those nerves whose anterior roots supply the diaphragm. Other areas of referred visceral pain include midthoracic levels for stomach, duodenum, pancreas, liver, and spleen; upper thoracic levels for the heart; upper and midthoracic levels for the lungs; and low thoracic and upper lumbar levels for the kidney. With some exceptions, the referred pain appears on the same side of the body in which the diseased organ is located.

The anatomy of the pain pathways influences the techniques for surgical management of chronic visceral pain. Because the visceral afferent fibers lie medial in the spinothalamic tracts, a cordotomy to control visceral pain must be carried out with a deeper incision than one for the relief of somatic pain. Also, because the afferent impulses from the viscera ascend for a greater distance before decussating, it must be done at a higher level. Because visceral pain may be carried in both crossed and uncrossed pathways, a cordotomy to control visceral pain may have to be bilateral.

Visceral sensation, although clinically important, cannot be adequately evaluated by the routine neurologic examination. There are special techniques that may give some information, such as tests for the appreciation of the sensations of distention, pain, heat, and cold in the bladder during cystometric examination.

BIBLIOGRAPHY

Gilman S. *Clinical Examination of the Nervous System*. New York: McGraw-Hill, 2000.

Gilman S, Newman SW. *Manter and Gatz's Essentials of Clinical Neuroanatomy and Neurophysiology*. 10th ed. Philadelphia: FA Davis, 2003.

Kandel ER. *Principles of Neural Science*. 5th ed. New York: McGraw-Hill, 2013.

Standring S, ed. *Gray's Anatomy: The Anatomical Basis of Clinical Practice*. 41st ed. New York: Elsevier Limited, 2016.

CHAPTER 35

Cerebral Sensory Functions

Cerebral sensory functions are those that involve the primary sensory areas of the cortex to perceive the stimulus and the sensory association areas to interpret the meaning of the stimulus and place it in context. These functions are also referred to as secondary or cortical modalities. The term combined sensation describes perception that involves integration of information from more than one of the primary modalities for the recognition of the stimulus. Cortical sensory processing is primarily a function of the parietal lobes. The parietal lobe functions to analyze and synthesize the individual varieties of sensation and to correlate the perception of the stimulus with memory of past stimuli that were identical or similar and with knowledge about related stimuli to interpret the stimulus and aid in discrimination and recognition.

The parietal cortex receives, correlates, synthesizes, and refines the primary sensory information. It is not concerned with the cruder sensations, such as recognition of pain and temperature, which are subserved by the thalamus. The cortex is important in the discrimination of the finer or more critical grades of sensation, such as the recognition of intensity, the appreciation of similarities and differences, and the evaluation of the gnostic, or perceiving and recognizing, aspects of sensation. It is also important in localization, in the recognition of spatial relationships and postural sense, in the appreciation of passive movement, and in the recognition of differences in form and weight and of two-dimensional qualities. These elements of sensation are more than simple perceptions, and their recognition requires integration of the various stimuli into concrete concepts as well as calling forth engrams.

Cortical sensory functions are perceptual and discriminative rather than the simple appreciation of information from the stimulation of primary sensory nerve endings. The cortical modalities of greatest clinical relevance include stereognosis, graphesthesia, two-point discrimination, sensory attention, and other gnostic or recognition functions. The loss of these varieties of combined sensation may be considered a variety of agnosia, or the loss of the power to recognize the meaning of sensory stimuli. The primary modalities must be relatively preserved before concluding that a deficit in combined sensation is due to a parietal lobe lesion. Only when the primary sensory modalities are normal can the unilateral failure to identify an object by feel be termed astereognosis and be attributed to a central nervous system lesion. Impairment of primary modalities too slight to account for the recognition difficulty can also properly be termed astereognosis; making this judgment requires experience.

Stereognosis is the perception, understanding, recognition, and identification of the form and nature of objects by touch. Inability to do this is astereognosis. Astereognosis can be diagnosed only if cutaneous and proprioceptive sensations are intact; if these are significantly impaired, the primary impulses cannot reach consciousness for interpretation. There are several steps in object recognition. First, the size is perceived, followed by appreciation of shape in two dimensions, form in three dimensions, and finally identification of the object. These steps may be analyzed individually. Size perception is tested by using objects of the same shape but different sizes, shape perception with objects of simple shape (circle, square, triangle), cut out of stiff paper or plastic, and form perception by using solid geometric objects (cube, pyramid, ball). Finally, recognition is evaluated by having the patient identify only by feel simple objects placed in his hand (e.g., key, button, coin, comb, pencil, safety pin, paper clip). For more refined testing, the patient may be asked to differentiate coins, identify letters carved from wood or fiberboard, or count the number of dots on a domino.

Obviously, stereognosis can be tested only in the hands. If weakness or incoordination prevents the patient from handling the test object, the examiner may rub the patient's fingers over the object. It is striking confirmation of the restricted nature of the deficit in pure motor stroke to demonstrate exquisitely preserved stereognosis in a paralyzed hand. When stereognosis is impaired, there may be a delay in identification or a decrease in the normal exploring movements as the patient manipulates the unknown object. Stereognosis testing normally compares the two hands, and any deficit will be unilateral. Inability to recognize objects by feel with either hand, if the primary modalities are intact, is tactile agnosia. Recognition of texture is a related type of combined sensation in which the patient tries to recognize similarities and differences between objects of varying textures, such as cotton, silk, wool, wood, glass, and metal. Astereognosis is usually accompanied by agraphesthesia and other cortical deficits; it may occur in isolation as the earliest sign of parietal lobe dysfunction.

Graphesthesia (traced figure discrimination, number writing) is the ability to recognize letters or numbers written on the skin with a pencil, dull pin, or similar object. It is a fine, discriminative variety of cutaneous sensation. Testing is often done over the finger pads, palms, or dorsum of the feet. Letters or numbers about 1 cm in height are written on the finger pads, larger elsewhere. Easily identifiable, dissimilar numbers should be used (e.g., 3 and 4 rather than 3 and 8). It really does not seem to matter whether the numbers are written as the patient would "read" them or "upside down," and, despite the temptation, it is not necessary to "erase" between stimuli. Loss of this sensory ability is known as agraphesthesia or graphanesthesia.

Even minimal impairment of primary sensory modalities may cause agraphesthesia. A related function is the ability to tell the direction of movement of a light scratch stimulus drawn for 2 to 3 cm across the skin (tactile movement sense, directional cutaneous kinesthesia), which may be a sensitive indicator of function of the posterior columns and primary somatosensory cortex. Loss of graphesthesia or the sense of tactile movement with intact peripheral sensation implies a cortical lesion, particularly when the loss is unilateral.

Two-point, or spatial, discrimination is the ability to differentiate, with eyes closed, cutaneous stimulation by one point from stimulation by two points. The best instrument for testing is a two-point discriminator designed for the purpose. Commonly used substitutes are electrocardiogram calipers, a compass, or a paper clip bent into a "V," adjusting the two points to different distances. There are two types of two-point discrimination: static and moving. To test static two point, the test instrument is held in place for a few seconds on the site to be tested. To test moving two point on a finger pad, the discriminator would be pulled from the crease of the distal interphalangeal joint toward the tip of the finger over several seconds.

Either one-point or two-point stimuli are delivered randomly, and the minimal distance that can be discerned as two points is determined. Accurate instructions are vital. It is best to start with a two-point stimulus, points relatively far apart ("this is two points"), then a single point ("this is one point"), and then two points close together ("this is two so close it feels like one"). Then one- and two-point stimuli are varied randomly, bringing the points closer and closer until the patient begins to make errors. The result is taken as the minimum distance between two points that can be consistently felt separately. This distance varies considerably in different parts of the body. Normal two-point discrimination is about 1 mm on the tip of the tongue, 2 to 3 mm on the lips, 2 to 4 mm on the fingertips, 4 to 6 mm on the dorsum of the fingers, 8 to 12 mm on the palm, 20 to 30 mm on the back of the hand, and 30 to 40 mm on the dorsum of the foot. Greater separation is necessary for differentiation on the forearm, upper arm, torso, thigh, and leg. The findings on the two sides of the body must always be compared. For moving two point, the technique is the same except the instrument is drawn slowly across the test area. Discrimination for two moving points is slightly better than for two stationary points. Moving two-point tests, the rapidly adapting mechanoreceptors and may have some advantages in the management of patients with peripheral nerve injuries.

Two-point discrimination requires keen tactile sensibility. The pathway is mainly through the posterior columns and medial lemniscus. Loss of two-point discrimination with preservation of other discriminatory tactile and proprioceptive sensation may be the most subtle sign of a lesion of the opposite parietal lobe. Loss of two-point discrimination limited to the distribution of a peripheral nerve or root is helpful in diagnosis and management. Two-point discrimination may also be used to demonstrate a sensory level on the trunk in myelopathy.

Sensory extinction, inattention, or neglect is loss of the ability to perceive two simultaneous sensory stimuli. It is a test of sensory attentional mechanisms rather than somatosensory function. It may occur in isolation with parietal lobe lesions or in company with other deficits of attention to hemispace with more extensive lesions. At its most extreme, there is inattention to all of contralateral hemispace (anosognosia, Chapter 10).

Testing for tactile extinction uses double simultaneous stimuli at homologous sites on the two sides of the body. Light touch is most often used. Extinction occurs when one of the stimuli is not felt. If using pinprick (with equally sharp pins), the stimulus on the abnormal side may feel blunt compared to the normal side. Extinction can also be done on one side, touching the face and hand simultaneously. In general, the more rostral area is the dominant one; when face and hand are stimulated, there is extinction of the hand percept (the face-hand test). It may be normal to extinguish the hand stimulus. The most subtle abnormality is for a hand stimulus on the normal side to extinguish a face stimulus on the abnormal side, but such testing pushes the limit of usefulness of the technique.

Sensory extinction may occur as the only manifestation of a lesion. The severity of extinction can be approximately quantitated by increasing the intensity of the stimulus on the abnormal side. Using one fingertip on the normal side, a patient with mild extinction will extinguish a two-fingertip stimulus on the abnormal side, but a one-fingertip/three-fingertip set will be felt as bilateral stimuli. With severe extinction, it may require a whole hand stimulus or even a firm squeeze on the abnormal side for the patient to appreciate that the stimulation was bilateral. Similar testing can be done with pinprick.

Tactile extinction is most likely to occur with a lesion of the parietal lobe but has been reported with lesions involving the thalamus or sensory radiations. Double simultaneous stimulation above and below the presumed level of a spinal cord lesion in which there is relative but not absolute sensory loss may aid in demonstrating the level of the lesion. If only the upper stimulus is perceived, the lower is moved more rostrally until the intensity of both is equal; this may indicate the segmental level of the lesion.

The ability to localize sensory stimuli also depends on the parietal lobes. To test this function, touch the patient on one side and ask him to point with the opposite index finger to the point touched by the examiner. When testing a hand, the patient should be able to localize the point touched precisely; with other body regions, the accuracy of localization may vary as occurs with two-point discrimination. A right parietal lesion interferes with touch localization on the left side of the body; a left parietal lesion causes localization deficits bilaterally.

Autotopagnosia (somatotopagnosia, body-image agnosia) is inability to identify body parts, orient the body, or understand the relation of individual parts—a defect in the body scheme. The patient may have complete loss of personal identification of one limb or one-half of the body. He may drop his hand from the table onto his lap and believe that some other object has fallen or feel an arm next to his body and not be aware that it is his own. Lack of awareness of one-half of the body is referred to as agnosia of the body half. Finger agnosia is an inability to name or recognize fingers. Finger agnosia occurs most commonly as part of Gerstmann's syndrome (finger agnosia, agraphia, acalculia, and right-left disorientation). Anosognosia is an absence of awareness, or denial of the existence, of disease. It is often used more or less synonymously with somatotopagnosia to refer to patients who deny the existence of hemiplegia or fail to recognize the paralyzed body parts as their own. Anosognosia is most often found in lesions of the right parietal lobe. These disorders are discussed in more detail in Chapter 10.

BIBLIOGRAPHY

Bender MB, Stacy C, Cohen J. Agraphesthesia. A disorder of directional cutaneous kinesthesia or a disorientation in cutaneous space. *J Neurol Sci* 1982;53:531–555.

Dellon AL. The moving two-point discrimination test: clinical evaluation of the quickly adapting fiber/receptor system. *J Hand Surg [Am]* 1978;3:474–481.

Fuller G. *Neurological Examination Made Easy*. 5th ed. Edinburgh: Churchill Livingstone, 2013.

Gardner EP, Sklar BF. Discrimination of the direction of motion on the human hand: a psychophysical study of stimulation parameters. *J Neurophysiol* 1994;71:2414–2429.

Gilman S. *Clinical Examination of the Nervous System*. New York: McGraw-Hill, 2000.

Gilman S, Newman SW. *Manter and Gatz's Essentials of Clinical Neuroanatomy and Neurophysiology*. 10th ed. Philadelphia: FA Davis, 2003.

Hankey GJ, Edis RH. The utility of testing tactile perception of direction of scratch as a sensitive clinical sign of posterior column dysfunction in spinal cord disorders. *J Neurol Neurosurg Psychiatry* 1989;52:395–398.

Hermann RP, Novak CB, Mackinnon SE. Establishing normal values of moving two-point discrimination in children and adolescents. *Dev Med Child Neurol* 1996;38:255–261.

Kandel ER. *Principles of Neural Science.* 5th ed. New York: McGraw-Hill Medical, 2013.

Lundborg G, Rosén B. The two-point discrimination test—time for a re-appraisal? *J Hand Surg Br* 2004;29:418–422.

Massey EW, Pleet AB, Scherokman BJ. *Diagnostic Tests in Neurology: A Photographic Guide to Bedside Techniques.* Chicago: Year Book Medical Publishers, Inc., 1985.

Robertson SL, Jones LA. Tactile sensory impairments and prehensile function in subjects with left-hemisphere cerebral lesions. *Arch Phys Med Rehabil* 1994;75:1108–1117.

Ross RT. *How to Examine the Nervous System.* 4th ed. Totowa: Humana Press, 2006.

Schwartzman RJ. *Neurologic Examination.* 1st ed. Malden: Blackwell Publishing, 2006.

Standring S, ed. *Gray's Anatomy: The Anatomical Basis of Clinical Practice.* 41st ed. New York: Elsevier Limited, 2016.

van Nes SI, Faber CG, Hamers RM, et al. Revising two-point discrimination assessment in normal aging and in patients with polyneuropathies. *J Neurol Neurosurg Psychiatry* 2008; 79:832–834.

Weibers DO, Dale AJD, Kokmen E, et al., eds. *Mayo Clinic Examinations in Neurology.* 7th ed. St. Louis: Mosby, 1998.

Wolf JK. *Segmental Neurology.* Baltimore: University Park Press, 1981.

Wolny T, Linek P, Michalski P. Inter-rater reliability of two-point discrimination in acute stroke patients. *Neurorehabilitation* 2017;41:127–134.

CHAPTER 36

Sensory Localization

Diminution or loss of sensation may occur because of lesions involving the peripheral nerves, nerve roots, spinal cord, brainstem, or higher centers of the brain, as may abnormal sensations, such as pain or paresthesia. Localization depends on the pattern and distribution of the sensory abnormality.

The primary modalities may be impaired because of disease involving peripheral nerve, spinal root, or sensory pathways within the central nervous system (CNS). When the primary modalities are normal in a particular body region, but the cortical modalities are impaired, a parietal lobe lesion may be responsible. When some primary modalities are involved more than others, the sensory loss is said to be "dissociated." The pathways conveying pain and temperature (the spinothalamic tracts) run in a different location than the pathways conveying touch, pressure, position, and vibration (the posterior columns, dorsolateral funiculus, and medial lemniscus). After running divergently through much of their central course, the sensory pathways converge again as they approach the thalamus and remain together in the thalamocortical projections. When the pathways are close together, such as in the peripheral nerve, spinal root, or thalamus, disease processes tend to affect all primary modalities to an approximately equal degree. When the pathways are remote from each other, such as in the spinal cord and brainstem, a disease process may affect one type of sensation and not another, producing dissociated sensory loss. A common example of dissociated sensory loss is lateral medullary stroke, or Wallenberg's syndrome. There is a very characteristic pattern of sensory loss, which only involves pain and temperature and completely spares light touch. The pain and temperature loss involves the ipsilateral face, because of involvement of the spinal tract of cranial nerve V, and the contralateral body, because of damage to the lateral spinothalamic tract, sparing the light touch pathways that are running in the midline in the medial lemniscus. A classic but not common cause of dissociated sensory loss is syringomyelia. The pain and temperature sensory fibers crossing in the anterior commissure are affected; light touch sensory fibers running in the posterior columns are well removed from the site of the pathology and remain intact. As a result, syringomyelia characteristically causes sensory loss to pain and temperature with preservation of light touch. Anterior spinal artery stroke is another example of dissociated sensory loss. The infarction involves the anterior two-thirds of the cord, sparing the posterior columns, which are perfused by the posterior spinal arteries. The patients have dense motor deficits and dense sensory loss to pain and temperature but normal touch, pressure, position, and vibration. Patients with Brown-Séquard syndrome have extreme dissociation of modalities, with loss of pain and temperature on one side of the body and loss of touch, pressure, position, and vibration on the other side of the body.

In contrast, disease processes affecting a peripheral nerve trunk or a spinal root tend to involve all of the sensory fibers traveling in that nerve or root. The sensory loss involves all modalities, but not necessarily to the same degree. Occasionally, generalized polyneuropathies may have a predilection for large or small fibers and can cause some differential involvement of pain and temperature as opposed to touch and pressure. These neuropathies are uncommon and tend to be generalized. When there is marked sensory dissociation affecting one body region, the pathology is virtually always going to be in the CNS, specifically in those regions where the different sensory pathways run in widely divergent locations.

The other consideration in elucidating the cause of sensory loss, in addition to the modalities involved, is the distribution of the abnormality. Deficits in a "hemi" distribution obviously suggest CNS disease, likely involving either the cortex or the thalamus.

Crossed deficits, affecting the face on one side and the body on the opposite side, suggest brainstem disease. Deficits involving both sides of the body below a certain level (e.g., T5) suggest spinal cord disease. A spinal cord level with "sacral sparing" suggests intraparenchymal spinal cord pathology rather than a myelopathy due to external pressure. Deficits due to generalized peripheral nerve disease typically involve the most distal body regions in a "stocking-glove" distribution. Sensory loss due to dysfunction of a peripheral nerve, nerve root, or nerve plexus follows the innervation pattern of that particular structure. Figure 36.1 depicts some of the commonly seen patterns of sensory loss. In hemidistribution sensory loss, there is a certain amount of side-to-side crossing or overlap of innervation along the anterior midline, which is greater on the trunk than on the face. Because of this midline overlap, organic sensory loss usually stops short of the midline, whereas nonorganic sensory loss may "split the midline" (see "Nonorganic Sensory Loss," below). Sacral sensation is not tested as part of a routine neurologic examination. In some instances, sensation in the saddle distribution should be examined (e.g., when a conus medullaris or cauda equina lesion is a possibility; when there is evidence of a myelopathy; or when there is bladder, bowel, or sexual dysfunction).

Sensory function and motor activity are interdependent, and severe motor disabilities may occur because of impaired sensation. This is particularly evident with parietal lobe lesions, but motor dysfunction may also occur with lesions involving the posterior roots, peripheral nerves, posterior columns of

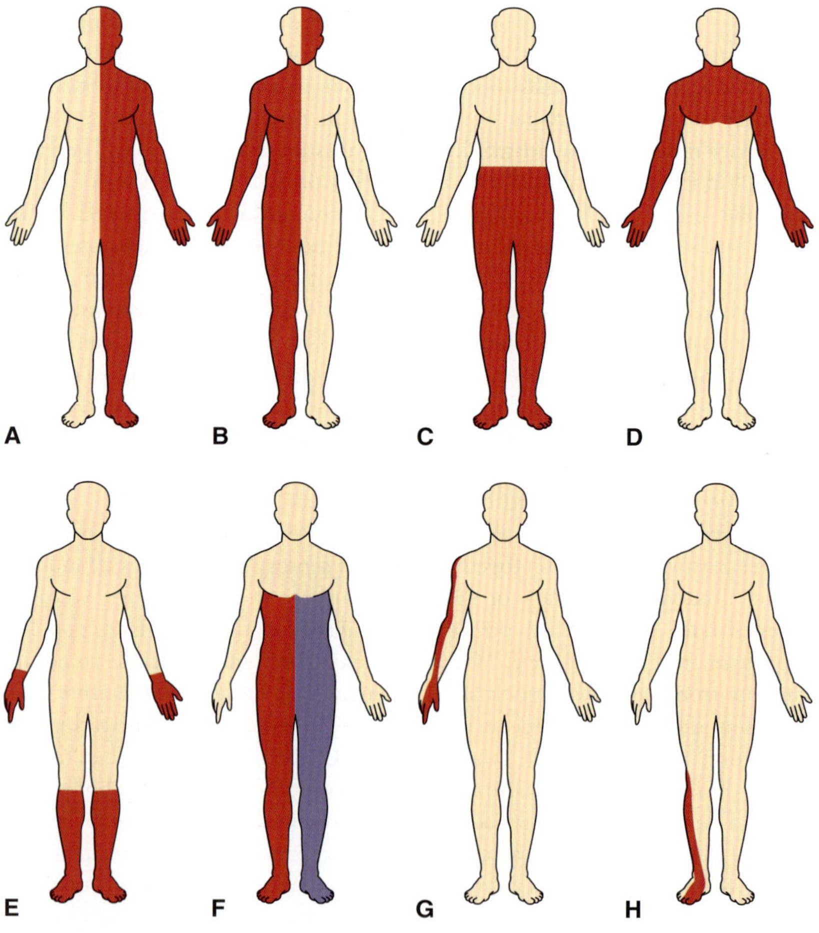

FIGURE 36.1 Some common patterns of sensory loss. **A.** Hemisensory loss due to a hemispheric lesion. **B.** Crossed sensory loss to pain and temperature due to a lateral medullary lesion. **C.** Midthoracic spinal cord level. **D.** Suspended, dissociated sensory loss to pain and temperature due to syringomyelia. **E.** Distal, symmetric sensory loss due to peripheral neuropathy. **F.** Crossed spinothalamic loss on one side with posterior column loss on the opposite side due to Brown-Séquard syndrome. **G.** Dermatomal sensory loss due to cervical radiculopathy. **H.** Dermatomal sensory loss due to lumbosacral radiculopathy.

the spinal cord, or the other central sensory pathways. Conversely, motor dysfunction may affect sensory discrimination. When equal weights are placed in a patient's hands, she may underestimate the weight on the side with cerebellar dysfunction and overestimate it on the side with extrapyramidal dysfunction.

Diminution or perversion of sensation may occur with pathology involving the *sensory receptors*, but this does not often arise in primary neurologic illnesses. Pain and pruritus due to skin irritation, traumatic denudements, and burns may result from abnormalities of the receptors or the nerve filaments to them, and decreased sensation in callosities and scars may result from involvement of the end organs and smaller filaments.

In *focal peripheral neuropathies*, the area of sensory abnormality corresponds to the distribution of the specific involved nerve. The areas of skin supplied by various nerves are shown in Figure 36.2. Within the involved area, all sensory modalities are affected

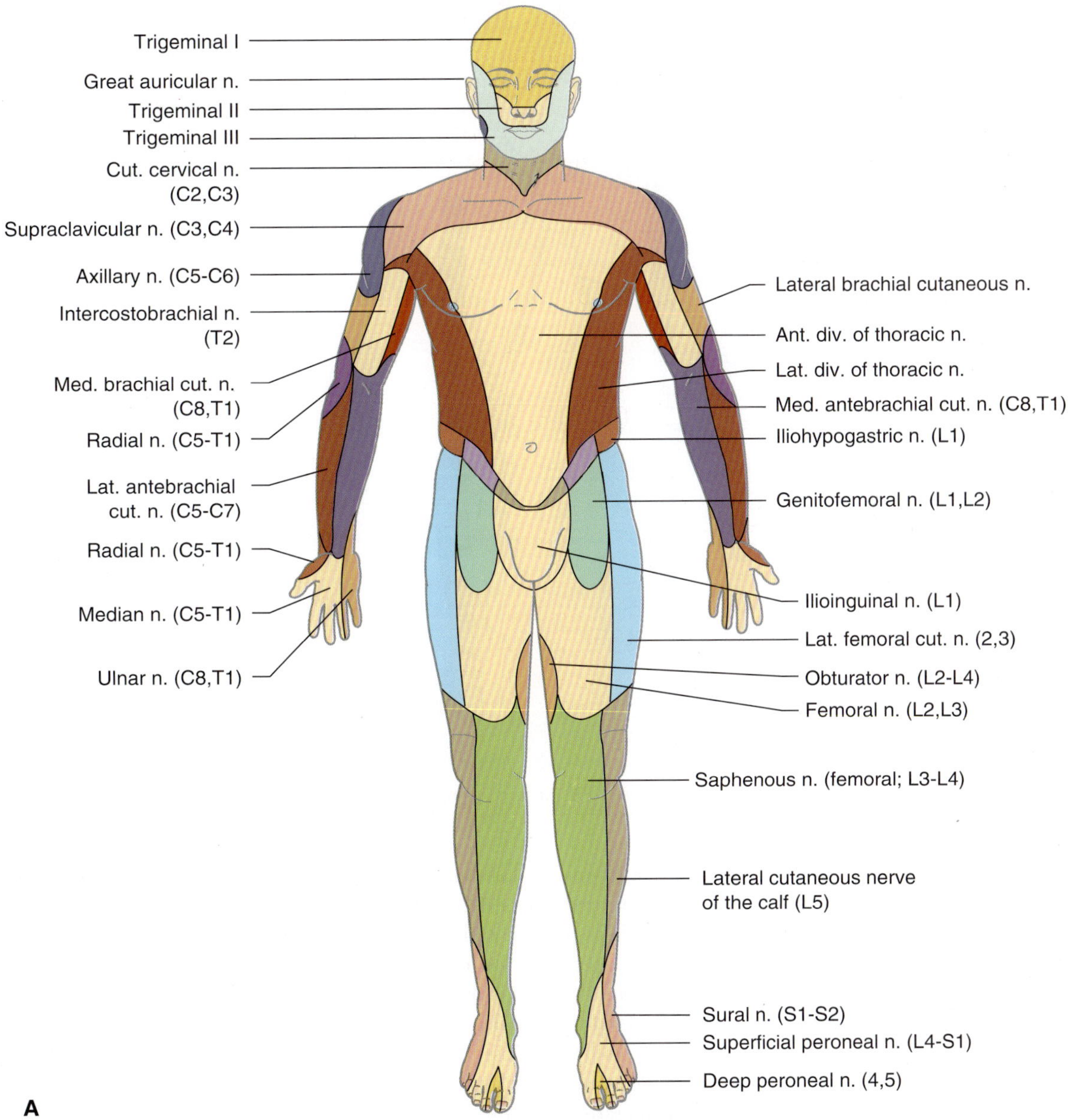

FIGURE 36.2 The cutaneous distribution of the peripheral nerves. **A.** On the anterior aspect of the body.

(continued)

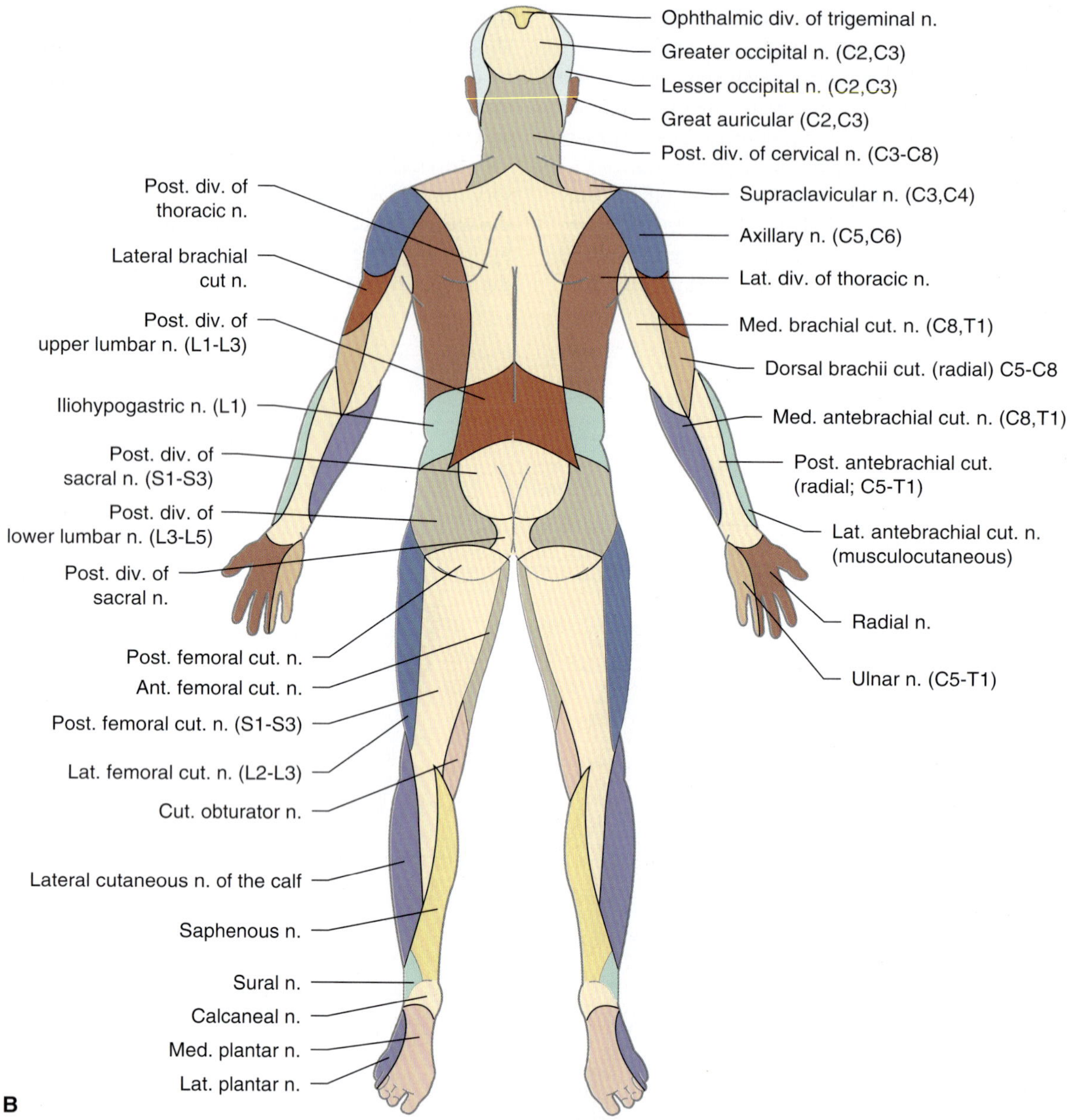

FIGURE 36.2 *(Continued)* **B.** On the posterior aspect of the body.

to a greater or lesser degree. Sensory distributions may vary slightly from individual to individual, and the mapped area may not correspond precisely to a published text or atlas. An excellent source for a pictorial/graphic demonstration of peripheral nerve distributions is http://www.neuroguide.com/nerveindex.html. Figure 36.3 demonstrates some of the variability in the cutaneous supply of the superficial radial nerve.

The demonstrable area of pain and temperature loss is typically smaller than the area of light touch loss, and smaller than the published peripheral nerve or dermatome distributions. The deficit to light touch usually corresponds more closely to a nerve distribution than the pinprick loss. In a patient with a focal nerve or root lesion, it may be possible with careful testing to identify a dense zone of severe sensory loss, corresponding to the area of autonomous supply, surrounded by areas of milder sensory loss in the zone of overlap with adjacent nerves (Figure 36.4). Occasionally, there is spread of sensory loss beyond the

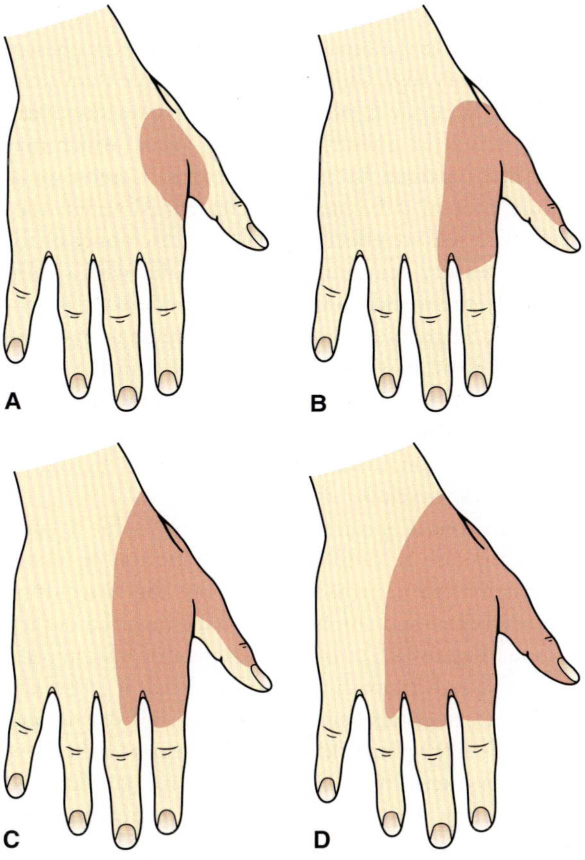

FIGURE 36.3 Variations in the cutaneous distribution of the radial nerve. **A.** Frequent distribution. **B.** Typical distribution. **C.** Frequent distribution. **D.** Anesthesia beyond the usual limit. (Modified from Tinel J. *Nerve Wounds*. Rothwell F [trans]. New York: William Wood & Co., 1917.)

field of an injured nerve. Patients may have allodynia or hyperpathia in the area of sensory loss. The sensory and other neurologic abnormalities associated with lesions of specific nerves are described in Chapter 46. The sensory examination is important in the diagnosis of peripheral nerve injuries and in the evaluation of progress in nerve regeneration. In disorders of the brachial and lumbosacral plexus, sensory loss follows the same principles as in focal neuropathy but is localized to some plexus component, for example, lateral shoulder in upper brachial plexopathy and medial forearm and hand in lower brachial plexopathy.

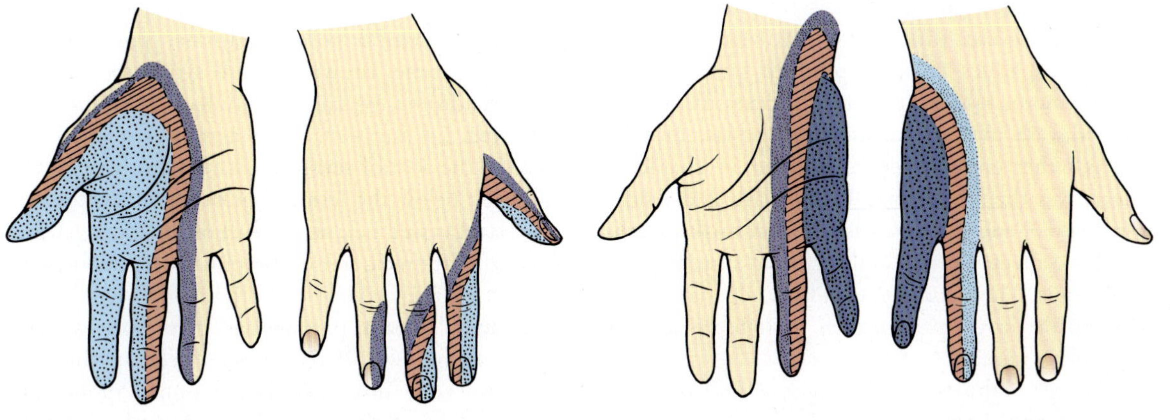

FIGURE 36.4 Transition in sensory changes with lesions of the median and the ulnar nerve. The smallest area is completely anesthetic, the next area has decreased sensation, and the surrounding area has only slight decrease in sensation. (Modified from Tinel J. *Nerve Wounds*. Rothwell F [trans]. New York: William Wood & Co., 1917.)

In *generalized peripheral neuropathies*, vibration is often the first modality affected, but in severe cases, all exteroceptive, proprioceptive, and combined modalities are impaired. Some generalized peripheral neuropathies are purely sensory and some purely motor, but most are sensorimotor. Most axonopathies are length dependent, and the distribution of sensory loss usually involves predominantly the distal segments, causing a stocking-glove distribution of blunted sensation. However, margins of the involved area may be poorly demarcated, with no sharp border between the normal and hypesthetic areas. When severe, length-dependent axonopathies cause sensory loss in a strip over the anterior trunk because of involvement of intercostal nerves (shield or cuirass pattern). Even more severe dying back may cause "beanie cap" sensory loss, or global sensory loss, sparing only a strip in the posterior midline. Leprosy sensory loss may be limited to acral, temperature-dependent regions. Axonopathies produce length-dependent reflex loss; ankle jerks first and then more proximal reflexes disappear as the disease progresses. Demyelinating neuropathies usually cause only slight sensory loss, and the reflexes are lost globally. Rare neuropathies, for example, Tangier's disease and porphyria, have a predilection for short fibers.

Some generalized neuropathies have a predilection to involve predominantly large or small fibers. Large fiber sensory neuropathies include uremia, Sjögren's syndrome, vitamin B_{12} deficiency, certain toxins (pyridoxine, cisplatin, metronidazole), and some cases of diabetes mellitus (pseudotabes). Small fiber neuropathies include amyloidosis, hereditary sensory autonomic neuropathy, and some cases of diabetes mellitus (pseudosyringomyelia). Large fiber neuropathies are typically associated with reflex loss and, when severe, with motor involvement. Small fiber neuropathies typically produce burning pain with no motor loss and preserved reflexes. Peripheral nerve disease may also cause paresthesias, or pain that is either constant or lancinating in character. The nerves themselves may be sensitive and tender to palpation, and there may be pain on brisk stretching of the affected nerves and increased susceptibility to ischemia. There sometimes is hyperalgesia or allodynia in the involved area, even though the sensory threshold is raised.

Disease of the *dorsal root ganglia* (*DRG*), or corresponding cranial nerve ganglia, is also associated with sensory changes. The sensory neurons of the DRG may be affected by autoimmune processes, causing degeneration and inflammation of the neurons. Patients have the subacute onset of pain, paresthesias, and sensory loss, which affects large more than small fibers. Strength is preserved, but reflexes disappear. There is often a disabling sensory ataxia, which may be accompanied by pseudoathetosis. Cerebrospinal fluid protein is frequently increased. Although classically a remote effect of small cell carcinoma of the lung, sensory neuronopathy is associated with a number of other conditions, including pyridoxine intoxication, Sjögren's syndrome, and lymphoma. In herpes zoster, there is severe, lancinating pain in the distribution of the affected ganglia. The now rare tabes dorsalis causes impairment of deep and superficial pain sensation. Transient, spontaneous "lightning" pains may develop.

Lesions of the *nerve root*, most often due to compression, are accompanied by diminution or loss of sensation, pain, or paresthesias, but the distribution is segmental and corresponds to the involved dermatome (Figure 36.5). As with focal neuropathy, in compressive radiculopathy, the touch deficit is larger and often corresponds better to the published dermatome than does the pinprick deficit. Pain may be either constant or intermittent and is often sharp, stabbing, and lancinating. It is increased by movement, coughing, or straining. There may be either hypalgesia or hyperalgesia. Examination may disclose root compression signs (see Chapter 47). Because of dermatome overlap, sensory changes may be difficult to demonstrate if only one root is involved.

With lesions of the *spinal cord* and *brainstem*, impairment of one or more modalities of sensation, or perversions of sensation in the form of either pain or paresthesias, may develop. Different sensory patterns may occur with myelopathy, for example, transverse syndrome, central cord syndrome, posterior column syndrome, Brown-Séquard syndrome, anterior cord syndrome, or conus medullaris syndrome (see Chapters 24 and 47). With a transverse cord syndrome, the area of sensory involvement may involve all levels below the lesion, but occasionally, the sensory level is well below the level of the lesion. A false localizing thoracic sensory level has been reported in lesions of the cervical spine and brainstem. Band-like radicular pain, paresthesias, or sensory loss may occur at the level of the lesion. Sacral sparing may be seen with intramedullary lesions. Spondylotic compression of the cervical spinal cord may cause glove-distribution sensory loss in the hands. Sensory loss is usually dissociated, with impairment of certain modalities and sparing of others. Because of the redundancy of the touch pathways, pain and temperature testing may be more useful than tactile sensation in evaluating CNS disease. Testing for the ability to detect the direction of skin movement above and below the level of the lesion and searching for a vibratory level may be helpful. Suspended dissociated sensory loss occurs in syringomyelia.

Lesions high in the cervical spinal cord and in the medulla may impair kinesthetic sensation in the upper extremities more than in the lower. As a result of the disturbance of proprioceptive sensations and a raised threshold for cutaneous senses, there may be stereoanesthesia, a term occasionally used when the difficulty results from infracerebral lesions, which is difficult to differentiate from astereognosis. Extinction and even autotopagnosia may be present with such lesions. Patients with pontine, medullary, or spinal cord lesions occasionally experience "central" pain. Lhermitte's sign, sudden electric-like or painful sensations spreading down the body or into the back or extremities on flexion of the neck due to involvement of the posterior columns, may occur with focal lesions of the cervical cord, multiple sclerosis, or other degenerative processes.

The pattern of sensory return with recovering spinal lesions is variable; the impairment may recede downward in a segmental manner; the return may start in the sacral distribution and ascend; or there may be a gradual recovery of function over the entire affected area. Pressure sensation returns first, and its recovery is usually the most complete, followed, in turn, by tactile, pain, cold, and heat sensibilities.

Sensory impulses that enter consciousness for interpretation by the parietal cortex must first pass through the *thalamus*. The thalamus is thought to be the end station for pain, heat, cold, and heavy contact, where sensory impulses produce a crude, uncritical form of perception. Thalamic lesions usually cause impairment of all sensory modalities on the opposite

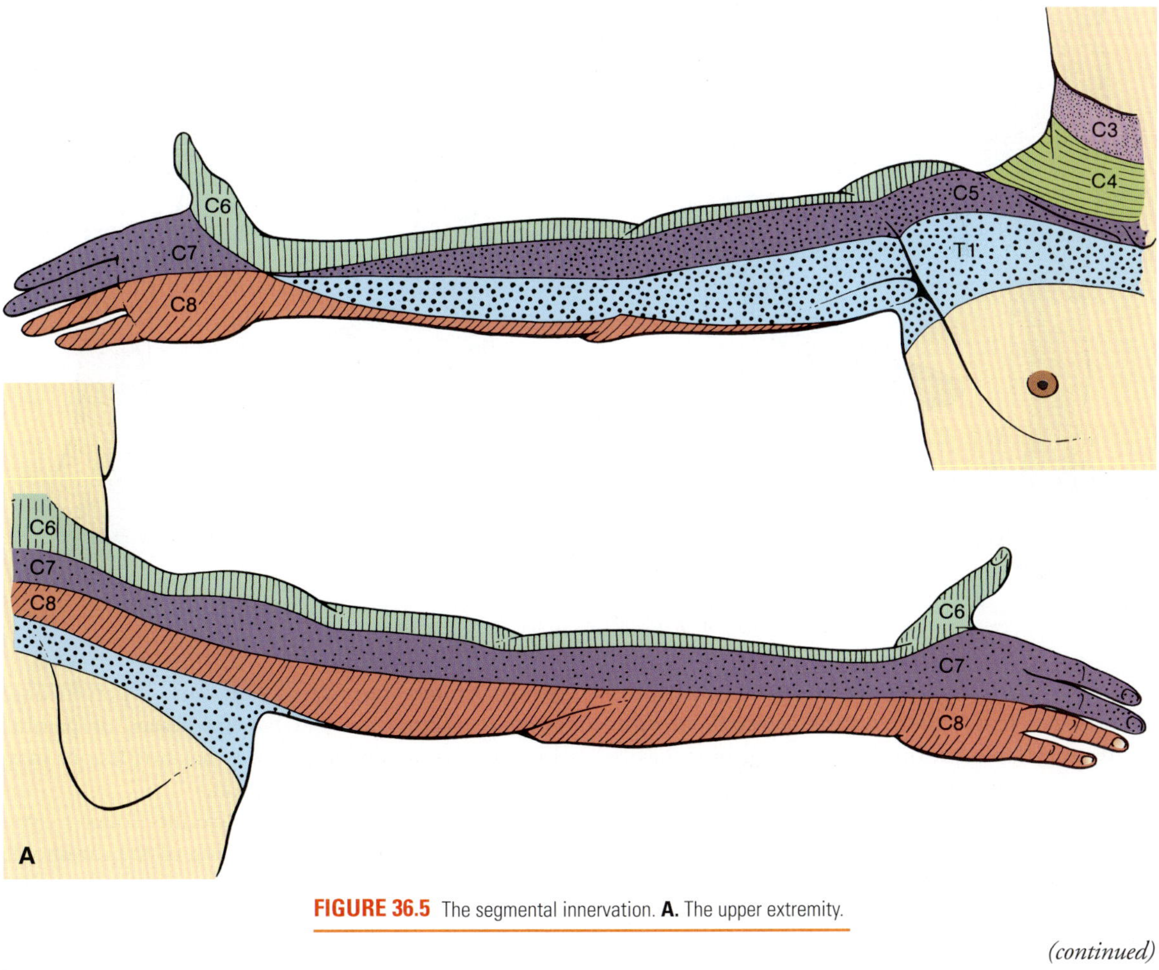

FIGURE 36.5 The segmental innervation. **A.** The upper extremity.

(continued)

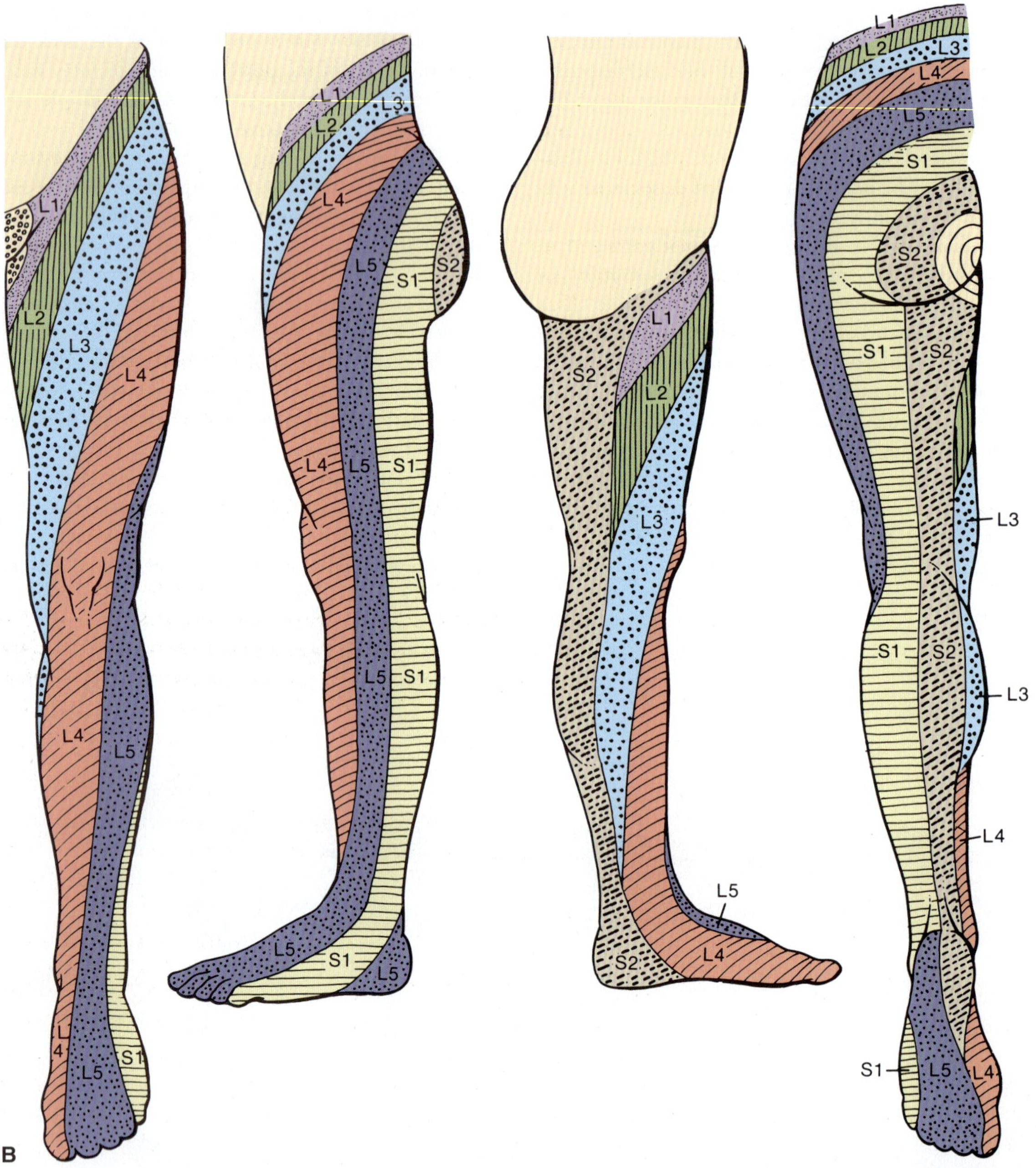

FIGURE 36.5 *(Continued)* **B.** The lower extremity.

side of the body. Small lesions limited to the ventral posterior lateral nucleus may cause paresthesias without demonstrable sensory loss. Severe and extensive lesions may cause gross impairment of all forms of sensation. Marked loss of appreciation of heavy contact, posture, passive movement, and deep pressure perception occurs, and the thresholds for light touch, pain, and temperature sensations are raised. Thalamic lesions are often associated with sensory perversions, such as paresthesias and hyperesthesias, or painful hyperpathia or allodynia. Some thalamic lesions may blunt cold but not heat sensation.

In the thalamic pain (Dejerine-Roussy) syndrome, there is blunting, or raising of the threshold, of all forms of sensation on the opposite side of the body, without complete anesthesia. The latency to

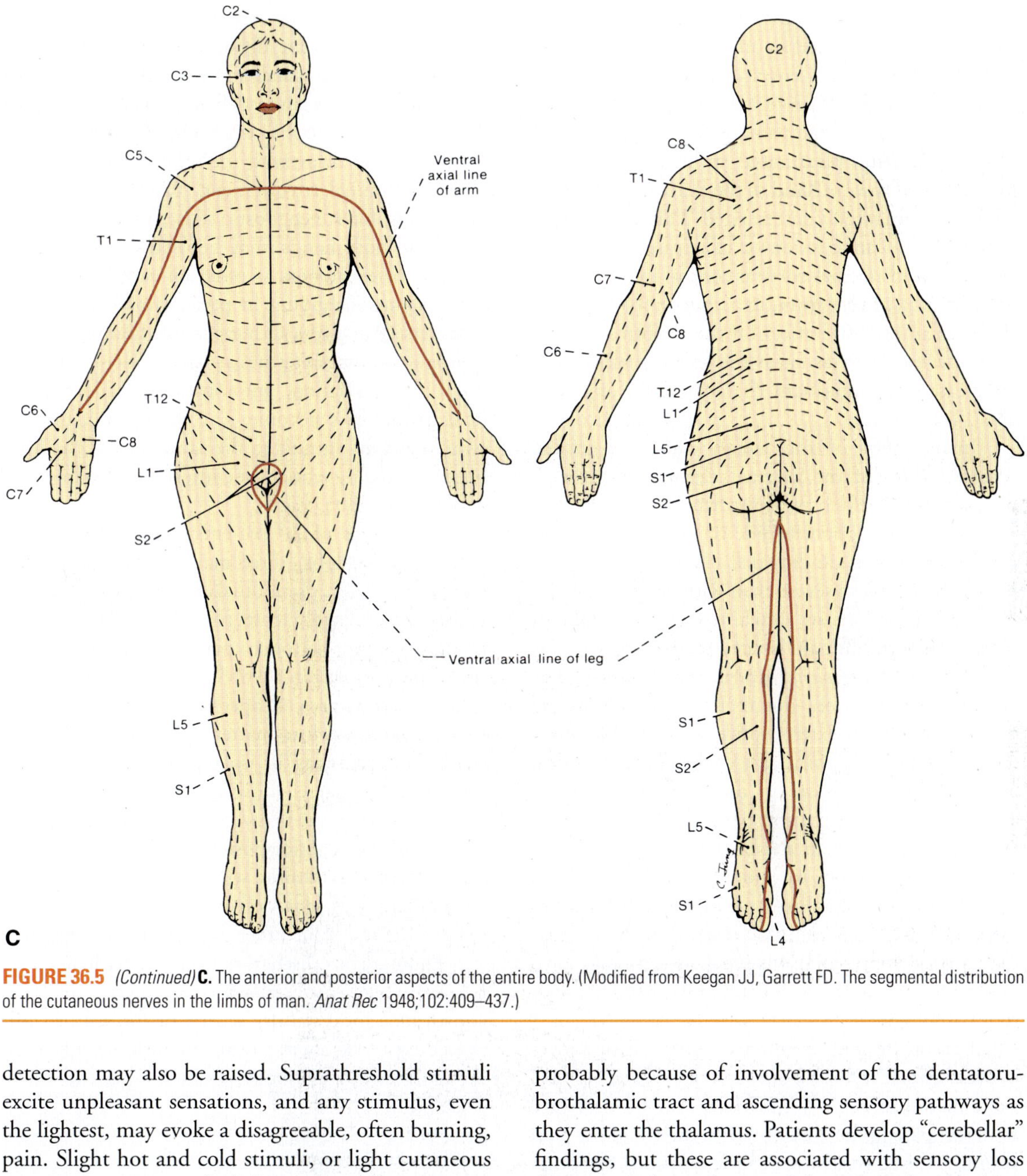

FIGURE 36.5 *(Continued)* **C.** The anterior and posterior aspects of the entire body. (Modified from Keegan JJ, Garrett FD. The segmental distribution of the cutaneous nerves in the limbs of man. *Anat Rec* 1948;102:409–437.)

detection may also be raised. Suprathreshold stimuli excite unpleasant sensations, and any stimulus, even the lightest, may evoke a disagreeable, often burning, pain. Slight hot and cold stimuli, or light cutaneous sensations, cause marked discomfort. The overreaction is termed hyperpathia, hyperalgesia, or allodynia depending on the stimulus. Impairment of sensation accompanied by intractable pain in the hypesthetic regions is called anesthesia dolorosa. In addition to the sensory changes, hemiparesis and hemianopia usually occur and, less frequently, hemiataxia, choreoathetosis, and unmotivated emotional responses. Thalamic ataxia refers to the incoordination that may develop because of a lesion involving the thalamus, probably because of involvement of the dentatorubrothalamic tract and ascending sensory pathways as they enter the thalamus. Patients develop "cerebellar" findings, but these are associated with sensory loss (hemiataxia-hypesthesia syndrome) and sometimes pain. In addition to ataxia and tremor, thalamic lesions may cause dystonia, myoclonus, and chorea. When these involve the hand, the condition is referred to as "thalamic hand" (see **Video Link 36.1**).

Pain of central origin is most often associated with thalamic lesions but may occasionally result from involvement of other central pain pathways. The posterior insula and adjacent medial operculum is an important receiving area for the spinothalamic system and has been proposed as a third somatosensory region (S3) devoted to processing spinothalamic inputs (Chapter 32). Central pain due to a parietal opercular lesion has been termed the pseudothalamic syndrome or parasylvian pain.

Occasionally, pleasurable stimulation, such as application of a warm hand to the skin on the affected side, may be markedly accentuated. This overreaction is due to a thalamic lesion or to release of thalamic function from normal cortical control by damage to higher centers. Every stimulus acting on the thalamus produces an excessive effect on the abnormal half of the body, especially as far as the affective element—the pleasant or unpleasant character in its appreciation—is concerned.

Involvement of the *sensory radiations* in the posterior limb of the internal capsule causes variable, sometimes extensive, impairment of all types of sensation on the opposite side of the body. Because the sensory fibers are crowded closely together, the sensory loss is more severe than with isolated cortical lesions. The changes are similar to those that follow a thalamic lesion, but pain is rare.

Lesions of the *parietal cortex* rarely cause complete loss of sensation, but there is a raising of the threshold for both exteroceptive and proprioceptive sensations of the opposite side of the body. Sensation is often disturbed more in the upper than in the lower extremity. The distal parts of the extremities are affected more than the proximal portions, with a gradual transition to more normal perception approaching the shoulder and hip. Involvement of the hand and face is common because of their extensive cortical representation. Small lesions may produce restricted deficits simulating peripheral nerve or root pathology.

Parietal lesions primarily cause disturbances in discriminatory sensation. Detailed and critical examination of sensory functions may be necessary to detect parietal lobe lesions. The threshold for pain stimuli is raised very little in parietal lesions, although a prick may feel less sharp than on the normal side; with deeper lesions, the threshold is more definitely raised. Qualitative appreciation of heat and cold are present, but there is loss of discrimination for slight variations in temperature, especially in the intermediate ranges. Light touch perception is little disturbed, but tactile discrimination and localization may be profoundly affected. There often is severe impairment of position sense resulting in sensory ataxia and pseudoathetosis, but vibratory sensation is only rarely affected (another instance where vibration and position sense loss are dissociated). Astereognosis is common, but both small and large objects may have to be used to detect the deficit; sometimes, a delay in answering when objects are placed in the affected hand, with no delay with the other hand, may be a clue to minimal involvement. Bilateral simultaneous testing for stereognostic sense, placing identical objects in both hands, may be useful. Sensory inattention, or extinction, is often an early and important diagnostic finding in parietal lobe lesions (see Chapters 10 and 35). Other possible findings include abarognosis, agraphesthesia, impairment of two-point discrimination, autotopagnosia, anosognosia, or Gerstmann's syndrome. The ability to distinguish two cutaneous stimuli to the same side of the body but separated by a brief time interval is also impaired with parietal lobe lesions.

In a series of 20 patients with stroke limited to the parietal lobe, three main sensory syndromes were found: (a) a pseudothalamic sensory syndrome consisting of faciobrachiocrural impairment of elementary sensation (touch, pain, temperature, vibration) due to a lesion involving the inferior-anterior parietal cortex, parietal operculum, posterior insula, and underlying white matter; (b) a cortical sensory syndrome consisting of isolated loss of discriminative sensation (stereognosis, graphesthesia, position sense) involving one or two parts of the body due to a lesion of the superior-posterior parietal cortex; and (c) an atypical syndrome with sensory loss involving all modalities of sensation in a partial distribution, likely a variant of the other two sensory syndromes.

Spontaneous discharges from the parietal cortex frequently cause contralateral paresthesias that may constitute a focal sensory seizure or the sensory aura preceding a jacksonian motor convulsion. Only rarely do spontaneous discharges from the parietal cortex cause pain.

NONORGANIC (FUNCTIONAL) SENSORY LOSS

One of the obvious clues that sensory loss is nonorganic is failure to follow any sort of anatomical distribution. The demarcation between normal and abnormal often occurs at some strategic anatomical point that has no neurologic significance, such as a joint or skin crease, causing a finding such as numbness circumferentially below the elbow, wrist, shoulder, ankle, or knee. Functional facial sensory loss often stops at the hairline and the angle of the jaw, a nonanatomic distribution. A real spinal sensory level on the trunk slants downward from back to front, but a psychogenic level may be perfectly horizontal; nonorganic sensory loss may be much different on the front and back.

The term stocking glove is used to describe both nonorganic sensory loss and peripheral neuropathy. The key to understanding this confusing usage is the type of stocking. When sensory loss due to length-dependent peripheral neuropathy extends to about the level of the knees, it appears in the hands, causing loss in a glove-knee sock distribution; with nonorganic sensory loss, the impairment may be distal to the wrists and ankles: a glove-ankle sock distribution.

With functional sensory loss, the border between normal and abnormal is usually abrupt and well demarcated, more discrete than in organic sensory loss, and may vary from examination to examination, or even from minute to minute. Responses are typically inconsistent. In spite of complete loss of cutaneous sensibility, the patient may have intact stereognosis and graphesthesia, or in spite of complete loss of position sense may be able to perform skilled movements and fine acts without difficulty and have no Romberg sign. On finger-to-nose testing, the examiner may touch one finger of the "anesthetic" hand and ask the patient to touch her nose with it. A patient with organic exteroceptive sensory loss will not know which finger was touched; a patient with functional sensory loss uses the correct finger but has trouble finding the nose. The hand wandering widely before eventually finding the nose suggests histrionic tendencies. In the search test, the patient holds the involved hand in the air and searches for it with the unaffected hand. In nonorganic loss, the patient may have no difficulty with this task, but with bona fide proprioceptive loss, performance is poor with either hand.

Sensory changes along the midline may provide useful clues. On the trunk, organic sensory loss typically stops short of midline because of the overlap from the opposite side and splitting of the midline suggests nonorganicity. With psychogenic sensory loss, the change may take place abruptly at the midline or even beyond it. This finding is not reliable on the face because there is less midline overlap on the face, so organic facial sensory loss may extend to the midline. With functional hemianesthesia, the midline change may include the penis, vagina, and rectum, a finding rare with organic lesions. There may even be midline splitting of vibration, so that the patient claims to perceive a difference in the intensity of vibration when the fork is placed just to right or left of the midline over the mandible, skull, sternum, or symphysis pubis, each a single bony structure, or comparing the medial ends of the clavicles or the medial incisor teeth. In all these locations, the vibration is transmitted to both sides, and patients with organic hemianesthesia do not perceive any difference in vibration along the midline. The reliability of this sign has not been validated; it can be misleading. Other signs reportedly suggestive of nonorganicity include a dissociation between pinprick and temperature, variability from trial to trial, history of hypochondriasis, secondary gain, nonanatomical sensory loss, and changing boundaries of hypalgesia.

Clinical subterfuge is often used to establish that sensory loss is nonorganic, such as asking the patient to respond "Yes if you feel it, no if you don't" (yes-no or touch-no touch test). It is often possible to confuse the patient and confirm the absence of organic changes by checking sensation while the hands are in some bewildering position where it is difficult to tell which side is which, such as crossed behind the back or rotated with fingers interlocked (Bowlus-Currier test; Figure 36.6).

The authors have seen all of these "tricks" fail (i.e., indicate the sensory loss is not real when it is), at one time or another, save one: the SHOT syndrome. In the SHOT syndrome, the patient claims to have no Sight in the eye, no Hearing in the ear, no Olfaction in the nose, and no Touch sensation on the body, all on the same side. This pattern is of course utterly impossible on an anatomic basis, and its presence reliably indicates that hemibody numbness is nonorganic.

Techniques to prove a deficit is psychogenic have held a cherished place in neurology since the days of Charcot. But many of the examination techniques touted as proof of nonorganicity are fallible, particularly for sensory findings. Most of the history and examination findings purported as helpful in separating functional and organic deficits have not been studied. The attitude of la belle indifference is not of value in discriminating real from nonorganic disease. Either things such as apparent secondary gain, nonanatomic deficits, and variability of findings on examination have not been studied or investigations have shown they are neither sensitive nor specific for functional disorders. A study of 30 consecutive neurology service admissions with acute structural nervous system damage were evaluated for the

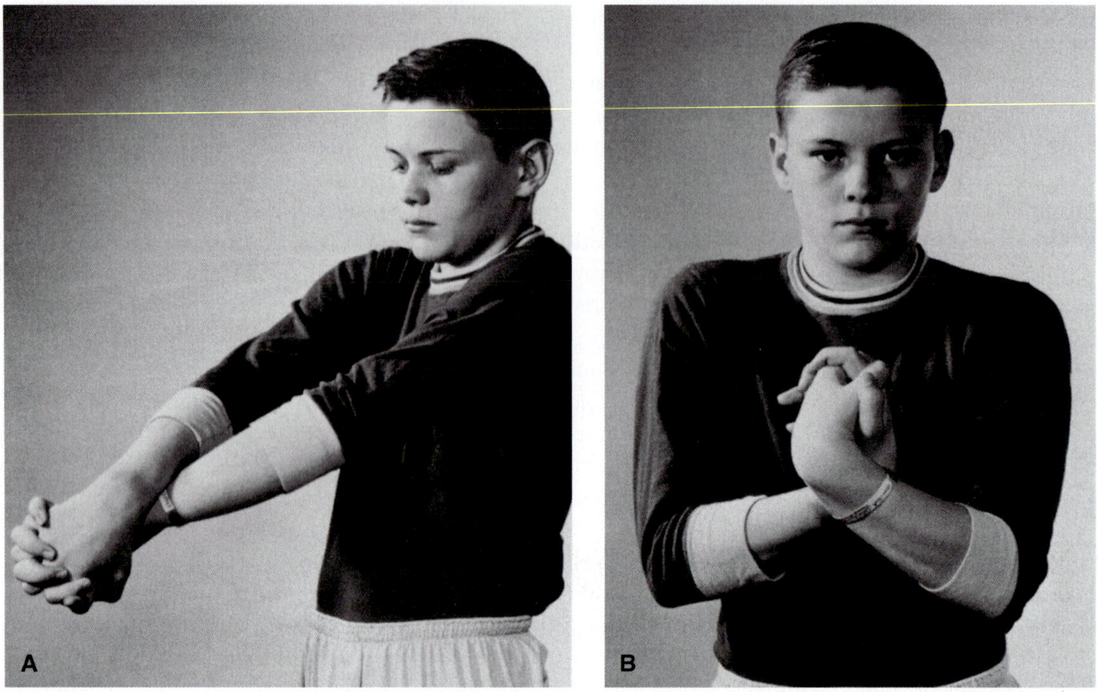

FIGURE 36.6 A and B. Maneuver used in testing for hysterical hemianesthesia.

presence of seven of the most accepted features of nonorganicity: history of hypochondriasis, secondary gain, la belle indifference, nonanatomical sensory loss, midline splitting of pain or vibration, changing boundaries of hypalgesia, and giveaway weakness. All subjects showed at least one of these findings, and most had three or four. Of these patients, 29 had at least one "nonphysiologic" sensory finding on examination, including 23% with nonanatomical sensory loss and 70% with midline splitting.

Video Links

Video Link 36.1. Thalamic hand. http://neurosigns.org/wiki/Thalamic_hand

BIBLIOGRAPHY

Adams KK, Jackson CE, Rauch RA, et al. Cervical myelopathy with false localizing sensory levels. *Arch Neurol* 1996;53:1155–1158.

Bassetti C, Bogousslavsky J, Regli F. Sensory syndromes in parietal stroke. *Neurology* 1993;43:1942–1949.

Bogousslavsky J, Regli F, Uske A. Thalamic infarcts: clinical syndromes, etiology, and prognosis. *Neurology* 1988;38:837–848.

Booij HA, Hamburger HL, Jöbsis GJ, et al. Stroke mimicking conversion disorder: two young women who put our feet back on the ground. *Pract Neurol* 2012;12:179–181.

Bowlus WE, Currier RD. A test for hysterical hemianalgesia. *N Engl J Med* 1963;269:1253–1254.

Bowsher D, Leijon G, Thuomas KA. Central poststroke pain: correlation of MRI with clinical pain characteristics and sensory abnormalities. *Neurology* 1998;51:1352–1358.

Brazis PW, Masdeu JC, Biller J. *Localization in Clinical Neurology*. 7th ed. Philadelphia: Wolters Kluwer/Lippincott Williams & Wilkins, 2017.

Crimlisk HL, Bhatia K, Cope H, et al. Slater revisited: 6 year follow up study of patients with medically unexplained motor symptoms. *Br Med J* 1998;316:582–586.

Deleu D, Lagopoulos M, Louon A. Thalamic hand dystonia: an MRI anatomoclinical study. *Acta Neurol Belg* 2000;100:237–241.

Espay AJ, Aybek S, Carson A, et al. Current concepts in diagnosis and treatment of functional neurological disorders. *JAMA Neurol* 2018;75(9):1132–1141.

Fisher CM. Pure sensory stroke and allied conditions. *Stroke* 1982;13:434–447.

Fuller G. *Neurological Examination Made Easy*. 5th ed. Edinburgh: Churchill Livingstone, 2013.

Garcia-Larrea L. The posterior insular-opercular region and the search of a primary cortex for pain. *Neurophysiol Clin* 2012;42:299–313.

Ghika J, Bogousslavsky J, Henderson J, et al. The "jerky dystonic unsteady hand": a delayed motor syndrome in posterior thalamic infarctions. *J Neurol* 1994;241:537–542.

Gilman S. *Clinical Examination of the Nervous System*. New York: McGraw-Hill, 2000.

Gilman S, Newman SW. *Manter and Gatz's Essentials of Clinical Neuroanatomy and Neurophysiology*. 10th ed. Philadelphia: FA Davis, 2003.

Gould R, Miller BL, Goldberg MA, et al. The validity of hysterical signs and symptoms. *J Nerv Ment Dis* 1986;174:593–597.

Gutrecht JA, Zamani AA, Slagado ED. Anatomic-radiologic basis of Lhermitte's sign in multiple sclerosis. *Arch Neurol* 1993;50:849–851.

Hellmann MA, Djaldetti R, Luckman J, et al. Thoracic sensory level as a false localizing sign in cervical spinal cord and brain lesions. *Clin Neurol Neurosurg* 2013;115:54–56.

Kandel ER. *Principles of Neural Science.* 5th ed. New York: McGraw-Hill Medical, 2013.

Kim JS. Pure sensory stroke. Clinical-radiological correlates of 21 cases. *Stroke* 1992;23:983–987.

Kim JH, Greenspan JD, Coghill RC, et al. Lesions limited to the human thalamic principal somatosensory nucleus (ventral caudal) are associated with loss of cold sensations and central pain. *J Neurosci* 2007;27:4995–5004.

Lanska DJ. Functional weakness and sensory loss. *Semin Neurol* 2006;26:297–309.

Lempert T, Dieterich M, Huppert D, et al. Psychogenic disorders in neurology: frequency and clinical spectrum. *Acta Neurol Scand* 1990;82:335–340.

Mace CJ, Trimble MR. Ten-year prognosis of conversion disorder. *Br J Psychiatry* 1996;169:282–288.

Massey EW, Pleet AB, Scherokman BJ. *Diagnostic Tests in Neurology: A Photographic Guide to Bedside Techniques.* Chicago: Year Book Medical Publishers, Inc., 1985.

Matsumoto S, Okuda B, Imai T. A sensory level on the trunk in lower lateral brainstem lesions. *Neurology* 1988;38:1515–1519.

Mauguière F, Desmedt JE. Thalamic pain syndrome of Dejérine-Roussy. Differentiation of four subtypes assisted by somatosensory evoked potentials data. *Arch Neurol* 1988;45:1312–1320.

Ochiai H, Yamakawa Y, Minato S, et al. Clinical features of the localized girdle sensation of mid-trunk (false localizing sign) appeared in cervical compressive myelopathy patients. *J Neurol* 2002;249:549–553.

Paciaroni M, Bogousslavsky J. Pure sensory syndromes in thalamic stroke. *Eur Neurol* 1998;39:211–217.

Rafael H. False localizing signs in upper cervical spinal cord compression. *Neurosurgery* 1997;40:217–218.

Ross RT. Dissociated loss of vibration, joint position and discriminatory tactile senses in disease of spinal cord and brain. *Can J Neurol Sci* 1991;18:312–320.

Ross RT. *How to Examine the Nervous System.* 4th ed. Totowa: Humana Press, 2006.

Schmahmann JD, Leifer D. Parietal pseudothalamic pain syndrome. Clinical features and anatomic correlates. *Arch Neurol* 1992;49:1032–1037.

Schwartzman RJ. *Neurologic Examination.* 1st ed. Malden: Blackwell Publishing, 2006.

Simmons Z, Biller J, Beck DW, et al. Painless compressive cervical myelopathy with false localizing sensory findings. *Spine (Phila Pa 1976)* 1986;11:869–872.

Slater ET, Glithero E. A follow-up of patients diagnosed as suffering from "hysteria". *J Psychosom Res* 1965;9:9–13.

Sonstein WJ, LaSala PA, Michelsen WJ, et al. False localizing signs in upper cervical spinal cord compression. *Neurosurgery* 1996;38(3):445–448.

Standring S, ed. *Gray's Anatomy: The Anatomical Basis of Clinical Practice.* 41st ed. New York: Elsevier Limited, 2016.

Stone J, Smyth R, Carson A, et al. La belle indifference in conversion symptoms and hysteria: systematic review. *Br J Psychiatry* 2006;188:204–209.

Stone J, Reuber M, Carson A. Functional symptoms in neurology: mimics and chameleons. *Pract Neurol* 2013;13:104–113.

Stone J, Vermeulen M. Functional sensory symptoms. *Handb Clin Neurol* 2016;139:271–281.

Voskuhl RR, Hinton RC. Sensory impairment in the hands secondary to spondylotic compression of the cervical spinal cord. *Arch Neurol* 1990;47:309–311.

Weibers DO, Dale AJD, Kokmen E, et al., eds. *Mayo Clinic Examinations in Neurology.* 7th ed. St. Louis: Mosby, 1998.

Wolf JK. *Segmental Neurology.* Baltimore: University Park Press, 1981.

SECTION G The Reflexes

CHAPTER 37

Introduction to the Reflexes

The reflex examination is important for several reasons. Reflex changes may be the earliest and most subtle indication of a disturbance in neurologic function. The testing of reflexes is the most objective part of the neurologic examination. Reflexes are under voluntary control to a lesser extent than most other parts of the neurologic examination, and reflex abnormalities are difficult to simulate. They are not as dependent on the attention, cooperation, or intelligence of the patient and can be evaluated in patients who cannot or will not cooperate with other parts of the examination. In such circumstances, the integrity of the motor and sensory systems can sometimes be appraised more adequately by the reflex examination than by other means. Although the reflex examination is an essential component, it is only one part of the neurologic examination and must be evaluated in the context of the other findings.

A reflex is an involuntary response to a sensory stimulus. Afferent impulses arising in a sensory organ produce a response in an effector organ. There are segmental and suprasegmental components. The segmental component is a local reflex center in the spinal cord or brainstem and its afferent and efferent connections. The suprasegmental component is made up of the descending central pathways that control, modulate, and regulate the segmental activity. Disease of the suprasegmental pathways may increase the activity of some reflexes, decrease the activity of others, and cause reflexes to appear that are not normally seen. A reflex response may be motor, sensory, or autonomic.

The stimulus is received by the receptor, which may be a sensory ending in the skin, mucous membranes, muscle, tendon, or periosteum, or, in special types of reflexes, in the retina, cochlea, vestibular apparatus, olfactory mucosa, gustatory bulbs, or viscera. Receptor stimulation initiates an impulse that travels along the afferent pathway to the central nervous system (CNS), where there is a synapse in a reflex center that activates the cell body of the efferent neuron. The efferent neuron transmits the impulse to the effector: the cell, muscle, gland, or blood vessel that then responds. A disturbance in function of part of the reflex arc—the receptor, afferent limb, reflex center, efferent limb, or effector apparatus—will disrupt the reflex arc, causing a decrease or loss of the reflex.

Most reflexes investigated clinically are more complex than the primitive reflex response just described. All parts of the nervous system are intimately connected; it is rare for one part to react without affecting or being affected by other parts. Almost immediately on entering the CNS, the afferent fiber sends collaterals to cells at higher and lower levels on the same and opposite side. Activation of an agonist muscle group is accompanied by inhibition of the antagonist muscle group (Sherrington's law of reciprocal innervation); when the extensors of a limb are contracted, the flexors are relaxed. Association pathways may carry the impulse to the cerebral cortex for either reflex or voluntary modification of the response. Complex reflexes involve connections between various segments on the same and opposite sides of the spinal cord, brainstem, and brain. The more complex the reflex, the greater the number of associated neurons and mechanisms involved. Stronger stimuli cause the excitation of a greater number of neurons: the phenomenon of irradiation.

Reflex activity is essential to normal functioning. Nociceptive reflexes help avoid injurious stimuli. Reflex activity is important in maintaining the body in its daily environment, in sustaining an upright position, in standing and walking, and in moving the extremities. It is an integral part of the response to visual, gustatory, auditory, and vestibular stimulation, and it is important in visceral functions.

Reflexes have been named in various ways: according to the site of elicitation, the body part stimulated, the muscles involved, the part of the body that responds, the ensuing movements, the joint acted on, or the nerve involved. Many carry the names of one or more individuals who are said to have first described them. Hundreds of reflexes have been identified. Because many are not clinically important and it is impractical to test all the reflexes routinely, only those more important for clinical diagnosis will be described. The majority of these are muscle responses. Reflex abnormalities due to disease involving the descending motor pathways are often clinically referred to as upper motor neuron, corticospinal, or pyramidal signs, but the abnormalities likely result from dysfunction of related motor pathways rather than the corticospinal tract proper (see Chapter 25).

CHAPTER 38

The Deep Tendon or Muscle Stretch Reflexes

When a normal muscle is passively stretched, its fibers resist the stretch by contracting. The stretch may be caused by gravity, manipulation, or other stimuli. In reflex responses, the contraction results from stimulation of the sensory organs in the muscle, either directly or indirectly through a stimulus applied to its tendons, the bone to which it is attached, or the overlying skin. In the monosynaptic stretch reflex, sudden lengthening stretches the muscle spindles, which send impulses via the primary spindle afferents into the spinal cord. The spindle afferents synapse directly, without participation of any interneuron, on the alpha motor neurons innervating the muscle, causing a reflex contraction of the muscle (Figure 32.1). This sequence of lengthening, contraction, and then relaxation is a stretch (tendon, deep tendon, muscle stretch, myotatic, or proprioceptive) reflex. Some muscles react more strongly than do others.

Stretch reflexes serve a protective function, particularly in standing and walking; they help to counter any sudden unexpected forces. Because of their critical roles in maintaining an erect posture, the extensor muscles of the legs, quadriceps, and calf muscles have better developed stretch reflexes than do the flexors. This important physiology is exploited clinically by applying an artificial stretch by striking the tendon of the muscle with a reflex hammer.

Reflexes elicited by application of a stretch stimulus to either tendons or periosteum or occasionally to bones, joints, fascia, or aponeurotic structures are usually referred to as muscle stretch or deep tendon reflexes (DTRs). The reflex is caused by sudden muscle stretch brought about by percussion of its tendon. Occasionally, the tendon is stretched by percussing a structure to which it is attached, as in the jaw jerk. The term deep helps separate these reflexes from the superficial or cutaneous reflexes, which are quite different.

Some authorities criticize the term deep tendon reflex, contending it implies the receptor is in the tendon, which is of course inaccurate. This link between the term and the location of the receptor is in the mind and opinion of the critic. Erb introduced the term tendon reflex in 1875 when he and Westphal published papers addressing the subject in the same issue of the same journal. In 1885, Gowers recommended the term be discarded. So, for over 100 years, it has been fashionable to rail against the term DTR. It is difficult to pick up a text on the neurologic examination without encountering at least a barb if not a screed on this point. In fact, the term DTR is in much wider use than muscle stretch reflex (MSR). Many more physicians are familiar with the acronym DTR than with MSR. Most physicians encountering the abbreviation MSR would think it was some Chinese cooking spice, but nearly everyone recognizes DTR, neurologist and nonneurologist alike. Gowers offered the term myotatic (Gr. myo, "muscle" + tatic "to stretch"), but many neurologists, not to mention other physicians, would pause and puzzle over this formal, obfuscatory term. For both pragmatic and antipedantic reasons, the abbreviation DTR is preferred in this text.

The primary problem areas in eliciting DTRs are poor tools and poor technique. These reflexes are best tested using a high-quality rubber percussion hammer. To properly obtain a reflex, a crisp blow must be delivered to quickly stretch the tendon. A heavy, high-quality reflex hammer is immensely helpful for this task, but many physicians use the cheapest hammer they can find, usually poor, pitiable, and inferior instruments.

A genuine, high-quality, purchased Taylor is the lowest level of acceptable hammer, and these are often inadequate in the hands of novices. A variety of good hammers are available at reasonable prices. Other objects are sometimes used, and it seems a point of honor among some physicians to use anything but a reflex hammer. They substitute fingers, the edge of a stethoscope, or anything else handy, sometimes to the point of absurdity. The reliability of such a reflex examination mirrors the effort put into using a proper instrument. A soft rubber hammer is most desirable. A blow with an ancient, desiccated, stony hard hammer may cause pain for the patient and interfere with the response. The hammer should never leave bruises on either the patient or the examiner. The first 10 minutes of the video *Demonstration of Teaching the Reflex Exam* by Dr. Abraham Verghese, from the 2015 Stanford 25 Skills Symposium (see **Video Link 38.1**), features an excellent discussion of reflex hammers, worthy of any neurologist, delivered by an internist.

Proper technique is much more difficult to describe than to demonstrate. The hammer strike should be quick, direct, crisp, and forceful but no greater than necessary. The most effective blow is delivered quickly with a flick of the wrist, holding the handle of the hammer near its end and letting it spin through loosely held fingertips. Putting the index finger on top of the handle and using primarily elbow motion, common faults, make it much harder to achieve adequate velocity at the hammer head. Another common mistake is "pecking:" striking the tendon with a timid, decelerating blow, pulling back at the last instant.

The patient should be comfortable, relaxed, and properly positioned. It may help relaxation to divert the patient's attention with light conversation. The optimal position is usually about midway in the range of motion of the muscle to be tested. Sometimes, as in the ankle reflex, positioning includes passively stretching the muscle slightly. An adequate stimulus must be delivered to the proper spot. Reinforcement methods are necessary if the reflex is not obtainable in the usual way. The part of the body to be tested should be in an optimal position for the response. In order to compare the reflexes on the two sides of the body, the position of the extremities should be symmetric. During the reflex examination, the patient should keep the head straight because looking to one side, as is the temptation, may alter reflex tone, especially in the arms (tonic neck reflex). The DTRs may be influenced to some degree by voluntary mental effort. Merely by concentrating, some individuals are able to somehow alter reflex excitability. Mentally induced reflex asymmetry is possible and may be clinically relevant in some cases.

The examiner can feel as well as see the contraction. Placing one hand over the muscle is often useful, especially when responses are sluggish. A reflex quadriceps contraction can sometimes be felt even when insufficient to produce visible contraction or knee movement. The activity of a reflex is judged by the speed and vigor of the response, the range of movement, and the duration of the contraction. An absent reflex often makes a dull, thudding sound when the tendon is struck.

The DTRs usually examined include the biceps, triceps, brachioradialis, knee (quadriceps), and ankle (Achilles) tendon reflexes **(Video 38.1)**. Other DTRs are occasionally useful **(Video 38.2)**. Table 38.1 summarizes the reflex levels. Reflexes may be graded as absent, sluggish or diminished, normal, exaggerated, and markedly hyperactive. For the purposes of clinical note-taking, most neurologists grade the DTRs numerically as follows: 0 = absent; 1+ (or +) = present but diminished; 2+ (or ++) = normal; 3+ (or +++) = increased but not necessarily to a pathologic degree; and 4+ (or ++++) = markedly hyperactive, pathologic, often with extra beats or accompanying sustained clonus (see Chapter 40). The "+" after the number is more traditional than informative and is sometimes omitted. Signs are sometimes used to indicate subtle asymmetry, but generally, a grade of 2 means the same as 2+. Another level, trace (or +/−), is frequently added to refer to a reflex, most often an ankle jerk, that appears absent to routine testing but can be elicited with reinforcement. Some add a grade of 5+ for the patient with extreme spasticity and clonus. In the 0 to 4 scale, level 1+ DTRs are still normal but somewhat sluggish and

TABLE 38.1 The Commonly Elicited Deep Tendon (Muscle Stretch) Reflexes

Reflex	Segmental Level	Peripheral Nerve
Biceps	C5-C6	Musculocutaneous
Triceps	C7-C8	Radial
Brachioradialis	C5-C6	Radial
Quadriceps	L3-L4	Femoral
Achilles	S1	Sciatic

TABLE 38.2 Method of Recording the Commonly Tested Muscle Stretch Reflexes

	Right	Left
Biceps	2+	2+
Triceps	2+	2+
Brachioradialis	2+	2+
Patellar	2+	2+
Achilles	2+	2+
Plantar	Down	Down

Grades 0 to 4+ (see text) used for all plantar reflex, which is down (normal), absent (0), equivocal (+/−), or up (abnormal). Other reflexes may be added and charted as needed.

difficult to elicit and hypoactive but, in the examiner's opinion, not pathologic. Grade 3+ reflexes are "fast normal," quicker than 2+, sometimes very quick, but not accompanied by any other signs of upper motor neuron pathology such as increased tone, upgoing toes, or sustained clonus. Normality of the superficial reflexes, normal lower-extremity tone, and downgoing toes are reassuring evidence of fast normal rather than pathologically quick reflexes. Some use 3+ to indicate the presence of spread or unsustained clonus, with all other normal reflexes, even very fast ones, labeled as 2+. Grade 4+ reflexes are unequivocally pathologic. The speed of the response is very fast, the threshold is low, the reflexogenic zone is wide, and there are accompanying signs of corticospinal tract dysfunction. Other scales are in use but not widely. The Mayo Clinic utilizes a scale in which 0 is normal and reflexes are either increased (1+ to 4+) or decreased (1− to 4−). Reflexes may be charted in several ways, for example, as shown in Table 38.2, or as in Figure 38.1. When reflexes are very active, responses may occur from muscles that have not been directly stretched, even in normal patients. The response may involve adjacent or even contralateral muscles, and the contraction of one muscle may be accompanied by contraction of other muscles. This is referred to as spread, or irradiation, of reflexes. It is normal for percussion of the brachioradialis tendon to also cause slight finger flexion. In the presence of spasticity and hyperreflexia, contraction of the biceps or brachioradialis may be accompanied by pronounced flexion of the fingers and adduction of the thumb. Extension of the knee may be accompanied by adduction of the hip, or there may be bilateral knee extension. Judging how much spread is still within normal limits can be difficult. Under some circumstances, the expected response to

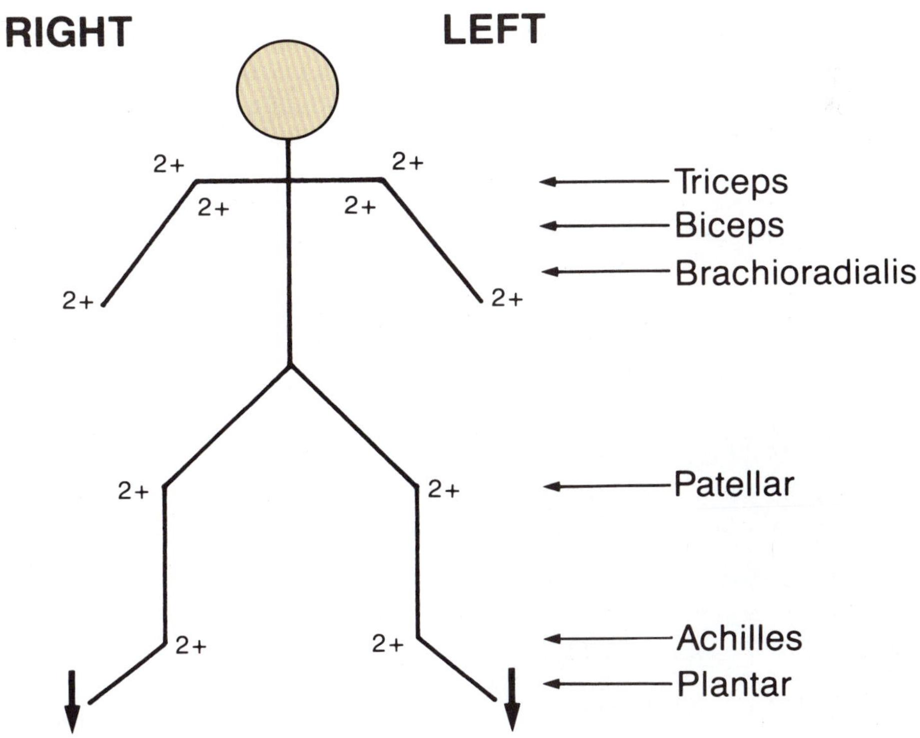

FIGURE 38.1 Alternate method of recording the commonly tested muscle stretch reflexes. For grading, see text and Table 38.2.

percussion of a tendon is absent, but muscles innervated by adjacent spinal cord segments contract instead (e.g., inverted brachioradialis reflex) (see Inverted and Perverted Reflexes). On other occasions, a reflex is absent and percussion of the tendon causes an inverted or paradoxical contraction (e.g., elbow flexion on attempted elicitation of the triceps reflex).

In some patients, DTRs may be markedly diminished, or even apparently absent, although there is no other evidence of nervous system disease. Under such circumstances, reinforcement techniques are often useful. Reflex reinforcement probably involves supraspinal, fusimotor, and long-loop mechanisms. A reflex can be reinforced or brought out using several methods. In the Jendrassik maneuver, the patient attempts to pull the hands apart with the fingers flexed and hooked together, palms facing, as the tendon is percussed (Figure 38.2). The effect is very brief, lasting only 1 to 6 seconds, and is maximal for only 300 ms. The Jendrassik maneuver is obviously useful only for lower-extremity reflexes. Other techniques include having the patient clench one or both fists or firmly grasp the arm of the chair, side of the bed, or the arm of the examiner. Reinforcement may also be carried out by having the patient look at the ceiling, grit the teeth, cough, squeeze the knees together, take a deep breath, count, read aloud, or repeat verses at the time the reflex is being tested. A sudden loud noise, a painful stimulus elsewhere on the body—such as the pulling of a hair or a bright light flashed in the eyes—may also be a means of reinforcement.

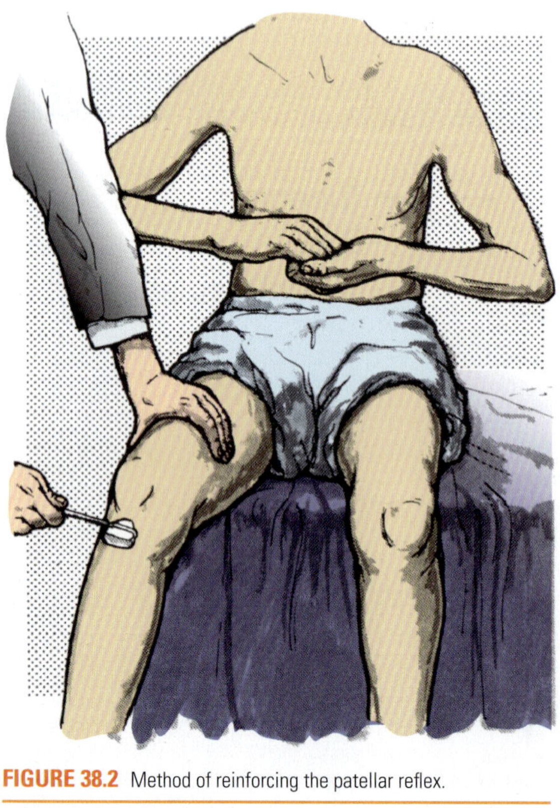

FIGURE 38.2 Method of reinforcing the patellar reflex.

Procedures other than distraction are also helpful in reflex reinforcement. A slight increase in tension of the muscle being tested may reinforce the reflex response. A simple and effective method to reinforce a knee or ankle jerk is to have the patient maintain a slight, steady contraction of the muscle whose tendon is being tested (e.g., slight plantar flexion by pushing the ball of the foot against the floor or the examiner's hand to reinforce the ankle jerk). The patient may tense the quadriceps by extending the knee slightly against resistance as the knee jerk is being elicited. Reinforcement may increase the amplitude of a sluggish reflex or bring out a latent reflex not otherwise obtainable. Reflexes that are normal on reinforcement, even though not present without reinforcement, may be considered normal. Slight muscle contraction due to inability to relax may be one reason for the slightly hyperactive reflexes often seen in patients who are tense or anxious.

The DTRs are instrumental in the evaluation of weakness. Under most circumstances, weakness accompanied by hyporeflexia is of lower motor neuron origin, and weakness accompanied by hyperreflexia is of upper motor neuron origin. The presence of pathologic reflexes (see Chapter 40) and abnormalities of associated movements (see Chapter 42) are also helpful in the differential diagnosis (Table 38.3). The following sections discuss the upper-extremity, trunk, and lower-extremity reflexes. The masseter or mandibular reflex (jaw jerk) is covered in Chapter 15.

THE UPPER-EXTREMITY REFLEXES

The biceps, triceps, brachioradialis, and finger flexor reflexes are the most important upper-extremity reflexes. Less often useful reflexes are summarized in Table 38.4.

The Biceps Reflex

With the arm relaxed and the forearm slightly pronated and midway between flexion and extension, the examiner places the palmar surface of her extended

TABLE 38.3 Reflex Patterns with Different Neurologic Disorders

Site or Type of Lesion	Muscle Stretch Reflexes	Superficial Reflexes	Pathologic Reflexes	Associated Movements
Neuromuscular junction	Normal or decreased	Normal	Absent	Normal
Muscle	Usually normal; may be decreased in proportion to weakness	Normal	Absent	Normal
Peripheral nerve	Decreased to absent	Normal, or decreased to absent in distribution of involved nerve(s)	Absent	Normal
Corticospinal tract (upper motor neuron syndrome)	Hyperactive (especially in speed of response)	Decreased to absent	Present	Pathologic associated movements present
Extrapyramidal system	Normal; occasionally slightly increased or decreased	Normal or slightly increased	Absent	Normal associated movements absent
Cerebellum	Pendular	Normal	Absent	Normal
Psychogenic	Normal or increased (especially in range of response)	Normal or increased	Absent	Normal or bizarre

thumb or finger on the patient's biceps tendon and then strikes the extensor surface with the reflex hammer (Figure 38.3). Pressure on the tendon should be light; too much pressure exerted with the thumb or finger against the tendon makes the reflex much harder to obtain. The hands may lie in the patient's lap, or the examiner may hold the patient's arm with the elbow resting in her hand. The major response is a contraction of the biceps muscle with flexion of the elbow. Because the biceps is also a supinator, there is often a certain amount of supination. If the reflex is exaggerated, the reflexogenic zone is increased and the reflex may even be obtained by tapping the clavicle; there may be abnormal spread with accompanying flexion of the wrist and fingers and adduction of the thumb.

TABLE 38.4 Less Often Useful Deep Tendon Reflexes

Reflex	Method	Response
Scapulohumeral reflex	Tapping over the vertebral border of the scapula, either at the tip of its spine or at its base near the inferior angle	Retraction of the scapula (rhomboids); possible elevation of the scapula and adduction and external rotation of the humerus (trapezius, latissimus, infraspinatus, and teres minor)
Wrist extension reflex	With the forearm pronated and the wrist hanging down, tapping the extensor tendons of the wrist	Contraction of the extensor muscles and extension at the wrist. Under certain circumstances, there may be flexion of the wrist and fingers (the carpometacarpal reflex, see Chapter 40).
Wrist flexion reflex	With the hand supinated and the fingers slightly flexed, tapping the flexor tendons of the wrist on the volar surface of the forearm at or above the transverse carpal ligament	Contraction of the flexor muscles of the hand and fingers
Thumb reflex	Tapping the flexor pollicis longus tendon just above the pronator quadratus	Flexion of the distal phalanx of the thumb
Gluteal reflexes	Tapping the lower portion of the sacrum or the posterior aspect of the ilium near the origin of the gluteus maximus muscle	Contraction of the muscle and extension of the thigh. Reflex best elicited with patient recumbent and weight on opposite side with moderate flexion of ipsilateral thigh; may also be elicited with patient prone
Extensor hallucis longus reflex	Using a finger, examiner pushes down on dorsal surface of great toe	Tapping finger causes toe extension more felt than seen
Tibialis posterior reflex	Tapping tendon of tibialis posterior just above and behind medial malleolus	Inversion of the foot

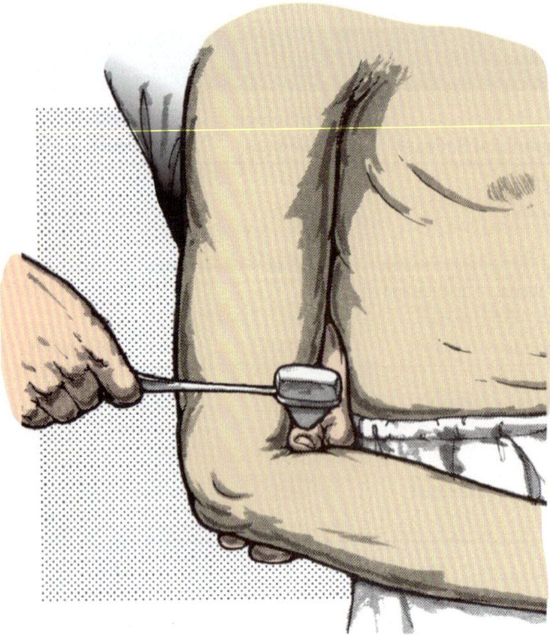

FIGURE 38.3 Method of obtaining the biceps reflex.

The Triceps Reflex

This reflex is elicited by tapping the triceps tendon just above its insertion on the olecranon process of the ulna. The arm is placed midway between flexion and extension and may be rested in the patient's lap, on her thigh or hip, or on the examiner's hand (Figure 38.4). The response is contraction of the triceps muscle with extension of the elbow. The most common error in eliciting the triceps jerk is simply too timorous a blow. The paradoxical or inverted triceps jerk consists of flexion of the elbow with percussion of the triceps tendon. This response appears when the afferent arc of the triceps reflex is damaged, as in lesions of the seventh and eighth cervical segments, particularly when there is an element of spasticity, as in cervical spondylosis with radiculomyelopathy.

The Brachioradialis (Radial Periosteal or Supinator) Reflex

Tapping just above the styloid process of the radius with the forearm in semiflexion and semipronation causes flexion of the elbow, with variable supination (Figure 38.5). The supination is more marked with the forearm extended and pronated, but there is less flexion. The principal muscle involved is the brachioradialis. The tendon can be percussed not only at its insertion on the lateral aspect of the base of the styloid process of the radius but also at about the junction of the middle and distal thirds of the forearm or at its tendon of origin above the lateral epicondyle of the humerus. The most common error is hitting the muscle belly rather than the tendon. The muscle becomes tendinous at about midforearm. A local contraction can be elicited from any muscle by directly striking the muscle belly. The point in eliciting a DTR is to lengthen the muscle by stretching its tendon. An idiomuscular contraction can be obtained by striking

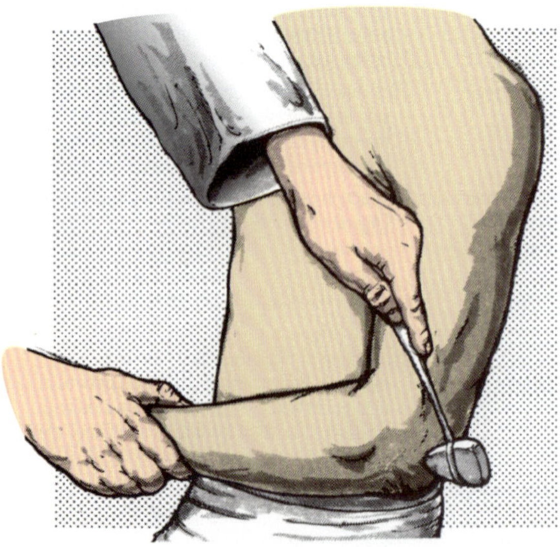

FIGURE 38.4 Method of obtaining the triceps reflex.

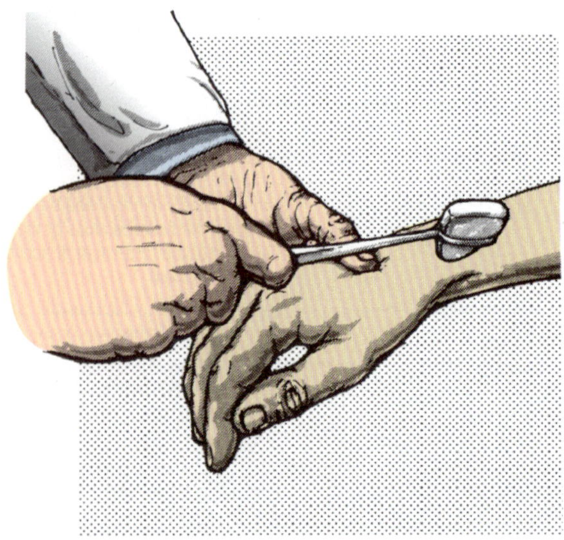

FIGURE 38.5 Method of obtaining the brachioradialis reflex.

the brachioradialis muscle belly in the proximal third of the forearm; this is not a DTR. If the reflex is exaggerated, there is associated flexion of the wrist and fingers, with adduction of the forearm. When the afferent limb of the reflex is impaired, there may be a twitch of the flexors of the hand and fingers without flexion and supination of the elbow; this is termed inversion of the reflex.

The biceps, triceps, and brachioradialis reflexes should be obtained without difficulty in normal individuals. The following upper-extremity reflexes may be elicited only to a slight extent in normal persons. They may become conspicuous when there is hyperreflexia.

The Finger Flexor Reflex (Wartenberg's Sign)

This is one of several signs attributed to Robert Wartenberg. To elicit the finger flexor reflex, the patient's hand is in supination, resting on a table or a solid surface, with the fingers slightly flexed. The examiner places her fingers against the patient's fingers and taps the backs of her own fingers lightly with the reflex hammer (Figure 38.6). The response is flexion of the patient's fingers and the distal phalanx of the thumb **(Video 38.2)**. The reflex may be reinforced by having the patient flex her fingers slightly as the blow is delivered. An alternate technique is for the patient to hold the hand in the air, palm down, and the examiner to touch fingers with palm up, with the blow delivered in an upward direction from below. The nerve supply, as in the wrist flexion reflex, is through the median and ulnar nerves (C8-T1). This reflex is difficult for the inexperienced examiner to elicit, and it is often absent in normals. However, Wartenberg considered it one of the most important upper-extremity reflexes. The Hoffmann and Trömner signs, which are pathologic variations of this response, are described in Chapter 40.

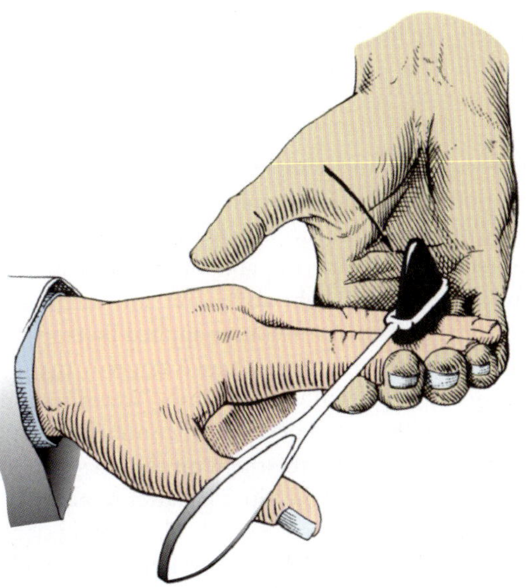

FIGURE 38.6 Method of obtaining the finger flexor reflex.

The Deltoid Reflex

Tapping over the insertion of the deltoid muscle at the junction of the upper and middle third of the lateral aspect of the humerus results in slight abduction of the upper arm (axillary nerve, C5-C6).

The Pectoralis Reflex

With the patient's arm in midposition between abduction and adduction, the examiner places her finger as nearly as possible on the tendon of the pectoralis major muscle near its insertion on the greater tuberosity of the humerus (Figure 38.7). Tapping the finger causes adduction and slight internal rotation of the arm at the shoulder **(Video 38.2)**. The contraction of the muscle may be felt but usually not seen in the normal individual. In patients with cervical spondylotic myelopathy, a hyperactive pectoralis reflex indicates spinal cord compression at the C2-C3 and/or C3-C4 levels. This reflex is mediated by the medial and lateral pectoral (anterior thoracic) nerves (C5-T1).

The Clavicle Reflex

In patients with upper-extremity hyperreflexia, a tap over the lateral aspect of the clavicle is followed by extensive contraction of various muscle groups in the upper limb (see **Video Link 38.2**). There are individual variations, but normally, the response should be the same on each side. This is not a specific reflex, but an indication of spread of the reflex response. The response is minimal, usually absent, except in the face of upper-extremity hyperreflexia. It is useful in comparing the reflex activity of the two upper limbs.

FIGURE 38.7 Method of obtaining the pectoralis reflex.

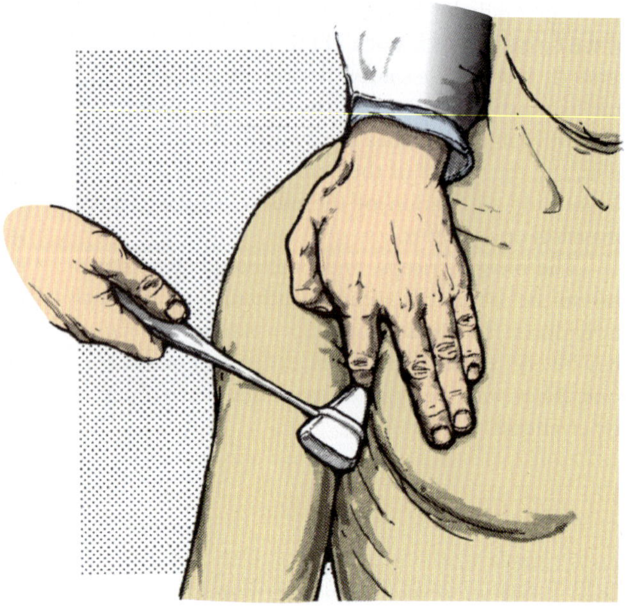

The Pronator Reflex

With the elbow in semiflexion and the forearm semipronated, tapping over either the volar surface of the distal radius or the dorsal aspect of the styloid process of the ulna may produce brief supination followed by pronation of the forearm **(Video 38.2)**. There may also be flexion of the wrist and fingers. The major muscles participating in this response are the pronator teres and pronator quadratus. This reflex may be exaggerated early when corticospinal tract lesions develop.

TRUNK REFLEXES

Reflexes from trunk muscles are obtained minimally or not at all in normal individuals.

The Abdominal Muscle (Deep Abdominal) Reflexes

The best responses are obtained by pressing down slightly with the fingers and then tapping briskly with a reflex hammer (see **Video Link 38.3**). The response is contraction of the abdominal muscles, and a deviation of the umbilicus toward the site of the stimulus. The innervation is by the intercostal nerves (anterior divisions of T5-T12), as well as the ilioinguinal and iliohypogastric nerves. The abdominal muscle reflexes are only minimally present in normal individuals. They are most significant if exaggerated or if there is dissociation between the deep and superficial abdominal reflexes (see Chapter 39). Brisk deep abdominal reflexes with absent superficial abdominal reflexes suggest a corticospinal tract lesion.

The Iliac Reflexes

Tapping over the iliac crest is followed by contraction of the lower abdominal muscles. This reflex is mediated by the lower intercostal nerves (T10-T12).

The Symphysis Pubis Reflexes

Tapping over the symphysis pubis is followed by a contraction of the abdominal muscles and a downward movement of the umbilicus. The patient should be recumbent, with the abdominal muscles relaxed and the thigh in slight abduction and internal rotation. If a unilateral stimulus is applied by tapping 1.5 to 2 cm from the midline, there is not only the "upper response" just described but also a "lower response," or puboadductor reflex, with contraction of the adductor muscles of the thigh on the side stimulated and some flexion of the hip. The latter response is also seen if the reflex is exaggerated. The symphysis pubis reflex is innervated by the lower intercostal, ilioinguinal, and iliohypogastric nerves (T11-T12 and upper lumbar segments). When there is spasticity, percussion over the symphysis may cause adduction of both legs. The costal periosteal, iliac, and symphysis pubis reflexes may be considered variations of the deep abdominal muscle reflexes in which the stimulus is directed toward the site of insertion.

THE LOWER-EXTREMITY REFLEXES

The Patellar Reflex (Quadriceps Reflex, Knee Jerk)

The patellar reflex is contraction of the quadriceps femoris muscle, with resulting extension of the knee, in response to percussion of the patellar tendon. A firm tap on the tendon draws the patella down, stretching the quadriceps and provoking reflex contraction. If the reflex is brisk, the contraction is strong and the amplitude of the movement is large. If the examiner places one hand over the muscle, and with the other hand taps the patellar tendon just below the patella, she can palpate the contraction as well as observe the rapidity and range of response. When the reflex is hypoactive, it may be better felt than seen. Palpation helps in judging the latency between the time of the stimulus and the resulting response.

The knee jerk can be elicited in various ways. The patient may sit in a chair with the knees slightly extended and the heels resting on the floor or sit on an examination table with the legs dangling (Figure 38.8). If the patient is lying in bed, the examiner should partially flex the knee by placing one hand beneath it and then tap the tendon (Figure 38.9). The responses on the two sides can be compared by lifting both knees simultaneously, supporting them on one forearm as the patient's heels rest lightly on the bed, before tapping the tendons. If the patient is wearing loose pajamas, the examiner can suspend both legs by holding the pajamas, as she uses the other hand to strike the tendon. Another technique is having the patient sit with one leg crossed over the other and tapping the patellar tendon of the uppermost leg, but this method does not facilitate side-to-side comparison. Figure 38.10 shows a physician using this method. The patellar reflex is mediated by the femoral nerve (L2-L4).

If there is reflex spread, extension of the knee may be accompanied by adduction of the hip, which on occasion is bilateral, or there may be bilateral knee extension. If the reflex is exaggerated, the response may be obtained by tapping the tendon not only in the usual spot but also just above the patella

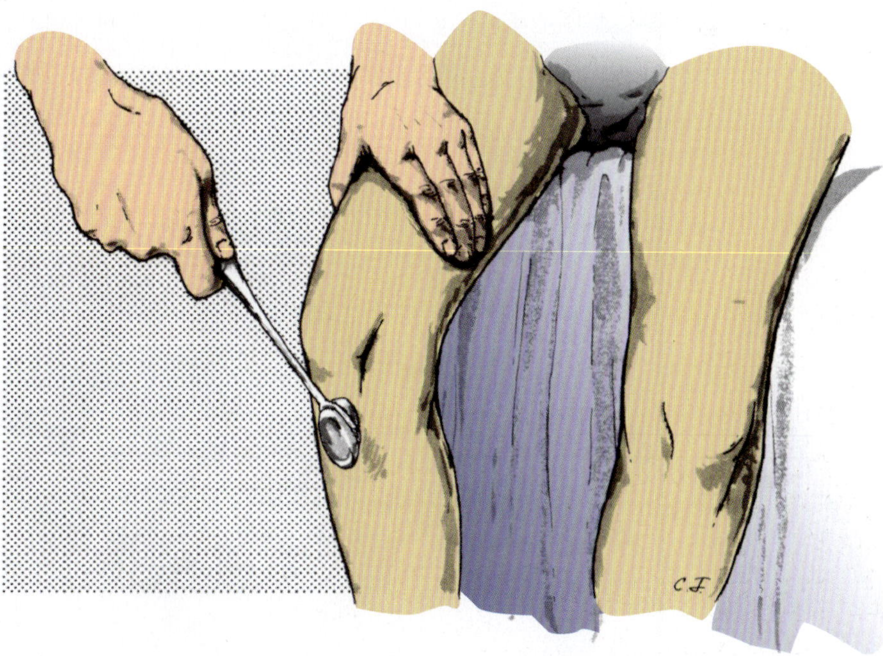

FIGURE 38.8 Method of obtaining the patellar (quadriceps) reflex with the patient seated.

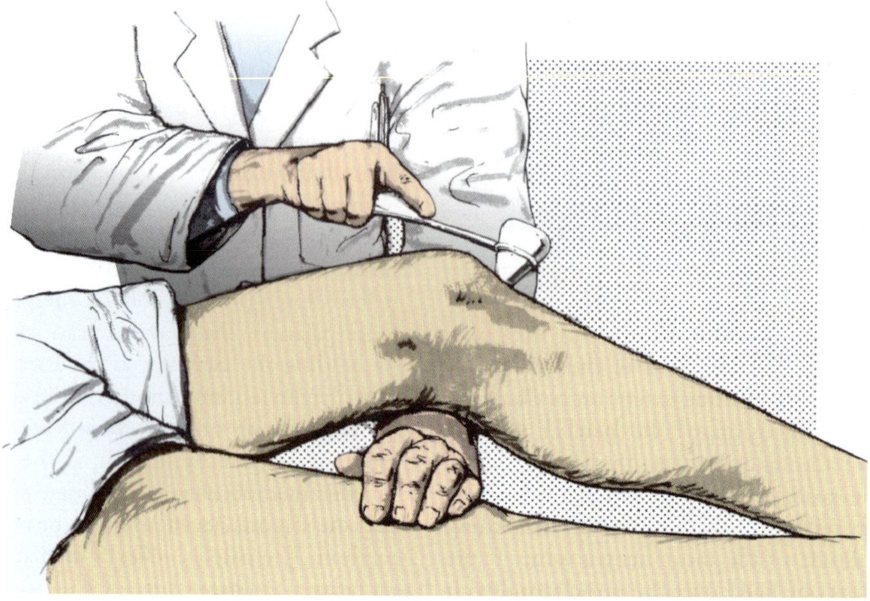

FIGURE 38.9 Method of obtaining the patellar (quadriceps) reflex with the patient recumbent.

FIGURE 38.10 Eliciting the knee jerk with one leg crossed over the other, using a Babinski hammer. (Reprinted from Lanska DJ. The Babinski reflex hammer. *Neurology* 1999;53[3]:655, with permission.)

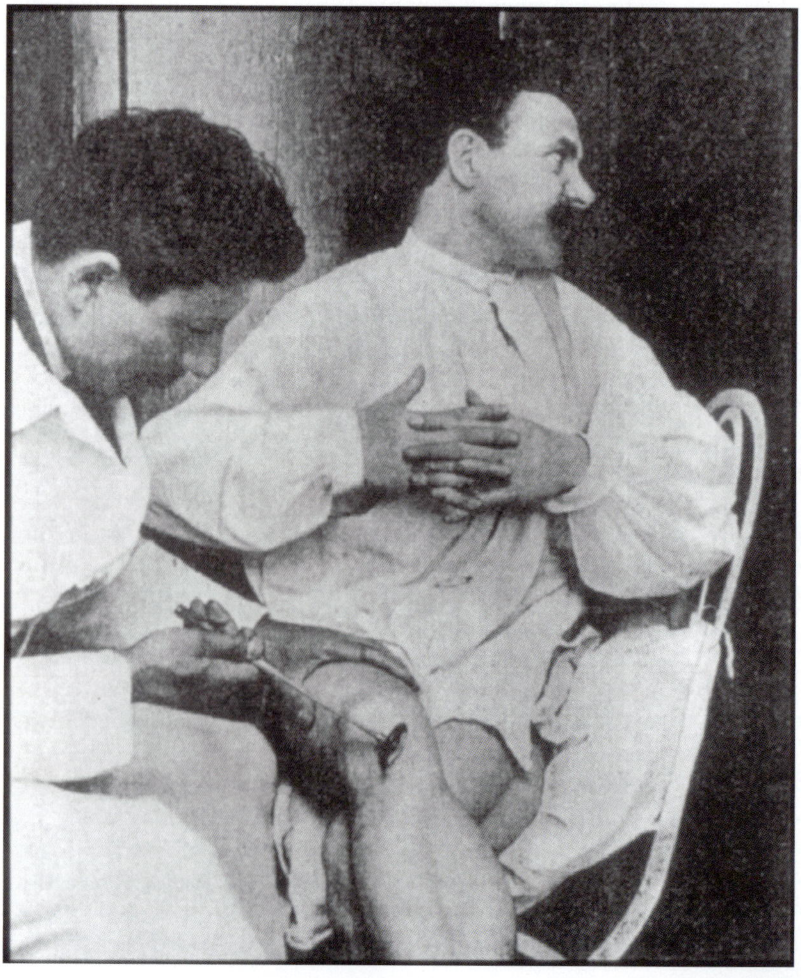

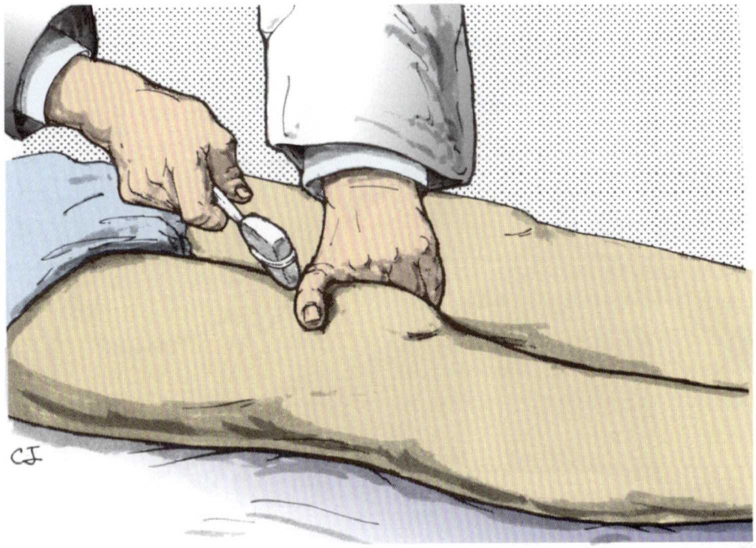

FIGURE 38.11 Method of obtaining the suprapatellar reflex.

(suprapatellar reflex); the tendon can be tapped directly, or, with the patient recumbent, the examiner can place her index finger on the upper border of the patella and tap the finger to push down the patella. Contraction of the quadriceps causes a brisk upward movement of the tendon, together with extension of the leg (Figure 38.11). Marked exaggeration of the patellar reflex may be accompanied by patellar clonus (see Chapter 40). An inverted patellar reflex may be seen with lesions of the nerve or nerve roots supplying the quadriceps: Tapping the patellar tendon results in contraction of the hamstrings and flexion of the knee.

The Achilles Reflex (Ankle Jerk, Triceps Surae Reflex)

The ankle jerk is obtained by striking the Achilles tendon just above its insertion on the calcaneus. The resulting contraction of the posterior crural muscles, the gastrocnemius, soleus, and plantaris, causes plantar flexion of the foot at the ankle. If the patient is seated or lying in bed, the thigh should be held in moderate abduction and external rotation and the knee flexed. If the patient is supine, access to the tendon requires placing the legs into a frog-leg position with the knees apart and the ankles close together. Some prefer to have the patient cross the leg to be examined atop the other shin or ankle ("figure-four position," as the legs form a 4). The examiner should place one hand under the foot and pull upward slightly to passively dorsiflex the ankle to about a right angle (Figure 38.12). The Achilles reflex is mediated by the tibial nerve (S1).

The ankle jerk is by far the most difficult reflex to master. There are two critical variables: proper stretch and efficient striking. Of the two, proper stretch is the more difficult to learn. Too little dorsiflexion leaves the tendon slack and able to absorb the blow without stretching the muscle. Too much passive dorsiflexion makes the tendon too taut and unable to be stretched. If the reflex is difficult to obtain, the patient may be asked to press her foot lightly against the examiner's hand in order to tense the muscle and reinforce the reflex. Using a driving analogy and asking the patient to imagine pressing on an accelerator enough to go "17 mph" communicates the need for a low-level but precisely graded contraction, which is then easy to adjust up or down to the proper level. The reflex may also be elicited by having the patient kneel on a chair or similar surface, with the feet projecting at right angles; the Achilles tendons are percussed while the patient is in this position (Figure 38.13). This method, introduced by Babinski, is particularly useful for comparing reflex activity on the two sides. Another method for supine examination is to strike the ball (sole) of the foot or strike the examiner's hand placed flat against the sole.

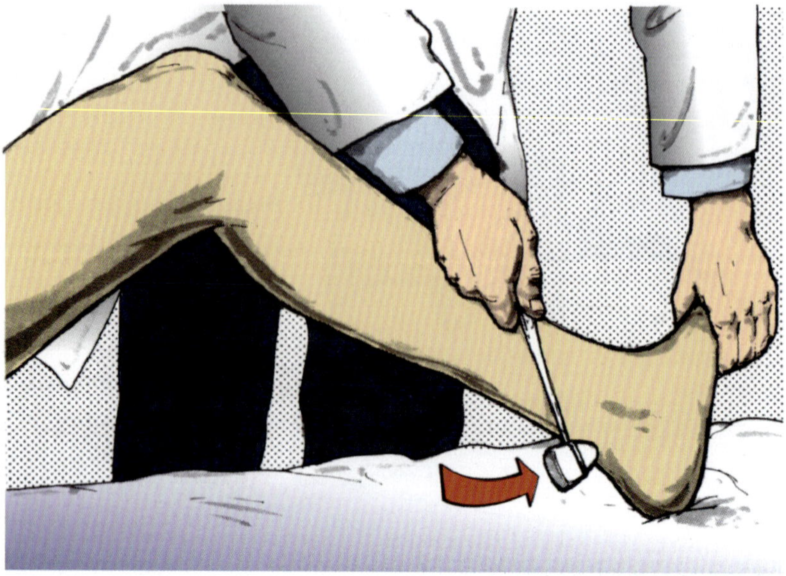

FIGURE 38.12 Method of obtaining the Achilles (triceps surae) reflex with the patient recumbent.

This plantar stretch reflex is considered equivalent to the ankle jerk for clinical purposes.

If the ankle jerk is hyperactive, it may be elicited by tapping other areas of the sole of the foot, the medioplantar reflex, or by tapping the anterior aspect of the ankle, the paradoxical ankle reflex. A hyperactive reflex may also result in extra beats or even clonus when the tendon is percussed. When there is reflex spread, striking the Achilles tendon may cause flexion of the knee. Although the Achilles reflex, when carefully elicited, should be present in normal individuals, it tends to diminish with age, and its bilateral absence in elderly individuals is not necessarily of clinical significance. Although it is common wisdom that the normal elderly may have absent ankle reflexes, of 200 consecutive patients admitted to a geriatric unit, 188 had ankle jerks using plantar rather than Achilles tendon strike; only 1.5% had absent ankle jerks attributable only to age. Another study comparing plantar strike and tendon strike in elderly patients found better intraobserver and interobserver agreement with the plantar strike. Differences in technique may explain some of the discrepancy between studies examining the prevalence of absent ankle jerks in elderly people.

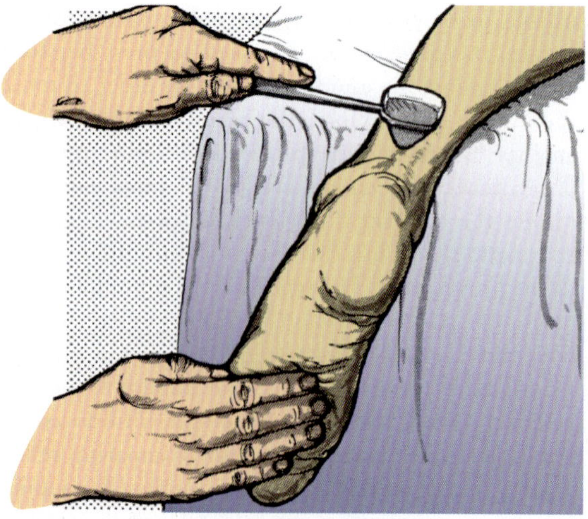

FIGURE 38.13 Method of obtaining the Achilles (triceps surae) reflex with the patient kneeling.

The knee and ankle reflexes are the most important DTRs in the lower extremities. The following reflexes are less significant. The response may be minimal or even absent in normal individuals. Because the responses may be difficult to elicit even in normal subjects, side-to-side comparison is critical. To be significant, absence must be unilateral. Exaggeration of these difficult-to-obtain reflexes suggests the presence of corticospinal tract disease.

The Adductor Reflex (Obturator Nerve, L2-L4)

With the thigh in slight abduction, tapping over either the medial epicondyle of the femur in the vicinity of the adductor tubercle or the medial condyle of the tibia results in contraction of the adductor muscles of the thigh and inward movement of the extremity. If the reflex is exaggerated, there may be crossed, or bilateral, adduction. A slightly crossed adductor response is not necessarily abnormal, but strong crossed adduction, or adduction of the opposite leg when obtaining the knee jerk, suggests corticospinal tract disease. When there is hyperreflexia, an adductor response may also be obtained while the patient is seated by tapping the spinous processes of the sacral or lumbar vertebrae (the spinal adductor reflex) or by tapping the crest or the superior spines of the ilium. An absent adductor reflex with a normal patellar reflex has been described as a sign of strangulated obturator hernia (Hannington-Kiff sign). The puboadductor reflex was described with the symphysis pubis reflex.

The Medial Hamstring (Internal Hamstring) Reflex

This reflex is elicited by striking the semitendinosus and semimembranosus tendons just above their insertions on the tibia. This may be done with the patient seated or recumbent, with the leg abducted and slightly rotated externally and the knee flexed. The examiner's fingers are placed over the tendons on the medial posterior aspect of the knee and the fingers tapped with the reflex hammer. The response is knee flexion **(Video 38.2)**. This reflex is mediated by tibial portion of the sciatic nerve, primarily by the L5 nerve root. It may be useful in the evaluation of suspected L5 radiculopathy. For a video of the medial hamstring reflex, see Perloff et al.

The Lateral Hamstring (External Hamstring) Reflex

This reflex is elicited by striking the biceps femoris tendon just above its insertion. With the patient sitting, recumbent, or lying on the opposite side and the knee moderately flexed, the examiner's fingers are placed over the tendon on the lateral posterior aspect of the knee and tapped (Figure 38.14). The response is knee flexion **(Video 38.2)**. The reflex may also be elicited by tapping the head of the fibula (fibular reflex). This reflex is mediated by tibial portion of the sciatic nerve, primarily by the S1 nerve root. The external hamstring reflex is sometimes helpful in sorting out whether an absent ankle jerk is due to peripheral neuropathy or radiculopathy. If due to neuropathy, the external hamstring will usually be preserved, but in radiculopathy, it may be depressed in concert with the ankle reflex.

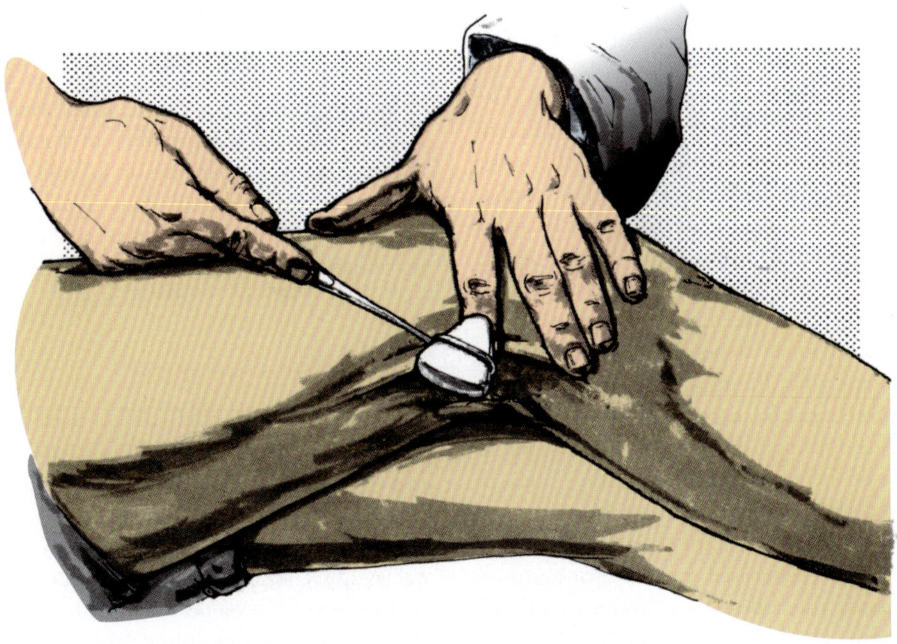

FIGURE 38.14 Method of obtaining the biceps femoris reflex.

The Peroneal (Tibialis Anterior) Reflex

With the patient's foot plantar flexed and inverted, the examiner presses a finger firmly over the distal ends of the first and second metatarsal bones. A brisk tap to the finger is followed by eversion and dorsiflexion of the foot. The reflex is due to contraction of muscles supplied by the deep and superficial peroneal nerves (L4-S1). The peroneal reflex may be useful in the evaluation of suspected L5 radiculopathy (see **Video Link 38.4**).

The Plantar Muscle Reflexes

There are numerous reflexes in which the response is flexion of the toes. These are difficult to elicit in normal individuals, of limited clinical significance, and of importance only when exaggerated. They are discussed with the pathologic reflexes in Chapter 40.

INTERPRETATION OF THE DEEP TENDON (MUSCLE STRETCH) REFLEXES

The most valuable DTRs for clinical diagnosis are the biceps, triceps, brachioradialis, patellar, and Achilles (see Table 38.1); under most circumstances, and using good technique, these are elicitable in every normal person. One or more of these reflexes may be absent in occasional individuals with no other evidence of disease of the nervous system. They are present even in the majority of premature infants. The activity of a DTR is judged by the threshold, latency, speed, vigor, and duration of contraction; the range of movement; and whether there is spread or irradiation of the reflex. Of these, the latent period between the time the stimulus is applied and the time the response occurs is most important for clinical evaluation of disease states. Accurate evaluation of the reflex responses obviously depends on the experience of the examiner. By far, the most important factor is the diligence and practice expended in learning the techniques. The appraisal depends on the individual interpretation of the examiner. There is no standard, and there is a certain amount of normal variation in reflex activity. What is normal for one individual may be an increased or a decreased response for another. In some persons, the reflexes are lively; in others, they are sluggish. Under normal circumstances, the reflexes should be equal on the two sides.

ABNORMALITIES OF THE DEEP TENDON (MUSCLE STRETCH) REFLEXES

Abnormal DTRs are either hypoactive or hyperactive. When hypoactive, the response varies from diminished or sluggish to complete absence of the reflex. Hyperactive reflexes are characterized by varying degrees of decreased latency, increased speed and vigor of response, increased range of movement, decrease in threshold, extension of the reflexogenic zone, and prolongation of the muscular contraction. The pathologic conditions in which these various changes occur are discussed in the following sections. Table 38.3 summarizes the patterns of reflex responses seen with lesions at various sites.

Reflexes are judged in both absolute and relative terms. Clearly hyperactive or hypoactive reflexes speak for themselves. But a reflex that is normal in absolute terms may be judged abnormal in comparison to the patient's other reflexes. The reflexes should be compared on the two sides of the body, the arms to the legs, and the knees to the ankles. The DTRs are normally symmetric, and reflexes otherwise normal may be abnormal if different from expected. For example, a 1+ biceps jerk in a patient with suspected cervical radiculopathy, although "normal," may be judged abnormal if the opposite biceps jerk is 2+. The DTRs are usually comparable in the upper and lower extremities. Slight differences are permissible, but a pronounced difference may be significant (e.g., in thoracic myelopathy, the DTRs in the legs may be much brisker than in the arms, even though not clearly pathologic). A proximal to distal gradient may also be significant. Symmetric 1+ ankle jerks when all of the other reflexes are 2+ may signal mild peripheral neuropathy. When asymmetry is the main finding, it is sometimes difficult to tell whether one side is increased or the other side decreased.

Hypoactive Reflexes

When a reflex is hypoactive, there is a sluggish response and/or a diminution in the range of response. An increase in stimulus intensity may be necessary to elicit the reflex, or repeated blows may be necessary, for a single stimulus may be subliminal. A DTR is absent if it is not obtained even with reinforcement. A depressed or absent reflex results from dysfunction of some component of the reflex arc. Interference with the afferent limb may be caused by lesions involving the sensory nerve, posterior root, dorsal root ganglion, or intramedullary pathways between the dorsal root entry zone and the anterior horn (e.g., syringomyelia). Abnormalities of the motor unit and final common pathway that make up the efferent limb of the reflex arc occur in many conditions, but particularly with radiculopathy and peripheral nerve lesions. In neurogenic processes, DTRs are lost out of proportion to atrophy and weakness. With a peripheral nerve lesion, a reflex may not return until much of the motor function has been recovered. Sometimes there is persistent areflexia following lesions of the nerve root or peripheral nerve, even after complete return of both motor and sensory functions. In myasthenia gravis, the reflexes are affected only when there is severe and extensive involvement, but in Lambert-Eaton syndrome, depressed reflexes are common. In periodic paralysis, DTRs may be temporarily absent during attacks. In myopathies, reflexes are lost in proportion to the atrophy and weakness. When atrophy and weakness are severe, reflexes may disappear. In many forms of muscular dystrophy, the proximal reflexes disappear early, whereas the distal reflexes may persist until the later stages of the disease.

The DTRs may also be decreased or absent in various other conditions. They are often absent in deep coma, narcosis, heavy sedation, and deep sleep. They are characteristically absent during nerve block, caudal anesthesia, and spinal anesthesia. They are absent in spinal shock following a sudden transverse lesion of the spinal cord but reappear below the level of the lesion after a period of 3 to 4 weeks and usually become hyperactive. In Adie's syndrome, the tonic pupils are accompanied by depressed or absent reflexes.

A prolonged relaxation phase causing a "hung-up" reflex, especially of the ankle jerk, is a classical finding of hypothyroidism (Woltman's sign); the reflexes return to normal with treatment **(Video Link 38.5)**. But most patients with seemingly hung-up ankle jerks are euthyroid. Cold legs and feet may cause hung-up ankle jerks. Relaxation slows with advancing age, more so in females. Slow contraction and relaxation times may also occur with other conditions, including lower motor neuron disease. Delayed relaxation may also occur in myotonic disorders. In diabetic neuropathy, there may be either prolongation of the reflex time or decrease or absence of the reflexes before there is other evidence of nervous system involvement. The reflexes may appear to be decreased or absent in neurologic disorders in which there is marked spasticity or rigidity with contractures and in diseases of the joints causing inflammation, contractures, and ankylosis. The apparent hyporeflexia is due to lack of motility at the joint or pain on moving the joint; careful observation may disclose a muscle contraction even though there is no movement at the joint.

Hyperactive Reflexes

Reflex hyperactivity is characterized by the following: a decrease in reflex threshold; a decrease in the latency, the time between tendon percussion and the reflex contraction; an exaggeration of the power and range of movement; prolongation of the reflex contraction; extension of the reflexogenic zone; and spread of the reflex response. When the reflex threshold is decreased, a minimal stimulus may evoke the reflex, and reflexes that are not normally obtained may be elicited with ease. Very hyperactive DTRs may sometimes be elicited with extremely slight percussion. Another manifestation of decreased reflex threshold may be a widening of the area from which the reflex may be elicited, and application of the stimulus to sites at some distance from the usual one may evoke the response; the patellar reflex may be elicited by tapping the tibia or dorsum of the foot, and the biceps and other arm reflexes by tapping the clavicle or scapula. There may also be abnormal spread of the response. One stimulus may provoke repetitive responses and sometimes elicit sustained clonus.

The DTRs become hyperactive with lesions of the corticospinal system. Spasticity and hyperreflexia are likely related to involvement of a variety of structures in the descending motor pathways at cortical, subcortical, midbrain, and brainstem levels. Hyperreflexia results from a lowering of the reflex threshold due to increased excitability of the lower motor neuron pool related to dysfunction of some or all of these structures. From a clinical point of view, the terms pyramidal, corticospinal, or upper motor neuron are used to encompass these changes. A lesion at any level of the corticospinal system or other related upper motor neuron components, from the motor cortex to just above the segment of origin of a reflex arc, will be accompanied by spasticity and hyperreflexia. The characteristic posture in hemiplegia is flexion of the upper extremities, with more marked weakness of the extensors, and extension of the lower extremities, with more marked weakness of the flexors. Consequently, the flexor reflexes are exaggerated to a greater degree in the upper extremities, and the extensor reflexes in the lower. The reflexes may be present in spinal cord lesions in spite of the absence of sensation. A reflex may be increased if the tone of the antagonist muscle is diminished (e.g., an increased knee jerk may occur if there is weakness of the hamstrings).

Exaggeration of the DTRs may occur in psychogenic disorders and in anxiety, fright, and agitation (Table 38.3). The reflexes vary in these conditions; they may be normal, or they may be decreased owing to voluntary or involuntary tension of the antagonistic muscle, but they are most frequently increased. Some normal individuals, particularly young women, have physiologically brisk reflexes. Hyperactivity may be marked, but it is an exaggeration not in the speed or threshold of the response but in the excursion or range of response. The foot may be kicked far into the air and held extended for a time after the patellar tendon is tapped, but the contraction and relaxation take place at a normal rate. There is often a bilateral response with extraneous and superfluous jerking of remote parts, including whole body jerks, when a reflex is tested. There is no increase in the reflexogenic zone in psychogenic lesions, and although there may be irregular repeated jerky movements (spurious clonus), no true clonus is present. Furthermore, there are no other signs of organic disease of the corticospinal system. To help distinguish physiologically brisk from pathologic reflexes, it is particularly useful to pay careful attention to lower extremity tone, to the status of the abdominal reflexes, and to the plantar responses. If the toes are down, the abdominals intact, and lower extremity tone normal, it is unlikely the DTRs are pathologic.

In lesions of the extrapyramidal system, there are no consistent reflex changes (Table 38.3). The activity of the response depends on the level of muscle tone and the amount of rigidity that is present. Usually, the reflexes are slightly exaggerated, owing to increased muscle tone, but this is not a consistent finding. Rigidity may cause depression or absence of the reflexes. In diseases of the cerebellum, the reflexes may be diminished (Table 38.3) and pendular: Eliciting the patellar reflex while the foot is hanging free may elicit a series of to-and-fro pendular movements of the foot and leg before the limb finally comes to rest. The increased swinging may result from hypotonia of the extensor and flexor muscles and a lack of the restraining influence they normally exert on each other. The pendular response may also be observed in chorea, but there is more frequently a "hung" reflex: If the patellar tendon is tapped while the foot is hanging free, the knee may be held in extension for a few seconds before relaxing because of prolonged contraction of the quadriceps. In chorea, the response may not be obtained until the stimulus has been applied a number of times.

Inverted (Paradoxic, Indirect) Reflexes

Occasionally, percussion of a tendon produces unexpected results. When reflexes are very active, responses may occur from muscles that have not been directly stretched, even in normal patients. The response may involve adjacent or even contralateral muscles, as in the crossed adductor response. It is normal for percussion of the brachioradialis tendon to also cause slight finger flexion as well as biceps contraction in some patients. This is referred to as spread, or irradiation, of reflexes.

Inverted reflexes are responses more bizarre than simple spread. The term inversion was first used by Babinski in describing "inversion of the radial reflex." These responses are most often seen when the segmental reflex is absent or impaired and there is also underlying hyperreflexia lowering the threshold for activation of other muscles. These responses have also been referred to as "indirect" reflexes because the reflex occurs without direct stretch of the muscle that contracts. The bulk of the evidence suggests these inverted and paradoxical reflexes are mediated by vibration in the periphery.

There are many examples of these inverted or paradoxical reflexes: contraction of the finger flexors on percussion of the distal radius (inverted brachioradialis reflex), contraction of the biceps on eliciting the triceps reflex (paradoxical triceps jerk), contraction of the hamstring on eliciting the knee reflex (inverted knee jerk), and contraction of the hamstring on eliciting the ankle reflex. These responses occur most commonly in the face of segmental central hyperexcitability combined with impairment of the local reflex arc, such as an inverted brachioradialis reflex in cervical spondylotic radiculomyelopathy.

The easiest paradoxical reflexes to understand are the inverted triceps jerk and the inverted knee jerk, which are truly "inverted" because the response is the opposite of that expected: flexion of the elbow or knee with percussion of the triceps or patellar tendon. An inverted triceps reflex appears when the afferent arc of the reflex is damaged, as in C7 or C8 radiculopathy, particularly when accompanied by an element of spasticity. Care must be taken not to strike too distally; a blow delivered over the olecranon may cause the elbow to flex because of the biomechanics and force vectors involved, simulating an inverted triceps reflex when one is not actually present. This response has been referred to as the olecranon reflex but is more of a technical error in the point of the strike than a true reflex. With an inverted knee jerk there is knee flexion instead of extension.

The inverted triceps and knee reflexes are straightforward: the response is the opposite of that expected. Other "inverted" reflexes are related to activation of muscles other than the antagonist. In the presence of spasticity and hyperreflexia, reflex contraction of the biceps or brachioradialis may be accompanied by pronounced flexion of the fingers and adduction of the thumb. The inverted brachioradialis reflex (often referred to as an inverted radial periosteal or inverted supinator reflex) does not result in true inversion, that is, elbow extension, but instead produces a perverted or aberrant response with thumb and finger flexion, perhaps because the vibration wave activates the finger flexor reflex arc.

In the paradoxical ankle reflex, plantar flexion of the foot is produced by tapping the anterior aspect of the ankle in patients with hyperreflexia. The ankle reflex is not necessarily depressed, as with other inverted or perverted reflexes, and the response is the normal one but is due to spread of the reflexogenic zone. Vibration transmitted to the gastrosoleus has been invoked as an explanation.

Video Links

Video Link 38.1. Discussion of reflex hammer. https://www.youtube.com/watch?v=1-0Gq6s_Eoo&t=374s

Video Link 38.2. The clavicle reflex. http://neurosigns.org/wiki/Clavicle_reflex

Video Link 38.3. Dissociation of the abdominal reflexes. http://neurosigns.org/wiki/Dissociation_of_the_abdominal_reflexes

Video Link 38.4. The peroneal reflex. http://neurosigns.org/wiki/Peroneal_reflex

Videl Link 38.5. Delayed ankle jerks in hypothyroidism. https://www.nejm.org/doi/10.1056/NEJMicm1713796?url_ver=Z39.88-2003&rfr_id=ori:rid:crossref.org&rfr_dat=cr_pub%3dwww.ncbi.nlm.nih.gov

BIBLIOGRAPHY

Berlin L. A peroneal muscle stretch reflex. *Neurology* 1971;21:1177.

Bhattacharyya KB. Deep tendon reflex: the background story of a simple technique. *Neurol India* 2017;65:245–249.

Boes CJ. The history of examination of reflexes. *J Neurol* 2014;261:2264–2274.

Boyle RS, Shakir RA, Weir AI, et al. Inverted knee jerk: a neglected localising sign in spinal cord disease. *J Neurol Neurosurg Psychiatry* 1979;42:1005.

Carel RS, Korczyn AD, Hochberg Y. Age and sex dependency of the Achilles tendon reflex. *Am J Med Sci* 1979;278:57–63.

Chandrasekhar A, Abu Osman NA, Tham LK, et al. Influence of age on patellar tendon reflex response. *PLoS One* 2013;8:e80799.

Dick JP. The deep tendon and the abdominal reflexes. *J Neurol Neurosurg Psychiatry* 2003;74:150–153.

Esene IN, Meher A, Elzoghby MA, et al. Diagnostic performance of the medial hamstring reflex in L5 radiculopathy. *Surg Neurol Int* 2012;3:104.

Estanol BV, Marin OS. Mechanism of the inverted supinator reflex. A clinical and neurophysiological study. *J Neurol Neurosurg Psychiatry* 1976;39:905–908.

Felsenthal G, Reischer MA. Asymmetric hamstring reflexes indicative of L5 radicular lesions. *Arch Phys Med Rehabil* 1982;63:377–378.

Fuller G. *Neurological Examination Made Easy*. 5th ed. Edinburgh: Churchill Livingstone, 2013.

Gilman S. *Clinical Examination of the Nervous System*. New York: McGraw-Hill, 2000.

Gregory JE, Wood SA, Proske U. An investigation into mechanisms of reflex reinforcement by the Jendrassik manoeuvre. *Exp Brain Res* 2001;138:366–374.

Hannington-Kiff JG. Absent thigh adductor reflex in obturator hernia. *Lancet* 1980;1:180.

Impallomeni M, Kenny RA, Flynn MD, et al. The elderly and their ankle jerks. *Lancet* 1984;1:670.

Jensen OH. The medial hamstring reflex in the level-diagnosis of a lumbar disc herniation. *Clin Rheumatol* 1987;6:570–574.

Kiely P, Baker JF, O'hEireamhoin S, et al. The evaluation of the inverted supinator reflex in asymptomatic patients. *Spine (Phila Pa 1976)* 2010;35:955–957.

Kochar DK, Agarwal N, Sharma BV, et al. Paradoxical triceps jerk, a neglected localising sign in clinical neurology. *Neurol India* 2001;49:213.

Lanska DJ. The history of reflex hammers. *Neurology* 1989;39:1542–1549.

Lanska DJ. The Babinski reflex hammer. *Neurology* 1999;53:655.

Louis ED. Erb and Westphal: simultaneous discovery of the deep tendon reflexes. *Semin Neurol* 2002;22:385–390.

Martinelli P, Minardi C, Ciucci G, et al. Neurophysiological evaluation of areflexia in Holmes-Adie syndrome. *Neurophysiol Clin* 1999;29:255–262.

Massey EW, Pleet AB, Scherokman BJ. *Diagnostic Tests in Neurology: A Photographic Guide to Bedside Techniques*. Chicago: Year Book Medical Publishers, Inc., 1985.

O'Keeffe ST, Smith T, Valacio R, et al. A comparison of two techniques for ankle jerk assessment in elderly subjects. *Lancet* 1994;344:1619–1620.

Perloff MD, Leroy AM, Ensrud ER. Teaching video neuroimages: the elusive L5 reflex. *Neurology* 2010;75:e50.

Pryse-Phillips W. *Companion to Clinical Neurology*. 3rd ed. Oxford: Oxford University Press, 2009.

Ross RT. *How to Examine the Nervous System*. 4th ed. Totowa: Humana Press, 2006.

Schwartz RS, Morris JGL, Crimmins D, et al. A comparison of two methods of eliciting the ankle jerk. *Aust NZ J Med* 1990;20:116.

Stam J. The tibialis anterior reflex in healthy subjects and in L5 radicular compression. *J Neurol Neurosurg Psychiatry* 1988;51:397–402.

Stam J, Speelman HD, van Crevel H. Tendon reflex asymmetry by voluntary mental effort in healthy subjects. *Arch Neurol* 1989;46:70.

Vrancken AF, Kalmijn S, Brugman F, et al. The meaning of distal sensory loss and absent ankle reflexes in relation to age: a meta-analysis. *J Neurol* 2006;253:578–589.

Wartenberg R. *The Examination of Reflexes: A Simplification.* Chicago: Year Book Medical Pub, 1945.

Watson JC, Broaddus WC, Smith MM, et al. Hyperactive pectoralis reflex as an indicator of upper cervical spinal cord compression. Report of 15 cases. *J Neurosurg* 1997;86:159–161.

Zabelis TN, Karandreas NT, Constantinidis TS, et al. The effect of Jendrassik manoeuvre on the latency, amplitude and left-right asymmetry of tendon reflexes. *Electromyogr Clin Neurophysiol* 1998;38:19–23.

Ziff M, Stark RJ. How to assess tendon reflexes of the lower limb in the elderly. *J Neurol Sci* 2017;372:196–200.

CHAPTER 39

The Superficial (Cutaneous) Reflexes

Superficial reflexes are responses to stimulation of either the skin or mucous membrane. Cutaneous reflexes are elicited by a superficial skin stimulus, such as a light touch or scratch. The response occurs in the same general area where the stimulus is applied (local sign). Too painful a stimulus may call forth a defensive reaction rather than the desired reflex. Superficial reflexes are polysynaptic, in contrast to the stretch reflexes, which are monosynaptic. The superficial reflexes respond more slowly to the stimulus than do the stretch reflexes; their latency is longer, they fatigue more easily, and they are not as consistently present as tendon reflexes. The primary utility of superficial reflexes is that they are abolished by pyramidal tract lesions, which characteristically produce the combination of increased deep tendon reflexes and decreased or absent superficial reflexes. The superficial reflexes obtained most often are the abdominal and cremasteric. Unilateral absence of the superficial abdominal reflexes may be an early and sensitive indicator of a corticospinal tract lesion. Many of the superficial reflexes are arcane, of minor clinical significance, and primarily of historical interest.

THE SUPERFICIAL REFLEXES OF THE UPPER EXTREMITIES

The Palmar Reflex

Gentle stroking across the palm of the hand is followed by flexion of the fingers or a closing of the hand. The response is minimal or absent in normal individuals beyond the first few months of life. When exaggerated, this response is referred to as a grasp reflex; it is discussed in more detail in Chapter 40. Sensory and motor innervation is C6-T1 via the median and ulnar nerves.

The Scapular or Interscapular Reflex

Scratching the skin over the scapula or in the interscapular space causes contraction of the scapular muscles with retraction and sometimes elevation of the scapula; there may be associated adduction and external rotation of the arm. The reflex is related to the deep scapulohumeral reflex (see Chapter 38), and the innervation is similar.

THE SUPERFICIAL ABDOMINAL REFLEXES

The superficial abdominal reflexes consist of contraction of the abdominal muscles, elicited by a light stroke or scratch of the anterior abdominal wall, pulling the linea alba and umbilicus in the direction of the stimulus (Figure 39.1). The response can be divided into the upper abdominal and lower abdominal reflexes. The umbilicus is at the level of T10. The anterior abdominal wall can be divided into four quadrants by vertical and horizontal lines through the umbilicus. Light stroking or scratching in each quadrant elicits the response, pulling the umbilicus in the direction of the stimulus. The stimulus may be directed toward, away, or parallel to the umbilicus; stimuli directed toward the umbilicus seem more effective. The response is a quick, flicking contraction followed by immediate relaxation. The response is mediated in the upper quadrants (supraumbilical reflexes) by the intercostal nerves (T7-T10) and in the lower quadrants (infraumbilical or suprapubic reflexes) by the intercostal, iliohypogastric, and ilioinguinal nerves (T10 to upper lumbar segments). In Bechterew's hypogastric reflex, stroking the skin on the inner surface of the thigh causes contraction of the homolateral lower abdominal muscles.

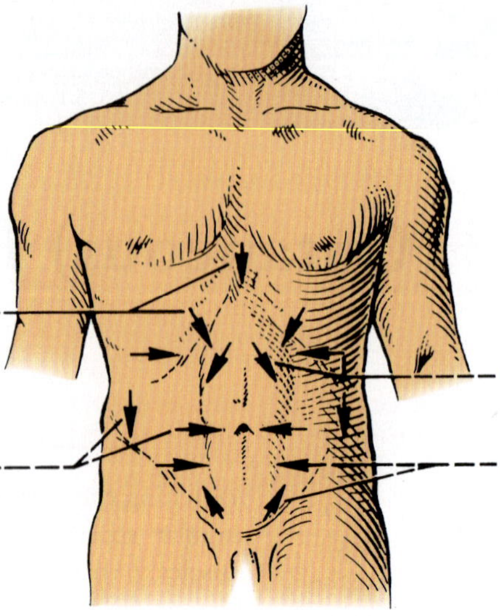

FIGURE 39.1 Sites of stimulation employed in eliciting the various superficial abdominal reflexes.

The responses are typically brisk and active in young individuals with good anterior abdominal tone. They may be sluggish or absent in normal individuals with lax abdominal tone, in those who are obese, or in women who have borne children. The epigastric reflex is similar but elicited by a stimulus moving from the xiphoid toward the umbilicus; there is usually no retraction or movement of the umbilicus.

The superficial abdominal reflexes may be difficult to obtain or evaluate in ticklish individuals. They may be absent in acute abdominal disorders (Rosenbach's sign) and with abdominal or bladder distension. They may be absent on the side of an incision from abdominal surgery or posterolateral thoracotomy. The latency is longer and the responses are slower in children and the elderly than in young adults. In a study of 65 adolescents and young adults, 14% of the subjects had asymmetric abdominal reflexes; in 15%, responses were absent in all quadrants; and 11% had no reflex in at least one quadrant; no subjects had reflexes present on one side and absent on the other. Dissociation of the abdominal reflexes, with absent superficial and exaggerated deep reflexes, suggests a corticospinal tract lesion (see **Video Link 39.1**). If the superficial abdominal reflexes are physiologically diminished or absent, the lower quadrant reflexes are usually affected first. In unilateral abdominal paralysis, there may be inversion of the reflex, with deviation of the umbilicus to the opposite side. Absence of superficial abdominal reflexes in patients with scoliosis has been suggested as an indicator of underlying syringomyelia. An abdominal reflex can be elicited electrophysiologically; its characteristics resemble the blink reflex.

THE SUPERFICIAL REFLEXES OF THE LOWER EXTREMITIES

The Cremasteric Reflex

This reflex is elicited by stroking or lightly scratching or pinching the skin on the upper, inner aspect of the thigh. The response consists of a contraction of the cremasteric muscle with a quick elevation of the homolateral testicle. The innervation is through the ilioinguinal and genitofemoral nerves (L1-L2). The cremasteric reflex must not be confused with the scrotal, or dartos, reflex, which produces a slow, writhing, vermicular contraction of the scrotal skin on stroking the perineum or thigh or applying a cold object to the scrotum. The cremasteric reflex may be absent in elderly males, in individuals who have a hydrocele or varicocele, in those with torsion of the testicle, and in those who have had orchitis or epididymitis.

The Gluteal Reflex

A contraction of the gluteal muscles may follow stroking the skin over the buttocks. The gluteus maximus is innervated by the inferior gluteal nerve (L4-S2), and the skin of this area is innervated by the cutaneous branches of the posterior rami of the lumbar and sacral nerves.

The Plantar Reflex

Stroking the plantar surface of the foot from the heel forward is normally followed by plantar flexion of the foot and toes (Figure 39.2). There is individual variation in the response and some variability dependent upon the site of maximal stimulation. Flexion is the normal response after the first 12 to 18 months of life. The pathologic variation of the plantar reflex is the Babinski sign (see Chapter 40). The normal plantar response may be difficult to obtain in individuals with plantar callosities. In ticklish patients, there may be voluntary withdrawal with flexion of the hip and knee, but in every normal individual, there is a certain amount of plantar flexion of the toes on stimulation of the sole of the foot. A tonic plantar reflex with slow, prolonged contraction has been described as a sign of frontal lobe and extrapyramidal disease. This reflex is innervated by the tibial nerve (L4-S2).

The Superficial Anal Reflex

The cutaneous anal reflex (anal wink) consists of contraction of the external sphincter in response to stroking or pricking the skin or mucous membrane in the perianal region. The reflex is mediated by the inferior hemorrhoidal nerve (S2-S5). Assessment of the superficial anal reflex is particularly important when a cauda equina or conus medullaris lesion is suspected. The internal anal sphincter reflex is discussed in Chapter 45.

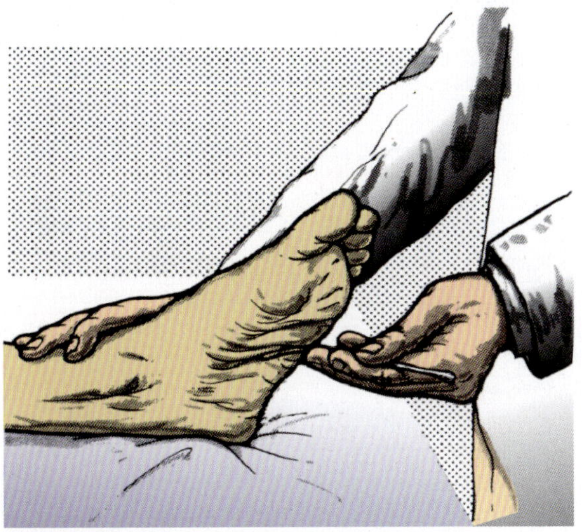

FIGURE 39.2 Method of obtaining the plantar reflex.

Bulbocavernosus Reflex

The bulbocavernosus reflex (BCR) is related to the anal reflex in that both cause contraction of the anal sphincter, but in the BCR, the stimulus is delivered to the glans penis or clitoris (clitoroanal reflex). The response is best palpated with a gloved finger in the rectum. Some forewarning and preliminary explanation is necessary, but the stimulus should still come as a surprise. In the male, a grabbing, pinching, or tweaking of the glans evokes the response, felt as a tightening of the sphincter on the finger. The response is much more difficult to elicit in females and the significance of its absence more dubious. The BCR is primarily useful is assessing the integrity of the cauda equina, lower sacral roots, and conus medullaris. It may be altered in some instances of multisystem atrophy.

ABNORMALITIES OF THE SUPERFICIAL REFLEXES

The effect on the superficial reflexes of lesions at various sites is summarized in Table 38.3. The superficial reflexes, like the deep reflexes, are impaired or absent with a lesion that disturbs the continuity of the reflex arc. In addition, a lesion anywhere along the corticospinal pathway will usually cause either diminution or absence of the superficial reflexes. The reflex change is contralateral to a lesion above the pyramidal decussation, and ipsilateral to a lesion below the pyramidal decussation. Corticospinal tract disease causes dissociation of reflexes, absence of superficial reflexes, and exaggerated deep reflexes. So, the superficial reflexes, especially the abdominal and cremasteric reflexes, have a special significance when their absence is associated with increased deep tendon reflexes or when they are absent when signs of corticospinal tract involvement are present. Dissociation of abdominal reflexes alone may be of diagnostic importance. Occasionally with apparent corticospinal tract disease, the superficial abdominal reflexes are intact. Superficial reflexes are absent in infants and appear after about 6 months to 1 year; their appearance may depend on myelination of the corticospinal tracts. When abdominal reflexes can be elicited in infants, they differ from the normal adult response, with a diffuse reaction often with associated movement of the legs. The abdominal and the cremasteric reflexes may occasionally be absent in persons without other evidence of neurologic disease.

The superficial reflexes, including the abdominal reflexes, are occasionally moderately exaggerated in parkinsonism and other extrapyramidal disorders. The abdominal reflexes may also be increased, often to a marked degree, with tension and anxiety. On occasion, this overactivity is so extreme that the umbilicus is said to "chase the pin" when the stimulating instrument is drawn in a circular manner over the surface of the abdomen. The superficial reflexes may help distinguish physiologic from pathologic hyperreflexia. In physiologic hyperreflexia, the abdominal and cremasteric reflexes are usually present and active, but in pathologic hyperreflexia due to an upper motor neuron lesion, they are usually absent. The superficial reflexes are normal with cerebellar lesions. Changes in the superficial reflexes must be interpreted in light of all other findings on the neurologic examination and related neurodiagnostic studies. Definite corticospinal tract signs (see Chapter 40) are of greater importance than changes in the superficial reflexes.

Video Links

Video Link 39.1. Dissociation of the abdominal reflexes. http://neurosigns.org/wiki/Dissociation_of_the_abdominal_reflexes

BIBLIOGRAPHY

Cai ZY, Niu XT, Pan J, et al. The value of the bulbocavernosus reflex and pudendal nerve somatosensory evoked potentials in distinguishing between multiple system atrophy and Parkinson's disease at an early stage. *Acta Neurol Scand* 2017;136:195–203.

Fujimori T, Iwasaki M, Nagamoto Y, et al. The utility of superficial abdominal reflex in the initial diagnosis of scoliosis: a retrospective review of clinical characteristics of scoliosis with syringomyelia. *Scoliosis* 2010;5:17.

Gosavi TD, Lo YL. Images in clinical medicine. Superficial abdominal reflex. *N Engl J Med* 2014;370:e29.

Huang HJ, Zhu XY, Wang X, et al. The Bulbocavernosus reflex in the differential diagnosis of multiple system atrophy with predominant parkinsonism and Parkinson's disease. *Front Neurol* 2018;8:697.

Lehoczky T, Fodors T. Clinical significance of the dissociation of abdominal reflexes. *Neurology* 1953;3:453.

Madonick MJ. Statistical control studies in neurology VIII. The cutaneous abdominal reflex. *Neurology* 1957;7:459.

Pryse-Phillips W. *Companion to Clinical Neurology*. 3rd ed. Oxford: Oxford University Press, 2009.

Saifuddin A, Tucker S, Taylor BA, et al. Prevalence and clinical significance of superficial abdominal reflex abnormalities in idiopathic scoliosis. *Eur Spine J* 2005;14:849–853.

Satomi K, Horai T, Hirakawa S. Electrophysiological study of superficial abdominal reflexes in normal men. *Electroencephalogr Clin Neurophysiol* 1993;89:113–119.

Schmitz D, Safranek S. Clinical inquiries. How useful is a physical exam in diagnosing testicular torsion? *J Fam Pract* 2009;58:433–434.

Schwarz GM, Hirtler L. The cremasteric reflex and its muscle—a paragon of ongoing scientific discussion: a systematic review. *Clin Anat* 2017;30:498–507.

Teasdall RD. Asymmetry of the superficial abdominal reflex in normal subjects. *Johns Hopkins Med J* 1970;126:276–278.

Wang ZY, Chen YH, Xu YY, et al. Altered bulbocavernosus reflex in patients with multiple system atrophy. *Neurol Res* 2016;38:138–143.

Wester C, FitzGerald MP, Brubaker L, et al. Validation of the clinical bulbocavernosus reflex. *Neurourol Urodyn* 2003;22(6):589–591.

Yngve D. Abdominal reflexes. *J Pediatr Orthop* 1997;17:105–108.

Zadeh HG, Sakka SA, Powell MP, et al. Absent superficial abdominal reflexes in children with scoliosis. An early indicator of syringomyelia. *J Bone Joint Surg Br* 1995;77:762–767.

CHAPTER 40

Pathologic Reflexes

Pathologic reflexes are responses not generally found in the normal individual. Some are responses that are minimally present and elicited with difficulty in normals but become prominent and active in disease, whereas others are not seen in normals at all. Many are exaggerations and perversions of normal muscle stretch and superficial reflexes. Some are related to postural reflexes or primitive defense reflexes that are normally suppressed by cerebral inhibition but become enhanced when the lower motor neuron is separated from the influence of the higher centers. Others are responses normally seen in the immature nervous system of infancy, then disappear only to reemerge later in the presence of disease. A decrease in threshold or an extension of the reflexogenic zone plays a role in many pathologic reflexes.

Descending motor influences normally control and modulate the activity at the local, segmental spinal cord level to ensure efficient muscle contraction and proper coordination of agonists, antagonists, and synergists. Disease of the descending motor pathways causes loss of this normal control so that activity spills from the motor neuron pool responsible for a certain movement to adjacent areas, resulting in the recruitment into the movement of muscles not normally involved. Some pathologic reflexes may also be classified as "associated movements," related to such spread of motor activity. Whether a certain abnormal response would be best classified as a reflex or an associated movement (see Chapter 42) is not always clear. Responses that are more in the realm of an associated movement are sometimes referred to clinically as reflexes (e.g., the Wartenberg thumb adduction sign, an associated movement, is sometimes called a Wartenberg reflex, see Chapter 42).

Most pathologic reflexes are related to disease involving the corticospinal tract and associated pathways. They also occur with frontal lobe disease and occasionally with disorders of the extrapyramidal system. There is a great deal of confusion regarding names of reflexes and methods of elicitation, and in many cases there has been significant drift away from the original description. Many of the responses are merely variations in the method of eliciting the same responses, or modifications of the same reflex. Some of these responses are arcane, seldom used, and primarily of historical interest; these are summarized in Tables 40.1 to 40.3. The typical reflex pattern with lesions involving the corticospinal tract, the upper motor neuron syndrome, is exaggeration of deep tendon reflexes (DTRs), disappearance of superficial reflexes, and emergence of pathologic reflexes (see Table 38.3).

The terms frontal release signs (FRS) and primitive, fetal, developmental, or atavistic reflexes refer to responses that are normally present in the developing nervous system but disappear to a greater or lesser degree with maturation. Although normal in infants and children, when present in an older individual they may be evidence of neurologic disease, although some may reappear in normal senescence. Many of these are exaggerations of normal reflex responses. Responses often included as FRS include the palmomental reflex (PMR), grasp, snout, suck, and others.

FRS occur most often in patients with severe dementias, with diffuse encephalopathy (metabolic, toxic, postanoxic), after head injury, and in other states in which the pathology is usually diffuse but involves particularly the frontal lobes or the frontal association areas. The significance and usefulness of some of these release signs or primitive reflexes have been questioned. Jacobs and Grossman, investigating the palmomental, snout, and corneomandibular reflexes, found that at least one of these was present in 50.5% of normal subjects in the third through ninth decades of life. The PMR appeared earliest and was the most frequent reflex at all ages, occurring in 20% to 25% of normal individuals in the third and fourth decades. In 20% of the group, more than one of the reflexes were elicited, and in about 2% all three were present. The Hoffman finger flexor reflex and its variants, which are sometimes classified as FRS and sometimes as corticospinal signs, are similarly present in a significant proportion of normal individuals. Clearly, these reflexes are a normal phenomenon in a significant proportion of the healthy population. They must be interpreted with caution and kept in clinical context. Even when such reflexes are briskly active in an appropriate clinical setting, the primitive reflexes do not have great localizing value, suggesting instead the presence of diffuse and widespread dysfunction of the hemispheres.

PATHOLOGIC REFLEXES IN THE LOWER EXTREMITIES

Pathologic reflexes in the lower extremities are more constant, more easily elicited, more reliable, and more clinically relevant than those in the upper limbs. The most important of these responses may be classified as (a) those characterized in the main by dorsiflexion of the toes and (b) those characterized by plantar flexion of the toes. The most important pathologic reflex by far is the Babinski sign, and a search for an upgoing toe has traditionally been part of every neurologic examination. There are, in addition, a few miscellaneous responses. Searching for upper-extremity pathologic reflexes is much less productive and often omitted.

Corticospinal Responses Characterized in the Main by Extension (Dorsiflexion) of the Toes

The Babinski Sign

In the normal individual, stimulation of the skin of the plantar surface of the foot is followed by plantar flexion of the toes (see Figure 39.2). In the normal plantar reflex, the response is usually fairly rapid, the small toes flex more than the great toe, and the reaction is more marked when the stimulus is along the medial plantar surface. In disease of the corticospinal system, there may instead be extension (dorsiflexion) of the toes, especially the great toe, with variable separation or fanning of the four lateral toes: the Babinski sign or extensor plantar response (Figure 40.1, **Video 40.1**). Babinski worked in a clinical arena dominated by Charcot and a focus on psychogenic symptoms. His primary aim was in trying to find reliable clinical signs to distinguish organic from nonorganic disease of the nervous system. Babinski described two components of the abnormal plantar reflex. He first described toe extension (1896) as *phénomène des orteils* (the dorsiflexion of the toes): "pricking of the sole... results in flexion of the thigh on the pelvis, of the leg on the thigh, and of the foot

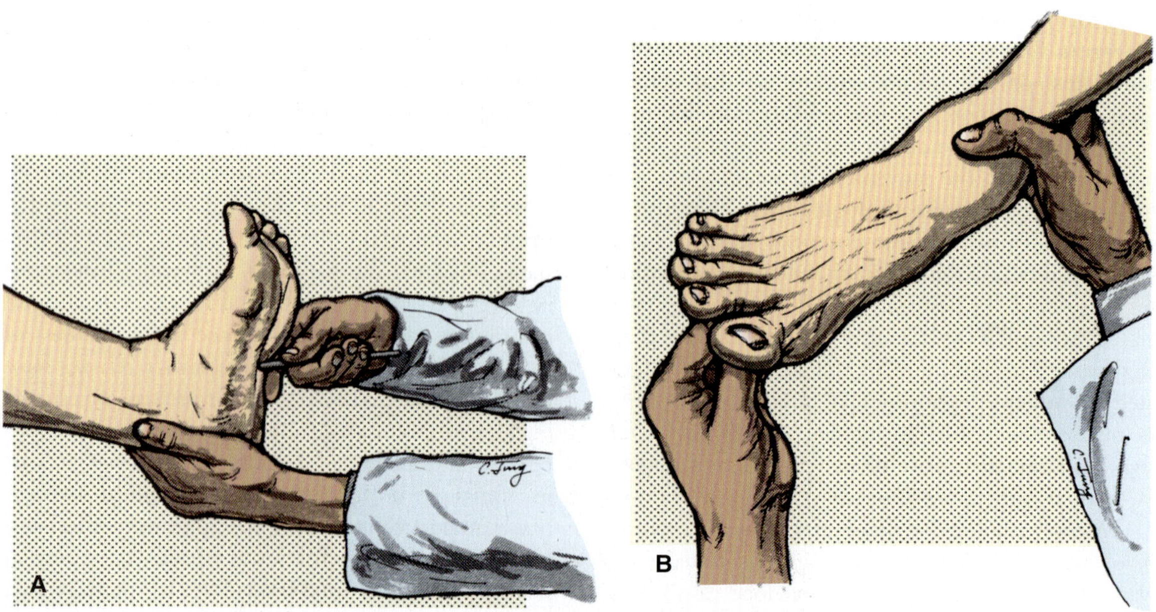

FIGURE 40.1 Method of eliciting the Babinski sign **(A)** with a sharp instrument and **(B)** with the thumb.

on the leg, but the toes, instead of flexing, execute a movement of extension upon the metatarsus." This is in fact a description of a triple flexion response. He also pointed out that the extension response was most easily elicited on stimulation of the outer aspect of the sole, in contrast to the normal plantar response. In 1903, he described abduction of the smaller toes, later labeled by others as the *signe de l'éventail* (the fanning). The Babinski sign has been called the most important sign in clinical neurology. It is one of the most significant indications of disease of the corticospinal system at any level from the motor cortex through the descending pathways.

The Babinski sign is obtained by stimulating the plantar surface of the foot with a blunt point, such as an applicator stick, handle of a reflex hammer, a broken tongue blade, the thumbnail, or the tip of a key. Much has been written about the best tools for eliciting the plantar response. Henry Miller, a legendary English neurologist, contended that the only proper instrument was a Bentley key. In the United States, the different types of keys used by neurologists as opposed to neurosurgeons are a source of tiresome levity. Babinski allegedly favored a goose quill.

Strength of stimulus is an important variable. It is not true that the stimulus must necessarily be deliberately "noxious," although most patients find it at least somewhat uncomfortable even if the examiner is trying to be considerate. It has been stated that eliciting the plantar responses brings out doctors' masochistic tendencies. Every physician should undergo plantar stimulation in order to appreciate the discomfort. When the response is strongly extensor, only minimal stimulation is required. Babinski observed the extensor plantar response when the wind blew the curtains across the feet of spinal cord–injured patients. Some reports have Babinski using a feather. The stimulus should be firm enough to elicit a consistent response, but as light as will suffice. Some patients are very sensitive to plantar stimulation, and only a slight stimulus will elicit a consistent response; stronger stimuli may produce confusing withdrawal. If the toe is briskly upgoing, merely a fingertip stimulus may elicit the response. If no response is obtained, progressively sharper objects and firmer applications are necessary. Although some patients require a very firm stimulus, it is not necessary to aggressively rake the sole as the opening gambit. Both tickling, which may cause voluntary withdrawal, and pain, which may bring about a reversal to flexion as a nociceptive response, should be avoided.

Plantar stimulation must be carried out far laterally, in the S1 root/sural nerve sensory distribution. More medial plantar stimulation may fail to elicit a positive response when one is present. Far medial stimulation may actually elicit a plantar grasp response, causing the toes to flex strongly. The stimulus should begin near the heel and be carried up the side of the foot at a deliberate pace, not too quickly, usually stopping at the metatarsophalangeal joints. The response has usually occurred by the time the stimulus reaches the midportion of the foot. If the response is difficult to obtain, the stimulus should continue along the metatarsal pad from the little toe medially, but stopping short of the base of the great toe. The most common mistakes are insufficiently firm stimulation, placement of the stimulus too medially, and moving the stimulus too quickly so that the response does not have time to develop. The only movements of significance are those of the great toe. Fanning of the lateral toes without an abnormal movement of the great toe is seldom of any clinical significance, and an absence of fanning does not negate the significance of great toe extension. The location of the lesion may influence the pattern of movement of the small toes.

The patient should be relaxed and forewarned of the potential discomfort. The knee must be extended; an upgoing toe may be abolished by flexion of the knee. The best position is supine, with hips and knees in extension and heels resting on the bed. Some neurologists will only check the plantar responses with the patient recumbent. If the patient is seated, the knee should be extended, with the foot held either in the examiner's hand or on her knee. The response may sometimes be reinforced by rotating the patient's head to the opposite side. It may be inhibited when the foot is cold and increased when the foot is warm.

Usually, the upward movement of the great toe is a quick, flicking motion, sometimes mistaken for withdrawal by the inexperienced. The response may be a slow, tonic, sometimes clonic, dorsiflexion of the great toe, and the small toes with fanning, or separation, of the toes. The slow great toe movement has been described as a "majestic rise." The nature of the stimulus may be related to the speed of the toe movement. Primarily proprioceptive stimuli (e.g., Gonda, Stransky, Szapiro) are more apt to be followed by a slow, tonic response; exteroceptive stimuli, by a brief, rapid extension (for video of the Stransky reflex, see Amir and Helsen). There may occasionally be initial extension, followed by flexion; less often brief flexion precedes extension. There may be extension of only the great toe, or extension of the great toe with flexion of the small toes. Puusepp's sign is tonic, slow abduction of the little toe on plantar stimulation and may be present when great toe extension is absent.

The Babinski sign is a part of the primitive flexion reflex. The central nervous system is organized according to movement patterns, and one of the most basic patterns is avoidance or withdrawal from a noxious stimulus. In higher vertebrates, the flexion response includes flexion of the hip and knee, and dorsiflexion of the ankle and toes, all serving to remove the threatened part from danger. Although the relevant muscles are anatomical extensors, and have extensor names (e.g., extensor hallucis longus [EHL]), physiologically flexors serve to shorten a limb, so toe "extension" is in fact part of the flexion response. In human infants, the primitive flexion response persists, and an extensor plantar response is normal up to about 1 year of age. The plantar response in infancy has been studied on several occasions, with variable results; Gingold et al. found extensor responses at birth in 100% of infants, at 6 months in 10.9%, at 1 year in none. There are several examples of infantile upgoing toes in Renaissance Madonna and child paintings (Boticelli recorded the extensor plantar response 400 years before Babinski). Maturation of the descending motor systems suppresses the primitive flexion response. This may be necessary for normal ambulation, or else our legs and feet might be whipping into flexion unexpectedly, just from stepping on a pebble. The corticospinal tract is myelinated by about the end of the first year of life, about the time babies begin to walk.

When there is disease involving the corticospinal tract, the primitive flexion response may reappear, and the first clinical evidence of this is the Babinski sign. With more severe and extensive disease, the entire flexion response emerges, so that stimulation of the sole causes dorsiflexion not only of the toe but also of the ankle, as well as flexion of the hip and knee (the "triple flexion" response, which for some perplexing reason has four parts). In addition, there is often contraction of the tensor fascia lata causing slight internal rotation at the hip and more rarely abduction of the hip (Brissaud's reflex). The Brissaud reflex may be useful for the rare patient whose great toe is missing or paralyzed, as may Puusepp's sign. These movements are all part of a spinal defense reflex mechanism, also known as the reflex of spinal automatism (Marie), the pathologic shortening reflex, reflex flexor synergy, the withdrawal reflex, and the mass flexion reflex. The dorsiflexion of the toes may be the only visible effect, but the contraction of the thigh and leg muscles is also present and may be detected by palpation. The response may be bilateral and is then called the crossed flexor reflex.

There are many other corticospinal tract responses in the lower extremities characterized by dorsiflexion of the toes. With severe corticospinal tract disease, the threshold for eliciting an upgoing toe is lower, the reflexogenic zone is wider, and more and more of the other components of the primitive flexion reflex appear as part of the response. This has led to a profusion of variations on the Babinski method of eliciting the extensor plantar response. Foster Kennedy referred to the 30 years around the turn of the 20th century as "open season for the hunting of the reflex." Grant referred to it as the "assault on the great toe." Many clinicians sought eponymic immortality by describing different ways of making the toe go up, other components of the reflex, and other variations on the theme. There are too many modifications to mention all. The most useful variation is the Chaddock sign, and the Oppenheim is also often done. Other responses have been relegated to the category of minor toe signs, which now amount to clinical parlor tricks (Table 40.1).

TABLE 40.1 Minor Extensor Toe Signs (Alternate Methods for Eliciting the Toe Dorsiflexion in Lesions of the Corticospinal Tract)

Sign	Stimulus
Gordon's sign	Squeezing of calf muscles
Schaefer's sign	Deep pressure on Achilles tendon
Bing's sign	Pricking dorsum of foot with a pin
Moniz' sign	Forceful passive plantar flexion at ankle
Throckmorton's sign	Percussing over dorsal aspect of metatarsophalangeal joint of great toe just medial to EHL tendon
Strümpell's phenomenon	Forceful pressure over anterior tibial region
Cornell response	Scratching dorsum of foot along inner side of EHL tendon
Gonda (Allen)	Forceful downward stretching or snapping of second, third, or fourth toe; if response is difficult to obtain, flex toe slowly, press on nail, twist the toe, and hold it for a few seconds
Stransky	Small toe forcibly abducted, then released
Allen and Cleckley	Sharp upward flick of second toe or pressure applied to ball of toe
Szapiro	Pressure against dorsum of second through fifth toes, causing firm passive plantar flexion while stimulating plantar surface of foot

EHL, extensor hallucis longus.

Some may occasionally be useful in cases where, for some reason, the plantar surface of the foot cannot be stimulated.

The Chaddock sign is elicited by stimulating the lateral aspect of the foot, not the sole, beginning about under the lateral malleolus near the junction of the dorsal and plantar skin, drawing the stimulus from the heel forward to the small toe **(Video 40.1)**. The reflex was described first by Yoshimura, but in Japanese so the observation was lost. In the "reverse Chaddock," the stimulus moves from the small toe toward the heel. The Chaddock is the only alternative toe sign that is truly useful (according to Sapira, in his time the best neurologist in St. Louis was C.G. Chaddock; the second best was C.G. Chaddock drunk). It may be more sensitive than the Babinski but is less specific. It produces less withdrawal than plantar stimulation. The two reflexes are complementary; each can occur without the other, but both are usually present. The Oppenheim sign is usually elicited by dragging the knuckles heavily down the anteromedial surface of the tibia from the infrapatellar region to the ankle **(Video 40.1)**. The response is slow and often occurs toward the end of stimulation. Oppenheim allegedly did this by raking the handle of his reflex hammer down the shin. A common ploy is to combine the Oppenheim and the Babinski to make a suspicious toe declare itself, but this is more painful and less useful than the Chaddock.

When the response is very active and the reflexogenic zone wide, the toe may go up with such minor stimuli as pulling back the bed sheets (the "bed sheet Babinski") or rapid removal of the sock or shoe. Occasionally, there is a "spontaneous Babinski," occurring with no apparent manipulation of the foot. There may even be contralateral or bilateral responses. The response may occur with passive extension of the knee or passive flexion of the hip and knee. Sometimes, the toes are held in a tonic position of dorsiflexion and fanning. Such a tonic toe may become problematic, causing skin breakdown on the dorsum of the great toe from friction against the shoe (an example of the maladaptive effect of an unsuppressed primitive flexion reflex). Botulinum toxin is sometimes injected into the EHL to control the tenacious toe extension. A tonic extensor plantar response must be distinguished from a "striatal toe" (see Figure 30.2).

The complete primitive flexion reflex can become tonic and permanent. This occurs most often in patients with severe myelopathy, usually traumatic, and produces a posture referred to as paraplegia in flexion. The exaggeration of the flexion reflex causes involuntary flexor spasms that hold the legs intensely flexed with increasing frequency and for longer and longer periods until they can no longer be actively or even passively extended. This terminates eventually in a tonic flexion posture, with permanent fixed flexion of the hips and knees and dorsiflexion of the ankles and toes. Secondary joint contractures are common. In the severest cases, the legs and thighs are completely flexed and the knees pressed against the abdomen. Even after the development of a fixed flexion posture, any additional stimulus may aggravate the degree of flexion.

Problems in Interpreting the Plantar Response

The extensor plantar response is one of the most reliable, dependable, and consistent signs in clinical neurology. Many studies have examined the interrater reliability of the Babinski and reached widely different conclusions, but it has generally good interobserver reliability, and its presence is, with rare exception, credible evidence of organic neurologic disease (as Babinski had originally hoped). A small but provocative study questioned whether the Babinski sign should be part of the routine neurologic examination, contending that its validity and interobserver reliability was limited. The authors suggested that slowed foot tapping was a more useful clinical sign. The article provoked an editorial and a flurry of correspondence challenging the conclusions and the methodology. A recent, small study using surface EMG and high-speed videography showed substantial interrater agreement.

Van Gijn and Bonke investigated the biasing effect of other signs and symptoms on the interpretation of plantar reflexes. They found that physicians place the toe in clinical context and this affects interpretation. The history and other examination findings have a significant influence, and many neurologists have a significant bias about the expected direction of toe movement before touching the foot. It appears preknowledge makes it easier to call an equivocal response extensor.

The Babinski is a valuable clinical sign, but it is not perfect, and the response to plantar stimulation may at times be difficult to evaluate. The most common problem is distinguishing an upgoing toe from voluntary withdrawal, especially when the plantar surface of the foot is unusually sensitive. Occasionally, even a seasoned clinician cannot be sure or makes the wrong interpretation. The Babinski sign is part of a withdrawal reflex, so flexion of the hip and knee are by no means reliable indicators that the withdrawal movement is voluntary. Voluntary withdrawal rarely causes dorsiflexion of the ankle, and there is usually plantar flexion of the toes. Voluntary withdrawal is more likely when the stimulus is too intense and uncomfortable. It helps if the patient understands the importance of holding still and receives some explanation of the relevance of this seemingly inane and cruel test. Some patients have ticklish feet and will pull away from even a light stimulus. If the patient is ticklish, it may help to simply hold the ankle firmly. Some believe withdrawal is less if the patient performs the plantar stimulation himself (an auto-Babinski); others (author included) have not found this useful. Some contend that pressure over the base of the great toe will inhibit the withdrawal extensor response but not eliminate the extension associated with corticospinal tract disease. Internal rotation of the leg during the "withdrawal" signals recruitment of the tensor fascia lata into the movement (the Brissaud reflex component) and makes it more likely the response is reflex and not voluntary.

The most important observation is the initial movement of the great toe. With repeated stimulation of the sole, the extensor plantar response may decrease and then disappear. So, the crucial observation is the first toe movement on the first stimulation. Occasionally, withdrawal makes it impossible to be certain whether the toe was truly extensor or not; these are equivocal plantar responses. Some patients have no elicitable plantar response, in which case the plantars are said to be mute or silent. An extensor plantar response may also show itself in formes frustes. There can be flexion of the hip and knee with no movement of the toes. Asymmetry of the plantar responses may be significant; a toe that does not go down as crisply as its fellow may be suspect, even if it does not frankly go up. A toe is more likely to go up late in the day or when the patient is tired.

A toe may occasionally fail to go up when expected, despite good technique. It is occasionally possible to elicit one or more of the other extensor toe signs, especially the Chaddock, when the Babinski cannot be obtained. A more extensive lesion may be necessary for production of the Oppenheim or Gordon sign than for the Babinski or Chaddock. It is occasionally useful to try two maneuvers simultaneously (e.g., Babinski and Oppenheim or Babinski and Gordon) to bring forth a latent extensor response by means of reinforcement. In a study of the consistency of the Babinski reflex and its variants, the combination of the Babinski and Chaddock reflexes was the most reliable.

Toe extension may occasionally fail to occur because of disruption of the lower motor neuron innervation to the EHL (e.g., radiculopathy, peroneal nerve palsy, peripheral neuropathy, amyotrophic lateral sclerosis [ALS]), in which case the toe is paralyzed for voluntary contraction as well. Contraction of the other muscles involved in the primitive flexion reflex may betray the upper motor neuron pathology. Frontal lobe lesions may cause a hyperactive plantar grasp reflex (see next section), driving the toes downward. The toe may not go up during the neural shock phase of acute insults to the corticospinal tract. Sometimes, the plantar response remains inexplicably flexor despite an abundance of other corticospinal tract signs. This may happen in ALS, in part because of lower motor neuron involvement of the toe extensors. In other instances, the absence of a toe sign remains a curious paradox. With pes cavus and high-arched feet, the response is difficult to evaluate because of fixed dorsiflexion of the toes.

An extensor plantar response may occasionally occur in patients with no other evidence of corticospinal tract disease and in a small percentage of individuals who appear otherwise neurologically normal. It may be the only residual sign of previous disease. With extensive disease involving both the basal ganglia and the corticospinal tract, there may be no extensor response. In all probability, intact extrapyramidal pathways are essential to its production. The extensor plantar response does not occur in lesions of the basal ganglia alone; its presence in some extrapyramidal disorders, such as Parkinson's disease, suggests associated corticospinal tract involvement. Paralysis of the toe flexors may cause a false-positive extensor plantar response.

An extensor plantar response does not always signify structural disease; it may occur as a transient manifestation of physiologic dysfunction of the corticospinal pathways. A Babinski sign may sometimes be found in deep anesthesia and narcosis, in drug and alcohol intoxication, in metabolic coma such as hypoglycemia, in deep sleep, postictally, and in other conditions of altered consciousness. The plantar response returns to normal with recovery of consciousness. During Cheyne-Stokes respirations, an upgoing toe may appear during the apneic phase and disappear during the phase of active respiration.

Corticospinal Tract Responses Characterized by Plantar Flexion of the Toes

In the newborn infant, there is a grasp reflex in the foot as well as the hand, with flexion and adduction of the toes in response to light pressure on the plantar surface of the foot, especially its distal and medial portions. The plantar grasp normally disappears by the end of the first year. A grasp reflex of the foot may reappear in adults, along with a grasp reflex of the hand, in disease of the opposite frontal lobe. The plantar grasp may be elicited by drawing the handle of a reflex hammer from the midsole toward the toes, causing the toes to flex and grip the hammer (Figure 40.2).

In addition to the superficial plantar reflex, there is a plantar muscle reflex consisting of contraction of the toe flexors following sudden stretching. This response is barely, if at all, perceptible normally, but becomes more obvious with reflex hyperactivity and, therefore, with corticospinal tract lesions. Plantar flexion of the toes may also be elicited by application of the stimulus to other portions of the foot and ankle. The best known of this group of reflexes is the Rossolimo sign (Table 40.2, Figure 40.3, **Video 40.1**). The presence of Rossolimo's sign is sometimes helpful in distinguishing an extensor plantar response from withdrawal. Many others have been described, all variations on the same reflex elicited by striking slightly different parts of the foot (Figure 40.4). In describing

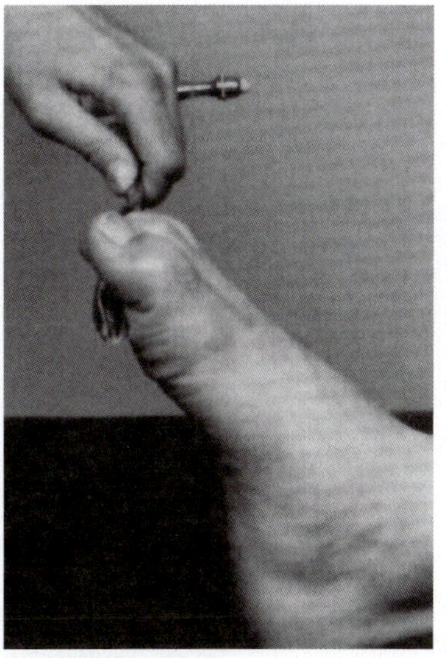

FIGURE 40.2 Plantar grasp reflex. Brisk bending of toes to grasp reflex hammer handle. (Reprinted from Massey EW, Pleet AB, Scherokman BJ. *Diagnostic Tests in Neurology: A Photographic Guide to Bedside Techniques*. Chicago: Year Book Medical Publishers, 1985. Copyright © 1985 Elsevier. With permission.)

TABLE 40.2 Other Lower-Extremity Pathologic Reflexes

Reflex	Stimulus	Response
Marie-Foix sign	Squeezing the toes or strongly plantar flexing toes or foot	Extension of toes, especially great toe, plus dorsiflexion of ankle and flexion at hip and knee (triple flexion)
Rossolimo's sign	Tapping ball of foot, or plantar surfaces of toes; giving a quick, lifting snap to tips of toes (Figure 40.3, Video 40.1)	Quick plantar flexion of toes, especially smaller ones; in normals there is no movement or slight dorsiflexion of toes
Mendel-Bechterew (dorsocuboidal, tarsophalangeal) reflex	Tapping or stroking outer aspect of dorsum of foot in region of cuboid bone, or over fourth and fifth metatarsals	Same as Rossolimo's
Bechterew's reflex	Percussion of middle of sole or heel	Plantar flexion response
Medioplantar reflex of Guillain and Barré	Tapping the midplantar region of the foot	Plantar flexion with fanning of the toes
Heel reflex of Weingrow	Tapping on base of heel	Plantar flexion with fanning of the toes
Antagonistic anterior tibial reflex of Piotrowski	Tapping belly of anterior tibial muscle	Plantar flexion of the ankle and sometimes of the toes
Paradoxical ankle reflex of Bing	Tapping the anterior aspect of the ankle joint	Plantar flexion of the foot
Adductor reflex of the foot (Hirschberg sign)	Stroking inner border of foot (not sole), from great toe to heel	Adduction, inversion, and slight plantar flexion of foot (posterior tibial contraction)
Balduzzi's sign	Same as adductor reflex	Same as adductor reflex but with contralateral or bilateral response
von Monakow's sign	Stroking lateral margin of foot	Foot eversion and abduction
Little toe reflex of Puusepp	Light stroking of outer border of foot	Slow abduction of little toe

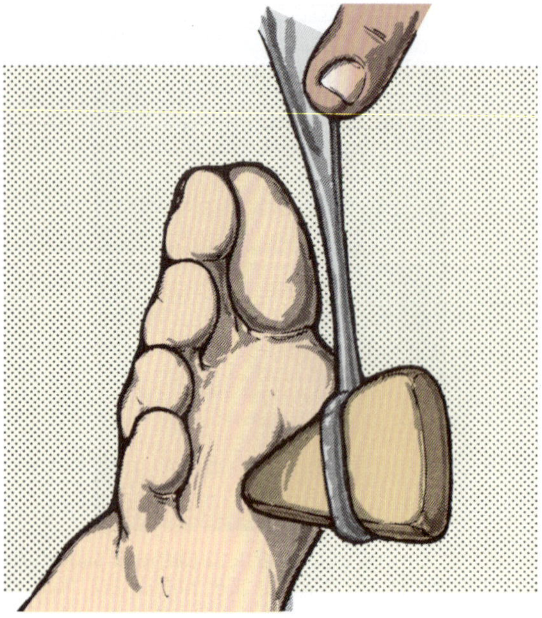

FIGURE 40.3 Method of eliciting the Rossolimo sign.

Figure 40.4 in his foreword to Wartenberg's monograph The Examination of Reflexes, Foster Kennedy said, "… a welter of the names of reflex describers has been placed in appropriate positions around a foot, like a litter at suck. And all describing small distinctions without differences, of no true significance and usually of little help." These variations are primarily manifestations of an exaggerated plantar muscle reflex, comparable to the variations of the finger flexor reflex in the upper extremities (see "The Hoffman and Trömner Signs and the Flexor Reflexes of the Fingers and Hand" below). Some correspond to alternate methods of eliciting the ankle reflex and may reflect spread of the reflexogenic zone.

Other Lower-Extremity Pathologic Reflexes

In the crossed extensor reflex, stimulation of the foot or leg on one side causes flexion of that extremity with extension of the other leg (Phillipson's reflex).

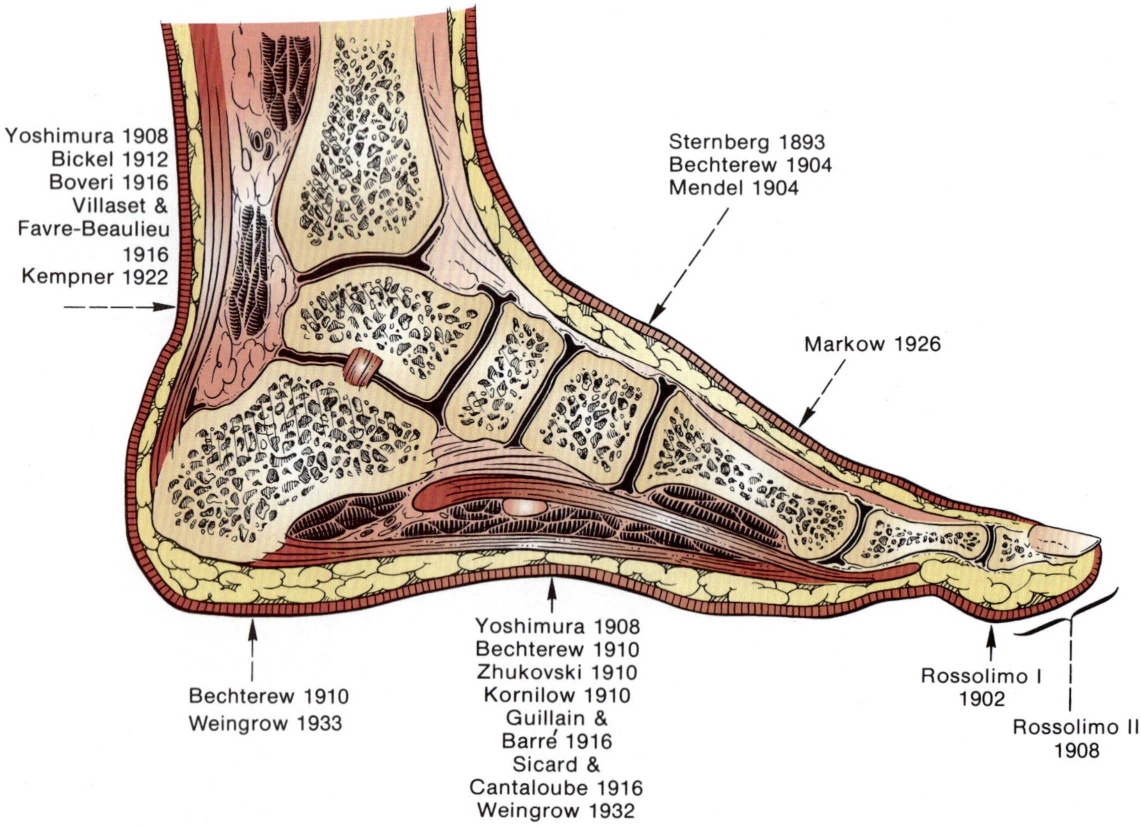

FIGURE 40.4 Plantar muscle reflex: sites on the surface of the foot where a tap with a reflex hammer will be followed by plantar flexion of the toes. Names of authors who described these reflexes and dates of publication are shown. Many of these reflexes are named for their discoverers. Dr. Wartenberg believed that all of the 20 reflexes indicated here represent the same reflex. (Modified from Wartenberg R. Studies in reflexes: III. History, physiology, synthesis and nomenclature. *Arch Neurol Psychiatry* 1944;52:359–382; figure also appears in Wartenberg R. *The Examination of Reflexes: A Simplification.* Chicago: Year Book Medical Publishers, 1945.)

The response is similar to the crossed extensor reflex of the spinal animal. Clinically, it is usually present in patients with severe spinal cord lesions. In the extensor thrust response, pressure applied to the foot of the passively flexed leg causes reflex extension. It also occurs with severe myelopathy. Similar extension may occur if a leg paralyzed by a spinal lesion is placed in flexion, and the skin in the lumbar or perineal area or in the adductor region of the thigh is pinched. The extension may be followed by flexion. At times, alternate extension and flexion occur, producing a stepping or marching movement of the legs. The mass reflex occurs in patients with severe myelopathy after the stage of spinal shock. Stimulation below the level of the lesion causes a massive response, including not only leg flexion but also muscular contractions of the abdominal wall, often evacuation of the bladder and bowel, sweating, reflex erythema, pilomotor responses, and hypertension. The reflexogenic zone may extend to the bladder, so that bladder distention may precipitate the entire reflex complex. Priapism and even ejaculation may be a part of the response.

PATHOLOGIC REFLEXES IN THE UPPER EXTREMITIES

Abnormal reflex responses in the upper extremities are less constant, more difficult to elicit, and usually less significant diagnostically than those found in the lower extremities. A great deal of confusion exists concerning the nomenclature of these reflexes, with many variations and modifications of the same response. The upper-extremity pathologic reflexes primarily fall into two categories: FRS and exaggerations of or variations on the finger flexor reflex. The grasp and PMRs are usually classified as FRS. The finger flexor–related responses are usually a manifestation of the spasticity and hyperreflexia that occur in lesions involving the corticospinal tract, so the Hoffman and Trömner signs are usually classified as corticospinal tract signs. These responses occur only with lesions above the C5 or C6 segment of the cervical spinal cord.

The Grasp (Forced Grasping) Reflex

The grasp reflex is usually classified as an FRS. Forced grasping is an involuntary flexor response of the fingers and hand following stimulation of the skin of the palmar surface of the fingers or hand. The patient is instructed not to hold on to the examiner's hand. There are four variations and modifications: (a) If the examiner's fingers are placed in the patient's hand, especially between the thumb and forefinger, or if the palmar skin is stimulated gently, there is slow flexion of the digits. The patient's fingers may close around the examiner's fingers in a gentle grasp that can be relaxed on command. This is the simple grasp reflex, an exaggeration of the normal palmar reflex. (b) If the patient's flexed fingers are gently extended by the fingers of the examiner, they will flex against the examiner's fingers in a "hooking" or traction response. (c) With a more marked grasp response, the strength of the grasp increases with attempts to withdraw the examiner's hand or to extend the patient's fingers passively and there is loss of ability to relax the grasp voluntarily or on command. The grip may be so firm that the patient can be lifted from the bed by the examiner. This is the forced grasping reflex and is a part of the counterholding, or gegenhalten, phenomenon, in which muscle contraction develops in response to contact and as a resistance to changes in position and posture. (d) The sight of the observer's hand near but not touching the patient's hand, or even a very light touch on the patient's hand between the thumb and forefinger while her eyes are closed, leads to groping movements, termed the groping response. Other things may be substituted for the examiner's fingers to elicit the grasp response (e.g., the handle of the reflex hammer).

The palmar grasp is normally present at birth and may be strong enough to suspend the infant by her own grasp. The response begins to diminish at the age of 2 to 4 months. It reappears primarily in association with extensive neoplastic or vascular lesions of the frontal lobes or with cerebral degenerative processes, usually contralaterally but occasionally ipsilaterally. Although the grasp reflex is usually classified as an FRS or primitive reflex, it may also occur as evidence of corticospinal tract dysfunction in spastic hemiplegia. The grasping responses are exaggerations of normal reactions and occur as release phenomena; the groping response is a more complicated reaction that is modified by visual and tactile integration at the cortical level. Some patients who have bilateral grasp responses exhibit the phenomenon of self-grasping, with one hand grasping the contralateral forearm. When this sign is present unilaterally, it suggests a contralateral frontal or parietal lobe lesion. When it occurs bilaterally, there is no localizing value.

The Palmomental Reflex of Marinesco-Radovici

The PMR, or palm-chin reflex, is contraction of the mentalis and orbicularis oris muscles causing wrinkling of the skin of the chin with slight retraction and sometimes elevation of the angle of the mouth in response to scratching or stroking the palm of the ipsilateral hand. The reflex is best elicited by stroking a blunt point over the thenar eminence, either from wrist toward thumb or vice versa, or by tapping this area. The PMR is so frequently present in normal persons that significance can only be attached to a marked exaggeration of the response or a conspicuous asymmetry between the two sides. If the response is marked, the reflexogenic zone may be wide, including the hypothenar area. A trigger area outside the palm probably does not occur in healthy people. In neurologic patients, the reflex can sometimes be elicited by stimulation of the forearm, chest, abdomen, or even the sole; and changing the name to "mentalis reflex" has been suggested. Spread of the reflex response beyond the chin region may also occur; involvement of the platysma has been termed the palmocervical reflex. The PMR is weak and fatigable in normals and stronger and more persistent in disease. The PMR can help in the differential diagnosis of facial palsy—it is absent in peripheral facial palsy and may be exaggerated in central facial paresis. The pollicomental reflex is the same response to stroking the palmar surface of the thumb. The localizing value and clinical significance of these reflexes are limited. A unilateral PMR may occur with bilateral, contralateral, or ipsilateral lesions. The pathways involved in the PMR remain uncertain, but it is clear that a unilateral PMR does not have localizing value. The PMR has been reviewed in detail by Owen and Mulley.

The Hoffmann and Trömner Signs and the Flexor Reflexes of the Fingers and Hand

The finger flexor reflex (Wartenberg's sign, one of many) is flexion of the patient's fingers and distal phalanx of the thumb in response to a stretch stimulus delivered with a reflex hammer (Figure 38.6). The Hoffmann and Trömner signs are alternative methods of delivering the stretch stimulus. They are prominent when the other upper-extremity DTRs are hyperactive, as in corticospinal tract lesions. These signs are not necessarily pathologic and are often present to some degree in normal individuals. As with the PMR, they are only of clinical significance when markedly active or very asymmetric. A very active, complete Hoffmann or Trömner sign, especially if unilateral or associated with other reflex abnormalities or a consistent history, is certainly suggestive if not diagnostic of corticospinal tract involvement.

To elicit the Hoffmann sign, the patient's relaxed hand is held with the wrist dorsiflexed and fingers partially flexed. With one hand, the examiner holds the partially extended middle finger between her index finger and thumb or between her index and middle fingers. With a sharp, forcible flick of the other thumb, the examiner nips or snaps the nail of the patient's middle finger, forcing the distal finger into sharp, sudden flexion followed by sudden release (Figure 40.5). The rebound of the distal phalanx stretches the finger flexors. If the Hoffmann sign is present, this is followed by flexion and adduction of the thumb and flexion of the index finger, and sometimes flexion of the other fingers as well. If only the thumb or only the index finger responds, the sign is "incomplete." In the Trömner sign, the examiner holds the patient's partially extended middle finger, letting the hand dangle, then, with the other hand, thumps or flicks the finger pad (Figure 40.6). The response is the same as that in the Hoffmann test. The two methods are equivalent, and either manner of testing may be used; both are sometimes referred to as the Hoffmann test.

Many other flexor reflexes of the fingers and hand have been described. Most are variations or exaggerations of the finger flexor reflex or of the finger flexor together with the wrist flexor reflex; some are related to forced grasping. These reflexes are not of great clinical utility and are summarized

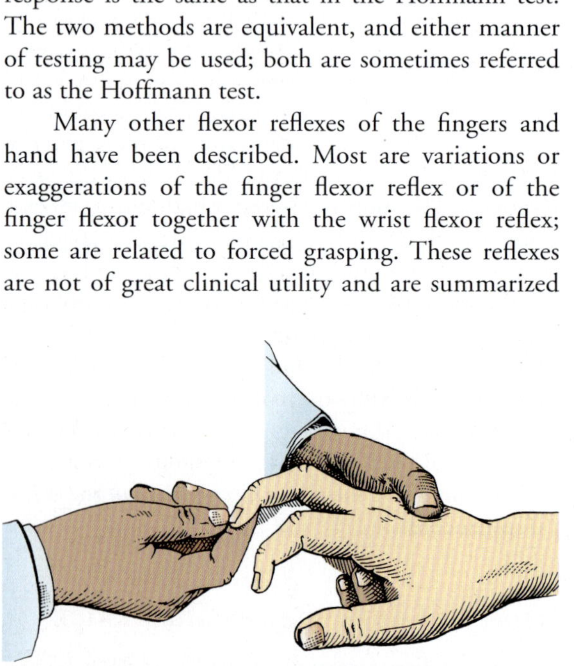

FIGURE 40.5 Method of eliciting the Hoffmann sign.

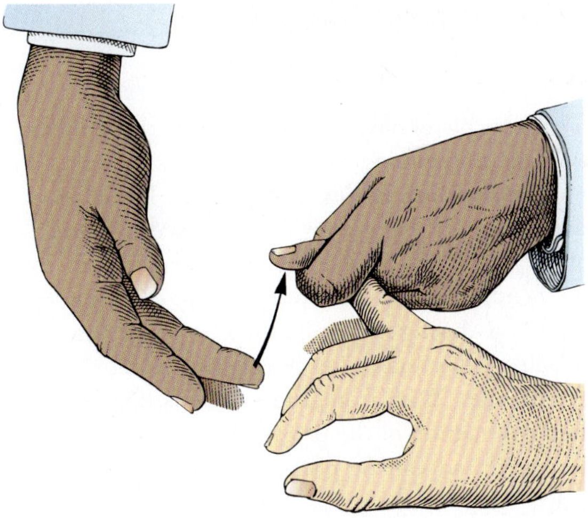

FIGURE 40.6 Method of eliciting the Trömner sign.

in Table 40.3. In some reflexes, hand flexion may be followed by extension, or extension responses occur instead of flexion. These extension reflexes, like the flexor reflexes, are evidence of reflex hyperactivity and suggest corticospinal tract involvement only if they are unilateral or associated with other reflex changes. These reflexes, although unique and interesting, probably have little clinical significance and are also summarized in Table 40.3.

Other Upper-Extremity Corticospinal Reflexes

Certain other reflexes may be found in the upper extremities in the presence of corticospinal tract pathology. These include the Klippel-Feil sign, the Leri sign, the Mayer sign, the bending reflex, and the

TABLE 40.3 Other Upper-Extremity Pathologic Reflexes

Reflex	Stimulus	Response
Rossolimo's of the hand	Percussion of palmar aspect of MCP joints or tapping volar surface of fingertips	Flexion of the fingers and supination of the forearm
Mendel-Bechterew of the hand (carpometacarpal or carpophalangeal reflex of Bechterew)	Percussion of dorsal aspect of carpal and metacarpal areas, or tapping dorsum of either hand or fingers	Flexion of the fingers and hand
Flexion reflex (Dejerine hand phenomenon)	Percussion of flexor tendons on volar surface of forearm (see https://www.youtube.com/watch?v=SAopdNT4-4E)	Flexion of fingers and hand
Thumb-adductor reflex of Marie-Foix	Superficial stroking of palm of hand in hypothenar region, or scratching ulnar side of palm	Adduction and flexion of thumb, sometimes with flexion of adjacent digits, more rarely with extension of little finger
Foxe reflex	Pinching hypothenar region	Same as Marie-Foix
Oppenheim's sign	Rubbing external surface of forearm	Same as Marie-Foix
Schaefer sign	Pinching flexor tendons at wrist	Same as Marie-Foix
Gordon's flexion sign	Squeezing muscles of forearm	Same as Marie-Foix
Ulnar adduction reflex of Pool	Stimulation of any portion of palm innervated by ulnar nerve	Adduction of the thumb
Chaddock's wrist sign	Pressure or scratching in depression at ulnar side of FCR and PL tendons at wrist, or pressure on PL tendon; at times stimulation almost anywhere on ulnar side of volar forearm as high as elbow	Flexion of wrist and simultaneous extension and separation of digits
Gordon's extension sign	Pressure on radial side of pisiform bone	Extension and occasionally fanning of the flexed fingers
Extension-adduction reflex of Dagnini	Percussion on radial aspect of dorsum of hand	Extension and slight adduction of wrist
Bachtiarow sign	Stroking downward along radius with thumb and index finger	Extension and slight adduction of thumb
Tonic extensor reflex of digits (Vernea and Botez)	Superficial stimulation of dorsum of fingers in patients with a grasp reflex	Tonic extension of the fingers; may be followed by grasp response

FCR, flexor carpi radials; MCP, metacarpophalangeal; PL, palmaris longus.

BOX 40.1

Other Upper-Extremity Corticospinal Reflexes

The Klippel-Feil Sign. Involuntary flexion, opposition, and adduction of the thumb on passive extension of the fingers when there is some degree of contracture in flexion.

The Leri Sign. The examiner holds the patient's supinated and slightly flexed forearm in one hand, and with the other forcibly flexes the patient's fingers and wrist. In normals, this causes biceps contraction and elbow flexion. This response is absent with lesions of the corticospinal system; the absence is known as the Leri sign.

The Mayer Sign. The patient's hand is held in the examiner's hand, palm up, fingers slightly bent, and thumb in slight flexion and abduction. The examiner places slow but firm pressure on the proximal phalanges of the fingers, especially the third and fourth fingers, flexing them at the metacarpophalangeal joints and pressing them against the palm. Normally, this causes adduction and opposition of the thumb with flexion at the metacarpophalangeal joint and extension at the interphalangeal joint (finger-thumb reflex). Absence of the response is the Mayer sign, seen in corticospinal tract lesions. It is occasionally absent in normals, but the absence should be bilateral.

The Leri and Mayer signs have little clinical significance, as the normal response may be difficult or impossible to elicit in individuals without other evidence of neurologic disease.

The Bending Reflex of Seyffarth. Forced passive flexion of the wrist is accompanied by flexion of the elbow in normal subjects (Leri's sign). In the bending reflex, attempted passive extension of the elbow during its phase of flexion reinforces the bending reflex and causes it to spread to the shoulder muscles. With frontal lobe lesions, the associated contraction of the proximal muscles is greatly increased and can be obtained even with passive radial flexion of the wrist.

The Nociceptive Reflexes of Riddoch and Buzzard. In spastic hemiplegia, scratching or pinching the medial upper extremity, walls of the axilla, or upper chest causes mass upper-extremity movements, with abduction and external rotation of the shoulder, and flexion of the elbow, wrist, and finger joints. In quadriplegia, especially due to a high cervical lesion, the same stimuli evoke an extensor response with adduction and internal rotation of the shoulder, elbow extension and pronation of the forearm. The flexor response is most easily elicited by stimulation of the hand or forearm; the extensor response is most easily initiated by a stimulus to the upper arm or axillary wall. These are postural reactions related to the reflexes of spinal automatism.

nociceptive reflexes of Riddoch and Buzzard. These are all of marginal clinical significance and are discussed briefly in Box 40.1.

OTHER FRONTAL RELEASE SIGNS

In addition to the PMR and grasp reflexes discussed above, other responses often included as FRS include the orbicularis oculi, or glabellar, snout, suck, head retraction, and corneomandibular. The orbicularis oculi reflex is discussed in Chapter 16 and the head retraction reflex in Chapter 15. The orbicularis oris (snout) reflex is puckering and protrusion of the lips in response to pressing firmly backward on the philtrum of the upper lip, a minimal tap to the lips, or sweeping a tongue blade briskly across the lips. When exaggerated, the response may include not only puckering and protrusion of the lips but also sucking and even tasting, chewing, and swallowing movements. The sucking reflex is normal in infants; stimulation of the perioral region is followed by sucking movements of the lips, tongue, and jaw. The response may be elicited by lightly touching, striking, or tapping the lips. A rooting (searching) reflex is when the lips, mouth, and even head deviate toward a tactile stimulus delivered beside the mouth or on the cheek. A grossly exaggerated response may include automatic opening of the mouth, smacking, chewing, and even swallowing movements, even when the object fails to touch the lips and is only brought near them. This exaggerated response is also known as the Atz, mastication, or "wolfing" reflex. The sucking reflex disappears after infancy, when sucking becomes a voluntary rather than reflex phenomenon. Like the other FRS, it may reappear in some patients with diffuse cerebral disease. In the bulldog or chewing reflex, a tongue blade inserted into the mouth produces a reflex clenching of the jaw that holds the blade so tightly that pulling it free is difficult. The patient may sit nonchalantly with the blade sticking out of her mouth as if it were an ordinary state of affairs. Tapping the end of the blade may then produce further snouting movements. In the corneomandibular reflex, stimulation of cornea causes contralateral movement of the mandible. It may be an associated movement rather than a true reflex and indicates supranuclear interruption of the ipsilateral corticotrigeminal tract. It is said to be the only eye sign in ALS.

CLONUS

Clonus is a series of rhythmic involuntary muscular contractions induced by the sudden passive stretching of a muscle or tendon. It often accompanies the spasticity and hyperactive DTRs seen in corticospinal tract disease. Clonus occurs most frequently at the ankle, knee, and wrist, occasionally elsewhere. Ankle clonus consists of a series of rhythmic alternating flexions and extensions of the ankle **(Video 40.2)**. It is easiest to obtain if the examiner supports the leg, preferably with one hand under the knee or the calf, grasps the foot from below with the other hand, and quickly dorsiflexes the foot while maintaining slight pressure on the sole at the end of the movement (Figure 40.7). The leg and foot should be well relaxed, the knee and ankle in moderate flexion, and the foot slightly everted. The response is a series of alternating contractions. Unsustained clonus fades away after a few beats; sustained clonus persists as long as the examiner continues to hold slight dorsiflexion pressure on the foot. Unsustained symmetric ankle clonus may occur in normal individuals with physiologically fast DTRs. Sustained clonus is never normal. In severe spasticity, clonus may occur spontaneously or with the slightest stimulus. Slight plantar flexion pressure, as in stepping on the accelerator of a car, may cause violent, uncontrollable, repetitive jerking of the foot. A single tap on the tendon to elicit the ankle jerk will occasionally provoke clonus.

Patellar clonus consists of a series of rhythmic up-and-down movements of the patella. It may be elicited if the examiner grasps the patella between index finger and thumb and executes a sudden, sharp,

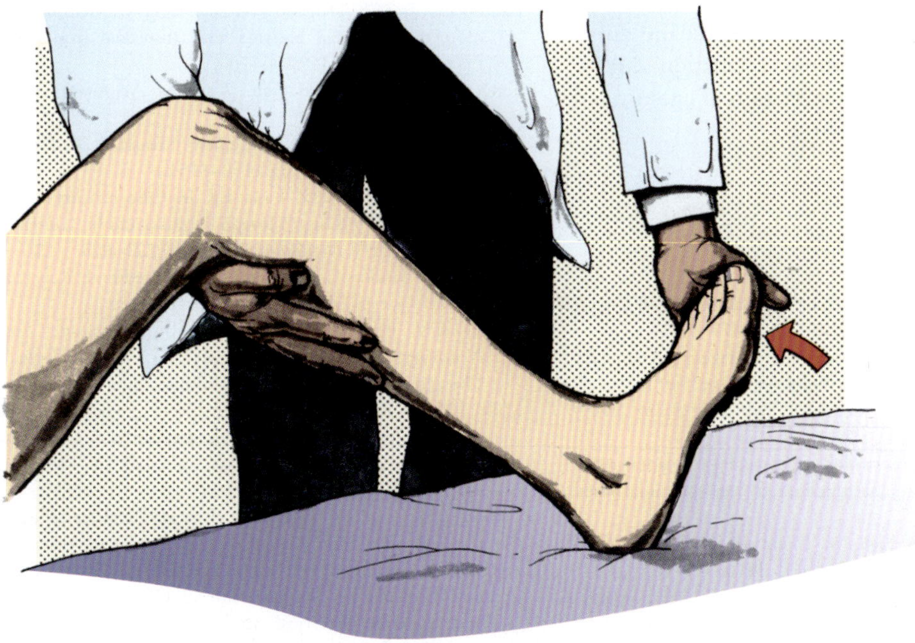

FIGURE 40.7 Method of eliciting ankle clonus.

downward thrust, holding downward pressure at the end of the movement. The leg should be extended and relaxed. Patellar clonus may appear when eliciting the patellar or suprapatellar reflex. Clonus of the wrist or of the fingers may be produced by a sudden passive extension of the wrist or fingers. Sudden supination of the forearm may elicit pronator clonus. Clonus of the jaw occurs occasionally. Nonorganic clonus occurs rarely. False clonus (pseudoclonus) in psychogenic disorders is poorly sustained and irregular in rate, rhythm, and excursion. At the ankle, true clonus can usually be stopped by sharp passive plantar flexion of the foot or the great toe; false clonus is not altered by such a maneuver.

At least two mechanisms may be involved in the production of clonus. For ankle clonus, the sudden stretch of the gastrosoleus muscle elicits a contraction essentially analogous to a stretch reflex that causes a contraction with resultant plantar flexion of the foot. The foot goes down. This contraction increases tension in the Golgi tendon organs in the gastrosoleus tendon, sending a volley of impulses via the Ib fibers that then inhibit the contraction of the gastrosoleus and facilitate contraction of its antagonist, the tibialis anterior muscle. The foot goes up. This in turn passively stretches the gastrosoleus, and the cycle is repeated. A simpler explanation is alternating stretch reflexes. Sharp dorsiflexion of the foot may initiate a stretch reflex in the plantarflexors, the plantar flexion then provoking a stretch reflex in the dorsiflexors, resulting in a rhythmic oscillation due to alternating contraction and relaxation of agonist and antagonist.

BIBLIOGRAPHY

Ambesh P, Paliwal VK, Shetty V, et al. The Babinski sign: a comprehensive review. *J Neurol Sci* 2017;372:477–481.

Amir R, Helsen G. Teaching video NeuroImages: the Stransky sign: a forgotten clinical sign. *Neurology* 2010;75:e11.

Berger JR, Fannin M. The "bedsheet" Babinski. *South Med J* 2002;95:1178–1179.

Brain R, Wilkinson M. Observation on the extensor plantar reflex and its relationship to the functions of the pyramidal tract. *Brain* 1959;82:297.

Campbell WW. *Clinical Signs in Neurology: A Compendium.* Philadelphia: Wolters Kluwer Health, 2016.

Chansakul C. Palmocervical reflex: a hyperactive palmomental reflex? *Neurology* 2010;74:91.

Cone TE Jr, Khoshbin S. Botticelli demonstrates the Babinski reflex more than 400 years before Babinski; pediatrics in art. *Am J Dis Child* 1978;132:188.

Dafkin C, Green A, Kerr S, et al. The interrater reliability of subjective assessments of the Babinski reflex. *J Mot Behav* 2016;48:116–121.

Deng T, Jia JP, Zhang T, et al. Cortical versus non-cortical lesions affect expression of Babinski sign. *Neurol Sci* 2013;34:855–859.

Ditunno JF, Bell R. The Babinski sign: 100 years on. *Br Med J* 1996;313:1029–1030.

Fuller G. *Neurological Examination Made Easy*. 5th ed. Edinburgh: Churchill Livingstone, 2013.

Gilman S. *Clinical Examination of the Nervous System*. New York: McGraw-Hill, 2000.

Goetz CG. History of the extensor plantar response: Babinski and Chaddock signs. *Semin Neurol* 2002;22:391–398.

Gotkine M, Haggiag S, Abramsky O, et al. Lack of hemispheric localizing value of the palmomental reflex. *Neurology* 2005;64:1656.

Grant R. The neurological assault on the great toe (1893–1911). *Scott Med J* 1987;32:57–59.

Heliopoulos I, Vadikolias K, Tsivgoulis G, et al. Corneomandibular reflex (Wartenberg reflex) in coma: a rarely elicited sign. *JAMA Neurol* 2013;70:794–795.

Hindfelt B, Rosen I, Hanko J. The significance of a crossed extensor hallucis response in neurologic disorders: a comparison with the Babinski sign. *Acta Neurol Scand* 1976;53:241–250.

Isaza Jaramillo SP, Uribe Uribe CS, García Jimenez FA, et al. Accuracy of the Babinski sign in the identification of pyramidal tract dysfunction. *J Neurol Sci* 2014;343:66–68.

Jacobs L, Gossman MD. Three primitive reflexes in normal adults. *Neurology* 1980;30:184–188.

Koehler PJ, Bruyn GW, Pearce JMS, eds. *Neurological Eponyms.* Oxford: Oxford University Press, 2000.

Kumar SP, Ramasubramanian D. The Babinski sign—a reappraisal. *Neurol India* 2000;48:314–318.

Ladino LD, Isaza S, Delgado J, et al. Diagnostic yield of the palmomental reflex in patients with suspected frontal lesion. *J Neurol Sci* 2015;359:156–160.

Lance JW. The Babinski sign. *J Neurol Neurosurg Psychiatry* 2002;73:360–362.

Landau WM. Plantar reflex amusement: misuse, ruse, disuse, and abuse. *Neurology* 2005;65:1150–1151.

Lanzino G, diPierro CG, Laws ER Jr. One century after the description of the "sign": Joseph Babinski and his contribution to neurosurgery. *Neurosurgery* 1997;40:822–828.

Massey EW, Sanders L. Babinski's sign in medieval, Renaissance, and baroque art. *Arch Neurol* 1989;46:85–88.

Massey EW, Pleet AB, Scherokman BJ. *Diagnostic Tests in Neurology: A Photographic Guide to Bedside Techniques.* Chicago: Year Book Medical Publishers, Inc., 1985.

Miller TM, Johnston SC. Should the Babinski sign be part of the routine neurologic examination? *Neurology* 2005;65:1165–1168.

Neelon FA, Harvey EN. Images in clinical medicine. The Babinski sign. *N Engl J Med* 1999;340:196.

Okuda B, Kawabata K, Tachibana H, et al. Primitive reflexes distinguish vascular parkinsonism from Parkinson's disease. *Clin Neurol Neurosurg* 2008;110:562–565.

Okun MS, Koehler PJ. Babinski's clinical differentiation of organic paralysis from hysterical paralysis: effect on US neurology. *Arch Neurol* 2004;61:778–783.

Owen G, Mulley GP. The palmomental reflex: a useful clinical sign? *J Neurol Neurosurg Psychiatry* 2002;73:113–115.

Pérez-Bovet J, Rimbau-Muñoz J. Dejerine hand phenomenon. *JAMA Neurol* 2015;72:940.

Pryse-Phillips W. *Companion to Clinical Neurology*. 3rd ed. Oxford: Oxford University Press, 2009.

Rayner PH. The Babinski sign. Eliciting the sign brings out doctors' masochistic tendencies. *Br Med J* 1997;314:374.

Rehman HU. Babinski sign. *Neurology* 2002;8:316–318.

Ross RT. *How to Examine the Nervous System*. 4th ed. Totowa: Humana Press, 2006.

Shibasaki H, Hallett M. *The Neurological Examination: Scientific Basis for Clinical Diagnosis*. Oxford/New York: Oxford University Press, 2016.

Singerman J, Lee L. Consistency of the Babinski reflex and its variants. *Eur J Neurol* 2008;15:960–964.

Tacik P, Krasnianski M, Zierz S. Puusepp's sign—clinical significance of a forgotten pyramidal sign. *Clin Neurol Neurosurg* 2009;111:919–921.

Tashiro K. Kisaku Yoshimura and the Chaddock reflex. *Arch Neurol* 1986a;43:1179–1180.

Tashiro K. Reversed Chaddock method: a new method to elicit the upgoing great toe. *J Neurol Neurosurg Psychiatry* 1986b;49:1321.

Tatu L. A newly discovered Babinski sign in a renaissance painting. *Eur Neurol* 2017;77:195.

van Gijn J. The Babinski reflex. *Postgrad Med J* 1995;71: 645–648.

van Gijn J. The Babinski sign: the first hundred years. *J Neurol* 1996;243:675–683.

Van Gijn J, Bonke B. Interpretation of plantar reflexes: biasing effect of other signs and symptoms. *J Neurol Neurosurg Psychiatry* 1977;40:787–789.

Wartenberg R. *The Examination of Reflexes: A Simplification*. Chicago: Year Book Medical Publishers, 1945.

Whittle IR, Miller JD. Clinical usefulness of the palmomental reflex. *Med J Aust* 1987;146:137–139.

Wilkins RH, Brody IA. Babinski's sign. *Arch Neurol* 1967;17: 441–445.

Willoughby EW, Eason R. The crossed upgoing toe sign: a clinical study. *Ann Neurol* 1983;14:480–482.

CHAPTER 41

Postural and Righting Reflexes

The postural and righting reflexes are a complex group of reactions that are relevant primarily in pediatric neurology. Posture is largely reflex in origin, with involuntary muscle contraction creating the necessary tone, especially in the antigravity muscles, to maintain the erect posture and normal position. The vestibular nuclei, especially the lateral, are particularly important for maintaining contraction in the antigravity muscles. Standing may be thought of as a postural reflex, and any interference with the mechanisms mediating postural reflexes may interfere with the act of normal standing. The postural and righting reflexes are difficult to study. Much of our knowledge comes from experimental neurology, but the clinical applicability is limited because of the differences in neurophysiology between the upright biped and the experimental quadruped.

Maintaining the orientation of the head to the body and of the head and body in space are basic functions. The complex reflex mechanisms of standing and righting involve the vestibular system, principally the utricle; proprioceptive impulses from muscles, tendons, and joints; exteroceptive impulses from the body surface; and visual stimuli. Righting reactions involve at least five separate types of reflexes: (a) labyrinthine righting reflexes acting on the neck muscles, (b) neck righting reflexes acting upon the body, (c) body righting reflexes acting upon the head, (d) body righting reflexes acting upon the body, and (e) visual righting reflexes acting upon the head and body. Vestibular input arises from otoliths of the utricles, and to a lesser extent the saccules; these organs respond to changes in head position that then influences body tone. The proprioceptive stimuli involved in neck righting reflexes originate in the muscles, tendons, and other deep structures of the neck and are mediated through the upper two or three cervical nerves and segments, and possibly through the spinal accessory nerve. They act principally on the head, but through the head act on the body as a whole. Afferents subserving body righting reflexes are analogous and arise from tissues in the trunk and extremities. The visual righting reflexes are mediated by the midbrain and the vestibular centers. When the eyes turn toward an object, the head and body follow. Although vision plays a role in posture, lack of vision does not impair postural or righting reflexes if the other mechanisms are intact. Conversely, loss of proprioception, as in posterior column disease, can be compensated for in part by visual input.

Abnormalities of the postural and righting reflexes are clinically relevant in pediatric patients; in certain adult patients, particularly those with extrapyramidal disorders, disturbances of gait and balance, and vestibular disorders; and in the aged. Loss of postural reflexes is an important feature of Parkinson's disease, and similar impairment is likely related to the tendency of the elderly to fall.

POSTURAL AND RIGHTING REFLEXES IN INFANCY AND CHILDHOOD

Myelination of the nervous system begins during the second trimester and continues for a long period of time, well after birth and perhaps into adolescence. The most rapid phase of myelination occurs during the first 6 months after birth. Different systems myelinate at different times, and the order of myelination is related to the appearance and disappearance of the postural and righting reflexes seen in pediatric patients. Demonstration of these reflexes helps to establish gestational age and assess the function of the immature nervous system.

Reflexes that are usually demonstrable in the normal neonate include the Moro, tonic neck reflex, rooting and sucking, grasp, placing, stepping, and trunk incurvation.

The Moro Reflex

This is the body startle reflex. A sudden stimulus, such as a loud noise or quick movement, directed toward the body causes abduction and extension of all four extremities, extension of the spine, and extension and fanning of the digits, followed by flexion and adduction of the extremities. The reflex is prominent during the first 3 months of life, and then the response gradually disappears, probably with the development of myelination. Children with motor deficits of cerebral origin may show the reflex in a fully developed form for years; the response may be unilateral if only one side is affected.

Landau Reflex

This is present in normal infants during the first 1 to 2 years of life. If an infant is held prone in the examiner's hand with the body parallel with the floor, there is extension of the head and spine so that the body forms an arc with the convexity downward. With the body in this position, passive flexion of the head causes flexion of the vertebral column, arms, and legs, and the body forms an arc with the convexity upward. If the child is placed supine, there is flexion of the neck, spine, arms, and legs. This posture is probably a combination of otolith and tonic neck reflexes.

Tonic Neck Reflexes

Passively turning the head toward one shoulder causes increased extensor tonus on that side and increased flexor tonus on the opposite side (Figure 41.1). The arm on the side toward which the head is turned goes into extension while the opposite arm flexes. The posture has been likened to that of a fencing thrust. If the head and neck are flexed, the arms flex and the legs extend. If the head and neck are extended, the arms extend and the legs flex. Reflexes of this type are often found in an incomplete form in normal infants but disappear by the age of 4 to 6 months. In later life, they may be demonstrable in patients who have "high" decerebration, or decortication, because of disease involving the upper brainstem or thalamodiencephalic level. The patient lies with the arms semiflexed over the chest and the legs in extension, but turning, flexion, or extension of the head causes the responses just described. These reflexes may contribute to the associated movements found in spastic hemiplegia and cerebral diplegia.

The Neck Righting Response

This is a variation of the tonic neck reflex. With the infant supine, its head is turned toward one side. A positive response results in rotation of the shoulder, trunk, and pelvis toward that side, occasionally followed by a turn of the entire body. The response should be approximately equal on each side. The reflex appears at about the time the tonic neck reflexes disappear and can be obtained in nearly all infants by the age of 10 months; it disappears at about the time the child can arise directly without first turning on its abdomen.

The Parachute Response

The parachute response appears at the age of 8 to 9 months and persists. To elicit it, the infant is held prone in the air and then suddenly thrust headfirst toward the examining table or floor. When the response is present, the arms immediately extend and adduct slightly, and the fingers spread as if to attempt to break the fall. Asymmetry of the response indicates unilateral upper-extremity weakness or spasticity.

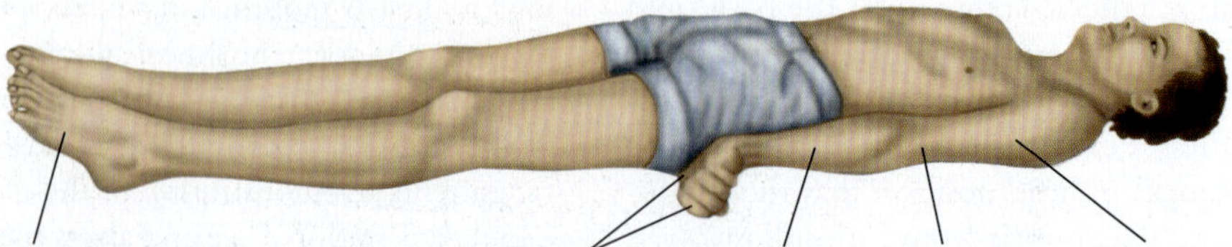

FIGURE 41.1 In decerebrate rigidity, the arms are adducted and extended at the elbows, with the forearms pronated and the wrists and fingers flexed. The legs are extended at the knees and internally rotated with the feet plantar flexed. The posture may occur spontaneously or in response to external stimuli such as light, noise, or pain. (Reprinted with permission from Bickley LS, Szilagyi P. *Bates' Guide to Physical Examination and History Taking*. 8th ed. Philadelphia: Lippincott Williams & Wilkins, 2003.)

Absence of the response is seen in severe motor disorders. The response does not depend upon vision and may occur in blindfolded children.

The Placing Reaction

With the infant held vertically, touching the dorsum of each foot to the side of the examining table causes placement of the foot on top of the table. The response usually disappears by the end of the first year of life.

Supporting and Stepping Reactions

Holding the infant vertically and allowing its feet to make firm contact with the top of the examining table produces contraction of the lower extremities as if to support the weight. This is usually followed by automatic stepping or walking movements. These responses are usually present at birth and gradually disappear.

DECEREBRATE AND DECORTICATE RIGIDITY

Severe lesions of the brainstem often produce increased tone in the extensor, or antigravity, muscles of the limbs and the spine. This phenomenon is known as decerebrate rigidity. In patients with extreme decerebrate rigidity, there is opisthotonos, with all four limbs stiffly extended, the head back, and the jaws clenched. The arms are internally rotated at the shoulders, extended at the elbows, and hyperpronated, with the fingers extended at the metacarpophalangeal joints and flexed at the interphalangeal joints. The legs are extended at the hips and knees while the ankles and toes are plantar flexed (Figure 41.1). The position is an exaggeration or caricature of the normal standing position. The deep tendon reflexes are exaggerated, the tonic neck and labyrinthine reflexes are present, and the righting reflexes abolished.

Decerebrate rigidity may follow severe insults to the brainstem at any level between the superior colliculi or the decussation of the rubrospinal pathway and the rostral portion of the vestibular nuclei. The vestibular nuclei enhance extensor tone, and integrity of the vestibular nuclei is necessary for decerebrate rigidity to occur. These nuclei are intact, but isolated from the midbrain, specifically from the red nuclei and rubrospinal tracts. Activity in the reticular formation is also important, particularly the pontine reticular nuclei and the medial reticulospinal tract, which also facilitates extensor muscle tone. Experimentally, decerebrate rigidity is abolished by section of the vestibulospinal pathways. In patients, when the process extends to involve the medulla, the decerebration disappears. The most common cause of decerebrate rigidity in humans is trauma, and the presence of extensor posturing is a poor prognostic indicator. The incidence of decerebrate rigidity in severe TBI is as high as 40%, and the presence of extensor posturing increases the mortality dramatically. An MRI investigation showed a significant correlation between decerebrate rigidity and the presence of midbrain lesions.

Decorticate rigidity is characterized by flexion of the elbows and wrists with extension of the legs and feet (Figure 41.2). The causative lesion is higher than that causing decerebrate rigidity, preserving the function of the rubrospinal tracts, which enhance flexor tone in the upper extremities.

The functional significance of the rubrospinal and vestibulospinal tracts can be best appreciated by observing a patient progress from decorticate rigidity to decerebrate rigidity to the flaccidity of brain death. After rostrocaudal deterioration to a certain level, the patient lies with arms flexed and legs

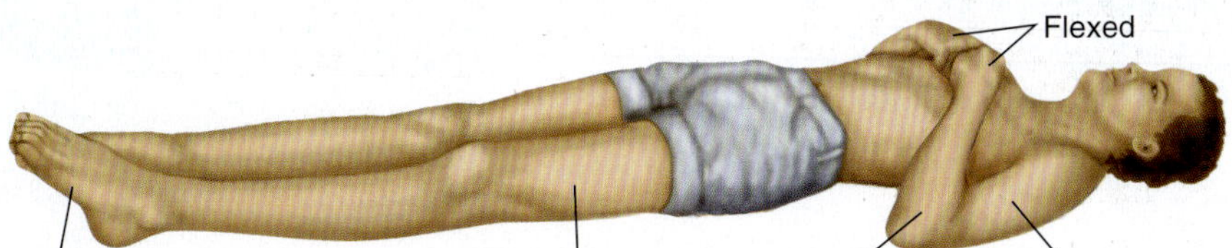

FIGURE 41.2 In decorticate rigidity, the elbows, wrists, and fingers are flexed with the legs extended and internally rotated. (Reprinted with permission from Bickley LS, Szilagyi P. *Bates' Guide to Physical Examination and History Taking*. 8th ed. Philadelphia: Lippincott Williams & Wilkins, 2003.)

extended—decorticate rigidity. This is due to the fact that the rubrospinal pathways are still intact and are enhancing flexor tone to the upper extremities, producing a flexed arm posture with an extended leg posture. With further rostrocaudal deterioration, the rubrospinal tracts cease to function, but the vestibulospinal tracts remain intact, facilitating extensor tone to all four extremities and resulting in an extension posture of both arms and legs. This is decerebrate rigidity. With further rostrocaudal deterioration, the vestibulospinal tracts cease to function and the patient becomes flaccid in all four extremities, an agonal condition.

BIBLIOGRAPHY

Bricolo A, Turazzi S, Alexandre A, et al. Decerebrate rigidity in acute head injury. *J Neurosurg* 1977;47:680–689.

Capute AJ, Wachtel RC, Palmer FB, et al. A prospective study of three postural reactions. *Dev Med Child Neurol* 1982; 24:314–320.

Carey JH, Crosby EC, Schnitzlein HN. Decorticate versus decerebrate rigidity in subhuman primates and man. *Neurology* 1970;20:396–397.

Carey JH, Crosby EC, Schnitzlein HN. Decorticate versus decerebrate rigidity in subhuman primates and man. *Neurology* 1971;21:738–744.

Davis RA, Davis L. Decerebrate rigidity in humans. *Neurosurgery* 1982;10:635–642.

Feldman MH. The decerebrate state in the primate. II. Studies in man. *Arch Neurol* 1971;25:517–525.

Kawai Y, DeMonbrun AG, Chambers RS, et al. A previously healthy adolescent with acute encephalopathy and decorticate posturing. *Pediatrics* 2017;139. pii: e20153779.

Nawashiro H, Wada K, Kita H. Decerebrate posture following bilateral middle cerebral artery occlusion. *Intern Med* 2011;50:2063.

Pryse-Phillips W. *Companion to Clinical Neurology*. 3rd ed. Oxford: Oxford University Press, 2009.

Woischneck D, Skalej M, Firsching R, et al. Decerebrate posturing following traumatic brain injury: MRI findings and their diagnostic value. *Clin Radiol* 2015;70:278–285.

Wehbe E, Saad D, Delgado F, et al. Reversible hepatic decerebration: a case report and review of the literature. *Eur J Gastroenterol Hepatol* 2010;22:759–760.

Zafeiriou DI, Tsikoulas IG, Kremenopoulos GM. Prospective follow-up of primitive reflex profiles in high-risk infants: clues to an early diagnosis of cerebral palsy. *Pediatr Neurol* 1995;13:148–152.

Zafeiriou DI. Primitive reflexes and postural reactions in the neurodevelopmental examination. *Pediatr Neurol* 2004;31:1–8.

CHAPTER 42

Associated Movements

An associated movement (AM) is an unintentional, involuntary, spontaneous, automatic movement that accompanies some other voluntary (or involuntary) movement. The associated, or synkinetic, movement is often one that serves to fix a part of the body as another part is voluntarily activated. AMs often occur because of activation of the synergistic and fixation muscles involved in a particular motion or spread of the activation to nearby motor neuron pools. This activity is normally suppressed by the descending motor pathways, but in the face of disease becomes clinically apparent. The corticospinal pathways are concerned primarily with fine, fractionated, discrete movements of the distal extremities. Disease in the corticospinal pathways may eliminate discrete distal movement but not affect mass movements of the proximal muscles. The mass movements usually play a secondary, supportive role, particularly in fixation of the part to be moved. However, when the distal movements are paralyzed, the primary movement left may be the associated mass movement. AMs are, to a certain extent, postural or righting reflexes that have a peculiarly widespread distribution. They may be clinical homologues of movements seen in decerebrate animals.

AMs are more complex manifestations of motor function than the simple reflexes but are more primitive than voluntary movements. They are probably initiated and largely controlled by the extrapyramidal system and its connections, although the corticospinal system also plays a role. Because they are motor responses, in many instances abnormal ones, they might be considered in the discussion of the motor system rather than the reflexes, but their physiologic relationship to various reflex responses and their correlation with various abnormalities in the reflexes are reasons for their inclusion in the present section.

PHYSIOLOGIC ASSOCIATED MOVEMENTS

Many AMs are present physiologically; in fact, they play a part in all normal motor activity. The activity of the antagonists, synergists, and muscles of fixation in any motor response may be considered AMs. Generally, the term is used for more widespread responses. Common examples of normal AMs include the following: pendular swinging of the arms when walking; the play of the muscles of facial expression when talking; facial contortions or grimaces with violent exertion; movements of the head and neck with movements of the eyes; contraction of the frontalis muscle with elevation of the eyes; turning of the eyes, head, or body in response to vestibular or auditory stimulation; normal extension of the wrist with flexion of the fingers; and generalized bodily accompaniments of yawning, stretching, coughing, and mental efforts. In some disease states, normal AMs may decrease or disappear. The normal AMs are lost in diseases of the extrapyramidal system, especially in the parkinsonian syndromes, where masking of facial expression and absence of arm swing when walking are prominent manifestations. In other conditions, normal AMs may be exaggerated, and abnormal AMs may be present. With lesions of the corticospinal system, a number of AMs may appear that are not present normally. Table 38.3 correlates the site of a lesion with the pattern of AMs. The AMs not usually present in the normal individual are discussed in the following paragraphs.

PATHOLOGIC ASSOCIATED MOVEMENTS

Abnormal or pathologic AMs are usually activity in paretic muscle groups that are brought out by active movement of other groups and seen predominantly in disease of the corticospinal pathways. They may be present at all times, be brought out by special examinations, or become evident only during physical activity or periods of emotional stress. They usually accompany vigorous voluntary movements of another part and occur on the hemiplegic side. AMs are slow, forceful movements of the already spastic parts that lead to the adoption of new postures. They have a longer latent period than do primary movements. The greater the spasticity, the greater the extent and duration of the AMs.

Generalized Associated Movements

Generalized AMs occur in hemiplegia, where they tend to emphasize or enhance the characteristic hemiplegic posture. The AMs often occur with exertion. Straining and attempts to grip with the paretic hand may cause an increase in the spasticity, with increased flexion of the wrist, elbow, and shoulder; this is sometimes accompanied by associated facial movements on the involved side. The new posture may be maintained until the grip is relaxed. An involuntary, automatic movement such as a yawn may cause the affected arm to extend at the elbow, wrist, and fingers, remaining rigidly in this new attitude until the yawn passes off. Movements such as coughing or stretching may cause similar reactions. These movements may arouse in the patient or others false hope of improvement. Tonic neck reflexes may also influence these generalized AMs. Turning the head toward the hemiplegic side may cause increased extensor tonus on that side and turning it to the normal side may be followed by either increased flexor tonus on the paretic side or flexion of the arm and extension of the leg.

Symmetric (Imitative or Contralateral) Associated Movements (Mirror Movements)

In the normal infant, there is a tendency for movements of one limb to be accompanied by similar involuntary movements of the opposite limb; this disappears as coordination and muscle power are acquired. These movements may persist to a certain extent in children, most frequently in the form of transient mirror movements, or involuntary imitative movements of the contralateral portions of the body; they may be present only as mirror writing. Similar movements are sometimes observed in adults who are in the process of acquiring new patterns of movement or who are exerting excessive physical or mental effort. Mirror movements usually disappear or become inconspicuous at adolescence; their persistence to any marked degree should be considered pathologic (see **Video Link 42.1**). They may occur in patients with brain injuries, disturbances of cerebral development, and dysplasias of the upper portion of the spinal cord; under such circumstances, there are usually associated abnormalities of motor function, tone, and reflexes. Occasionally, persisting mirror movements are familial and not accompanied by other signs of neurologic disease.

In certain neurologic disorders, forceful voluntary movements of one limb may be accompanied by identical involuntary movements of the same limb on the other side. They are usually seen in the paretic limb when the opposite healthy one is forcefully moved, although occasionally such movements may appear in the healthy limb on extreme attempts to move the affected extremity (especially in extrapyramidal disease). They appear particularly during exertion to carry out a quick or strenuous movement. When squeezing the examiner's hand with the healthy hand, the paretic hand may flex. Any forceful movement on the normal side may be followed by a similar but slow tonic duplication of the movement on the paretic side. There may be a spreading of the response, evolving into a generalized AM with assumption of the characteristic positions. Imitation synkinesias by themselves have little localizing significance, occurring with lesions in various portions of the neuraxis. Their value in neurologic assessment is in conjunction with other findings.

Coordinated Associated Movements

Coordinated AMs are involuntary movements of synergistic muscle groups that accompany a voluntary movement of a paretic limb. They are exaggerations or perversions of ordinary synergistic and cooperative movements and may be classified into three groups: (a) movements, not present normally, which accompany movements of a paretic limb; (b) contralateral coordinated AMs; and (c) AMs, normally present, which are abolished in cerebral hemiplegia. These responses may be useful in the differentiation between organic and nonorganic deficits.

Coordinated Associated Movements in the Paretic Limb

Coordinated AMs that accompany voluntary motion of involved extremities in patients with hemiparesis are characterized by a spread of movement from one muscle or group of muscles to others. They do not appear in the normal individual or in nonorganic weakness. The best known of these are Wartenberg's thumb adduction sign, the Babinski trunk-thigh sign, and the tibialis sign of Strümpell; others are listed in Table 42.1. Pronator drift (Barré's sign) is sometimes

TABLE 42.1 Other Associated Movement (AM) Signs

	Name	Sign
Coordinated AMs in the paretic limb		
	Finger sign (interosseous phenomenon) of Souques	Active elevation and extension of paretic arm is followed by involuntary hyperextension and abduction of the fingers (see Chapter 27).
	Strümpell's pronator sign	Active flexion of paretic forearm is followed by pronation and flexion of the hand; if patient can bring hand to shoulder, dorsum of hand strikes shoulder; if the forearm is flexed in supination or passively flexed and supinated by examiner, it immediately assumes a position of pronation.
	Radialis sign of Strümpell	Attempts to close fingers or make a fist on paretic side are accompanied by dorsiflexion of wrist.
	Flexion response of the forearm	Flexion of hips and knees to squatting position causes increased flexion of paretic forearm; flexion of forearm also increased by flexion and decreased by extension of the neck.
	Quadrupedal extensor reflex	On leaning forward or bending over, as if to place hands to floor, flexed hemiparetic arm extends.
	Combined extension of trunk and thigh	Patient, seated on edge of examining table, holding on to edge, leans backward as far as arms will stretch. Normally, no change in position of dependent feet and legs; in corticospinal paresis, hip and knee extend and ankle flexes.
	Raimiste leg sign	With forceful abduction or adduction of the sound leg against resistance, paretic leg executes an identical movement (see Chapter 27 on abductor sign).
	Abduction response at hip joint	If patient with corticospinal weakness stands erect and marks time, there is abduction movement at hip as hip and knee on paretic side are flexed.
	Coughing sign of Huntingdon	Coughing and straining cause hip flexion, knee extension, and elevation of paretic lower extremity.
	Reinforcement sign of Babinski	In patient seated with legs hanging free, Jendrassik maneuver causes knee extension on paretic side.
Contralateral coordinated AMs		
	Brachioradial response	Extension of flexed elbow on normal side causes flexion of the elbow on paretic side.
	Sterling's sign	In upper motor neuron facial weakness, platysma fails to contract as it normally does when patient opens mouth as widely as possible, grimaces, or touches chin to chest.
	Grip sign	Examiner's fingers inserted into patient's fist; grip relaxes when wrist is passively flexed but tightens as wrist is extended.
Other changes in motor function		
	Raimiste's arm sign	Patient's elbow is placed on a table, hand and forearm held upright by examiner; when sound hand is released, it remains upright; when paretic hand is released, it flexes to an angle of about 130 degrees; a sign of flaccidity rather than spasticity; may be present immediately after the onset of an organic hemiparesis.
	Pronation sign of Neri	Patient supine, upper extremities extended and pronated; when forearm is flexed and supinated by examiner, paretic arm returns to pronation; similar to Strümpell's and Babinski's pronator signs.
	Claude's sign of reflex hyperkinesia	Reflex movements, either extension or retraction, following painful stimulus to an extremity, even though the part seems totally paralyzed.
	Phenomenon of Grasset and Gaussel	Normal supine patient can raise either leg separately or raise both together. In pyramidal lesions, she may still be able to raise either one separately but cannot raise them together. If she first raises the paretic one, it falls on attempting to lift the normal one.

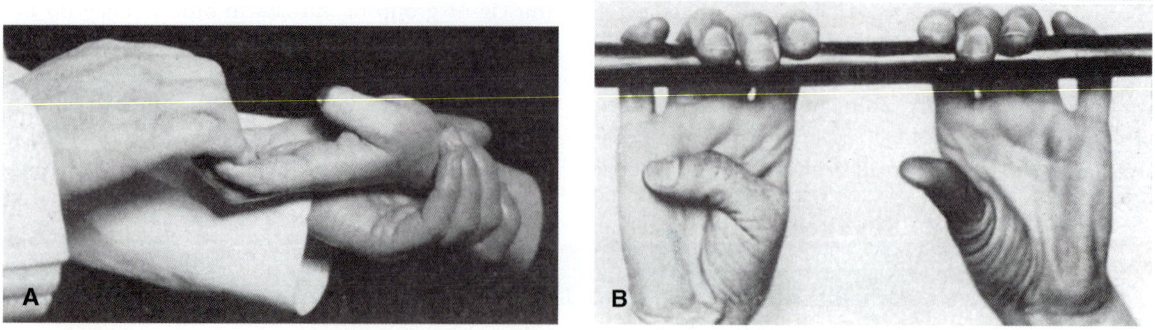

FIGURE 42.1 Wartenberg's thumb adduction sign. **A.** The patient bends his last four fingers against resistance of four hooked fingers of the examiner. Thumb moves toward palm. Mild spastic paralysis of hand. **B.** With his fingers hooked over a horizontally fastened rod, the patient is asked to pull down. Right thumb performs an associated movement toward the palm. Right-sided spastic hemiplegia. (Reprinted from Wartenberg R. *Diagnostic Tests in Neurology*. Chicago: Year Book Medical Publishers, 1953. Copyright © 1953 Elsevier. With permission.)

included as an AM but is better understood as an indication of corticospinal tract distribution weakness (see Chapter 27). The Klippel-Feil sign, the Marie-Foix phenomenon, and the reflex responses of Riddoch, Buzzard, and others are sometimes classified as abnormal AMs, but they are all characterized by a response to a specific stimulus and therefore are described in Chapter 40.

Wartenberg's Thumb Adduction Sign

Active flexion of the terminal phalanges of the four fingers of a paretic hand about a firm object, or against resistance offered by the examiner's fingers similarly flexed, is followed by adduction, flexion, and opposition of the thumb (Figure 42.1, **Video 42.1**). In a normal extremity, the thumb remains in abduction and extension.

The Trunk-Thigh Sign of Babinski, or Combined Flexion of the Trunk and Thigh

The patient, lying supine with legs abducted, attempts to sit up while holding the arms crossed on the chest. Normally, the legs remain motionless and the heels down. In corticospinal hemiparesis, the hip flexes as the trunk flexes, and there is an involuntary elevation of the paretic limb off the bed (Figure 42.2). The toes may spread out in a fan-like fashion. The normal limb remains on the bed or rises slightly, but not as high as the paretic one. In paraparesis, both legs rise equally. In nonorganic weakness, the normal leg rises and the paretic one does not, or neither leg rises. The same phenomenon occurs if the standing patient bends over (Figure 42.3).

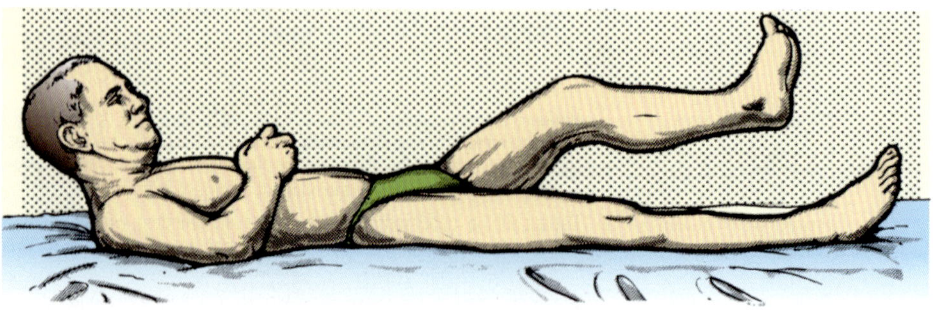

FIGURE 42.2 Trunk-thigh sign in patient with left hemiparesis.

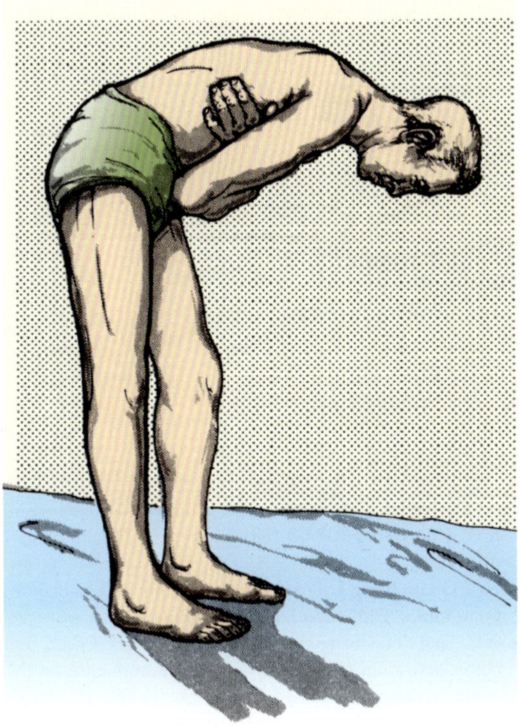

FIGURE 42.3 Combined flexion of the thigh and leg in a patient with left hemiparesis.

The Tibialis Sign of Strümpell

Normally, vigorous flexion of the hip and knee is accompanied by plantar flexion of the foot. In lower extremity weakness due to a corticospinal tract lesion, voluntary flexion of the hip and knee is accompanied by involuntary dorsiflexion and inversion of the paretic foot; there may also be dorsiflexion of the great toe or of all the toes. The patient is unable to flex the hip and knee without dorsiflexing the foot (Figure 42.4). The response is accentuated if the movement is carried out against resistance. The sign may also be elicited by flexing the knee with the patient lying prone (Figure 42.5).

Contralateral Coordinated Associated Movements

Coordinated AMs in which the response is contralateral are similar to the symmetric AMs, but the response is not always imitative and may involve muscles other than those used in the primary movement.

Associated Contralateral Contraction of the Triceps

Normally, biceps muscle contraction in one arm is associated with contraction of the contralateral triceps and extension of the opposite elbow. In organic hemiparesis, this contralateral extension is present in the normal arm on forceful flexion of the paretic arm, but absent in the paretic arm on flexion of the normal arm.

Hoover's sign exploits an automatic walking AM of the legs to detect nonorganic weakness (see Chapter 27). Other contralateral AMs are described in Table 42.1.

Loss of Coordinated Associated Movements

Certain coordinated AMs normally present are abolished in pyramidal lesions. Normal associated and automatic movements, such as swinging of the arms in walking and synergistic movements used in rising and sitting down, are also lost in disorders of the extrapyramidal system, especially parkinsonian syndromes.

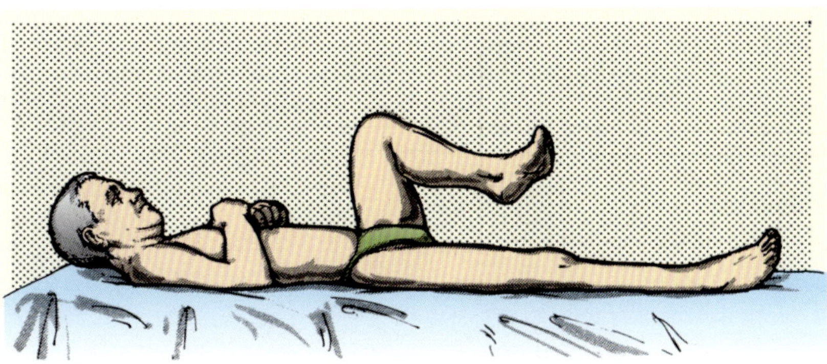

FIGURE 42.4 Tibialis sign in a patient with left hemiparesis.

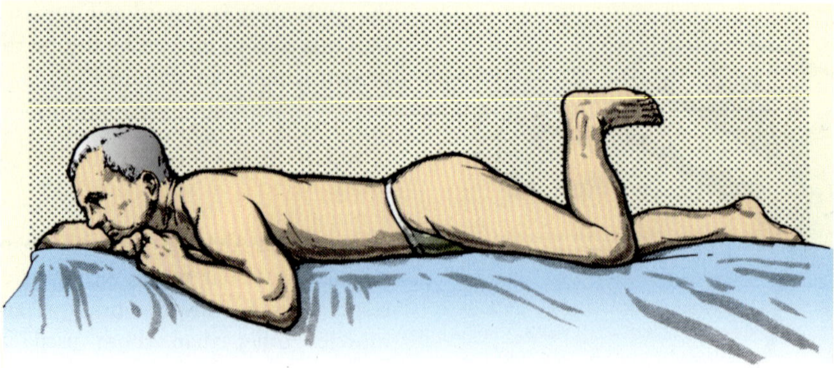

FIGURE 42.5 Tibialis sign elicited with the patient in the prone position.

OTHER CHANGES IN MOTOR FUNCTION

The Leri and Mayer signs are discussed in Box 40.1; the Babinski platysma sign and the grip sign are summarized in Table 42.1. Other changes in motor function that may be considered abnormalities of AM are summarized in Table 42.1.

Video Links

Video Link 42.1. Mirror movements. https://www.youtube.com/watch?v=pkZuK7tfv9k

BIBLIOGRAPHY

Archibald KC, Weichec CF. A reappraisal of Hoover's test. *Arch Phys Med Rehabil* 1970;51:234.

Cincotta M, Borgheresi A, Balzini L, et al. Separate ipsilateral and contralateral corticospinal projections in congenital mirror movements: neurophysiological evidence and significance for motor rehabilitation. *Mov Disord* 2003;18:1294–1300.

Farmer SF, Ingram DA, Stephens JA. Mirror movements studied in a patient with Klippel-Feil syndrome. *J Physiol* 1990;428:467–484.

Kaulen LD, Baehring JM. Mirror movements in a patient with brain tumor. *JAMA Neurol* 2018;75:512.

Kim YH, Jang SH, Chang Y, et al. Bilateral primary sensori-motor cortex activation of post-stroke mirror movements: an fMRI study. *Neuroreport* 2003;14:1329–1332.

Koehler PJ, Okun MS. Important observations prior to the description of the Hoover sign. *Neurology* 2004;63:1693–1697.

Largo RH, Caflisch JA, Hug F, et al. Neuromotor development from 5 to 18 years. Part 2: associated movements. *Dev Med Child Neurol* 2001;43:444–453.

Mehndiratta MM, Kumar M, Nayak R, et al. Hoover's sign: clinical relevance in neurology. *J Postgrad Med* 2014;60:297–299.

Pearce JM. A note on Hoover's sign. *J Neurol Neurosurg Psychiatry* 2003;74:432.

Sonoo M. Abductor sign: a reliable new sign to detect unilateral non-organic paresis of the lower limb. *J Neurol Neurosurg Psychiatry* 2004;75:121–125.

Vidal JS, Derkinderen P, Vidailhet M, et al. Mirror movements of the non-affected hand in hemiparkinsonian patients: a reflection of ipsilateral motor overactivity? *J Neurol Neurosurg Psychiatry* 2003;74:1352–1353.

Wartenberg R. *Diagnostic Tests in Neurology*. Chicago: Year Book Medical Publishers, 1953.

SECTION H Coordination and Gait

CHAPTER 43

Cerebellar Function

The cerebellum is tasked with bringing finesse to the motor system. Although not primarily involved in the mechanisms for production of muscle power, it is necessary for normal control and regulation of muscle contraction. The major function of the cerebellum, from a clinical point of view, is the coordination of movement. The cerebellum is the portion of the brain through which the cerebral motor cortex achieves the synthesis and coordination of individual muscle contractions required for normal voluntary movements. Without it, movements are gross, uncoordinated, clumsy, and tremulous, and precise movements become impossible. Lesions of the cerebellum do not cause weakness, but rather loss of coordination and inability to gauge and regulate, as Gordon Holmes said, the "rate, range, and force" of movement. Although motor strength and power are preserved, active movements are severely compromised.

In order to perform any movement—especially a complex act involving many muscle groups—contractions of the agonists, antagonists, synergists, and muscles of fixation must be adequately coordinated. To begin a movement, the agonists contract to execute the movement; the antagonists relax or modify their tone to facilitate it; the synergists reinforce the movement; and the fixating muscles prevent displacements and maintain the appropriate posture of the limb. To terminate the movement, the antagonists contract and the agonists relax. The individual muscles that enter into the act must be controlled and coordinated, as a conductor would direct an orchestra, precisely regulating the action of the individual parts. The cerebellum is the conductor. It is essential to the synergy of muscle contraction and is the center of coordination for voluntary movement. It does not provide power and does not play an instrument, but without it the symphony of normal movement degenerates into a cacophony of disorganized muscle contractions.

A major manifestation of cerebellar lesions is ataxia (Gr. a "without," taxis "order"); a rough translation is "not orderly." The essential feature in ataxia is that movements are not normally organized. Although the term is a general one, indicating chaotic and disorganized movement, it is used clinically primarily to refer to the motor control abnormalities—including incoordination, tremor, and impaired rapid alternating movements (RAMs)—that occur with cerebellar lesions. Ataxia is not specific for cerebellar disease, and lesions in other parts of the nervous system must be excluded before attributing ataxia to cerebellar disease. Impaired proprioception may cause sensory ataxia, and lesions involving pathways that originate in the frontal lobe may cause frontal lobe ataxia. Other common manifestations of cerebellar disease include nystagmus, impaired balance, and difficulty walking.

ANATOMY

The cerebellum is located in the posterior fossa, beneath the tentorium cerebelli. Below and anteriorly, it is separated from the dorsal pons by the fourth ventricle and from the medulla and the dura mater covering the atlanto-occipital membrane by the cisterna magna. Grossly, there are three parts: (a) the cerebellar hemispheres, two larger, lateral masses; (b) the vermis, a small, unpaired median portion that connects the hemispheres (Figures 43.1 and 43.2); and (c) the flocculonodular (FN) lobe, a small, midline structure that lies on the anterior part of the inferior surface. The FN lobe consists of the paired lateral flocculi and the midline nodulus (Figure 43.3). The vermis is separated from the hemispheres by the paramedian sulci. The cerebellar tonsils are small, rounded lobules on the inferior aspect of the cerebellar hemispheres, just above the foramen magnum.

Gross Anatomy

Anatomically, the cerebellum is divided into three lobes: anterior, posterior, and FN. Each has a vermis and hemisphere portion (Figure 43.3). The deep transverse primary fissure divides the cerebellum into anterior and posterior lobes. The posterolateral fissure separates the FN lobe from the posterior lobe. Anatomists further divide the cerebellum by fissures and sulci into 10 lobules that bear arcane names of no clinical relevance (Figure 43.4). In terms of afferent and efferent connections, the cerebellum can also be organized into three parallel, sagittal zones: vermian, paravermian, and lateral. As mentioned previously, clinicians divide the cerebellum functionally into three parts: (a) the hemispheres, responsible for appendicular coordination; (b) the anterior, superior vermis (or simply the vermis), responsible for gait and other axial functions; and (c) the FN lobe, or vestibulocerebellum. The FN lobe is phylogenetically the oldest and is referred to as the archicerebellum. The FN lobe has extensive connections with the vestibular nuclei and is concerned primarily with eye movements and gross balance. It also receives visual afferents from the superior colliculi and the visual cortex. The primary concerns of the archicerebellum are eye movement control and gross orientation in space, such as up and down. The next area of the cerebellum to evolve was the paleocerebellum or spinocerebellum. In humans, the paleocerebellum consists of the anterior, superior vermis and adjacent paravermal cortex; it corresponds approximately to the anatomical anterior lobe. The paleocerebellum developed during a period of evolution when extremity control was not a concern; it is

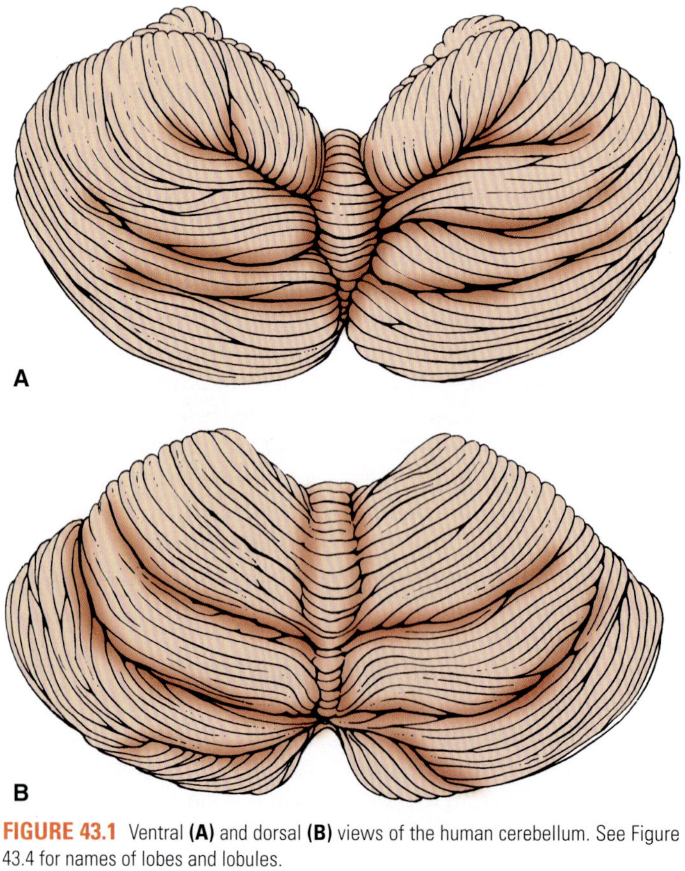

FIGURE 43.1 Ventral **(A)** and dorsal **(B)** views of the human cerebellum. See Figure 43.4 for names of lobes and lobules.

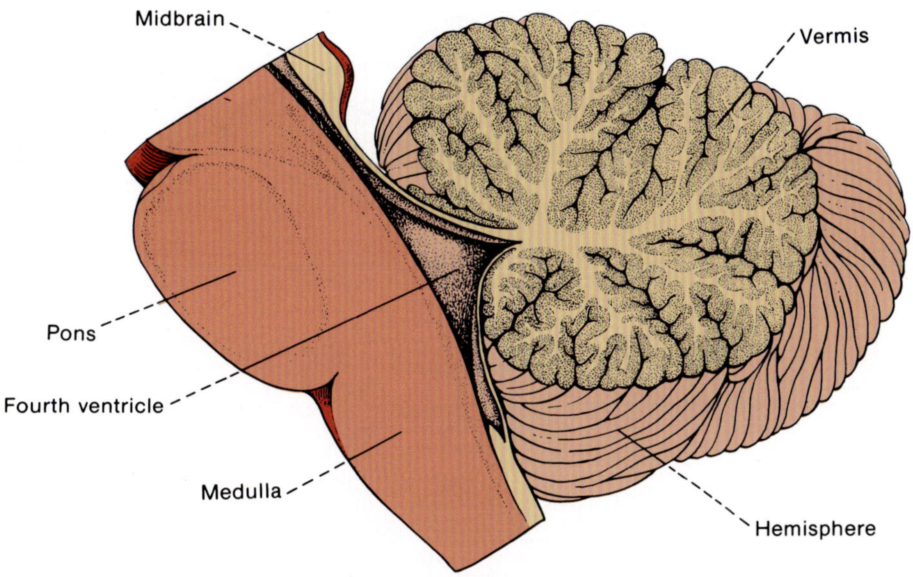

FIGURE 43.2 Median longitudinal section through the human cerebellum, pons, and medulla.

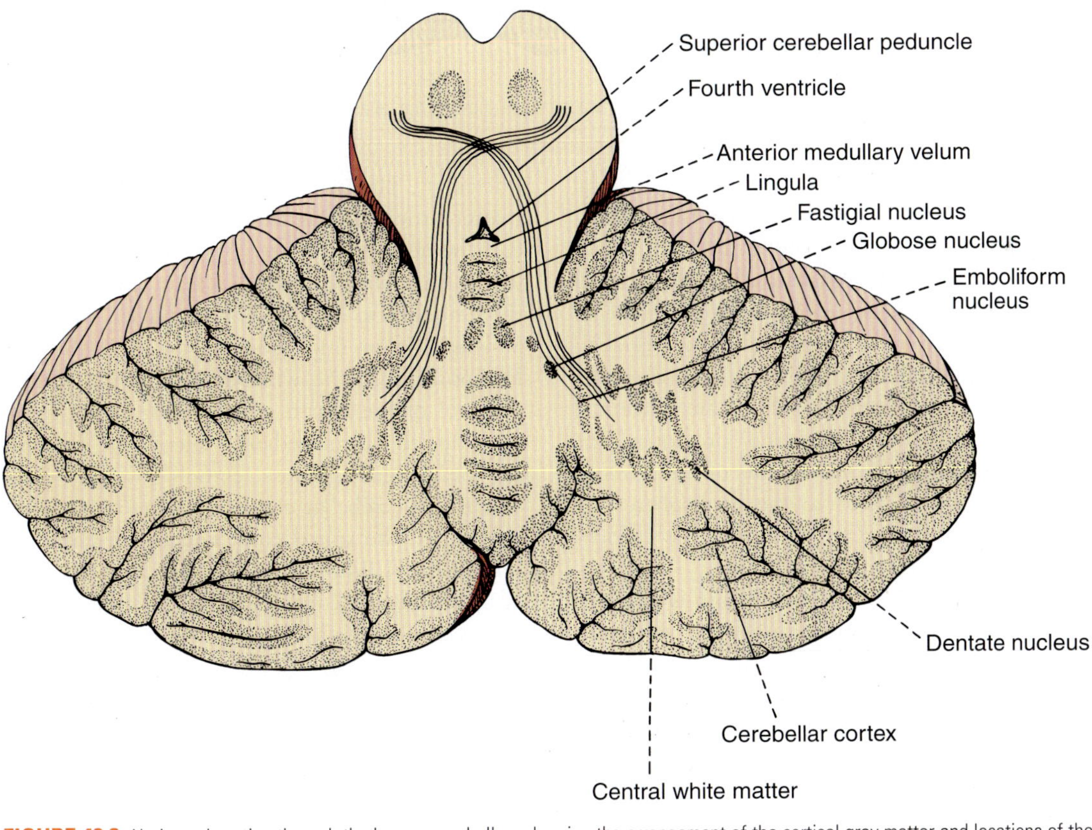

FIGURE 43.3 Horizontal section through the human cerebellum showing the arrangement of the cortical gray matter and locations of the nuclei within the white matter.

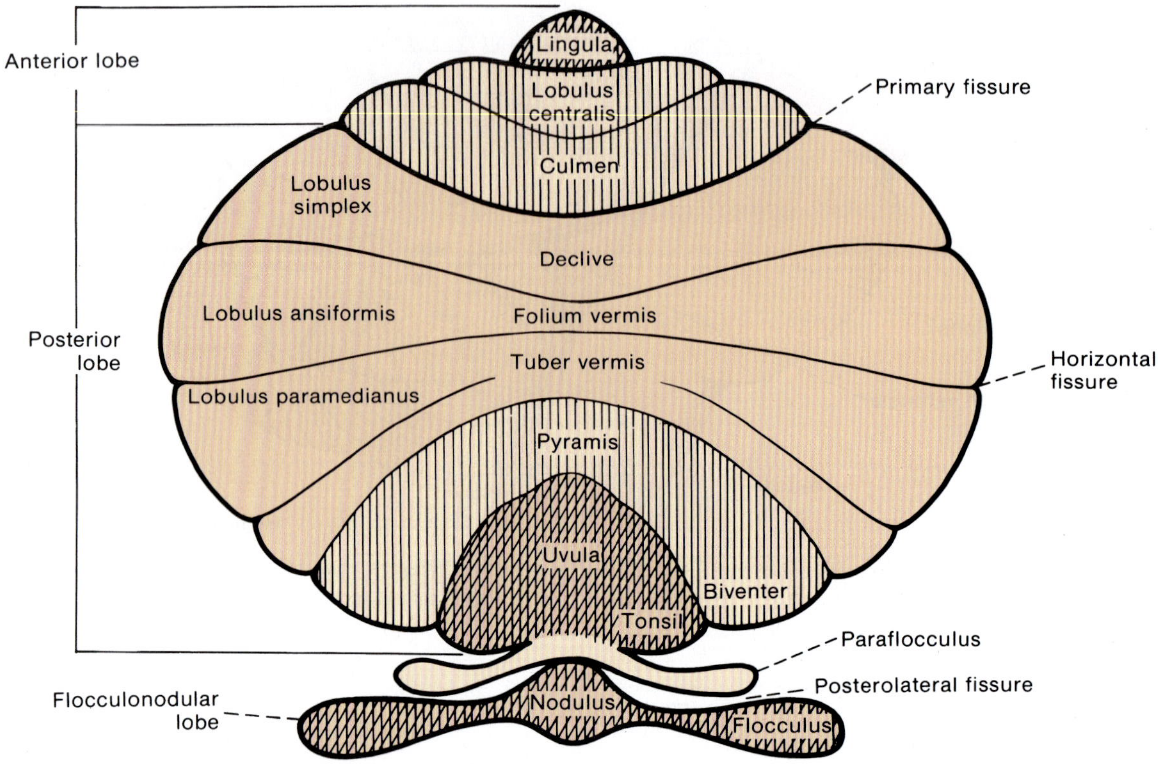

FIGURE 43.4 Diagram of the cerebellum showing the lobes and lobules.

concerned primarily with posture, muscle tone, axial muscle control, and locomotion. There are extensive connections between the vermis and spinal cord pathways. The most phylogenetically recent part of the cerebellum is the neocerebellum, or the cerebellar hemispheres, which make up the bulk of the cerebellum. The neocerebellum corresponds approximately to the posterior lobe. The hemispheres are concerned with coordinating movement and providing fine motor control for precise movements of the extremities. The primary afferents to the hemispheres are from the pontine nuclei, which receive the corticopontine fibers from the cerebral cortex.

Another way to view the cerebellum is in terms of its primary afferent connections: the vestibulocerebellum (input from vestibular nuclei to the FN lobe), the spinocerebellum (input from the spinocerebellar tracts to the anterior vermis), and the pontocerebellum (input from the pontine nuclei to the hemispheres).

The cerebellum is made up of a white matter core, covered with a thin layer of gray matter, the cerebellar cortex. Deep in the white matter are several gray masses, the cerebellar nuclei. The dentate nuclei, the largest of the cerebellar nuclei, are gray matter structures situated deep in the white matter of each hemisphere (Figure 43.3). In the hilus of each dentate nucleus lie the emboliform nuclei; medial to the emboliform are the globose nuclei. The globose and emboliform nuclei together are called the nucleus interpositus. In the white matter of the vermis, at the roof of the fourth ventricle, are the fastigial, or roof, nuclei. From medial to lateral, the deep nuclei are the fastigial, globose, emboliform, and dentate. The major cerebellar connections are to the vestibular system, the spinal cord, and the cerebral cortex (Figure 43.5). Microscopically, the cortex is made up of three layers: the outer, nuclear, or molecular layer; the layer of Purkinje cells; and the inner, or granular, layer (Figure 43.6).

The FN lobe is a primitive part of the cerebellum primarily concerned with vestibular function. The connections of the FN lobe are primarily, if not entirely, vestibular. The FN lobe receives afferent impulses from the labyrinths and vestibular centers, spinal cord, and brainstem—including the reticular formation and olivary bodies—and projects to the vestibular nuclei, vestibulospinal tracts, and reticular

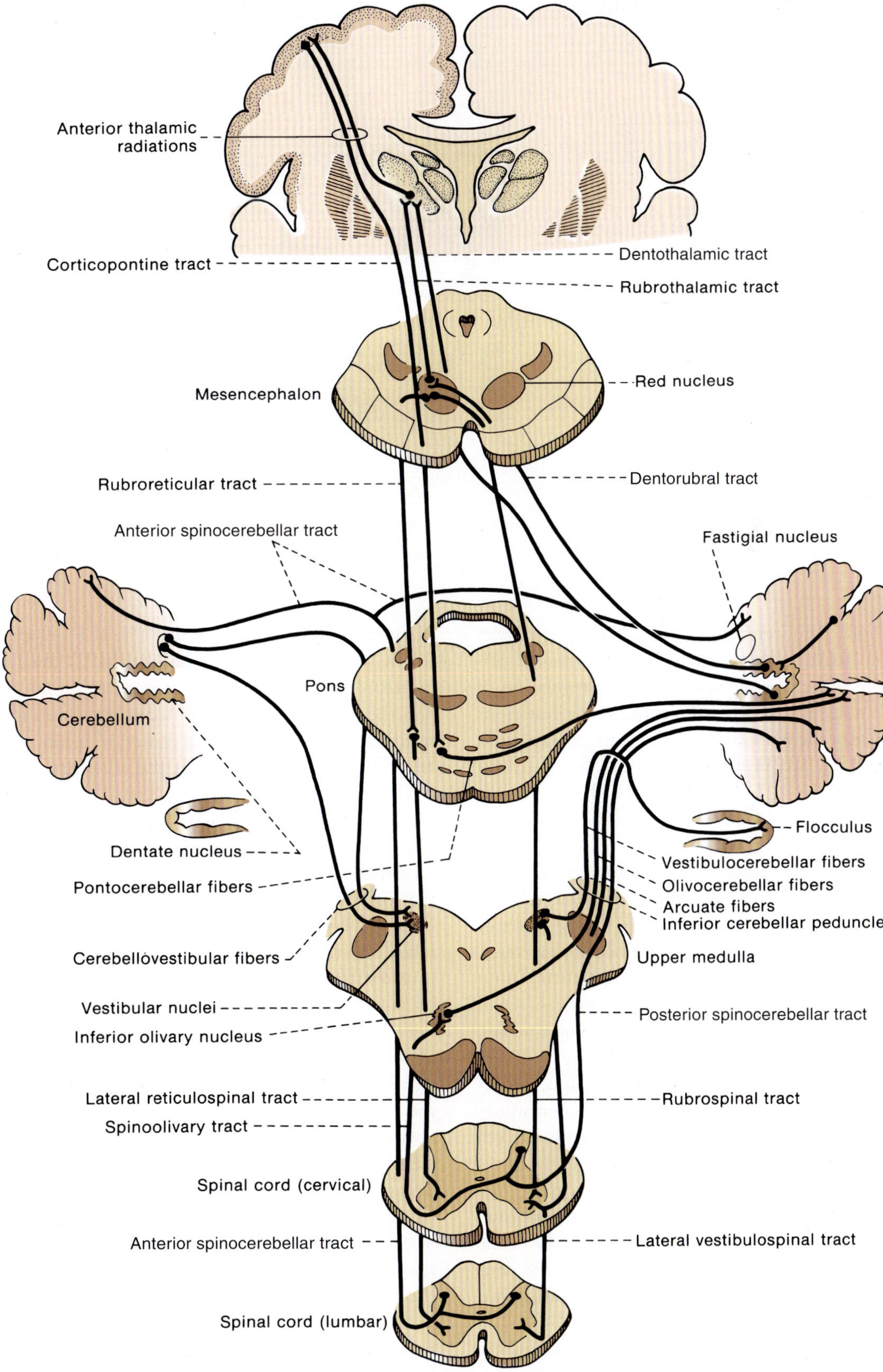

FIGURE 43.5 Principal afferent and efferent connections of the cerebellum.

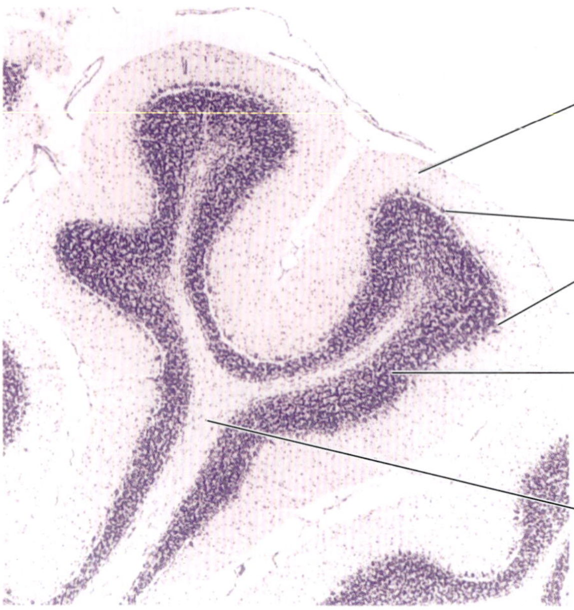

FIGURE 43.6 Transverse section of cerebellar folia showing the three layers of the cortex and the underlying white matter (*cresyl violet*). (Reprinted from Kiernan JA. *Barr's The Human Nervous System: An Anatomical Viewpoint*. 9th ed. Philadelphia: Wolters Kluwer Health/ Lippincott Williams & Wilkins, 2009, with permission.)

formation. The cerebellum and vestibular centers function together to maintain equilibrium, the orientation of the body in space, and the regulation of muscle tone and posture. The clinical manifestations of disease of the FN lobe are difficult to separate from the invariably accompanying vestibular findings, primarily nystagmus. Isolated FN lobe dysfunction is usually caused by ependymomas and medulloblastomas in children.

The paleocerebellum communicates with the spinal cord, brainstem, and vestibular centers. The principal afferent connections of the anterior lobe come from the anterior spinocerebellar tract, although it receives trigeminocerebellar fibers, input from the vestibular nuclei, and some corticocerebellar fibers. The discharges are to the vestibular nuclei, brainstem, and spinal cord.

The neocerebellum (pontocerebellum) communicates with the cerebral cortex. It is enormously developed in mammals in association with growth of the cerebral hemispheres. In primates, the hemispheres overshadow the rest of the cerebellum. Its afferent connections are principally corticopontine, or corticopontocerebellar, although there are some spinocerebellar fibers; it discharges through the dentate nucleus to the red nucleus and thalamus, and thus to the cerebral cortex.

The cerebellum is connected to the brainstem by the three cerebellar peduncles. The inferior cerebellar peduncle (ICP) connects the cerebellum with the spinal cord and the medulla. The ICP lies medial to the middle cerebellar peduncle (MCP, brachium pontis). The ICP has two parts: the restiform body and the juxtarestiform body. Ascending fibers in the restiform body include the posterior spinocerebellar and cuneocerebellar (from the accessory cuneate nucleus) tracts, the dorsal and ventral external arcuate fibers from the nuclei gracilis and cuneatus, and the olivocerebellar, trigeminocerebellar, and reticulocerebellar pathways. Lying just medial to ICP is the juxtarestiform body, made up of fibers traveling directly between the vestibular nuclei and the FN lobe. The restiform body is an afferent system; the juxtarestiform body contains both vestibulocerebellar and cerebellovestibular fibers. The juxtarestiform body is mainly efferent. Although it carries primary afferent vestibulocerebellar fibers from the vestibular nerve and secondary vestibulocerebellar fibers from the vestibular nuclei, its primary component is cerebellovestibular fibers from the vermis and the FN lobe (fastigiobulbar tract). Other cerebellovestibular fibers run from the fastigial nucleus to the vestibular nuclei in the uncinate fasciculus, which enters the brainstem adjacent to the ICP. The MCP connects the cerebellum with the pons, and through it run the pontocerebellar tracts; these are the final neurons of the corticopontocerebellar pathway that comes mainly from the frontal, temporal, and other areas of the cortex to communicate with the contralateral cerebellar hemisphere.

The superior cerebellar peduncle (SCP, brachium conjunctivum) contains the principal efferent fibers of the cerebellum and the dentatorubral and the dentatothalamic pathways. It also carries the afferent anterior spinocerebellar tract, as well as cerebellovestibular fibers in the uncinate fasciculus. The cerebellotegmental, cerebellotectal, and tectocerebellar tracts also travel in the SCP. The afferent fibers to the cerebellar cortex arrive primarily by tracts that enter through the middle and inferior peduncles, but the anterior spinocerebellar tract enters via the SCP.

Microscopic Anatomy

The molecular layer of the cerebellar cortex contains the dendritic arborizations of the Purkinje cells, radial fibers of the Bergmann glial cells, basket cells, stellate cells, climbing fibers, and parallel fibers (Figure 43.6). The flattened dendritic trees of the Purkinje cells spread out perpendicular to the long axis of the cerebellar folium. Climbing fibers are the terminal ramifications of fibers from the inferior olivary nucleus that ascend through the granular layer to contact Purkinje dendrites in the molecular layer. Each climbing fiber forms an excitatory synapse with a single Purkinje cell. Climbing fibers also synapse on the neurons of the deep cerebellar nuclei. Parallel fibers are granule cell axons that extend upward into the molecular layer where they bifurcate to send branches in opposite directions along the axis of a folium to terminate on the Purkinje cell dendrites. The parallel fibers intersect the Purkinje cell dendrites like telephone wires over the cross pieces of a telephone pole.

The Purkinje cell layer contains the perikarya of the large Purkinje cells and the smaller Bergmann (epithelial) glial cells. The granule cell layer lies between the white matter and the Purkinje cell layer; it contains granule cells, Golgi cells, brush cells, and the cerebellar glomeruli (Figure 43.7). The granule cells send their axons to the molecular layer where they branch to form parallel fibers. Mossy fibers are the predominant afferent system to the cerebellum. They arise from the spinal cord, the trigeminal, reticular formation, vestibular and pontine nuclei of the brainstem. The mossy fibers terminate as mossy fiber rosettes that lie at the center of each cerebellar glomerulus. Like the climbing fibers, mossy fibers are excitatory. The mossy fibers primarily use glutamate; the climbing fibers release glutamate or aspartate. Cerebellar glomeruli are synaptic formations with mossy fiber rosettes at the center, surrounded by granule and Golgi cell dendrites (Figure 43.8).

The Purkinje cells are excited by the parallel and climbing fibers and send inhibitory GABA-ergic

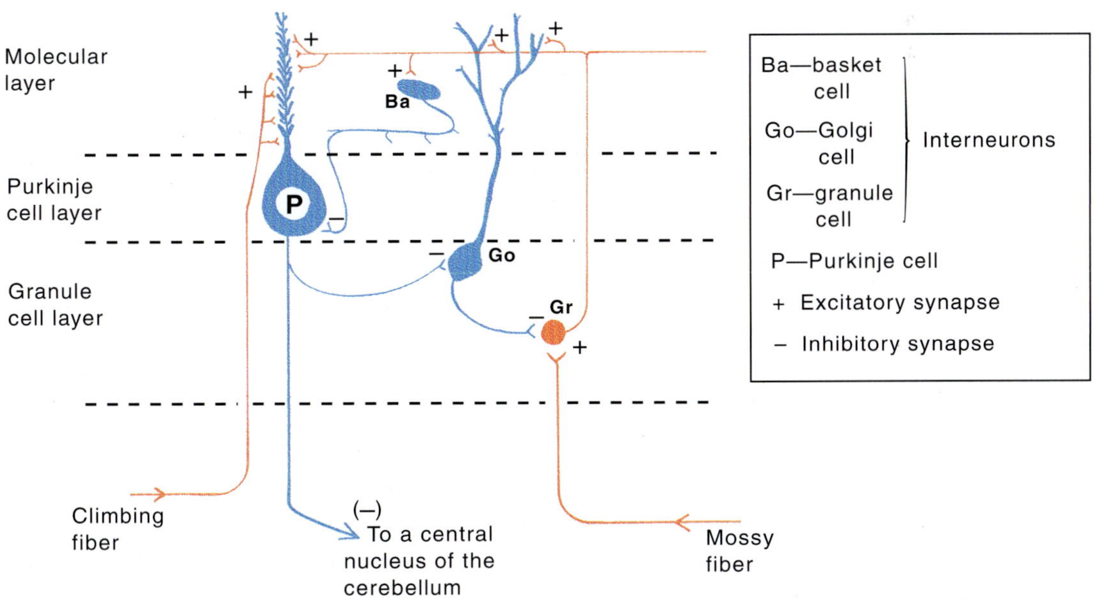

FIGURE 43.7 Neurons in the cerebellar cortex showing excitatory and inhibitory synapses. The diagram represents a longitudinally sectioned folium, with an edge-on view of the dendritic tree of the Purkinje cell. Glutaminergic (excitatory) neurons are *red*; GABA-ergic (inhibitory) neurons are *blue*. (Reprinted from Kiernan JA. *Barr's The Human Nervous System: An Anatomical Viewpoint*. 9th ed. Philadelphia: Wolters Kluwer Health/Lippincott Williams & Wilkins, 2009, with permission.)

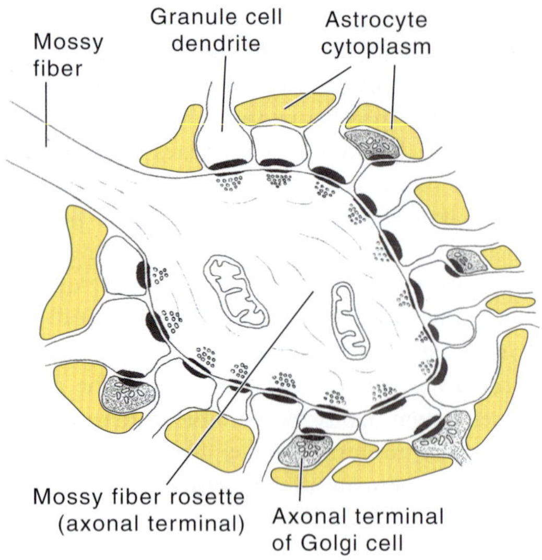

FIGURE 43.8 Ultrastructure of a synaptic glomerulus in the granule cell layer. The astrocytic processes (*yellow*) prevent diffusion of neurotransmitters to adjacent synapses. (Reprinted from Kiernan JA. *Barr's The Human Nervous System: An Anatomical Viewpoint*. 9th ed. Philadelphia: Wolters Kluwer Health/Lippincott Williams & Wilkins, 2009, with permission.)

projections to the deep cerebellar and the vestibular nuclei. Input from the basket and stellate cells inhibit the Purkinje cells. The granule cells are excitatory, glutaminergic neurons. The parallel fibers that arise from the granule cells excite the Purkinje, basket, stellate, and Golgi cells. The granule cell is excited by mossy fiber input at the cerebellar glomerulus and inhibited by Golgi cells. The mossy fiber input excites Purkinje cells indirectly through the granule cell–parallel fiber system and produces simple spikes from the Purkinje cell. The climbing fibers are entwined around the Purkinje cell, like a vine around a tree trunk, and excite it directly, producing complex spikes. The cerebellar cortex also receives noradrenergic fibers from the locus coeruleus, dopaminergic fibers from the substantia nigra, and serotonergic fibers from the raphe nuclei. All the aminergic afferents are probably inhibitory. Afferents to the cerebellar cortex and deep nuclei generally produce an increase in excitability. The Purkinje cells impose inhibitory control over the cells of the deep nuclei. Mossy fiber input causes strong direct excitation of the deep nuclei; the additional input via the granule cell-parallel fiber system provides inhibitory control and modulation of the direct excitatory pathway. The climbing fibers modulate the activity of the Purkinje cells by controlling the influence of the different systems that converge on it.

The efferent fibers from the Purkinje cells in the cerebellar cortex are nearly all relayed to the deep nuclei, where the cerebellar outflow originates (Figure 43.5). The output from the deep cerebellar nuclei is excitatory and glutaminergic except for the projection to the inferior olive, which uses gamma-aminobutyric acid. The fastigial nucleus, the oldest of the cerebellar nuclei, receives afferent fibers from the paleocerebellum and also from the vestibular nuclei and the eighth cranial nerve. Its efferent impulses, many of them crossing in the roof, pass into the brainstem to the vestibular nuclei—especially the lateral vestibular nucleus—and to the reticular formation. Some of these go through the ICP; others travel in the SCP in the uncinate fasciculus. The fastigial nucleus also projects to the ventral lateral (VL) nucleus of the thalamus, which in turn projects to the trunk area of the motor strip. The interposed nuclei receive afferents primarily from the paravermal cortex and project to VL and to the magnocellular part of the contralateral red nucleus, which gives rise to the rubrospinal tract. The dentate nuclei, the most important of the nuclear masses in terms of clinical function, receive afferents principally from the Purkinje cells of the neocerebellum. The dentate projects to the ipsilateral VL and intralaminar thalamic nuclei and to the contralateral red nucleus and inferior olivary nucleus.

The cerebellum is part of complex feedback loops that are involved in the coordination of motor activity (Figures 43.9 to 43.11). Large myelinated muscle spindle and Golgi tendon organ afferents travel to the cerebellum via the spinocerebellar tracts and enter primarily through the ICP. This information is processed in the hemispheres and influences the activity of Purkinje cells in the deep, midline (primarily dentate) nucleus. The Purkinje cells send axons via the SCP to the contralateral VL nucleus of the thalamus, which in turn projects to the motor cortex. Descending corticopontine fibers then synapse on pontine nuclei in the basis pontis, which in turn send pontocerebellar axons via the MCP to the cerebellar hemispheres. Other descending corticomotor fibers actually execute the task at hand. The cerebellum can thereby communicate the need for fine adjustment of movement to the cortex, and the cortex can take corrective action while simultaneously informing the cerebellum of the extent of the correction so further adjustments can be made (see Chapter 22). The motor thalamus serves to integrate cerebellar, basal ganglia, and cortical activity. Another loop consists of fibers that arise from the inferior olive and travel via the ICP to the dentate nucleus, with

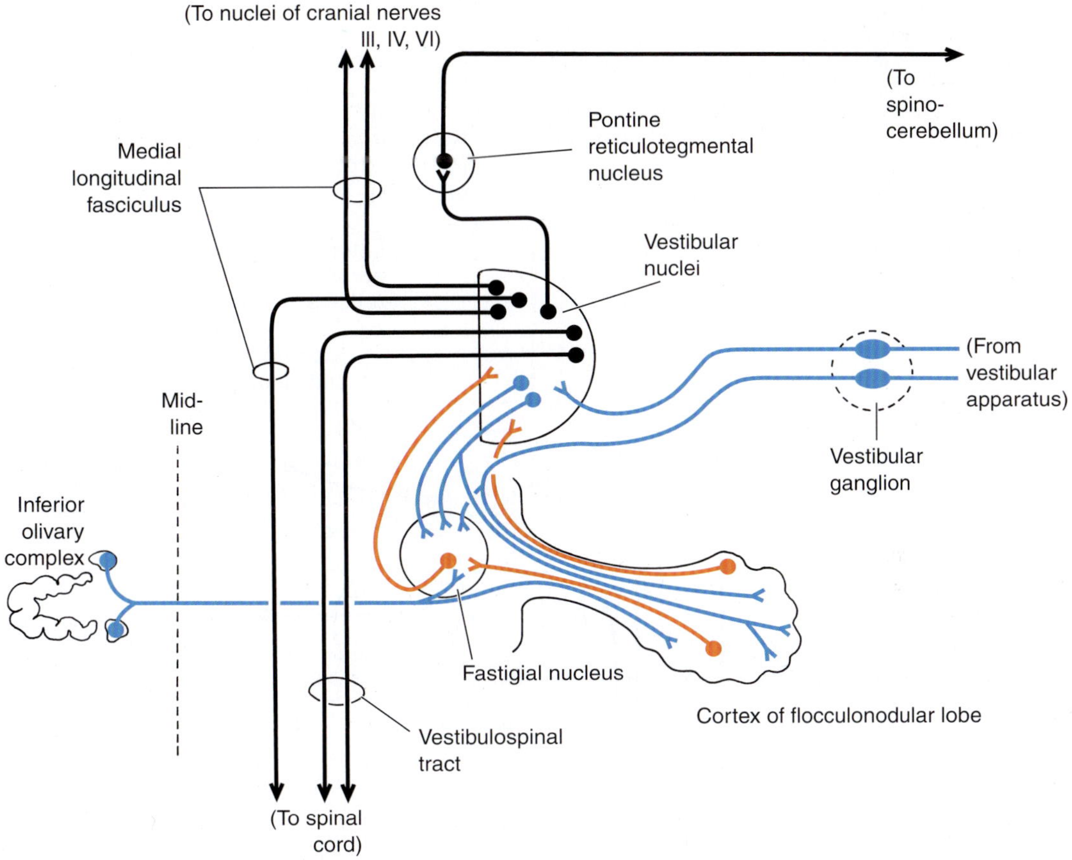

FIGURE 43.9 Connections of the vestibulocerebellum and vestibular nuclei. Afferents to the cerebellum are *blue*, cerebellar efferents are *red*, and other neurons are *black*. (Reprinted from Kiernan JA. *Barr's The Human Nervous System: An Anatomical Viewpoint*. 9th ed. Philadelphia: Wolters Kluwer Health/Lippincott Williams & Wilkins, 2009, with permission.)

projections from the dentate going to the red nucleus, which then projects to the inferior olive (Guillain-Mollaret triangle, see Chapter 30). The direct vestibulocerebellar and returning cerebellovestibular fibers form yet another circuit. The cerebellum also receives input from the hypothalamus.

CLINICAL MANIFESTATIONS OF CEREBELLAR DYSFUNCTION

Patients with cerebellar dysfunction suffer from various combinations of tremor, incoordination, difficulty walking, dysarthria, and nystagmus, depending on the parts of the cerebellum involved (see Table 22.1). Ataxia is the cardinal sign of cerebellar disease; it consists of varying degrees of dyssynergia, dysmetria, lack of agonist-antagonist coordination, and tremor. Ataxia may affect the limbs, the trunk, or the gait. Cerebellar disease may also cause hypotonia, asthenia or slowness of movement, and deviation or drift of the outstretched limbs. Disease involving the cerebellar connections in the brainstem causes abnormalities indistinguishable from disease of the cerebellum itself. When cerebellar ataxia results from dysfunction of the cerebellar connections in the brainstem, there are usually other brainstem signs.

Dyssynergia

The essential disturbance in cerebellar disease is dyssynergia. Normally, there is harmonious, coordinated action between the various muscles involved in a movement so that they contract with the proper force, timing, and sequence of activation to carry out the movement smoothly and accurately. Cerebellar disease impairs the normal control mechanisms that organize and regulate the contractions of the different participating muscles and muscle groups to insure smooth, properly coordinated movement. There is a

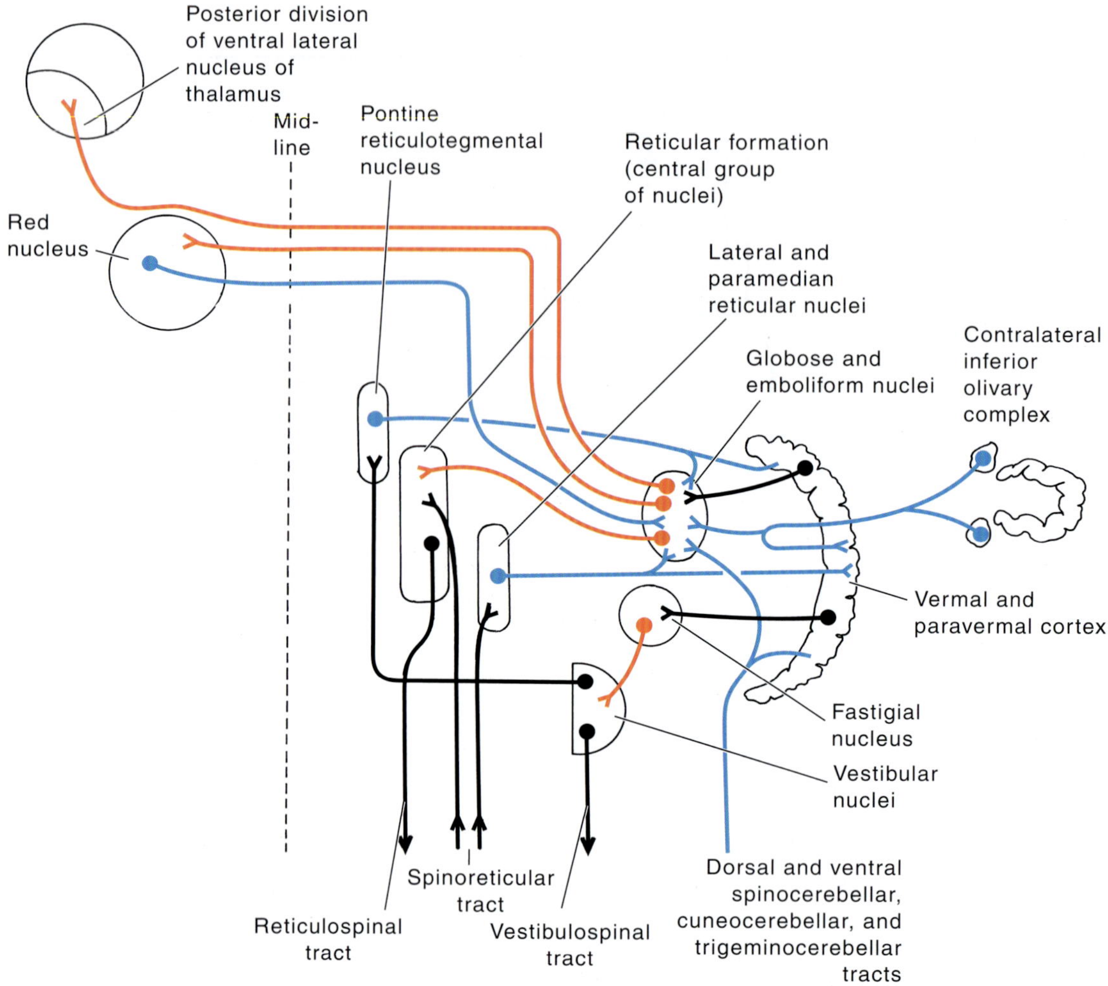

FIGURE 43.10 Connections of the spinocerebellum. Afferents to the cerebellum are *blue*, cerebellar efferents are *red*, and other neurons are *black*. (Reprinted from Kiernan JA. *Barr's The Human Nervous System: An Anatomical Viewpoint*. 9th ed. Philadelphia: Wolters Kluwer Health/Lippincott Williams & Wilkins, 2009, with permission.)

lack of speed and skill in performing movements that require the coordinated activity of several groups of muscles or of several movements. The cerebellum is instrumental in timing the activation of the different muscles involved in a movement. Lack of integration of the components of the act results in decomposition of movement—the act is broken down into its component parts and carried out in a jerky, erratic, awkward, disorganized manner. The cerebellum is particularly important in coordinating multijoint movements.

Dysmetria

Dysmetria refers to errors in judging distance and gauging the distance, speed, power, and direction of movement. Cerebellar dysfunction leads to loss of the normal collaboration between agonist and antagonist. When reaching for an object 50 cm away, the hand shoots out 55 cm, overshooting the target (hypermetria), or fails to reach the target (hypometria). Hypermetria is more common. The movement may be carried out too slowly or too rapidly with too much or too little force. The patient with dysmetria does not make a movement along a straight line between two points but erratically deviates from the intended track. Electromyographic studies have shown that dysmetria is associated with abnormalities of the timing and force of antagonist contraction necessary to decelerate the movement. Hypermetria is

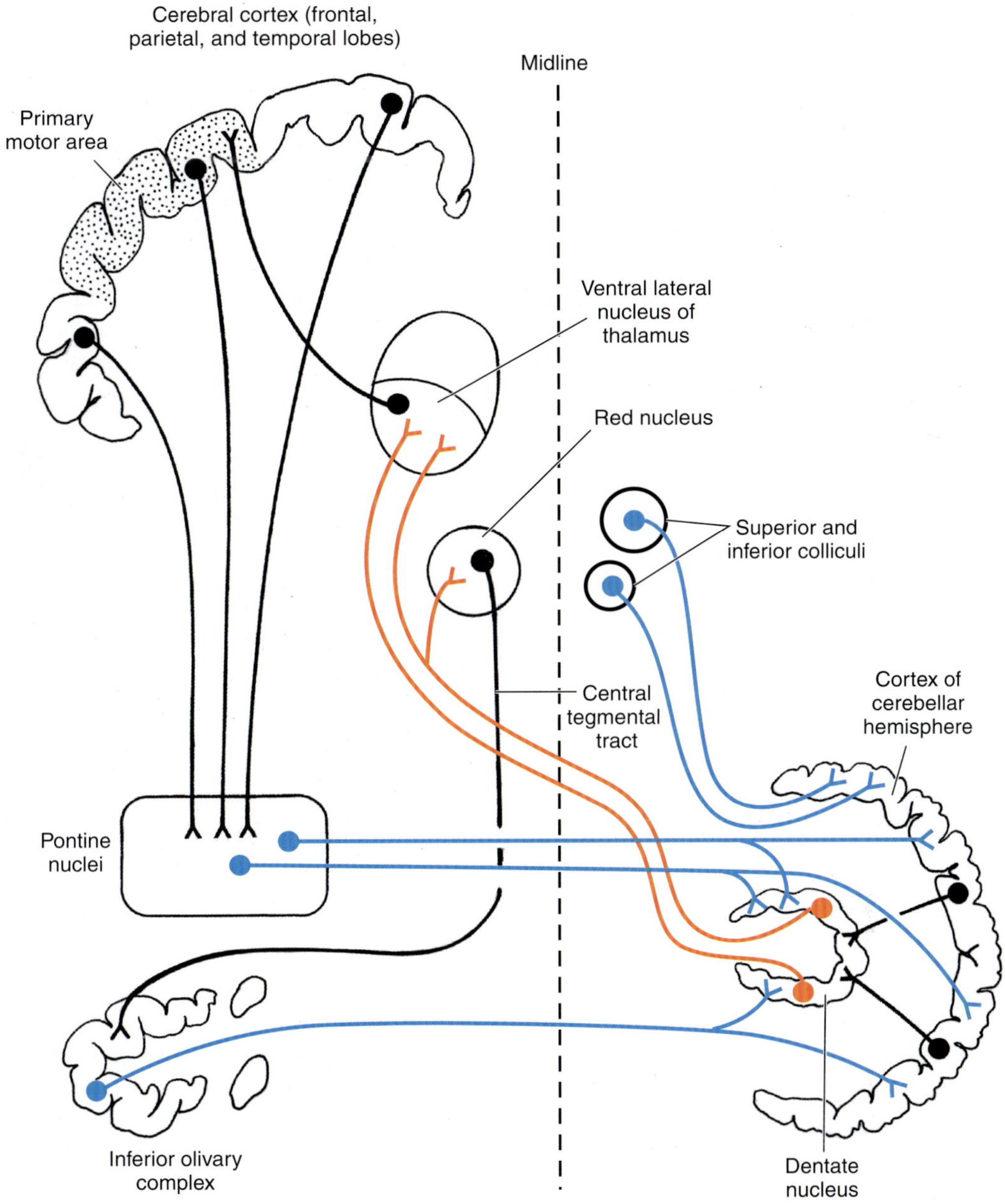

FIGURE 43.11 Connections of the pontocerebellum and vestibular nuclei. Afferents to the cerebellum are *blue*, cerebellar efferents are *red*, and other neurons are *black*. (Reprinted from Kiernan JA. *Barr's The Human Nervous System: An Anatomical Viewpoint*. 9th ed. Philadelphia: Wolters Kluwer Health/Lippincott Williams & Wilkins, 2009, with permission.)

associated with a more gradual buildup and prolongation of agonist activity with a delayed onset of antagonist activity or with a slower rate of rise of activity in the antagonists. Evidence suggests that different mechanisms may underlie dysmetria, depending on the anatomical location of the cerebellar lesion.

Agonist-Antagonist Coordination

A disturbance in reciprocal innervation results in a loss of the ability to stop the contraction of the agonists and rapidly contract the antagonists to control and regulate movement. In patients with cerebellar deficits attempting to make rapid, voluntary movements, the first agonist burst is frequently prolonged, the acceleration time is longer than normal, and the acceleration time may exceed the deceleration time. The normal triphasic agonist-antagonist-agonist sequence of activity is disturbed by a too long or too short agonist burst, or an agonist burst that continues into the antagonist activity. Impairment of the ability to carry out successive movements and to stop one act and follow it immediately by its diametric opposite causes dysdiadochokinesia, loss of checking movements, and the rebound phenomenon. Dysdiadochokinesia (or adiadochokinesia) is a clumsy term (coined by Babinski) that means inability to make rapid alternating movements or RAMs. The patient with impaired RAMs has difficulty with such tests as patting the palm of one hand alternately with the palm and dorsum of the other hand, rapid tapping of the fingers, tapping out a complex rhythm, or tapping the foot in steady beat. Inability to rapidly reverse an action also causes impairment of the check response, producing the Holmes rebound phenomenon (see section on "Impaired Check and the Rebound Phenomenon").

Tremor

The most common type of cerebellar tremor is an intention (active, kinetic, or terminal) tremor that is not present at rest but becomes evident on purposeful movement. In the upper extremity, when the patient reaches to touch an object, there are irregular, to-and-fro, jerky movements perpendicular to the path of movement that increase in amplitude as the hand approaches the target. A postural tremor of the outstretched limbs may also occur, without the patient reaching for a target. Cerebellar tremor often involves the proximal muscles. When severe, cerebellar tremor may involve not only the extremities but also the head or even the entire body. Severe cerebellar tremor may at times take on an almost myoclonic character. The tremors and other movements probably result from disease involving the cerebellar efferent pathways or their connections with the red nucleus and thalamus (dentatorubral and dentatothalamic pathways, or SCP) and are sometimes referred to as a cerebellar outflow tremor. A rubral tremor is present at rest but worsens with action and probably also results from a lesion involving the cerebellar outflow tracts (see Chapter 30).

Hypotonia

Hypotonia, or muscle flaccidity, with a decrease in resistance to passive movement, is often seen in cerebellar disease. Cerebellar dysfunction results in a decrease in the tonic output of the cerebellar nuclei, causing loss of cerebellar facilitation to the motor cortex. The muscles are flabby and assume unnatural attitudes; the parts of the body can be moved passively into positions of extreme flexion or extension. The stretch reflexes are normal or diminished in disease limited to the cerebellum. Occasionally, the tendon reflexes are "pendular." Tapping the patellar tendon with the foot hanging free results in a series of to-and-fro movements of the foot and leg before the limb finally comes to rest. Pendular reflexes are caused by muscle hypotonicity and the lack of normal checking of the reflex response. The superficial reflexes are unaffected by cerebellar disease. Cerebellar disease may also cause a characteristic position of the extended hand, probably because of hypotonia. The wrist is flexed and arched dorsally, with the fingers hyperextended, and a tendency toward overpronation. The hand is similar to that seen in Sydenham's chorea. A cerebellar lesion may cause a decrease in the normal pendular movement of the affected arm when walking. A decreased arm swing may also occur with extrapyramidal disorders and with mild hemiparesis. In the shoulder-shaking test, a cerebellar lesion causes an increase in the range and duration of swinging of the involved arm, although the movements may be irregular and nonrhythmic (see Chapter 28).

Dysarthria

Cerebellar disease often affects speech. Articulation may be slow, ataxic, slurred, drawling, jerky, or explosive in type because of dyssynergy of the muscles of phonation. A scanning type of dysarthria is particularly characteristic of cerebellar disease (see Chapter 9). The scanning speech of multiple sclerosis and the staccato speech of Friedreich's ataxia (FA) are probably the result of cerebellar dysfunction. Dysarthria may be an isolated manifestation of paravermal cerebellar infarction.

Nystagmus

Nystagmus and other disturbances of ocular motility may occur with lesions of the cerebellum. Nystagmus often indicates involvement of vestibulocerebellar pathways. The ocular abnormalities often result from involvement of the connections of the cerebellum with other centers rather than actual cerebellar dysfunction. Cerebellar disease may cause gaze paretic nystagmus. The patient is unable to sustain eccentric gaze and requires repeated saccades to gaze laterally. With a lesion of one hemisphere, the eyes at rest may be deviated 10 to 30 degrees toward the unaffected side. When the patient attempts to gaze elsewhere, the eyes saccade toward the point of fixation with slow return movements to the resting point. The movements are more marked and of greater amplitude when the patient looks toward the affected side. When a tumor of the cerebellopontine angle is present, the nystagmus is coarse on looking toward the side of the lesion and fine and rapid on gaze to the opposite side (Bruns' nystagmus). Other ocular motility disturbances seen with cerebellar disease include skew deviation, ocular dysmetria, ocular flutter, opsoclonus, ocular tilt reaction, and saccadic intrusions. Rebound nystagmus is a type of nystagmus that may be unique to cerebellar disease; the fast component is in the direction of lateral gaze but transiently reverses direction when the eyes come back to primary position (see Chapter 14). For a detailed discussion of cerebellar eye signs, see *Cerebellar Eye Signs* from Dr. Robert B. Darroff, Neuro-ophthalmology Virtual Education Library (NOVEL), University of Utah, **Video Link 43.1.**

Other Abnormalities

Abnormalities of posture and gait with abnormal attitudes and spontaneous deviation of the head and parts of the body may be seen in cerebellar disease. In unilateral cerebellar disease, there may be deviation of the head and body toward the affected side, with past pointing of the extremities toward the affected side. When standing, there is an inclination to fall, and when walking a tendency to deviate, toward the side of the lesion. The outstretched extremities deviate laterally, toward the affected side. There may be a decrease or absence of the normal pendular movement of the arm in walking. In midline, or vermis, lesions, the patient may not be able to stand erect and may fall either backward or forward. The gait is staggering, reeling, or lurching in character, without laterality. "Cerebellar fits" is an antiquated term, referring to episodes of decerebrate rigidity because of brainstem dysfunction due to mass effect from lesions in the cerebellum.

EXAMINATION OF COORDINATION AND CEREBELLAR FUNCTION

Clinical tests for cerebellar dysfunction are basically designed to detect dyssynergia, decomposition of movement, and dysmetria. The combination of incoordination, awkwardness, errors in the speed, range and force of movement, along with dysdiadochokinesia, and intention tremor is referred to as cerebellar ataxia. Simple observation can be as informative as a detailed clinical examination. Watching as the patient is standing, walking, dressing and undressing, buttoning and unbuttoning clothing, and tying shoelaces may reveal tremor, incoordination, clumsiness, and disturbed postural fixation. The patient may be asked to write, use simple tools, drink from a glass, and trace lines with a lightweight pen while no support is given at the elbow. The examination of infants and children may be limited to simple observation, noting the child's ability to reach for and use toys and objects. Tests for coordination may be divided into those concerned with equilibratory and nonequilibratory functions.

Equilibratory Coordination

Equilibratory coordination refers to the maintenance of balance and the coordination of the body as a whole. The examination of station and gait assesses equilibratory coordination; these are discussed further in Chapter 44.

Nonequilibratory Coordination

Tests of nonequilibratory coordination assess the patient's ability to carry out discrete, oftentimes relatively fine, intentional movements with the extremities. Although these are primarily tests of coordination, other neural systems must be intact for normal performance. The other components affecting fine motor control are discussed in Chapter 27. It is important to consider handedness in judging coordination and to allow for the normal slight clumsiness of the nondominant side. Patients who are fatigued or sedated may have incoordination that is not normal for the individual. Fine motor skills may also be assessed functionally by asking the patient to do such things as thread a needle, pick up a pin, string beads, pour water, or draw circles.

The Finger-to-Nose (Finger-Nose-Finger) Test

There are several variations on the theme of having the patient touch the index finger to the nose, all of which will be included as the finger-to-nose (FTN) test. All may be carried out with the patient lying, seated, or standing. The patient extends the arm completely and then touches the tip of the index finger to the tip of the nose, slowly at first, then rapidly, with the eyes open and then closed. The examiner may place the outstretched extremity in various positions and have the test carried out in different planes and from various angles. The patient may be asked to touch the tip of his index finger to his nose, then touch the tip of the examiner's finger, and then back to the tip of his nose. It is helpful to demonstrate the requested movement, lest the patient make some odd interpretation of the verbal request; an occasional patient will attempt to put his index finger on the examiner's finger without removing it from his own nose. The examiner's finger may be moved about during the test, and the patient asked to try to touch the moving target as the finger is placed in different locations at different distances and to move both slowly and quickly. The examiner may pull his finger away and make the patient chase it (finger chase test). Fully extending the arm in this way can bring out mild intention tremor.

During these movements, note the smoothness and accuracy with which the act is executed and look for oscillations, jerkiness, and tremor. An intention tremor becomes more marked, coarse, and irregular as the finger approaches the target. There may be little tremor during the midrange of the movement, but near the end, the tremor erupts; when the finger contacts the target, the tremor stops. In cerebellar ataxia, the difficulty may vary from slight incoordination, with a blundering type of movement, to wild oscillations causing complete inability to execute the act. A patient with severe appendicular ataxia may not be able to touch hand to head, much less finger to nose.

Video 43.1 demonstrates a patient with appendicular ataxia.

With dysmetria, the patient may stop before he reaches his nose, pause and then complete the act slowly and unsteadily, or overshoot the mark and bring the finger to the nose with too much speed and force. With dyssynergy, the act is not carried out smoothly and harmoniously; there may be irregular stops, accelerations, and deflections, or the movement may disintegrate into its component parts. Performing the FTN test against slight resistance may cause mild ataxia to become more obvious, or latent ataxia evident. The examiner may apply resistance by placing his fingers against the patient's forearm and exerting slight pressure as the patient moves his arm toward the nose, or by placing a long rubber band around the patient's wrist and pulling gently on it during the test. Another test is to have the patient draw a line, starting and then stopping at fixed points. He may have difficulty in starting at the correct point and may either stop short of the second point or overshoot the mark. This may also demonstrate tremor, with side-to-side oscillations along the intended tract. The patient with cerebellar disease may have macrographia, using large characters that become larger across the page, the opposite of the writing disturbance seen in Parkinson's disease.

In the finger-to-finger (fingertips in the midline) test, the patient abducts the arms widely to the horizontal and then brings in the tips of the index or middle fingers through a wide arc to touch them exactly in the midline. This is done slowly and rapidly, with the eyes first open and then closed. With unilateral cerebellar disease, the finger on the involved side may fail to reach the midline, and the finger on the normal side may cross the midline to reach it. Also, the arm on the affected side may sag or rise, causing the finger on that side to be below or above the one on the normal side.

In patients with functional neurologic presentations, there may be bizarre responses of various types. The patient may act as if unable to touch the finger to the nose, or circle around it with widespread, wandering movements but eventually touch the very tip. Or the patient may repeatedly but precisely touch some other part of the face, implying there is no loss of sensation or coordination.

Similar tests may be used to evaluate the lower extremities. In the heel-to-shin (heel-knee-shin/toe) test, the patient is asked to place the heel of one foot on the opposite knee, tap it up and down on the knee several times, push the point of the heel (not the instep) along the shin in a straight line to the great toe, and then bring it back to the knee. The patient with cerebellar disease is likely to raise the foot too high, flex the knee too much, and place the heel down above the knee. The excursions along the shin are jerky and unsteady. With sensory ataxia, the patient may have difficulty locating the knee with the heel, groping around for it; there is difficulty keeping the heel on the shin, and it may slip off to either side while sliding down the shin. In the toe-to-finger test, the patient tries to touch his great toe, knee bent, to the examiner's finger. If there is dysmetria, the patient will undershoot or overshoot the mark; intention tremor and oscillations may also be evident. The patient may be asked to draw a circle or a figure eight with his foot, either in the air or on the floor; in ataxia, the movement will be unsteady and the figure irregular.

Rapid Alternating Movements

With dysdiadochokinesia, one act cannot be immediately followed by its diametric opposite; the contraction of one set of agonists and relaxation of the antagonists cannot be followed immediately by relaxation of the agonists and contraction of the antagonists. Patients with cerebellar ataxia may have great difficulty making these kinds of movements **(Video 43.1)**. A common test for dysdiadochokinesia is to have the patient alternately pronate and supinate his hands, as in patting alternately with the palm and dorsum of the hand on the thigh or on the palm or dorsum of the other hand, or imitating screwing in a light bulb or turning a doorknob. The movements are performed repetitively and as rapidly as possible. Any movement involving reciprocal innervation and alternate action of agonists and antagonists can be used, such as alternate opening and closing of the fists, quickly flexing and extending individual fingers, touching the tip of the index finger to the tip or extended interphalangeal joint of the thumb, or patting rapidly against a table top with hand or fingertips. A good test is to have the patient touch the tip of his thumb with the tip of each finger rapidly and in sequence—starting with the index finger and proceeding to the little finger, repeating with the little finger and going to the index finger, and so forth. Another good test is to have the patient tap out a simple rhythm with each hand (e.g., 1-2-3/pause in steady beat), and then a more complex but familiar rhythm (e.g., Happy Birthday song). Testing RAMs in the lower extremity is much more limited. The patient may be asked to pat the foot steadily, against the floor if standing, and against the examiner's palm if recumbent or to repetitively touch the heel up and down to the knee if supine. RAMs of the tongue may be tested by having the patient move the tongue in and out or from side to side as rapidly as possible.

In all of these tests, note the rate, rhythm, accuracy, and smoothness of the movements. In patients with ataxia, the RAMs are carried out either slowly and hesitantly, with pauses during transition between the opposing motions, or unsteadily and irregularly, with loss of rhythm. There may be a rapid fatigability: The movements may be executed satisfactorily in the beginning, but after a few attempts, they become awkward and clumsy. The two extremities are usually compared, but patients with bilateral abnormalities are common, and the examiner must rely on experience or use another control. Demonstrating the movements to the patient provides an opportunity for the examiner to be the control. For some maneuvers, such as rapid, repetitive finger movements, the two extremities can be examined simultaneously and one side compared with the other. Simultaneous testing may also cause accentuation of the abnormality on the affected side.

Impaired Check and the Rebound Phenomenon

Checking movements involve contraction of the antagonists after a load is unexpectedly removed during strong contraction of the agonists. The agonists must immediately relax and the antagonists must contract to provide braking after the sudden release of resistance. Because cerebellar dysfunction causes impairment of the reciprocal relationship between agonist and antagonist, patients may have impairment of the checking response.

In the Holmes (Stewart-Holmes) rebound test, the patient holds the arm adducted at the shoulder and flexed at the elbow, with the forearm supinated and the fist firmly clenched. The elbow may rest on a table or be held unsupported close to the body. The examiner pulls on the wrist, and the patient strongly resists the examiner's attempt to extend the elbow. The examiner then suddenly releases his grip on the wrist. Normally, with the sudden unloading, the contraction of the elbow flexors immediately ceases and is rapidly followed by contraction of the elbow extensors to arrest the sudden flexion movement and stop the patient from hitting himself. The normal patient is able to control the unexpected flexion movement of the elbow. In cerebellar disease, when the strongly flexed extremity is suddenly released, the patient cannot stop the flexor contraction and engage the extensors to stop the elbow movement. Because of loss of the checking response, the fist flies up to the shoulder or mouth, often with considerable force. The examiner's free arm should be placed between the patient's fist and face to block the blow. The prevalent description of this as the Holmes rebound phenomenon is not precisely correct. Stewart and Holmes used rebound to refer to the jerk back in the opposite direction, the recoil, on release of the restraint. The rebound phenomenon is present normally and exaggerated in spastic limbs. It is the absence of rebound (usually accompanied by impaired checking) in limbs affected by cerebellar disease that is abnormal. It is the loss of rebound that is abnormal and characteristic of cerebellar disease, not its presence.

The rebound test may be carried out in other ways. Elbow extension against resistance may be tested instead of flexion. With both arms outstretched in front of the patient, the examiner may press either down or up on them as the patient resists and then suddenly lets go. This allows comparison of the rebound phenomenon and loss of checking movements on the two sides. In the lower extremities, rebound can be tested by sudden release after the patient has been resisting either flexion or extension at the knee, hip, or ankle. Impaired checking and loss of rebound are not invariably present in cerebellar disease and may sometimes be present in normal limbs. Loss of rebound is more significant unilaterally than bilaterally. In the arm-stopping test, the patient holds both arms overhead or by his sides, the examiner holds his arms outstretched horizontally, and then the patient tries to quickly bring his arms up or down so that his fingertips are at the exact same level as the examiner's. With a unilateral hemispheric lesion, the good arm will stop on target, the affected arm often overshoots and then corrects in the opposite direction, oscillating around the target before eventually coming to rest.

Deviation and Past Pointing

Patients with cerebellar disease often have difficulty maintaining normal alignment of the limbs or body when performing a task such as holding the arms outstretched or walking, especially with eyes closed. The patient may miss when trying to reach out to touch a target (past pointing), drift to one side when walking eyes closed, or have drift of the outstretched arm **(Video 43.2)**. Similar findings may occur with vestibular lesions.

To perform the traditional test for past pointing, the patient and examiner should be facing, either seated or standing, the outstretched upper extremity of each held horizontally with the index fingers in contact. The patient raises his arm to a vertical position, finger pointed directly upward, and then returns to horizontal to again touch the examiner's finger. The maneuver should be tried a few times with the eyes open and then executed with the eyes closed. The arms may be tested sequentially or simultaneously. The test is less commonly done with the patient raising the arm from below up to the horizontal. Normally, the patient will return to the starting position fairly accurately, without any drift or deviation. In labyrinthine disease or with a cerebellar hemispheric lesion, the arm will deviate to the involved side on the return track, more so with the eyes closed. This deviation is called past pointing. A simpler way to test for past pointing is to have the patient close his eyes while doing the finger-nose-finger test. With eyes open, the pointing is accurate, but with eyes closed, the patient points off to the side of the target. Repeating the test several times may produce greater deviation. With severe lesions, past pointing may occur even with eyes open. The pattern is different in vestibular as opposed to cerebellar past pointing. In vestibular disease, past pointing occurs with both upper extremities toward the involved side; in unilateral cerebellar disease, past pointing occurs toward the side of the lesion, or erratically to either side, but only in the ipsilateral arm. Past pointing is discussed further in Chapter 17.

A cerebellar lesion may also cause drift of the outstretched upper extremities. Three types of drift may occur when the patient attempts to hold the arms outstretched with eyes closed: pyramidal drift, parietal drift, and cerebellar drift. In pronator drift (Barré's sign) due to a pyramidal lesion, the arm sinks downward and there is accompanying pronation of the forearm (see Chapter 27). In parietal drift, the arm usually rises and strays outward (updrift). With cerebellar drift, the arm drifts mainly outward, either at the same level, rising, or less often sinking. Testing is done with arms outstretched and eyes closed. With disease involving one cerebellar hemisphere, the arm drifts toward the side of the lesion. The deviation may be accentuated by tapping the patient's outstretched wrists. Tapping on the wrists may also create an up-and-down oscillation because of impaired checking, so that the arm swings up and down a few times and gradually drifts laterally and often upward.

Position holding can also be tested in the lower extremities. The patient, lying supine, raises the legs one at a time. When there is ataxia, the leg cannot be lifted steadily or in a straight line. There may be adduction, abduction, rotation, oscillations, or jerky movements from one position to another. When the limb is lowered, the patient may throw it down heavily, and it may not return to its original position beside its mate but may be deviated across it or away from it. When the seated patient extends the legs without support and attempts to hold them steady, a unilateral cerebellar lesion may cause oscillations and lateral deviation of the ipsilateral extremity. If the prone patient bends the knees and tries to maintain the shins vertically, there may be marked oscillations and lateral deviation of the leg on the side of the lesion.

Deviation and drift may also occur when the patient tries to walk with eyes closed. As in vestibulopathy, the patient drifts to the side of the lesion (see Chapter 17). Walking back and forth with eyes closed may reveal a "compass" or "star" gait due to deviation toward the involved side. When walking around a chair, the patient shows a tendency to fall toward the affected side.

CEREBELLAR SYNDROMES

Cerebellar disease may affect all or only a specific part of the cerebellum. There are two clearly defined cerebellar syndromes: a midline or vermis syndrome and a lateral or hemispheric syndrome. With the vermis, or midline, syndrome, the outstanding symptoms are abnormalities of station and gait, with abnormalities ranging from slight widening of the base on walking in mild disease (gait ataxia) to total inability to sit or walk in severe disease. Disease of the cerebellar hemispheres produces appendicular ataxia, disturbance in coordination of the ipsilateral extremities, the arm more than the leg. The primary clinical manifestations of dysfunction of the FN lobe or its connections are disturbances of equilibrium; nystagmus, often positional; and other abnormalities of extraocular movement. There is no limb ataxia. Table 43.1 summarizes the clinical manifestations of disease of these parts of the cerebellum.

TABLE 43.1 Clinical Manifestations of Disorders of the Cerebellum (Related to the Different Zones of the Cerebellum)

Zone of Cerebellum	Clinical Manifestation	Possible Disorder
Flocculonodular lobe (archicerebellum)	Nystagmus; extraocular movement abnormalities	Medulloblastoma
Vermis (paleocerebellum)	Gait ataxia	Alcoholic degeneration
Hemisphere (neocerebellum)	Appendicular ataxia	Tumor; stroke
Pancerebellar	All of the above	Paraneoplastic

The manifestations of cerebellar disease differ markedly in severity, depending upon the acuteness or chronicity of the process. The ability of the nervous system to compensate for a cerebellar lesion can be remarkable. If the lesion is acute, the symptoms are profound; if it is slowly progressive, they are much less severe. There may be considerable recovery from an acute lesion. If a lesion develops insidiously, there may be extensive involvement of the hemispheres without much in the way of clinical findings. The neural plasticity and compensation are such that some patients with little remaining cerebellar tissue can eventually function quite well. The symptoms of cerebellar disease are similar regardless of the etiology of the disease process, and whether the lesion is congenital or acquired.

Midline Syndrome

The vermis is important in the control of axial structures, or those that are bilaterally innervated; vermian lesions primarily affect midline functions, such as walking and coordination of the head and trunk. A patient with mild vermian disease has gait ataxia. The base is widened, tandem gait is particularly difficult, and there may be decompensation on turning. The Romberg test is negative—the imbalance does not worsen significantly with eyes closed. With severe dysfunction of the vermis, there may be gross postural and locomotor disturbances of the entire body. There is no lateralization, and the tendency to fall may be either backward or forward. The gait is wide based and characterized by swaying and staggering; the patient may reel in a drunken manner to either side. Cerebellar ataxia is discussed further in Chapter 44.

With truncal ataxia, there is swaying and unsteadiness when standing, and the patient may be unable to maintain an upright position. There may be loss of the ability to remain erect when seated or to hold the neck and head steady and upright; when severe, the standing and sitting balance disturbance leads to constant, to-and-fro swaying, nodding, and weaving movements of the head and trunk when the patient is upright known as titubation. The head movements in titubation are primarily anteroposterior (yes-yes) at 3 to 4 Hz. Vermis dysfunction causes little or no abnormality of the extremities, especially the upper extremities, although all coordinated movements may be poorly performed. Muscle tone and reflexes are normal. Nystagmus may be present but is usually not marked. Ocular dysmetria, rebound nystagmus, and pursuit abnormalities may also occur. Lesions involving the vermis may cause upbeat nystagmus. Dysarthria is often present. There is sometimes an abnormal rotated or tilted head posture.

Common causes of a midline cerebellar syndrome are alcoholic cerebellar degeneration and medulloblastoma. Alcohol preferentially poisons the vermis, leading to a characteristic syndrome of gait ataxia with sparing of the limbs. Such patients may have no demonstrable lower-extremity ataxia while lying supine, yet be totally unable to walk. Unwary examiners may conclude such findings represent hysteria. Medulloblastomas occur most often in the cerebellar vermis.

Hemispheric Syndrome

With a lesion involving one cerebellar hemisphere, the manifestations are appendicular rather than axial. Cerebellar hemispheric deficits are unilateral and ipsilateral to the lesion, as the pathways are uncrossed (or, more correctly, double crossed). There is a disturbance of skilled movements of the extremities, with ataxia, dysmetria, dyssynergy, dysdiadochokinesia, and hypotonicity affecting the arm and hand more than the leg and foot. Distal movements are affected more than proximal and fine movements more than gross ones. Movements are performed irregularly, and there may be intention tremor or other hyperkinesias if the dentate nucleus or its efferent pathways are involved.

Posture and gait are not impaired as severely as in the vermis syndrome, but abnormalities do occur. There may be swaying and falling toward the side of the lesion. The patient may be able to stand one legged using the contralateral but not the ipsilateral foot. He may be unable to bend his body toward the involved side without falling. The abnormalities often resemble those of a unilateral vestibular lesion. On walking, there may be unsteadiness, with deviation or rotation toward the involved side. There may be drift and past pointing toward the involved side. Dysarthria may occur, although disturbances of articulation are not as severe as in vermis lesions. Nystagmus is a common finding, usually horizontal but sometimes rotatory. It is usually more prominent when looking toward the side of the lesion. Common causes of a cerebellar hemispheric syndrome include cerebellar astrocytoma, multiple sclerosis, and lateral medullary stroke.

Diffuse Cerebellar Dysfunction

Some conditions affect the cerebellum diffusely, causing midline and bilateral hemispheric abnormalities. Patients may have nystagmus, gait and truncal ataxia, and appendicular incoordination. Etiologies include the hereditary spinocerebellar ataxia (SCA) syndromes, drugs (especially phenytoin), toxins, and paraneoplastic cerebellar degeneration.

Sensory Ataxia

Incoordination may also result from a lack of proprioceptive input from the limbs. Sensory ataxia results from peripheral nerve disease affecting primarily sensory fibers; pathology involving the dorsal root ganglia, dorsal roots, or posterior columns of the spinal cord; interruption of the proprioceptive pathways in the brainstem; or disease of the parietal lobe. Incoordination due to sensory ataxia can closely mimic that of cerebellar ataxia (Table 43.2). With cerebellar ataxia, it makes little difference whether the patient's eyes are open or closed. In sensory ataxia, performance is not normal with eyes open but worsens markedly with eyes closed. The different components of the abnormality may behave slightly differently when visual input is removed. Some of the tremor in sensory ataxia is due to visually guided voluntary corrections of deviations from the intended track. Because of loss of appreciation of limb position in space, with eyes closed, the patient may be unable to find his nose or the examiner's finger, but the tremor may actually abate because the patient cannot

TABLE 43.2 Associated Findings Helpful in Distinguishing Sensory from Cerebellar Ataxia

Sensory Ataxia	Cerebellar Ataxia
Sensory loss, especially for joint position and vibration	Nystagmus, ocular dysmetria, and other eye movement abnormalities
Steppage gait	Reeling, ataxic gait
Decreased reflexes	Other signs of cerebellar disease (dyssynergia, dysmetria, dysdiadochokinesia, hypotonia, rebound, impaired check response)

see that a deviation is occurring and does not attempt to correct it. He may be wildly off target but move in a straighter line. The distinction between cerebellar and sensory ataxia is also made by the associated findings (Table 43.2).

Other Abnormalities

There are many potential causes for a lack of coordination of movement. All of the levels of the motor system are involved in performing smooth and accurate movement. Weakness of any origin may interfere with skill and precision. Abnormalities of tone of any type may interfere with coordination. Diseases of the extrapyramidal system may impair motor control because of rigidity, akinesia or bradykinesia, lack of spontaneity, and loss of associated movements. A corticospinal tract lesion may cause jerkiness and clumsiness of movement, loss of motor control, and poor integration of skilled acts. Nonorganic illness may cause difficulty with coordination simulating true ataxia. Hyperkinetic movement disorders may cause irregularity in the timing and excursion of successive movements. Proprioceptive abnormalities may impair motor performance. To always attribute ataxia to cerebellar disease is an oversimplification because many conditions can cause incoordination and clumsiness. Often, the cause is multifactorial. A good general rule is to avoid drawing conclusions about the meaning of "cerebellar signs" in the face of any significant degree of weakness, spasticity, rigidity, or sensory loss. When the examination shows no other abnormalities, incoordination and awkwardness of movement are usually due to cerebellar disease.

Frontal lobe ataxia refers to disturbed coordination due to dysfunction of the contralateral frontal lobe; it may resemble the deficits due to abnormalities of the ipsilateral cerebellar hemisphere. Frontal lobe ataxia results from disease involving the frontopontocerebellar fibers en route to synapse in the pontine nuclei. Frontal lobe lesions may produce other abnormalities, such as hyperreflexia, increased tone, and pathologic reflexes, whereas purely cerebellar lesions typically cause hypotonia, diminished or pendular reflexes, and no pathologic reflex responses. Pressure on the brainstem by a cerebellar mass lesion may cause corticospinal tract findings that can confuse the picture. Bruns' ataxia refers to a gait disturbance seen primarily in frontal lobe lesions (see Chapter 44).

A variety of other functions have been attributed to the cerebellum, and there has been increasing awareness of its nonmotor functions. Roles for the cerebellum in learning, planning, emotion, and cognition have been proposed. It may play a role in sensory-motor integration, motor coordination, motor learning, and timing. A cerebellar cognitive affective syndrome has been described, characterized by disturbed executive function, visuospatial disorganization and impaired visuospatial memory, personality change, and linguistic difficulties such as dysprosodia, agrammatism, and mild anomia. The cerebellum has considerable influence in language processing. Children with cerebellar malformations have a high prevalence of nonmotor developmental and functional disabilities including cognitive, language, and social-behavioral deficits. The cerebellar mutism syndrome (posterior fossa syndrome) consists of diminished speech progressing to mutism, emotional lability, hypotonia, and ataxia. It is common following resection of a midline posterior fossa tumor in children, particularly medulloblastoma. Dysarthria may occur as a sequela. Nonmotor dysfunction of the cerebellum has been implicated in conditions as diverse as autism, dyslexia, and schizophrenia.

CEREBELLAR DISORDERS

Conditions causing a relatively acute ataxia include metabolic disorders, infections, toxins, neoplasms, infarction, hemorrhage, and demyelinating disease. An idiopathic condition, acute cerebellar ataxia or "cerebellitis," is most common in children. Autoimmunity may account for some cases of idiopathic sporadic cerebellar ataxia. The metabolic disorders include Wernicke's encephalopathy, biotinidase deficiency, and hyperammonemia. Conditions causing episodic or recurrent ataxia include channelopathies, such as the episodic ataxia syndromes, basilar artery migraine, recurrent toxin exposure (alcohol is the archetypal cerebellar toxin), and metabolic disorders such as Hartnup's disease, Leigh's syndrome, and organic acidurias.

Chronic ataxia may be relatively fixed or progressive. Static forms include alcoholic cerebellar degeneration and malformations, such as the Dandy-Walker and Chiari malformations. The Chiari I malformation is relatively common. It is often asymptomatic and discovered incidentally on neuroimaging. When symptomatic, typical other manifestations include headache and neck pain (worsened by cough or Valsalva maneuver), evidence of lower brainstem dysfunction (e.g., dysarthria, dysphagia, downbeat nystagmus),

TABLE 43.3 The Common Forms of Spinocerebellar Ataxia (SCA)

Name	Genetics	Phenotype
SCA1	6p22–p23; CAG repeats; ataxin-1	Ataxia; ophthalmoparesis; pyramidal and extrapyramidal findings
SCA2	12q23–q24.1; CAG; ataxin-2	Ataxia; slow saccades; minimal pyramidal and extrapyramidal findings
SCA3 (Machado-Joseph disease)	14q24.3–q32; CAG repeats; ataxin-3	Ataxia; ophthalmoparesis; variable pyramidal, extrapyramidal, and amyotrophic signs
SCA6	19p13.2; CAG repeats; CACNA1A protein, P/Q-type calcium channel subunit	Ataxia; dysarthria; nystagmus; mild proprioceptive sensory loss
SCA7	3p14.1–p21.1; CAG repeats; ataxin-7 binding protein	Ophthalmoparesis; visual loss; ataxia; dysarthria; extensor plantar response; pigmentary retinal degeneration
SCA8	13q21 with CTG repeats; noncoding; 3′ untranslated region of transcribed RNA	Gait ataxia; dysarthria; nystagmus; leg spasticity; reduced vibratory sensation

Modified from Rosenberg RN. Ataxic disorders. In: Longo D, Fauci AS, Kasper DL, et al., eds. *Harrison's Principles of Internal Medicine*. 18th ed. New York: McGraw-Hill, 2011.

myelopathy, and syringomyelia. Causes of chronic progressive ataxia include the hereditary SCAs and acquired disorders such as hypothyroidism, paraneoplastic cerebellar degeneration, and multiple sclerosis.

The inherited ataxias may be transmitted through autosomal dominant, autosomal recessive, or maternal (mitochondrial) modes of inheritance. A genomic classification has now largely superseded previous ones based on clinical expression alone. The clinical manifestations and neuropathologic findings of cerebellar disease dominate the clinical picture; there may also be characteristic changes in the basal ganglia, brainstem, spinal cord, optic nerves, retina, and peripheral nerves. The conditions clinically range from purely cerebellar syndromes to mixed cerebellar and brainstem disorders, cerebellar and basal ganglia syndromes, and spinal cord or peripheral nerve disease.

The most common form of hereditary ataxia is the autosomal recessive condition called FA. The most common molecular abnormality in FA is a trinucleotide repeat expansion in the gene encoding *frataxin*. The condition is characterized by progressive gait and limb ataxia with associated limb muscle weakness, absent lower limb reflexes, extensor plantar responses, dysarthria, decreased vibratory and proprioception sense, scoliosis, pes cavus, hammer toes, and cardiac abnormalities. Onset is usually in the first or second decade, before the end of puberty. The triad of hypoactive knee and ankle jerks, signs of progressive cerebellar dysfunction, and preadolescent onset is commonly regarded as sufficient for diagnosis. Uncommon features and atypical forms have been recognized. As many as one-quarter of the patients, even homozygotes, have atypical features, including older age at presentation and intact tendon reflexes. Smaller trinucleotide repeat expansions correlate with later onset and longer times to loss of ambulation.

The autosomal dominant SCAs include SCA types 1 through 47 (at this writing). The most common disorders are SCA 1, 2, 3 (Machado-Joseph disease), 6, 7, and 8 (Table 43.3). Many of the conditions are nucleotide repeat disorders; others are channelopathies. Most of the CAG repeat disorders result in proteins, termed *ataxins*, that produce a toxic gain of function. Although the phenotype is variable for any given disease gene, a pattern of neuronal loss with gliosis is produced that is relatively unique for each ataxia.

Video Links

Video Link 43.1. Cerebellar eye signs. https://collections.lib.utah.edu/details?id=188448

BIBLIOGRAPHY

Almeida J, Afonso JG. Cerebellum and schizophrenia: from concepts to clinical practice. *Eur Psychiatry* 2011;26:1340.

Amarenco P, Chevrie-Muller C, Roullet E, et al. Paravermal infarct and isolated cerebellar dysarthria. *Ann Neurol* 1991;30:211–213.

Andreasen NC, Pierson R. The role of the cerebellum in schizophrenia. *Biol Psychiatry* 2008;64:81–88.

Angel RW. The rebound phenomenon of Gordon Holmes. *Arch Neurol* 1977;34:250.

Baier B, Dieterich M. Ocular tilt reaction: a clinical sign of cerebellar infarctions? *Neurology* 2009;72:572–573.

Bertini E, des Portes V, Zanni G, et al. X-linked congenital ataxia: a clinical and genetic study. *Am J Med Genet* 2000;92:53–56.

Bolduc ME, Du Plessis AJ, Sullivan N, et al. Spectrum of neurodevelopmental disabilities in children with cerebellar malformations. *Dev Med Child Neurol* 2011;53:409–416.

Campbell WW. *Clinical Signs in Neurology: A Compendium*. Philadelphia: Wolters Kluwer Health, 2016.

Cruz-Marino T, Gonzalez-Zaldivar Y, Laffita-Mesa JM, et al. Uncommon features in Cuban families affected with Friedreich ataxia. *Neurosci Lett* 2010;472:85–89.

Daum I, Ackermann H. Cerebellar contributions to cognition. *Behav Brain Res* 1995;67:201–210.

Diehl B, Lee MS, Reid JR, et al. Atypical, perhaps under-recognized? An unusual phenotype of Friedreich ataxia. *Neurogenetics* 2010;11:261–265.

Diener HC, Dichgans J. Pathophysiology of cerebellar ataxia. *Mov Disord* 1992;7:95–109.

Durr A, Cossee M, Agid Y, et al. Clinical and genetic abnormalities in patients with Friedreich's ataxia. *N Engl J Med* 1996;335:1169–1175.

Fenichel GM, Phillips JA. Familial aplasia of the cerebellar vermis. Possible X-linked dominant inheritance. *Arch Neurol* 1989;46:582.

Fine EJ, Ionita CC, Lohr L. The history of the development of the cerebellar examination. *Semin Neurol* 2002;22:375–384.

Fogel BL, Perlman S. Clinical features and molecular genetics of autosomal recessive cerebellar ataxias. *Lancet Neurol* 2007;6: 245–257.

Fuller G. *Neurological Examination Made Easy*. 5th ed. New York: Churchill Livingstone, 2013.

Gilman S. *Clinical Examination of the Nervous System*. New York: McGraw-Hill, 2000.

Gilman S, Newman SW. *Manter and Gatz's Essentials of Clinical Neuroanatomy and Neurophysiology*. 10th ed. Philadelphia: FA Davis, 2003.

Goldstein BH, Birk CL, Van HM, et al. Ovarian cancer and late onset paraneoplastic cerebellar degeneration. *Arch Gynecol Obstet* 2009;280:99–101.

Gomez CM, Subramony SH. Dominantly inherited ataxias. *Semin Pediatr Neurol* 2003;10:210–222.

Gould DJ, Fix JD. *Neuroanatomy*. 5th ed. Philadelphia: Wolters Kluwer/Lippincott Williams & Wilkins, 2014.

Gudrunardottir T, Sehested A, Juhler M, et al. Cerebellar mutism: review of the literature. *Childs Nerv Syst* 2011;27:355–363.

Hallett M, Berardelli A, Matheson J, et al. Physiological analysis of simple rapid movements in patients with cerebellar deficits. *J Neurol Neurosurg Psychiatry* 1991;54:124–133.

Hallett M, Massaquoi SG. Physiologic studies of dysmetria in patients with cerebellar deficits. *Can J Neurol Sci* 1993;20(Suppl 3):S83–S92.

Hore J, Wild B, Diener HC. Cerebellar dysmetria at the elbow, wrist, and fingers. *J Neurophysiol* 1991;65:563–571.

Iannicelli M, Brancati F, Mougou-Zerelli S, et al. Novel TMEM67 mutations and genotype-phenotype correlates in meckelin-related ciliopathies. *Hum Mutat* 2010;31:E1319–E1331.

Inhoff AW, Diener HC, Rafal RD, et al. The role of cerebellar structures in the execution of serial movements. *Brain* 1989;112:565.

Ivry RB, Keele SW, Diener HC. Dissociation of the lateral and medial cerebellum in movement timing and movement execution. *Exp Brain Res* 1988;73:167.

Karmon Y, Inbar E, Cordoba M, et al. Paraneoplastic cerebellar degeneration mimicking acute post-infectious cerebellitis. *Cerebellum* 2009;8:441–444.

Kiernan JA, Rajakumar N. *Barr's The Human Nervous System: An Anatomical Viewpoint*. 10th ed. Philadelphia: Wolters Kluwer/ Lippincott Williams & Wilkins, 2014.

Klockgether T, Ludtke R, Kramer B, et al. The natural history of degenerative ataxia: a retrospective study in 466 patients. *Brain* 1998;121(Pt 4):589–600.

Landau WM. Ataxic hindbrain thinking: the clumsy cerebellum syndrome. *Neurology* 1989;39:315.

Lechtenberg R, Gilman S. Speech disorders in cerebellar disease. *Ann Neurol* 1978;3:285–290.

Lee H, Sohn SI, Cho YW, et al. Cerebellar infarction presenting isolated vertigo: frequency and vascular topographical patterns. *Neurology* 2006;67:1178–1183.

Leiner HC, Leiner AL, Dow RS. Reappraising the cerebellum: what does the hindbrain contribute to the forebrain? *Behav Neurosci* 1989;103:998–1008.

Manto M, Godaux E, Jacquy J, et al. Cerebellar hypermetria associated with a selective decrease in the rate of rise of antagonist activity. *Ann Neurol* 1996;39:271–274.

Manto MU, Setta F, Jacquy J, et al. Different types of cerebellar hypometria associated with a distinct topography of the lesion in cerebellum. *J Neurol Sci* 1998;158:88–95.

Massey EW, Pleet AB, Scherokman BJ. *Diagnostic Tests in Neurology: A Photographic Guide to Bedside Techniques*. Chicago: Year Book Medical Publishers, Inc., 1985.

Masur H, Elger CE, Ludolph AC, et al. Cerebellar atrophy following acute intoxication with phenytoin. *Neurology* 1989;39:432.

Miquel M, Toledo R, García LI, et al. Why should we keep the cerebellum in mind when thinking about addiction? *Curr Drug Abuse Rev* 2009;2:26–40.

Morrison PJ. Paediatric and adult autosomal dominant ataxias (update 6). *Eur J Paediatr Neurol* 2010;14:261–263.

Narabayashi H. Analysis of intention tremor. *Clin Neurol Neurosurg* 1992;94(Suppl):S130–S132.

Oberdick J, Sillitoe RV. Cerebellar zones. History, development, and function. *Cerebellum* 2011;10:301–306.

Pernet CR, Poline JB, Demonet JF, et al. Brain classification reveals the right cerebellum as the best biomarker of dyslexia. *BMC Neurosci* 2009;10:67.

Pestronk A. Hereditary ataxias. http://neuromuscular.wustl.edu/ataxia/aindex.html. Accessed May 28, 2018.

Piven J, Saliba K, Bailey J, et al. An MRI study of autism: the cerebellum revisited. *Neurology* 1997;49:546–551.

Pollack IF, Polinko P, Albright AL, et al. Mutism and pseudobulbar symptoms after resection of posterior fossa tumors in children: incidence and pathophysiology. *Neurosurgery* 1995;37: 885–893.

Pryse-Phillips W. *Companion to Clinical Neurology*. 3rd ed. Oxford: Oxford University Press, 2009.

Ropper AH, Samuels MA, Klein J. *Adams and Victor's Principles of Neurology*. 10th ed. New York: McGraw-Hill Education Medical, 2014.

Rosenberg RN. Ataxic disorders. In: Longo D, Fauci AS, Kasper DL, et al., eds. *Harrison's Principles of Internal Medicine*. 18th ed. New York: McGraw-Hill, 2011.

Ross RT. *How to Examine the Nervous System*. 4th ed. Totowa: Humana Press, 2006.

Sabater L, Bataller L, Suarez-Calvet M, et al. ZIC antibodies in paraneoplastic cerebellar degeneration and small cell lung cancer. *J Neuroimmunol* 2008;201–202:163–165.

Sacchetti B, Scelfo B, Strata P. Cerebellum and emotional behavior. *Neuroscience* 2009;162:756–762.

Schmahmann JD, MacMore J, Vangel M. Cerebellar stroke without motor deficit: clinical evidence for motor and non-motor domains within the human cerebellum. *Neuroscience* 2009;162:852–861.

Schmahmann JD, Sherman JC. The cerebellar cognitive affective syndrome. *Brain* 1998;121(Pt 4):561–579.

Schols L, Bauer P, Schmidt T, et al. Autosomal dominant cerebellar ataxias: clinical features, genetics, and pathogenesis. *Lancet Neurol* 2004;3:291–304.

Serrao M, Pierelli F, Ranavolo A, et al. Gait pattern in inherited cerebellar ataxias. *Cerebellum* 2011;11:194–211.

Spencer RM, Zelaznik HN, Diedrichsen J, et al. Disrupted timing of discontinuous but not continuous movements by cerebellar lesions. *Science* 2003;300:1437–1439.

Subramony SH. Approach to ataxic diseases. *Handb Clin Neurol* 2011;103:127–134.

Subramony SH. Overview of autosomal dominant ataxias. *Handb Clin Neurol* 2011;103:389–398.

Timmann D, Drepper J, Frings M, et al. The human cerebellum contributes to motor, emotional and cognitive associative learning. A review. *Cortex* 2010;46:845–857.

Turgut M. Cerebellar mutism. *J Neurosurg Pediatr* 2008;1:262.

Wartenberg R. *Diagnostic Tests in Neurology, A Selection for Office Use*. Chicago: Year Book Medical Publishers, 1953.

Weibers DO, Dale AJD, Kokmen E, et al., eds. *Mayo Clinic Examinations in Neurology*. 7th ed. St. Louis: Mosby, 1998.

Wild B, Klockgether T, Dichgans J. Acceleration deficit in patients with cerebellar lesions. A study of kinematic and EMG-parameters in fast wrist movements. *Brain Res* 1996;713:186–191.

Wu JP, Jedynak CP, Pidoux B, et al. Quantitative study of Stewart-Holmes test. *Electromyogr Clin Neurophysiol* 1998;38:237–245.

Zanni G, Barresi S, Travaglini L, et al. FGF17, a gene involved in cerebellar development, is downregulated in a patient with Dandy-Walker malformation carrying a de novo 8p deletion. *Neurogenetics* 2011;12:241–245.

Zanni G, Bertini ES. X-linked disorders with cerebellar dysgenesis. *Orphanet J Rare Dis* 2011;6:24.

Zanni G, Bertini E, Bellcross C, et al. X-linked congenital ataxia: a new locus maps to Xq25–q27.1. *Am J Med Genet A* 2008;146:593–600.

Zanni G, Saillour Y, Nagara M, et al. Oligophrenin 1 mutations frequently cause X-linked mental retardation with cerebellar hypoplasia. *Neurology* 2005;65:1364–1369.

Zhang N, Ottersen OP. In search of the identity of the cerebellar climbing fiber transmitter: immunocytochemical studies in rats. *Can J Neurol Sci* 1993;20(Suppl 3):S36–S42.

CHAPTER 44

Gait and Station

It is likely possible to learn more about neurologic status from watching a patient walk than from any other single procedure, and observation of gait should always be part of a neurologic examination. Abnormalities of gait are a common clinical problem with numerous causes, both neurologic and nonneurologic. A careful general evaluation is always necessary to exclude a nonneurologic cause.

Station is the way a patient stands and gait the way she walks. Standing and walking are active processes that depend upon a number of factors and reflex responses. The mechanisms are complex, especially in the human, whose biped gait and erect position over a narrow base require more efficient maintenance and control of equilibrium than is necessary in quadrupeds. Normal resting tone, especially in the antigravity muscles, is essential. The postural and righting reflexes described in Chapter 41 are particularly important. Standing may be considered a postural reflex that is dependent on reflexes mediated through the brainstem and influenced to a major degree by tonic neck and labyrinthine reflexes. If the mechanisms mediating static and postural reflexes are impaired, normal standing and walking will be impaired. In addition, proprioceptive sensation must be received, the skeletal system must be intact, the muscles must be functioning normally, and coordination must be adequate. Gait and station may be affected by abnormalities of proprioception, abnormalities of muscle power or tone, and abnormalities of vestibular function and by dysfunction of the basal ganglia, the cerebellum, or their connections.

Neurologic causes of an abnormal gait include conditions as varied as footdrop due to peroneal nerve palsy, myopathy, hydrocephalus, and cerebellar degeneration. The various gait abnormalities have different findings on physical examination in regard to the gait itself, such as a steppage pattern as opposed to a pelvic waddle. The differential diagnosis of the gait abnormality is also very dependent on the history and the other clinical signs present. Some of the more common abnormal gait patterns are summarized in Table 44.1.

EXAMINATION OF STATION

Station is the patient's attitude, posture, or manner of standing. The healthy individual stands erect with her head up, chest out, and abdomen in. Abnormality of station may be an important indicator of neurologic disease. Station is tested by having the patient stand, feet closely together, noting any unsteadiness or swaying. More rigorous testing includes having the patient stand eyes open and eyes closed, on one foot at a time, on toes and heels, and tandem with one heel in front of the toes of the other foot. She may be given a gentle push to see whether she falls to one side, forward, or backward.

Patients with unsteadiness standing often attempt to compensate by placing the feet wide apart in order to stand on a broader and steadier base. In cerebellar disease, the patient usually stands on a broad base and there is swaying, to more or less an equal degree, with eyes open and closed. With a lesion of the vermis, the patient may sway backward, forward, or to either side. With a lesion of one hemisphere, she sways or falls toward the affected side. Unilateral vestibular disease also causes falling toward the affected side. In a unilateral, cerebellar hemispheric lesion, or in a unilateral vestibulopathy, the patient may tilt the head toward the involved side with the chin rotated toward the sound side, with the shoulder on the involved side somewhat higher than the other and slightly in front of it. If the patient with a cerebellar hemispheric lesion is given

TABLE 44.1 Some of the More Common Neurologic Abnormalities of Gait

Gait Disorder	Gait Characteristics	Usual Associated Findings
Spastic	Stiff legged, scissoring (wooden soldier)	Hyperreflexia, extensor plantar responses
Cerebellar ataxia	Wide based, reeling, careening (drunken sailor)	Heel-to-shin ataxia, other cerebellar signs
Sensory ataxia	Wide based, steppage	Positive Romberg, impaired joint position sense
Hemiparetic	Involved leg spastic, circumduction, often with footdrop	Weakness, hyperreflexia, extensor plantar response
Parkinsonian	Small steps, flexed posture, shuffling, festination	Tremor, rigidity, bradykinesia
Marche à petits pas	Small steps, slow shuffling	Dementia, frontal lobe signs
Footdrop (unilateral or bilateral)	High steppage pattern to clear the toes from the floor, double tap with toe strike before heel strike	Foot dorsiflexion weakness
Myopathic	Exaggerated "sexy" hip motion, waddling, lumbar hyperlordosis	Hip girdle weakness

a light push—first toward one side and then toward the other—she will lose balance more easily when pushed toward the involved side. If asked to stand on one foot at a time, the patient with a cerebellar hemispheric lesion may be unable to maintain equilibrium standing on the ipsilateral foot but may stand without difficulty on the contralateral foot.

Other abnormalities may be apparent during station testing, particularly movement disorders. Patients with chorea seem unusually fidgety and often have small adventitial finger movements **(Video 30.4)**. Skeletal changes (such as kyphosis, scoliosis, or lordosis); abnormalities in the position of the head, shoulders, hips, or extremities; asymmetries; anomalies of development; and abnormalities of contour may be apparent. Patients who are weak or debilitated may need support to stand erect. If the patient is unable to stand alone, or unable to stand at all, document how much support and assistance is required (e.g., stands with a walker, chair bound). If the patient is chair bound or bed bound, describe the sitting or recumbent posture. The patient with a hemiparesis may stand with the upper extremity flexed and pronated and the lower extremity extended. Patients with Parkinson's disease stand in a flexed posture, stooped over with head and shoulders bent forward and arms and knees flexed. Pelvic girdle weakness may cause pronounced lordosis, especially in muscular dystrophy (Figure 4.5). Depressed patients may appear stooped and dejected; in manic states, an erect, domineering, aggressive posture may be present. In schizophrenia, the patient may assume bizarre postures and hold them for long periods of time. Hyperkinesias, such as athetoid and choreic movements, may become evident during the evaluation of station.

The Romberg Sign

When proprioception is disturbed, the patient may be able to stand with eyes open but sways or falls with eyes closed (Romberg sign). The Romberg sign is often misunderstood and misinterpreted. The essential finding is a difference between standing balance with eyes open and closed. In order to test this function, the patient must have a stable stance eyes open and then demonstrate a decrease in balance with eyes closed when visual input is eliminated, and the patient must rely on proprioception to maintain balance (see **Video Link 44.1**). Romberg described this sign in patients with tabes dorsalis and thought it was pathognomonic. He said, "If he is ordered to close his eyes while in the erect posture, he at once commences to totter or swing from side to side; the insecurity of his gait also exhibits itself more in the dark." Romberg did not state that the feet should be placed together; that was a later addition. Nor did he comment on where the arms were to be positioned. It is common practice to have the patient hold the arms outstretched in front, but this is in order to check simultaneously for pronator drift or to perform finger-to-nose testing; it is not what Romberg described. Some authorities recommend the arms be held at the sides, others that the arms be crossed on the chest. Whether arm position makes any difference in test sensitivity is unknown. Turning the head side to side eliminates vestibular clues and increases the reliance on proprioception (Ropper's refined Romberg test).

The Romberg test can be difficult to interpret. There is some variability, even among expert examiners, in how the Romberg test is performed and interpreted. Many patients sway slightly with eyes closed, and minimal amounts of sway, especially in elderly patients, are seldom significant. Minor, normal swaying may stop if the patient is simply asked to stand perfectly still. Most clinicians discount sway at the hips and insist on seeing sway at the ankles before calling the test positive, some require the patient take a corrective step to the side, and others that the patient nearly fall. Some require the patient be barefoot. The "sharpened" or tandem Romberg is done by having the patient stand in tandem position with eyes open and closed; the limits of normality for this variation are conjectural.

The Romberg sign is used primarily as a test of proprioceptive, not cerebellar, function. The pioneering 19th-century clinicians thought it was particularly useful in separating tabes dorsalis from cerebellar disease. In fact, patients with cerebellar disease, particularly disorders of the vestibulocerebellum or spinocerebellum, may have some increase in instability with eyes closed, but not usually to the degree seen with impaired proprioception. A patient with an acute unilateral vestibulopathy may fall toward the side of the lesion when standing with eyes closed. Patients with cerebellar disease, or those with severe weakness, may not have a stable base eyes open. It may help to have the patients widen stance to the point where they are stable eyes open, then close the eyes, and check for any difference. Only a marked worsening of balance with eyes closed qualifies as a positive Romberg sign. A patient who cannot maintain balance feet together and eyes open does not have a positive Romberg.

Some patients will sway with eyes closed in the absence of any organic neurologic impairment (false Romberg sign) indicating a psychogenic gait disorder. The swaying is usually from the hips and may be exaggerated. If the patient takes a step, the eyes may remain closed, which never happens with a bona fide Romberg. The instability can often be eliminated by diverting the patient's attention. Effective distracters are to ask the patient to detect numbers the examiner writes with her finger on the forehead, to wiggle the tongue, or to perform the finger-to-nose testing. Having the shoes off and watching the toe movements may be very informative. The toes of the patient with histrionic sway are often extended; the patient with organic imbalance flexes the toes strongly and tries to grip the floor.

PHYSIOLOGY OF GAIT

The brainstem and spinal cord in lower forms contain "central pattern generators," which are groups of interneurons that coordinate the activity in pools of motor neurons to produce patterned movements. Although the existence of such cell groups in humans is unproven, locomotion likely depends on activity in pattern generators. The pattern generators control the activity in lower motor neurons that execute the mechanics of walking. Higher centers in the subthalamus and midbrain, particularly the pedunculopontine nucleus, modulate the activity in the spinal cord pattern generators through the reticulospinal tracts.

The gait cycle refers to the events that transpire between the time that one heel strikes the ground and the time the same heel strikes the ground again (see **Video Link 44.2**). The gait cycle begins when the forward foot hits the ground (heel strike or initial contact). During the stance phase, the stance leg supports all or most of the weight. At the end of the stance phase, there is a push off (toe-off or preswing phase) after which the leg swings forward to contact the ground again. The stance period is divided into four phases: initial contact, loading, midstance, and terminal stance. The swing phase is also divided into four parts: preswing, initial swing, midswing, and terminal swing. The functional task during the stance phase is to bear weight; the functional task during swing phase is to advance the limb. Periods of single limb support (one foot on the ground) alternate with periods of double limb support (two feet on the ground).

Various parameters are used to measure and characterize gait, including gait velocity, stride time, step time, stride length, step width, and step length. Stride length is the distance covered by a gait cycle; step length is the distance covered by the swing phase of one leg. When walking, at least one foot is in contact with the ground at all times, and there are two periods of double limb support. When there is no longer a moment in time when both limbs are in contact with the ground, walking has become running. A typical adult walking comfortably on a level surface walks at a velocity of about 80 m/min, taking about 113 steps per minute, with a stride length of 1.41 m. About 60% of the gait cycle is spent in stance, 40% in swing, and 10% in double limb support. Periods of double limb increase quickly to compensate for instability.

The body's center of mass is located just anterior to the S2 vertebral body. An efficient gait minimizes the displacement of the center of mass by rotating and tilting the pelvis and flexing and extending the various joints involved. Gait disturbances that increase the normal displacement of the center of mass are less efficient and require an increased expenditure of energy. Patients typically compensate by walking more slowly and employing compensatory maneuvers to regain lost efficiency. In addition to the increased energy requirement, abnormal gaits increase the risk of falling and the susceptibility to biomechanical injury.

EXAMINATION OF GAIT

The first step in analyzing gait is to check the width of the base, or the step width. The wider the base, the better the balance, and spreading the feet farther apart is the first compensatory effort in most gait disorders. Under normal circumstances, the medial malleoli pass within about 2 in of each other during the stride phase, a narrow and well-compensated gait. Any spread more than this may signal some problem with gait or balance.

The forefoot on each side should clear the ground to about the same degree; asymmetry of toe lift may be the earliest evidence of footdrop. A shortened stride length may be early evidence of bifrontal or extrapyramidal disease. Excessive movement of the hips may occur with any process causing proximal muscle weakness. Note the reciprocal arm swing; a decreased swing on one side is sometimes an early indicator of hemiparesis or hemiparkinsonism. Watch the hands for tremor or chorea.

Tandem walking stresses the gait and balance mechanisms even further. Elderly patients may have difficulty with tandem gait because of obesity or deconditioning. In relatively young patients with a low likelihood of neurologic disease, a quick and effective substitute for the Romberg is simply to have the patient close her eyes while walking tandem. This is a difficult maneuver and has high value as a screening test. Having the patient walk briskly and then stop abruptly on command, or make quick turns, first in one direction and then in the other, may bring out ataxia and incoordination not noticeable on straightaway walking. Rather than turning easily, the patient may have to turn in small, staccato steps. The patient may be asked to walk sideways, backward, and overstep, or cross one foot over the other. Having the patient walk on heels and toes may bring out weakness of dorsiflexion or plantar flexion. An excellent screening test is to have the patient hop on either foot. This simultaneously assesses lower-extremity strength, especially of the gastrosoleus, plus balance functions. Individuals who can hop adroitly on either foot are unlikely to have significant neurologic disease. Note if the patient is able to maintain balance with a sudden push or pull backward, forward, or to the side. This can be done by gently tapping the upper chest or pulling on the shoulders while standing behind the patient, reassuring the patient, "I will catch you if you begin to fall." Note whether the patient has any obvious orthopedic limitations, such as a varus deformity of the knee, genu recurvatum, pelvic tilt, or any other abnormalities. Also note whether there is any difficulty rising from a chair or initiating gait. Note posture, arm swing, extraneous movements, step height, and any side to side lurching.

ABNORMAL GAITS

A nosology has been suggested that classifies abnormal gait syndromes into low-, mid-, and high-level disorders. Low-level disorders are due to peripheral motor or sensory abnormalities; mid-level disorders include hemiplegic, paraplegic, cerebellar ataxic, parkinsonian, choreic, and dystonic disorders. Highest-level disorders include cautious gait, subcortical and frontal disequilibrium, isolated gait ignition failure, frontal gait disorder, and psychogenic gait disorder (PGD). Description of the clinical semiology of gait disorders continues to be the most common approach.

Cerebellar Ataxia

The gait of cerebellar disease is caused by involvement of the coordinating mechanisms in the cerebellum and its connecting systems **(Video 44.1)**. The only sign of mild ataxia may be the inability to walk tandem. Sudden stopping or turning may bring out a stagger. With more severe disease, there is a clumsy, staggering, unsteady, irregular, lurching, titubating, and wide-based gait, and the patient may sway to either side, back, or forward. Leg movements are erratic, and step length varies unpredictably. The patient may compensate by avoiding periods of single limb support, creating a shuffling gait. The patient is unable to walk tandem or follow a straight line on the floor. There may be tremors and oscillatory movements involving the entire body.

Ataxia of the lower extremities when tested separately usually accompanies cerebellar gait ataxia, except when disease is limited to the vermis (see below). With a lesion of the cerebellar vermis, the patient will exhibit a lurching, staggering gait, but without laterality, the ataxia will be as marked toward one side as the other. Cerebellar ataxia is present with eyes both open and closed; it may increase slightly with eyes closed, but not so markedly as in sensory ataxia. A gait resembling cerebellar ataxia is seen in acute alcohol intoxication. With a cerebellar hemispheric lesion, the patient will stagger and deviate toward the involved side. In disease localized to one cerebellar hemisphere or in unilateral vestibular disease, there is persistent swaying or deviation toward the abnormal side. As the patient attempts to walk a straight line or to walk tandem, she deviates toward the side of the lesion. Walking a few steps backward and forward with eyes closed may bring out "compass deviation" or a "star-shaped gait" (see Chapter 17). When attempting to walk a fixed circle around a chair, clockwise then counterclockwise, the patient will tend to fall toward the chair if it is on the side of the lesion, or to spiral out away from the chair if on the opposite side.

Either unilateral cerebellar or vestibular disease may cause turning toward the side of the lesion on the Unterberger-Fukuda stepping test (Chapter 17). For all the tests that bring out deviation in one direction, other findings must be used to differentiate between vestibulopathy and a cerebellar hemispheric lesion. Unilateral ataxia may be demonstrated by having the patient attempt to jump on one foot, with the eyes either open or closed. The patient with bilateral vestibular disease may seek to minimize head movement during walking, holding the head stiff and rigid; having the patient turn the head back and forth during walking may bring out ataxia. Cerebellar gait ataxia is common in multiple sclerosis (MS), alcoholic cerebellar degeneration, cerebellar tumors, stroke, and cerebellar degenerations. With alcoholic cerebellar degeneration, pathology is restricted to the vermis. Nystagmus, dysarthria, and appendicular ataxia, even of the legs, are typically absent.

Sensory Ataxia

Sensory ataxia occurs when the nervous system is deprived of the sensory information, primarily proprioceptive, necessary to coordinate walking **(Video 44.1)**. Deafferentation may result from disease of the posterior columns (e.g., tabes dorsalis or subacute combined degeneration) or disease affecting the peripheral nerves (e.g., sensory peripheral neuropathy). The term "spinal ataxia" is sometimes used, but the pathology is not always in the spinal cord. The patient loses awareness of the position of the lower extremities in space, or even of the body as a whole, except as provided by the visual system. The patient is extremely dependent on visual input for coordination. When deprived of visual input, as with eyes closed or in the dark, the gait deteriorates markedly. The difference in walking ability with and without visual input is the key feature of sensory ataxia. If the condition is mild, locomotion may appear normal when the patient walks eyes open; more commonly, it is wide based and poorly coordinated.

The term "steppage gait" refers to a manner of walking in which the patient takes unusually high steps. Sensory ataxia is one of the causes of a steppage gait. The patient takes a high step, throws out her foot, and slams it down on the floor in order to increase the proprioceptive feedback. The heel may land before the toe, creating an audible "double tap." An additional sound effect may be the tapping of a cane, creating a "slam, slam, tap" cadence. The sound effects may be so characteristic that the trained observer can make the diagnosis by listening to the footfalls. The patient with sensory ataxia watches her feet and keeps her eyes on the floor while walking. With eyes closed, the feet seem to shoot out, the staggering and unsteadiness are increased, and the patient may be unable to walk. There is less reeling and lurching in sensory ataxia than with a comparable degree of cerebellar ataxia. The difficulty is even worse walking backward, because the patient cannot see where she is going. The patient with bilateral footdrops, however, also has a steppage gait and a double tapping sound (see "Steppage Gait" below). For a striking illustration of a tabetic gait in sequential photographs by Eadweard Muybridge in 1887, see Lanska and Goetz.

In all of these tests, sensory ataxia can be differentiated from predominantly cerebellar ataxia by accentuation of the difficulty with eyes closed; and unilateral cerebellar or vestibular disease from vermis involvement by laterality of unsteadiness. Ropper and Samuels point out the similarity of the wide based, stamping gait of sensory ataxia to film depictions of Frankenstein.

The Gait of Spastic Hemiparesis

The gait of spastic hemiparesis may be caused by a lesion interrupting the corticospinal pathways to one-half of the body, most commonly stroke. The patient stands with a hemiparetic posture, arm flexed, adducted, and internally rotated, and leg extended. There is plantar flexion of the foot and toes, either due to foot dorsiflexion weakness or to heel cord shortening, rendering the lower extremity on the involved side functionally slightly longer than on the normal side, referred to as an equinus deformity. (A horse's foot is digitigrade; horses stand on the tips of their toes. The human foot is normally plantigrade, with the whole plantar surface in contact with the ground. The human foot with a footdrop or shortened heel cord resembles a horse's, hence the term.) When walking, the patient holds the arm tightly to the side, rigid and flexed, extends it with difficulty, and does not swing it in a normal fashion **(Video 44.1)**. The leg is held stiffly in extension and the patient drags or shuffles the foot and scrapes the toes. With each step, the pelvis tilts upward on the involved side to aid in lifting the foot off the floor (hip hike), and during swing phase, the entire extremity sweeps around in a semicircle from the hip (circumduction). The stance phase is shortened because of weakness, and the swing phase shortened because of spasticity and slowing of movement. The sound produced by the scraping of the toes, as well as the wear of the shoe at the toe, may be quite characteristic. The patient is able to turn toward the paralyzed side more easily than toward the normal side. Loss of normal arm swing and slight circumduction of the leg may be the only gait abnormalities in very mild hemiparesis.

Spastic Gait, Scissoring

This gait pattern occurs in patients who have severe spasticity of the legs. It occurs in patients who have congenital spastic diplegia (Little's disease, cerebral palsy) and related conditions and in chronic myelopathies due to conditions such as MS and cervical spondylosis. It is essentially a bilateral hemiplegic gait affecting the legs. There is characteristic tightness of the hip adductors causing adduction of the thighs, so that the knees may cross, one in front of the other, with each step (scissors gait). The patient walks on an abnormally narrow base, with a stiff shuffling gait, dragging both legs and scraping the toes **(Video 44.1)**. The steps are short and slow; the feet seem to stick to the floor. There may be a marked compensatory sway of the trunk away from the side of the advancing leg. Swaying and staggering may suggest an element of ataxia, but usually there is no true loss of coordination. The shuffling, scraping sound—together with worn areas at the toes of the shoes—are characteristic. The equinus position of the feet and heel cord shortening often cause the patient to walk on tiptoe.

The Spastic-Ataxic Gait

Some neurologic disorders cause involvement of both the corticospinal and the proprioceptive pathways (e.g., combined system disease due to vitamin B_{12} deficiency, or MS), resulting in a gait that has features of both spasticity and ataxia. The relative proportion of each abnormality depends on the particulars of the case. The ataxic component may be either cerebellar or sensory. In vitamin B_{12} deficiency, it is predominantly sensory; in MS, both components may be present.

The Parkinsonian Gait

The gait in most akinetic-rigid, parkinsonian syndromes is characterized by rigidity, bradykinesia, and loss of associated movements. The patient is stooped, with head and neck forward and knees flexed; the upper extremities are flexed at the shoulders, elbows, and wrists, but the fingers are usually extended (Figure 30.1). The gait is slow, stiff, and shuffling; the patient walks with small, mincing steps. Other features include involuntary acceleration (festination), decreased arm swing, en bloc turning, start hesitation, and freezing when encountering obstacles such as doorways **(Video 30.2)**.

The patient loses balance easily with a gentle shove or pull. Difficulty walking may be one of the earliest symptoms of the disease. The gait of Parkinson's disease is further described in Chapter 30. The same gait disorder can occur with any condition causing parkinsonism, such as drug side effects. Gait difficulty and a tendency to fall is particularly prominent in progressive supranuclear palsy (PSP).

Frontal Lobe Gait Disorders

A number of gait disorders have been ascribed to dysfunction of the frontal lobes. Lesions of the frontal lobe, or of the frontal lobe connections with the basal ganglia and cerebellum, may lead to a gait disorder characterized by a slightly flexed posture, short, shuffling steps, a widened base, and an inability to integrate and coordinate lower-extremity movements to accomplish normal ambulation. There is particular difficulty with starts and turns. Some of these are poorly understood and the relationship between them unclear. In some, the frontal lobe "dysfunction" has been attributed to normal aging. Many terms have been used, which refer to more or less the same phenomenon, including gait apraxia, frontal disequilibrium or ataxia, Bruns' apraxia/ataxia, magnetic gait, and lower half/body or vascular (arteriosclerotic) parkinsonism. Some of the gait disorders often included under this rubric include gait apraxia, the gait of normal pressure hydrocephalus (NPH), marche à petits pas, and the cautious (senile) gait.

Marche à Petits Pas

The marche à petits pas (walk of little steps) gait resembles that of parkinsonism but lacks the rigidity and bradykinesia. Locomotion is slow, and the patient walks with very short, mincing, shuffling, and somewhat irregular footsteps. The length of the step may be less than the length of the foot. There is often a loss of associated movements. This type of gait may be seen in normal elderly persons but also occurs in patients who have diffuse cerebral hemispheric dysfunction, particularly involving the frontal lobes. It may also occur as part of the syndrome of NPH and in other types of hydrocephalus. The same gait disturbance is typical of multi-infarct dementia or lacunar state. In some patients with marche à petits pas, there are bizarre movements such as dancing or hopping. There may be generalized weakness of the lower extremities or of the entire body, with the patient fatiguing easily.

Gait Apraxia

Apraxia of gait is the loss of the ability to use the legs properly in walking, without demonstrable sensory impairment, weakness, incoordination, or other apparent explanation. The term has been criticized as not being loss of a learned skill. Gait apraxia is seen in patients with extensive cerebral lesions, especially of the frontal lobes. It is a common feature of NPH and may occur in frontal lobe neoplasms, Binswanger's disease, frontotemporal dementia, and other conditions that cause diffuse frontal lobe dysfunction. The patient cannot carry out purposeful movements with the legs and feet, such as making a circle or kicking an imaginary ball. In rising, standing, and walking, there is difficulty in initiating movement, and the automatic sequence of component movements is lost. The gait is slow and shuffling, with short steps. The patients may have the greatest difficulty initiating walking, making small, feeble, stepping movements with minimal forward progress. Eventually, the patient may be essentially unable to lift the feet from the floor, as if they were stuck or glued down, or may raise them in place without advancing them (magnetic gait, gait ignition failure, start hesitation). After a few hesitant shuffles, the stride length may increase (slipping clutch gait). When trying to turn, the patient may freeze (turn hesitation). The patient may be able to imitate normal walking movements when sitting or lying down, but eventually, even this ability is often lost. In addition, perseveration, hypokinesia, rigidity, and stiffness of the limb in response to contact (gegenhalten) are often seen. In the syndrome of isolated gait ignition failure, or freezing of gait, patients have difficulty starting to walk, but with continued stepping, the gait improves. They may again freeze when turning or encountering an obstacle.

Gait of Normal Pressure Hydrocephalus

Gait difficulty is typically the initial and most prominent symptom of NPH. The primary changes are slow walking, widened base, short steps, and shuffling, all nonspecific features and natural compensations seen in patients with various gait disorders. It may range from mild, with only a cautious gait or difficulty with tandem walking, to severe, when unaided gait is impossible **(Video 44.1)**. It has been referred to as a gait apraxia. Features in common with other frontal lobe gait disorders include reduced velocity, stride length, and step height. NPH causes more widening of the base and outwardly rotated feet and is less responsive to external cues such as marching to a cadence or in step with the examiner. As with other disorders of frontal lobe function, patients may mimic stepping motions while supine or sitting.

Cautious (Senile) Gait

A cautious gait is seen in older patients who have no neurologic disease but are uncertain of their balance and postural reflexes. The gait takes on the characteristics seen when a healthy person walks on an icy surface: velocity slows, steps shorten, double support time increases, and the base widens. The foot-floor clearance is not decreased, and the patient does not shuffle. There is no difficulty with gait initiation, nor is there freezing.

There is an ostensible "multimodal" gait disorder in the elderly, attributed to aging of the vestibular system, impaired proprioceptive function caused by distal neuropathy in the elderly, and impaired vision. Baloh et al. found that age-related decreases in vestibular, visual, auditory, and somatosensation occurred in normal older people but were only weakly correlated with changes in gait and balance. White matter hyperintensities on magnetic resonance imaging were more highly correlated with changes in gait.

Steppage Gait

A problem arises with the use of the term "steppage," which means that the patient is lifting one or both legs high during her respective swing phases, as though she were walking up steps though the surface is level. Patients with footdrop may do this in order to help the foot clear the floor and avoid tripping. Patients with sensory ataxia, classically tabes dorsalis, may also lift the feet up high and then slap them down smartly to improve proprioceptive feedback. Because both of these gaits are "high stepping," both have been referred to as steppage gaits, but the causes and mechanisms are quite different.

A patient with footdrop has weakness of the dorsiflexors of the foot and toes. When mild, this may be manifest only as a decrease in toe clearance during the swing phase. With more severe footdrop, the patient is in danger of tripping, and may drag the toe when she walks, characteristically wearing out the toe of her shoe. When footdrop is severe, the foot dangles uncontrollably during the swing phase. To compensate, she lifts the foot as high as possible, hiking the hip and flexing the hip and knee **(Video 44.1)**. The foot is thrown out and falls to the floor, toe first. The touching of the toe, followed by the heel creates a "double tap" that has a different sound than the heel first double tap of sensory ataxia. The patient is unable to stand on her heel, and when standing with her foot projecting over the edge of a step, the forefoot drops. The footdrops and steppage gait may be unilateral or bilateral. Common causes of unilateral footdrop and steppage gait include peroneal nerve palsy and L5 radiculopathy. Causes of bilateral footdrop and steppage gait include amyotrophic lateral sclerosis, Charcot-Marie-Tooth disease and other severe peripheral neuropathies, and certain forms of muscular dystrophy. In severe polyneuropathies, the steppage gait may have components of both sensory ataxia and footdrop.

The Myopathic (Waddling) Gait

Myopathic gaits occur when there is weakness of the hip girdle muscles, most often due to myopathy and most characteristically due to muscular dystrophy. If the hip flexors are weak, there may be a pronounced lordosis (Chapter 27). The hip abductor muscles are vital in stabilizing the pelvis, while walking. Trendelenburg's sign is an abnormal drop of the pelvis on the side of the swing leg because of hip abductor weakness (Chapter 27). When the weakness is bilateral, there is an exaggerated pelvic swing that results in a waddling gait. The patient walks with a broad base, with an exaggerated rotation of the pelvis, rolling or throwing the hips from side to side with every step to shift the weight of the body. In the extreme forms, this gait pattern has a bizarre appearance. The patient walks with a pronounced waddle, shoulders thrown back and pelvis thrust forward (see **Video Link 44.3**). This form of gait is particularly common in facioscapulohumeral muscular dystrophy. The myopathy patient has marked difficulty climbing stairs, often needing to pull herself up with the hand rail. Patients also have difficulty going from a lying to standing position without placing the hands on the knees and hips to push themselves up (Gower's sign, Figure 29.4). For a vintage motion picture showing a myopathic gait with calf pseudohypertrophy, toe walking, and Gower's sign in a boy with Duchenne's dystrophy, see **Video Link 44.4**).

Hyperkinetic Gait

In conditions such as Sydenham's chorea, Huntington's disease, other forms of transient or persistent chorea, athetosis, and dystonia, the abnormal movements may become more marked while the patient is walking, and the manifestations of the disease more evident. Walking may accentuate not only the hyperkinesias but also the abnormalities of power and tone that accompany them. In Huntington's disease, the gait may be grotesque, dancing or prancing with abundant extraneous movement. It may look psychogenic but is all too real **(Video Link 44.5)**. The distal movements in athetosis and the proximal movements in dystonia may be marked during walking, and in both, there are accompanying grimaces. Some movement disorders may present as a gait disturbance. Oppenheim termed the walking pattern in dystonia musculorum deformans "dromedary" because of the exaggerated lumbar lordosis and hip flexion.

Gaits Associated with Focal Weakness

In addition to the steppage gait that accompanies footdrop, weakness limited to other muscle groups may cause gait difficulties. With paralysis of the gastrocnemius and soleus muscles, the patient is unable to stand on the toes, and unable to push off to enter the swing phase with the affected leg. This may cause a shuffling gait that is devoid of spring. In weakness of the quadriceps muscle (e.g., femoral neuropathy), there is weakness of knee extension, and the patient can only accept weight on the affected extremity by bracing the knee. When walking, the knee is held stiffly, and there is a tendency to fall if the knee bends. The patient has less difficulty walking backward than forward. Lumbosacral radiculopathy may cause either footdrop or a unilateral Trendelenburg's gait, or both (see Chapters 27 and 47). In addition, the patient with acute radiculopathy may walk with a list or pelvic tilt, accompanied by flattening of the normal lumbar lordosis because of low back muscle spasm. The patient may walk with small steps; if the pain is severe, she may place only the toes on the floor, because dorsiflexion of the foot aggravates the pain. Patients commonly use a cane to avoid bearing weight on the involved leg.

Other Gait Disorders

Patients with unilateral thalamic lesions may have an inability to stand or sit out of proportion to weakness or sensory loss, with a tendency to fall backward or to the side contralateral to the lesion (thalamic astasia). A toppling gait refers to a tendency to totter and fall seen with brainstem and cerebellar lesions, perhaps due to a failure of righting reflexes and slow motor responses. Primary progressive freezing gait causes early and progressive gait freezing; it is not a distinct disorder but a syndrome with diverse causes.

NONNEUROLOGIC GAIT DISORDERS

Abnormalities of gait may occur for many other reasons and may be confused with neurologic disorders. An antalgic gait is one in which walking is disordered because of pain. Pain in a lower extremity, for whatever reason, causes a shortening of the stance phase on the involved limb as the patient seeks to avoid bearing weight. On more than one occasion, neurologic consultation has been requested in a patient who ultimately proved to have acute podagra or a hip fracture. An antalgic gait may also occur with peripheral neuropathy causing painful dysesthesias and allodynia of the feet. The patient walks as if on hot coals. Arthritis may cause difficulties with gait that are secondary to both pain and deformity. In pregnancy, ascites, and abdominal tumors, there may be a lordosis that resembles that seen in the muscular dystrophies. With dislocation of the hips, there may be waddling suggestive of a myopathic gait. A waddling gait is also typical of advanced pregnancy. Patients with severe orthostatic hypotension may complain of difficulty walking rather than dizziness. Marked stooping in ankylosing spondylitis may resemble parkinsonism. A gait abnormality due to generalized weakness may occur after a period of bed rest, or in wasting and debilitating diseases. It is characterized mainly by unsteadiness and the wish for support. The patient staggers and sways from side to side with a suggestion of ataxia. She moves slowly, and the knees may tremble. If the difficulty is marked, she may fall.

NONORGANIC (FUNCTIONAL) GAIT ABNORMALITIES

Derangements of station and gait on a nonorganic basis are common. Affected patients may be unable either to stand or walk, despite the absence of weakness or other objective neurologic abnormalities. Testing for strength, tone, and coordination is normal if carried out supine. Astasia-abasia is an old term meant largely to describe the gait in conversion disorders. PGD is preferable and includes gait changes related to depression, anxiety, and phobic states.

The gait may suggest the presence of a monoparesis, hemiparesis, or paraparesis, yet the limbs can be used in an emergency. In Keane's series of 60 patients, 23 mimicked paresis and most of the remainder had various ataxic or histrionic patterns. Several authors have noted that knee buckling is a common type of PGD. The histrionic type of PGD is nondescript and bizarre and may take any number of forms that do not conform to a specific organic disease pattern (see **Video Link 44.6**). The gait is irregular and variable, with a great deal of superfluous movement and often marked swaying from side to side. The patient may appear to be in great danger of falling but rarely does so, often demonstrating superb balance during the contortions. If she does fall, it is in a theatrical manner without injury. The bizarre movements often require better than normal coordination. The patient may balance on the stance leg for a prolonged period of time, while bringing up the swing leg with a great show of effort. The gait may show skating, hopping, dancing, or zigzag characteristics; the legs may be thrown out wildly, or there may be a tendency to kneel every few steps. Tremulousness of the extremities or tic-like or compulsive features may be present. Although the patient cannot walk forward, she may be able to walk backward or to one side or to run without difficulty. Better ability to propel a wheeled, swivel chair than to walk ("chair test") favors PGD. In most patients with PGD, the similarity to neurologic disease is slight. Hyperkinetic gait disorders are most likely to be confused with functional conditions.

The term astasia-abasia originated in an 1888 monograph by Blocq, and the condition is sometimes referred to as Blocq's syndrome. Blocq described patients who were able to jump, or walk on all fours, but unable to stand upright (astasia) or to walk (abasia). There is normal lower-extremity function when recumbent, yet an inability to walk. This same pattern can occur in lesions involving the cerebellar vermis, such as alcoholic cerebellar degeneration or medulloblastoma, and in frontal lobe disorders. Astasia-abasia is sometimes used to refer to any inability to either stand or walk normally but generally refers to a histrionic and dramatic gait disturbance with wild lurching and near falls.

Video Links

Video Link 44.1. The Romberg sign. http://neurosigns.org/wiki/Romberg%27s_sign
Video Link 44.2. Physiology of Gait. www.youtube.com/watch?v=5j4YRHf6Iyo
Video Link 44.3. Myopathic gait. http://neurosigns.org/wiki/Myopathic_gait
Video Link 44.4. Myopathic gait in DMD. http://www.nejm.org/doi/full/10.1056/NEJMicm1007790
Video Link 44.5. Choreic gait. http://neurosigns.org/wiki/Hyperkinetic_gait_disorders
Video Link 44.6. Psychogenic gait disorders. https://journals.lww.com/continuum/Pages/videogallery.aspx?videoId=46&autoPlay=true

BIBLIOGRAPHY

Alexander NB. Gait disorders in older adults. *J Am Geriatr Soc* 1996;44:434–451.

Allali G, Laidet M, Armand S, et al. A combined cognitive and gait quantification to identify normal pressure hydrocephalus from its mimics: the Geneva's protocol. *Clin Neurol Neurosurg* 2017;160:5–11.

Atchison PR, Thompson PD, Frackowiak RS, et al. The syndrome of gait ignition failure: a report of six cases. *Mov Disord* 1993;8:285–292.

Baik JS, Lang AE. Gait abnormalities in psychogenic movement disorders. *Mov Disord* 2007;22:395–399.

Baker JM. Gait Disorders. *Am J Med* 2018;131:602–607.

Beckmann H, Bohlen S, Saft C, et al. Objective assessment of gait and posture in premanifest and manifest Huntington disease—a multi-center study. *Gait Posture* 2018;62:451–457.

Benson RR, Guttmann CR, Wei X, et al. Older people with impaired mobility have specific loci of periventricular abnormality on MRI. *Neurology* 2002;58:48–55.

Berlot R, Gregorič Kramberger M, Dreo J, et al. Blurred boundaries between organic and functional etiology: a man with a jerky leg. *J Neurol Sci* 2015;354:122–123.

Bloem BR, Haan J, Lagaay AM, et al. Investigation of gait in elderly subjects over 88 years of age. *J Geriatr Psychiatry Neurol* 1992;5:78–84.

Campbell WW. *Clinical Signs in Neurology: A Compendium.* Philadelphia: Wolters Kluwer Health, 2016.

Chambers HG, Sutherland DH. A practical guide to gait analysis. *J Am Acad Orthop Surg* 2002;10:222–231.

Della SS, Francescani A, Spinnler H. Gait apraxia after bilateral supplementary motor area lesion. *J Neurol Neurosurg Psychiatry* 2002;72:77–85.

Diener HC, Dichgans J. Pathophysiology of cerebellar ataxia. *Mov Disord* 1992;7:95–109.

Ebersbach G, Sojer M, Valldeoriola F, et al. Comparative analysis of gait in Parkinson's disease, cerebellar ataxia and subcortical arteriosclerotic encephalopathy. *Brain* 1999;122 (Pt 7):1349–1355.

Elble RJ, Hughes L, Higgins C. The syndrome of senile gait. *J Neurol* 1992;239:71–75.

Espay AJ, Narayan RK, Duker AP, et al. Lower-body parkinsonism: reconsidering the threshold for external lumbar drainage. *Nat Clin Pract Neurol* 2008;4:50–55.

Espay AJ, Aybek S, Carson A, et al. Current concepts in diagnosis and treatment of functional neurological disorders. *JAMA Neurol* 2018;75(9):1132–1141.

Factor SA, Higgins DS, Qian J. Primary progressive freezing gait: a syndrome with many causes. *Neurology* 2006;66:411–414.

Fasano A, Bloem BR. Gait disorders. *Continuum (Minneap Minn)* 2013;19(5 Movement Disorders):1344–1382.

Ferrandez AM, Pailhous J, Durup M. Slowness in elderly gait. *Exp Aging Res* 1990;16:79–89.

Fisher CM. Hydrocephalus as a cause of disturbances of gait in the elderly. *Neurology* 1982;32:1358–1363.

Fung VS. Functional gait disorder. *Handb Clin Neurol* 2016;139: 263–270.

Hausdorff JM, Cudkowicz ME, Firtion R, et al. Gait variability and basal ganglia disorders: stride-to-stride variations of gait cycle timing in Parkinson's disease and Huntington's disease. *Mov Disord* 1998;13:428–437.

Hausdorff JM, Schaafsma JD, Balash Y, et al. Impaired regulation of stride variability in Parkinson's disease subjects with freezing of gait. *Exp Brain Res* 2003;149:187–194.

Hennerici MG, Oster M, Cohen S, et al. Are gait disturbances and white matter degeneration early indicators of vascular dementia? *Dementia* 1994;5:197–202.

Jankovic J, Nutt JG, Sudarsky L. Classification, diagnosis, and etiology of gait disorders. *Adv Neurol* 2001;87:119–133.

Keane JR. Hysterical gait disorders: 60 cases. *Neurology* 1989;39: 586–589.

Koehler PJ, Bruyn GW, Pearce JMS, eds. *Neurological Eponyms*. Oxford: Oxford University Press, 2000.

Koller WC, Glatt SL, Fox JH. Senile gait. A distinct neurologic entity. *Clin Geriatr Med* 1985;1:661–669.

Kuba H, Inamura T, Ikezaki K, et al. Gait disturbance in patients with low pressure hydrocephalus. *J Clin Neurosci* 2002;9:33–36.

Lanska DJ, Goetz CG. Romberg's sign: development, adoption, and adaptation in the 19th century. *Neurology* 2000;55:1201.

Lau B, Welter ML, Belaid H, et al. The integrative role of the pedunculopontine nucleus in human gait. *Brain* 2015;138 (Pt 5):1284–1296.

Lim MR, Huang RC, Wu A, et al. Evaluation of the elderly patient with an abnormal gait. *J Am Acad Orthop Surg* 2007; 15:107–117.

Liston R, Mickelborough J, Bene J, et al. A new classification of higher level gait disorders in patients with cerebral multi-infarct states. *Age Ageing* 2003;32:252–258.

Mahlknecht P, Kiechl S, Bloem BR, et al. Prevalence and burden of gait disorders in elderly men and women aged 60-97 years: a population-based study. *PLoS One* 2013;8:e69627.

Maranhao-Filho P, Maron RM, de Rosso AL. Teaching video NeuroImage: waddling-steppage gait secondary to spinal arachnoid cyst: an exceptional surgical outcome. *Neurology* 2008;70:e85.

Margolesky J, Singer C. How tandem gait stumbled into the neurological exam: a review. *Neurol Sci* 2018;39(1):23–29.

Marshall FJ. Approach to the elderly patient with gait disturbance. *Neurol Clin Pract* 2012;2:103–111.

Masdeu JC, Alampur U, Cavaliere R, et al. Astasia and gait failure with damage of the pontomesencephalic locomotor region. *Ann Neurol* 1994;35:619–621.

Masdeu JC, Sudarsky L, Wolfson L, eds. *Gait Disorders of Aging. Falls and Therapeutic Strategies*. Philadelphia: Lippincott-Raven, 1997.

Morris M, Iansek R, Matyas T, et al. Abnormalities in the stride length-cadence relation in parkinsonian gait. *Mov Disord* 1998;13:61–69.

Nadeau SE. Gait apraxia: further clues to localization. *Eur Neurol* 2007;58:142–145.

Nutt JG. Higher-level gait disorders: an open frontier. *Mov Disord* 2013;28:1560–1565.

Nutt JG, Marsden CD, Thompson PD. Human walking and higher-level gait disorders, particularly in the elderly. *Neurology* 1993;43:268–279.

Okun MS, Koehler PJ. Paul Blocq and (psychogenic) astasia abasia. *Mov Disord* 2007;22:1373–1378.

Okun MS, Rodriguez RL, Foote KD, et al. The "chair test" to aid in the diagnosis of psychogenic gait disorders. *Neurologist* 2007;13:87–91.

Pahapill PA, Lozano AM. The pedunculopontine nucleus and Parkinson's disease. *Brain* 2000;123(Pt 9):1767–1783.

Palliyath S, Hallett M, Thomas SL, et al. Gait in patients with cerebellar ataxia. *Mov Disord* 1998;13:958–964.

Pyo SJ, Kim H, Kim IS, et al. Quantitative gait analysis in patients with Huntington's disease. *J Mov Disord* 2017;10:140–144.

Reynolds NC Jr, Myklebust JB, Prieto TE, et al. Analysis of gait abnormalities in Huntington disease. *Arch Phys Med Rehabil* 1999;80:59–65.

Ropper AH. Refined Romberg test. *Can J Neurol Sci* 1985;12:282.

Ropper AH, Samuels MA, Klein J. *Adams and Victor's Principles of Neurology*. 10th ed. New York: McGraw-Hill Education Medical, 2014.

Rubino FA. Gait disorders in the elderly. Distinguishing between normal and dysfunctional gaits. *Postgrad Med* 1993;93: 185–190.

Snijders AH, van de Warrenburg BP, Giladi N, et al. Neurological gait disorders in elderly people: clinical approach and classification. *Lancet Neurol* 2007;6:63–74.

Solomon DH, Barohn RJ, Bazan C, et al. The thalamic ataxia syndrome. *Neurology* 1994;44:810–814.

Stolze H, Kuhtz-Buschbeck JP, Drucke H, et al. Comparative analysis of the gait disorder of normal pressure hydrocephalus and Parkinson's disease. *J Neurol Neurosurg Psychiatry* 2001;70:289–297.

Sudarsky L. Geriatrics: gait disorders in the elderly. *N Engl J Med* 1990;322:1441–1446.

Sudarsky L. Psychogenic gait disorders. *Semin Neurol* 2006; 26:351–356.

Sudarsky L, Ronthal M. Gait disorders among elderly patients. A survey study of 50 patients. *Arch Neurol* 1983;40: 740–743.

Sudarsky L, Tideiksaar R. The cautious gait, fear of falling, and psychogenic gait disorders. In: Masdeu JC, Sudarsky L, Wolfson L, eds. *Gait Disorders of Aging. Falls and Therapeutic Strategies*. Philadelphia: Lippincott-Raven, 1997.

Takahashi K, Osaka A, Tsuda H, et al. Isolated astasia caused by a localized infarction in the suprathalamic white matter. *J Gen Fam Med* 2017;18:275–278.

Tanaka A, Okuzumi H, Kobayashi I, et al. Gait disturbance of patients with vascular and Alzheimer-type dementias. *Percept Mot Skills* 1995;80:735–738.

Vachranukunkiet T, Esquenazi A. Pathophysiology of gait disturbance in neurologic disorders and clinical presentations. *Phys Med Rehabil Clin N Am* 2013;24:233–246.

Verghese J, Lipton RB, Hall CB, et al. Abnormality of gait as a predictor of non-Alzheimer's dementia. *N Engl J Med* 2002;347:1761–1768.

Viswanathan A, Sudarsky L. Balance and gait problems in the elderly. *Handb Clin Neurol* 2011;103:623–634.

SECTION I The Autonomic and Peripheral Nervous Systems

CHAPTER 45

The Autonomic Nervous System

The autonomic nervous system (ANS) is the system that controls nonstriated muscles and glands. There are three divisions of the ANS: sympathetic (thoracolumbar), parasympathetic (craniosacral), and enteric. The sympathetic and parasympathetic divisions are characterized by a two-neuron chain with two anatomic elements: a preganglionic (first-order) neuron within the central nervous system (CNS) that terminates in a ganglion outside the CNS and a postganglionic (second-order) neuron that carries impulses to a destination in the viscera. An overview of the anatomy of the sympathetic and parasympathetic division is shown in Figure 45.1. The enteric nervous system is located in the walls of the gastrointestinal tract. In addition, dorsal root ganglion neurons convey afferent visceral impulses that arise in both sympathetic and parasympathetic fibers. There are also autonomic neurons within the CNS at various levels from the cerebral cortex to the spinal cord. Autonomic functions are beyond voluntary control and for the most part beneath consciousness.

THE PERIPHERAL AUTONOMIC NERVOUS SYSTEM

The parasympathetic division is composed of the general visceral efferent fibers of cranial nerves III, VII, IX, X, and bulbar portion of XI (the cranial outflow), together with fibers arising in the S2-S4 segments of the spinal cord (the sacral outflow). The parts of the parasympathetic division are widely separated, but because of anatomic characteristics, similarity in function, and similar pharmacologic responses, they are classified as parts of one system rather than as separate divisions. The parasympathetic nerves have long preganglionic fibers that end in peripheral ganglia near or in the viscera they supply, and short postganglionic fibers that arise in proximity to or within the viscus innervated. One preganglionic fiber usually synapses with only one postganglionic neuron.

The anatomy of the cranial portion of the parasympathetic division is discussed with the individual cranial nerves. In brief, it consists of the Edinger-Westphal nucleus, the superior and inferior salivatory nuclei, the dorsal motor nucleus of the vagus, and neurons in the vicinity of the nucleus ambiguus. The sacral parasympathetic fibers arise from cells in the intermediolateral cell column at the S2-S4 levels of the sacral spinal cord, travel through the sacral nerves, and are collected into the pelvic splanchnic nerves (nervi erigentes), which proceed to the pelvic plexuses and their branches. Some postganglionic fibers may travel from these plexuses to the pelvic viscera, but most preganglionic fibers continue to small ganglia in or near the viscera, from where postganglionic fibers supply the bladder, descending colon, rectum, anus, and genitalia. The greatest parasympathetic outflow is via the vagus nerves. Peripheral parasympathetic ganglia include the ciliary, otic, submandibular, and sphenopalatine (Figure 45.2).

The sympathetic division is composed of preganglionic fibers that arise from cells in the

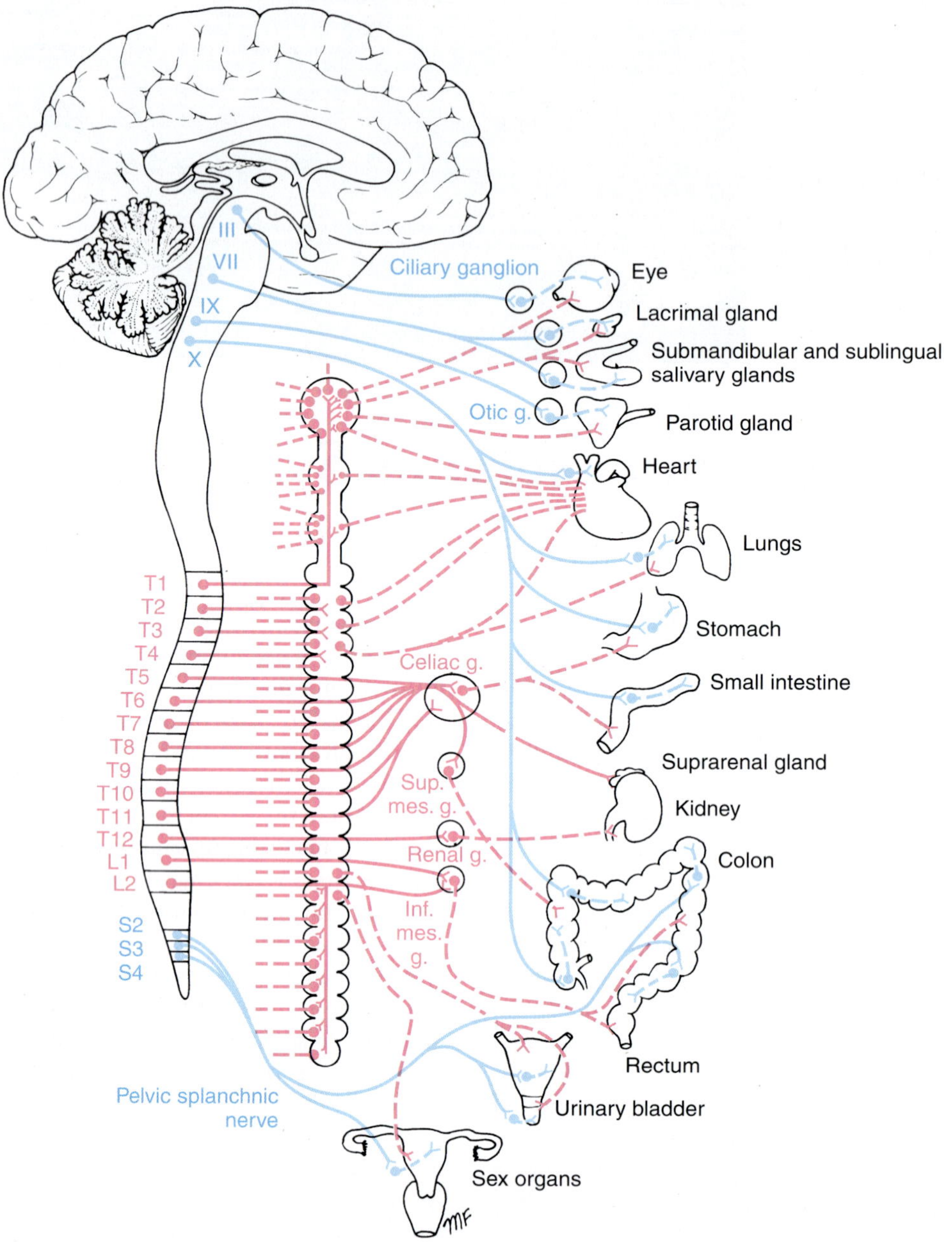

FIGURE 45.1 General arrangement of the autonomic nervous system. The sympathetic components are shown in *red* and the parasympathetic component in *blue*. (Reprinted with permission from Snell R. *Clinical Neuroanatomy*. 7th ed. Philadelphia: Wolters Kluwer Health/Lippincott Williams & Wilkins, 2009.)

intermediolateral columns from the T1 to the L3 segments of the spinal cord. The fibers exit through the ventral roots of the corresponding segmental nerves (Figure 24.3). These fibers terminate in the paravertebral ganglionic chain, prevertebral plexuses, and collateral ganglia, or occasionally in terminal ganglia (Figure 45.3). Postganglionic fibers go to the viscera. The sympathetic preganglionic fibers are typically short and terminate on ganglia some distance from the viscera they supply, with long postganglionic fibers that travel from the ganglia to the viscera. One preganglionic fiber may synapse with many postganglionic neurons.

The sympathetic ganglia are arranged into two plexuses: paravertebral and prevertebral. The paravertebral ganglia lie alongside the vertebral column;

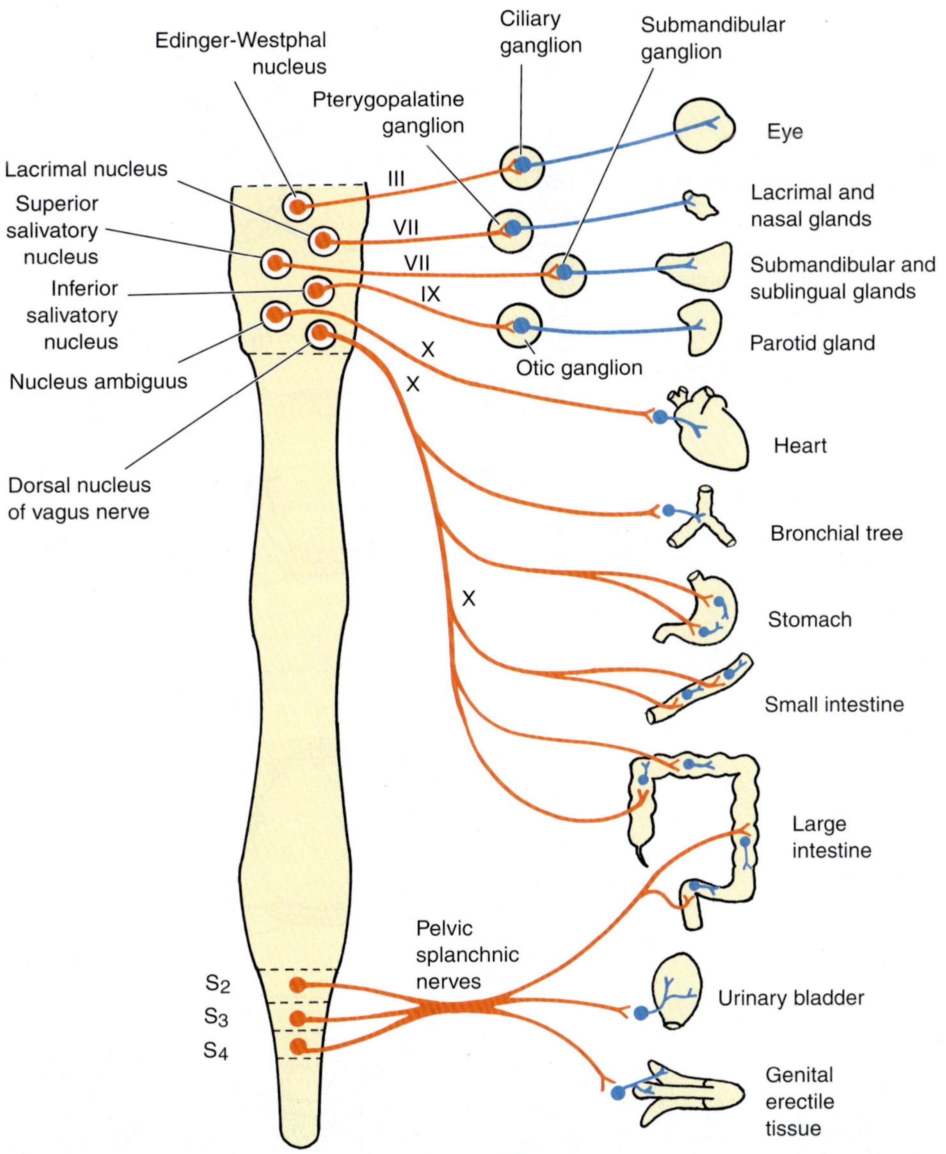

FIGURE 45.2 The parasympathetic division. Preganglionic neurons are *red*, and postganglionic neurons are *blue*. (Reprinted with permission from Kiernan JA. *Barr's The Human Nervous System: An Anatomical Viewpoint.* 9th ed. Philadelphia: Wolters Kluwer Health/Lippincott Williams & Wilkins, 2009.)

the prevertebral ganglia lie anterior to the vertebral column. The prevertebral ganglia innervate the viscera of the abdomen and pelvis. The paravertebral sympathetic chain consists of two elongated plexuses, each composed of a series of ganglia that are segmentally arranged and bound together by ascending and descending nerve fibers. The sympathetic trunks have from 22 to 24 ganglia and extend from the level of C2 to the coccyx. There are 3 cervical, 10 to 12 thoracic, 4 lumbar, and 4 to 5 sacral ganglia. The chains usually join at the level of the coccyx in an unpaired coccygeal ganglion (ganglion impar). Preganglionic fibers leave the spinal cord through the anterior root and mixed spinal nerve to reach the anterior primary ramus and then exit as finely myelinated fibers (white rami communicantes) to enter the ganglionic chain. They may synapse immediately or ascend or descend before synapsing. The postganglionic fibers return to the anterior primary ramus as unmyelinated fibers (gray rami communicantes). The T1-T3 segments innervate the head and neck, the T3-T11 segments innervate the upper

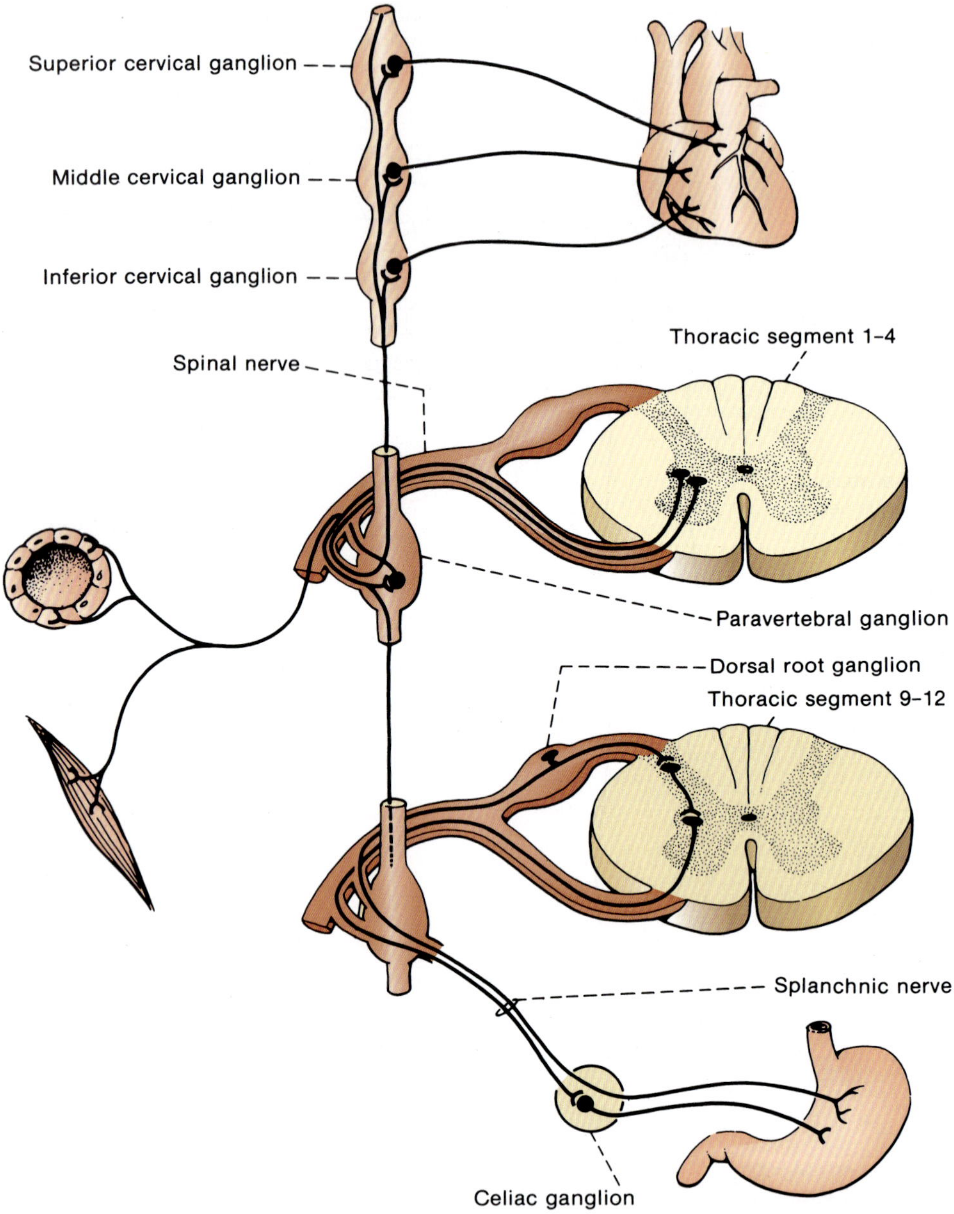

FIGURE 45.3 The sympathetic outflow, showing connections with the paravertebral ganglionic chain, splanchnic nerves, and collateral ganglia.

extremities and viscera in the thorax and abdomen, and the T12-L2 segments innervate the lower extremities and pelvic viscera.

The cervical portion of the sympathetic chain consists of the superior, middle, and inferior cervical ganglia. These innervate structures within the head, upper extremities, and thorax. The superior cervical ganglion, the largest, lies opposite the C2-C3 vertebrae and behind the internal carotid artery. It is primarily supplied by the first two thoracic segments. The internal carotid nerve, a direct continuation of the superior cervical ganglion, gives rise to postganglionic filaments that supply the internal carotid, and terminates as the internal carotid and cavernous plexuses. Anterior branches from the ganglion form plexuses around the middle meningeal and external carotid and maxillary arteries. The sympathetic innervation of the ciliary ganglia travels through the long ciliary nerves from the cavernous plexus. The sphenopalatine ganglion is supplied by the internal carotid plexus through the deep petrosal and vidian nerves. The otic ganglion receives its sympathetic innervation from the plexus around the middle meningeal artery, and the submaxillary ganglion from that around the external maxillary artery. There are other connections from the superior cervical ganglion to other cranial nerves and the upper four cervical nerves, the pharyngeal plexus, the carotid sinus and body, the heart, and the superior cardiac nerves. The middle cervical ganglion communicates with the fifth and sixth cervical nerves to begin the middle cardiac nerve and sends other branches to the thyroid gland. The inferior cervical ganglion communicates with the seventh and eighth cervical nerves to form the inferior cardiac nerve and nerves to the blood vessels.

The paravertebral ganglia provide long unmyelinated axons to all sympathetically innervated tissues and organs except those in the abdomen, pelvis, and perineum. The superior cervical ganglion (T1-T2) provides pupillodilator and sudomotor fibers to the face. The stellate ganglion (T2-T6) innervates the upper limb through branches of the brachial plexus, and the lumbar sympathetic ganglia (T9-L1) innervate the lower limb through branches of the lumbosacral plexus. The postganglionic sympathetic fibers join the peripheral somatic nerves via the gray rami communicantes, and thus their distribution is similar to that of the corresponding somatic nerve.

The thoracic portion of the sympathetic trunk rests against the heads of the ribs. Occasionally the first thoracic ganglion is blended with the inferior cervical ganglion to form the stellate ganglion. The stellate ganglion receives preganglionic fibers from the T2-T6 levels, and its postganglionic fibers are distributed with the nerves of the brachial plexus to provide autonomic innervation to the upper extremity. The sympathetic fibers traveling in somatic nerves innervate vasomotor, sudomotor, and pilomotor structures in the distribution of the nerve in which they are carried.

The upper five ganglia provide branches to the cardiac and pulmonary plexuses. The abdominal portion of the sympathetic trunk is situated in front of the vertebral column along the medial margin of the psoas major muscle, and the pelvic portion is in front of the sacrum. All of these ganglia send gray rami communicantes to the corresponding spinal nerves and many branches to the various plexuses and collateral ganglia. The postganglionic fibers terminate on blood vessels, sweat glands, and other smooth muscle and glandular structures.

Branches of the lower seven thoracic ganglia unite to form the three splanchnic nerves that penetrate the diaphragm and supply the abdomen and the pelvic viscera. These branches are white in color and primarily carry preganglionic fibers that pass through the ganglia without synapsing and terminate in the prevertebral plexuses or the collateral ganglia. The greater splanchnic nerve is formed by branches of the 5th through the 9th or 10th thoracic ganglia; it terminates in the celiac ganglion. The lesser splanchnic nerve is formed by branches of the 9th, 10th, and sometimes the 11th thoracic ganglia; it ends in the aorticorenal ganglion. The lower splanchnic nerve arises from the last thoracic ganglion; it ends in the renal plexus.

Within the thoracic, abdominal, and pelvic cavities are aggregations of nerves and ganglia known as the prevertebral plexuses and their collateral ganglia. These are composed of both parasympathetic and sympathetic fibers. The parasympathetic fibers are preganglionic and may synapse in the plexuses or go through without synapse to terminal ganglia. The sympathetic fibers, mainly from the splanchnic nerves, usually synapse in the plexuses. From these plexuses, branches are given off to the abdominal and pelvic viscera. The cardiac plexus is supplied by the cardiac branches of the vagus nerves and the cardiac nerves arising from the cervical and upper thoracic sympathetic ganglia. The cardiac plexus also communicates with the pulmonary and the esophageal plexuses, all supplied by the vagus nerve as well as the thoracic sympathetic ganglia.

The celiac plexus is the largest of the three sympathetic plexuses and innervates all the abdominal viscera except for the descending colon. The thoracic splanchnic nerves, carrying preganglionic fibers from the T5-T12 levels, perforate the diaphragm and form the celiac plexus, which lies in the abdomen at the level of the upper part of the first lumbar vertebra, behind the stomach and omental bursa, in front of the diaphragm and abdominal aorta, and between the adrenal glands. It is composed of the two celiac ganglia that are supplied by the greater splanchnic nerves and filaments from the right vagus nerve, and the aorticorenal ganglia, which receive the lesser splanchnic nerves. Other plexuses arise from or are connected with the celiac plexus, including phrenic, hepatic, splenic, and others. The superior (anterior) gastric plexus and the hepatic plexus also receive branches from the left vagus nerve. The renal and inferior mesenteric plexuses and their branches are also supplied by the lowest splanchnic nerve.

The hypogastric plexus is located in front of the last lumbar vertebra and the promontory of the sacrum, between the two common iliac arteries, and is formed by the union of many elements from the aortic plexus and the lumbar sympathetic chain, together with some fibers from the inferior mesenteric plexus. It is divided into the two pelvic plexuses formed by fibers from the hypogastric plexus; preganglionic sympathetic fibers from the second, third, and fourth sacral nerves; and a few filaments from the sacral sympathetic ganglia. Branches are distributed to the pelvic viscera and the internal and external genitalia through the middle hemorrhoidal, vesical, prostatic, vaginal, and uterine plexuses.

The enteric nervous system consists of intrinsic and extrinsic components. The intrinsic component consists of Meissner's submucosal and Auerbach's myenteric plexi. The extrinsic component consists of preganglionic sympathetic, from prevertebral ganglia, and parasympathetic, from the dorsal motor nucleus of the vagus and the sacral parasympathetic centers, inputs that control peristalsis and secretion.

Autonomic Afferents

General visceral afferent fibers convey both conscious and unconscious sensations from the viscera and are involved in autonomic reflexes. Small myelinated and unmyelinated fibers carry impulses from visceral receptors to cell bodies in the dorsal root and cranial nerve ganglia. The visceral afferents that enter the spinal cord synapse on neurons in the dorsal horn and intermediolateral gray column. Centrally, sensation from the viscera travels mainly in the spinothalamic and spinoreticular tracts, but some visceral afferents—especially those related to bowel and bladder control—are carried in the posterior columns. After a synapse in the thalamus, visceral sensory fibers project to areas of the cortex involved in autonomic function. Afferent autonomic fibers in the vagus nerve synapse in the nodose ganglion, and those in the glossopharyngeal nerve synapse in the petrosal ganglion. The vagal afferents transmit impulses from the heart, great vessels, lungs, and gastrointestinal (GI) tract; the glossopharyngeal afferents convey information from the carotid sinus. These afferents synapse in the nucleus of the solitary tract and are involved in autonomic reflexes as well as such functions as coughing and swallowing.

Neurotransmitters

Acetylcholine is the neurotransmitter at sympathetic and parasympathetic preganglionic neurons, and at postganglionic parasympathetic neurons. Norepinephrine is the primary postganglionic sympathetic neurotransmitter, except at sweat glands, which are cholinergic. There are two subtypes of acetylcholine receptor: nicotinic and muscarinic. Most of the postganglionic acetylcholine receptors are muscarinic. They mediate the cardiac effects and cause pupillary constriction, lacrimal and salivary secretion, bronchoconstriction, and erection. They also stimulate GI tract motility and cause evacuation of the bladder and rectum. There are two main subtypes of adrenergic receptors: alpha and beta. The alpha-adrenergic receptors mediate pupillary dilatation, vasoconstriction, and ejaculation, and they also control the internal sphincters of the bladder and rectum. Beta-adrenergic receptors control the heart, cause vasodilation and bronchial dilatation, and mediate metabolic effects. Some postganglionic sympathetic neurons also utilize adenosine triphosphate and neuropeptide Y, and some postganglionic parasympathetic endings may use vasoactive intestinal polypeptide or nitric oxide.

The Physiology of the Peripheral Autonomic Nervous System

The ANS governs the activities of cardiac and smooth muscle, including the smooth muscle of the blood vessels and the functions of most glandular structures. It regulates such important functions as respiration, circulation, digestion, temperature adjustment, and metabolism—all vital to normal existence—and combats forces acting from within or without that would tend to cause undesirable changes in the normal function of the body. By homeostasis the constancy of the internal environment of the body and the uniformity and stability of the organism are maintained.

The sympathetic division supplies all parts of the body. Its functions are catabolic and directed toward the utilization of energy. It prepares the organism for combat or escape (fight-or-flight response). It acts whenever rapid adjustment to the environment is required. It accelerates the heart, dilates the coronary vessels, increases the arterial blood pressure, empties the blood reservoirs, dilates the bronchi, liberates glucose, and inhibits GI activity. It is an emergency protective mechanism that is called into action under emotional stress and causes the individual to react strongly to stimuli of rage and fear. The parasympathetic division supplies special structures, such as the pupils, salivary glands, heart, lungs, GI tract, bladder, and portions of the genital system. In certain

TABLE 45.1 Effects of Sympathetic and Parasympathetic Systems on Various Effector Organs

Organ	Sympathetic Effect	Parasympathetic Effect
Pupil	Pupillodilation (alpha)	Pupilloconstriction
Accommodation	Decreased	Increased
Heart	Positive chronotropic effect (beta)	Negative chronotropic effect
	Positive inotropic effect (beta)	Negative inotropic effect
Arteries	Vasoconstriction (alpha)	Vasodilation
	Vasodilation (beta)	
Veins	Vasoconstriction (alpha)	
	Vasoconstriction (beta)	
Tracheobronchial tree	Bronchodilation (beta)	Bronchoconstriction
		Increased bronchial gland secretions
Gastrointestinal tract	Decreased motility (beta)	Increased motility
	Contraction of sphincters (alpha)	Relaxation of sphincters
Bladder	Detrusor relaxation (beta)	Detrusor contraction
	Contraction of sphincter (alpha)	Relaxation of sphincter
Salivary glands	Scant, thick, viscid saliva (alpha)	Copious, thin, watery saliva
Skin	Piloerection (cutis anserina)	No piloerection
Sweat glands	Increased secretion (cholinergic)	Decreased secretion
Genitalia		Erection
	Ejaculation	Ejaculation
Adrenal medulla	Catecholamine release	
Glycogen	Glycogenolysis (alpha and beta)	Glycogen synthesis
	Lipolysis (alpha and beta)	

parasympathetic functions, as in bladder, rectal, and genital activity, contraction of striated muscles is closely integrated with that of smooth muscle. The parasympathetic division conserves energy. It controls anabolic, excretory, and reproductive functions, and conserves and restores bodily resources and energy.

The viscera receive a dual autonomic supply, both sympathetic and parasympathetic. In general these two divisions are antagonistic and reciprocal in their functions, but there are exceptions. Table 45.1 compares the functions of the two divisions in the innervation of various effector organs.

THE CENTRAL REGULATION OF AUTONOMIC FUNCTION

The peripheral ANS is under the control of higher centers in the cerebral cortex, especially the amygdala, hypothalamus, basal forebrain, ventral striatum, brainstem, and spinal cord that regulate and influence the function of its peripheral components. The centers in the CNS that are involved in autonomic function are referred to as the central autonomic network. The neurons of the central autonomic network are interconnected and make up a functional unit. The most important of these centers is the hypothalamus.

The Hypothalamus

The hypothalamus (Figure 45.4) is part of the ventral diencephalon, lying just below the thalamus and above the pituitary gland. The entire area measures only about 14 × 18 × 20 mm and weighs only 4 g. It forms most of the floor and part of the lateral wall of the third ventricle, extending from the level of the chiasm to the interpeduncular fossa. From a strictly anatomic point of view it includes the optic chiasm, neurohypophysis (posterior pituitary), infundibulum, pars supraoptica, tuber cinereum, and mammillary bodies, but from a physiologic point of view the first three structures are not included. The supraoptic nucleus is located just above the optic chiasm. The mammillary bodies are a pair of small spherical gray matter masses that lie in the interpeduncular

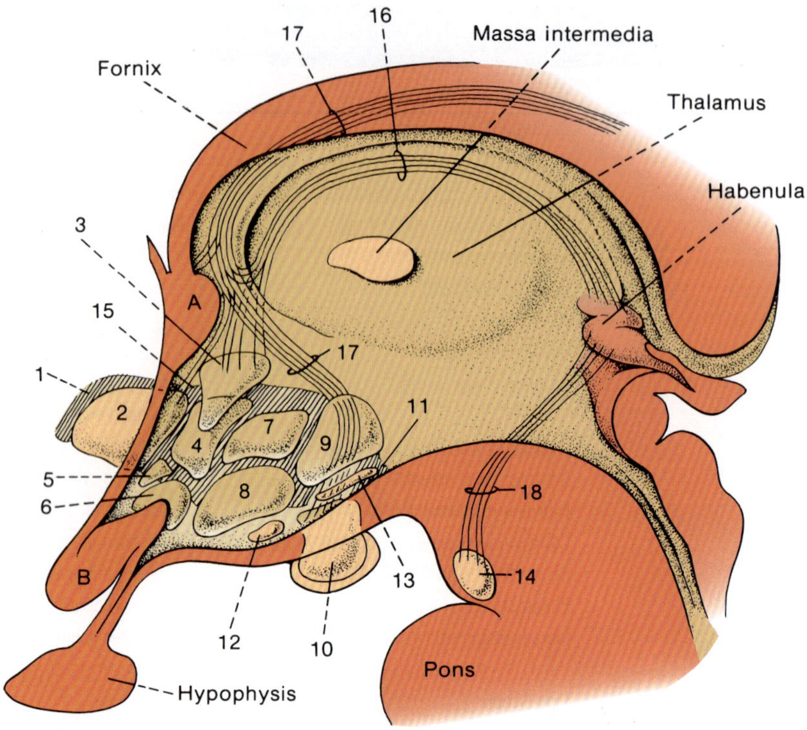

FIGURE 45.4 Diagrammatic sketch of the human hypothalamus. **A.** Anterior commissure. **B.** Optic nerve. (*1*) Lateral preoptic area, permeated by the median forebrain bundle. (*2*) Medial preoptic area. (*3*) Paraventricular nucleus. (*4*) Anterior hypothalamic area. (*5*) Suprachiasmatic nucleus. (*6*) Supraoptic nucleus. (*7*) Dorsomedial hypothalamic nucleus. (*8*) Ventromedial hypothalamic nucleus. (*9*) Posterior hypothalamic area. (*10*) Medial mammillary nucleus. (*11*) Lateral mammillary nucleus. (*12*) Premammillary area. (*13*) Supramammillary area. (*14*) Interpeduncular nucleus. (*15*) Lateral hypothalamic area. (*16*) Stria habenularis. (*17*) Fornix. (*18*) Habenulopeduncular tract.

fossa rostral to the posterior perforated substance and contain the mammillary nuclei; they form the caudal portion of the hypothalamus. Beneath the hypothalamus a hollow, conical process, the infundibulum, or pituitary stalk, projects downward and forward and is attached to the posterior lobe of the hypophysis. The infundibulum contains the supraopticohypophyseal and tuberohypophyseal tracts. The tuber cinereum is a prominence that lies between the mammillary bodies and the infundibulum.

The boundaries of the hypothalamus are not sharply defined. Anteriorly it merges with the basal olfactory and preoptic areas, and caudally it is continuous with the central gray matter and tegmentum of the midbrain. Laterally it is continuous with the subthalamic region; superiorly it is separated from the thalamus proper by the hypothalamic sulcus. The preoptic area is the region just above and anterior to the chiasm, extending to the lamina terminalis and anterior commissure.

The hypothalamus is composed of numerous nerve cells, not uniformly distributed but arranged into more or less definite regions or nuclear groups. It can be divided into three longitudinal zones: periventricular, medial, and lateral, all of which send descending fibers to the brainstem and spinal cord. The paraventricular and supraoptic hypothalamic nuclei give rise to the supraopticohypophyseal tract and are important in osmotic balance. The paraventricular nucleus has subpopulations of neurons that produce vasopressin, oxytocin, corticotropin-releasing hormone, and other hormones involved in pituitary function. Destruction of the paraventricular and supraoptic nuclei causes diabetes insipidus. The paraventricular nucleus is important in cardiovascular regulation. Afferents to the paraventricular nucleus come from the medial prefrontal cortex, amygdalae, and insular and other hypothalamic nuclei.

The medial zone of the hypothalamus contains the medial preoptic nucleus, which controls gonadotropin release and is involved in thermoregulation, and the anterior nucleus, which is also involved in thermoregulation. The lateral zone contains the lateral preoptic and lateral hypothalamic nuclei and is traversed by the medial forebrain bundle. Stimulation of the lateral nucleus causes eating, whereas ablation causes starvation. The lateral zone is also involved in arousal and sleep mechanisms. The arcuate (infundibular) nucleus lies in the periventricular region of the tuber cinereum and gives rise to the tuberohypophyseal tract. It contains releasing factors that control release of hormones from the anterior pituitary. It also contains dopaminergic neurons that act to inhibit the release of prolactin.

The autonomic pathways that descend from the hypothalamus run primarily in the ipsilateral brainstem tegmentum. In the spinal cord the descending autonomic fibers are in the anterolateral fasciculus. They are widely distributed but run primarily in the reticulospinal tracts. Some fibers, especially those subserving bladder control, lie close to the lateral corticospinal tracts. Impulses carried through these pathways terminate at appropriate levels in the intermediolateral column of the spinal cord.

Despite its small size, the hypothalamus has extensive and complex connections, some organized into definite bundles or tracts, others diffuse and difficult to trace (Figure 45.5). It is involved in the functions of the ANS, the endocrine system, and the limbic system. The hypothalamus receives impulses from the primary olfactory area, septal area, and orbitofrontal cortex through the medial forebrain bundle; from the amygdaloid nucleus through the stria terminalis; from the hippocampal formation through the fornix; and from the raphe nuclei, locus caeruleus, and tegmental nuclei of the brainstem. It sends efferent fibers through the medial forebrain bundle to the septal area and brainstem, via the mamillothalamic tract to the anterior nucleus of the thalamus, by the stria terminalis to the amygdala, and to the dorsomedial nucleus of the thalamus. The tuberohypophyseal tract and hypophyseal portal system connect the hypothalamus to the adenohypophysis and the supraopticohypophyseal tract connects it to the neurohypophysis.

Other Components of the Central Autonomic Network

Other important centers involved in autonomic control include the periaqueductal gray matter (PAG) in the midbrain, other brainstem nuclei, the cerebral cortex, and the amygdala. The PAG is important in the micturition reflex, pain mechanisms—including opiate responsiveness—and the fight-or-flight response. Descending pathways from the PAG modulate, primarily inhibit, pain. The nucleus of the solitary tract (NST) in the medulla is involved in cardiopulmonary and GI function. It receives afferents from arterial baroreceptors and chemoreceptors, and mediates important autonomic reflexes. The medullary cardiorespiratory centers consist of cells in the reticular formation of the ventral medulla that control blood pressure and respiration and mediate cardiorespiratory reflexes. Afferents from baroreceptors, chemoreceptors, and cardiac and pulmonary receptors travel into the brainstem through the glossopharyngeal and vagus nerves and synapse in the NST. Projections from the NST activate the nucleus ambiguus and dorsal motor nucleus of the vagus, which send parasympathetic fibers to the heart and lungs. Bilateral lesions of the NST cause acute neurogenic hypertension. There are also projections from the NST to the reticular formation neurons involved in respiratory rhythmogenesis, and to cells that send sympathetic fibers to the intermediolateral column of the spinal cord. Reticular formation interneurons, along with the NST, are also involved in such functions as coughing, sneezing, and vomiting. The reticulospinal pathways involved in cardiovascular and respiratory function descend in the ventral part of lateral columns of the spinal cord.

Neurons in the nucleus ambiguus are part of the system of cardiac parasympathetic innervation and are involved in the automatic control of respiration. The parabrachial nuclear complex lies in the dorsolateral pontine tegmentum. It includes the medial and lateral parabrachial nuclei and the Kölliker-Fuse nucleus. The parabrachial complex is involved in the processing of visceral information, pain modulation, and automatic control of respiration.

The primary cortical areas involved in autonomic function include the cortex of the insula, the medial prefrontal cortex, the cingulate gyrus, and the nucleus of the amygdala. The medial prefrontal cortex is activated by stress and is involved in autonomic and affective responses. Sensory input from the viscera project to the insula. It connects with the limbic system and projects to the amygdalae. There are wide connections with other cortical regions. It is an important area in cardiovascular regulation. Damage to the insula in cerebrovascular disease may mediate hypertension, arrhythmias, myocardial injury, and an increased risk of sudden death. The amygdala communicates with the hypothalamus, PAG, and the brainstem autonomic nuclei.

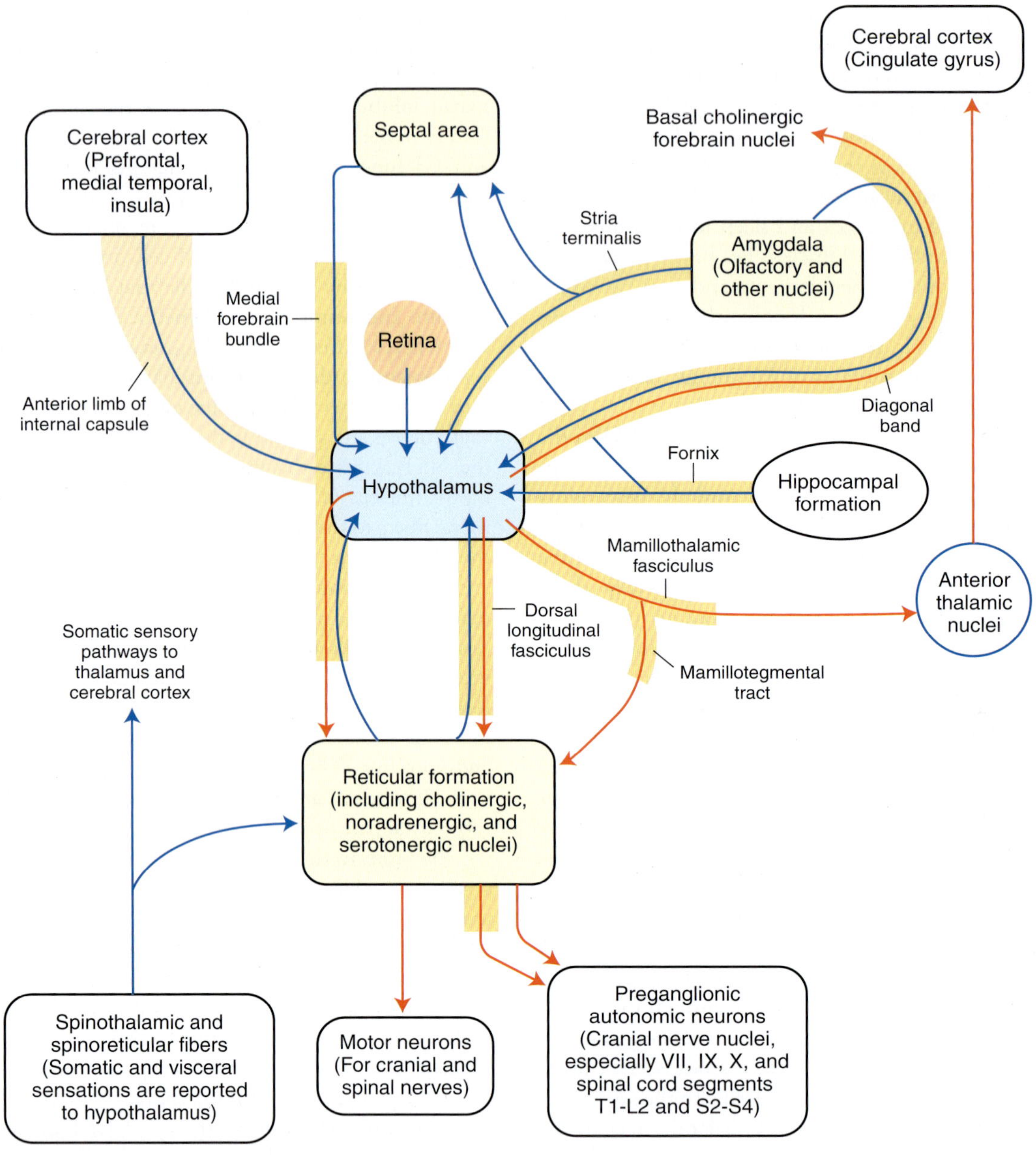

FIGURE 45.5 Direct and indirect neural connections of the hypothalamus with other parts of the brain and spinal cord. (Reprinted with permission from Kiernan JA. *Barr's The Human Nervous System: An Anatomical Viewpoint*. 9th ed. Philadelphia: Wolters Kluwer Health/Lippincott Williams & Wilkins, 2009.)

It is important in regulating vigilance, memory modulation, emotional learning, and fear mechanisms.

EXAMINATION

The history in patients with autonomic insufficiency may reveal symptoms related to orthostatic hypotension, abnormalities of sweating, or dysfunction of the GI or genitourinary tracts. Symptoms of orthostasis include dizziness or light-headedness, feelings of presyncope, syncope, palpitations, tremulousness, weakness, confusion, or slurred speech, all worse with standing. Occasional patients complain only of difficulty walking. The symptoms of orthostasis are often worse postprandially, after a hot bath or ingestion of alcohol, or following exercise. Sweating abnormalities may produce abnormal dryness of the skin, sometimes with excessive sweating in uninvolved regions. Other symptoms include constipation, dysphagia, early satiety, anorexia, diarrhea (particularly at night), weight loss, erectile dysfunction, ejaculatory failure, retrograde ejaculation, urinary retention, urinary urgency, recurrent urinary tract infections, and urinary or fecal incontinence.

The general physical and neurologic examinations may reveal a variety of abnormalities in patients with disorders of the ANS. Acromegaly, dwarfism, or signs of endocrine imbalance or sexual immaturity may indicate a hypothalamic abnormality. Abnormal dryness of the skin may be a sign of sudomotor failure and could occur in a localized distribution, as with a peripheral nerve injury, or be generalized, as in diffuse dysautonomia. Lack of normal moisture in the socks may indicate deficient sweating. A simple bedside test to demonstrate the distribution of abnormal skin dryness related to loss of sweating is to note the resistance to stroking of the skin with a finger or an object such as the barrel of a pen or a spoon. When a spoon is drawn over the skin, it pulls smoothly over dry (sympathectomized) skin but irregularly and unevenly over moist, perspiring skin. It is often possible to see the sweat droplets on the skin, especially on the papillary ridges of the fingers, using the +20 ophthalmoscope lens. Other cutaneous signs of autonomic dysregulation include changes in skin temperature or color, mottling, alopecia, hypertrichosis, thickening or fragility of the nails, absent piloerection, decreased hand wrinkling in water, and skin atrophy. Acral vasomotor dysregulation may lead to pallor, acrocyanosis, mottling, erythema, or livedo reticularis. Patients with dysautonomia associated with a regional pain syndrome may have allodynia and hyperalgesia in addition to the autonomic changes.

Assessment of orthostatic changes in blood pressure (BP) and heart rate (HR) are basic tests of cardiovascular autonomic function. At the bedside, BP and pulse are taken with the patient supine and after standing for variable periods; typically the BP is determined at 1, 3, and 5 minutes after standing. Tilt table testing is more precise. Normally, systolic blood pressure (SBP) on standing does not decrease by more than 20 mm Hg, and the diastolic blood pressure (DBP) by not more than 10 mm Hg. There are more stringent diagnostic criteria that permit a 30-point drop in SBP or a 15-point drop in DBP in normals. When BP measurement is done with a standard sphygmomanometer, the cuff should be kept at heart level to minimize hydrostatic influence on the measurement. When routine measurements are unrevealing, orthostatic blood pressure declines can sometimes be detected by having the patient perform 5 to 10 squats and then repeating the measurements.

The HR should not increase by more than 30 beats per minute above baseline on standing. In hypovolemia, the most common cause of orthostasis, a reflex tachycardia develops in response to the fall in standing blood pressure. When autonomic cardiovascular reflexes are impaired, the reflex tachycardia may not occur. Patients with the postural tachycardia syndrome will develop a brisk tachycardia without orthostatic hypotension (increased pulse rate more than 30 beats per minute above baseline or more than 120 beats per minute). The sustained hand grip, mental stress, and cold pressor tests all look for increases in DBP of at least 15 mm Hg or an increase in HR of greater than 10 beats per minute in response to peripheral vasoconstriction induced, respectively, by isometric hand exercise, mental arithmetic, or immersion of the hand in cold water. The cold face test assesses the trigeminovagal (diving) reflex. Resting tachycardia may be a sign of parasympathetic dysfunction.

Clinical assessment of bladder function is done by looking for evidence of distension by palpation and percussion, and by checking the anal wink and bulbocavernosus reflexes. The bulbocavernosus and superficial anal reflexes are somatic motor reflexes; the internal anal and scrotal reflexes are autonomic reflexes. The internal anal sphincter reflex is contraction of the internal sphincter on insertion of a gloved finger into the anus. If the reflex is impaired there is decreased sphincter tone and the anus does not close immediately after withdrawal. Postvoid residual urine volume is determined by catheterization after voiding.

Tear production by the lacrimal glands can be evaluated in a number of ways by ophthalmologists. A convenient and simple bedside assessment can be obtained with the Schirmer test, done by placing a strip of sterile filter paper in the lower conjunctival sac and measuring the degree of wetting over 5 minutes. Additional eye findings include excessive dryness with redness and itching, and ptosis. Examination of the pupil is discussed in Chapter 14. When autonomic failure occurs as part of a neurologic illness, there may be findings related to the underlying condition such as extrapyramidal or cerebellar signs, abnormal eye movements, weakness, sensory loss, or reflex abnormalities.

Autonomic Function Testing

Many different procedures have been developed to test the sympathetic and parasympathetic nervous systems. Tests of cardiac vagal tone include assessment of heart rate variability to deep breathing, standing, and performing Valsalva. The beat-to-beat changes in heart rate in response to autonomic reflexes occur quickly, often too quickly for bedside assessment to be accurate. It is possible at the bedside to determine if heart rate variability with respiration or to Valsalva is present and obvious (probably normal), present but minimal (possibly abnormal), or absent (abnormal). More precise testing requires equipment, and may include an indwelling arterial catheter to follow BP changes.

Normal sinus arrhythmia is the beat-to-beat variability in heart rate that occurs with respiration. It is most prominent in healthy young people. Sinus arrhythmia normally becomes less prominent with age, and it may be markedly impaired or abolished when vagal innervation of the heart is compromised. The heart rate response to deep breathing (HR_{DB}) shows maximal variability at a breathing rate of 5 to 6 per minute. The HR_{DB} can be assessed at the bedside simply by noting pulse variability; it can be measured more quantitatively by measuring the R-R interval with cardiac monitoring. The expiratory-to-inspiratory ratio quantitates the variability in HR_{DB}. The heart rate response to standing (30:15 ratio) is another method of evaluating the baroreflex arc. The most dramatic changes in HR normally occur in the first 30 seconds after standing, with an initial tachycardia, followed by bradycardia about 20 seconds later. The 30:15 (tachycardia:bradycardia) ratio is the ratio of the R-R interval at beat 30/R-R interval at beat 15; normal is >1.04.

The respiratory variability in heart rate is exaggerated when a Valsalva maneuver is performed. The cardiovascular responses to Valsalva are divided into four phases. Phases I and II occur during breath holding and phases III and IV after release. The BP and HR responses are mirror images: when BP increases, HR reflexly decreases. Measuring HR alone is adequate for some aspects of the Valsalva response, but a complete evaluation requires measurement of BP. In phase I there is a brief rise in BP because of increased intrathoracic pressure constricting the great vessels; in phase II, there is a gradual fall in BP because of impaired venous return that reaches a plateau because of peripheral vasoconstriction, with a compensatory tachycardia; in phase III, there is a brief fall in BP because of removal of the intrathoracic pressure constricting the great vessels. Phase IV occurs after the Valsalva is released and the patient resumes normal breathing; the BP begins to recover and slowly rises. About 15 to 20 seconds after release, there is a rebound overshoot of BP to a level above baseline, accompanied by a reflex bradycardia with an HR below baseline, lasting for approximately 1 minute. The Valsalva ratio is the ratio of the fastest HR during phase II to the slowest HR during phase IV, or the longest R-R interval during phase IV to the shortest R-R interval during phase II. Normal is approximately ≥1.45, but age specific reference values are more precise. A lack of rebound overshoot of BP during phase IV is an early indicator of autonomic dysfunction. A lack of overshoot can also occur in some non-neurologic conditions, such as congestive heart failure. The BP changes occur quickly, and it is not possible to follow the complete cycle at the bedside with a BP cuff. The rebound overshoot in phase IV, however, can be detected by inflating a cuff to just at SBP and then having the patient Valsalva. Without changing the cuff pressure, the sounds will disappear during breath holding, and on release the sounds will return and can be followed up to detect the rebound overshoot in BP.

Tilt-table testing evaluates the integrity of autonomic reflexes. Autonomic laboratories use different degrees of tilt, but usually in the range of 60 to 80 degrees and for different durations. In neurocardiogenic (vasovagal, vasodepressor) syncope, or fainting, hypotension is accompanied by bradycardia, rather than the tachycardia that should occur. It occurs in response to emotional upsets such as fear, stress, or the sight of blood; occasionally in relation to micturition (micturition syncope) or coughing (cough syncope); and sometimes without identifiable provocation. Tilt-table testing has shown that a neurocardiogenic mechanism is responsible for a large proportion of the patients with recurrent, unexplained syncope.

Tests for thermoregulatory and sudomotor function include the sympathetic skin response (SSR), QSART (Quantitative Sudomotor Axon Reflex Test), sweat imprint, and thermoregulatory sweat test (TST). The SSR assesses peripheral sympathetic function by detecting changes in skin resistance in response to sudomotor discharges. The TST assesses both the central and peripheral sympathetic components by analyzing the sweating response to a rise in body temperature. The QSART assesses the postganglionic sudomotor fibers by measuring the sweat output in response to iontophoresis into the skin of acetylcholine. The sweat imprint test quantitates sweat output by visualizing the imprints sweat droplets make on a plastic or silicone mold. A TST combined with a test of postganglionic function can localize the site of a process producing anhidrosis. If the postganglionic function test is abnormal, the cause is postganglionic. But if the postganglionic test is normal and the TST is abnormal, the cause is preganglionic. Sudoscan measures electrochemical skin conductance of the hands and feet through reverse iontophoresis. This technique is another method for measuring sudomotor function in small fiber neuropathy.

DISORDERS OF THE AUTONOMIC NERVOUS SYSTEM

Autonomic disorders can be divided into those that affect the central autonomic elements and are typically associated with other evidence of CNS disease and those that affect the peripheral autonomic nervous system. Disorders may be local or generalized, and primary or secondary. Adie's pupil is an example of localized and acute pandysautonomia an example of generalized dysfunction. Pure autonomic failure is an example of primary and amyloid neuropathy an example of secondary dysautonomia. Autonomic dysfunction is usually manifest by underactivity, but hyperactivity occurs under some circumstances. Paroxysmal dysautonomia is common in spinal cord injury. Orthostatic hypertension occurs because of overactive pressor reflexes. A massive trigeminal-parasympathetic discharge causes the lacrimation and nasal secretion during attacks of cluster headache.

Multiple system atrophy (MSA) is a degenerative neurologic disorder, which is usually accompanied by prominent dysautonomia (Chapter 30). The autonomic failure in MSA results from involvement of preganglionic neurons in the brainstem and spinal cord in the degenerative process. Autonomic failure produces orthostatic hypotension, impotence, constipation, and urinary incontinence; it may be associated with respiratory symptoms such as laryngeal stridor and sleep apnea. Autonomic dysfunction may also occur in patients with Parkinson's disease, but usually late in the illness and not to the degree typical of MSA. Autonomic disturbances may accompany seizures, including cardiovascular changes, flushing, pallor, sweating, shivering, piloerection, vomiting, and respiratory abnormalities. Seizure-induced cardiovascular abnormalities include sinus tachycardia, bradyarrhythmia, sinus arrest, and ventricular tachyarrhythmias, including ventricular fibrillation. Autonomic dysfunction may also be a major feature of dementia with Lewy bodies, MS, and Wernicke's encephalopathy.

Hypothalamic disorders may cause many abnormalities of autonomic function, including deficiencies in osmoregulation and thermoregulation; abnormalities of appetite and body weight; sleep disturbances; changes in carbohydrate, fat, and water metabolism; and respiratory abnormalities together with, in many instances, behavioral abnormalities and personality changes. Hypothalamic lesions may cause either hyperthermia or hypothermia. Hyperthermia generally results from involvement of the tuberal region, especially the supraoptic nuclei or the rostral portion of the anterior hypothalamus. It is a common manifestation of third ventricular tumors, and may occur after head trauma or cranial surgery; terminal hyperthermia is a frequent manifestation of neurologic disease. Hypothermia tends to occur with involvement of the posterior hypothalamic area and mammillary bodies. Disorders of the anterior hypothalamus tend to cause loss of the ability to regulate against heat and disorders of the posterior hypothalamus, loss of the ability to regulate against cold.

The hypothalamus is closely related anatomically and physiologically to the pituitary gland (Figure 45.6). Because the hypothalamus controls the release of many of the anterior pituitary hormones, abnormalities of hypothalamic function may have a close relationship to some endocrine disorders. Lesions of the supraoptic nuclei or the supraoptico-hypophyseal tract cause diabetes insipidus. Diabetes insipidus is a common manifestation of tumors in the parasellar region, encephalitis, and meningitis, and it may develop after intracranial surgery or head injury. Lesions involving the hypothalamus may also cause disturbances of fat metabolism. The Froehlich, or adiposogenital, syndrome was the first hypothalamic syndrome described. It is characterized by disturbances of fat metabolism and sexual underdevelopment.

Abnormalities of respiration may be caused by hypothalamic dysfunction. These include hyperpnea, apnea, Cheyne-Stokes respirations, and Biot breathing. Disturbances of the sleep cycle may occur with hypothalamic lesions, especially those involving its posterior portions, including the mammillary bodies.

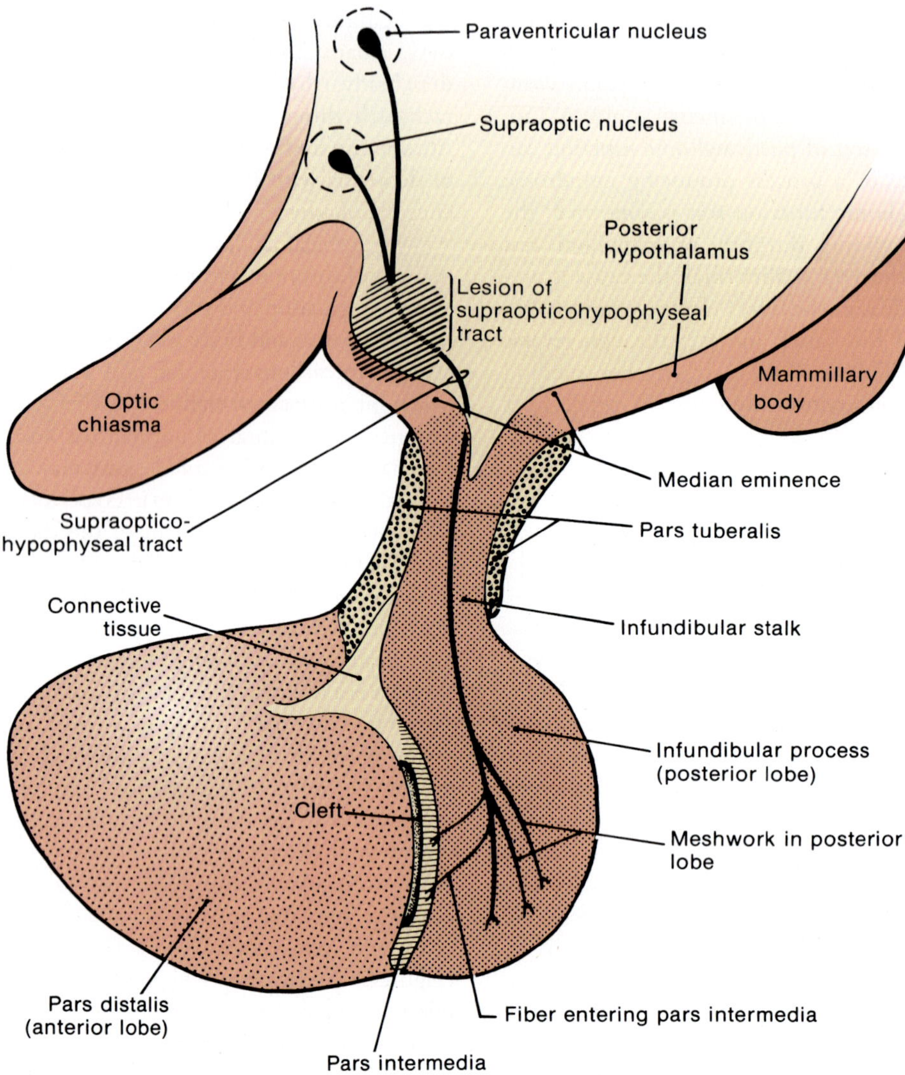

FIGURE 45.6 Longitudinal section through the human hypothalamus and hypophysis.

There may be hypersomnolence, inversion of the sleep cycle, or insomnia. In the Kline-Levin syndrome there are periodic attacks of hypersomnolence, accompanied by bulimia, irritability, behavioral changes, and uninhibited sexuality. Neurons in the lateral hypothalamus synthesize hypocretin, a chemical involved in the pathogenesis of narcolepsy, and project to brainstem regions involved in rapid-eye-movement sleep. Disturbances of sexual function and sexual development occur with hypothalamic lesions, including precocious puberty and sexual infantilism.

The hypothalamus is involved with emotions. It is the center that coordinates the neural and humoral mechanisms of emotional expression. Hypothalamic lesions in animals may cause "sham rage," with pupillary dilatation, increased pulse rate and BP, piloerection, and other signs of sympathetic overactivity. These physical manifestations suggest an intense emotional reaction is taking place, but there is no change in affect.

Brainstem disorders commonly cause autonomic dysfunction, including paroxysmal hypertension, profound bradycardia, intractable vomiting, central hypo- and hyperventilation, neurogenic pulmonary edema, and Horner's syndrome. The automatic and the voluntary breathing pathways are separated in the brainstem and upper spinal cord. Selective damage of the pathways subserving automatic breathing may cause respiratory insufficiency during sleep, with preserved respiration during wakefulness (Ondine's curse).

The Cushing reflex, or Cushing triad, is bradycardia, hypertension, and slow, irregular respirations due to brainstem compromise and has ominous prognostic implications. Myelopathy, particularly spinal cord injury, is often associated with severe dysautonomia.

Peripheral autonomic failure results from disorders that involve the autonomic ganglia or postganglionic nerve fibers. The syndrome of pure autonomic failure is a slowly progressive, degenerative disorder of the ANS in which dysautonomia occurs in isolation, without other evidence of neurologic disease. Dysautonomia occurs commonly in some peripheral nerve disorders. It may develop acutely in Guillain-Barré syndrome, porphyria, and some paraneoplastic neuropathies. Acute pandysautonomia is a condition probably akin to Guillain-Barré syndrome but in which dysautonomia occurs in isolation. Chronic neuropathies often associated with major autonomic dysfunction include diabetes mellitus, alcoholism, amyloidosis, hereditary sensory autonomic neuropathy type III (Riley-Day syndrome), Fabry's disease, and vincristine toxicity. The most common cause of autonomic neuropathy is diabetes mellitus. Patients typically develop orthostatic hypotension, impotence, gastroparesis, constipation alternating with diarrhea, nocturnal diarrhea, and difficulty voiding. Autoimmune attack on autonomic ganglia may cause severe autonomic failure.

Dysautonomia may accompany disorders of neuromuscular transmission, particularly Lambert-Eaton syndrome and botulism, in which the defect is presynaptic and acetylcholine release is impaired at autonomic synapses as well as at neuromuscular junctions. Some autonomic disorders occur in a restricted distribution or involve a particular organ system. Autonomic disorders of the pupil include Argyll Robertson and Adie's pupils, Horner's syndrome, and third cranial nerve palsy. Dysautonomia primarily involving the vascular system may cause Raynaud's phenomenon, acrocyanosis, erythromelalgia (Weir Mitchell syndrome), and livedo reticularis. Autonomic dysfunction of the genitalia causing erectile dysfunction and other abnormalities is common, especially in diabetes mellitus. Abnormalities of sweating occur frequently and are sometimes the only manifestation of the autonomic disturbance. Autonomic dysregulation is a common component of complex regional pain syndromes (reflex sympathetic dystrophy) and occurs in the same distribution as the pain.

The Bladder

Bladder function involves both the autonomic and the voluntary nervous systems, and disorders of bladder function may follow lesions of the paracentral lobule, hypothalamus, descending pathways in the spinal cord, pre- or postganglionic parasympathetic nerves, or pudendal nerve. The detrusor muscle of the bladder is innervated by parasympathetic neurons located in the S2-S4 intermediolateral column (Figure 45.7). Onuf's nucleus consists of additional motor neurons located in the nearby anterior horn at the same levels. The axons from Onuf's nucleus innervate the external urethral sphincter. There is a curious preservation of the Onuf nucleus neurons in amyotrophic lateral sclerosis. The internal urethral sphincter at the neck of the bladder receives its innervation from the intermediolateral column at the T12-L1 level, via the sympathetic prevertebral plexus and the hypogastric nerve.

Micturition is a spinobulbospinal reflex. In response to stretch, afferent impulses are carried to the sacral spinal cord. Sacral cord projections to the PAG are relayed to the pontine micturition center (Barrington's nucleus) in the dorsomedial pontine tegmentum, near the locus caeruleus, which sends descending fibers to the preganglionic parasympathetic motoneurons in the sacral cord innervating the bladder. The pontine micturition center is under the control of centers in the forebrain. Descending impulses activate the efferent centers in the sacral cord, causing contraction of the detrusor muscle and relaxation of the internal sphincter. In the infant, bladder function is purely reflex, but with cortical maturation and the completion of myelination inhibitory control over this reflex develops, as well as voluntary regulation of the external sphincter. Normal micturition requires intact autonomic and spinal pathways, and cerebral inhibition and control of the external sphincter must be normal.

Forebrain lesions may cause loss of voluntary bladder control, but do not affect the spinobulbospinal reflex mechanisms. Disruption of the bulbospinal pathway from the pontine micturition center to the sacral cord, and lesions affecting the afferent and efferent connections between the bladder and the conus medullaris, may cause severe disturbances in bladder function.

The term neurogenic bladder refers to bladder dysfunction caused by disease of the nervous system.

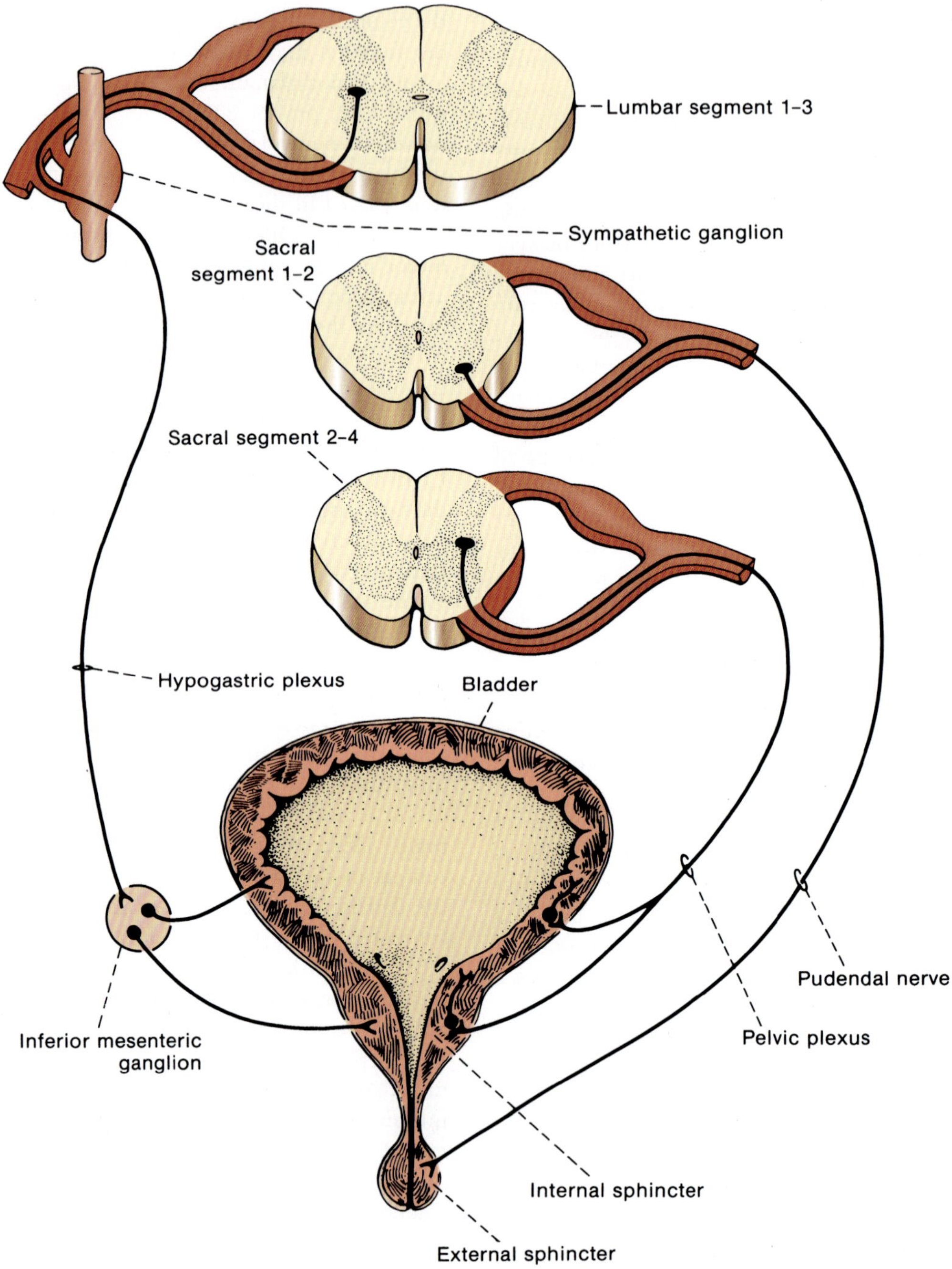

FIGURE 45.7 Innervation of the urinary bladder.

Symptoms of bladder dysfunction are often among the earliest manifestations of nervous system disease. Frequency, urgency, precipitate micturition, massive or dribbling incontinence, difficulty in initiating urination, urinary retention, and loss of bladder sensation may occur. One practical classification of neurogenic bladder dysfunction is based on urodynamic criteria and includes the following types: uninhibited, reflex, autonomous, sensory paralytic, and motor paralytic.

In the uninhibited neurogenic bladder, there is a loss of the cortical inhibition of reflex voiding, although bladder tone remains normal. Bladder distention causes contraction in response to the stretch reflex. There is frequency, urgency, and incontinence that are not associated with dysuria. Hesitancy may precede urgency. Bladder sensation is usually normal. There is no residual urine. The reflex neurogenic bladder occurs with severe myelopathy or extensive brain lesions causing interruption of both the descending autonomic tracts to the bladder and the ascending sensory pathways above the sacral segments of the cord. The bladder capacity is small, and micturition is reflex and involuntary. The residual urine volume is variable. An autonomous neurogenic bladder is one without external innervation. It is caused by neoplastic, traumatic, inflammatory, and other lesions of the sacral spinal cord, conus medullaris or cauda equina, S2-S4 motor or sensory roots, or the peripheral nerves, and with congenital anomalies such as spina bifida. There is destruction of the parasympathetic supply. Sensation is absent, and there is no reflex or voluntary control of the bladder; contractions occur as the result of stimulation of the intrinsic neural plexuses within the bladder wall. The amount of residual urine is large, but the bladder capacity is not greatly increased. A sensory paralytic bladder is found with lesions that involve the posterior roots or posterior root ganglia of the sacral nerves, or the posterior columns of the spinal cord. Sensation is absent, and there is no desire to void. There may be distention, dribbling, and difficulty both in initiating micturition and in emptying the bladder. There is a large amount of residual urine. A motor paralytic bladder develops when the motor nerve supply to the bladder is interrupted. The bladder distends and decompensates, but sensation is normal. The residual urine and bladder capacity vary.

Sexual Function

Disturbed sexual function is common in dysautonomia. In the genital (sex, ejaculatory, coital) reflex, arousal causes penile erection and sometimes ejaculation. Erection is a parasympathetic function mediated through S2-S4; ejaculation is a largely sympathetic function mediated by the lumbar nerves. Autonomic insufficiency usually causes impotence, but pathologic exaggeration of the sexual reflex may occur as part of the mass reflex, a spinal defense reflex seen in severe myelopathy (see Chapter 40), and may produce priapism and occasionally ejaculation after minimal stimulation. In autonomic neuropathy, especially from diabetes, retrograde ejaculation may precede the development of impotence. Because the internal vesical sphincter does not close, semen goes into the bladder rather than externally through the urethra. The patient with retrograde ejaculation may notice milky-appearing urine.

BIBLIOGRAPHY

Adkisson WO, Benditt DG. Syncope due to autonomic dysfunction: diagnosis and management. *Med Clin North Am* 2015;99:691–710.

Alexander MS. Autonomic function and spinal cord injury: are we at a crossroads? *Spinal Cord* 2008;46:402–405.

Ay H, Koroshetz WJ, Benner T, et al. Neuroanatomic correlates of stroke-related myocardial injury. *Neurology* 2006;66:1325–1329.

Baguley IJ. Autonomic complications following central nervous system injury. *Semin Neurol* 2008;28:716–725.

Baranchuk A, Nault MA, Morillo CA. The central nervous system and sudden cardiac death: what should we know? *Cardiol J* 2009;16:105–112.

Benarroch EE. The central autonomic network: functional organization, dysfunction, and perspective. *Mayo Clin Proc* 1993;68:988–1001.

Benarroch EE. Brainstem respiratory control: substrates of respiratory failure of multiple system atrophy. *Mov Disord* 2007;22:155–161.

Benarroch EE, Chang FI. Central autonomic disorders. *J Neurophysiol* 1993;10:39–50.

Benarroch E, Freeman R, Kaufmann H. Autonomic nervous system. In: Goetz CG, ed. *Textbook of Clinical Neurology*. Philadelphia: Saunders, 2003.

Blok BF, Holstege G. Direct projections from the periaqueductal gray to the pontine micturition center (M-region). An anterograde and retrograde tracing study in the cat. *Neurosci Lett* 1994;166:93–96.

Blok BF, Holstege G. The central nervous system control of micturition in cats and humans. *Behav Brain Res* 1998;92:119–125.

Cheshire WP. Autonomic disorders and their management. In: Goldman L, Schafer AI, eds. *Goldman-Cecil Medicine*. 25th ed. Philadelphia: W.B. Elsevier/Saunders, 2016.

Cheshire WP Jr, Saper CB. The insular cortex and cardiac response to stroke. *Neurology* 2006;66:1296–1297.

Drummond PD. Mechanisms of autonomic disturbance in the face during and between attacks of cluster headache. *Cephalalgia* 2006;26:633–641.

Duchesne M, Richard L, et al. Assessing sudomotor impairment in patients with peripheral neuropathy: comparison between electrochemical skin conductance and skin biopsy. *Clin Neurophysiol* 2018;129:1341–1348.

England JD, Gronseth GS, Franklin G, et al. Practice parameter: the evaluation of distal symmetric polyneuropathy: the role of autonomic testing, nerve biopsy, and skin biopsy (an evidence-based review). Report of the American Academy of Neurology, the American Association of Neuromuscular and Electrodiagnostic Medicine, and the American Academy of Physical Medicine and Rehabilitation. *PM R* 2009;1:14–22.

Elmquist JK, Elias CF, Saper CB. From lesions to leptin: hypothalamic control of food intake and body weight. *Neuron* 1999;22:221–232.

Etienne M, Weimer LH. Immune-mediated autonomic neuropathies. *Curr Neurol Neurosci Rep* 2006;6:57–64.

Fessel J, Robertson D. Orthostatic hypertension: when pressor reflexes overcompensate. *Nat Clin Pract Nephrol* 2006;2:424–431.

Freeman R. Autonomic peripheral neuropathy. *Neurol Clin* 2007;25:277–301.

Freeman R, Chapleau MW. Testing the autonomic nervous system. *Handb Clin Neurol* 2013;115:115–136.

Freeman R, Dover JS. Autonomic neurodermatology (Part I): erythromelalgia, reflex sympathetic dystrophy, and livedo reticularis. *Semin Neurol* 1992;12:385–393.

Freeman R, Schachter SC. Autonomic epilepsy. *Semin Neurol* 1995;15:158–166.

Freeman R, Waldorf HA, Dover JS. Autonomic neurodermatology (Part II): disorders of sweating and flushing. *Semin Neurol* 1992;12:394–407.

Goldstein DS, Robertson D, Esler M, et al. Dysautonomias: clinical disorders of the autonomic nervous system. *Ann Intern Med* 2002;137:753–763.

Haensch CA, Jorg J. Autonomic dysfunction in multiple sclerosis. *J Neurol* 2006;253(suppl 1):I3–I9.

Jones PK, Gibbons CH. Autonomic function testing: an important diagnostic test for patients with syncope. *Pract Neurol* 2015;15:346–351.

Kandel ER. *Principles of Neural Science*. 5th ed. New York: McGraw-Hill Medical, 2013.

Kaufmann H. Neurally mediated syncope and syncope due to autonomic failure: differences and similarities. *J Clin Neurophysiol* 1997;14:183–196.

Kimpinski K, Iodice V, Sandroni P, et al. Sudomotor dysfunction in autoimmune autonomic ganglionopathy. *Neurology* 2009;73: 1501–1506.

Klein CM. Evaluation and management of autonomic nervous system disorders. *Semin Neurol* 2008;28:195–204.

Klein CM, Vernino S, Lennon VA, et al. The spectrum of autoimmune autonomic neuropathies. *Ann Neurol* 2003;53:752–758.

Leone M, Bussone G. Pathophysiology of trigeminal autonomic cephalalgias. *Lancet Neurol* 2009;8:755–764.

Low PA, Opfer-Gehrking TL, Textor SC, et al. Postural tachycardia syndrome (POTS). *Neurology* 1995;45:S19–S25.

Low PA, Vernino S, Suarez G. Autonomic dysfunction in peripheral nerve disease. *Muscle Nerve* 2003;27:646–661.

Luigetti M, Primiano G, Cuccagna C, et al. Small fibre neuropathy in mitochondrial diseases explored with sudoscan. *Clin Neurophysiol* 2018;129:1618–1623.

Mehr SE, Barbul A, Shibao CA. Gastrointestinal symptoms in postural tachycardia syndrome: a systematic review. *Clin Auton Res* 2018;28:411–421.

Pasnoor M, Dimachkie MM. Chronic autonomic neuropathies. In: Roos RP, Editor-in-Chief. *MedLink Neurology*. San Diego: MedLink Corporation. www.medlink.com. Accessed January 7, 2016.

Perkes I, Baguley IJ, Nott MT, et al. A review of paroxysmal sympathetic hyperactivity after acquired brain injury. *Ann Neurol* 2010;68:126–135.

Pischik E, Kauppinen R. Neurological manifestations of acute intermittent porphyria. *Cell Mol Biol (Noisy-le-grand)* 2009;55:72–83.

Rajan S, Campagnolo M, Callaghan B, et al. Sudomotor function testing by electrochemical skin conductance: does it really measure sudomotor function? *Clin Auton Res* 2018. [Epub ahead of print].

Ravits JM. AAEM minimonograph #48: autonomic nervous system testing. *Muscle Nerve* 1997;20:919–937.

Ropper AH, Samuels MA, Klein J. *Adams and Victor's Principles of Neurology*. 10th ed. New York: McGraw-Hill Education Medical, 2014.

Saper CB. "All fall down": the mechanism of orthostatic hypotension in multiple systems atrophy and Parkinson's disease. *Ann Neurol* 1998;43:149.

Sedy J, Zicha J, Kunes J, et al. Mechanisms of neurogenic pulmonary edema development. *Physiol Res* 2008;57:499–506.

Shields RW. Functional anatomy of the autonomic nervous system. *J Neurophysiol* 1993;10:2–13.

Shivaprasad C, Amit G, Anish K, et al. Clinical correlates of sudomotor dysfunction in patients with type 2 diabetes and peripheral neuropathy. *Diabetes Res Clin Pract* 2018;139: 188–194.

Tabbaa MA, Leshner RT, Campbell WW. Malignant thymoma with dysautonomia and disordered neuromuscular transmission. *Arch Neurol* 1986;43:955–957.

Vernino S. Antibody testing as a diagnostic tool in autonomic disorders. *Clin Auton Res* 2009;19:13–19.

Vernino S, Sandroni P, Singer W, et al. Invited article: autonomic ganglia: target and novel therapeutic tool. *Neurology* 2008;70:1926–1932.

Vianna DM, Brandao ML. Anatomical connections of the periaqueductal gray: specific neural substrates for different kinds of fear. *Braz J Med Biol Res* 2003;36:557–566.

Weimer LH. Autonomic testing: common techniques and clinical applications. *Neurologist* 2010;16:215–222.

Zilliox L, Russell JW, Weimer LH. Acute autonomic neuropathies. In: Weimer LH, Editor-in-Chief. *MedLink Neurology*. San Diego: MedLink Corporation. www.medlink.com. Accessed May 24, 2018.

Zimmerman M, Pourhamidi K, Rolandsson O, et al. Autonomic neuropathy-a prospective cohort study of symptoms and *E/I* ratio in normal glucose tolerance, impaired glucose tolerance, and type 2 diabetes. *Front Neurol* 2018;9:154.

CHAPTER 46

Peripheral Neuroanatomy and Focal Neuropathies

Focal neuropathies may result from compression, entrapment, ischemia, stretch, direct trauma such as lacerations and missile wounds, involvement in fractures or dislocations, and other processes. Although carpal tunnel syndrome (CTS), ulnar neuropathy at the elbow (UNE), peroneal neuropathy at the knee, retrohumeral radial neuropathy, and facial neuropathy constitute the majority of focal neuropathies, virtually any nerve in the body can be compressed or entrapped. This chapter reviews the gross anatomy of the peripheral nervous system and some of the more common focal neuropathies. The microanatomy and physiology of peripheral nerve are discussed in Chapter 23.

PERIPHERAL NEUROANATOMY

Cervical Plexus

The cervical plexus is formed by the anterior primary rami of C1-C4. These divide into anterior and posterior branches or divisions that unite to form three anastomotic loops. The cervical plexus is situated in the lateral neck, adjacent to the upper four cervical vertebrae deep to the sternocleidomastoid muscle. The phrenic nerve is the most important nerve derived from the cervical plexus; it arises from C3, C4, and sometimes C5 and innervates the diaphragm. Other motor branches innervate the paravertebral muscles, scalenus medius, and levator scapulae; join with CN IX to supply portions of the trapezius muscle; or connect with CN XII (Figure 20.2). The most notable cutaneous nerves are the greater occipital (primarily C2) and the great auricular. Postganglionic sympathetic nerve fibers that originate in the superior cervical ganglion also traverse the cervical plexus.

Damage to the cervical plexus may occur from surgical trauma (e.g., radical neck dissections or carotid endarterectomy) or penetrating injuries. Nonpenetrating violent trauma occurs from motor vehicle, especially motorcycle, accidents. Other processes that may damage the cervical plexus include invasion by neoplasm, usually metastases or lymphomas and squamous cell carcinomas of the head and neck, and iatrogenic causes, for example, radiation therapy or intraoperative positioning. The most serious manifestation of cervical plexopathies is involvement of the phrenic nerve (see below).

Brachial Plexus

The brachial plexus (BP) arises from the anterior primary rami of C5-T1 (Figure 46.1). The posterior primary rami leave the spinal nerves just after they exit to innervate the paraspinal muscles. Assessment of the paraspinal muscles by needle electromyography is essential in localizing a disease process to the brachial or lumbosacral plexus (LSP) and excluding radiculopathy. The phrenic, long thoracic, and dorsal scapular nerves come off at root level, and this feature can sometimes help in localization of plexus lesions. The plexus is made up of upper, middle, and lower trunks; anterior and posterior divisions; medial, lateral, and posterior cords; and terminal branches. The C5 and C6 roots join to form the upper trunk. The suprascapular nerve to the supraspinatus and infraspinatus comes off the upper trunk, making the spinati the most proximal muscles innervated by the plexus proper. The C7 anterior primary ramus continues as the middle trunk. The C8 and T1 rami combine to form the lower trunk. The trunks are named for their relationship to one another.

The three trunks slope laterally and then split into anterior and posterior divisions, from which

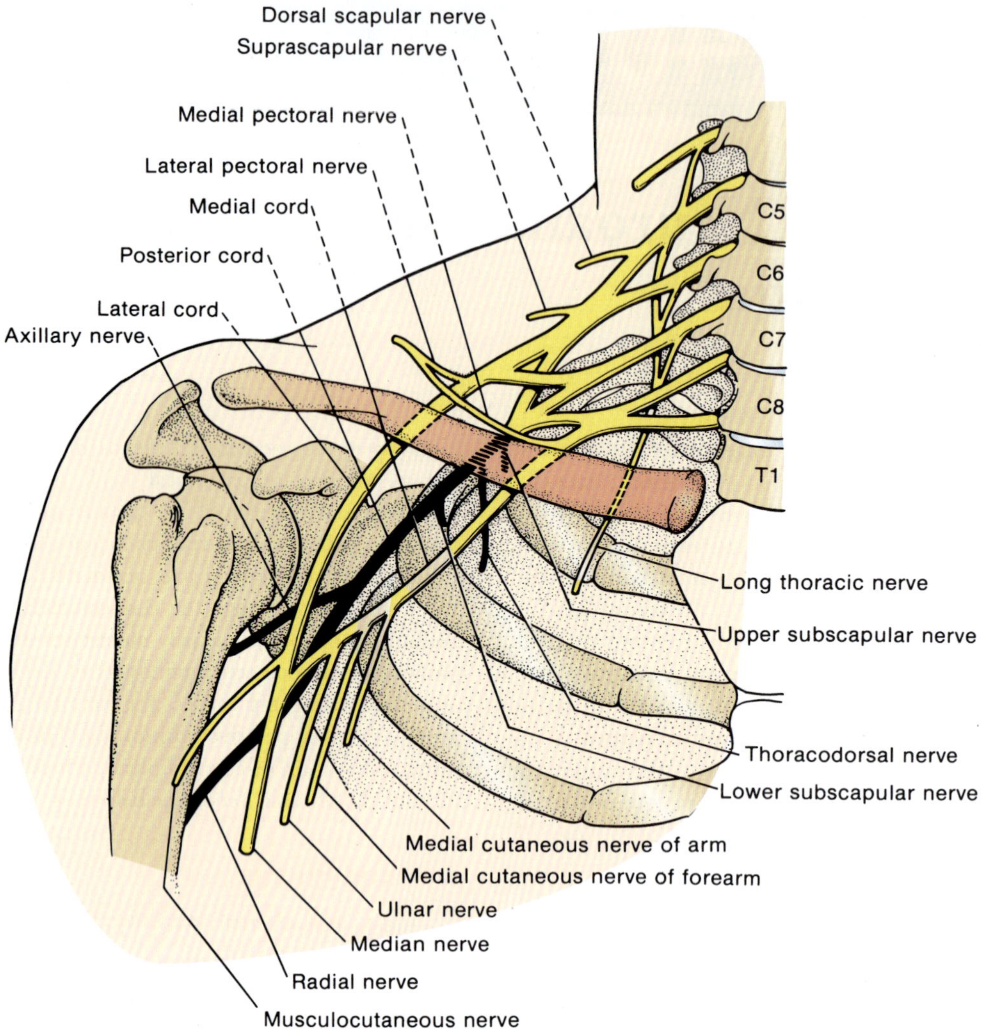

FIGURE 46.1 Brachial plexus showing its various constituents and their relationship to structures in the region of the upper chest, axilla, and shoulder.

the three cords are derived. The lower trunk is adjacent to the apex of the lung. The cords of the BP are named for their anatomical relationships to the axillary artery. All the posterior divisions come together to form the posterior cord, which lies posterior to the artery. It is smaller than the other cords and contains little if any contribution from T1. It divides into two major terminal branches: the radial and axillary nerves. The anterior divisions form the medial and lateral cords. The anterior divisions of the upper and middle trunk combine to form the lateral cord, which lies lateral to the artery and terminates in two major branches: the musculocutaneous nerve and the lateral head of the median nerve. The lateral head of the median carries all median sensory functions and the motor innervation to the pronator teres and flexor carpi radialis. The anterior division of the lower trunk continues as the medial cord, which lies medial to the artery, and also terminates in two major branches: the medial head of the median nerve and the ulnar nerve. The medial head of the median nerve carries all of the other median motor functions but has no cutaneous sensory component. After giving off the medial head to the median nerve, the medial cord continues as the ulnar nerve. As a generalization, the posterior cord supplies the extensor muscles, and the lateral and medial cords the flexor muscles.

The roots and trunks of the plexus lie in the posterior triangle of the neck, in the angle between the clavicle and the posteroinferior border of the sternocleidomastoid; the cords lie in the axilla; the divisions span the gap and lie approximately beneath the medial two-thirds of the clavicle, between the clavicle and the first rib. The cords are the longest component of the plexus. In the lower axilla, the BP divides into its terminal branches. The plexus is sometimes divided into a supraclavicular portion (roots and trunks) and an infraclavicular portion (divisions, cords, and terminal branches). In other schemes, the divisions are said to join the supra- and infraclavicular portions of the plexus. The BP is also broadly divided into the upper plexus (upper trunk and lateral cord) and lower plexus (lower trunk and medial cord). Some pathologic processes have a predilection for different parts of the plexus. Trauma is particularly likely to affect the upper plexus (e.g., Erb's palsy); lower plexopathies are often nontraumatic (e.g., Pancoast tumor or thoracic outlet syndrome). The terminal branches of the BP may be divided into a supraclavicular and an infraclavicular group. The clinically important supraclavicular nerves are the phrenic, long thoracic, suprascapular, and dorsal scapular. The other terminal branches are infraclavicular.

The BP can be involved in a plethora of disease processes. The most common and clinically important of these include neuralgic amyotrophy (NA); trauma, such as with missile and stab wounds or motor vehicle (especially motorcycle) accidents; neoplasms; postradiation plexopathy; obstetrical palsies; postsurgical plexopathy; the "stinger" or "burner" phenomenon that frequently affects football players, which is likely a mild form of plexus injury; and thoracic outlet syndrome.

NA (brachial plexitis, acute BP neuropathy, acute brachial plexopathy, Parsonage-Turner syndrome) is a fairly stereotyped clinical syndrome characterized by the acute onset of pain in the shoulder and upper arm, followed by weakness, then atrophy, of variable severity, primarily affecting upper arm and shoulder muscles. The BP can sustain injury in a number of ways: missile and stab wounds, motor vehicle (especially motorcycle) accidents, football, and iatrogenically. Stretch injuries of the plexus occur during childbirth and usually involve the upper plexus (Erb's palsy), much less often the lower plexus (Klumpke's palsy) or the entire plexus. Neoplasms, especially breast and lung, may invade the plexus. Radiation plexopathy may complicate treatment of such tumors and appears after a delay of months to years. This is also the time frame in which the radiation therapy may have kept a tumor at bay. Distinguishing recurrent tumor from radiation plexopathy is often difficult.

Other etiologies of brachial plexopathy include external compression (e.g., backpack or rucksack palsy), compression from an internal process (e.g., encroachment on the lower BP from a Pancoast tumor), or involvement in systemic processes such as systemic lupus erythematosus (SLE) or sarcoid, or iatrogenic plexopathy during cardiac surgery. The plexus may rarely be involved in a number of other conditions, including lupus, lymphoma, Ehlers-Danlos syndrome, and infectious or parainfectious disorders. Some of these processes are by nature progressive.

With pressure injuries, the same general rules apply as for other nerves. Mild lesions produce primarily demyelination and can cause severe clinical deficits but have an excellent prognosis. With plexopathies, there may be the additional complication of disease progression. Many of the conditions that affect the plexi are not static. Pancoast tumors continue to grow, radiation damage tends to progress, and systemic diseases such as SLE continue their activity. All these mechanisms of injury make the pathophysiology of plexopathies complex and the clinical evaluation challenging.

The Phrenic Nerve

The phrenic nerve arises from the phrenic nucleus at C3-C5; it also carries some sensory filaments from the diaphragm, pericardium, and pleura. The fibers of the phrenic nerve arise from root level. Unilateral diaphragmatic paralysis is frequently asymptomatic, except for orthopnea and exertional dyspnea. With bilateral paralysis, there is dyspnea on the slightest exertion, a scaphoid abdomen that does not protrude on expiration, absence of Litten's sign, increased excursion of the costal margins, retraction of the epigastrium on inspiration, overactivity of the accessory respiratory muscles, and difficulty in coughing, sneezing, or making quick forceful inspiratory movements such as sniffing.

The nerve may be involved in NA, damaged by surgical procedures on the neck or chest, or compressed in the mediastinum by enlarged nodes, aneurysms, or neoplasms. The segmental supply to the diaphragm is frequently compromised in upper spinal cord injuries and determines whether the quadriplegic patient will or will not be able to live without a ventilator. Involvement of phrenic motor neurons is common in amyotrophic lateral sclerosis. Other causes of phrenic neuropathy include diabetes mellitus, mediastinal irradiation, sarcoidosis, tuberculosis, Lyme disease, and acute and chronic inflammatory demyelinating polyneuropathies. Idiopathic bilateral phrenic neuropathies causing diaphragmatic paralysis may occur.

The Long Thoracic Nerve

This nerve is derived from the C5-C7 roots and supplies the serratus anterior muscle. Paralysis of the serratus anterior muscle causes winging of the scapula (Figure 27.8). The long thoracic nerve (LTN) may be injured by pressure from carrying heavy objects or packs on the shoulder (backpack or rucksack palsy) or by penetrating wounds. It may be involved in NA, sometimes in isolation. Iatrogenic LTN palsy may follow anesthesia or local invasive procedures on the anterolateral aspect of the thorax. Paralysis may also occur with myopathic processes, such as facioscapulohumeral (FSH) dystrophy and the scapuloperoneal syndromes.

The Dorsal Scapular Nerve

The dorsal scapular nerve arises directly from the C5 nerve root to innervate the rhomboid muscles. Weakness causes lateral displacement of the vertebral border of the scapula and lateral displacement of the inferior angle. Atrophy may be obscured by the overlying trapezius. Isolated lesions have been reported in bodybuilders. It is occasionally of importance, especially electromyographically, in distinguishing between C5 radiculopathy and upper trunk brachial plexopathy.

The Suprascapular Nerve

This nerve is derived from C5-C6 and arises from the upper trunk. It runs posteriorly through the suprascapular notch, beneath the suprascapular ligament, to innervate the supraspinatus muscle, and then around the glenoid process of the spine of the scapula in the spinoglenoid notch to reach the infraspinous fossa and innervate the infraspinatus. The nerve may be entrapped at the suprascapular notch, causing pain and weakness of both supraspinatus and infraspinatus, or at the spinoglenoid notch, causing weakness of only the infraspinatus. Because of selective fascicular vulnerability, a lesion at the suprascapular notch may also involve only the infraspinatus branch. A common cause of suprascapular neuropathy is NA.

The most common causes of suprascapular neuropathy are occupational overuse, sports-related injury, direct trauma, and ganglion cysts. Suprascapular neuropathy may occur after scapular fracture or by direct pressure (mobile telephone user's shoulder droop). Repetitive motion injuries in sports that particularly involve strenuous overhead activity pose a particular hazard. The prevalence of infraspinatus muscle atrophy in the hitting shoulders of professional beach volleyball players is 30%.

The Axillary Nerve

The axillary (circumflex) nerve is a terminal branch of the posterior cord of the BP derived from C5-C6. It accompanies the posterior humeral circumflex artery through the quadrangular space and then divides into anterior and posterior branches. The anterior branch supplies the anterior part of the deltoid muscle; the posterior branch supplies the posterior part of the deltoid and the teres minor muscles and sends sensory twigs to a small circular area of skin over the deltoid muscle just above the deltoid attachment. Axillary nerve lesions are usually due to trauma or NA. The nerve may be injured by fracture or dislocation of the humeral head, penetrating wounds, misplaced therapeutic injections, arthroscopy, or direct blows to the shoulder. It is also prone to injury by overhead activity in sports, especially volleyball, tennis, and baseball. There is weakness and wasting of the deltoid, often profound, and a small patch of sensory loss over the shoulder. Isolated lesions of the anterior branch may spare sensation. Conversely, isolated involvement of the sensory branch has been reported after shoulder arthroscopy. Preservation of dorsal scapular and suprascapular nerve function helps distinguish axillary neuropathy from C5 radiculopathy and upper trunk plexopathy, but the evaluation of suprascapular nerve function must usually be made electromyographically, as both the deltoid and supraspinatus are shoulder abductors, and both the teres minor and infraspinatus are external rotators.

The Musculocutaneous Nerve

This nerve is derived from C5-C7 and is a terminal branch of the lateral cord. It passes into the upper arm in the groove between the deltoid and pectoral muscles, sends a branch to the coracobrachialis muscle, then traverses a foramen in the muscle, after which it descends and innervates the biceps and most of the brachialis. At the elbow, it pierces the deep fascia just lateral to the biceps tendon and continues as the lateral antebrachial cutaneous nerve (lateral cutaneous nerve of the forearm) to supply sensation to the lateral

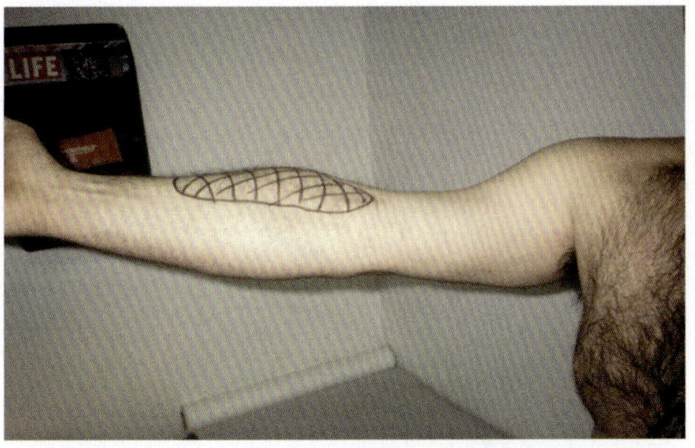

FIGURE 46.2 Musculocutaneous neuropathy after performing one-armed pull-ups. Note the striking biceps atrophy and sensory loss in the distribution of the lateral antebrachial cutaneous nerve.

aspect of the forearm from the elbow to the thenar eminence. The musculocutaneous may be injured by overly vigorous elbow flexion (weight lifter's palsy, Figure 46.2). There is weakness of elbow flexion with the forearm supinated and marked weakness of supination. The semipronated forearm can still be flexed by the brachioradialis. There is a relatively small area of sensory loss on the lateral surface of the forearm. The biceps reflex is diminished or absent. Preservation of axillary, dorsal scapular, and suprascapular nerve functions differentiates musculocutaneous palsy from an upper trunk lesion and C5 radiculopathy, and preservation of forearm pronation and lateral hand sensation, median nerve functions, distinguishes from a lateral cord lesion and C6 radiculopathy.

The Median Nerve

The median nerve has two components: a lateral division and a medial division. The lateral cord of the BP divides into two terminal branches: One becomes the musculocutaneous nerve, and the other becomes the lateral division of the median nerve. The medial cord of the BP also divides into two terminal branches: One forms the medial division of the median nerve, and the other continues as the ulnar nerve. The medial and lateral divisions of the median nerve join to form a single trunk, which passes through the upper arm without branching down to the region of the elbow (Figure 46.3). There, the branches begin to separate. Innervating twigs are given off from the lateral head to the pronator teres and flexor carpi radialis muscles.

The main trunk passes through the two heads of the pronator teres muscle and beneath an aponeurosis connecting the two heads of the flexor digitorum superficialis (the sublimis bridge). Just distal to the pronator teres, the nerve gives off the anterior interosseous nerve (AIN), which runs along the interosseous membrane and innervates the median head (lateral portion) of the flexor digitorum profundus (FDP), the flexor pollicis longus, and the pronator quadratus. The AIN has no cutaneous sensory component. The main trunk of the median nerve continues down the forearm, giving off muscular branches to the palmaris longus and flexor digitorum superficialis.

The median nerve crosses from the distal forearm to the hand through the carpal tunnel. The walls and floor of the tunnel are formed by the carpal bones and the roof by the transverse carpal ligament (TCL). The TCL evolves from the antebrachial fascia at about the level of the wrist crease and extends 4 to 6 cm into the palm. The passageway is narrowest 2.0 to 2.5 cm distal to its origin, which corresponds to the usual site of median nerve compression in CTS (Figure 46.4). Lying with the median nerve in the canal are the eight deep and superficial finger flexor tendons and the tendon of the flexor pollicis longus surrounded by a complex synovial sheath.

The palmar cutaneous branch of the median nerve leaves the main trunk 5 to 8 cm proximal to the wrist crease. It travels through its own separate passageway in the TCL and provides sensation to the thenar eminence; it does not traverse the carpal tunnel. Loss of sensation over the thenar eminence is not part of CTS and suggests a lesion proximal to the wrist. After exiting the carpal tunnel, the median nerve gives off its recurrent thenar motor branch, which curves backward and radially to innervate the median thenar muscles (abductor pollicis brevis, opponens pollicis, and lateral head of the flexor pollicis brevis). The nerve ends by giving off terminal motor branches to innervate the first and second lumbricals and then dividing into common digital sensory branches that carry sensory fibers from the palmar surfaces of the thumb and index and middle fingers, palmar aspect of the radial half of the ring finger, and the dorsal aspect of the middle and distal phalanges of the index and middle fingers and radial half of the ring finger. The finger flexor reflex is mediated in part by the median nerve. The pronator reflex, pronation of the forearm after tapping in the region of the radial styloid on the volar surface of the forearm, is also median innervated.

Carpal Tunnel Syndrome

Entrapment of the median nerve beneath the TCL is often brought on or exacerbated by excessive hand/wrist/finger movements; the combination of

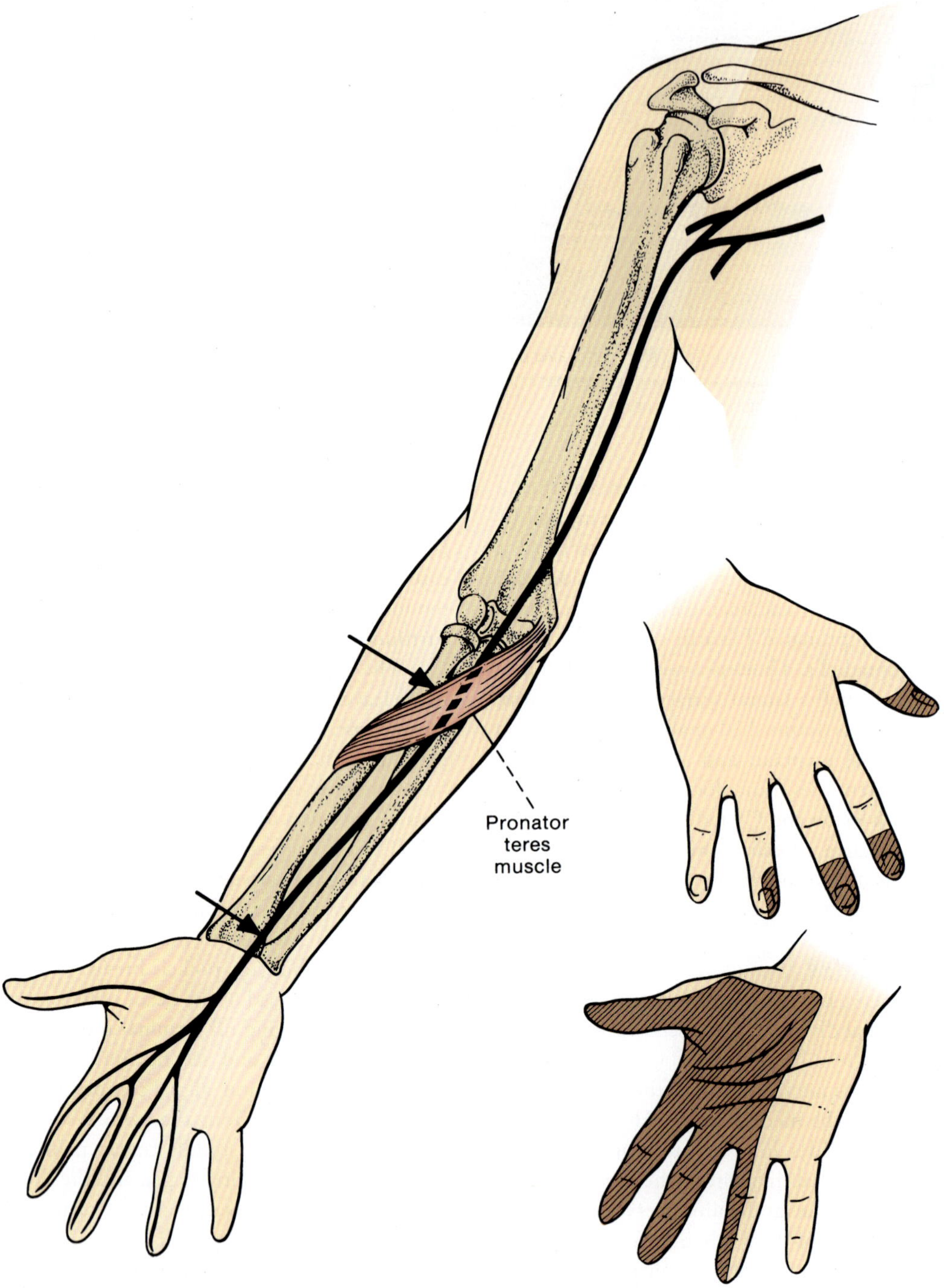

FIGURE 46.3 Common sites for injury to the median nerve and the distribution of sensory loss with a proximal median nerve lesion. In carpal tunnel syndrome (CTS), sensation over the thenar eminence is spared.

repetitive finger flexion with wrist motion seems to be the most hazardous ergonomic stress. Both vocational and recreational activities can incite or aggravate the condition. Although keyboarding is often blamed, the frequency of CTS in computer users is similar to that in the general population. CTS can rarely result from mass lesions narrowing the passageway (e.g., ganglion, osteophyte, lipoma, aneurysm, anomalous

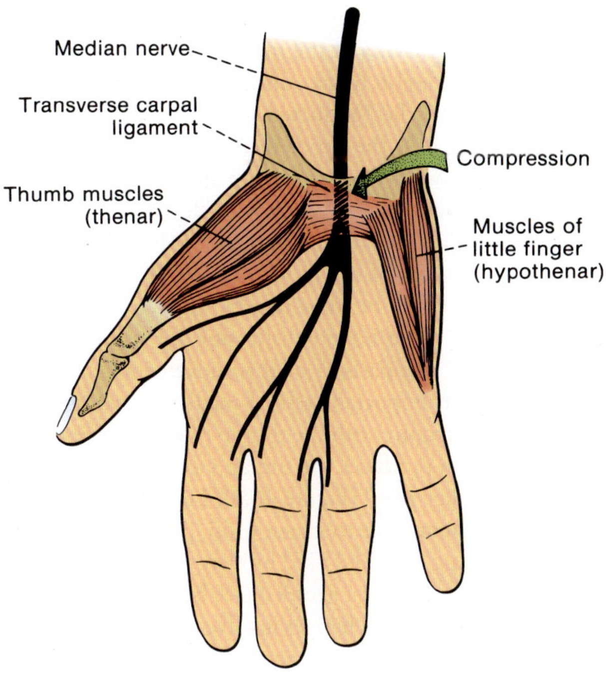

FIGURE 46.4 The relationship of the median nerve to the transverse carpal ligament and the site of compression in CTS.

muscle). Numerous systemic conditions predispose to CTS, including rheumatoid arthritis, diabetes mellitus, chronic renal insufficiency and hemodialysis, hypothyroidism, amyloidosis, myeloma, acromegaly, and pregnancy. Constriction within the carpal tunnel is often due to nonspecific tenosynovitis of the flexor tendons. A congenitally narrow canal may predispose some patients.

CTS produces a characteristic clinical picture of hand pain, numbness, and paresthesias, all usually more severe at night. Patients often claim relief by shaking or flicking (see below) the hand. The reason for the nocturnal exacerbation of symptoms remains obscure, but the diagnosis should remain suspect in the absence of this feature. Proximal upper-extremity pain, usually in the forearm but sometimes as far as the shoulder, is less typical but not uncommon. Many patients complain of "whole hand" numbness, and rarely, for unclear reasons, a patient with CTS may present with ulnar or even radial distribution paresthesias. In a survey of 100 patients with electrodiagnostically confirmed CTS and no other pathology, symptoms were most commonly reported in both median and ulnar digits, followed by median digits only and a glove distribution. Unusual sensory patterns were reported by some patients. In another study, over 50% of patients with exclusive CTS had tingling or numbness involving the whole hand, ulnar or radial nerve distributions. Some patients reported symptoms proximal to the wrist.

Findings on examination vary with the severity of the condition. Patients with mild CTS may have a normal physical exam or trivial sensory loss over the fingertips. The earliest sensory loss seems to occur over the volar tip of the middle finger. Patients with more advanced disease have more easily demonstrable sensory loss and frequently have weakness of the thenar muscles. The opponens pollicis is occasionally, and the abductor pollicis brevis rarely, innervated by the ulnar nerve and may be spared in some patients. The lumbrical muscles are usually spared. Although there may be sensory complaints in unusual distributions, sensory signs do not extend beyond the median nerve territory, recalling of course that there may be variations in the territory of cutaneous nerves (Figure 36.3).

Patients with severe involvement demonstrate thenar weakness and atrophy and dense sensory loss (Figure 29.2). Tinel's sign is paresthesias produced by percussion over a peripheral nerve that may indicate focal nerve pathology. Eliciting a Tinel's sign can be useful, but many normal patients "Tinel" over all their nerves; only the presence of a disproportionately active Tinel's sign over the clinically suspect nerve has any localizing value. Phalen's (wrist flexion) test is numbness or paresthesias in the median distribution produced by forceful flexion of the wrist for 1 minute.

The reverse Phalen's (prayer) test is the same but with the wrist hyperextended. In the carpal compression maneuver, the examiner applies firm thumb pressure over the median nerve at the wrist crease, seeking to reproduce CTS symptoms. These provocative tests have proven disappointing, with high proportions of false positives and false negatives. The "flick" sign, in which the patients flick the wrist to demonstrate what they do to "restore the circulation" at night, is more useful but still imperfect. The rare "reverse Tinel's sign" with paresthesias radiating retrograde up the forearm may be more specific for CTS. The tourniquet test (cuff compression test) seeks reproduction of pain and paresthesias with compression above systolic pressure. The elevated arm stress test (Roos test) has been touted as useful in both thoracic outlet syndrome and CTS but has a high incidence of false positives in both.

The most common differential diagnostic exercise is between CTS and cervical radiculopathy, most often C6. Neck and shoulder pain, weakness in C6 innervated muscles, reflex changes, sensory loss restricted to the thumb, the absence of nocturnal paresthesias, and reproduction of the paresthesias with root compression maneuvers all favor cervical radiculopathy. Other conditions occasionally meriting consideration include proximal median neuropathy, neurogenic thoracic outlet syndrome, and upper brachial plexopathy. Various musculoskeletal conditions, especially de Quervain's tendonitis, can cause hand and wrist pain suggestive of CTS.

Proximal Median Neuropathy

The proximal median nerve is well protected by soft tissues and, accordingly, is injured less frequently than either the radial or the ulnar nerve. It may be involved in dislocations of the shoulder, injuries of the elbow joint, fractures of the humerus or radius, penetrating wounds, or compression injuries. The usual etiology is a supracondylar fracture. Proximal median neuropathy may be a complication of shunt placement for hemodialysis. Median neuropathy proximal to the carpal tunnel may occur in wheelchair athletes. A triad neuropathy is involvement of median, ulnar, and radial nerves, usually from a lesion in the axilla, for example, crutch palsy, or of the BP distal branches.

A complete proximal median nerve lesion causes paralysis of flexion of the wrist and radial fingers, forearm pronation, and thumb abduction, opposition, and flexion. Finger flexion at the metacarpophalangeal (MCP) joints may be partially preserved because of preserved interosseous function. Loss of ability to flex the distal phalanx of the index finger, without a bone or tendon lesion to account for it, is pathognomonic. The thumb lies adducted and extended; it cannot be opposed to the tip of the little finger or abducted at right angles to the palm (palmar abduction), and the terminal phalanx cannot be flexed (Figure 46.5). Many of the lost movements, except for flexion of the distal phalanx of the index finger and movements of the thumb, can be substituted for by ulnar-innervated muscles. There is no substitution for palmar abduction, and comparison of this movement on the two sides is an important test of median nerve function. Thenar atrophy with the thumb rotated and resting in adduction produces the simian (ape) hand deformity, or "monkey paw" (Figure 46.6). Loss of finger flexion when attempting to make a fist produces a posture resembling the hand used by clergy in making a benediction, a term best avoided (see below).

The sensory changes involve the radial side of the palm, including the thenar region (palmar cutaneous distribution), the index and middle fingers, and the radial half of the ring finger. They are less complete on the dorsum of the hand than on the palmar surface, and usually involve only the distal (or middle

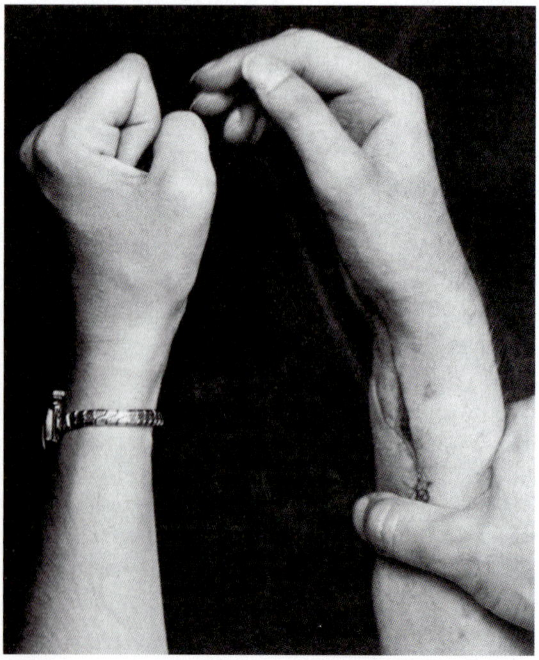

FIGURE 46.5 Motor changes secondary to a lesion of the median nerve, showing loss of flexion of the distal phalanges of the radial fingers.

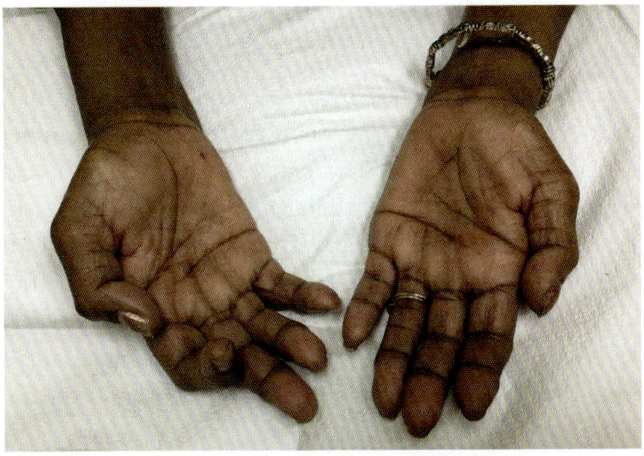

FIGURE 46.6 Simian hands in a patient with long-standing CIDP.

and distal) phalanges of the index and middle fingers, and sometimes part of the thumb and radial half of the ring finger (Figure 36.4). There are no significant reflex changes. Median nerve paralysis is often accompanied by vasomotor and trophic changes and by intractable, burning pain (causalgia, reflex sympathetic dystrophy, complex regional pain syndrome) especially if the lesion is incomplete. The skin may be flushed, cyanotic, and either wet or dry; the nails are brittle or striated, and there may be changes in hair growth.

The median nerve may rarely be entrapped by the ligament of Struthers, an anomalous fibrous band running from a distal humeral supracondylar spur to the medial epicondyle (ME). In the pronator teres syndrome, the median nerve is entrapped at the point where it passes through the two heads of the pronator teres; it may affect the main trunk, causing both motor and sensory dysfunction; more often, only the AIN is involved (Kiloh-Nevin syndrome). Hypertrophy of the pronator teres has been implicated. There is often pain in the proximal forearm, and there may be tenderness and/or a Tinel's sign over the pronator muscle. Depending on the individual anatomy and the origin of the branch to the pronator teres, the pronator teres may or may not be involved in a pronator syndrome. The pronator quadratus is involved with either proximal median neuropathy or the AIN syndrome; distinguishing between pronator teres and pronator quadratus requires careful elbow positioning (see Chapter 27).

Complete AIN paralysis causes inability to flex the distal phalanx of either the thumb or index finger. The patient cannot make a circle by touching the tip of the thumb to the tip of the index finger, making a triangle instead by touching the finger pads (pinch sign, or OK sign [the patient is unable to make the OK sign with the involved hand]) (Figure 46.7). There are no cutaneous sensory changes in AIN palsy, but there may be pain carried by afferent fibers innervating joints. AIN palsy often occurs as an isolated manifestation of NA. Recent magnetic resonance imaging (MRI) evidence indicates the process in many cases predominantly involves AIN fascicles in the main trunk of the median nerve in the upper arm. Other etiologies include strenuous exertion, especially when involving flexion and pronation of the forearm, and trauma, for example, fracture, venipuncture, penetrating injury, and intraoperative positioning.

The Ulnar Nerve

The ulnar nerve arises as a continuation of the medial cord of the BP. As it exits from the thorax, it passes through the axilla and into the upper arm lying medial to the brachial artery in a common

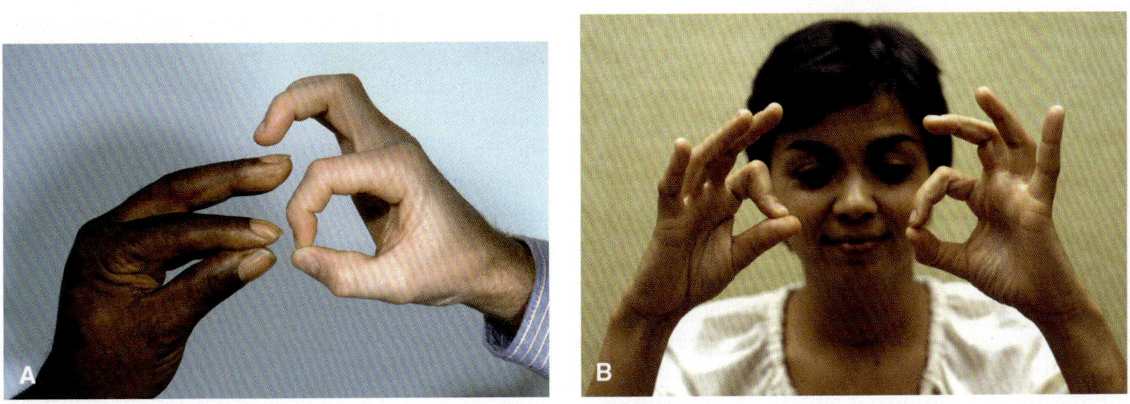

FIGURE 46.7 Anterior interosseous neuropathy; the patient is unable to flex the distal phalanx of the thumb or index finger and is thus unable to make the "OK sign." **A.** Patient on the left, control on the right. **B.** Involved side is the patient's right.

neurovascular sheath with the median nerve and the medial brachial and antebrachial cutaneous nerves. At about the level of the insertion of the coracobrachialis, the ulnar leaves the common neurovascular bundle and pierces the medial intermuscular septum to gain the posterior compartment of the arm. The nerve then descends toward the elbow in a groove alongside the medial head of the triceps. The point of the ulnar nerve's penetration of the medial intermuscular septum and the nearby deep fascia binding the nerve in the triceps groove are sometimes referred to as the arcade of Struthers, a potential entrapment site (not to be confused with the ligament of Struthers). Whether the arcade of Struthers actually exists remains a point of disagreement. After piercing the medial intermuscular septum, the nerve slants distally and medially and then traverses the retroepicondylar (RTC) (ulnar) groove between the ME and olecranon process (OP). It then passes beneath the humeroulnar aponeurotic arcade (HUA), a dense aponeurosis joining the humeral and ulnar heads of origin of the flexor carpi ulnaris (FCU) muscle, which typically lies 1.0 to 2.5 cm distal to a line connecting the ME and the OP.

After passing under the HUA, the nerve runs through the belly of the FCU, then exits through the deep flexor-pronator aponeurosis lining the deep surface of the muscle 4.0 to 6.0 cm beyond the ME, and then runs distally toward the wrist. The ulnar palmar cutaneous branch arises in the mid to distal forearm and pursues a separate course to the hand. It enters the hand superficial to Guyon's canal and supplies sensation to the skin of the hypothenar region. The large dorsal ulnar cutaneous (DUC) branch leaves the main trunk 5 to 10 cm proximal to the wrist to wind posteriorly and emerge on the dorsal surface of the wrist to provide sensation to the dorsal, ulnar aspect of the hand, as well as the small and ring fingers.

The ulnar nerve enters the hand through Guyon's canal. The TCL, which forms the roof of the carpal tunnel, dips downward as it spans medially and forms the floor of Guyon's canal. The pisohamate ligament, which runs from the pisiform bone to the hook of the hamate, forms the distal part of the floor of the canal. The volar carpal ligament, a thin investment that is basically a continuation of the deep forearm fascia, arches over and forms the roof of Guyon's canal along with the thin palmaris brevis muscle. The hook of the hamate forms the lateral, and the pisiform bone and FCU tendon the medial, boundaries.

As it emerges from beneath the volar carpal ligament, the ulnar gives a branch to the palmaris brevis and then branches into the superficial terminal sensory division and the deep palmar division. The deep branch exits Guyon's canal, passes through the pisohamate hiatus, and then arches laterally beneath the flexor tendons, innervating the interossei and breaking up into terminal branches on reaching the adductor pollicis and first dorsal interosseous. The deep head of the flexor pollicis brevis is usually supplied by a short twig from the terminal branch to the adductor pollicis.

Ulnar Neuropathy at the Elbow

UNE is most often due to compression in the RTC groove, but may be due to entrapment beneath the HUA, other entrapment sites are rare. UNE was originally described in patients with elbow deformities because of remote fracture and/or dislocation. The UNE occurred because of chronic compression and stretch and typically followed the injury by months or years (tardy ulnar palsy). Gradually, the term tardy ulnar palsy became a generic for any UNE, even without a history or evidence of elbow joint pathology. Compression at the HUA was actually recognized in the 1920s by Buzzard and Sargent, but it was not until the landmark Canadian papers of the 1950s that it became widely known. Fiendel and Stratford proposed the term *cubital tunnel syndrome* (cubit is Latin for elbow) to refer to compression by the HUA. The title of their paper is telling: "The role of the cubital tunnel in tardy ulnar palsy." Gradually, cubital tunnel syndrome has replaced tardy ulnar palsy as a generic referring to any UNE. The term is thus used very inconsistently, and has outlived its usefulness, but is very entrenched. Although rare cases of UNE are caused by ganglia, tumors, fibrous bands, or accessory muscles, most are caused by external compression, repeated trauma, or repetitive elbow flexion. Chronic minor trauma and compression, including leaning on the elbow, can result in UNE at the groove. It can also occur in patients who suffer compression during anesthesia or coma.

In the majority of patients with UNE, the initial symptoms are intermittent numbness and tingling in the ulnar nerve distribution, often associated with elbow flexion. Occasionally, the initial problems may be motor dysfunction, such as a feeling of weakness of grasp and pinch, or a loss of dexterity. Patients may not see a physician until the initially small degrees of intrinsic muscle atrophy become difficult to overlook.

A history of elbow fracture or dislocation, acute blunt trauma, chronic occupational trauma, or arthritis may be important. When there is no relevant history, entrapment at the HUA should be considered. An early motor symptom sometimes noted is loss of adduction of the small finger, which may cause the finger to get caught when the patient is trying to place the hand in a pocket, and examination may show an abducted posture of the small finger (Wartenberg's sign), both due to weakness of the third palmar interosseous muscle.

Examination usually discloses weakness of ulnar-innervated hand intrinsics. Not all intrinsics are necessarily involved to an equal degree; the first dorsal interosseous is the most commonly affected. Weakness of the adductor pollicis interferes with thumb adduction; impaired adduction is often tested by trying to elicit Froment's sign (Figure 46.8). The patient is asked to hold a piece of paper between palm and thumb, and the examiner attempts to withdraw it. With weak thumb adduction, the patient will substitute the flexor pollicis longus and flex the interphalangeal (IP) joint of the thumb. Weakness of the FCU and or the FDP to the ring and small fingers reliably point to an elbow lesion. However, the ulnar forearm muscles are frequently spared in UNE, so the lack of clinical, or even electromyographic, abnormality in these muscles in no way excludes a lesion at the elbow. Non–ulnar-innervated hand and forearm muscles should be systematically assessed in suspected ulnar neuropathy. Weakness of nonulnar muscles is the usual clue to disease involving the lower BP or C8 root. In the elbow flexion test, the elbow is held fully flexed and pressure applied just distal to the ulnar groove to elicit paresthesias. A variant is to hold the elbow flexed and the wrist flexed in ulnar deviation.

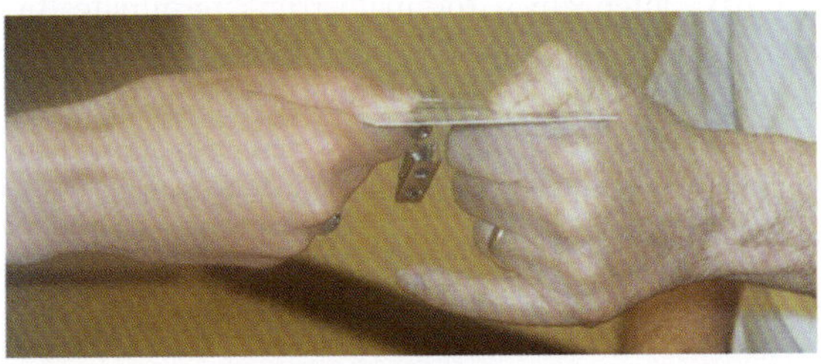

FIGURE 46.8 Froment's sign. The patient attempts to grasp a piece of paper between the thumb and the radial border of the hand. In ulnar neuropathy, the IP joint flexes to compensate for weakness of the adductor pollicis. (Reprinted with permission from Berg D, Worzala K, eds. *Atlas of Adult Physical Diagnosis*. Philadelphia: Lippincott Williams & Wilkins, 2006.)

The lumbricals flex the MCP joints and extend the IP joints. The lumbricals for the ring and small fingers are normally supplied by the ulnar nerve and those for the index and middle fingers by the median. In ulnar lesions, unopposed extensor tone at the fourth and fifth MCP joints and unopposed flexor tone at the IP joints produce the ulnar griffe or claw deformity (Figure 46.9). Clawing varies, depending upon the amount of muscle weakness, the laxity of the MCP joints, and the level of the lesion. A "low" (distal) ulnar lesion with preserved function of the FDP induces more clawing than a "high" (proximal) ulnar lesion, where the accompanying FDP weakness creates less of the unopposed flexor pull deforming the ring and small fingers. The term benediction hand (preacher's hand, papal hand) is sometimes used to refer to an ulnar griffe with the hand at rest, and sometimes to a high median neuropathy when the patient is attempting to make a fist. The hand posture is somewhat similar in that the ring and small fingers are flexed and the index and middle fingers are not. Usage favors median neuropathy in the neuroscience literature, ulnar neuropathy in the non-neuroscience literature. There is conjecture that a medieval pope had this hand deformity, and his successor learned it as the proper hand position for blessing the masses, passing it down as tradition.

Ulnar sensory loss is usually easiest to establish over the distal two phalanges of the little finger, as this is the autonomous zone of the ulnar nerve. Sensory abnormality is more often observed for tactile as opposed to pinprick and thermal sensations; two-point

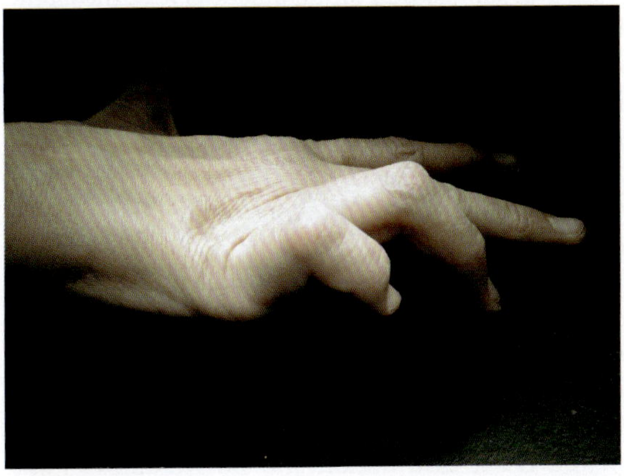

FIGURE 46.9 Clawing of the ulnar digits in low ulnar nerve palsy. (Reprinted with permission from Rayan GM, Akelman E, eds. *The Hand: Anatomy, Examination, and Diagnosis*. 4th ed. Philadelphia: Wolters Kluwer Health/Lippincott Williams & Wilkins, 2012.)

discrimination and ability to feel textures and light touch may constitute the most revealing tests. On the volar finger surface, the median and ulnar distributions usually split the ring finger, and such splitting fairly reliably excludes plexopathy and radiculopathy. However, in about 20% of cases, the ulnar nerve supplies the entire ring and ulnar half of the middle finger, or only the small finger. The DUC supplies the dorsal skin over the fifth and the ulnar half of the fourth metacarpal, and the same area of the fourth and fifth digits. The palmar cutaneous branch supplies the hypothenar eminence. There are many variations of this sensory distribution. The cutaneous field of the ulnar nerve does not extend more than a few centimeters proximal to the wrist crease. The medial antebrachial cutaneous nerve (medial cutaneous nerve of the forearm) arises as a separate branch from the BP and travels with the ulnar to just above the ulnar groove, where it diverts to run anterior to the ME to supply the skin of the medial forearm; involvement of this distribution excludes UNE. Impaired sensation over the dorsum of the hand establishes the location of the lesion as proximal to the takeoff of the DUC, but sparing of the DUC territory does not exclude UNE because of possible selective sparing of its fascicles. Involvement of the palmar cutaneous branch distribution likewise suggests a lesion proximal to the distal forearm.

Impaired elbow range of motion or a valgus deformity strongly suggests UNE. Reproduction of symptoms with elbow flexion and ulnar groove pressure can be informative. Examining for subluxation is seldom helpful, as this is a common phenomenon in normal individuals. The best current evidence indicates that subluxation of the ulnar nerve at the elbow bears no relation to UNE.

Ulnar nerve lesions can also occur at several sites in the distal forearm and hand. Compression most frequently occurs in the palm or wrist (ulnar neuropathy at the wrist [UNW]), but involvement in the forearm and isolated lesions of the DUC branch (handcuff neuropathy, pricer palsy) have also been reported. The clinical presentation of UNW depends on which fibers are compressed. If the lesion affects the main ulnar nerve at the wrist and all its branches, the clinical syndrome will closely resemble an UNE. However, examination will show normal sensation in the DUC distribution and no weakness of the FCU or FDP. The more common presentation of UNW involves the deep palmar branch alone or the deep palmar branch in conjunction with the motor branches to the hypothenar muscles. In these cases, sensation will be normal. This pattern occurs in 75% of patients with UNW. Patients present with painless weakness and atrophy of ulnar intrinsic hand muscles, sparing sensation (another Ramsay Hunt syndrome, Box 16.2). Motor neuron disease is often suspected because of the complete absence of sensory loss or symptoms. The branch to the palmaris brevis muscle arises proximal to Guyon's canal. The palmaris brevis sign is wrinkling of the hypothenar skin on small finger abduction due to contraction of the palmaris brevis; it reliably indicates that the lesion is at the wrist.

Pseudoulnar neuropathy refers to isolated hand weakness in an ulnar distribution due to a lesion of the contralateral angular gyrus. Pseudoulnar sensory loss can also occur with contralateral hemispheric lesions.

The Radial Nerve

The radial nerve arises as a direct continuation of the posterior cord of the BP. It exits through the axilla and then runs down the medial aspect of the upper arm. Just after passing the teres major muscle, it enters the triceps muscle. At about the mid-upper arm, it curves around the mid-humerus in the spiral groove. Branches innervating the long head of the triceps muscle arise before the nerve enters the spiral groove; those to the medial and lateral heads frequently arise in the groove. The nerve pierces the lateral intermuscular septum and then descends through the lateral upper arm, giving off a branch to the brachioradialis muscle. It runs between the brachialis, to which it sends an innervating branch in many individuals, and brachioradialis muscles just anterior to the lateral epicondyle and then enters the forearm in the groove between the biceps tendon and the brachioradialis. Innervating twigs are given off to the brachioradialis and the extensor carpi radialis longus and brevis (ECRB), after which the main trunk terminates by dividing into the posterior interosseous nerve (PIN, deep motor branch) and the superficial radial nerve.

The superficial radial nerve descends along the lateral aspect of the forearm; however, it does not supply the skin in this region, which is instead supplied by the lateral antebrachial cutaneous nerve. The superficial radial branch terminates as sensory fibers that supply the radial aspect of the dorsum of the hand and the radial three and one-half digits. At its takeoff, the PIN sends a branch to the supinator muscle and then passes over the fibrous edge of the ECRB and through a slit in the supinator muscle (the arcade of Frohse), a potential site of compression.

It continues along the interosseous membrane supplying the extensor carpi ulnaris, extensor muscles of the fingers and thumb, and the abductor pollicis longus; it has no cutaneous sensory component.

The radial nerve may be injured anywhere along its course (Figure 46.10). In the axilla, it may be traumatized by crutches (triad neuropathy), shoulder dislocation, fractures of the humerus, or penetrating injuries. Severe radial nerve injury may occur due to the "windmill" pitching motion of competitive softball. Radial nerve "entrapment" in the upper arm at the lateral head of the triceps muscles may occur after continuous repetitive arm exercise with sudden forceful contraction.

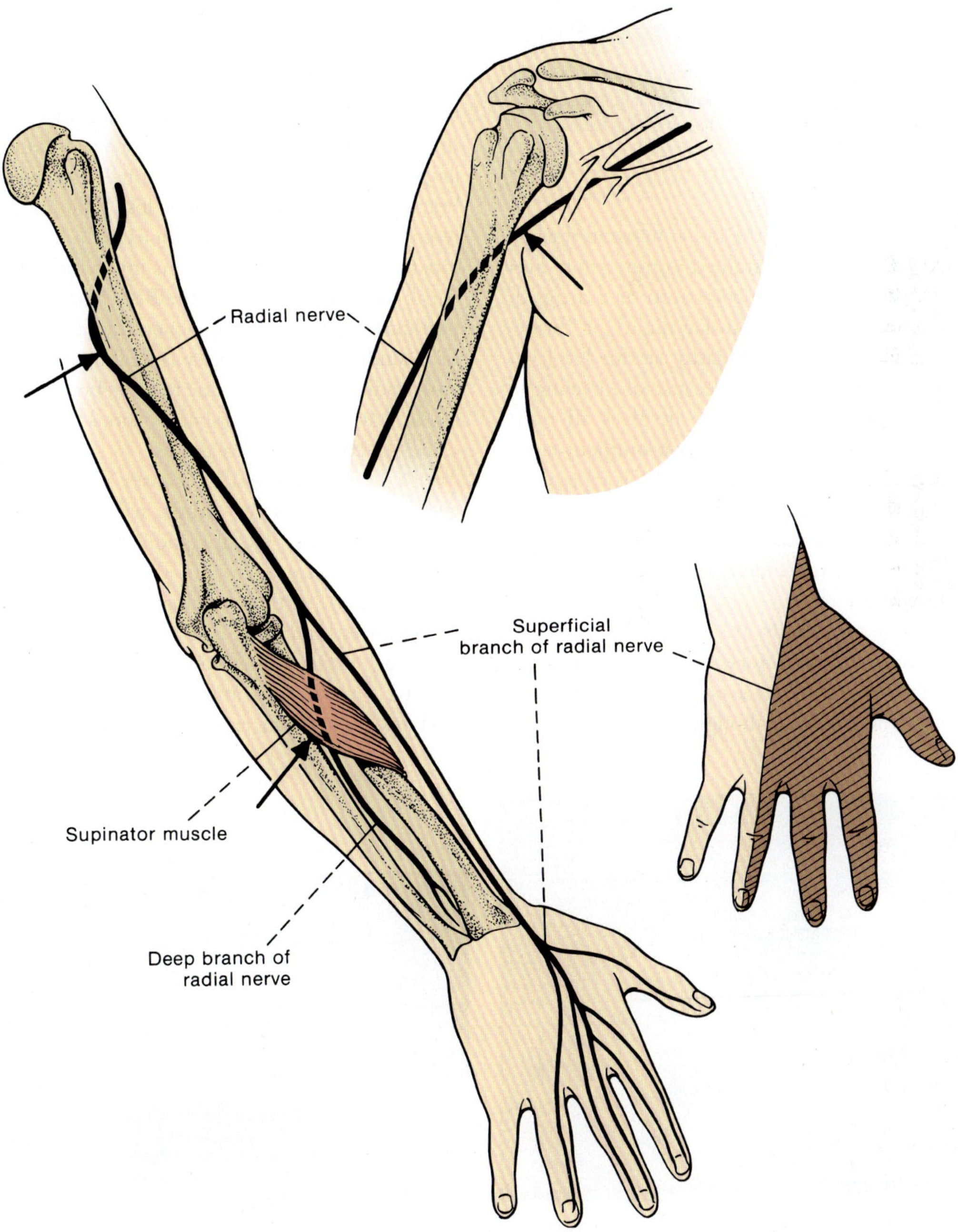

FIGURE 46.10 Common sites for injury to the radial nerve and the distribution of sensory loss with a radial nerve lesion.

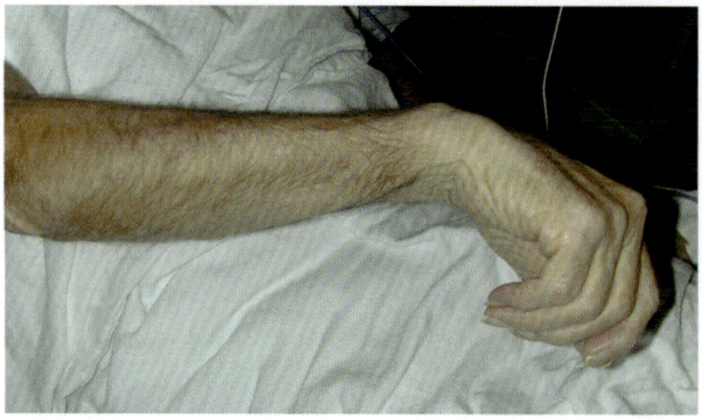

FIGURE 46.11 High radial nerve palsy with paralysis of wrist, finger, and thumb extension. (Reprinted with permission from Maschke S, Graham TJ, Evans P, eds. *Master Techniques in Orthopaedic Surgery: The Hand.* 3rd ed. Philadelphia: Wolters Kluwer, 2016.)

Acute compression of the radial nerve in the spiral groove results from sustained compression over a period of several hours during sleep or a drug- or alcohol-induced stupor ("Saturday night" or "bridegroom's" palsy). Radial neuropathy at this level has also been reported in soldiers because of kneeling in the shooting position. Weakness involves all muscles distal to the triceps. The most prominent complaint and finding in radial neuropathy is wrist drop (Figure 46.11). There is weakness of finger extension at the MCP joints. Extension of the IP joints is preserved because this movement is carried out by the lumbricals and interossei.

Confusion commonly arises on two points: (a) because of mechanical factors, the interossei cannot exert normal power in the face of finger drop and may seem weak—the patient is thought to also have ulnar neuropathy; and (b) weakness of thumb abduction occurs due to dysfunction of the radial-innervated abductor pollicis longus—the patient is thought to also have median neuropathy.

If the lesion is above the branch to the brachioradialis, there is weakness of flexion of the semipronated forearm. In a lesion still higher, there is also involvement of the triceps. Sensory loss is variable and often minimal because of overlapping of cutaneous nerves (Figure 36.3). The involved area is usually limited to the dorsum of the thumb, although it may involve the dorsum of the radial half or two-thirds of the hand, the first interosseous space and the index finger, and the dorsum of the adjacent proximal phalanges. Trophic changes are minimal. The triceps and brachioradialis reflexes may be lost. The primary differential diagnostic considerations include C7 radiculopathy, PIN palsy, and lesions involving the middle trunk or posterior cord of the BP. The radial nerve is particularly prone to involvement in systemic vasculitis. Pseudoradial nerve palsy is weakness in an apparently radial distribution due to a cerebral hemispheric lesion. Myasthenia gravis has a curious predilection to cause selective triceps weakness.

A lesion of the PIN causes weakness of finger extension (finger drop) without wrist drop (Figure 46.12A). Compression may occur at the arcade of Frohse or within the supinator (supinator channel). Other etiologies include penetrating injuries, fractures, use of Canadian (forearm) crutches, local masses, and overuse syndrome in athletes, musicians, and upholsterers. The wrist deviates radially on extension because of weakness

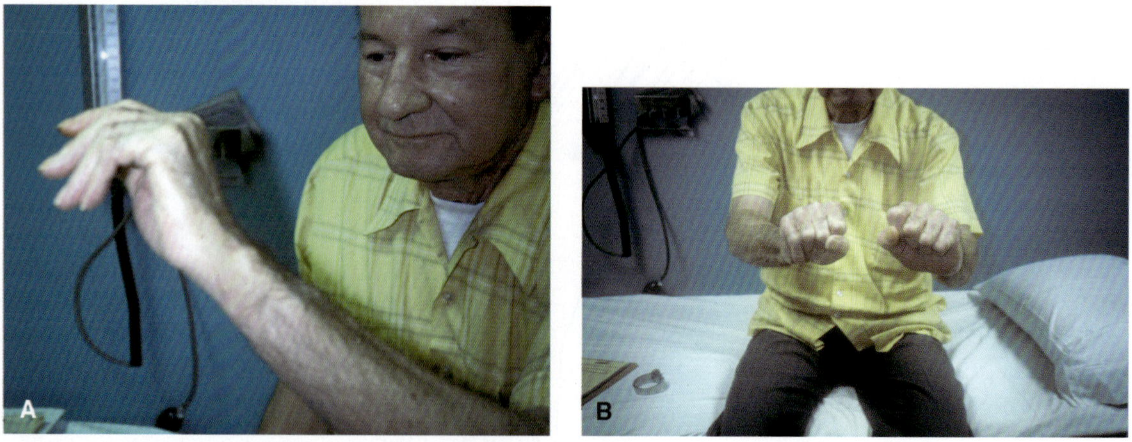

FIGURE 46.12 Posterior interosseous neuropathy causing **(A)** finger drop without wrist drop and **(B)** radial deviation on wrist extension (patient's left hand).

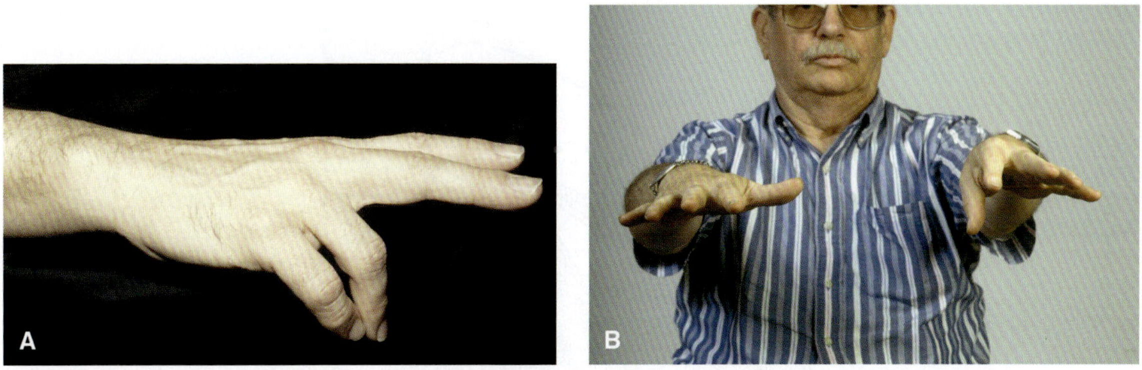

FIGURE 46.13 Posterior interosseous neuropathy causing selective finger drop **(A)** involving primarily the fourth and fifth fingers (pseudoulnar claw) and **(B)** involving primarily the thumb and index finger.

of the PIN-innervated extensor carpi ulnaris with preservation of the main trunk-innervated extensor carpi radialis longus (Figure 46.12B). The supinator may or may not be involved. Some fingers may be affected more than others; most often, the ring and small fingers are selectively dropped, producing a posture that superficially resembles an ulnar griffe (pseudoulnar claw hand, Figure 46.13A). A selective thumb drop may occur (Figure 46.13B). Occasionally, cervical radiculomyelopathy will selectively drop the ring and small fingers (Ono's hand, myelopathy hand, pseudopseudoulnar claw hand, Figure 46.13A). A PIN lesion causes no cutaneous sensory changes, but as with AIN palsy, there may be pain carried by afferent fibers innervating joints. Rarely, focal myopathy of the forearm extensors may mimic a PIN lesion. Selective vulnerability of the posterior interosseous fascicles in retrohumeral radial neuropathy may cause confusion with a PIN lesion. Multifocal motor neuropathy and related conditions are prone to involve radial-innervated muscles and cause weakness of the wrist and finger extensors. Neuropathy of the superficial radial nerve will cause pain and alterations of sensation in its distribution (Wartenberg's syndrome or cheiralgia paresthetica); it may be injured by tight bands around the wrist (handcuff neuropathy).

The radial tunnel syndrome (RTS) is a dubious entity allegedly due to compression of radial nerve branches in a nebulous anatomical passageway variously said to consist of the fibrous edge of the ECRB, distal border of the supinator muscle, or fibrous adhesions between the brachialis and brachioradialis. The contention is that nerve entrapment causes chronic lateral elbow pain in the absence of any objective neurologic dysfunction. Descriptions of clinical manifestations of RTS in the surgical literature are often identical to descriptions of lateral epicondylitis.

LOWER-EXTREMITY NERVES

The Lumbosacral Plexus

The nerves innervating the lower extremity and hip region arise from the LSP, which is in fact two plexi, even three if the coccygeal plexus is counted as a component (Figures 46.14 and 46.15). The lumbar portion of the plexus originates from the anterior primary rami of L1-L4. It lies within the substance of the psoas major muscle. The L4 and L5 roots give rise to the lumbosacral trunk, which joins the lumbar plexus to the sacral plexus. Roots from S1-S3 join the lumbosacral trunk to complete the plexus; the sacral portion lies along the posterolateral wall of the pelvis, between the piriformis muscle and the major vessels.

The major motor nerves arising from the LSP are the femoral, obturator, sciatic, common fibular (peroneal), tibial, superior gluteal, inferior gluteal, and pudendal. The major sensory branches are the saphenous, a continuation of the femoral nerve, the iliohypogastric, ilioinguinal, genitofemoral, and the lateral femoral cutaneous (LFC) nerve, which arises from the lumbar plexus, courses around the pelvic brim, and exits beneath the inguinal ligament adjacent to the anterior superior iliac spine.

Conditions affecting the LSP include diabetes, neoplasms, retroperitoneal hemorrhage, and postradiation plexopathy. Diabetic lumbosacral radiculoplexus neuropathy (diabetic amyotrophy) is common; it causes a syndrome of pain, proximal bilateral but usually very asymmetric leg weakness,

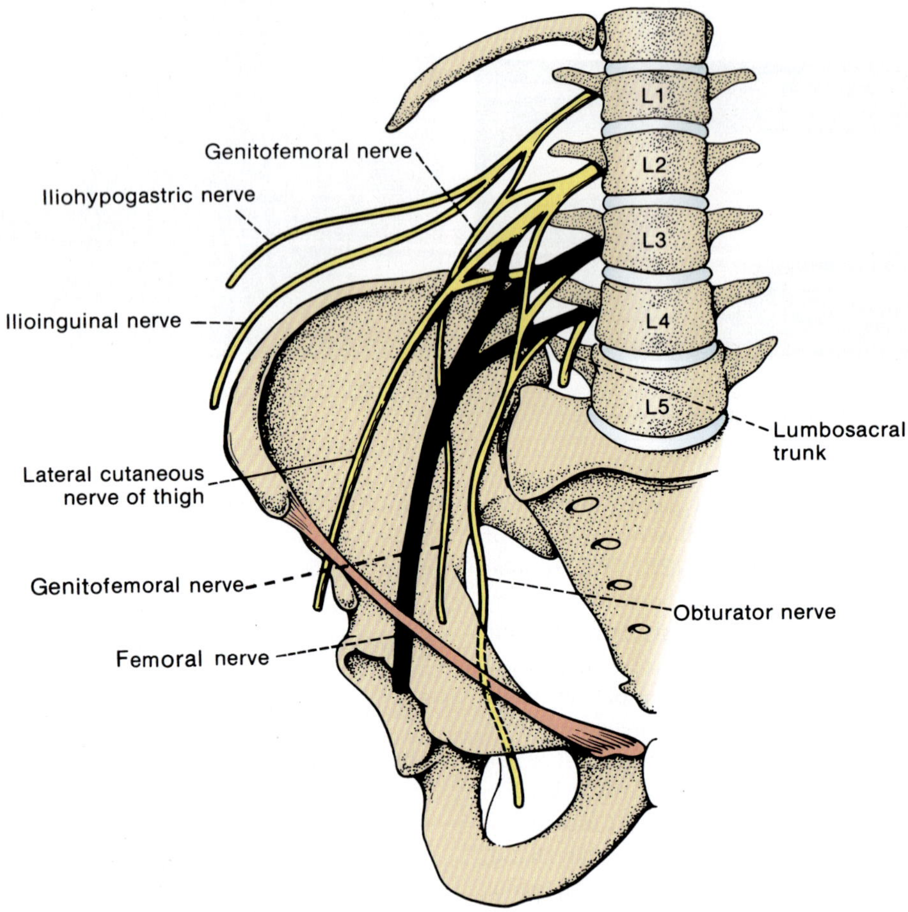

FIGURE 46.14 Constituents of the lumbar plexus.

and weight loss. Neoplasms may metastasize to the LSP, or directly invade it, and radiation therapy given as treatment for the tumor may itself damage the plexus. Whether there is a primary, spontaneous plexitis affecting the LSP analogous to the entity of NA of the BP has been a matter of conjecture. Hemorrhage into the psoas muscle, a feared complication of anticoagulation, may severely damage the LSP.

The Femoral Nerve

The femoral nerve is the largest branch of the lumbar plexus. It forms within the belly of the psoas muscle from the posterior divisions of the anterior primary rami of the L2-L4 roots. Leaving the cover of the psoas, it runs between the psoas and the iliacus muscle and exits from the pelvis beneath the inguinal ligament, lateral to the femoral vessels. Its motor branches innervate the psoas, iliacus, sartorius, pectineus, and quadriceps muscles. Its sensory branches, the intermediate (anterior) and medial femoral cutaneous nerves, innervate the skin of the anterior thigh. The femoral nerve terminates as a large sensory branch, the saphenous nerve, which supplies an extensive cutaneous field along the medial aspect of the lower leg and the medial aspect of the foot.

The femoral nerve may be involved in pelvic tumors, psoas abscesses or hematomas, fractures of the pelvis and upper femur, aneurysms of the femoral artery, and penetrating wounds; it may be affected in diabetic mononeuropathy and injured during labor or abdominal or pelvic surgery (Figure 46.16). A substantial number of femoral nerve palsies are iatrogenic, from the lithotomy position or surgical trauma. Femoral neuropathies may result from stretch as a result of hip hyperextension (see hanging leg syndrome below).

Femoral nerve motor dysfunction always causes impairment of knee extension. Walking forward and

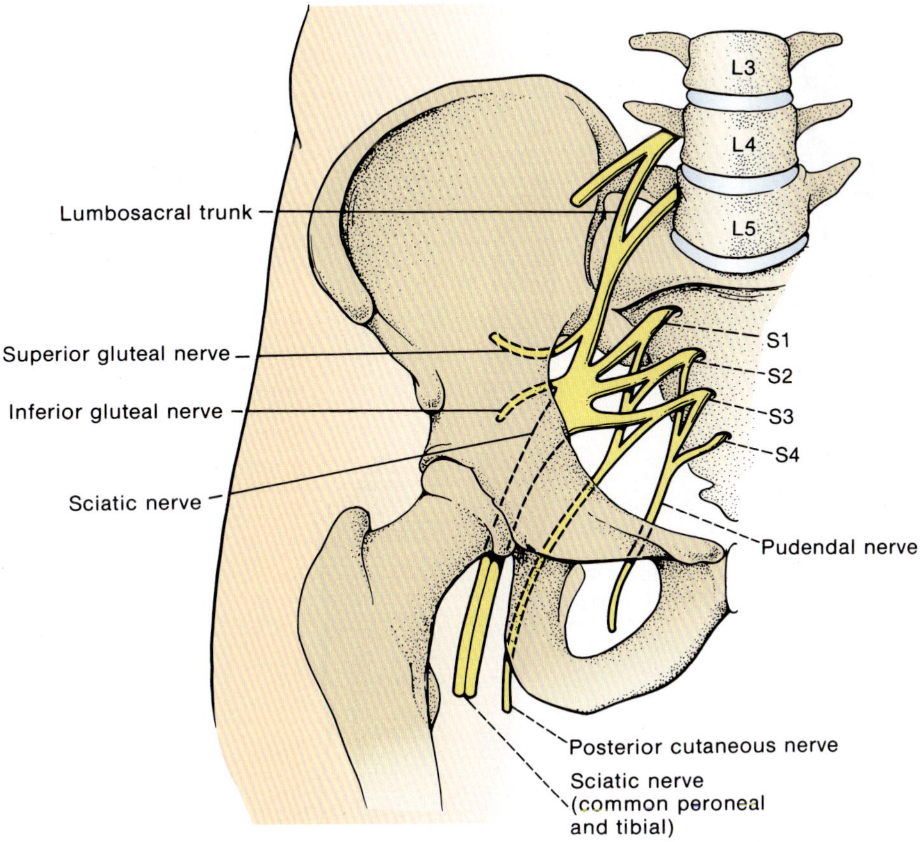

FIGURE 46.15 Constituents of the sacral plexus.

climbing stairs is difficult, although the patient may walk backward with ease. The patient may walk holding the knee stiff, and if the knee bends, the patient may fall. Involvement within the pelvis or abdomen may also affect the function of the psoas major, causing weakness of hip flexion. Femoral nerve lesions impair the patellar reflex and cause sensory loss over the anterior and medial aspects of the thigh and the medial aspect of the leg.

The Obturator Nerve

This nerve arises from the lumbar plexus from the anterior divisions of the anterior primary rami of L2-L4. It supplies the adductor muscles of the thigh, the gracilis, and the obturator externus and transmits sensation from a small area on the medial aspect of the thigh. Obturator lesions are rare, but when they occur, there is weakness of adduction and external rotation of the thigh, with a small area of anesthesia over the inner surface of the thigh. Causes include orthopedic, gynecologic, or urologic surgery or injuries; obturator hernia; iliopsoas hemorrhage; and rarely diabetes.

The Lateral Femoral Cutaneous Nerve (Lateral Cutaneous Nerve of the Thigh)

The LFC is a sensory nerve formed by the posterior divisions of the L2-L3 anterior primary rami. It transmits sensation from the skin of the anterolateral aspect of the thigh. Pain, paresthesias, and sensory loss in the distribution of the LFC (meralgia paresthetica) are a very common clinical syndrome. The nerve probably becomes entrapped where it passes under or through the inguinal ligament just medial to the anterior superior iliac spine, or where it pierces the fascia lata. Precipitating causes include weight gain, pregnancy, ascites, trauma, pressure by a belt or other tight abdominal garment, and possibly diabetes mellitus. The primary differential point is to exclude an upper lumbar radiculopathy.

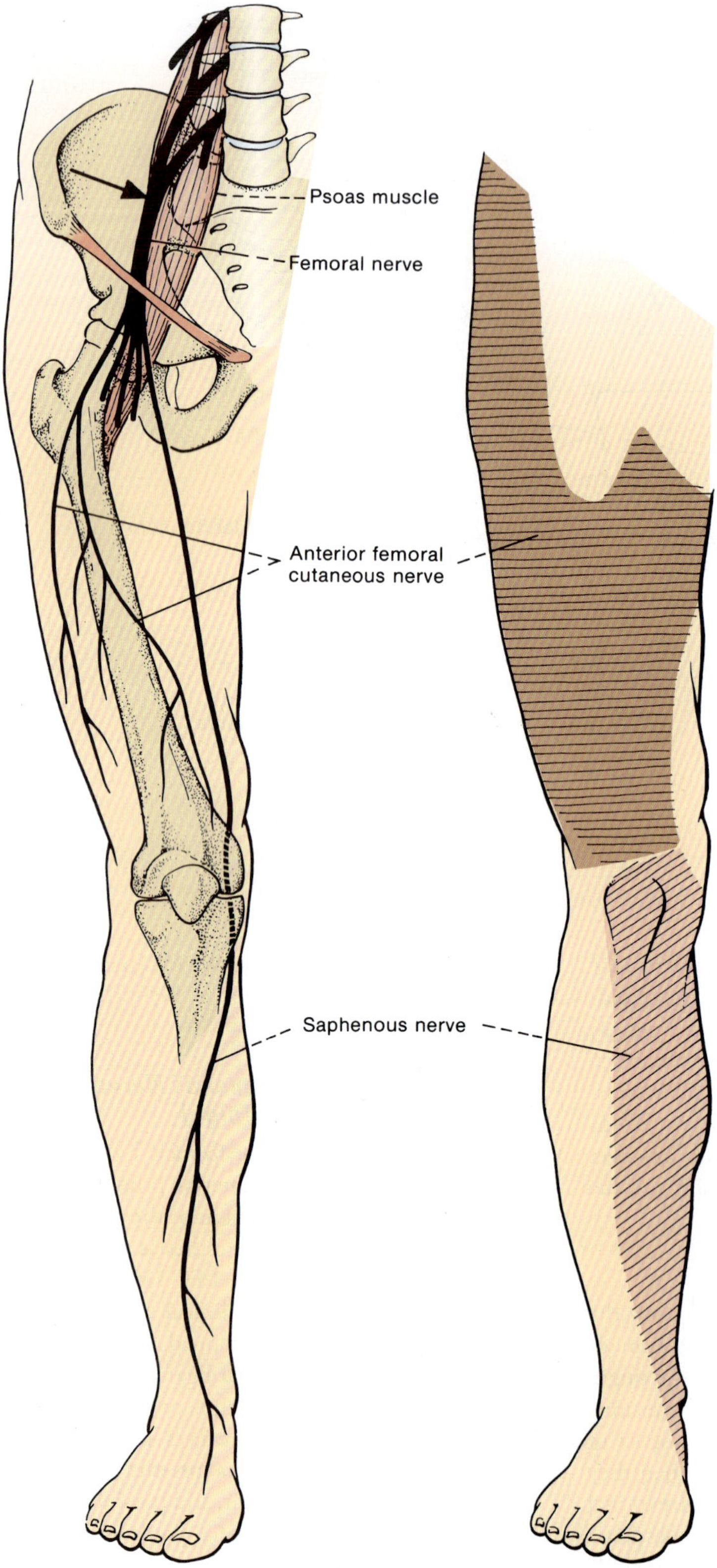

FIGURE 46.16 Common sites for injury to the femoral nerve and distribution of sensory loss with a lesion of the femoral nerve and its branches.

The Sciatic Nerve

The lumbosacral trunk arises from the lower part of the lumbar plexus and fuses with elements of the sacral plexus to form the sciatic nerve. The sciatic, superior gluteal, and inferior gluteal nerves all exit the pelvis through the greater sciatic foramen. The sciatic usually exits beneath the piriformis muscle but may pierce it or rarely pass above it. The nerve courses in close proximity to the posterior aspect of the hip joint and then enters the thigh. In its course through the thigh, it innervates the hamstring muscles and also sends a twig to the adductor magnus.

From its beginnings, the sciatic nerve is made up of two divisions: the fibular (peroneal, lateral) and the tibial (medial). The tibial division arises from the anterior divisions of the LSP, and the fibular, or peroneal, from the posterior divisions. The fibular and tibial divisions run together in a common sheath, forming the sciatic nerve, until the level of the knee where they divide and pursue separate courses. The only portion of the hamstring muscle mass innervated by the fibular division is the short head of the biceps femoris; all other hamstring muscles are innervated by the tibial division.

After the bifurcation in the popliteal fossa, the peroneal (fibular) nerve moves laterally and winds around the fibular head (FH) and then descends toward the foot. The tibial nerve descends in the midline down the posterior aspect of the leg to innervate the gastrosoleus. In its proximal course, it gives off a sural communicating branch, which joins its fellow from the common peroneal nerve to form the sural nerve proper. The sural then moves laterally as it runs distally, pierces the deep fascia to emerge into a superficial position about 15 cm proximal to the lateral malleolus, and then curves around and beneath the lateral malleolus to supply the skin of the lateral aspect of the foot and toes. Distally, the tibial nerve passes beneath the medial malleolus, under the flexor retinaculum, which forms the roof of the tarsal tunnel. The tibial nerve terminates by dividing into the medial and lateral plantar nerves, which innervate the abductors and short flexors of the toes and supply sensation to the skin of the sole.

Injury to the main trunk of the sciatic nerve may result in weakness of both the common peroneal- and tibial-innervated muscles, but often the deficit involves predominantly or solely one division, most often the peroneal. Hamstring muscle weakness clearly indicates that the lesion involves the main trunk of the sciatic nerve. When the deficit is limited to the peroneal division, the only way to prove the lesion involves the sciatic nerve rather than the peroneal is to demonstrate abnormality in the short head of the biceps femoris by needle electromyography.

With complete sciatic lesions, sensory loss involves all but the anteromedial aspect of the leg (saphenous distribution). Knee flexion is greatly impaired, the only muscles participating in this movement being the sartorius and gracilis. Flexion and extension of the ankle and toe joints and inversion and eversion of the foot are lost. The patient cannot stand on either heel or toes. Trophic disturbances and neuropathic pain are frequent.

The sciatic nerve may be injured in pelvic fractures, hip fracture or dislocation, total hip arthroplasty and other orthopedic procedures on the hip, intragluteal injections, gluteal hemorrhage or compartment syndrome, and penetrating wounds. It may be entrapped by heterotopic ossification or impinged by a methylmethacrylate spur. The nerve may be compressed by prolonged sitting in the lotus position (lotus neuropathy) or prolonged pressure from a toilet seat, both termed "another Saturday night palsy." In the hanging leg syndrome, sciatic neuropathy, with accompanying femoral neuropathy, develops from having the legs hanging off the bed with hips hyperextended while intoxicated or in coma. The piriformis syndrome is sciatic compression by the piriformis muscle as the sciatic nerve exits the pelvis. The existence of this syndrome is controversial. External compression of the nerve in the hip may occur with pressure due to a fat wallet or coins or a pistol in the hip pocket (pistol packer's palsy). Such instances do not qualify as piriformis syndrome. In a series of 380 patients with sciatic nerve injuries, 60% were at the buttock level and 40% were in the thigh. Injection injuries made up more than half of the buttock-level cases. In future case series, the incidence of injection injuries is likely to fall dramatically because of the advent of patient-controlled anesthesia.

Common Peroneal (Fibular) Neuropathy at the Fibular Head

The primary root origin of the peroneal nerve is L5, with lesser contributions from L4 (primarily to the tibialis anterior) and from S1 (primarily to the small foot muscles). After traversing the LSP, the peroneal joins the posterior tibial nerve to form the sciatic nerve. In the mid-thigh, the peroneal division sends a twig to the short head of the biceps femoris. Just distal to the sciatic bifurcation, the common peroneal gives off its sural communicating branch and the lateral cutaneous nerve of the calf, which sends sensory innervation to the lateral lower leg. The common peroneal nerve then winds around the FH, pierces the peroneus longus muscle (the "fibular tunnel"), and divides into superficial and deep branches (Figure 46.17). The superficial branch innervates the peroneus longus and brevis and terminates as the superficial sensory branch, which provides sensation to the dorsum of the foot (Figure 46.18). The deep

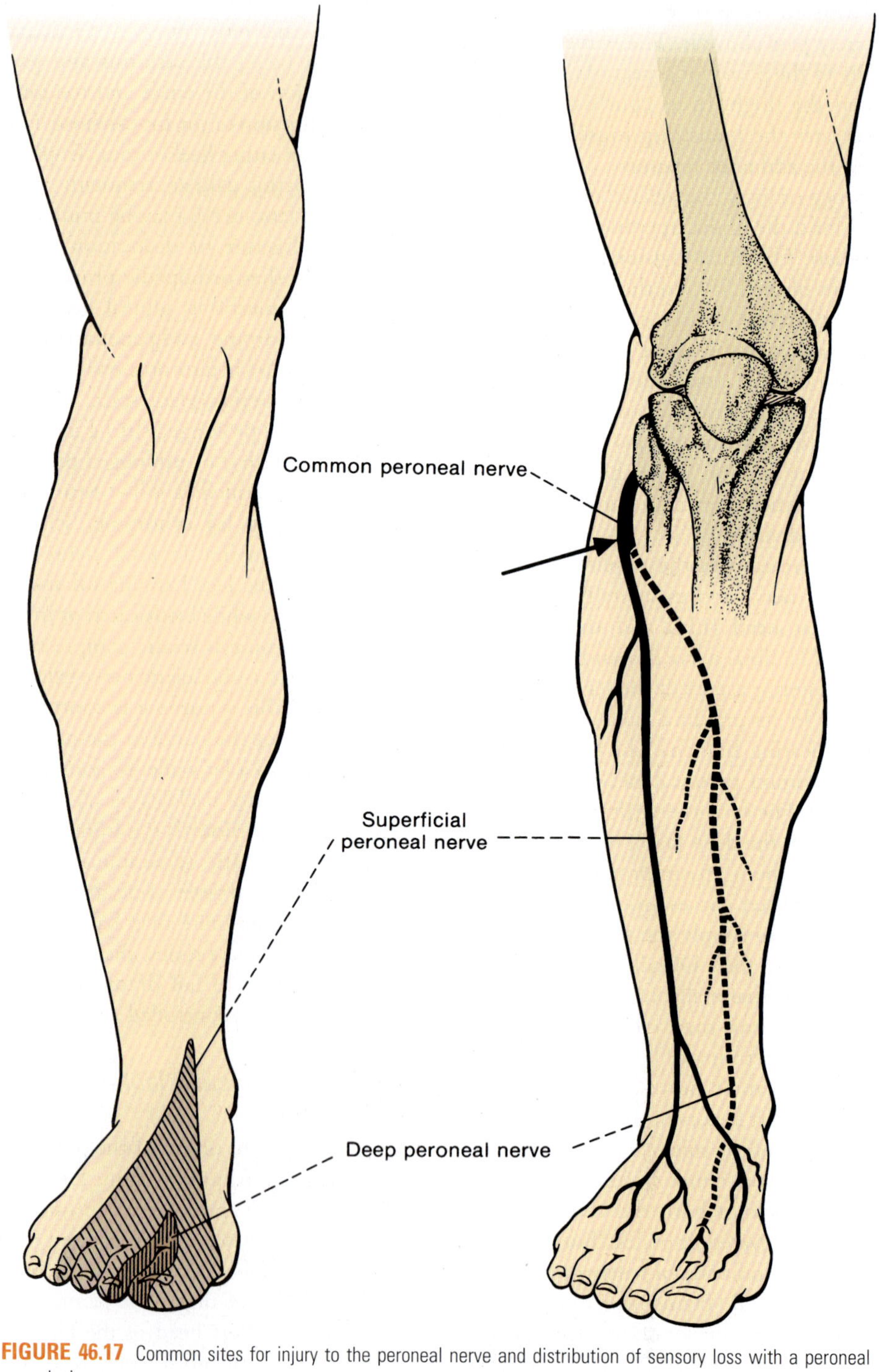

FIGURE 46.17 Common sites for injury to the peroneal nerve and distribution of sensory loss with a peroneal nerve lesion.

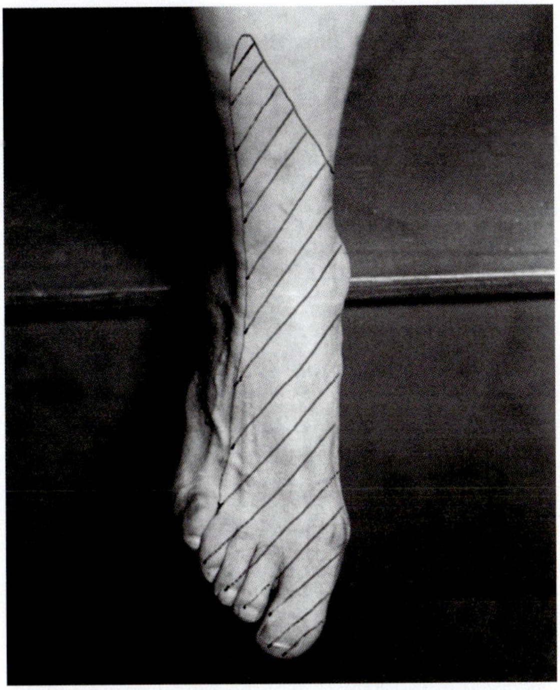

FIGURE 46.18 Distribution of sensory loss in a right common peroneal neuropathy.

peroneal branch innervates the tibialis anterior, peroneus tertius, and long and short toe extensors and provides sensation to the web space between the first and second toes. An accessory peroneal is a common anomaly, affecting about 20% of the population; the branch arises from the superficial peroneal, passes behind the lateral malleolus, and innervates the lateral portion of the extensor digitorum brevis. Common peroneal mononeuropathy at the FH causes weakness of dorsiflexion of the foot and toes and weakness of ankle eversion. Severe peroneal neuropathy causes a foot drop. Sensation is lost over the dorsum of the foot.

The peroneal nerve at the FH is superficial, covered only by skin and subcutaneous tissue, making it exceptionally vulnerable to external compression. The nerve is also tethered at its point of passage through the peroneus longus muscle, making it susceptible to stretch as well. Habitual leg crossing is a classical cause of common peroneal neuropathy at the fibular head (CPNFH). Occasionally, a skin dimple marks the precise site of compression. This type of CPNFH is particularly common in slender or depressed patients or those who have recently lost weight (slimmer's palsy). Any number of external forces may substitute for the patient's opposite kneecap as the agent of compression, including plaster casts, knee braces, or tight bandages. In immobile, comatose, paralyzed, or anesthetized patients, an ordinary mattress can exert enough force to injure the nerve. Prolonged squatting is another common cause of CPNFH, possibly from a combination of stretch, compression, and kinking—a particular hazard for roofers, carpet layers, women who squat in labor (pushing palsy), and farmers (strawberry picker's palsy). Sudden, forceful plantar flexion or inversion of the ankle may stretch the nerve and cause focal damage at the point where it is tethered in its passage through the peroneus longus. CPNFH is surprisingly common in patients with severe ankle injuries. Transient foot drop is reportedly common in NFL kickers (punter's palsy). Rare causes of CPNFH include true entrapment in the fibular tunnel, Baker's cyst, nerve tumor, ganglion, and lipoma. In a study of 318 cases of CPNFH that underwent surgery, 44% were due to stretch or contusion without fracture or dislocation and 7% to stretch or contusion with fracture or dislocation, 12% were due to lacerations, 9% to entrapments, 4% were iatrogenic injuries, and 4% were due to gunshot wounds.

The most common differential diagnostic exercise is between CPNFH and L5 radiculopathy in the patient with foot drop. The presence of back and leg pain, weakness of foot inversion, positive root stretch signs, and depression of the medial hamstring reflex favor radiculopathy. The absence of pain, weakness limited to ankle eversion and foot/toe dorsiflexion, and preservation of the medial hamstring reflex favor CPNFH. The pattern of sensory changes is rarely helpful. Inspection for a skin dimple, discoloration or callus over the FH, percussion to elicit Tinel's sign, and careful palpation of the popliteal fossa and FH are likewise important. In most patients with CPNFH, a meticulous history will uncover an explanatory mechanism through external pressure or stretch. In rare patients, sciatic neuropathy, deep peroneal neuropathy, or lumbosacral plexopathy may simulate CPNFH. A number of generalized conditions may require consideration, especially if foot drop is bilateral, including polyneuropathy, motor neuron disease, and several types of primary muscle disease (e.g., distal myopathy, inclusion body myositis, myotonic dystrophy, and scapuloperoneal syndromes).

The Tibial Nerve

The tibial nerve is the larger of the two terminal branches of the sciatic nerve. It is formed by a fusion of all five of the anterior divisions of the sacral plexus (L4-S2 or S3). It supplies the long head of the biceps femoris and the semimembranosus, semitendinosus, gastrocnemius, popliteus, soleus, plantaris, tibialis posterior, and flexors digitorum longus and hallucis longus muscles and, through the medial and lateral plantar nerves, the plantar flexors of the toes and the small muscles of the foot. Through the sural nerve, it transmits sensation from the posterolateral aspects of the leg and ankle and the lateral aspects of the heel and foot. Calcaneal nerves supply sensation to the posterior and medial aspects and plantar surface of the heel; the medial and lateral plantar nerves supply the plantar surface of the foot.

If the tibial nerve is injured, there is weakness distal to the lesion, with sensory loss over the plantar and lateral aspects of the foot, the heel, and the posterolateral aspects of the leg and ankle. The patient may be unable to plantar flex or invert the foot or to flex, adduct, or abduct the toes. Trophic changes and pain are common. The Achilles reflex is lost. Tibial nerve injuries are relatively infrequent because of its deep location and protected course, but it may be involved in lesions in or below the popliteal space.

Etiologies of tibial neuropathy in the popliteal fossa include trauma, especially when associated with hemorrhage, synovial (Baker's) cyst, intraneural ganglion, nerve tumors, idiopathic hypertrophic neuropathy, and entrapment by a tendinous arch at the origin of the soleus muscle or by fibrous bands between the heads of the gastrocnemius muscle. Popliteal fossa lesions cause pain and tenderness and a positive Tinel's sign in the popliteal fossa, helpful in distinguishing clinically from tibial nerve compression at the ankle and from S1 radiculopathy. Proximal main trunk tibial neuropathies are most often due to trauma or ischemia.

Compression by the flexor retinaculum behind the medial malleolus (lancinate ligament) may cause burning pain and sensory loss in the toes and sole of the foot and paresis or paralysis of the small muscles of the foot (tarsal tunnel syndrome [TTS]). TTS is sometimes seen as the lower-extremity analog of CTS and the diagnosis made to explain pain of no other apparent origin even in absence of any neurologic deficit, for which division of the lancinate ligament may be performed. The condition has been attributed to tenosynovitis of the long flexor tendons, bony prominences in the tunnel, external trauma, poor shoes, stretch injury with ankle sprain or dislocation, and space-occupying lesions (lipoma, varicosities, ganglion, anomalous muscles). Patients may have sensory symptoms provoked by weight bearing and relieved by rest. Physical findings are few. There is seldom, if ever, weakness of intrinsic foot muscles. In bona fide TTS, there may be sensory loss over the sole, especially in the medial plantar distribution, usually sparing the heel (calcaneal branch); tenderness behind medial malleolus; and a Tinel's sign over the tarsal tunnel. A test similar to Phalen's, passively holding the ankle maximally everted and dorsiflexed with the toes pulled up to elicit paresthesias, is said to be useful. Rarely, individual nerve branches may be damaged in the foot. Medial plantar neuropathy has been attributed to compression at the entrance to a fibromuscular tunnel behind the navicular tuberosity, distal to the tarsal tunnel. Selective lateral plantar neuropathy has also been described.

Other Lower-Extremity Nerves

Focal neuropathies occasionally involve other nerves. The iliohypogastric nerve arises from L1 and is mainly sensory. It supplies the skin of the gluteal region and the hypogastric region, just above the symphysis pubis. The ilioinguinal nerve is also a branch of L1. Like the iliohypogastric nerve, it is mainly sensory, innervating the skin of the upper, medial thigh, upper part of the root of the penis and the scrotum in the male, and the mons pubis and the labia majora in the female. The genitofemoral nerve arises from L1-L2. It supplies the cremaster muscle and transmits sensation from the skin of the scrotum or labia and from a small area on the upper thigh. The posterior femoral cutaneous nerve arises from the posterior divisions of S1-S2 and the anterior divisions of S2-S3. It transmits sensation from the posterior aspect of the thigh and upper leg. Its gluteal branches supply the skin of the lower gluteal region; the perineal branches are distributed to the upper and medial aspect of the thigh; the inferior pudendal branch supplies the skin of the perineal region together with the scrotum in the male and the labia majora in the female. Lesions of these nerves may cause pain and loss of sensation in their areas of distribution.

The superior gluteal nerve arises from the posterior divisions of L4-S1 and innervates the gluteus medius, gluteus minimus, and tensor fascia lata muscles. The inferior gluteal nerve arises from posterior divisions of L5-S2 and innervates the gluteus maximus. The pudendal nerve arises from the anterior divisions of S2-S4 and exits through the lesser sciatic foramen. It has three major divisions. The inferior rectal (hemorrhoidal) nerve is distributed to the external anal sphincter and to the skin and mucosa about the anus. The perineal nerve divides into deep (muscular) and superficial branches. The deep branches supply the bulbocavernosus, ischio-cavernosus, and other perineal muscles, together with the external urethral sphincter; the superficial branches form the posterior scrotal (or labial) nerves that transmit sensation from the scrotum in the male and the labia in the female. The dorsal nerve of the penis (or clitoris) supplies the corpus cavernosum and the skin and mucous membrane of the dorsum of the penis (or clitoris), including the glans. The pudendal nerve also transmits sensation from the bladder.

BIBLIOGRAPHY

Akane M, Iwatsuki K, Tatebe M, et al. Anterior interosseous nerve and posterior interosseous nerve involvement in neuralgic amyotrophy. *Clin Neurol Neurosurg* 2016;151:108–112.

Al-Qattan MM, Robertson GA. Pseudo-anterior interosseous nerve syndrome: a case report. *J Hand Surg [Am]* 1993;18:440–442.

Almeida DF, Scremin L, Zuniga SF, et al. Focal conduction block in a case of tarsal tunnel syndrome. *Muscle Nerve* 2010;42:452–455.

Amirfeyz R, Clark D, Parsons B, et al. Clinical tests for carpal tunnel syndrome in contemporary practice. *Arch Orthop Trauma Surg* 2011;131:471–474.

Anto C, Aradhya P. Clinical diagnosis of peripheral nerve compression in the upper extremity. *Orthop Clin North Am* 1996;27:227–236.

Arnold WD, Elsheikh BH. Entrapment neuropathies. *Neurol Clin* 2013;31:405–424.

Baima J, Krivickas L. Evaluation and treatment of peroneal neuropathy. *Curr Rev Musculoskelet Med* 2008;1:147–153.

Bäumer P, Kele H, Xia A, et al. Posterior interosseous neuropathy: supinator syndrome vs fascicular radial neuropathy. *Neurology* 2016;87:1884–1891.

Bhanushali MJ, Muley SA. Diabetic and non-diabetic lumbosacral radiculoplexus neuropathy. *Neurol India* 2008;56:420–425.

Boonyapisit K, Katirji B. Multifocal motor neuropathy presenting with respiratory failure. *Muscle Nerve* 2000;23:1887–1890.

Borschel GH, Clarke HM. Obstetrical brachial plexus palsy. *Plast Reconstr Surg* 2009;124(1 Suppl):144e–155e.

Bouche P. Compression and entrapment neuropathies. *Handb Clin Neurol* 2013;115:311–366.

Brazis PW, Masdeu JC, Biller J. *Localization in Clinical Neurology.* 7th ed. Philadelphia: Wolters Kluwer/Lippincott Williams & Wilkins, 2017.

Brown WF, Watson BV. AAEM case report #27: acute retrohumeral radial neuropathies. *Muscle Nerve* 1993;16:706–711.

Burnham RS, Steadward RD. Upper extremity peripheral nerve entrapments among wheelchair athletes: prevalence, location, and risk factors. *Arch Phys Med Rehabil* 1994;75:519–524.

Busis NA. Femoral and obturator neuropathies. *Neurol Clin* 1999;17:633–653.

Buzzard EF. Some varieties of traumatic and toxic ulnar neuritis. *Lancet* 1922;199:317–319.

Campbell WW. Diagnosis and management of common compression and entrapment neuropathies. *Neurol Clin* 1997;15:549–567.

Campbell WW. Treatment and management of segmental neuromuscular disorders. In: Bertorini TE, ed. *Neuromuscular Disorders: Treatment and Management.* 1st ed. Philadelphia: Elsevier Saunders, 2011.

Campbell WW. Ulnar nerve subluxation. *Muscle Nerve* 2013;48:997–998.

Campbell WW. *Essentials of Electrodiagnostic Medicine.* 2nd ed. New York: Demos Medical, 2014.

Campbell WW. *Clinical Signs in Neurology: A Compendium.* Philadelphia: Wolters Kluwer Health, 2016.

Campbell WW, Buschbacher R, Pridgeon RM, et al. Selective finger drop in cervical radiculopathy: the pseudopseudoulnar claw hand. *Muscle Nerve* 1995;18:108–110.

Campbell WW, Landau ME. Controversial entrapment neuropathies. *Neurosurg Clin N Am* 2008;19:597, vii.

Cerrato P, Lentini A, Baima C, et al. Pseudo-ulnar sensory loss in a patient from a small cortical infarct of the postcentral knob. *Neurology* 2005;64:1981–1982.

Chariot P, Ragot F, Authier FJ, et al. Focal neurological complications of handcuff application. *J Forensic Sci* 2001;46:1124–1125.

Davidson JJ, Bassett FH III, Nunley JA. Musculocutaneous nerve entrapment revisited. *J Shoulder Elbow Surg* 1998;7:250–255.

Dawson DM. Entrapment neuropathies of the upper extremities. *N Engl J Med* 1993;329:2013–2018.

Dawson DM, Hallett M, Wilbourn AJ, eds. *Entrapment Neuropathies.* 3rd ed. Philadelphia: Lippincott Williams & Wilkins, 1999.

Domingo CA, Landau ME, Campbell WW. Selective triceps muscle weakness in myasthenia gravis is under-recognized. *J Clin Neuromuscul Dis* 2016;18:103–104.

Dramis A, Pimpalnerkar A. Suprascapular neuropathy in volleyball players. *Acta Orthop Belg* 2005;71:269–272.

England JD. Entrapment neuropathies. *Curr Opin Neurol* 1999;12:597–602.

Erdem S, Demirci M, Tan E. Focal myopathy mimicking posterior interosseous nerve syndrome. *Muscle Nerve* 2001;24:969–972.

Ferrante MA. The thoracic outlet syndromes. *Muscle Nerve* 2012;45:780–795.

Ferrante MA, Ferrante ND. The thoracic outlet syndromes: Part 1. Overview of the thoracic outlet syndromes and review of true neurogenic thoracic outlet syndrome. *Muscle Nerve* 2017a;55:782–793.

Ferrante MA, Ferrante ND. The thoracic outlet syndromes: Part 2. The arterial, venous, neurovascular, and disputed thoracic outlet syndromes. *Muscle Nerve* 2017b;56:663–673.

Gupta SK, Benstead TJ. Symptoms experienced by patients with carpal tunnel syndrome. *Can J Neurol Sci* 1997;24:338–342.

Hinchey JA, Preston DC, Logigian EL. Idiopathic lumbosacral neuropathy: a cause of persistent leg pain. *Muscle Nerve* 1996;19:1484–1486.

Hobson-Webb LD, Juel VC. Common entrapment neuropathies. *Continuum (Minneap Minn)* 2017;23(2, Selected Topics in Outpatient Neurology):487–511.

Hopkins A. A novel cause of a pressure palsy: mobile telephone user's shoulder droop. *J Neurol Neurosurg Psychiatry* 1996;61:346.

Ishaq S, Quinet R, Saba J. Phrenic nerve paralysis secondary to Lyme neuroborreliosis. *Neurology* 2002;59:1810–1811.

Iyer VG. Palmaris brevis sign in ulnar neuropathy 1998. *Muscle Nerve* 1998;21:675–677.

Jaeckle KA. Neurologic manifestations of neoplastic and radiation-induced plexopathies. *Semin Neurol* 2010;30:254–262.

Jamieson WG, Chinnick B. Thoracic outlet syndrome: fact or fancy? A review of 409 consecutive patients who underwent operation. *Can J Surg* 1996;39:321–326.

Kauppila LI, Vastamaki M. Iatrogenic serratus anterior paralysis. Long-term outcome in 26 patients. *Chest* 1996;109:31–34.

Kim DH, Murovic JA, Tiel RL, et al. Management and outcomes in 318 operative common peroneal nerve lesions at the Louisiana State University Health Sciences Center. *Neurosurgery* 2004;54:1421–1428.

Kim DH, Murovic JA, Tiel RL, et al. Management and outcomes of 42 surgical suprascapular nerve injuries and entrapments. *Neurosurgery* 2005;57:120–127.

Kitagawa R, Kim D, Reid N, et al. Surgical management of obturator nerve lesions. *Neurosurgery* 2009;65(4 Suppl):A24–A28.

Knossalla F, Nicolas V, Tegenthoff M. Suprascapular nerve entrapment in a canoeist. *Arch Neurol* 2006;63:781.

Kopell HP, Thompson WAL. *Peripheral Entrapment Neuropathies*. 2nd ed. Huntington: Robert E. Krieger, 1976.

Kornetzky L, Linden D, Berlit P. Bilateral sciatic nerve "Saturday night palsy". *J Neurol* 2001;248:425.

Kumar N, Folger WN, et al. Dyspnea as the predominant manifestation of bilateral phrenic neuropathy. *Mayo Clin Proc* 2004;79:1563–1565.

Lahrmann H, Grisold W, Authier FJ, et al. Neuralgic amyotrophy with phrenic nerve involvement. *Muscle Nerve* 1999;22:437–442.

Lajtai G, Pfirrmann CW, Aitzetmuller G, et al. The shoulders of professional beach volleyball players: high prevalence of infraspinatus muscle atrophy. *Am J Sports Med* 2009;37:1375–1383.

Levin KH. Common focal mononeuropathies and their electrodiagnosis. *J Clin Neurophysiol* 1993;10:181–189.

Lin PT, Andersson PB, Distad BJ, et al. Bilateral isolated phrenic neuropathy causing painless bilateral diaphragmatic paralysis. *Neurology* 2005;65:1499–1501.

Logigian EL, Busis NA, Berger AR, et al. Lumbrical sparing in carpal tunnel syndrome: anatomic, physiologic, and diagnostic implications. *Neurology* 1987;37:1499–1505.

Logigian EL, Villanueva R, Twydell PT, et al. Electrodiagnosis of ulnar neuropathy at the elbow (Une): a Bayesian approach. *Muscle Nerve* 2014;49:337–344.

Mastaglia FL. Musculocutaneous neuropathy after strenuous physical activity. *Med J Aust* 1986;145:153–154.

Mastaglia FL. Tibial nerve entrapment in the popliteal fossa. *Muscle Nerve* 2000;23:1883–1886.

Mastaglia FL, Venerys J, Stokes BA, et al. Compression of the tibial nerve by the tendinous arch of origin of the soleus muscle. *Clin Exp Neurol* 1981;18:81–85.

Mondelli M, Cioni R, Federico A. Rare mononeuropathies of the upper limb in bodybuilders. *Muscle Nerve* 1998;21: 809–812.

Miller RG. The cubital tunnel syndrome: diagnosis and precise localization. *Ann Neurol* 1979;6:56–59.

Nakano KK. Nerve entrapment syndromes. *Curr Opin Rheumatol* 1997;9:165–173.

Nord KM, Kapoor P, Fisher J, et al. False positive rate of thoracic outlet syndrome diagnostic maneuvers. *Electromyogr Clin Neurophysiol* 2008;48:67–74.

O'Brien M. *Aids to the Examination of the Peripheral Nervous System*. 5th ed. London: Saunders Elsevier, 2010.

O'Ferrall EK, Busche K, Dickhoff P, et al. A patient with bilateral sciatic neuropathies. *Can J Neurol Sci* 2007;34:365–367.

Oh SJ, Lee KW. Medial plantar neuropathy. *Neurology* 1987;37:1408–1410.

Paladini D, Dellantonio R, Cinti A, et al. Axillary neuropathy in volleyball players: report of two cases and literature review. *J Neurol Neurosurg Psychiatry* 1996;60:345–347.

Patijn J, Mekhail N, Hayek S, et al. Meralgia Paresthetica. *Pain Pract* 2011;11:302–308.

Pham M, Bäumer P, Meinck HM, et al. Anterior interosseous nerve syndrome: fascicular motor lesions of median nerve trunk. *Neurology* 2014;82:598–606.

Pleet AB, Massey EW. Palmaris brevis sign in neuropathy of the deep palmar branch of the ulnar nerve. *Ann Neurol* 1978;3:468–469.

Robinson LR, Henderson M. Handcuff neuropathy involving the dorsal ulnar cutaneous nerve. *Muscle Nerve* 1994;17:113–114.

Rosenbaum RB, Ochoa JL. *Carpal Tunnel Syndrome and Other Disorders of the Median Nerve*. Boston: Butterworth-Heinemann, 1993.

Scherer K, Skeen MB, Strine SA, et al. Hanging leg syndrome: combined bilateral femoral and sciatic neuropathies. *Neurology* 2006;66:1124–1125.

Schwartzman RJ. *Differential Diagnosis in Neurology*. Amsterdam: IOS Press, 2006.

Seror P, Seror R. Meralgia paresthetica: clinical and electrophysiological diagnosis in 120 cases. *Muscle Nerve* 2006;33:650–654.

Shapiro BE, Preston DC. Entrapment and compressive neuropathies. *Med Clin North Am* 2003;87:663–696.

Shyu WC, Lin JC, Chang MK, et al. Compressive radial nerve palsy induced by military shooting training: clinical and electrophysiological study. *J Neurol Neurosurg Psychiatry* 1993;56:890–893.

Sinson G, Zager EL, Kline DG. Windmill pitcher's radial neuropathy. *Neurosurgery* 1994;34:1087–1089.

Smith BE. Focal and entrapment neuropathies. *Handb Clin Neurol* 2014;126:31–43.

Sourkes M, Stewart JD. Common peroneal neuropathy: a study of selective motor and sensory involvement. *Neurology* 1991;41:1029–1033.

Spinner RJ, Amadio PC. Compressive neuropathies of the upper extremity. *Clin Plast Surg* 2003;30:155–173.

Spinner RJ, Tiel RL, Kline DG. Predominant infraspinatus muscle weakness in suprascapular nerve compression. *J Neurosurg* 2000;93:516.

Stevens JC, Smith BE, Weaver AL, et al. Symptoms of 100 patients with electromyographically verified carpal tunnel syndrome. *Muscle Nerve* 1999;22:1448–1456.

Stevens JC, Witt JC, Smith BE, et al. The frequency of carpal tunnel syndrome in computer users at a medical facility. *Neurology* 2001;56:1568–1570.

Stewart JD. *Focal Peripheral Neuropathies*. 4th ed. West Vancouver: JBJ Publishing, 2010.

Stewart JD. Magnificent MRI and fascinating selective nerve fascicle damage. *Neurology* 2014;82:554–555.

Stojkovic T, De Seze J, Hurtevent JF, et al. Phrenic nerve palsy as a feature of chronic inflammatory demyelinating polyradiculoneuropathy. *Muscle Nerve* 2003;27:497–499.

Streib E. Upper arm radial nerve palsy after muscular effort: report of three cases. *Neurology* 1992;42:1632–1634.

Subramony SH. AAEE case report #14: neuralgic amyotrophy (acute brachial neuropathy). *Muscle Nerve* 1988;11:39–44.

Thoma A, Levis C. Compression neuropathies of the lower extremity. *Clin Plast Surg* 2003;30:189–201.

Thomas JE, Cascino TL, Earle JD. Differential diagnosis between radiation and tumor plexopathy of the pelvis. *Neurology* 1985;35:1–7.

Tyrrell PJ, Feher MD, Rossor MN. Sciatic nerve damage due to toilet seat entrapment: another Saturday night palsy. *J Neurol Neurosurg Psychiatry* 1989;52:1113–1115.

van Alfen N. Clinical and pathophysiological concepts of neuralgic amyotrophy. *Nat Rev Neurol* 2011;7:315–322.

van Alfen N, Malessy MJ. Diagnosis of brachial and lumbosacral plexus lesions. *Handb Clin Neurol* 2013;115:293–310.

Van Den Berg PJ, Pompe SM, Beekman R, et al. Sonographic incidence of ulnar nerve (sub)luxation and its associated clinical and electrodiagnostic characteristics. *Muscle Nerve* 2013;47:849–855.

Van Slobbe AM, Bohnen AM, Bernsen RM, et al. Incidence rates and determinants in meralgia paresthetica in general practice. *J Neurol* 2004;251:294–297.

Wertsch JJ. Pricer palsy. *N Engl J Med* 1985;312:1645.

Wilbourn AJ. Thoracic outlet syndromes. *Neurol Clin* 1999;17:477–497.

Wilbourn AJ. Plexopathies. *Neurol Clin* 2007;25:139–171.

Witt JC, Stevens JC. Neurologic disorders masquerading as carpal tunnel syndrome: 12 cases of failed carpal tunnel release. *Mayo Clin Proc* 2000;75:409–413.

Yeremeyeva E, Kline DG, Kim DH. Iatrogenic sciatic nerve injuries at buttock and thigh levels: the Louisiana State University experience review. *Neurosurgery* 2009;65(4 Suppl): A63–A66.

Yilmaz C, Eskandari MM, Colak M. Traumatic musculocutaneous neuropathy: a case report. *Arch Orthop Trauma Surg* 2005;125:414–416.

Yuen EC, So YT. Sciatic neuropathy. *Neurol Clin* 1999;17: 617–631.

SECTION J Orthopedic Neurology

CHAPTER 47

Neck and Back Pain

Patients with primary orthopedic or musculoskeletal problems may have symptoms and signs that simulate neurologic disease. Such patients are frequently referred for neurologic consultation, particularly for electromyography (EMG). It is important to be able to recognize musculoskeletal disease in order to provide the appropriate evaluation. In addition, patients with neurologic disease, primarily radiculopathy, may present with pain patterns that can be confused with primary musculoskeletal processes. Patients with neck and arm pain, and back and leg pain, are frequent visitors to the neurologist. This chapter focuses on the clinical characteristics and differential diagnosis of cervical and lumbosacral radiculopathy (LSR), and the following chapter covers common musculoskeletal conditions that often arise in the differential diagnosis of neurologic illness.

CLINICAL PATHOANATOMY OF THE SPINE

The vertebrae are separated by intervertebral discs, which are composed of an outer fibrous ring, the annulus fibrosus, and an inner gelatinous core—the nucleus pulposus (NP). The "posterior elements" of the vertebral bodies spread out to encircle the spinal cord and form the spinal canal. Extending backward from the vertebral body, with varying degrees of slant, are the pedicles. The pedicles end in a bony mass, which has smooth upper and lower surfaces—the superior and inferior articulating facets, which are separated by the pars interarticularis. From the facet masses, the transverse processes jut laterally, and the laminae extend backward to join in the midline and complete the circle. From the junction point of the laminae, the spinous process extends backward a bit farther (Figure 47.1). The lateral recess is the corner formed by the pedicle, vertebral body, and superior articular facet (Figure 47.2).

The mixed spinal nerve passes outward from the spinal canal through the intervertebral foramen. The foramen is a passageway formed by the vertebral body anteriorly; pedicles above and below; and the facet mass and its articulation, the zygapophyseal joint, posteriorly. The neural foramen has an entrance, a middle zone, and an exit. The lateral recess of the spinal canal merges into the entry zone of the foramen. The dorsal root ganglion (DRG) occupies the midzone. The uncovertebral joints (of Luschka), which are not true joints, are the points where the posterolateral surface of a cervical vertebra comes into apposition with a neighboring vertebra. Degenerative osteophytes projecting into the intervertebral foramen from the uncovertebral "joints" may narrow it and cause radiculopathy (Figure 47.1). The uncovertebral joints are not present in the lumbosacral spine.

The tough anterior longitudinal ligament (ALL) extends lengthwise along the anterior aspect of the vertebral column, providing anterior reinforcement for the annulus. The posterior longitudinal ligament (PLL) extends along the posterior aspect of the

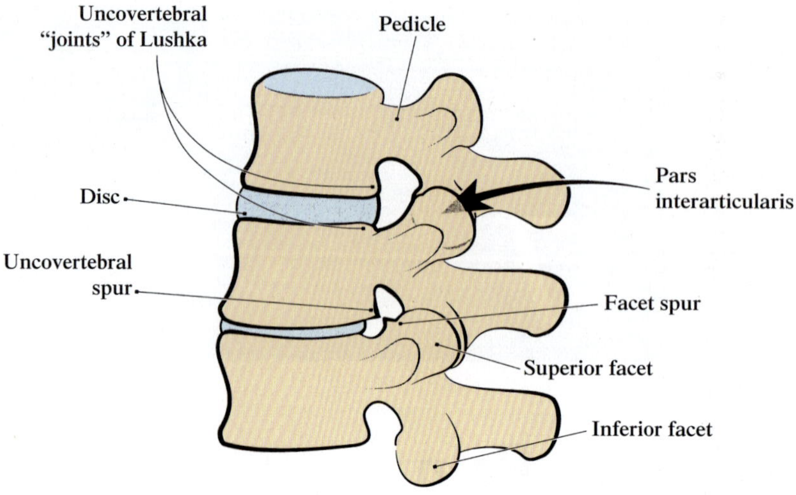

FIGURE 47.1 Lateral view of the cervical spine. Shows the vertebral bodies separated by intervertebral discs, the pedicles merging into the facet joint with its superior and inferior facets, and intervening pars interarticularis. The facets are oblique in the cervical region and more vertical in the lumbosacral spine. The uncovertebral joints are not true joints but just the opposing surfaces of the vertebral bodies. The uncovertebral processes may form osteophytes, or "spurs," which then project into the foramen. (From Campbell WW. *Essentials of Electrodiagnostic Medicine.* Philadelphia: Lippincott Williams & Wilkins, 1999. Reprinted with permission of Dr. William W. Campbell.)

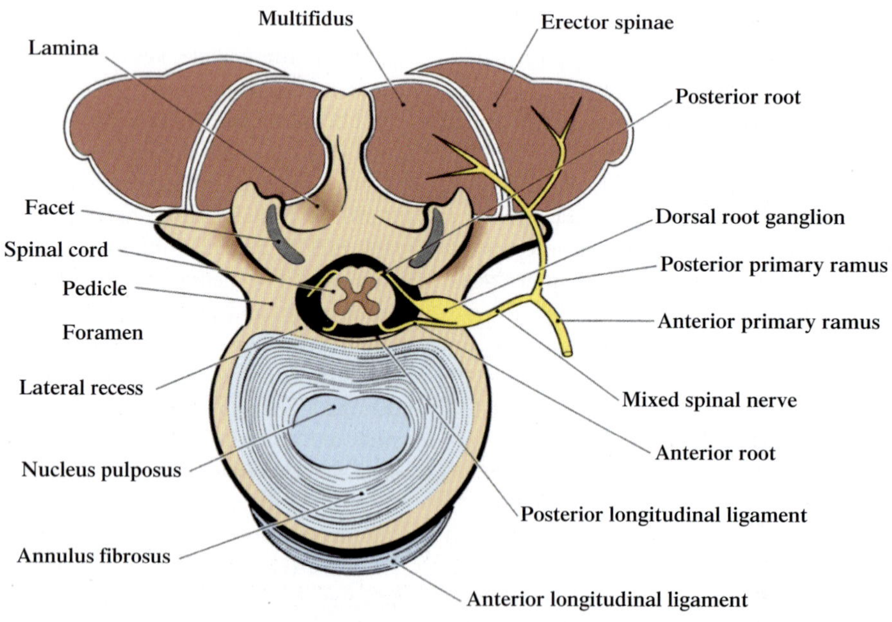

FIGURE 47.2 Cross section of a vertebral body with one pedicle cut away to show the contents of the intervertebral foramen, with the dorsal root ganglion lying in the midzone. Note the location of the multifidus muscle compartment and the innervation of the paraspinal muscles by the posterior primary ramus. The posterior longitudinal ligament is incomplete laterally, and disc ruptures tend to occur in a posterolateral direction. When a facet joint becomes enlarged because of osteoarthritis, it may encroach on the lateral recess, where the nerve root is entering the foramen. (From Campbell WW. *Essentials of Electrodiagnostic Medicine.* Philadelphia: Lippincott Williams & Wilkins, 1999. Reprinted with permission of Dr. William W. Campbell.)

vertebral bodies and reinforces the discs posteriorly. Compared with the ALL, the PLL is weak and flimsy and narrows as it descends. Disc herniations tend to occur posterolaterally, especially in the lumbosacral region, in part because of the lateral incompleteness of the PLL. In the cervical region, the PLL may ossify and contribute to spondylotic narrowing. The ligamentum flavum extends along the posterior aspect of the spinal canal. It buckles and folds during neck extension and may also contribute to canal narrowing.

The static anatomy of the spine provides only a partial understanding of the changes that occur on motion. Direct measurements have shown that the pressure within a lumbar disc varies markedly with different postures and activities. It is lowest when lying supine, increases by fourfold on standing, and increases a further 50% when leaning forward. The pressure is 40% higher sitting than standing. The higher pressure when sitting is clinically relevant, as patients with lumbosacral disc ruptures characteristically have more pain sitting than standing. The intradiscal pressure during a sit-up is astronomical.

The size of the intervertebral foramina decreases with extension and with ipsilateral bending. In extension, the facet joints draw closer together and the posterior quadrants of the spinal canal narrow. Cervical roots stretch with flexion and may angulate at the entrance to the foramen. The intraspinal subarachnoid pressure varies with respiration and increases markedly with Valsalva or restriction of venous outflow. The epidural and radicular veins change in size with posture and respiration. These dynamic changes, which are especially relevant in the presence of pathology, form the basis for clinical tests and historical questions useful for distinguishing the various causes for back and neck pain.

The Intervertebral Disc

The annulus provides circumferential reinforcement for the disc; the spherical NP allows the vertebral bodies above and below to glide and slip across it, like a ball bearing. The NP is eccentrically placed, closer to the posterior aspect of the disc (Figure 47.2). The relative thinness of the annulus posteriorly is another factor contributing to the tendency of disc herniations to occur in that direction. The great majority of the weight-bearing function of a normal disc is borne by the NP, which contains proteoglycans, macromolecules that heartily imbibe fluid. Early in life, the NP is 90% water, but it undergoes progressive desiccation over time. With desiccation of the nucleus and loss of compressibility, the annulus must assume more of the weight burden. This increased load, in the face of its own degenerative weakening, then makes the annulus prone to tears.

The Spinal Roots

The anatomy of the spinal nerve is shown in Figure 24.3. Myotomal anatomy is discussed in Chapter 27 and dermatomal anatomy in Chapters 31 and 36. In the cervical spine, the nerve root exits over the vertebral body of like number until the C8 root exits beneath C7; all subsequent roots exit beneath the vertebral body of like number (Figure 24.1). In contrast to LSR, where disease usually affects the spinal root exiting one vertebral level lower, that is, disease at the L4-L5 level affects the L5 root, cervical radiculopathy (CR) tends to affect the nerve root laterally at its level of exit. Disease at the C5-C6 vertebral level affects the C6 root and at the C6-C7 level, the C7 root. When the cord terminates at the level of L1-L2, the remaining roots drop vertically downward in the cauda equina to their exit foramina. The L5 nerve root exiting at the L5-S1 interspace has arisen as a discrete structure at L1-L2 and had to traverse the interspaces at L2-L3, L3-L4, and L4-L5 before exiting at L5-S1, sliding laterally all the while. The L5 root could be injured by a central disc at L2-L3 or L3-L4, a posterolateral disc at L4-L5, or a far lateral disc or lateral recess stenosis at L5-S1 (Figure 47.3). A posterolateral disc at L4-L5 is the most likely culprit but not the sole suspect. The clinician must correlate the clinical localization of a given root lesion with the radiographic and clinical information to deduce the vertebral level involved and the proper course of action.

With aging and recurrent micro- and macrotrauma, degenerative spine disease develops. This involves both the disc (degenerative disc disease or DDD) and the bony structures and joints (degenerative joint disease or DJD). These processes are separate but related. Together, DDD and DJD are referred to as spondylosis. Small tears in the annulus may cause nonspecific, nonradiating neck or back pain. More extensive tears lead to disc bulging or protrusion, in which the disc herniates but remains beneath the PLL. Frank ruptures breach the PLL and allow a full-blown herniation of the nucleus pulposus (HNP) into the epidural space. Most HNPs occur in a posterolateral direction; occasionally, they are directly lateral or central. Which nerve roots are damaged

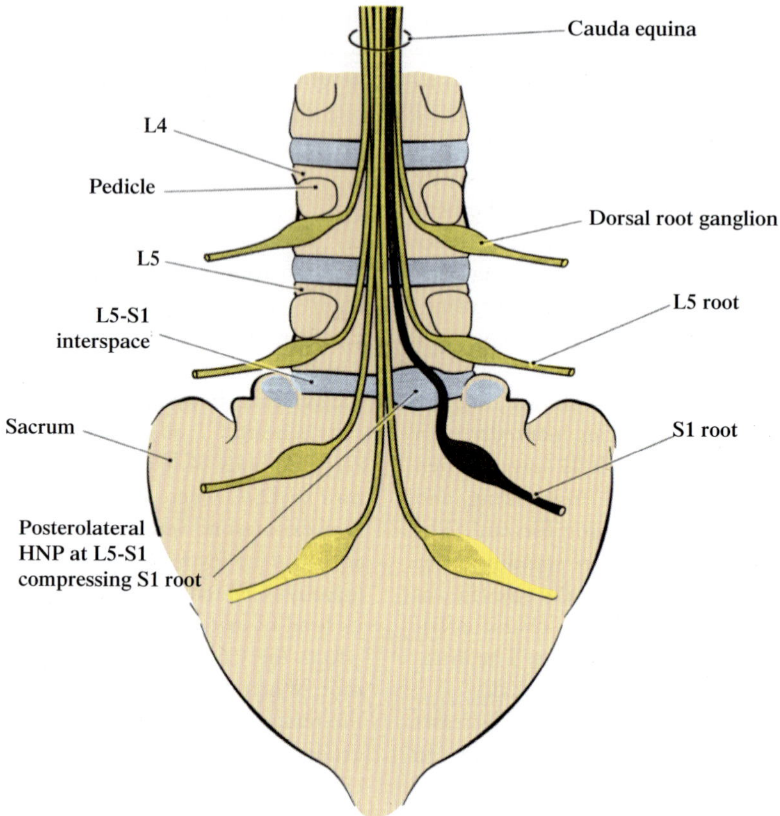

FIGURE 47.3 Posterior view of the cauda equina with exiting nerve roots. The nerve roots move laterally en route to their exit foramina. A posterolateral herniation of the nucleus pulposus (HNP) has compressed the S1 root as it passes by the L5-S1 interspace. A central HNP at any interspace could affect multiple roots. (From Campbell WW. *Essentials of Electrodiagnostic Medicine*. Philadelphia: Lippincott Williams & Wilkins, 1999. Reprinted with permission of Dr. William W. Campbell.)

depends largely on the direction of the herniation. In the face of disc herniation, the root may be damaged not only by direct compression but also by an inflammatory process induced by intradiscal proteoglycans, ischemia due to pressure, and adhesions and fibrosis.

The anterior elements, vertebral body and pedicles, normally bear 80% to 90% of the weight. As degenerative changes advance with desiccation and loss of disc height, the posterior elements (facets, pars, and laminae) may come to carry up to 50% of the weight-bearing function. This increases the work of the posterior elements and accelerates their degenerative changes. They react to the increased weight-bearing role by becoming hypertrophic and elaborating osteophytes. Osteoarthritis and synovitis of the facet joints is another point of pathology. In response to the increased loading attendant on loss of disc height and shift of weight bearing posteriorly, the facet joints develop degenerative changes: laxity of the capsule, instability, subluxation, and bony hypertrophy with osteophyte formation. The friction induced by minor instability and microtrauma leads to the formation of osteophytes. In the cervical spine, there is the added element of hypertrophy of the uncinate processes and the development of uncovertebral spurs. Degenerative osteophytes arising simultaneously from the uncus and from the vertebral body end-plate region may become confluent and create a spondylotic bar or ridge that stretches across the entire extent of the spinal canal. Like any arthritic joint, the facet may enlarge, impinging on the intervertebral foramen or the spinal canal, especially in the lateral recess. Loss of disc height causes the PLL and the ligamentum flavum to buckle and bulge into the canal. The degenerative changes in the discs and bony elements eventually produce cervical or lumbar spondylosis and may culminate in the syndrome of spinal stenosis.

All these degenerative changes leave less room for the neural elements. In the sagittal plane, the average cervical spinal cord is about 8 mm and the average cervical spinal canal about 14 mm. A sagittal canal diameter less than 10 mm may put the spinal cord at risk. The epidural space is normally occupied primarily by epidural fat and veins. When disc herniations and osteophytes intrude into the space, the resultant clinical manifestations depend in large part on how much room there is to accommodate them. Patients blessed by nature with capacious spinal canals can asymptomatically harbor a surprising amount of pathology. Patients with congenitally narrow canals and those who have undergone past spinal fusion procedures are at increased risk for developing spinal stenosis. Compression of vascular structures may introduce an additional complication of cord and/or root ischemia.

Several different clinical syndromes may ensue from degenerative spine disease, including the following: simple, single-level radiculopathy; multilevel radiculopathy; cauda equina syndrome; cervical myelopathy; cervical radiculomyelopathy; neurogenic claudication; lateral recess syndrome; and occasionally, a central cord or Brown-Séquard syndrome. Rarely, radiculopathy results from other processes, such as tumor (e.g., neurofibroma, meningioma, metastasis), arachnoid or synovial cysts, infection (e.g., Lyme disease, CMV, epidural abscess), infiltration (e.g., meningeal neoplasia, sarcoidosis), epidural block, irradiation, or ischemia (e.g., diabetes). A common cause of noncompressive radiculopathy is herpes zoster. Reactivation of a latent varicella-zoster virus resident in DRG cells triggers a herpes zoster outbreak ("shingles"). Affected patients develop an extremely painful vesicular rash in the distribution of the involved dorsal root ganglia, usually a single dermatome. Although thoracic segments are involved most often, zoster can strike anywhere. Severe myotomal weakness may result when herpes zoster strikes in the cervical or lumbar enlargements (Figure 4.7). Zoster may also cause plexopathy, mononeuropathy, or radiculoplexus neuropathy. Acute and chronic inflammatory demyelinating polyradiculoneuropathies produce marked abnormalities of the roots.

Because of the varied pathology involved, different types of radiculopathy occur in degenerative spine disease. The process is frequently multifactorial, involving some combination of disc herniation and spondylosis. The most straightforward clinical syndrome is unilateral "soft disc" rupture, an HNP. A similar clinical picture can result from a foraminal osteophyte, a "hard disc," or spur. Some patients have soft disc superimposed on hard disc. It is clinically, radiologically, and sometimes surgically difficult to distinguish between soft disc and hard disc. Osteophytes, spurs, and foraminal stenosis are more common than simple soft disc in the etiology of CR. In Radhakrishnan et al.'s series, soft disc (i.e., not present in association with significant spondylosis) was responsible in only 22%; the remainder had hard disc or a combination. As a general rule, soft disc is more likely in younger patients. A central HNP may compress the spinal cord or cauda equina.

In compressive radiculopathy, sensory loss occurs in a dermatomal distribution and weakness in a myotomal distribution. Dermatomal sensory loss is less than expected because of extensive overlap in the innervation zones of spinal roots. Investigators used very different techniques to obtain the available dermatome maps (see Chapter 31 and Figure 36.5). The maps of Keegan and Garrett most closely approximate clinical reality. Sensory loss is most readily demonstrated in the signature zones of the major roots. Weakness in radiculopathy is also usually less than expected for a given myotome because most muscles receive multisegmental innervation (see Chapter 27). Disease affecting multiple levels causes much more severe weakness.

NECK AND ARM PAIN

Pain in the neck or upper extremity is a common clinical problem. Pain may involve the neck, shoulder, arm, forearm, or hand in virtually any combination. Potential causes of neck and arm pain are many. Common neurologic etiologies are CR, degenerative spine disease, brachial plexopathy, and peripheral nerve entrapment. Neck and arm pain of musculoskeletal origin is also common. Neurologic and musculoskeletal etiologies may be difficult to separate.

CERVICAL RADICULOPATHY

The population-based study of CR by Radhakrishnan et al. provided a wealth of interesting information. The incidence was highest at ages 50 to 54, with a mean age of 47, a male predominance, and a decline in incidence after age 60. There was a history of physical injury or exertion in only 15%; the most common precipitants were shoveling snow or playing golf. The onset was acute in half, subacute in a

TABLE 47.1 Clinical Findings in 100 Cervical Radiculopathy (CR) Patients

Clinical Finding	Highly Localizing to	Suggestively Localizing to
Pain only in neck and shoulder		C5
Presence of scapular/interscapular pain		C7 or C8
No pain below elbow		C5
Pain involving the posterior upper arm		C7
Pain involving the medial upper arm		C7 or C8
Paresthesias limited to the thumb	C6	
Paresthesias limited to the index and middle fingers	C7	
Paresthesias limited to the ring and small fingers	C8	
Whole hand paresthesias		C7
Depressed triceps reflex	C7 or C8	
Depressed biceps and brachioradialis reflexes	C5 or C6	
Weakness of spinati	C5	
Weakness of deltoid	C5 or C6	
Weakness of triceps	C7	
Weakness of hand intrinsics	C8	
Sensory loss over thumb only		C6 or C7
Sensory loss involving middle finger	C7	
Sensory loss involving small finger	C8	

quarter, and insidious in a quarter, with the majority of patients symptomatic for about 2 weeks prior to diagnosis. Surgery was done in 26%. The disease tends to recur—some 31% of patients had a previous history of CR, and 32% had a recurrence during follow-up. At last follow-up, 90% of the patients had minimal to no symptoms. Others have noted this favorable long-term prognosis.

A number of clinical conditions may be confused with CR. These primarily include brachial plexopathies, entrapment neuropathies, and nonneuropathic mimickers. The more common musculoskeletal conditions causing confusion include shoulder pathology (bursitis, tendonitis, impingement syndrome), lateral epicondylitis, and de Quervain's tenosynovitis (see Chapter 48). Cervical myofascial pain, facet joint disease, and cervical vertebral body pathology can cause neck pain with referred pain to the arm. Pain can be referred to the neck, arm, or shoulder from the heart, lungs, esophagus, or upper abdomen.

Clinical Signs and Symptoms in Cervical Radiculopathy

The classic articles by Yoss et al. and Murphey et al. detail the history and examination findings in CR. Yoss et al. evaluated 100 patients with surgically confirmed single-level cervical radiculopathies. The highly and suggestively localizing findings from these 100 patients are summarized in Table 47.1. Murphey et al. reviewed 648 cases of surgically treated single-level cervical radiculopathies. Findings in terms of pain radiation and neurologic deficits were similar to Yoss et al. Murphey et al. emphasized the occurrence of pain in the pectoral region in 20% of their cases; they opined that neck, periscapular, and pectoral region pain was referred from the disc itself and that arm pain was the result of nerve root compression.

In the Radhakrishnan et al. series, cervicobrachial pain was present at the onset in 98% and was radicular in 65%. Paresthesias were reported by 90%, almost identical to the Yoss series. Pain on neck movement was present in 98%, paraspinal muscle spasm in 88%, decreased reflexes in 84% (triceps 50%, biceps or brachioradialis 34%), weakness in 65%, and sensory loss in 33%. In the Levin et al. series, 70% had motor and sensory symptoms, 12% had motor symptoms only, and 18% had sensory symptoms only.

The history, especially patterns of pain radiation and paresthesias, can provide localizing information in suspected CR. Radiating pain on coughing, sneezing, or straining at stool (Dejerine's sign) is significant but seldom elicited. Increased pain on shoulder motion suggests nonradicular pathology. Relief of pain by resting the hand atop the head is reportedly characteristic of CR, but the author has seen this phenomenon with a Pancoast tumor. Hand paresthesias at night suggest carpal tunnel syndrome, but carpal tunnel syndrome can occur in association with CR ("double crush syndrome"), so nocturnal acroparesthesias do not exclude coexistent radiculopathy.

Physical examination in patients with suspected CR should include an assessment of the range of motion of the neck and arm, a search for root compression signs, detailed examination of strength and reflexes, a screening sensory examination, and probing for areas of muscle spasm or trigger points **(Video 47.1)**. Patients with either weakness or reduced reflexes on physical examination are up to five times more likely to have an abnormal electrodiagnostic study. A normal physical examination by no means excludes CR (negative predictive value 52%).

The cervical spine range of motion is highly informative. Patients should be asked to put chin to chest and to either shoulder, each ear to shoulder, and to hold the head in full extension; these maneuvers all affect the size of the intervertebral foramen. Pain produced by movements that narrow the foramen suggests CR. Pain on the symptomatic side on putting the ipsilateral ear to the shoulder suggests radiculopathy, but increased pain on leaning or turning away from the symptomatic side suggests a myofascial origin. Radiating pain or paresthesias with the head in extension and tilted slightly to the symptomatic side is highly suggestive of CR (Spurling's sign or maneuver, foraminal compression test); brief breath holding or gentle Valsalva in this position will sometimes elicit the pain if positioning alone is not provocative. The addition of axial compression by pressing down on the crown of the head does not seem to add much. Spurling's test is specific but not very sensitive. Light digital compression of the jugular veins until the face is flushed and the patient is uncomfortable will sometimes elicit radicular symptoms: unilateral shoulder, arm, pectoral or scapular pain, or radiating paresthesias into the arm or hand (Viets' sign). A slight cough while the face is suffused may increase the sensitivity. In the past, clinicians sometimes went so far as to put a blood pressure cuff around the patient's neck to occlude the jugular veins (Naffziger's sign). The two eponyms are often used interchangeably, and more often Naffziger's sign is used for both techniques. Jugular compression is thought to engorge epidural veins or the cerebrospinal fluid reservoirs, which in the normal individual is harmless. But when some element of foraminal narrowing and nerve root pressure exists, the additional compression causes the acute development of symptoms. The same mechanism likely underlies the exacerbation of root pain by coughing, sneezing, and straining. Like Spurling's test, Viets/Naffziger's sign is specific but insensitive. It is less useful in LSR than in CR.

An occasional CR patient has relief of pain with manual upward neck traction, particularly with the neck in slight flexion (cervical distraction test). Likely related to the occasional relief of pain by resting the hand on top of the head, some patients have a decrease in pain with shoulder abduction (Bakody's sign, shoulder abduction relief test, arm abduction sign); this sign is more likely to occur with soft disc herniation. Flexion of the neck may cause Lhermitte's sign in patients with cervical spondylosis or large disc herniations. Pain or limitation of motion of any upper-extremity joint should signal the possibility of nonradicular pathology. The differentiation of CR from primary shoulder disease (e.g., bursitis, capsulitis, tendonitis, or impingement syndrome) can be particularly difficult (see Chapter 48).

A focused but detailed strength exam should at least assess the power in the deltoids, spinati, biceps, triceps, pronators, wrist extensors, finger extensors, thenar muscles, and interossei. Testing muscles in a position of mechanical disadvantage may help detect mild weakness (see Chapter 27). The sensory exam should concentrate on the hand, and particularly assess touch, because the large, myelinated fibers conveying light touch are more vulnerable to pressure injury than the smaller fibers carrying pain and temperature. Reflex exam should include not only the standard upper-extremity reflexes but the knee and ankle jerks and plantar reflexes as well. Increased lower-extremity reflexes and extensor plantar responses suggest myelopathy complicating the radiculopathy.

Based on the foregoing, Table 47.2 outlines the clinical data that favor the diagnosis of CR.

Individual Root Lesions

In the cervical spine, C7 root lesions are the most common (±60%), C6 next most common (±20%), with C5 and C8 lesions making up about equal proportions of the remainder. Involvement of the upper cervical roots is rare. In C5 lesions, weakness is most easily detected in the supra- and infraspinatus, deltoid, biceps, and brachioradialis. The rhomboids

TABLE 47.2 Clinical Signs and Symptoms That Favor a Diagnosis of Cervical Radiculopathy

- Age 35–60
- Acute/subacute onset
- Past history of cervical or lumbosacral radiculopathy
- Cervicobrachial pain radiating to shoulder, periscapular region, pectoral region, or arm
- Paresthesias in arm or hand
- Pain on neck movement—especially extension or ipsilateral bending
- Positive root compression signs
- Radiating pain with cough, sneeze, or bowel movement
- Myotomal weakness
- Decreased reflex(es)
- Dermatomal sensory loss
- Pain relief with hand on head
- Pain relief with manual upward traction

may also be weak but are difficult to examine. The biceps and brachioradialis reflexes may be depressed. The signature zone for sensory loss lies over the mid-deltoid region. In C6 lesions, weakness is most likely in the biceps, pronator teres, flexor carpi radialis, brachioradialis, and wrist extensors. The biceps and brachioradialis reflexes may be depressed. If there is concomitant myelopathy, along with reflex depression, spread to the finger flexors or frank "inversion" of the reflex may occur (see Chapter 38). The signature zone for sensory loss lies along the radial aspect of the forearm and the thumb. In C7 lesions, detectable weakness is most common in the triceps (use mechanical advantage), pronator teres, flexor carpi radialis, and wrist and finger extensors. Weakness of the triceps and pronator teres is pathognomonic, because C7 is their only common innervation. Depression of the triceps may be present, and with concomitant myelopathy, it may be inverted (i.e., elbow flexion occurs). The signature zone for sensory loss lies over the middle finger. In C8 lesions, expect weakness in the flexor digitorum profundus and superficialis, flexor pollicis longus, flexor carpi ulnaris, pronator quadratus, extensor indicis, extensor pollicis longus and brevis, and all hand intrinsics. The finger flexor reflex, and rarely the triceps, may be depressed. The signature zone for sensory loss is the small finger and medial forearm.

A study of 69 patients with magnetic resonance imaging (MRI) confirmed C6 and C7 nerve root compression found that arm pain and sensory symptoms were diffuse and not distinctly different for C6 or C7 radiculopathy. Weakness was reported by 41% of patients, and the specific pattern of weakness had only limited value in discriminating between the levels.

LUMBOSACRAL RADICULOPATHY

About 70% of humans suffer from at least an occasional episode of low back pain (LBP), but clinically significant radiculopathy occurs in only 4% to 6% of the population. Abnormalities on imaging studies are common in asymptomatic subjects and only loosely associated with symptoms and signs. Most benign self-limited episodes of LBP arise from musculoligamentous structures, and discomfort is localized to the low back region. There are numerous pain-sensitive structures that can underlie a clinical episode of LBP: the intervertebral disc, especially the outer fibers of the annulus; the facet joints; other bony structures; subcutaneous tissues; the meninges; the paravertebral muscles and ligaments; and spinal nerve roots. Pain can also be referred to the lower back from visceral structures in the abdomen and pelvis. The back may also be involved in systemic diseases, such as spondyloarthropathies.

Involvement of some of these pain-sensitive structures can produce referred pain that radiates to the extremity (buttock, hip, thigh) and can simulate the radiating pain of nerve root origin. In some patients, there is referred pain to one or both lower extremities that arises from within the disc or other structures, without actual nerve root compression. Considerable pain can be referred to the buttock and thigh with disease limited to the disc, the facet joint, or the sacroiliac joint. A study of 1,293 cases of LBP concluded that referred pain to the lower limb most often originated from sacroiliac and facet joints. Referred pain to the extremity occurred nearly twice as often as true radicular pain and frequently mimicked the clinical presentation of radiculopathies. A study of 92 patients with chronic LBP concluded that 39% had annular tears or other forms of internal disc disruption as the etiology of their pain.

Clinical Signs and Symptoms in Lumbosacral Radiculopathy

Deyo et al. reviewed the information that could be obtained from the history and physical examination in patients with LBP and suggested three basic questions: (a) is there a serious, underlying systemic disease present? (b) is there neurologic compromise that might require further evaluation? and (c) are there psychological factors leading to pain amplification? Things that suggest underlying systemic disease include the following: a history of cancer, unexplained weight loss, pain lasting longer than 1 month, pain unrelieved by bed rest, fever, focal spine tenderness, morning stiffness, improvement in pain with exercise, and failure of conservative treatment. Other symptoms suggesting serious pathology include bowel and bladder disturbances, perineal sensory loss, and a history of violent trauma.

Pain radiating below the knee is more likely of true radicular origin than pain radiating only to the posterior thigh. The relationship of the pain to position and exercise is important. The pain of an HNP is typically more severe when the patient is seated than when standing but is usually increased by activity, particularly bending, twisting, lifting, or stooping, especially when the knees are extended. Other common causes of LBP, such as muscle strain, osteoarthritis, and spinal stenosis cause pain that is worse when standing. Nonmechanical pain is unrelated to posture, position, or activity. Pain that is constant, progressive, and nonmechanical is more likely to indicate serious underlying pathology. Radicular pain is characteristically intensified by coughing, straining, and sneezing. The pain of a spinal cord tumor may also be aggravated by increasing the intracranial or intraspinal pressure but is typically more severe when the patient is lying down than when seated.

The utility, or lack thereof, of various physical examination findings has been studied. The straight leg raising (SLR, Lasègue) test remains the mainstay in detecting radicular compression. The test is performed by slowly raising the symptomatic leg with the knee extended (Figure 47.4, Video 47.2). Pain caused by flexing the hip with the knee bent is suggestive of hip disease. The FABERE or Patrick's test also checks for hip disease (see Chapter 48). During SLR, tension is transmitted to the nerve roots between about 30 and 70 degrees and pain increases. Pain at less than 30 degrees raises the question of nonorganicity, and some discomfort and tightness beyond 70 degrees is routine and insignificant. There are various degrees or levels of positivity. Ipsilateral leg tightness is the lowest level; pain in the back, more significant; and radiating pain in the leg, highly significant. When raising the good leg produces pain in the symptomatic leg (crossed SLR), the likelihood of a root lesion is very high. Rarely, SLR may even cause numbness and paresthesias in the distribution of the affected nerve root. The buckling sign is knee flexion during SLR to avoid sciatic nerve tension. Kernig's sign is an alternate way of stretching the root (see Chapter 52).

Various SLR modifications may provide additional information; all of these variations are referred to as root stretch signs. The pain may be more severe, or elicited sooner, if the test is carried out with the thigh and leg in a position of adduction and internal rotation (Bonnet phenomenon). The SLR can be enhanced by passively dorsiflexing the patient's foot (Bragard's sign) or great toe (Sicard's sign) just at the elevation angle at which the increased root tension begins to produce pain (Figure 47.5).

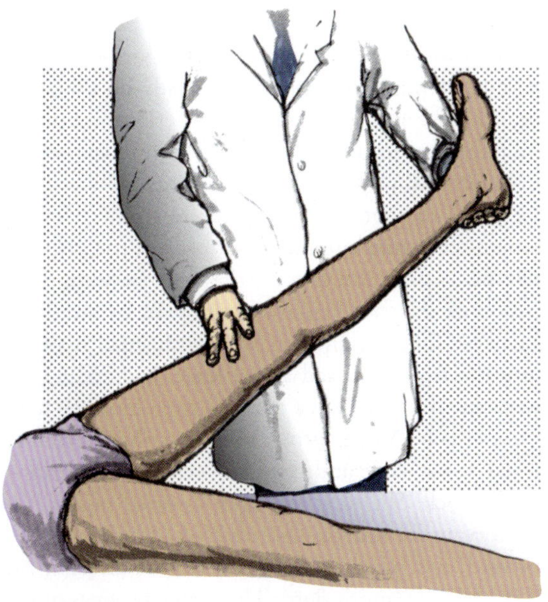

FIGURE 47.4 Method of eliciting straight leg raising (Lasègue's sign).

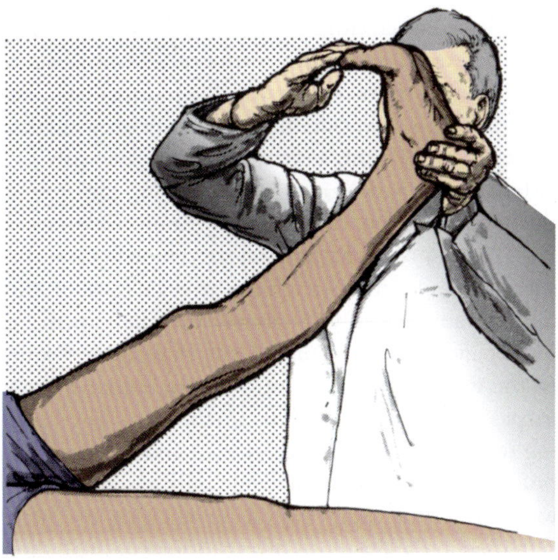

FIGURE 47.5 Accentuation of straight leg raising by dorsiflexion of either the foot or the great toe.

The term Spurling's sign is also used for either of these. A quick snap to the sciatic nerve in the popliteal fossa just as stretch begins to cause pain (bowstring sign or popliteal compression test) accomplishes the same end and may cause pain in the lumbar region, in the affected buttock, or along the course of the sciatic nerve. In severe cases, pain may be elicited merely by dorsiflexion of the foot or great toe as the patient lies supine with legs extended. A similar modification may be carried out by flexing the thigh to an angle just short of that necessary to cause pain and then flexing the neck; this may produce the same exacerbation of pain that would be brought about by further flexion of the hip (Brudzinski's sign). Occasionally, the pain may be brought on merely by passive flexion of the neck when the patient is recumbent with legs extended. The pain with SLR should be the same with the patient supine or seated. Failure of a patient with a positive supine SLR to complain or lean backward when the extended leg is brought up while in the seated position (e.g., under the guise of doing the planter response) suggests nonorganicity. In the sitting position, the patient may be able to extend each leg alone but extending both together causes radicular pain (Bechterew's test).

In O'Connell's test, SLR is first carried out on the sound limb, and the angle of flexion and site of pain are recorded; the pain may be on the opposite side. Then, SLR is carried out on the affected limb, and the angle and site of pain again noted. Then, both thighs are flexed simultaneously, keeping the knees extended. The angle of flexion permitted may be greater than that allowed when either the affected limb or the sound limb is flexed alone. Finally, with both thighs flexed to an angle just short of that which produces pain, the sound limb is lowered; this may result in a marked exacerbation of pain, sometimes associated with paresthesias. The patient may be able to do a sit-up with the knees flexed but not extended (Kraus-Weber test).

The reverse SLR (femoral stretch or Ely test) is a way of eliciting root stretch in the evaluation of high lumbar radiculopathy (Figure 47.6). The patient lies prone, and the knee is pulled into maximum flexion, or the examiner pulls upward on the extended knee to passively extend the hip. In the bent knee pulling test, the patient's knee is flexed and the examiner pulls upward on the ankle while pushing the buttock forward (in the same way as for eliciting the psoas sign used in the diagnosis of appendicitis). In all these variations, the normal individual should complain only of quadriceps tightness. With disc disease, there is pain in the back or in the femoral nerve distribution on the side of the lesion.

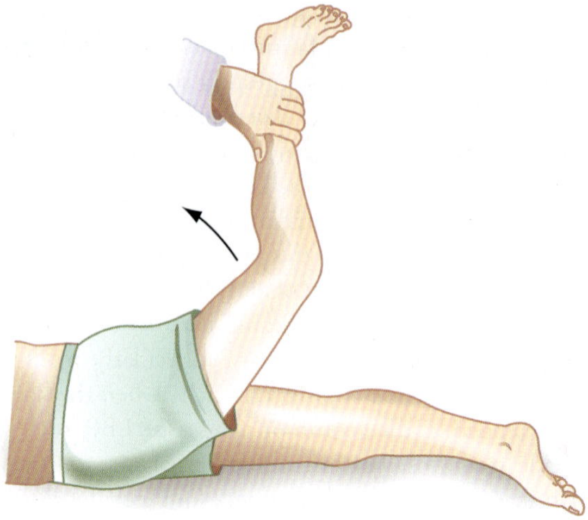

FIGURE 47.6 Reverse straight leg raising (femoral nerve stretch test) for evaluation of suspected high lumbar radiculopathy. (Modified with author's permission from Reeves AG, Swenson RS. *Disorders of the Nervous System: A Primer.* New Haven: Dartmouth Medical School, 2004. Retrieved on August 28, 2018. http://www.dartmouth.edu/~dons/index.html. Copyright © 2008 Reeves.)

The examiner should also look for abnormalities of posture, deformities, tenderness, and muscle spasm. With radiculopathy, there may be loss of the normal lumbar lordosis because of involuntary spasm of the paravertebral muscles. In addition, there is often a lumbar scoliosis, with a compensatory thoracic scoliosis. Most commonly, the list of the body is away from the painful side, and the pelvis is tilted so that the affected hip is elevated (Figure 47.7). The patient attempts to bear weight mostly on the sound leg. The list and scoliosis may sometimes be toward the painful side, and the patient's body may be bent forward and toward that side to avoid stretching the involved root. With very severe sciatic pain, the patient will avoid complete extension at the knee and may place only the toes on the floor because dorsiflexion of the foot aggravates the pain by stretching the nerve. The patient may walk with small steps and keep the leg semiflexed at the knee. In bending forward, she flexes the knee to avoid stretching the nerve (Neri's sign). When sitting, she keeps the affected leg flexed at the knee and rests her weight on the opposite buttock. She may rise from a seated position by supporting herself on the unaffected side, bending forward, and placing one hand on the affected side of the back (Minor's sign). There may be areas of tenderness in the lumbosacral region, and manipulation

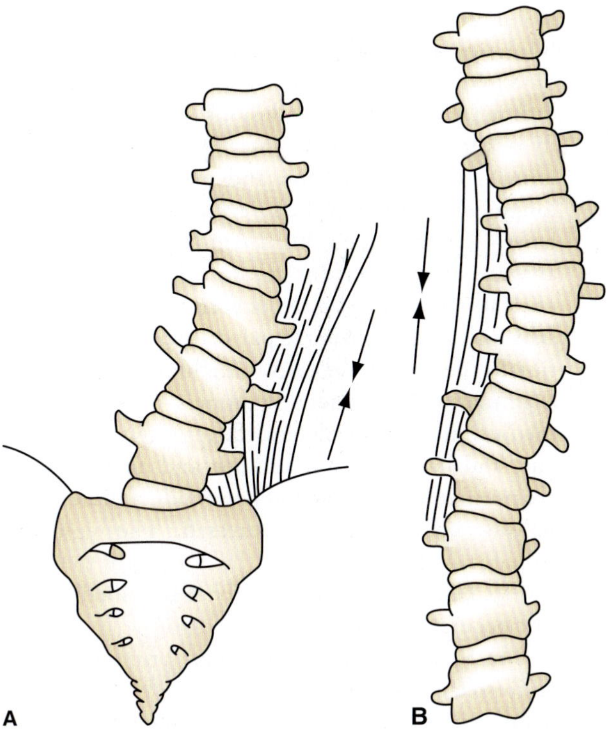

FIGURE 47.7 Curvature of the vertebral column associated with unilateral paraspinal muscle spasm. Unilateral spasm causes the spine to curve with the concavity toward the spasm **(B)**. Because of the broad attachment of the paraspinal muscles to the sacrum and the ilium at the lumbosacral junction, the convexity appears on the side of the spasm **(A)**. (Modified from Reeves AG, Swenson RS. *Disorders of the Nervous System: A Primer.* New Haven: Dartmouth Medical School, 2004. Retrieved on August 28, 2018. http://www.dartmouth.edu/~dons/index.html)

or percussion over the spinous processes, or pressure just lateral to them, may reproduce or exacerbate the pain. A sharp blow with a percussion hammer on or just lateral to the spinous processes while the patient is bending forward may bring out the pain. There may be spasm not only of the paravertebral muscles but also of the hamstrings and calf muscles. Flexion, extension, and lateral deviation of the spine are limited; the pain is usually accentuated with passive extension of the lumbar spine toward the affected side while the patient is standing erect. There may be localized tenderness at the sciatic notch and along the course of the sciatic nerve. Pelvic and rectal examination may be necessary in some instances.

The neurologic examination should include assessment of power in the major lower-extremity muscle groups, but especially the dorsiflexors of the foot and toes and the evertors and invertors of the foot. Plantar flexion of the foot is so powerful that manual testing rarely suffices. Having the patient do 10 toe raises with either foot is a better test. As the patient is standing on one leg, look for Trendelenburg's sign (Chapter 27). Normally, the pelvis remains level or slants upward toward the unsupported leg. With a positive Trendelenburg, the hip moves laterally and up and the shoulder moves down on the weight-bearing side, and the pelvis sags toward the unsupported leg (see **Video Link 47.1**). On walking, weakness of the hip abductors, primarily the L5-S1 innervated gluteus medius, causes the weight-bearing leg to adduct and the hip to jut laterally on the affected side (Trendelenburg gait, gluteus medius lurch). Trendelenburg's sign or gait may occur with other processes causing hip abductor weakness, for example, superior gluteal neuropathy or myopathy, and may also occur with musculoskeletal disease, such as hip dislocation, fracture of the femoral head, or coxa vara. The peroneal reflex is sometimes useful (see **Video Link 47.2**).

In addition to assessing power, it is important to look for atrophy and fasciculations. Sensation should be tested in the signature zones of the major roots. The status of knee and ankle reflexes reflects the integrity of the L3-L4 and S1 roots, respectively. There is no good reflex for the L5 root, but the hamstring reflexes are sometimes useful (see Chapter 38). An occasional L5 radiculopathy produces a clear selective diminution of the medial hamstring reflex.

Tests for nonorganicity are useful in the evaluation of LBP **(Video 47.2)**. Waddell et al. identified a set of eight nonorganic signs in 1980, and the overall Waddell score is considered positive if at least three of the signs are positive. The usefulness of the Waddell score remains controversial, and it suggests at least the possibility of somatic amplification and the contribution of psychosocial factors to the clinical picture. Imaging studies show that while there is more overall pathology in patients without Waddell signs, many of these patients have significant spinal pathology. Pain during simulated spinal rotation, pinning the patient's hands to the sides while rotating the hips (no spine rotation occurs as shoulders and hips remain in a constant relationship) suggests somatic amplification. Also useful are a discrepancy between the positivity of the SLR between the supine and seated position, pain in the back on pressing down on top of the head, widespread and excessive "tenderness" (touch-me-not sign), general overreaction during testing, and nondermatomal/nonmyotomal neurologic signs.

The major lumbosacral radicular syndromes include HNP, lateral recess stenosis, and spinal stenosis with cauda equina compression. Virtually all patients with radiculopathy have sciatica. The odds of a patient without sciatica having radiculopathy have been estimated at 1:1,000. With HNP or lateral recess stenosis, leg pain usually predominates over back pain. With HNP, the pain is typically worse when sitting, better when standing, better still when lying down, and generally worse in flexed than extended postures—all reflecting the known changes in intradiscal pressure that occur in these positions. With lateral recess stenosis, the pain is worse with standing or walking because of spinal extension, relieved by sitting with the torso flexed or by lying down. Patients with HNP tend to have a positive SLR, those with recess stenosis do not. The essence of the recess stenosis picture then is pain on standing, lack of pain on sitting, and a negative SLR. The essence of the HNP picture is pain worse on sitting, lessened with standing, and a positive SLR. Patients with HNP are usually in the 30 to 55 age range, and those with lateral recess stenosis are a bit older. As with CR, pain may exacerbate with cough, sneeze, or Valsalva.

Individual Root Lesions

In LSR, the root is most often compromised at the level above its level of exit, but foraminal pathology at the exit level or a central disc at levels above may cause damage as the root exits or passes by in its descent.

The most common LSRs involve either L5 or S1. Upper lumbar radiculopathies are rare. Disease of S2-S5 is usually part of a cauda equina syndrome (see below). In L5 lesions, weakness primarily occurs in the tibialis anterior, extensor hallucis longus, tibialis posterior, and extensor digitorum longus and brevis. When severe the patient may have a footdrop. In this setting, the presence or absence of involvement of the tibialis posterior is critical in distinguishing between an L5 radiculopathy and a peroneal nerve palsy. Involvement of the tibialis posterior suggests radiculopathy. Careful examination may reveal weakness of the gluteus medius, tensor fascia lata, flexor digitorum longus, and hamstrings. The knee and ankle reflexes are normal, but the medial hamstring and peroneal reflexes are sometimes depressed. The signature zone for sensory loss is over the dorsum of the foot. Rarely, neurogenic hypertrophy of the tibialis anterior occurs.

In S1 lesions, weakness occurs primarily in the gastrosoleus. Because this muscle is so powerful, hand strength testing often fails to detect weakness (see above). Further testing may reveal weakness of the gluteus maximus, hamstrings, and toe flexors. The ankle reflex and the plantar stretch reflex (see Chapter 38) are often depressed; the subtlest evidence is asymmetry of the ankle reflexes on very careful testing as by having the patient in a kneeling position. The signature zone for sensory loss is along the lateral border of the foot. Neurogenic hypertrophy of the calf happens rarely.

Spinal Stenosis

As patients mature into the seventh decade and beyond, the liability to disc rupture decreases, but degenerative spine disease attacks in a different form. Osteophytic spurs and bars; bulging discs; thickened laminae and pedicles; arthritic, hypertrophied facets; and thickened spinal ligaments all combine to narrow the spinal canal and produce the syndrome of spinal stenosis. Because of the diffuse involvement, there is commonly evidence of multilevel LSR. An extension posture contributes to spinal stenosis by causing narrowing of the foramina and dorsal quadrants and buckling of the ligamentum flavum. Narrowing of the canal compresses neural and possibly vascular structures.

Flexing the spine, as by leaning forward, stooping over, or sitting down opens the canal and decreases the symptomatology.

A common feature of lumbar spondylosis is neurogenic claudication (claudication of the cauda equina, pseudoclaudication), generally attributed to mechanical pressure on the nerve roots and blood vessels of the cauda equina. Such pain in the legs on walking can be easily confused with vascular claudication. Patients with spinal stenosis and neurogenic claudication experience pain, weakness, numbness, and paresthesias/dysesthesias when standing or walking. Prolonged standing, as at a cocktail party, often exacerbates the symptoms. An occasional patient will have a bizarre symptom, such as spontaneous erections or fecal incontinence brought on by walking. Differentiation from vascular claudication is made by the wide distribution of symptoms, the neurologic accompaniments, and the necessity to sit down for relief (Table 47.3). Vascular claudication tends to produce focal, intense, crampy pain in one or both calves, and the pain subsides if the patient just stops and stands. Patients with vascular claudication have even more symptoms walking uphill because of the increased leg work. Neurogenic claudication may decrease when walking uphill because of the increased spinal flexion in forward leaning. Patients with vascular claudication have as much trouble riding a bicycle as walking because of the leg work involved, whereas forward flexion on the bicycle opens up the spinal canal, allowing patients with neurogenic claudication to ride a bike with greater ease than they can walk. Vespers (L. "evening") curse, a rare but interesting manifestation of spinal stenosis, often with coincidental CHF, mimics restless legs syndrome (see Chapter 30). The essential difference between neurogenic and vascular claudication is the symptoms are evoked by spine extension in the former and leg exertion in the latter. Table 47.3 lists differential points helpful in distinguishing vascular from neurogenic claudication. Helpful points in the differential diagnosis of back and leg pain are summarized in Table 47.4.

Conus Medullaris and Cauda Equina Lesions

In conus medullaris lesions, the pathology is limited to the parenchyma of the terminal spinal cord; in cauda equina lesions, the pathology involves multiple nerve roots. A conus lesion is intramedullary; a cauda equina lesion is extramedullary. Some processes may involve both structures, and it is not always possible to make a clear clinical distinction, as many of the manifestations are similar. Favoring a lesion of the conus are prominent and early bowel, bladder, and sexual dysfunction; mild, symmetric lower-extremity motor involvement; and a relative lack of pain. In lesions of the cauda equina, pain is more prominent; bowel, bladder, and sexual dysfunction are less prominent; and motor, sensory, and reflex loss tend to be asymmetric and suggestive of nerve root involvement (Table 47.5).

TABLE 47.3 Differential Diagnostic Points in Neurogenic versus Vascular Claudication

Manifestation	Neurogenic Claudication	Vascular Claudication
Location of pain	Back, buttocks, legs; bilateral	Calf; unilateral
Associated symptoms	Paresthesias, weakness, priapism, incontinence	None
Provoking factors	Prolonged standing (cocktail party syndrome) walking downhill > uphill	Walking uphill > downhill
Relieving factors	Sitting, lying down, bending over	Stopping exertion
Time for relief	Minutes	Seconds
Effect of back hyperextension	Reproduces symptoms	No effect
Bicycle	No symptoms	Reproduces symptoms
Pulses	Normal	Decreased
Neurologic exam after exercise	Weakness, loss of reflexes	No change

TABLE 47.4 Differential Diagnostic Points in Patients with Low Back Pain Syndromes

Disorder	Site of Involvement	Local Pain	Referred Radiating Pain	Radicular Radiating Pain	Pain Increased By	Pain Decreased By	Positive SLR	Weakest Muscles	Decreased Reflex	Other
L5 radiculopathy—HNP	L5 root posterolateral HNP at L4-L5	Back	Buttock, posterior thigh	Buttock, posterior thigh, lower leg, dorsum of foot, big toe	Sitting, standing, cough, sneeze, spinal flexion	Standing, lying	Yes	TA, EHL, TP, EDL/EDB, PL	MHS (±)	
L5 radiculopathy—lateral recess syndrome	L5 root lateral recess stenosis	Back	Buttock, posterior thigh	Buttock, posterior thigh, lower leg, dorsum of foot, big toe	Standing, extension	Spinal flexion	No	TFL, GMD		Age 30–55 for HNP, older for lateral recess stenosis; generally leg pain > back pain
S1 radiculopathy—HNP	S1 root posterolateral HNP at L5-S1	Back	Buttock, posterior thigh	Buttock, posterior thigh, lower leg, heel, lateral foot/toes	Sitting > standing, cough, sneeze, spinal flexion	Standing, lying	Yes	Gastroc, FDL, short toe flexors, decreased	Ankle, LHS (±)	
S1 radiculopathy—lateral recess syndrome	S1 root lateral recess stenosis	Back	Buttock, posterior thigh	Buttock, posterior thigh, lower leg, heel, lateral foot/toes	Standing, extension	Spinal flexion	No	No. of toe raises		
Discogenic pain	Intervertebral disc torn annulus; internal disruption	Back	Buttock, posterior thigh	None	Sitting, spinal flexion	Lying	No	No weak muscles, possible splinting because of pain	None	
Facet pain	Facet joint	Back	Buttock, posterior thigh	None	Lying supine, extension, rotation	Walking, flexion	No	No weak muscles	None	Pain may decrease with facet block
Musculoligamentous pain	Musculoligamentous structures of low back	Back	Buttock, posterior thigh	None	Walking, bending, stooping, minor movements	Sitting or lying	Negative or equivocal, not radiating	No weak muscles	None	Frequently follows unaccustomed exertion of the back; trigger points
Spinal stenosis	Cauda equina, multilevel radiculopathy	Back	Buttock, posterior thigh	Depends on root and level	Walking, standing	Sitting, leaning forward	Variable	Depends on root	Depends on root	No signs of peripheral vascular insufficiency

High lumbar disc	L2, L3, L4, usually HNP	Back	Buttock	Anterior thigh	Sitting	Lying	No	Quads, adductors	Knee	+Reverse SLR
Hip disease	Hip joint, trochanteric bursa	Hip, buttock	Groin, anterior thigh, lateral thigh, knee	None	Standing, walking, hip rotation	Sitting or lying supine	No	None	None	+FABERE (see Chapter 48)
SI joint disease	SI joint	Back, buttock	Posterior thigh	None	Resting	Repetitive movement, exercise, activity	No	None	None	Age <30, male, history of pain >3 mo, morning stiffness, +SI joint maneuvers
Bony spine pain, for example, metastatic disease, osteomyelitis	Vertebral body	Back	Buttocks, thighs	None	Nothing specific	Nothing specific	No	None	None	Boring, relentless pain, worse at night, history of cancer, history of unexplained weight loss, age >50
Viscerogenic pain	Viscera, for example, colon, rectum, prostate, uterus and adnexa, aortoiliac vessels	Variable, sometimes none	Back	None	Nothing specific	Nothing specific	No	None	None	Evidence of visceral disease; pain unrelated to activity or posture
Nonorganic		Back and any other; often back + neck	None	None	No consistent pattern	No consistent pattern	Variable and nonorganic	None	None	Nonorganic physical signs, depression, disability, litigation

From Campbell WW. *Essentials of Electrodiagnostic Medicine.* Philadelphia: Lippincott Williams & Wilkins, 1999. Reprinted with permission of Dr. William W. Campbell.

The table outlines what is generally true; it is not a statement of absolutes.

AH, abductor hallucis; EDB, extensor digitorum brevis; EDL, extensor digitorum longus; EHL, extensor hallucis longus; FDL, flexor digitorum longus; GMD, gluteus medius; GMX, gluteus maximus; HNP, herniated nucleus pulposus; IP, iliopsoas; LHS, lateral hamstring; MHS, medial hamstring; PL, peroneus longus; RF, rectus femoris; SLR, straight leg raising; TA, tibialis anterior; TFL, tensor fascia lata; TP, tibialis posterior.

TABLE 47.5 Signs and Symptoms Differentiating Between Lesions of the Conus Medullaris and Cauda Equina

	Conus Medullaris	Cauda Equina
Spontaneous pain	Not common or severe; bilateral and symmetric; in perineum or thighs	May be most prominent symptom; severe; radicular in type; unilateral or asymmetric; in perineum, thighs, legs, or back; distribution of sacral nerves
Sensory deficit	Saddle distribution; bilateral, usually symmetric; dissociation of sensation	Saddle distribution; may be unilateral and asymmetric; all forms affected; no dissociation of sensation
Motor loss	Symmetric; not marked; fasciculations may be present	Asymmetric; more marked; atrophy may occur; usually no fasciculations
Reflex loss	Only Achilles reflex absent	Patellar and Achilles reflexes may be absent
Bladder and rectal symptoms	Early and marked	Late and less marked
Trophic changes	Decubiti common	Decubiti less marked
Sexual functions	Erection and ejaculation impaired	Less marked impairment
Onset	Sudden and bilateral	Gradual and unilateral

THORACIC RADICULOPATHY

Thoracic radiculopathy is most often due to either diabetes (diabetic truncal radiculoneuropathy or thoracoabdominal neuropathy) or herpes zoster. True neurogenic thoracic outlet syndrome primarily affects the T1 root fibers. Compressive radiculopathy occurs very rarely. A lesion of the T1 root may cause weakness of the hand intrinsics, especially the abductor pollicis brevis. The primary representation of the T1 myotome is in the APB. Sensory loss occurs over the medial forearm and in the axilla. Neoplastic invasion of the T1 root may present as relentless axillary pain. Depression of the finger flexor reflex and a Horner's syndrome may aid in localization. The primary neurologic manifestation of other thoracic radiculopathies is sensory loss in the distribution of the involved root. Rare motor manifestations include abdominal pseudohernia. Notalgia paresthetica causes pain, paresthesias, and pruritus in the distribution of the posterior primary rami of T2-T6 between the spine and the medial border of the scapula; it is relatively common.

MRI has shown that thoracic disc herniations occur much more frequently than previously thought. Still, compressive thoracic radiculopathies occur rarely.

Video Links

Video Link 47.1. Trendelenburg's sign. https://www.youtube.com/watch?v=DkSTr7K-eAo

Video Link 47.2. The peroneal reflex. http://neurosigns.org/wiki/Peroneal_reflex

BIBLIOGRAPHY

Alexander CE, Dulebohn SC. Lumbosacral Facet Syndrome. In: *StatPearls [Internet]*. Treasure Island: StatPearls Publishing, 2018. Last updated November 5, 2017. http://www.ncbi.nlm.nih.gov/books/NBK441906/

Apeldoorn AT, Bosselaar H, Blom-Luberti T, et al. The reliability of nonorganic sign-testing and the Waddell score in patients with chronic low back pain. *Spine (Phila Pa 1976)* 2008;33:821–826.

Bowen J, Gregory R, Squier M, et al. The post-irradiation lower motor neuron syndrome neuronopathy or radiculopathy? *Brain* 1996;119(Pt 5):1429–1439.

Brazis PW, Masdeu JC, Biller J. *Localization in Clinical Neurology*. 7th ed. Philadelphia: Wolters Kluwer/Lippincott Williams & Wilkins, 2017.

Brinjikji W, Luetmer PH, Comstock B, et al. Systematic literature review of imaging features of spinal degeneration in asymptomatic populations. *AJNR Am J Neuroradiol* 2015;36:811–816.

Campbell WW. *Clinical Signs in Neurology: A Compendium*. Philadelphia: Wolters Kluwer Health, 2016.

Campbell WW, Buschbacher R, Pridgeon RM, et al. Selective finger drop in cervical radiculopathy: the pseudopseudoulnar claw hand. *Muscle Nerve* 1995;18:108–110.

Cockerell OC, Ormerod IE. Focal weakness following herpes zoster. *J Neurol Neurosurg Psychiatry* 1993;56:1001–1003.

Corey DL, Comeau D. Cervical radiculopathy. *Med Clin North Am* 2014;98:791–799.

Cox JS, Blizzard S, Carlson H, et al. Lumbar magnetic resonance imaging findings in patients with and without Waddell signs. *Spine J* 2017;17:990–994.

Deyo RA, Mirza SK. Clinical practice: Herniated lumbar intervertebral disk. *N Engl J Med* 2016;374:1763–1772.

Deyo RA, Loeser JD, Bigos SJ. Herniated lumbar intervertebral disk. *Ann Intern Med* 1990;112:598–603.

Deyo RA, Rainville J, Kent DL. What can the history and physical examination tell us about low back pain? *JAMA* 1992;268:760–765.

Fast A, Parikh S, Marin EL. The shoulder abduction relief sign in cervical radiculopathy. *Arch Phys Med Rehabil* 1989;70:402–403.

Foris LA, Dulebohn SC. Spinal stenosis and neurogenic claudication.. In: *StatPearls [Internet]*. Treasure Island (FL): StatPearls Publishing; 2018. Last updated May 3, 2018. http://www.ncbi.nlm.nih.gov/books/NBK430872/

Gilliatt RW, Le Quesne PM, Logue V, et al. Wasting of the hand associated with a cervical rib or band. *J Neurol Neurosurg Psychiatry* 1970;33:615–624.

Goh KJ, Khalifa W, Anslow P, et al. The clinical syndrome associated with lumbar spinal stenosis. *Eur Neurol* 2004;52:242–249.

Haig AJ, Tzeng HM, LeBreck DB. The value of electrodiagnostic consultation for patients with upper extremity nerve complaints: a prospective comparison with the history and physical examination. *Arch Phys Med Rehabil* 1999;80: 1273–1281.

Helfgott SM, Picard DA, Cook JS. Herpes zoster radiculopathy. *Spine (Phila Pa 1976)* 1993;18:2523–2524.

Hosono N, Makino T, Sakaura H, et al. Myelopathy hand: new evidence of the classical sign. *Spine (Phila Pa 1976)* 2010;35:E273–E277.

Jensen MC, Brant-Zawadzki MN, Obuchowski N, et al. Magnetic resonance imaging of the lumbar spine in people without back pain. *N Engl J Med* 1994;331:69–73.

Jones LK Jr, Reda H, Watson JC. Clinical, electrophysiologic, and imaging features of zoster-associated limb paresis. *Muscle Nerve* 2014;50:177–185.

LaBan MM. "Vespers Curse" night pain—the bane of Hypnos. *Arch Phys Med Rehabil* 1984;65:501–504.

Lauder TD. Physical examination signs, clinical symptoms, and their relationship to electrodiagnostic findings and the presence of radiculopathy. *Phys Med Rehabil Clin N Am* 2002;13:451–467.

Levin KH. Neurologic manifestations of compressive radiculopathy of the first thoracic root. *Neurology* 1999;53: 1149–1151.

Magee DJ. *Orthopedic Physical Assessment*. 4th ed. Philadelphia: W.B. Saunders, 2002.

Manifold SG, McCann PD. Cervical radiculitis and shoulder disorders. *Clin Orthop* 1999;368:105–113.

Murphey F, Simmons JCH, Brunson B. Surgical treatment of laterally ruptured cervical disc: review of 648 cases, 1939–1972. *J Neurosurg* 1973;38:679–683.

Ono K, Ebara S, Fuji T, et al. Myelopathy hand. New clinical signs of cervical cord damage. *J Bone Joint Surg Br* 1987;69:215–219.

Ozgur BM, Marshall LF. Atypical presentation of C7 radiculopathy. *J Neurosurg* 2003;99(2 Suppl):169–171.

Pleet AB, Massey EW. Notalgia paresthetica. *Neurology* 1978;28:1310–1312.

Radhakrishnan K, Litchy WJ, O'Fallon WM, et al. Epidemiology of cervical radiculopathy. A population-based study from Rochester, Minnesota, 1976 through 1990. *Brain* 1994;117:325–335.

Rainville J, Jouve C, Finno M, et al. Comparison of four tests of quadriceps strength in L3 or L4 radiculopathies. *Spine* 2003;28:2466–2471.

Rainville J, Joyce AA, Laxer E, et al. Comparison of symptoms from C6 and C7 radiculopathy. *Spine (Phila Pa 1976)* 2017;42:1545–1551.

Ricker K, Rohkamm R, Moxley RT III. Hypertrophy of the calf with S1 radiculopathy. *Arch Neurol* 1988;45:660–664.

Rubin DI, Shuster EA. Axillary pain as a heralding sign of neoplasm involving the upper thoracic root. *Neurology* 2006;66:1760–1762.

Schwarzer AC, Aprill CN, Derby R, et al. Clinical features of patients with pain stemming from the lumbar zygapophysial joints. Is the lumbar facet syndrome a clinical entity? *Spine* 1994;19:1132–1137.

Stewart JD. Diabetic truncal neuropathy: topography of the sensory deficit. *Ann Neurol* 1989;25:233–238.

Tender GC, Thomas AJ, Thomas N, et al. Gilliatt-Sumner hand revisited: a 25-year experience. *Neurosurgery* 2004;55: 883–890.

Tong HC, Haig AJ, Yamakawa K. The Spurling test and cervical radiculopathy. *Spine* 2002;27:156–159.

van der Windt DA, Simons E, Riphagen II, et al. Physical examination for lumbar radiculopathy due to disc herniation in patients with low-back pain. *Cochrane Database Syst Rev* 2010;(2):CD007431.

Waddell G, McCulloch JA, Kummel E, et al. Nonorganic physical signs in low-back pain. *Spine (Phila Pa 1976)* 1980;5:117–125.

Wallace D. Disc compression of the eighth cervical nerve: pseudo ulnar palsy. *Surg Neurol* 1982;18:295–299.

Weeks RA, Thomas PK, Gale AN. Abdominal pseudohernia caused by diabetic truncal radiculoneuropathy. *J Neurol Neurosurg Psychiatry* 1999;66:405.

Wipf JE, Deyo RA. Low back pain. *Med Clin North Am* 1995;79:231–246.

Wolf JK. *Segmental Neurology: A Guide to the Examination and Interpretation of Sensory and Motor Function*. Baltimore: University Park Press, 1981.

Yoo JU, McIver TC, Hiratzka J, et al. The presence of Waddell signs depends on age and gender, not diagnosis. *Bone Joint J* 2018;100-B:219–225.

Yoss RE, Corbin KB, MacCarty CS, et al. Significance of symptoms and signs in localization of involved root in cervical disc protrusion. *Neurology* 1957;7:673–683.

CHAPTER 48

Other Musculoskeletal Disorders

There are many common musculoskeletal conditions that produce symptoms easily confused with neurologic conditions. Some of the conditions that often merit consideration in the differential diagnosis of radiculopathy or entrapment neuropathy include myofascial pain, and conditions affecting the shoulder and hip. The following discussion concentrates on primarily orthopedic conditions that are often seen by neurologists.

THE NECK

Neck pain related to disc disease and radiculopathy is discussed in Chapter 47. There are many other causes of neck pain. Most neck pain is benign, but it can result from serious pathologic processes, such as malignancy, inflammatory arthritis, meningitis, osteomyelitis, and diskitis. Other common causes of neck pain include fibromyalgia or myofascial pain, cervical osteoarthritis (OA), and diffuse idiopathic skeletal hyperostosis. Pain can be referred to the neck from the temporomandibular joint, heart, diaphragm, and gastrointestinal sources. In general, pain arising from deep structures of the neck is poorly localized and ill defined. Cervical spine disorders may cause pain that radiates to the upper thoracic spine, shoulders, arms, or periscapular regions, typically aggravated by neck movement. Pain due to disease of the articular structures of the vertebral columns may be accompanied by sensations of grating, clicking, and grittiness on movement of the neck. Disease arising from the upper cervical spine, particularly OA of the apophyseal joints of the upper three cervical vertebrae, may cause referred pain to the occipital and temporal regions, and even retro-orbitally (cervicogenic headache).

When neck pain is due to referred pain from other sources, there is often a clue from the history. Pain of cardiac origin is usually related to exertion and relieved by rest or nitroglycerin. Pain of esophageal origin is usually related to eating and relieved by antacids. Neither is accompanied by neurologic symptoms or findings. Pain from shoulder structures is usually referred to the area of the deltoid insertion and made worse by shoulder movement rather than neck movement. In myofascial neck pain, the discomfort is usually localized to the posterior neck region and is vague and diffuse, sometimes with a burning component. There is typically no specific injury, or the pain may begin days to weeks after minor trauma. The pain may first be noted following prolonged sitting or sleeping and may improve after activity. There are no neurologic symptoms. Neck pain due to malignancy is usually poorly localized and ill defined; not relieved by rest, supine position, or immobilization; and often associated with objective neurologic findings. Neck pain and limitation of motion due to meningismus is worse with neck flexion and is less and often nonexistent with bending or rotation.

On examination, the neck should be inspected for the presence of the normal cervical lordosis and any scars, masses, or other deformities. Palpation may be informative. Bony structures are best palpated with the patient supine to relax the neck muscles. The spinous processes should be normally aligned. The spinous process of C2 can be felt in the midline just beneath the external occipital protuberance. The C7 spinous process protrudes conspicuously, but the other spinous processes are indistinct. On deep palpation, the apophyseal joints feel like small mounds about 2.5 cm lateral to the spinous processes. The C4 and C5 joints are approximately at the level of the thyroid cartilage. Osteoarthritic apophyseal joints are frequently tender on palpation. OA tends to involve the upper cervical spine; cervical spondylosis more often involves the C5-C6 and C6-C7 levels. Paravertebral muscle spasm causes a feeling of tenseness and tightness of the involved muscles. The trapezius often has focal areas of pain and tenderness in myofascial neck pain, fibrositis, and fibromyalgia.

Examination of the range of motion (ROM) of the cervical spine is discussed in Chapter 47. Patients with arthritic necks usually have restricted motion, often painless. There may be palpable or audible crepitus. A single loud click on turning the head may indicate facet malalignment. Lateral flexion is affected earliest and to a greater degree in OA and degenerative spine disease; rotation is most impaired in rheumatoid arthritis because of involvement of the odontoid. Diffuse idiopathic skeletal hyperostosis and ankylosing spondylitis cause global restriction of neck motion in all directions.

In cervical myofascial pain, palpation may reveal a trigger point: a firm, discrete area of nodularity, particularly in the trapezius and neck extensor muscles. Pressure over the trigger point causes pain that may radiate distally. There is no muscle spasm. The muscle may twitch on palpation of the trigger point. Myofascial pain syndromes merge with fibrositis and fibromyalgia; all appear related and perhaps identical. The patient usually has pain on active movement of the neck, but passive ROM is normal. Neck pain is a common complaint in patients who are neurotic or depressed, malingering, or seeking compensation. Myofascial pain following a motor vehicle accident (whiplash) is very common. Patients with cervical strain due to whiplash rarely have radiculopathy. There were zero cases of herniation of the nucleus pulposus due to whiplash in the Radhakrishnan et al. cervical radiculopathy series.

THE SHOULDER

Shoulder pain is a common complaint, and disorders of the shoulder can be mistaken for neurologic disease, especially cervical spine disease and brachial plexopathy. In addition, pain is often referred to the shoulder from the internal organs, especially the heart, diaphragm, and subphrenic space. The shoulder is the most mobile joint in the body, but the price paid for this mobility is instability and susceptibility to strain, sprain, and a variety of diseases.

Anatomy

The shoulder is made up of the articulations of the humerus, scapula, and clavicle, joined by four joints (sternoclavicular, acromioclavicular [AC], scapulothoracic, and glenohumeral). The muscles acting at the shoulder are discussed in Chapter 27. The rotator cuff consists of the supraspinatus, infraspinatus, teres minor, and subscapularis, all of which insert into the greater and lesser tuberosities of the humerus. The rotator cuff muscles stabilize the humeral head and prevent upward translation during shoulder abduction, as well as keep the humeral head centered in the glenoid fossa. The tendon of the long head of the biceps passes through the intertubercular (bicipital) groove to insert on the superior rim of the glenoid. The greater tuberosity of the humerus makes up the outer wall of the bicipital groove and the lesser tuberosity the inner wall. Disease involving the biceps tendon in the bicipital groove (bicipital tendonitis) causes pain on motion and may damage, and even cause eventual rupture of, the biceps tendon.

The coracoacromial ligament joins the coracoid and the acromion, forming an arch over the rotator cuff tendons and the humeral head. In abduction, the space is narrow, and the room for the tendons is limited. The subacromial (subdeltoid) bursa lies between the tendon of the supraspinatus and the overhanging acromion, separating the rotator cuff from the coracoacromial arch and deltoid muscle; it allows for a smooth gliding movement. Bursitis decreases the lubrication and causes pain on movement.

The Painful Shoulder

Pain in the shoulder can occur for many reasons. A common condition is related to disease involving the tendons of the rotator cuff. Numerous terms have been used to describe the same basic process, including rotator cuff tendonitis, subacromial bursitis, subdeltoid bursitis, supraspinatus tendonitis, impingement syndrome, and calcific tendonitis. Most nontraumatic shoulder pain is related to disease of the rotator cuff. The condition usually begins as a tendonitis involving the supraspinatus tendon. With progression, other tendons may become involved, and the process may extend to involve the subacromial bursa and joint capsule and lead to tendon rupture or frozen shoulder. Pathologically, rotator cuff tendonitis is a spectrum of inflammation, degeneration, and damage by impact against the bony structures of the shoulder. The wear and tear may extend to involve the infraspinatus and long head of the biceps tendons. Rotator cuff tendonitis may be related to repetitive microtrauma, a degenerative process (tendinosis), or areas of decreased vascularity in the tendon. As rotator cuff degeneration progresses, calcium deposits may form in the tendons (calcific tendonitis).

In the early stages of rotator cuff disease, the primary manifestation is impingement syndrome. The tendons of the rotator cuff, primarily the supraspinatus tendon, become inflamed and edematous. The involved tendons are prone to become trapped beneath the coracoacromial arch with activities that involve raising the arm, particularly with the shoulder internally rotated, as in reaching forward and upward to place something on a shelf. As the condition progresses, the tendons suffer further damage that may progress to frank rotator cuff tear (RCT). The supraspinatus tendon is the structure most often involved, and the tear can be partial or full thickness. An acute RCT usually follows some trauma, such as a slip and fall. Chronic tears usually occur in older patients in the setting of preexistent rotator cuff pathology. The onset is typically gradual, with pain on performing overhead activities and conspicuous night pain. Examination usually discloses weakness of abduction and external rotation, often with disuse atrophy of the supraspinatus and deltoid. Isolated weakness of external rotation is often a sign of rotator cuff disease.

AC joint lesions cause pain in the superior aspect of the shoulder, and local joint tenderness exaggerated by adduction of the arm across the chest. Pain arising from the AC joint can sometimes be reproduced by horizontal adduction of the shoulder as if the patient were placing the hand on the opposite shoulder. Having the patient resist the examiner's downward pressure on the elbow may exacerbate the discomfort. Problems with the AC joint usually follow trauma, such as falling on the point of the shoulder, causing a ligamentous strain. An AC joint separation causes a step-off between the clavicle and acromion. Adhesive capsulitis is characterized by pain and decreased shoulder motion. Adhesions develop within the glenohumeral joint or its capsule. Both active and passive ROMs are limited, especially in abduction and external rotation. OA of the shoulder primarily involves either the glenohumeral or AC joints. There is pain, limitation of ROM, and often joint crepitus. Frozen shoulder is a general term describing all causes of loss of shoulder ROM. When severe, there may be essentially no motion at the glenohumeral joint. The exact cause of frozen shoulder is unknown but probably involves an inflammatory process similar to that causing rotator cuff tendonitis but affecting the joint capsule. Bicipital tendonitis is due to inflammation of the tendon of the long head of the biceps in the intertubercular groove. Patients typically have anterior shoulder pain that occasionally radiates down to the elbow. The pain is worsened by shoulder flexion or forearm supination and relieved by rest.

History

Relevant history in the patient with shoulder pathology includes any type of injury, location of initial pain, rapidity of onset, character and severity of pain, aggravating and relieving factors, effect of position, relationship to time of day or night, effect of passive and active movement, and any neurologic symptoms. Pain due to AC joint disease is located at the joint. With other shoulder disorders, pain may be located anywhere in the arm, neck, or shoulder. With severe shoulder pathology, the entire arm may be painful, but it is rare for pain from shoulder disease to extend below the elbow. With rotator cuff disease, pain is usually referred from the supraspinatus tendon to the area near the deltoid insertion, especially with active abduction. Pain caused by lying on the involved shoulder suggests supraspinatus tendonitis. In impingement syndrome, the pain initially occurs primarily after strenuous activity. With progression, the pain may become constant, exacerbated by arm-raising activities, and is particularly prone to occur at night. In dealing with a patient with shoulder pain, it is useful to ascertain the functional limitations. The patient may have difficulty dressing, especially reaching back to insert the arm into a coat sleeve, combing the hair, and reaching for a hip pocket wallet.

Examination

In addition to the neurologic portion of the physical examination, assessment of the shoulder should include inspection, palpation, full active ROM, and, if necessary, passive ROM. Inspection may reveal atrophy, swelling, or a change in contour. Looking down at the seated patient is useful for looking for deltoid atrophy. Palpation may reveal tenderness over inflamed or edematous structures. The posterior aspect of the rotator cuff is readily palpable with the arm adducted across the chest, and it may actually be possible to feel a torn rotator cuff through the deltoid (rent test). Palpation of the biceps tendon over the bicipital groove and moving the tendon from side to side (Lippman's test, Figure 48.1) causes pain in

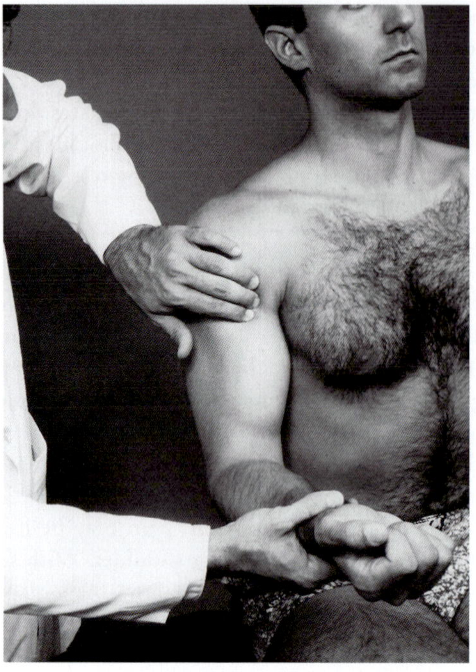

FIGURE 48.1 Lippman's test; moving the biceps tendon back and forth in the bicipital groove reproduces the pain in biceps tendonitis. (Reprinted with permission from Cipriano JJ. *Photographic Manual of Regional Orthopaedic and Neurological Tests.* 4th ed. Philadelphia: Lippincott Williams & Wilkins, 2003.)

patients with bicipital tendonitis. Vigorous palpation can cause some discomfort even in the absence of pathology, so it is useful to compare the pain produced on the symptomatic and asymptomatic sides.

Full active ROM should carry the shoulder through flexion, extension, adduction, abduction, and medial and lateral rotation. Note the motion of the scapula and the scapulohumeral rhythm (see Chapter 27). When severe shoulder pathology restricts glenohumeral motion, the patient abducts the arm primarily at the scapulothoracic joint. Excessive scapular motion during arm abduction signifies limited glenohumeral motion. Some or all of abduction may be accomplished by shrugging, and the scapula and humerus move as a unit (reversal of scapulohumeral rhythm). Limitation of active ROM could occur because of mechanical limitation (e.g., frozen shoulder) or because of pain or muscle weakness. Passive greater than active ROM excludes any mechanical limitation. Even when there is marked limitation of active ROM due to pain or a torn rotator cuff, gentle passive ROM may be normal. A convenient way to assess active ROM is the Apley scratch test, in which the patient makes three moves as if to scratch: (a) reaching to the opposite shoulder to touch it from the front, (b) from behind the neck as if to touch the upper vertebral border of the opposite scapula, and (c) from behind the lower back as if to touch the lower tip of the opposite scapula (Figure 48.2A and B). The latter two can be combined by having the patient try to touch the fingertips together in the interscapular space, one hand from above and the other from below.

To elicit the drop-arm sign, during passive ROM with the patient sitting, the examiner places the shoulder in 90 degrees of abduction then releases the arm and asks the patient to slowly lower it. This may cause severe pain, or the patient may not be able to lower the arm slowly and it may drop abruptly. A positive drop-arm sign suggests dysfunction of the supraspinatus tendon. In a large series of patients with suspected RCTs the clinical findings most closely associated were included infra- and supraspinatus atrophy, weakness with either elevation or external rotation, painful arc, and impingement sign. Age 65 years and above and night pain also correlated with the presence of RCT.

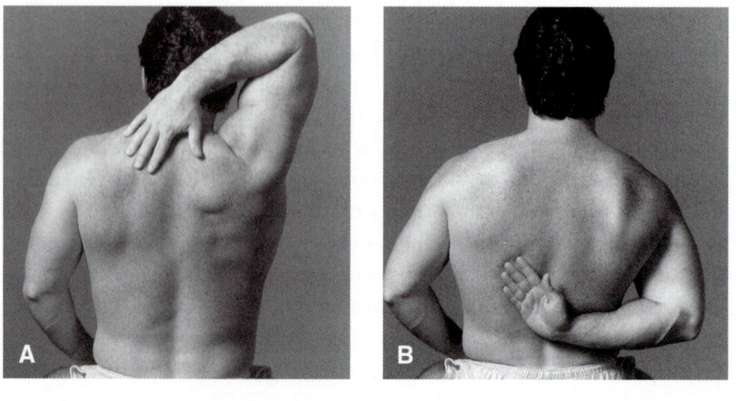

FIGURE 48.2 A,B. The Apley scratch test. Exacerbation of the patient's pain indicates degenerative tendinopathy of one of the rotator cuff tendons, usually the supraspinatus. (Reprinted with permission from Cipriano JJ. *Photographic Manual of Regional Orthopaedic and Neurological Tests.* 4th ed. Philadelphia: Lippincott Williams & Wilkins, 2003.)

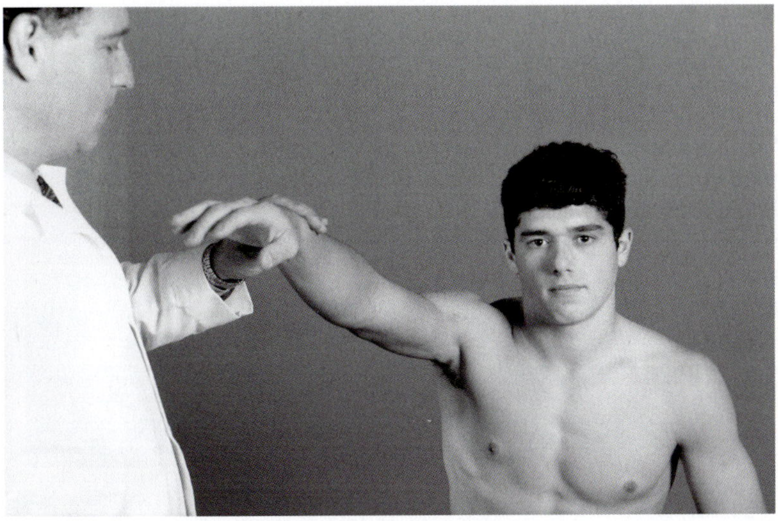

FIGURE 48.3 Elicitation of Neer's impingement sign. With the arm pronated, elevation entraps the supraspinatus tendon under the coracoacromial arch. (Reprinted with permission from Cipriano JJ. *Photographic Manual of Regional Orthopaedic and Neurological Tests.* 4th ed. Philadelphia: Lippincott Williams & Wilkins, 2003.)

A number of specific maneuvers may be useful to evaluate the shoulder.

Impingement Sign

Two different impingement signs are in common use; both produce pain by trapping the rotator cuff tendons between the humeral head and the acromion during passive movement of the shoulder. In the Neer impingement test, the extended arm is internally rotated and then raised directly overhead with the palm facing laterally (Figure 48.3). In the Hawkins (Hawkins-Kennedy) impingement test, the arm is held in abduction and external rotation, elbow flexed, and then forcefully rotated internally, driving the supraspinatus tendon through the subacromial space (Figure 48.4). In another method, the elbow is flexed and the shoulder internally rotated as if to lay the forearm across the abdomen; the arm is then raised so that the forearm passes in an arc in front of the face and overhead. Internal rotation is a key part of the maneuver in the impingement tests, as it rotates the greater tuberosity anteriorly and narrows the space beneath the acromion. Inflamed and tender tendons are then trapped between the greater tuberosity and the acromion, causing pain during the maneuver. The pain may also lessen when the patient bends forward and lets the arm hang limp, distracting the inflamed tendons from the point of impingement, or if the examiner supports the flexed forearm at the elbow and pulls gently downward. In impingement syndrome, the diseased tendons pass beneath the acromion in the arc between 60 and 120 degrees of abduction. Abduction out to 60 degrees may be painless, but the arc between 60 and 120 degrees is very uncomfortable; beyond 120 degrees, after the swollen and tender supraspinatus tendon has cleared the narrow confines of the subacromial space, motion is again painless. The "painful arc sign"

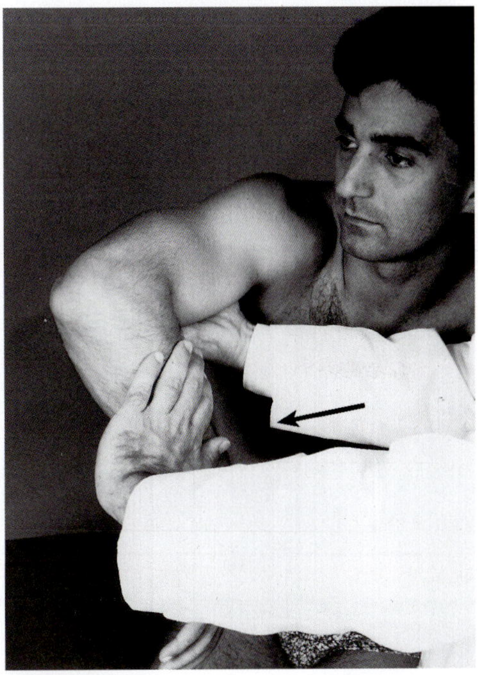

FIGURE 48.4 Elicitation of the Hawkins impingement sign. Rotation forces the rotator cuff tendons beneath the coracoacromial arch. (Reprinted with permission from Cipriano JJ. *Photographic Manual of Regional Orthopaedic and Neurological Tests.* 4th ed. Philadelphia: Lippincott Williams & Wilkins, 2003.)

is elicited either by having the examiner elevate the patient's arm passively to 180 degrees and then having the patient lower the arm actively or by having the patient actively abduct from 0 to 180 degrees. The sign is positive with pain in the 60 to 120 degrees range and not at the extremes. The painful arc sign has high sensitivity as a single finding, making it helpful in ruling out RCTs when absent.

The action of the supraspinatus can be relatively isolated by having the patient attempt to abduct the arm laterally with the shoulder internally rotated and forearm hyperpronated, as if to move the little finger toward the ceiling. The shoulder should be flexed about 30 degrees forward of the coronal plane of the body to line the humerus up in the plane of the scapula and isolate the supraspinatus. This is the same movement that would be made emptying a can and is sometimes referred to as the empty can test.

In Speed's test, the elbow is held extended and supinated, and the patient flexes the shoulder (not the elbow) against resistance (Figure 48.5). This movement causes the biceps tendon to move through the bicipital groove and causes anterior shoulder pain in patients with bicipital tendonitis. In Yergason's test, with the elbow flexed to 90 degrees and the forearm pronated, the patient attempts to simultaneously flex the elbow and supinate the hand against the examiner's resistance (Figure 48.6). The biceps is an elbow flexor and supinator, and this test uses both motions to cause the biceps to contract and its tendon to move in the bicipital groove, reproducing pain in the anterior shoulder in bicipital tendonitis.

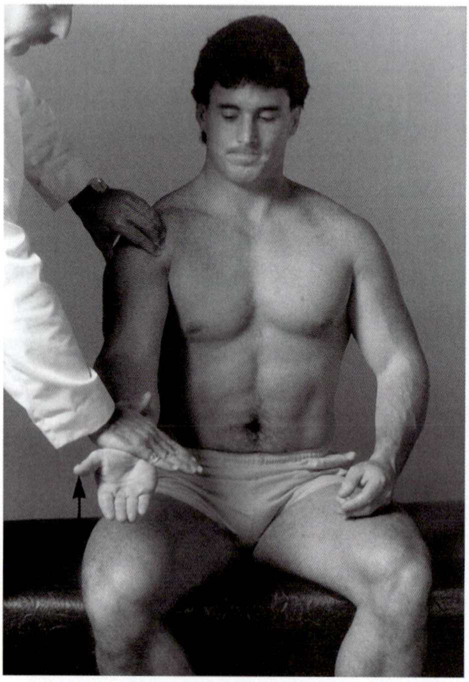

FIGURE 48.5 Elicitation of pain from the anterior shoulder in bicipital tendonitis by flexion of the shoulder against resistance. (Reprinted with permission from Cipriano JJ. *Photographic Manual of Regional Orthopaedic and Neurological Tests.* 4th ed. Philadelphia: Lippincott Williams & Wilkins, 2003.)

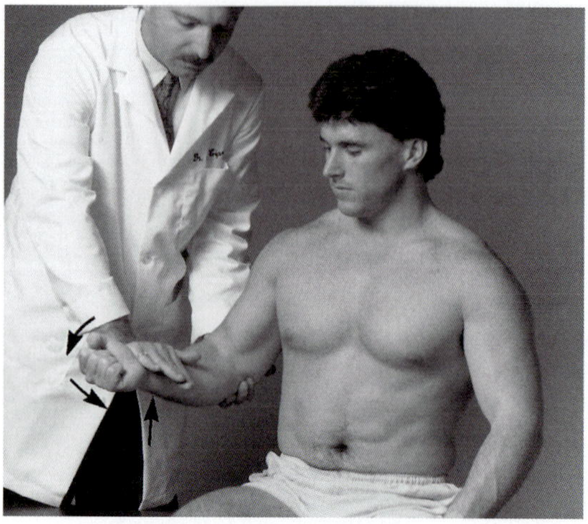

FIGURE 48.6 Elicitation of pain from the anterior shoulder in bicipital tendonitis by flexing and supinating the elbow against resistance, which stresses the biceps tendon in its groove (Yergason's sign). (Reprinted with permission from Cipriano JJ. *Photographic Manual of Regional Orthopaedic and Neurological Tests.* 4th ed. Philadelphia: Lippincott Williams & Wilkins, 2003.)

THE ELBOW

Patients with pain in the elbow are not often thought to have a neurologic process. There are a few conditions that merit discussion: lateral epicondylitis, medial epicondylitis, the radial tunnel syndrome, and ulnar neuropathy at the elbow.

The elbow joint has two articulations: humeroulnar and humeroradial. The possible movements are flexion/extension and pronation/supination. The lateral and medial epicondyles are nonarticular processes that surmount the respective humeral condyles. The supinator and common extensor tendons arise from the lateral epicondyle; the common extensor tendon is the origin of the extensor digitorum, extensor digiti minimi, and extensor carpi ulnaris. Lateral epicondylitis (tennis elbow) is a very common syndrome of pain over the lateral epicondyle that is

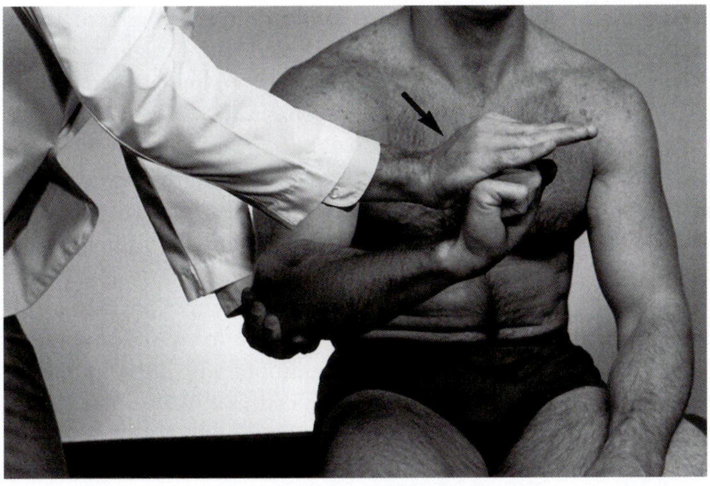

FIGURE 48.7 Elicitation of lateral epicondylar pain by forceful wrist extension (Cozen's sign). (Reprinted with permission from Cipriano JJ. *Photographic Manual of Regional Orthopaedic and Neurological Tests.* 4th ed. Philadelphia: Lippincott Williams & Wilkins, 2003.)

most often an overuse injury involving the extensor and supinator muscles that originate from the lateral epicondyle. It occurs most often in tennis players (up to 50%) but may result from other types of overuse from many activities. Examination typically discloses tenderness to palpation over the lateral epicondyle, with maximal tenderness just distal to the epicondyle. With the elbow extended, extension (Cozen's sign, Figure 48.7) or supination of the wrist against the examiner's resistance (Mill's test) reproduces the pain. Forceful passive wrist flexion or pronation may stretch the inflamed region and also cause pain. In the chair raise test, the patient stands behind a chair, grasps the chair back with the hand pronated and the elbow extended, and tries to pick it up, reproducing the pain.

Lateral epicondylitis usually responds to conservative treatment. When it does not, sometimes a diagnosis of "resistant tennis elbow" is made. There is a belief among some, primarily orthopedic surgeons, that some cases of resistant tennis elbow are due to entrapment of radial nerve branches in the "radial tunnel," an anatomical passageway that allegedly consists of various structures, such as the fibrous edge of the extensor carpi radialis brevis, the arcade of Frohse, the distal border of the supinator muscle, or fibrous bands in the supinator muscle. It is dubious whether a radial tunnel even exists. Proponents of radial tunnel syndrome believe that the nerve entrapment causes chronic lateral elbow pain in the absence of any objective neurologic dysfunction. The descriptions of the clinical manifestations of radial tunnel syndrome in the surgical literature are remarkably similar to, often identical with, the descriptions of lateral epicondylitis.

THE WRIST AND HAND

The motions of the wrist are flexion and extension and radial and ulnar deviation. The wrist (radiocarpal) joint is formed by articulation of the distal end of the radius with the carpal bones. There are eight carpal bones. The proximal row consists of the scaphoid, lunate, triquetral, and pisiform; the distal row is made up of the trapezium, trapezoid, capitate, and hamate. The pisiform bone forms an easily palpable hump on the palmar aspect of the wrist at the base of the hypothenar eminence. The hook of the hamate lies about 1 in distal to the pisiform, in line with the ulnar border of the ring finger and can be felt by deep palpation. The pisohamate ligament joins the pisiform to the hook of the hamate; it can compress the deep palmar branch of the ulnar nerve. The superficial division of the ulnar nerve can be rolled from side to side over the tip of the hook.

The "anatomical snuff box" is a small hollow seen just distal to the radial styloid on the lateral aspect of the wrist when the thumb is fully extended. The extensor pollicis brevis and abductor pulses longus tendons form the volar border of the snuff box; the extensor pollicis longus tendon forms the dorsal border. With the thumb forcefully extended, the tendon of the extensor pollicis longus can be seen standing out and running to its insertion on the distal phalanx of the thumb. The superficial radial nerve crosses the tendon of the extensor pollicis longus and can be palpated and rolled from side to side over the tendon.

A decrease in both active and passive ROM suggests pathology involving the joint or tendon, or contracture. When there is only loss of active ROM, disruption of a tendon may be responsible. de

Quervain's disease is an inflammatory tenosynovitis that involves the extensor muscles of the thumb, primarily the extensor pollicis brevis. Patients develop pain in the wrist and thumb, primarily involving the radial aspect of the wrist, with tenderness to palpation over the anatomical snuff box. Extension of the thumb against resistance causes pain, but passive extension is painless. In Finkelstein's test, the patient places the thumb in the palm and wraps the fingers around it. The examiner then slowly pushes the wrist in an ulnar direction (Figure 48.8). This stretching of the inflamed thumb extensor tendons reproduces the pain. Mild discomfort with forced ulnar deviation is expected. Patients with active de Quervain's disease have exquisite pain with Finkelstein's test.

Rupture of tendons can cause weakness easily mistaken for a neurologic process. Rupture of a finger extensor tendon causes isolated finger drop. A common type of extensor tendon injury involves the distal phalanx, causing the tip of the involved finger to droop (mallet finger, as the extended finger resembles a tiny mallet). Rupture of the extensor tendon to the proximal interphalangeal joint causes both middle and distal phalanges to droop (typewriter finger).

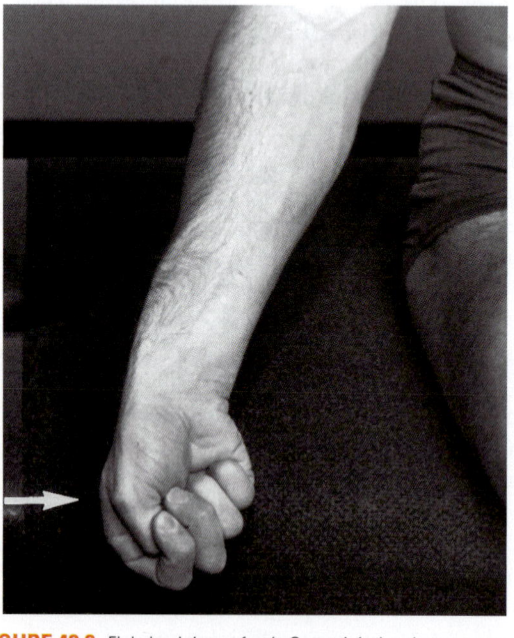

FIGURE 48.8 Finkelstein's test for de Quervain's thumb extensor tendonitis. With the thumb trapped, forceful ulnar deviation of the wrist stretches the thumb extensor tendons. (Reprinted with permission from Cipriano JJ. *Photographic Manual of Regional Orthopaedic and Neurological Tests.* 4th ed. Philadelphia: Lippincott Williams & Wilkins, 2003.)

When multiple tendons are involved, as sometimes happens in rheumatoid arthritis (Vaughan-Jackson syndrome), the appearance may simulate partial posterior interosseous neuropathy. Jersey (sweater) finger is an injury that usually occurs when a player grabs a running opponent's jersey, avulsing the flexor digitorum profundus tendon from the distal phalanx. The patient is then unable to flex the distal interphalangeal joint. This can be mistaken for flexor digitorum profundus weakness as might occur in anterior interosseous nerve palsy. There are many other interesting hand and finger conditions with colorful names, but few are likely to be confused with a neurologic process.

THE LOWER EXTREMITY

The musculoskeletal conditions most relevant in the differential diagnosis of lumbosacral radiculopathy are myofascial or musculoligamentous back pain, disease of the sacroiliac (SI) joints, and hip pathology. In musculoligamentous, myofascial or "mechanical" low back pain, the pain is usually episodic. During an attack there is low back pain that is often referred to the buttocks and thighs and often aggravated by any movement. Pain is present particularly when starting a movement. The pain is present on bending forward and also on standing back up, and is worsened by sitting, standing, walking, and activity in general. Morning stiffness is common, and the pain usually becomes worse over the course of the day. It may be relieved by a change of position, especially by lying down.

Hip pathology can be classified as anterior, lateral, or posterior based on the location of the pain. By "hip," patients often mean the buttock, so it is useful to have the patient point to the site of the pain. Pain arising from the hip joint is usually referred anteriorly to the groin and inguinal region. Causes of anterior hip pain include OA, fracture, and avascular necrosis. Pain in the posterior hip and buttock may occur from disease of the SI joint. This is also a common area for pain due to lumbosacral radiculopathy.

With the patient standing, compare the heights of the iliac crests, greater trochanters, and posterior superior iliac spine dimples to be certain they are level. Leg length discrepancy may result from many conditions, including hip fracture. Palpation may reveal areas of tenderness when bursitis involves the greater trochanter or ischial tuberosity. There may also be tender areas or trigger points due to myofascial pain.

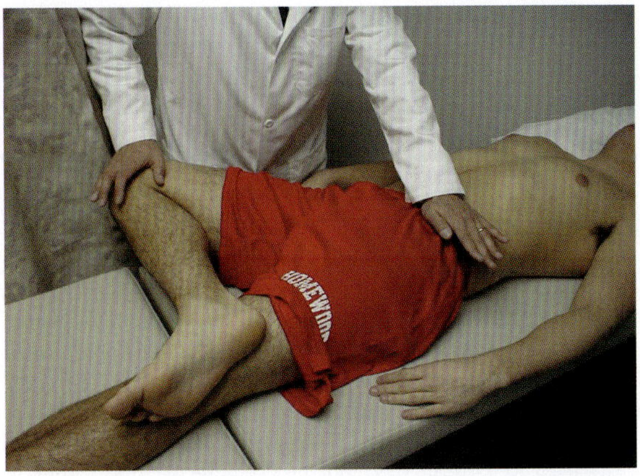

FIGURE 48.9 The FABER(E) or Patrick's test for hip disease. The figure-of-four maneuver forces the femoral head into the acetabulum. The thigh is flexed, abducted, and externally rotated. (Reprinted with permission from Boulware DW, Heudebert GR, eds. *Lippincott's Primary Care Rheumatology*. Philadelphia: Wolters Kluwer Health/Lippincott Williams & Wilkins, 2012.)

The gentlest test for disease of the hip joint is to rotate the hip internally and externally by rocking the leg back and forth with the patient supine or moving the foot medially and laterally with the patient sitting. Rotation can also be tested with the patient supine and the hip and knee flexed to 90 degrees. The leg-raising test is also useful in the evaluation of hip disease. Patients with hip disease have pain on raising the leg whether the knee is bent or straight; those with root stretch signs only have pain when the hip is flexed with the knee extended (positive straight leg raising). Pain from hip disease is maximal when the hip is flexed, abducted, and externally rotated by putting the patient's foot on the contralateral knee (figure-four position) and pressing down slightly on the flexed knee (FABER, FABERE, or Patrick's test, Figure 48.9). FABER(E) is an acronym: the hip is flexed, abducted, and externally rotated. Pain in the groin elicited in this position is suggestive of intra-articular pathology; pain posteriorly suggests SI joint disease. The most likely reason for hip joint pain is OA; other causes include hip fracture and avascular necrosis of the femoral head. Arthritis of the hip usually causes restricted motion, especially in flexion and internal rotation. SI joint pain may be reproduced by maneuvers that extend the hip. In Gaenslen's test, the patient clutches one knee to the chest to stabilize the pelvis, while the leg to be tested is extended. The test may be done with the patient lying on one side and the examiner forcefully pulling the test leg backward. Alternatively, the patient may lie supine with the buttock on the side to be tested partially off the table, allowing the leg to drop toward the floor (Figure 48.10). Reproduction of pain suggests SI joint disease.

Causes of pain in the lateral hip region include trochanteric bursitis, iliotibial band syndrome, and meralgia paresthetica. Trochanteric bursitis typically causes pain referred to the lateral hip over the region of the greater trochanter. Patients report pain on weight bearing or lying on the symptomatic side. There is usually tenderness to palpation over the affected bursa. The patient may have pain when attempting to abduct the involved leg against resistance or with passive external hip rotation. Patients with the iliotibial band syndrome often report a snapping sensation in the hip with flexion and extension. Patients with meralgia paresthetica typically have prominent sensory complaints in addition to the pain.

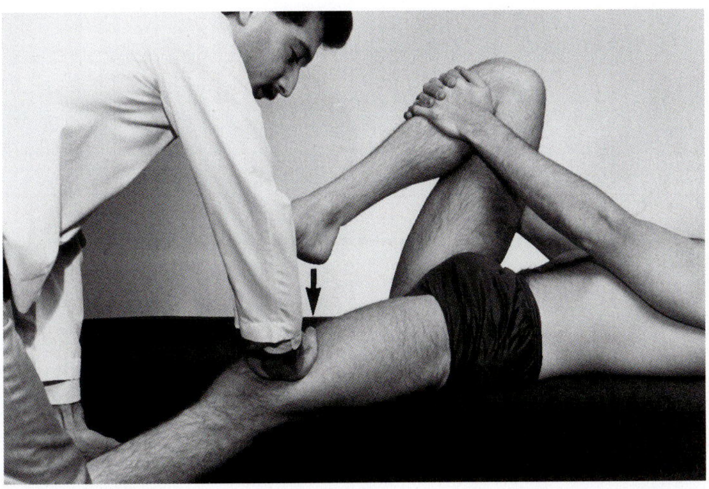

FIGURE 48.10 Gaenslen's test. Flexion of one thigh stabilizes the pelvis; dropping the other leg off the examination table stresses the sacroiliac joint (SI) and reproduces the pain in SI joint disease. (Reprinted with permission from Cipriano JJ. *Photographic Manual of Regional Orthopaedic and Neurological Tests*. 4th ed. Philadelphia: Lippincott Williams & Wilkins, 2003.)

BIBLIOGRAPHY

Cipriano JJ. *Photographic Manual of Regional Orthopaedic and Neurological Tests.* 4th ed. Philadelphia: Lippincott Williams & Wilkins, 2003.

Collee G, Dijkmans BA, Vandenbroucke JP, et al. Greater trochanteric pain syndrome (trochanteric bursitis) in low back pain. *Scand J Rheumatol* 1991;20:262–266.

Devereaux MW. Neck and low back pain. *Med Clin North Am* 2003;87:643–662.

Dick AG, Houghton JM, Bankes MJK. An approach to hip pain in a young adult. *BMJ* 2018;361:k1086.

Ebell MH. Diagnosing rotator cuff tears. *Am Fam Physician* 2005;71:1587–1588.

Gong HS, Lee JO, Baek GH, et al. Extensor tendon rupture in rheumatoid arthritis: a survey of patients between 2005 and 2010 at five Korean hospitals. *Hand Surg* 2012;17:43–47.

Hanchard NC, Lenza M, Handoll HH, et al. Physical tests for shoulder impingements and local lesions of bursa, tendon or labrum that may accompany impingement. *Cochrane Database Syst Rev* 2013;(4):CD007427.

Hardin J Jr. Pain and the cervical spine. *Bull Rheum Dis* 2001;50:1–4.

Hegedus EJ, Goode AP, Cook CE, et al. Which physical examination tests provide clinicians with the most value when examining the shoulder? Update of a systematic review with meta-analysis of individual tests. *Br J Sports Med* 2012;46:964–978.

Hsueh JH, Liu WC, Yang KC, et al. Spontaneous extensor tendon rupture in the rheumatoid wrist: risk factors and preventive role of extended tenosynovectomy. *Ann Plast Surg* 2016;76 Suppl 1:S41–S47.

Jain NB, Wilcox RB III, Katz JN, et al. Clinical examination of the rotator cuff. *PM R* 2013;5:45–56.

Litaker D, Pioro M, El Bilbeisi H, et al. Returning to the bedside: using the history and physical examination to identify rotator cuff tears. *J Am Geriatr Soc* 2000;48:1633–1637.

MacDonald PB, Clark P, Sutherland K. An analysis of the diagnostic accuracy of the Hawkins and Neer subacromial impingement signs. *J Shoulder Elbow Surg* 2000;9:299–301.

Magee DJ. *Orthopedic Physical Assessment.* 4th ed. Philadelphia: W.B. Saunders, 2002.

Mandell BF. Avascular necrosis of the femoral head presenting as trochanteric bursitis. *Ann Rheum Dis* 1990;49:730–732.

Mansour ES, Steingard MA. Anterior hip pain in the adult: an algorithmic approach to diagnosis. *J Am Osteopath Assoc* 1997;97:32–38.

Margo K, Drezner J, Motzkin D. Evaluation and management of hip pain: an algorithmic approach. *J Fam Pract* 2003;52:607–617.

Naam NH, Nemani S. Radial tunnel syndrome. *Orthop Clin North Am* 2012;43:529–536.

Roberts CS, Davila JN, Hushek SG, et al. Magnetic resonance imaging analysis of the subacromial space in the impingement sign positions. *J Shoulder Elbow Surg* 2002;11:595–599.

Rosenbaum R. Disputed radial tunnel syndrome. *Muscle Nerve* 1999;22:960–967.

Schwarzer AC, Aprill CN, Bogduk N. The sacroiliac joint in chronic low back pain. *Spine* 1995;20:31–37.

Shbeeb MI, Matteson EL. Trochanteric bursitis (greater trochanter pain syndrome). *Mayo Clin Proc* 1996;71:565–569.

Somerville LE, Willits K, Johnson AM, et al. Clinical assessment of physical examination maneuvers for rotator cuff lesions. *Am J Sports Med* 2014;42:1911–1919.

Tortolani PJ, Carbone JJ, Quartararo LG. Greater trochanteric pain syndrome in patients referred to orthopedic spine specialists. *Spine J* 2002;2:251–254.

Traycoff RB. "Pseudotrochanteric bursitis": the differential diagnosis of lateral hip pain. *J Rheumatol* 1991;18:1810–1812.

White H, Barrett M, Gooding C. Chronic hip pain. *BMJ* 2018;360:j5882.

Williams BS, Cohen SP. Greater trochanteric pain syndrome: a review of anatomy, diagnosis and treatment. *Anesth Analg* 2009;108:1662–1670.

Williamson L, Mowat A, Burge P. Screening for extensor tendon rupture in rheumatoid arthritis. *Rheumatology (Oxford)* 2001;40:420–423.

Wolf EM, Agrawal V. Transdeltoid palpation (the rent test) in the diagnosis of rotator cuff tears. *J Shoulder Elbow Surg* 2001;10:470–473.

Zacher J, Gursche A. Regional musculoskeletal conditions: 'hip' pain. *Best Pract Res Clin Rheumatol* 2003;17:71–85.

SECTION K Circulation and Cerebrospinal Fluid

CHAPTER 49

The Blood Supply of the Brain

THE CEREBRAL ARTERIES

The brain receives its blood supply from the vertebral and the internal carotid arteries. In general, branches derived from the vertebral arteries supply the caudal half of the brain, including the brainstem, midbrain, occipital lobes, inferior portion of the temporal lobes, and most of the thalamus, whereas branches of the internal carotid arteries supply the basal ganglia, frontal and parietal lobes, the lateral portion of the temporal lobes, and most of the internal capsule. Areas of perfusion are shown in Figure 49.1.

Carotid Artery

Each internal carotid artery (ICA) arises in the neck as one of the terminal branches of the common carotid artery. The cervical portion of the ICA ascends the neck (cervical segment) without branches and enters the skull through the carotid canal in the petrous portion of the temporal bone, courses through the petrous bone (petrous segment), and emerges intracranially within the cavernous sinus (intracranial segment). The vessel has an S-shaped course in the sinus, referred to as the carotid siphon. Within the cavernous sinus, the ICA lies in close proximity to cranial nerves (CNs) III, IV, $V_{1,2}$, and VI. Ascending sympathetic fibers surround the artery. Involvement of these structures may occur with intracavernous carotid disease, for example, aneurysm. The meningohypophyseal trunk arises from the presellar or juxtasellar ICA to supply the posterior lobe of the pituitary and adjacent meninges.

Immediately after exiting the sinus, the ophthalmic artery arises and then the posterior communicating artery, which connects the internal carotid and posterior cerebral arteries (PCAs), followed by the anterior choroidal artery. The ophthalmic artery gives rise to orbital, extraorbital, central retinal, anterior ciliary, and long and short posterior ciliary branches. The two carotids, their communicating branches, and the basilar artery make up the arterial circle of Willis at the base of the brain (Figures 49.2 to 49.5). The circle of Willis is subject to wide variations in configuration, with frequent anomalies. There may be hypoplasia of one or more components, which may have a string-like caliber, or duplication of vessels, absent vessels, or persistent embryonic origin of some of the constituents (Figure 49.6). The circle is normal and completely formed in only about half of individuals without evidence of nervous system disease. Anomalies occur in about 80% of patients with neural dysfunction.

Branches of the posterior communicating artery enter the base of the brain between the infundibulum and the optic tract and supply the anteromedial thalamus and the walls of the third ventricle. The anterior choroidal artery arises from the ICA just before its termination. It passes backward along the optic tract and around the cerebral peduncle as far as the lateral geniculate body, where its main branches turn to enter the inferior horn of

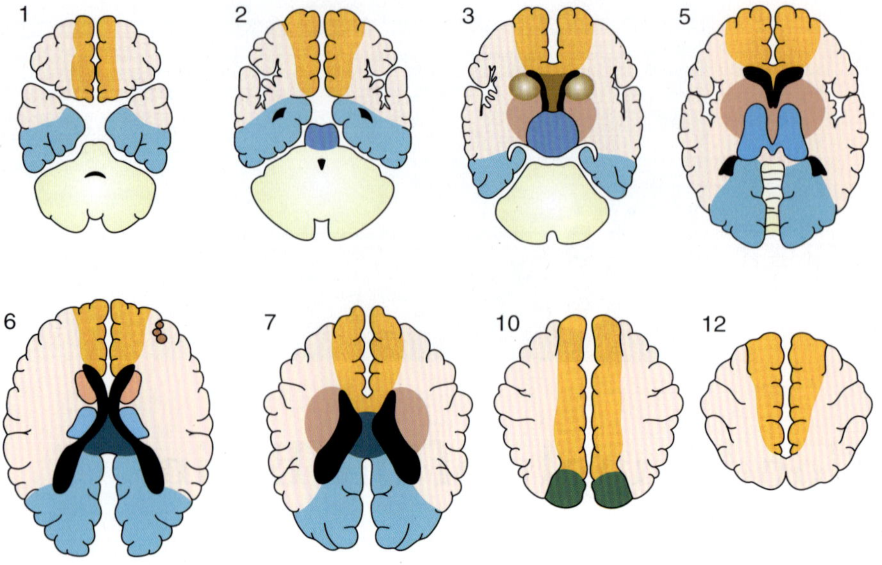

FIGURE 49.1 Vascular territories. *Gold*, anterior cerebral artery (ACA); *pink*, middle cerebral artery (MCA); *blue*, posterior cerebral artery (PCA). From https://medpix.nlm.nih.gov/home, courtesy Dr. James Smirniotopoulos.

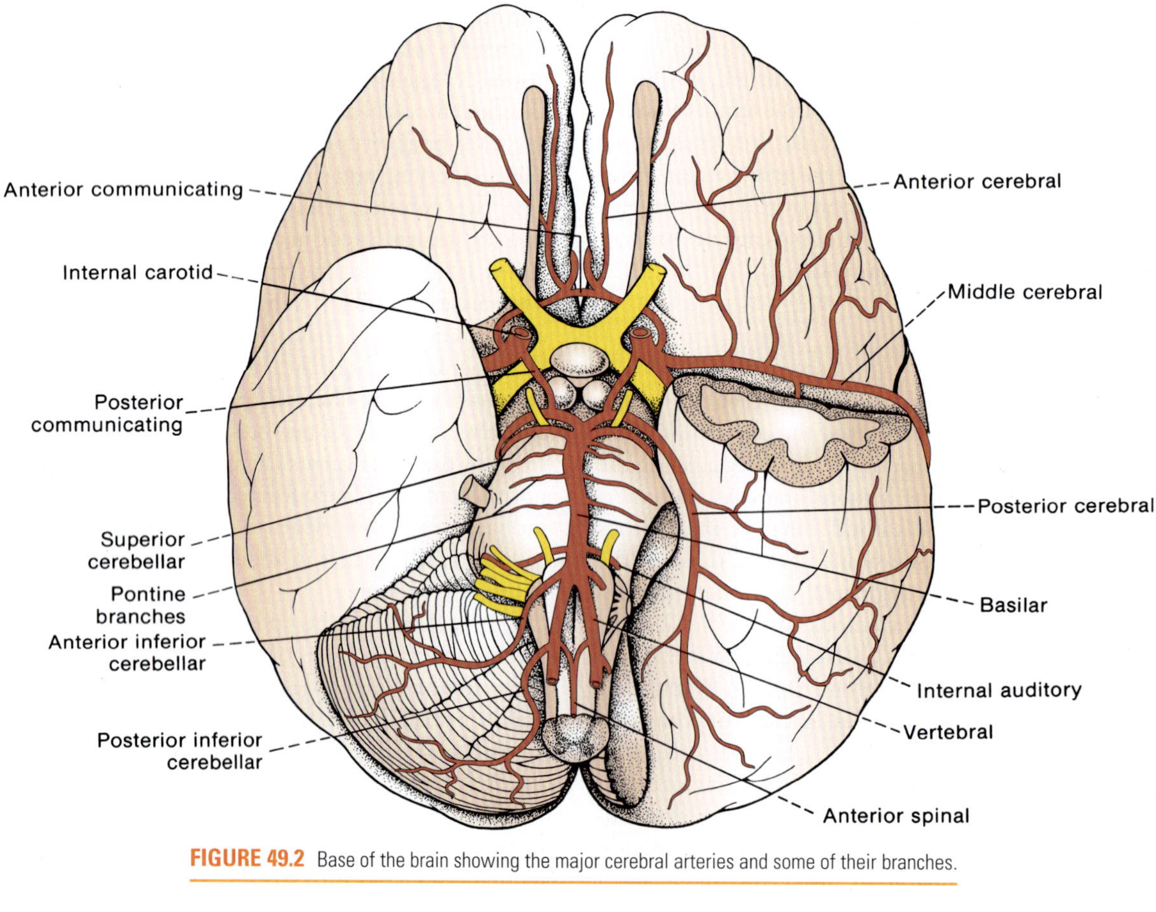

FIGURE 49.2 Base of the brain showing the major cerebral arteries and some of their branches.

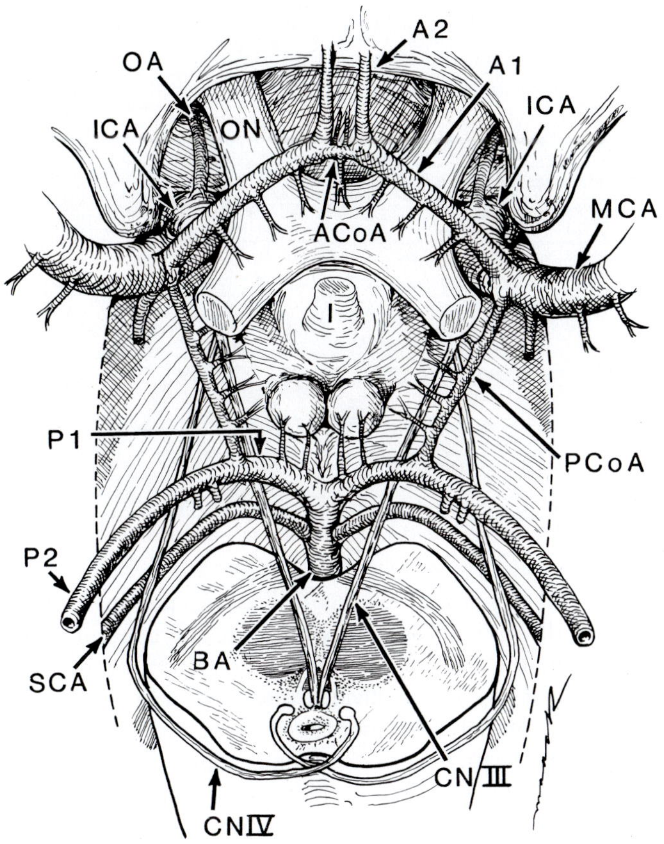

FIGURE 49.3 The circle of Willis and its relationship to adjacent structures. Note innumerable perforating branches arising from every part of the circle to supply the deep midline structures. A1, horizontal segment of ACA; A2, vertical segment of ACA; ACoA, anterior communicating artery; BA, basilar artery; CNIII, oculomotor nerve; CN IV, trochlear nerve; I, infundibulum; ICA, internal carotid artery; MCA, middle cerebral artery; OA, ophthalmic artery; ON, optic nerve; P1, horizontal segment of PCA; P2, ambient segment of PCA; PCoA, posterior communicating artery; SCA, superior cerebellar artery. (Reprinted with permission from Osborn AG. *Diagnostic Cerebral Angiography*. 2nd ed. Philadelphia: Lippincott Williams & Wilkins, 1999.)

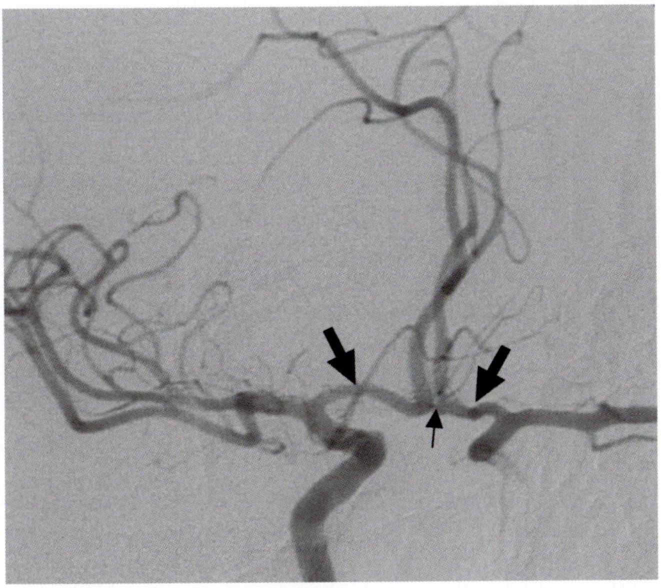

FIGURE 49.4 Right internal carotid arteriogram performed with temporary cross compression of the left common carotid. Both ACAs (*large arrows*) fill via the anterior communicating artery (*small arrow*). (Reprinted with permission from Osborn AG. *Diagnostic Cerebral Angiography*. 2nd ed. Philadelphia: Lippincott Williams & Wilkins, 1999.)

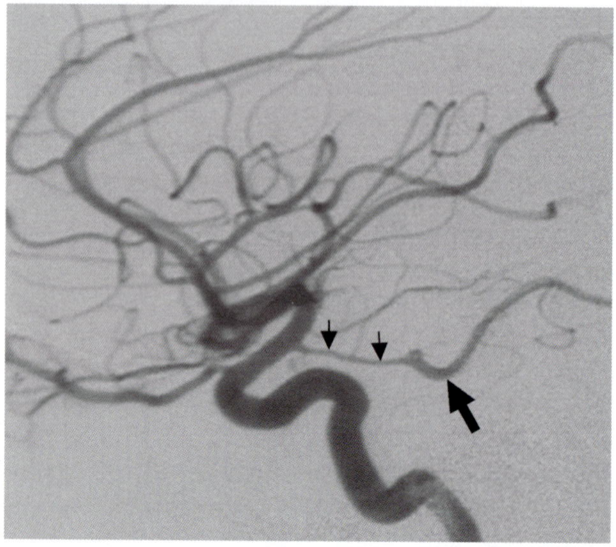

FIGURE 49.5 Lateral view of left internal carotid arteriogram showing filling of the posterior communicating (*small arrows*) and posterior cerebral (*large arrow*) arteries. (Reprinted with permission from Osborn AG. *Diagnostic Cerebral Angiography*. 2nd ed. Philadelphia: Lippincott Williams & Wilkins, 1999.)

the lateral ventricle; it supplies the choroid plexus of the lateral ventricle. During its course, it gives branches to the optic tract, hippocampus, tail of the caudate nucleus, medial and intermediate portions of the globus pallidus, posterior two-thirds of the posterior limb of the internal capsule, middle third of the cerebral peduncle, and outer part of the lateral geniculate body. The retrolenticular and sublenticular portions of the internal capsule are also supplied by this artery.

The ICA terminates just lateral to the optic chiasm, near the medial side of the temporal pole, and the medial and lower portion of the sylvian fissure by dividing into its major terminal branches: the anterior cerebral artery (ACA) and the middle cerebral artery (MCA). The deep, central, or lenticulostriate arteries, 2 to 12 in number, originate from the main trunk, terminal trunks, the bifurcation site, and/or leptomeningeal branches of the MCA, either separately or from common trunks. They dip perpendicularly into the brain substance to supply the basal ganglia and the genu, anterior limb, and superior part of the posterior limb of the internal capsule. They are terminal branches and do not anastomose with each other (end arteries), and occlusion produces localized infarction in the distribution of the involved vessel (lacunar infarction).

The Anterior Cerebral Artery

The ACA, normally the smaller of the two terminal ICA branches, crosses the anterior perforated space above the optic nerve and runs forward and medially to the medial longitudinal fissure; just in front of the optic chiasm, it is linked to the opposite ACA by the anterior communicating artery (Figures 49.4 and 49.7). It is divided into three segments angiographically: A1 (horizontal or precommunicating), A2 (vertical or postcommunicating), and A3 (distal and cortical branches). It then travels forward and rostrally within the interhemispheric fissure, lying on the medial surface of the hemisphere close to the corpus callosum (Figures 49.8 and 49.9). Along its course, the ACA artery gives off four primary cortical branches. The orbital or orbitofrontal artery arises proximally, where the main trunk turns upward, and spreads out over the orbital surface of the frontal lobe, supplying the olfactory lobe, gyrus rectus, and medial and inferior portions of the orbital gyri. Near the genu of the corpus callosum, the frontopolar artery arises to supply the medial surface of the prefrontal region as far forward as the frontal pole. The ACA arcs around the genu of the corpus callosum and then gives off the callosomarginal artery, which courses backward in the cingulate sulcus; it gives off the anterior internal frontal branch about the middle of the superior frontal gyrus, the middle internal frontal branch at the posterior extremity of the superior frontal gyrus, and the posterior internal frontal branch in the region of the paracentral lobule and then continues backward to the posterior parietal region. The ACA continues as the pericallosal artery, which follows the body and posterior part of the corpus callosum to end by anastomosing with branches of the PCA.

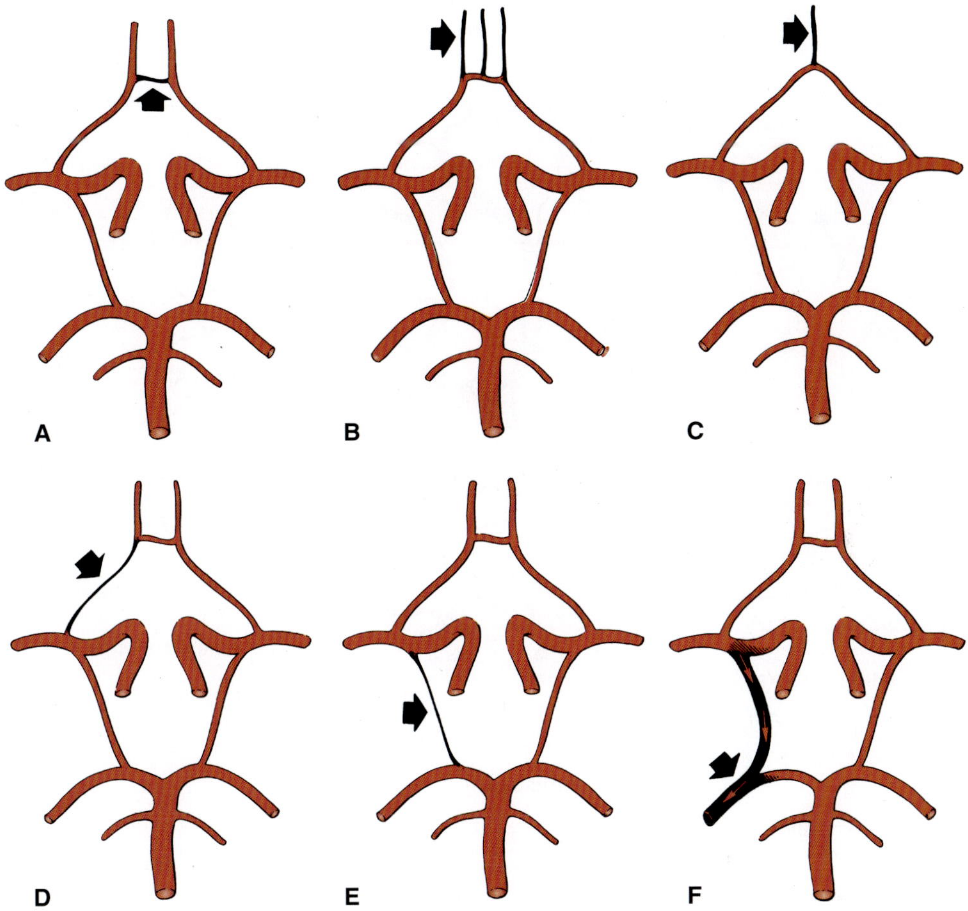

FIGURE 49.6 Variations in the circle of Willis. **A.** Hypoplasia of the anterior communicating artery. **B.** Anomalous ACAs. **C.** Fusion of the ACAs. **D, E.** Hypoplasia of branches of the internal carotid artery (ICA). **F.** PCA from the ICA. (Modified from Alpers BJ, Berry RG, Paddison RM. Anatomical studies of the circle of Willis in normal brain. *Arch Neurol Psychiatry* 1959;81:409–418.)

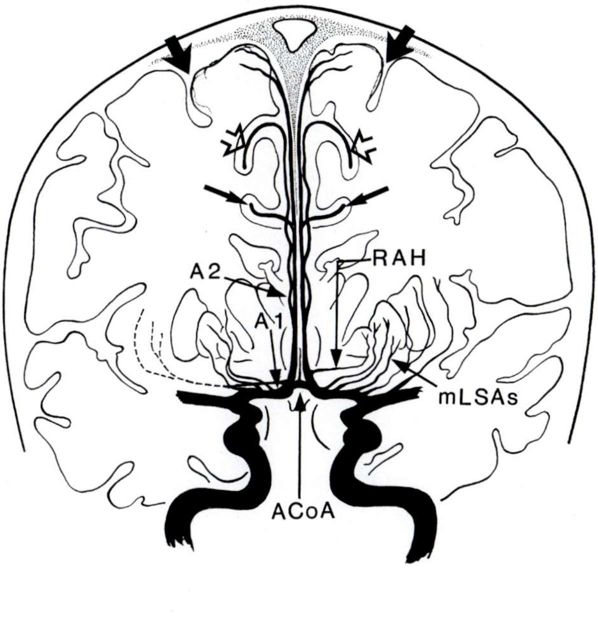

FIGURE 49.7 Drawing of the ACAs and branches. A1, horizontal segment; A2, vertical segment; ACoA, anterior communicating artery; mLSAs, medial lenticulostriate arteries; RAH, recurrent artery of Heubner. *Large arrows* indicate the vascular watershed or border zone between the anterior and middle cerebral arteries. (Reprinted with permission from Osborn AG. *Diagnostic Cerebral Angiography*. 2nd ed. Philadelphia: Lippincott Williams & Wilkins, 1999.)

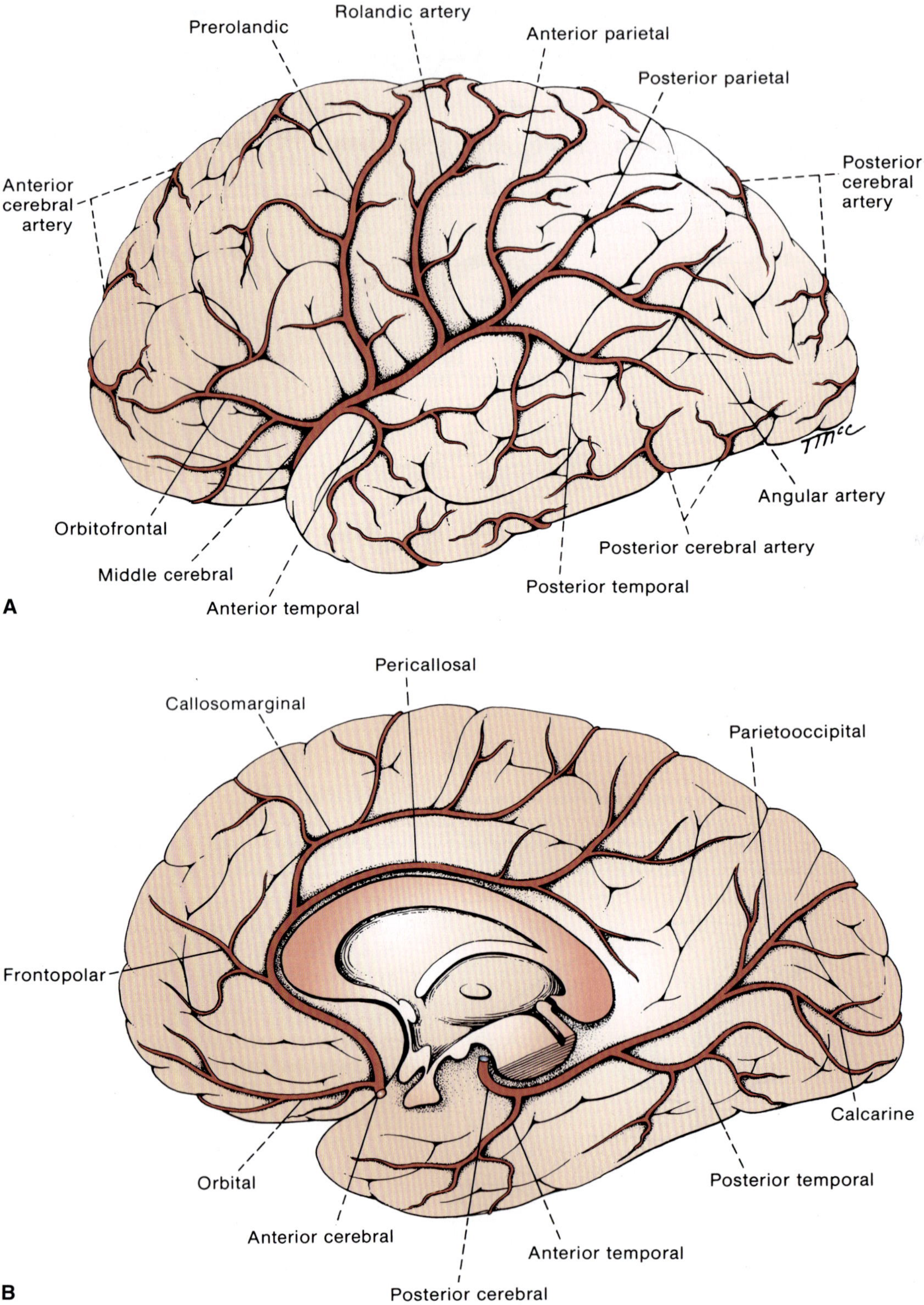

FIGURE 49.8 Blood supply of the cerebral cortex. **A.** Lateral surface of the brain. **B.** Medial surface of the brain.

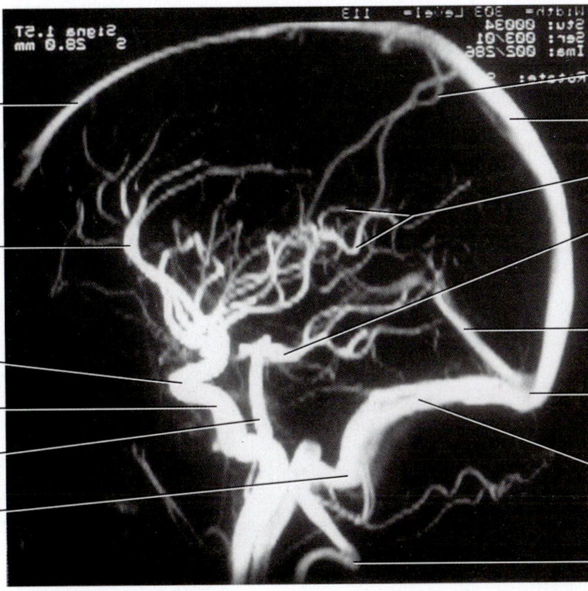

FIGURE 49.9 Lateral view of magnetic resonance angiogram, showing major arteries and venous sinuses. ICA, internal carotid artery; MCA, middle cerebral artery; PCA, posterior cerebral artery. (Reprinted with permission from Fix JD. *Neuroanatomy*. 4th ed. Philadelphia: Wolters Kluwer Health/Lippincott Williams & Wilkins, 2009.)

Numerous small branches of both the anterior cerebral and pericallosal arteries penetrate the corpus callosum. The cortical branches of the ACA supply the medial and orbital surfaces of the frontal lobe, the medial surface of the parietal lobe as far as the parietooccipital fissure, the cingulate gyrus, and the genu and anterior four-fifths of the corpus callosum; these areas include the motor and somesthetic centers in the paracentral lobule. The terminal branches, like those of the PCA, wind around to supply a small portion of the lateral surface of the hemisphere, in this case, of the frontal and parietal lobes.

The largest of the deep, or central, branches of the ACA is the recurrent artery of Heubner (medial striate artery). It takes a recurrent course, and after giving a few branches to the orbital cortex, passes through the anterior perforated space to join the deep branches of the MCA. It supplies the lower part of the head of the caudate nucleus, the lower part of the frontal pole of the putamen, the frontal pole of the globus pallidus, the adjacent frontal half of the anterior limb of the internal capsule, and the anterior portions of the external capsule and lateral ventricle. The anteromedial group of central arteries arises from the anterior cerebral and anterior communicating arteries and supplies the anterior hypothalamus, including the preoptic and suprachiasmatic regions, the genu of the corpus callosum, the septum pellucidum, the anterior pillars of the fornix, and part of the anterior commissure.

The Middle Cerebral Artery

The MCA is the largest of the cerebral arteries (Figures 49.8 and 49.9). It is divided into four segments angiographically: the M1 (horizontal), M2 (insular), M3 (opercular), and M4 (cortical branches). After giving off the posterior communicating artery, it turns laterally (its M1 segment) and along this segment gives off the lenticulostriate arteries (Figures 49.10 and 49.11). These pierce the anterior perforated substance and supply all of the putamen except for its anterior pole, the upper part of the head of the caudate nucleus and all of its body, the lateral part of the globus pallidus, and the posterior part of the anterior limb, the genu, and the anterior third of the posterior limb of the internal capsule. The lenticulostriate arteries are the vessels most often involved in hypertension-induced fibrinoid necrosis, leading to either occlusion (lacunar stroke) or hemorrhage. It is not usually possible to distinguish any dominant individual branch. Charcot thought there was such a vessel, the largest of the group, which he termed the "artery of cerebral hemorrhage" because of the frequent occurrence of cerebral hemorrhage in this region.

The MCA then travels first laterally to enter the sylvian fissure and then turns up and back to course in the depths of the fissure, laterally, posteriorly, and upward, over the surface of the insula and between the frontal and temporal lobes. The MCA gives off many cortical branches that supply the lateral surface

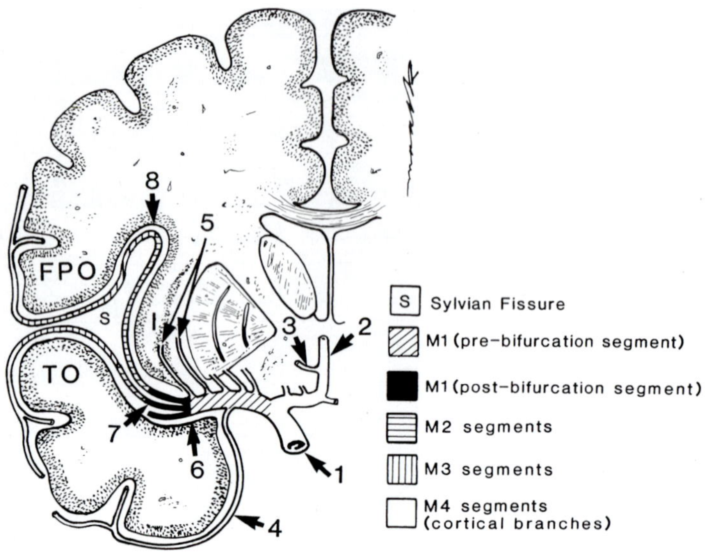

FIGURE 49.10 Drawing of the middle cerebral artery (MCA). Segments as indicated. *1*, Internal carotid; *2*, anterior cerebral; *3*, recurrent artery of Heubner; *4*, anterior temporal artery; *5*, lateral lenticulostriate arteries; *6*, MCA bifurcation/trifurcation; *7*, genu of MCA; *8*, top of the sylvian fissure. (Reprinted with permission from Osborn AG. *Diagnostic Cerebral Angiography*. 2nd ed. Philadelphia: Lippincott Williams & Wilkins, 1999.)

of the brain. The anterior temporal artery curves out of the sylvian fissure and runs over the temporal lobe to supply the temporal pole and the anterior third of the superior and middle temporal gyri. The orbitofrontal artery supplies the lateral part of the orbital surface of the frontal lobe, the lateral surface of the orbital gyri, and the lateral surface of the inferior frontal convolution. The prerolandic artery runs for a short distance in the central fissure and then curves over the precentral gyrus to enter the precentral fissure, supplying the lower and anterior portions of the precentral gyrus and the posterior portions of the middle and inferior frontal convolutions.

The rolandic artery runs over the opercular part of the postcentral gyrus and then enters the central sulcus; it supplies the posterior portion of the precentral gyrus and the anterior portion of the postcentral gyrus. The anterior parietal artery curves over the opercular portion of the parietal lobe and extends to the interparietal fissure, supplying the posterior border of the postcentral gyrus and the anterior parts of the other parietal convolutions. The posterior temporal artery descends from the sylvian fissure and supplies the posterior two-thirds of the superior and middle temporal convolutions. The posterior parietal (supramarginal) artery arises near the end of the

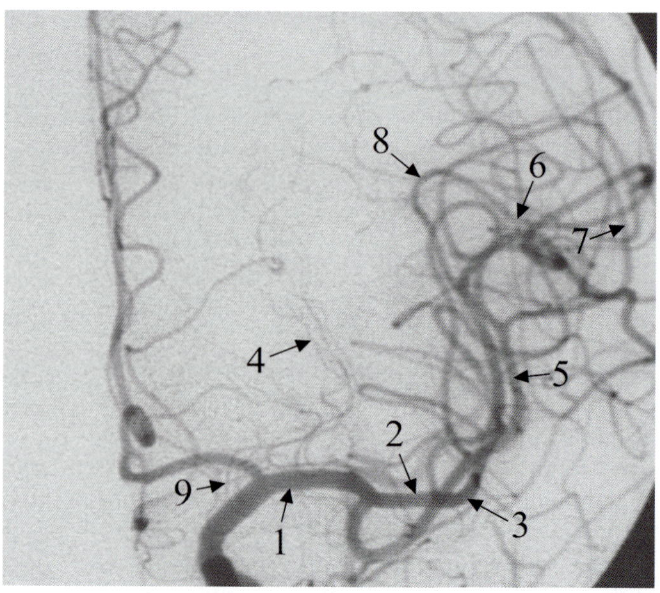

FIGURE 49.11 AP carotid arteriogram showing the middle cerebral artery (MCA) branches. *1*, M1 segment (prebifurcation); *2*, M1 segment (postbifurcation); *3*, MCA genu; *4*, lateral lenticulostriate arteries; *5*, M2 segment; *6*, M3 segment; *7*, M4 segment (cortical branches); *8*, apex of sylvian fissure (angiographic sylvian point); *9*, anterior choroidal artery. (Reprinted with permission from Osborn AG. *Diagnostic Cerebral Angiography*. 2nd ed. Philadelphia: Lippincott Williams & Wilkins, 1999.)

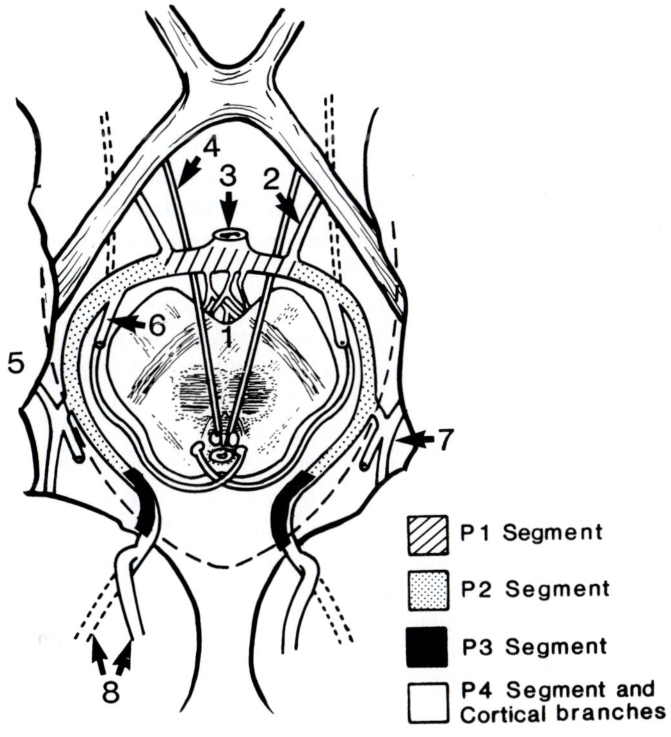

FIGURE 49.12 Drawing of the anatomy of the PCA and its relationship to nearby structures from above. PCA segments as indicated. *1*, Perforating branches; *2*, posterior communicating artery; *3*, basilar artery; *4*, oculomotor nerve; *5*, trochlear nerve; *6*, posterior choroidal arteries; *7*, temporal branches; calcarine (*solid line*) and parietooccipital (*dotted line*) terminal branches. (Reprinted with permission from Osborn AG. *Diagnostic Cerebral Angiography*. 2nd ed. Philadelphia: Lippincott Williams & Wilkins, 1999.)

sylvian fissure and supplies the supramarginal gyrus and the posterior part of the inferior parietal lobule. The MCA terminates as the angular artery, which supplies the angular gyrus and the adjoining parts of the parietal lobe.

The MCA breaks up into terminal cortical branches near the apex of the sylvian fissure. These enter the pia mater where they form a superficial plexus of anastomosing vessels; from these plexuses, smaller terminal branches enter the brain substance at right angles. These branches anastomose with branches of the ACAs and PCAs that project onto the lateral surface of the hemispheres. These anastomotic branches create a collateral blood supply that can compensate to a variable extent for occlusion of a particular vessel.

Vertebrobasilar System

The PCAs are formed by the bifurcation of the basilar artery. The PCA is divided into four segments angiographically: the P1 (precommunicating or mesencephalic), P2 (ambient), P3 (quadrigeminal), and P4 (calcarine). They arch backward and laterally around the cerebral peduncle, close to the upper border of the pons, parallel to the superior cerebellar artery (SCA), and above the oculomotor nerve (Figures 49.12 and 49.13). After receiving the posterior communicating branch from the ICA, the PCA continues along the medial surface of the corresponding cerebral hemisphere, beneath the splenium of the corpus callosum, to reach the medial and inferior surfaces of the temporal lobe and the medial surface of the occipital lobe (Figure 49.8), where it divides into its four cortical branches: (a) the anterior temporal artery supplies the uncus and the anterior parts of the inferior temporal, fusiform, and hippocampal gyri, except for the temporal pole, which is supplied by the MCA; (b) the posterior temporal artery supplies the rest of the fusiform and inferior temporal gyri; (c) the calcarine artery supplies the lingual gyrus and the inferior half of the cuneus; and (d) the parietooccipital, or posterior occipital, artery supplies the upper part of the cuneus, with branches to the splenium of the corpus callosum. The cortical branches of the PCA provide blood to the medial surface of the occipital lobe, including the entire visual cortex, the medial and inferior surfaces of the temporal lobe, and the splenium of the corpus callosum. Terminal branches wind around onto the lateral surfaces of the temporal and occipital lobes and a small part of the superior parietal lobule, where they anastomose with branches of the MCA and ACA.

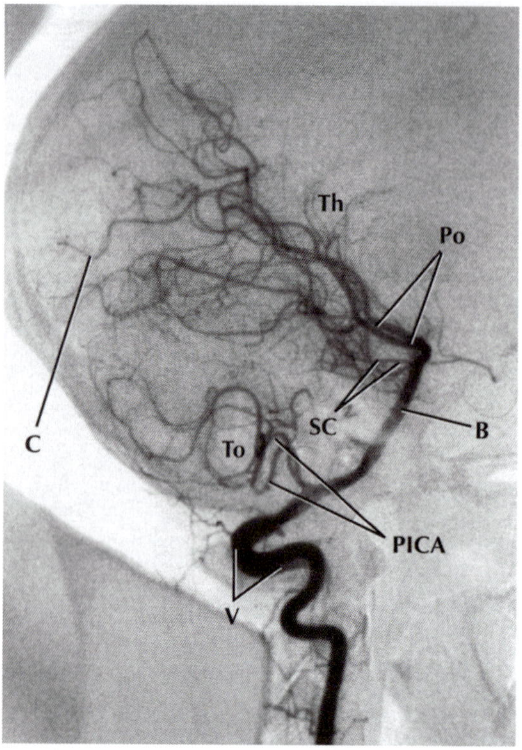

FIGURE 49.13 Lateral subtraction angiogram of the vertebral artery. B, basilar artery; C, calcarine branch of a PCA; PO, PCAs; PICA, posterior inferior cerebellar arteries of both sides; SC, superior cerebellar arteries; Th, position of the thalamus; TO, position of cerebellar tonsil; V, vertebral arteries. (Reprinted with permission from Kiernan JA. *Barr's: The Human Nervous System: An Anatomical Viewpoint.* 7th ed. Baltimore: Lippincott-Raven, 1998.)

The blood supply to the brainstem arises from the vertebral and basilar arteries (Figures 49.14 and 49.15). The two vertebral arteries enter the skull through the foramen magnum and run upward along the clivus. The vertebral artery is divided into four segments angiographically: the V1 (extraosseous), V2 (foraminal), V3 (extraspinal), and V4 (intradural). The medulla receives its blood supply from the vertebral arteries, the pons from the basilar, and the midbrain from the basilar and proximal posterior cerebrals (Figures 49.16 and 49.17). Although there is some normal variability, the right vertebral artery arises from the right subclavian and the left usually comes off the aortic arch proximal to the origin of the left subclavian artery. The relationship of the left vertebral to the subclavian is important in the pathophysiology of the subclavian steal syndrome. The two vertebral arteries are rarely the same size. The left is most often dominant; it is not uncommon for the right to be significantly smaller and occasionally completely atretic. The vertebrals ascend in the foramina transversaria of the transverse processes of the cervical vertebrae from C6 to C2, giving off muscular branches. At the craniocervical junction, they escape from the upper transverse foramina and form a loop before entering the skull through the foramen magnum. The two arteries converge as they climb the clivus anterior to the hypoglossal rootlets and then meet to form the basilar at the level of the pontomedullary junction. The posterior inferior cerebellar artery (PICA) arises from the midportion of each vertebral to supply the medulla and cerebellum (Figure 49.13). Just prior to joining, each vertebral gives off an anterior and a posterior spinal artery. The anterior spinal arteries join at the midmedulla and descend to supply the lower medulla, cervicomedullary junction, and upper spinal cord; the posterior spinal arteries remain separate. The anterior spinal arteries supply the pyramids, medial lemniscus, and emerging hypoglossal fibers.

At about the lower border of the pons, the two vertebrals join to form the basilar, a short (about 2 in long), thick artery that ends at the upper border of the pons (Figure 49.17). The basilar gives rise to three sets of vessels: paramedian perforators, short circumferential, and long circumferential arteries. The paramedian perforators are small arteries that arise from the main trunk of the basilar and dive deeply into the substance of the brainstem to supply the midline structures. The short circumferential arteries are larger vessels that supply slightly more lateral areas. The long circumferential vessels are the major named arteries: the PICA, anterior inferior cerebellar artery (AICA), and SCA. They supply the lateral brainstem and the cerebellum. Each of the long circumferential vessels is paired. Various brainstem vascular syndromes are related to disease of these different arteries (see Chapter 21).

The PICA occasionally arises directly from the basilar or shares a common origin with the AICA. It supplies the inferior cerebellar peduncle, the dorsolateral medullary tegmentum posterior to the inferior olive and lateral to the hypoglossal nucleus, and the inferior surface of the vermis and adjacent cerebellar hemisphere. The AICA is usually a branch of the basilar artery but is the most variable of the named posterior circulation arteries. It supplies the lateral tegmentum of the upper medulla and lower pons, the inferior cerebellar peduncle, lower portion of the middle cerebellar peduncle, flocculus, and inferior surface of the cerebellar hemisphere. The internal

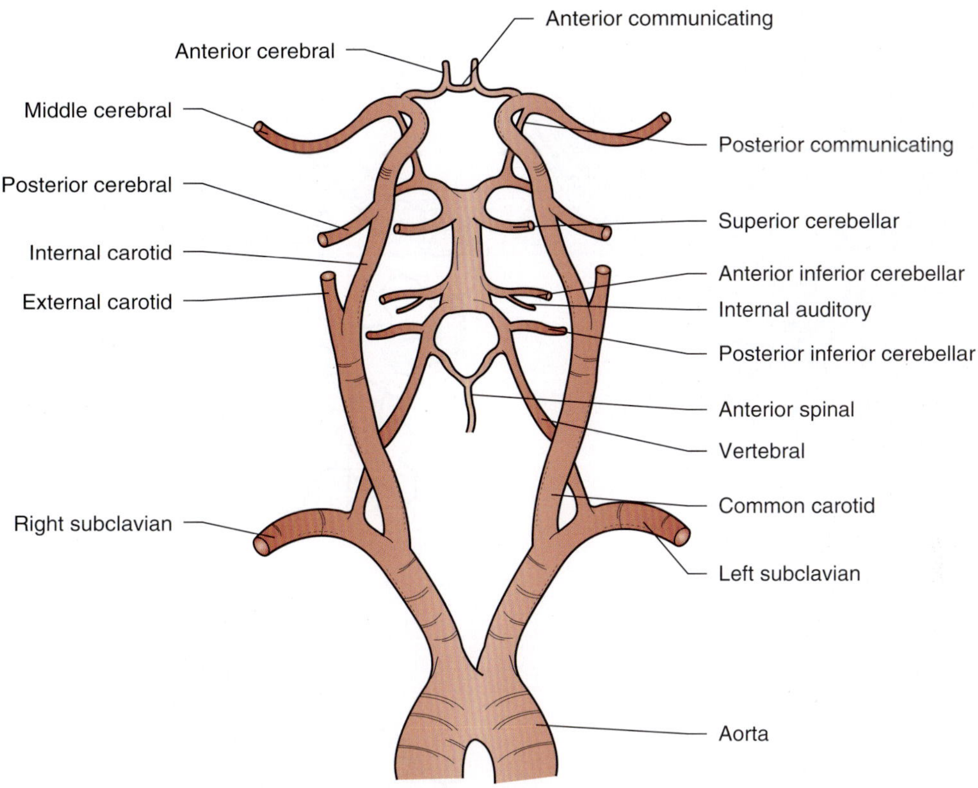

FIGURE 49.14 An overview of the vertebrobasilar arterial system (not to scale).

auditory (labyrinthine) artery usually arises from AICA but often comes directly off the basilar. The AICA often loops into the internal auditory meatus, and the internal auditory artery usually arises from this segment; it terminates as cochlear and vestibular branches, which supply the labyrinth.

The basilar terminates at the level of the pontomesencephalic junction by dividing into the two PCAs that supply the occipital and medial temporal lobes. Just prior to its termination, the basilar gives rise to the two SCAs, which supply the lateral part of the tegmentum of the pons and midbrain, upper portion of the middle cerebellar peduncle, the superior cerebellar peduncle, superior surface of the cerebellum, and the cerebellar nuclei, and sends branches to the cerebral peduncles. As it exits from the interpeduncular fossa, CN III runs between the SCA and the PCA. Interpeduncular branches supply the deep midline of the rostral brainstem, including the medial cerebral peduncles, red nuclei, decussation of the superior cerebellar peduncle, the nuclei of CNs III and IV, and the adjacent subthalamic region. Quadrigeminal branches supply the superior and inferior colliculi. From the top of the basilar and adjacent proximal PCAs, a thatch of deep perforating vessels arises: the medial and lateral posterior choroidals, thalamoperforators, and thalamogeniculates.

The posterior choroidal arteries encircle the cerebral peduncle and give off branches to the midbrain, the tela choroidea and choroid plexus of the third ventricle, and the superomedial surface of the thalamus. The posteromedial arteries, derived from the posterior communicating artery as well as the posterior cerebral, supply the hypophysis, infundibulum, tuberal and mammillary regions of the hypothalamus, walls of the third ventricle, medial and anteromedial portions of the thalamus, subthalamic structures, tegmentum of the midbrain, red nucleus, and medial portion of the cerebral peduncle. The posterolateral, or thalamogeniculate, arteries supply the caudal half of the thalamus, the posterior portion of the internal capsule, the superior cerebellar peduncle, the superior colliculus, and the geniculate bodies.

Border Zone (Watershed) Areas

Cortical branches arising from distal portions of the ACA, MCA, and PCA communicate in their

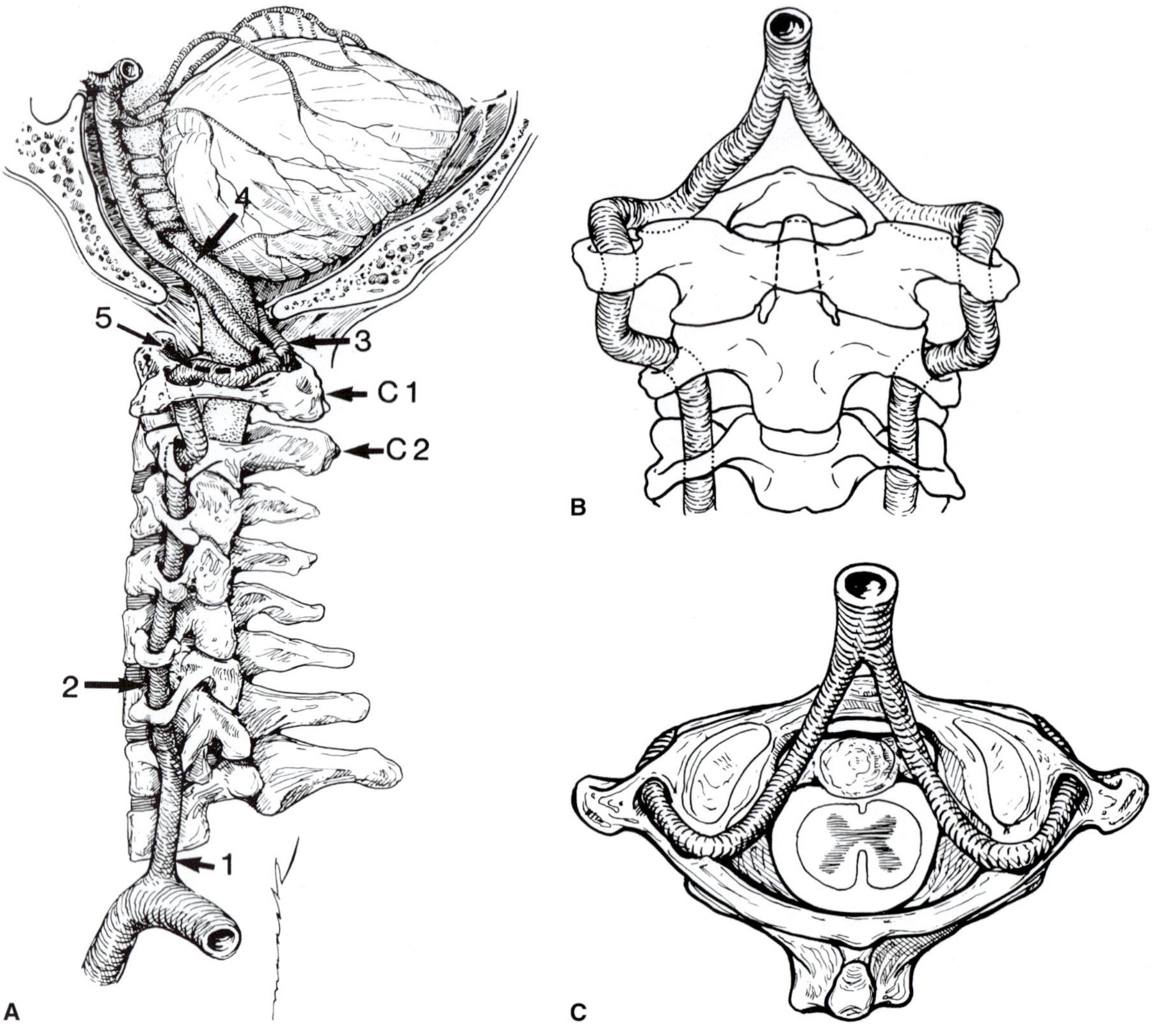

FIGURE 49.15 The proximal vertebral artery segments. **A.** Lateral. **B.** Anteroposterior. **C.** Submentovertex view. *1*, Extraosseous (V1) segment; *2*, foraminal (V2) segment; *3*, extraspinal (V3) segment; *4*, intradural (V4) segment; *5*, approximate location of the occipital condyle. (Reprinted with permission from Osborn AG. *Diagnostic Cerebral Angiography*. 2nd ed. Philadelphia: Lippincott Williams & Wilkins, 1999.)

terminal ramifications. Small collateral vessels enter the pia mater, where they form a superficial plexus of anastomosing vessels; from these plexuses, smaller terminal branches enter the brain substance at right angles. Because of these terminal anastomoses between larger cortical arteries, blood supply from neighboring branches may compensate to a variable extent for a vascular occlusion. Collateral vessels are better developed in some individuals than others. The areas between the major vessels are called watershed areas or border zones. The watershed areas are a cerebrovascular "no man's land," marginally perfused and susceptible to ischemic injury when the perfusion pressure falls.

Cerebral blood flow is studied with a variety of techniques. The least invasive include single photon emission computed tomography (CT), xenon clearance studies, and positron emission tomography. Both total and regional cerebral blood flow may be evaluated. The vessels themselves can be examined by conventional angiography or by digital subtraction techniques employing arterial or venous routes. Doppler and other ultrasonic tests detect the presence of occlusions or stenoses in the large neck vessels in a noninvasive manner, and transcranial Doppler studies help with evaluation of flow in the intracranial vessels. Magnetic resonance angiography (MRA), as well as CT angiography and conventional angiography,

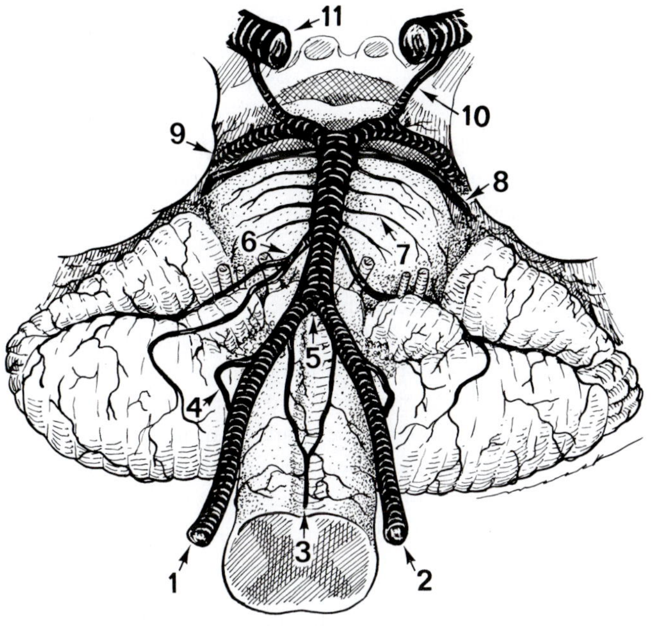

FIGURE 49.16 The vertebrobasilar system and its major branches. *1*, Right vertebral; *2*, left vertebral; *3*, anterior spinal; *4*, posterior inferior cerebellar; *5*, junction of vertebrals forming the basilar artery; *6*, anterior inferior cerebellar; *7*, lateral pontine arteries; *8*, superior cerebellar; *9*, posterior cerebral; *10*, posterior communicating; *11*, internal carotid. (Reprinted with permission from Osborn AG. *Diagnostic Cerebral Angiography*. 2nd ed. Philadelphia: Lippincott Williams & Wilkins, 1999.)

can demonstrate stenoses or other focal vascular abnormalities and can demonstrate intracranial vascular lesions such as aneurysms, angiomas, and malformations. CT identifies intracranial hemorrhagic lesions reliably. Magnetic resonance imaging provides evidence of cerebral infarction in various vascular territories. Diffusion- and perfusion-weighted imaging provides immediate evidence of focal ischemia.

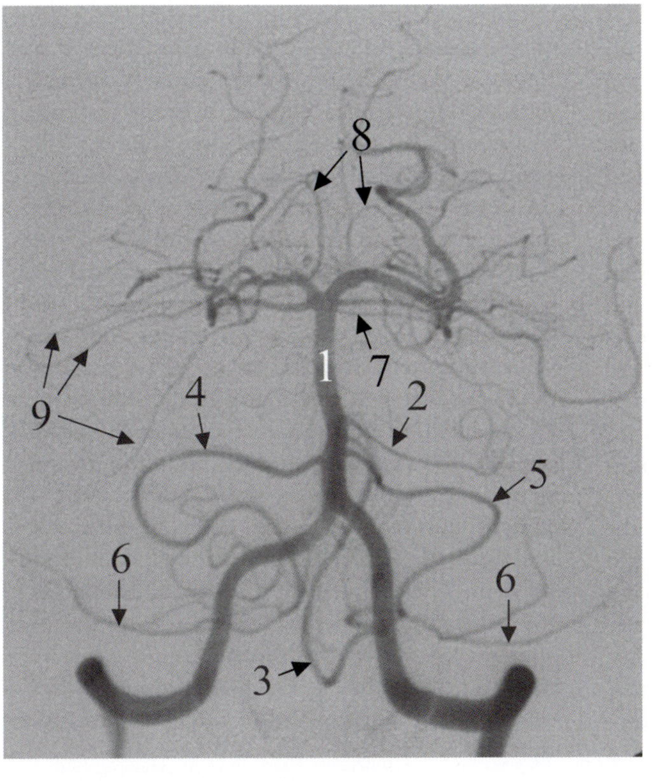

FIGURE 49.17 Left vertebral arteriogram. *1*, Basilar artery; *2*, left anterior inferior cerebellar (AICA); *3*, caudal loop of posterior inferior cerebellar (PICA); *4*, common trunk for right AICA-PICA; *5*, left PICA; *6*, hemispheric branches of PICA; *7*, superior cerebellar (SCA); *8*, hemispheric branches of SCA; *9*, superior vermian branches of SCA. (Reprinted with permission from Osborn AG. *Diagnostic Cerebral Angiography*. 2nd ed. Philadelphia: Lippincott Williams & Wilkins, 1999.)

THE CEREBRAL VEINS AND THE VENOUS SINUSES

The cerebral veins do not parallel the cerebral arteries; they possess no valves, and their walls are extremely thin. They may be divided into an external, superficial, or cortical group, and an internal, deep, or central group (Figure 49.18). The external veins arise from the cortex and medullary substance of the hemisphere. They anastomose freely and form a network of large trunks in the pia mater. The superior cerebral veins, 8 to 12 in number, drain the superior, lateral, and medial surfaces of the hemispheres above the sylvian and callosomarginal fissures. Most of them are lodged in the sulci between the gyri, although some of the larger trunks run across the convexity of the gyri. They pierce the arachnoid membrane and the inner layer of the dura mater and, after a short intradural course, terminate in the superior sagittal sinus (SSS) or its venous lacunae. The arrangement on the two sides is asymmetric, and a separation into anterior and posterior groups is usually evident. The anterior veins drain the upper parts of the frontal lobe and enter the SSS at right angles to its lateral wall. The larger posterior veins drain the parietal region and run forward before entering the sinus; some from the convex surface of the occipital lobe may terminate in the transverse sinus.

The inferior cerebral veins are small and drain the basal surfaces of the hemispheres and the lower portion of the lateral surfaces. Those on the orbital surface of the hemisphere enter the superior veins and then into the SSS. Those from the temporal lobes anastomose with the middle cerebral veins and enter the cavernous, sphenoparietal, transverse, and superior petrosal sinuses. The middle cerebral vein traverses the sylvian fissure and drains the insula and the opercular region. It terminates either in the cavernous or sphenoparietal sinus or occasionally in the transverse or superior petrosal sinus. It is connected with the SSS by the great anastomotic vein of Trolard and with the transverse sinus by the small, or posterior, anastomotic vein of Labbé.

The deep cerebral veins drain the interior of the hemispheres. The choroidal vein runs the entire length of the choroid plexus and receives branches from the hippocampus, fornix, and corpus callosum. The terminal vein runs in the groove between the caudate nucleus and thalamus and receives many tributaries from these structures as well as from the internal capsule. Near the interventricular foramen, the terminal and choroidal veins fuse to form the internal cerebral vein. The basal vein (of Rosenthal) is formed at the anterior perforated space by the union of a small anterior vein that accompanies the ACA, the deep middle cerebral vein, and the inferior striate vein; it passes backward around the cerebral peduncle to end in the internal cerebral vein and receives tributaries from the cingulate gyrus, anterior part of the corpus callosum, orbital surface of the frontal lobe, olfactory groove, optic chiasm, hypophysis, cerebral peduncle, interpeduncular fossa, inferior horn of the lateral ventricle, hippocampal gyrus, and midbrain. The internal occipital vein also enters the internal cerebral vein. The great cerebral vein of Galen is formed just behind the pineal body by the union of the two internal cerebral veins. It is a short midline trunk that curves backward and upward around the splenium of the corpus callosum and empties into the straight sinus. The deep venous system is the entire territory served by the great vein of Galen and the basal veins. The superficial venous system drains the rest of the hemisphere. A venous watershed exists between the territories of the deep and superficial venous systems.

The venous sinuses of the dura mater are channels that lie between the two layers of the dura; the cerebral veins terminate in them (Figure 49.19). The SSS occupies the convex, or attached, margin of the falx cerebri from the foramen cecum to the region of the internal occipital protuberance, where it continues as one of the transverse sinuses. In its middle portion, it gives off a number of lateral diverticula, or venous lacunae, into which protrude the arachnoid (pacchionian) granulations. The SSS receives the superior cerebral veins, veins from the diploë and dura mater, and, in the parietal region, emissary veins from the pericranium. The inferior sagittal sinus is located in the posterior half or two-thirds of the free, inferior margin of the falx cerebri and receives veins from the falx and from the medial surfaces of the hemispheres. It terminates in the straight sinus at the junction of the falx cerebri and tentorium cerebelli and runs backward to end in the transverse sinus opposite the one in which the SSS ends. The straight sinus receives, in addition to the inferior sagittal sinus, the vein of Galen and the superior cerebellar veins. The occipital sinus begins at the margin of the foramen magnum and courses through the lower attached margin of the falx cerebri to the transverse sinus. The superior sagittal, straight, and occipital sinuses come together at the confluence of sinuses (torcular herophili).

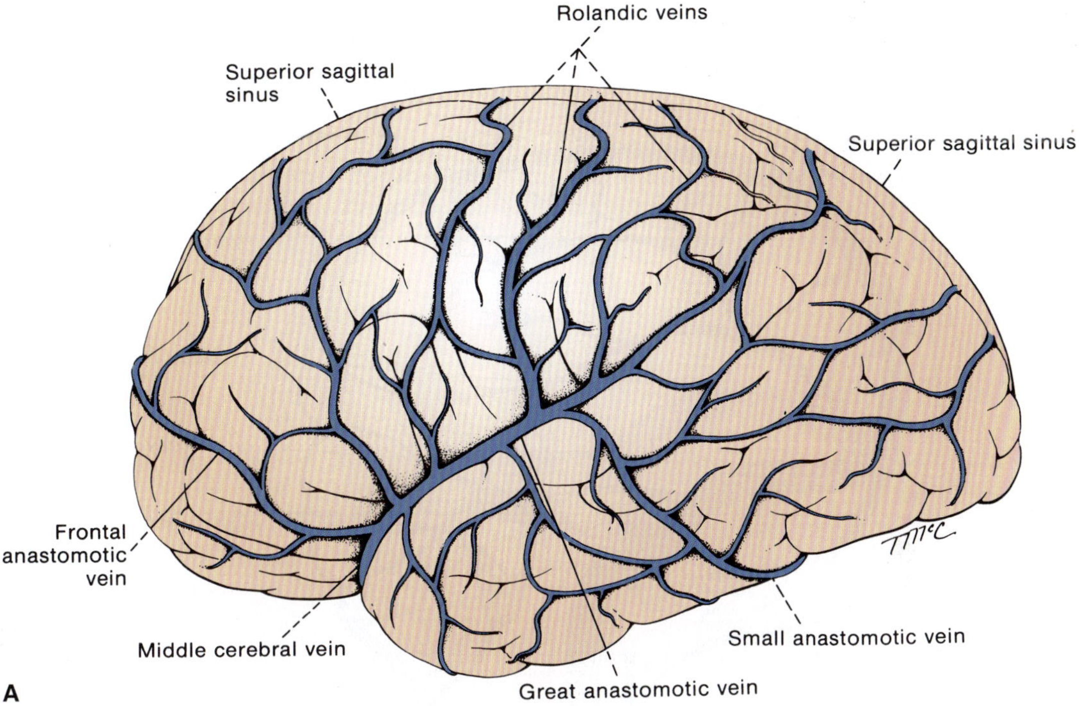

A

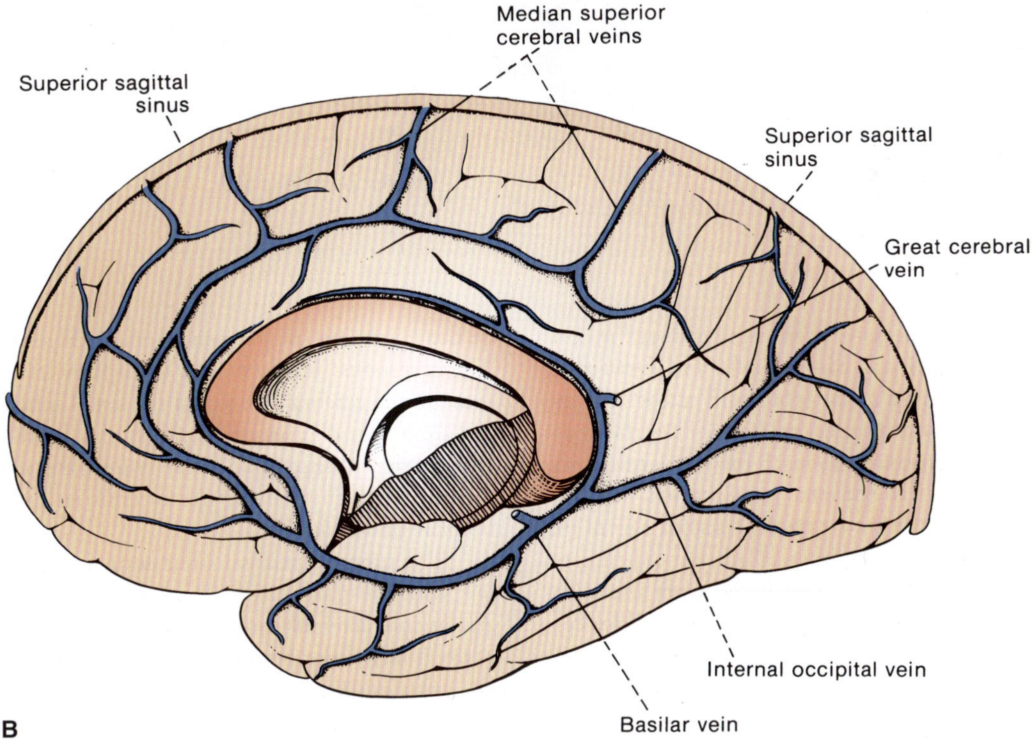

B

FIGURE 49.18 Venous drainage of the cerebral cortex. **A.** Lateral surface. **B.** Medial surface.

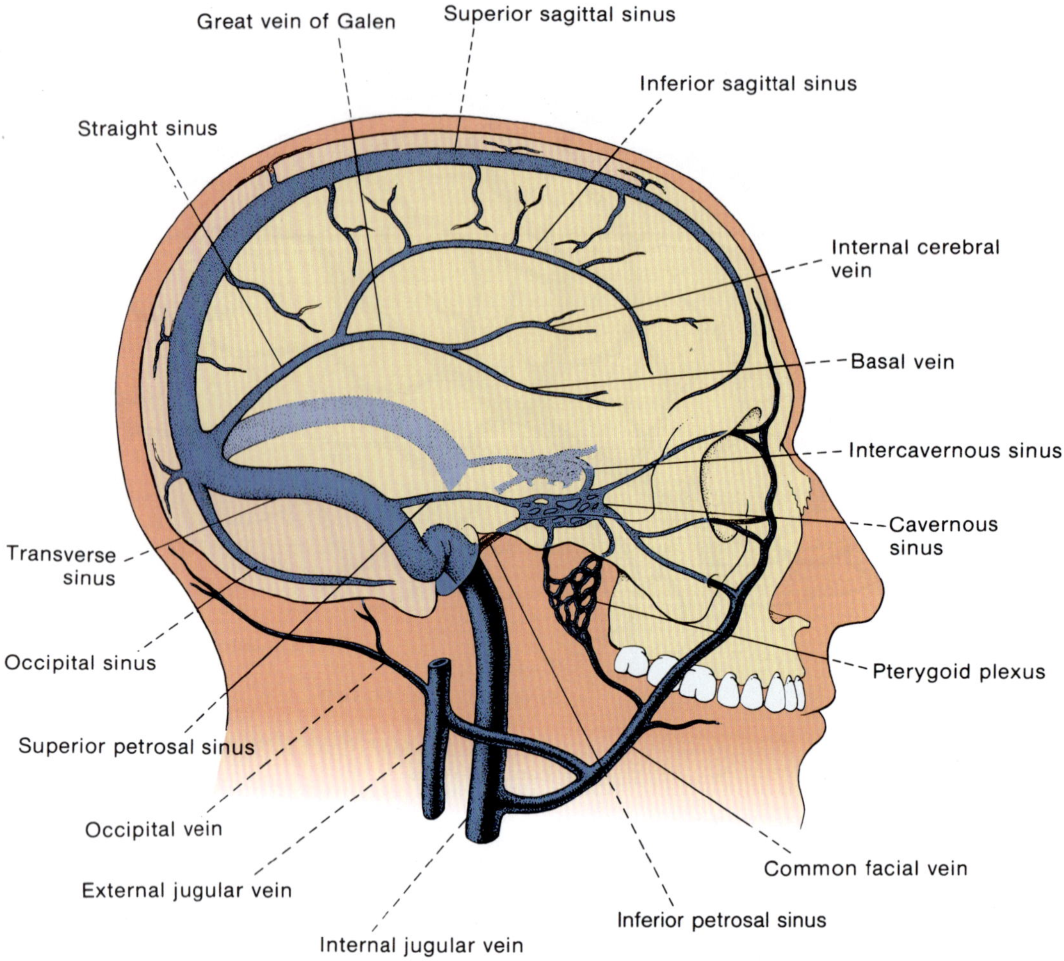

FIGURE 49.19 Venous drainage of the brain, showing the dural sinuses and their principal connections with extracranial veins.

The transverse (lateral) sinuses begin at the confluence of sinuses and pass laterally and forward in the attached margin of the tentorium cerebelli to the petrous portion of the temporal bone. They then pass downward and medially to reach the jugular foramen where they end in the internal jugular veins. The portions occupying the groove on the mastoid part of the temporal bone are sometimes called sigmoid sinuses. The transverse sinuses receive blood from the superior petrosal sinuses, inferior cerebral and inferior cerebellar veins, and emissary and diploic veins.

The cavernous sinuses lie on each side of the body of the sphenoid bone, lateral to the sella turcica, and extend from the superior orbital fissure to the petrous portion of the temporal bone. They open behind into the petrosal sinuses. The ICA lies medially in the sinus; the abducens, oculomotor, and trochlear nerves, and the ophthalmic and maxillary divisions of the trigeminal nerve, run laterally (Figure 14.6). The cavernous sinuses receive the ophthalmic veins, some of the cerebral veins, and the small sphenoparietal sinus that courses under the surface of the small wing of the sphenoid bone. The two sinuses communicate with each other by the anterior and posterior intercavernous sinuses.

The superior petrosal sinus connects the cavernous with the transverse sinus and receives cerebellar and inferior cerebral veins and veins from the tympanic cavity. The inferior petrosal sinus connects the cavernous sinus with the internal jugular vein and receives the internal auditory veins and veins from the cerebellum and medulla. The basilar plexus consists of several interlacing venous channels between the layers of the dura mater on the basilar part of the occipital bone; it connects the two inferior petrosal sinuses and communicates with the vertebral venous plexuses. Emissary veins pass through apertures in the cranial wall and establish communications between the sinuses inside the skull and veins external to it. Diploic veins occupy channels in the diploë of the cranial bones and communicate with the sinuses of the dura mater, veins of the pericranium, and meningeal veins.

The venous drainage from the medulla goes caudally into the venous plexus surrounding the spinal cord, the adjacent dural venous sinuses, or along the last four CNs via radicular veins to the inferior petrosal sinus or superior bulb of the jugular vein. Veins draining the pons and midbrain go cephalad into the basal vein, great cerebral veins, cerebellar veins, or the petrosal or transverse sinuses. Consequently, compression at either the foramen magnum or the tentorium may cause bleeding into the brainstem.

NEUROVASCULAR EXAMINATION

Examination of the vascular system is often included as part of the neurologic examination, especially in patients with suspected cerebrovascular disease. Blood pressure should be determined in both arms. A significant asymmetry may signify brachiocephalic occlusive disease on the side with the lower pressure. High-grade stenosis or occlusion may produce a palpable delay or loss of volume of the brachial or radial pulse on the involved side. Gentle and cautious palpation of the carotid pulse in the neck may give some information about the patency in certain cases. By careful palpation either low in the neck or just below the mandible, it may be possible to distinguish between common and internal carotid pulsations. Diminished, unequal, or absent pulsations may indicate either partial or complete obstruction. There is some risk to carotid palpation, and the useful information obtained is limited. An increase in the superficial temporal and facial artery pulses may reflect occlusive disease of the ICA with collateral perfusion through the external carotid artery. Occlusive disease of the common carotid may cause decreased facial pulses on the involved side. Evaluation of the peripheral pulses in the lower extremities may reveal evidence of generalized vascular disease.

Bruits heard over the carotid artery bifurcations in the neck, over the common carotids proximally, or in the supraclavicular fossae usually signify occlusive vascular disease, but the correlation between bruits and carotid occlusive disease is imprecise. Bruits may be heard diffusely in some patients, particularly those with a hyperdynamic circulation or increased cardiac output (e.g., hyperthyroidism or patients on hemodialysis) and in the young, especially children, without signifying occlusive vascular disease. In older patients and those with symptoms of vascular disease, diffuse or localized bruits, unilateral or bilateral, are equally predictive of moderate-to-severe atherosclerosis in the extracranial carotid artery. Mild stenosis does not often cause an audible bruit. Bruits correlate with moderate stenosis, approximately 50% or greater. Severe occlusive disease with high-grade stenosis may cause only a very soft, short, unimpressive systolic bruit because of the severely restricted flow through the stenotic vessel. In certain clinical circumstances, soft bruits are more ominous than loud bruits. A very high-pitched, whistling bruit is a fairly reliable indicator of severe underlying stenosis. With complete occlusion of one artery, a bruit may be heard on the opposite side because of increased flow, but no bruit may be heard on the occluded side. Bruits often arise from the external carotid, so the presence of a bruit does not reliably indicate that the ICA is patent. Bruits in asymptomatic patients are important as an indicator of underlying coronary artery disease as well as extracranial cerebrovascular disease. Magyar et al. found the sensitivity of carotid auscultation for the detection of a 70% to 99% stenosis of the common or extracranial ICA was 56% and specificity was 91%. The positive predictive value of a bruit was 27%, and the negative predictive value of a normal examination was 97%. Davies and Humphrey found that moderate (30% to 69%) or severe (70% to 99%) stenosis was present in 37% of patients with, and 17% of those without, a carotid bruit; 32% of patients with a bruit had normal carotid arteries.

It is often very difficult to distinguish a systolic murmur transmitted from the heart from a bruit due to occlusive cerebrovascular disease. It is sometimes possible to track a transmitted murmur from the base of the heart along the course of the proximal carotid and up to the angle of the mandible. Bruits due to carotid disease are usually limited to the bifurcation. A bruit arising from the carotid bifurcation may be transmitted to the mastoid process, but this rarely if ever occurs with a transmitted murmur. An orbital bruit is best heard using a stethoscope with a deep, narrow bell (Ford-Bowles type). The wide shallow bells best for cardiac auscultation work poorly for listening over the orbits. An orbital bruit usually signifies significant intracranial occlusive disease but does indicate that the carotid artery on the side of the bruit is patent. The most common cause is stenosis of the carotid siphon ipsilateral to the ocular bruit.

Compensatory increased flow through the nonoccluded carotid may account for an orbital bruit over the eyeball contralateral to a stenotic vessel. An ocular bruit was the only auscultatory finding in 28% in one series of patients with symptoms of atherothrombotic ischemic cerebrovascular disease. Ocular bruits, like other cephalic bruits, occasionally occur in the absence of demonstrable disease. See Smith for a podcast on orbital bruits.

Examination of the fundus is important in patients with cerebrovascular disease. Retinal changes of hypertension may be present. ICA occlusive disease may protect the ipsilateral eye and cause the hypertensive changes to be less severe than in the fellow eye. Fundus examination may also disclose retinal emboli or evidence of chronic ocular ischemia. A careful search for retinal emboli should always be made on the side of suspected carotid occlusive disease. There are two types of emboli commonly seen in carotid artery disease, particularly in the presence of ulcerated plaque: bright, yellow cholesterol emboli (Hollenhorst plaque) and white fibrin-platelet emboli (Figure 49.20). Emboli may be seen at arterial bifurcations over the disk, or more peripherally. They are particularly likely to be visible in the perimacular region. Calcific emboli may originate from the aortic valve. Roth spots are areas of focal retinal hemorrhage with a focal white center that may be seen with endocarditis and other conditions.

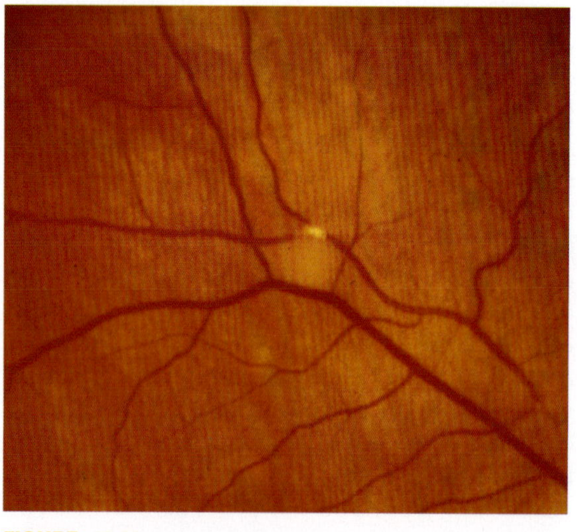

FIGURE 49.20 Branch retinal artery occlusion with Hollenhorst plaque. (Reprinted with permission from Gerstenblith AT, Rabinowitz MP, eds. *The Wills Eye Manual: Office and Emergency Room Diagnosis and Treatment of Eye Disease.* 6th ed. Philadelphia: Wolters Kluwer Health/Lippincott Williams & Wilkins, 2012.)

BIBLIOGRAPHY

Andeweg J. Consequences of the anatomy of deep venous outflow from the brain. *Neuroradiology* 1999;41:233–241.

Bisschops RH, Klijn CJ, Kappelle LJ, et al. Collateral flow and ischemic brain lesions in patients with unilateral carotid artery occlusion. *Neurology* 2003;60:1435–1441.

Caruso G, Vincentelli F, Giudicelli G, et al. Perforating branches of the basilar bifurcation. *J Neurosurg* 1990;73:259–265.

Chaynes P. Microsurgical anatomy of the great cerebral vein of Galen and its tributaries. *J Neurosurg* 2003;99:1028–1038.

Donzelli R, Marinkovic S, Brigante L, et al. Territories of the perforating (lenticulostriate) branches of the middle cerebral artery. *Surg Radiol Anat* 1998;20:393–398.

Floriani M, Giulini SM, Bonardelli S, et al. Value and limits of "critical auscultation" of neck bruits. *Angiology* 1988;39:967–972.

Ghika JA, Bogousslavsky J, Regli F. Deep perforators from the carotid system. Template of the vascular territories. *Arch Neurol* 1990;47:1097–1100.

Goldman L, Koller RL, Lebow SS, et al. Cervical bruits: clinical correlates of stenosis. *Angiology* 1991;42:491–497.

Hendrikse J, Hartkamp MJ, Hillen B, et al. Collateral ability of the circle of Willis in patients with unilateral internal carotid artery occlusion: border zone infarcts and clinical symptoms. *Stroke* 2001;32:2768–2773.

Hu HH, Liao KK, Wong WJ, et al. Ocular bruits in ischemic cerebrovascular disease. *Stroke* 1988;19:1229–1233.

Ingall TJ, Homer D, Whisnant JP, et al. Predictive value of carotid bruit for carotid atherosclerosis. *Arch Neurol* 1989;46:418–422.

Johnston DC, Goldstein LB. Clinical carotid endarterectomy decision making: noninvasive vascular imaging versus angiography. *Neurology* 2001;56:1009–1015.

Komiyama M, Nakajima H, Nishikawa M, et al. Middle cerebral artery variations: duplicated and accessory arteries. *Am J Neuroradiol* 1998;19:45–49.

Macchi V, Porzionato A, Parenti A, et al. The course of the posterior inferior cerebellar artery may be related to its level of origin. *Surg Radiol Anat* 2004;26(1):60–65.

Magyar MT, Nam EM, Csiba L, et al. Carotid artery auscultation—anachronism or useful screening procedure? *Neurol Res* 2002;24:705–708.

Mandell BF. It's not the noise, it's what you do with it. *Cleve Clin J Med* 2015;82:792–798.

Marinkovic S, Milisavljevic M, Kovacevic M. Interpeduncular perforating branches of the posterior cerebral artery. Microsurgical anatomy of their extracerebral and intracerebral segments. *Surg Neurol* 1986;26:349–359.

Marinkovic S, Gibo H, Milisavljevic M, et al. Anatomic and clinical correlations of the lenticulostriate arteries. *Clin Anat* 2001;14:190–195.

Osborn AG. *Diagnostic Cerebral Angiography.* 2nd ed. Philadelphia: Lippincott Williams & Wilkins, 1999.

Paraskevas KI, Hamilton G, Mikhailidis DP. Clinical significance of carotid bruits: an innocent finding or a useful warning sign? *Neurol Res* 2008;30:523–530.

Pickett CA, Jackson JL, Hemann BA, et al. Carotid bruits and cerebrovascular disease risk: a meta-analysis. *Stroke* 2010;41:2295–2302.

Phillips CD, Bubash LA. CT angiography and MR angiography in the evaluation of extracranial carotid vascular disease. *Radiol Clin North Am* 2002;40:783–798.

Ratchford EV, Jin Z, Di Tullio MR, et al. Carotid bruit for detection of hemodynamically significant carotid stenosis: the Northern Manhattan Study. *Neurol Res* 2009;31:748–752.

Ross JS, Masaryk TJ, Modie MT, et al. Magnetic resonance angiography of the extracranial carotid arteries and intracranial vessels: a review. *Neurology* 1989;39:369.

Smith JH. Pearls & Oy-sters: the orbital bruit: a poor man's angiogram. *Neurology* 2009;73:e81–e82.

Stahlfeld KR, Means JR, Didomenico P. Carotid artery fibromuscular dysplasia. *Am J Surg* 2007;193:71–72.

Stefani MA, Schneider FL, Marrone AC, et al. Anatomic variations of anterior cerebral artery cortical branches. *Clin Anat* 2000;13:231–236.

Takahashi S, Suzuki M, Matsumoto K, et al. Extent and location of cerebral infarcts on multiplanar MR images: correlation with distribution of perforating arteries on cerebral angiograms and on cadaveric microangiograms. *Am J Roentgenol* 1994;163: 1215–1222.

Ture U, Yasargil MG, Al Mefty O, et al. Arteries of the insula. *J Neurosurg* 2000;92:676–687.

Wiebers DO, Whisnant JP, Sandok BA, et al. Prospective comparison of a cohort with asymptomatic carotid bruit and a population-based cohort without carotid bruit. *Stroke* 1990;21:984–988.

Wiesmann M, Yousry I, Seelos KC, et al. Identification and anatomic description of the anterior choroidal artery by use of 3D-TOF source and 3D-CISS MR imaging. *Am J Neuroradiol* 2001;22:305–310.

CHAPTER 50

The Ventricular System and the Cerebrospinal Fluid

The gross anatomy of the ventricular system and subarachnoid cisterns is discussed in Chapter 2, and Figure 2.5 shows the cerebrospinal fluid (CSF) spaces. The CSF is produced by the choroid plexus, which lies within the atrium, body, and inferior horn of each of the lateral ventricles; in the third ventricle; and in the roof of the fourth ventricle. The bulk of the CSF is produced in the lateral ventricles. The two lateral ventricles come together in the midline, where they join the third ventricle. The slit-like interventricular foramina of Monro lie at the junction of the roof and the anterior wall of the third ventricle and connect the lateral ventricles with the third ventricle. The foramen of Monro is the site of the original outgrowth of the telencephalon to form the cerebral hemispheres. Although the majority of the CSF originates in the choroid plexus of the ventricles of the brain, there is also some production through the ependymal lining and in the subarachnoid and perivascular spaces. The CSF is discharged into and fills the ventricles, basal cisterns, and subarachnoid spaces.

The choroid plexus is a vascular invagination of the pia into the ventricles, forming a rich network of pial vessels, covered by a layer of ependymal cells that are continuous with the lining of the ventricles. The ependymal cells have tight junctions on their apical surface. The arterial supply to the choroid plexus in the lateral ventricle is provided by the anterior choroid artery, a branch of the internal carotid, and by the posterior choroidal arteries from the posterior cerebral artery. Arterial pulsations in the choroid plexus facilitate circulation of the CSF.

The CSF is formed by a combination of active secretion and filtration at a rate of 0.35 to 0.37 mL/min. The brain interstitial fluid (ISF) circulates between brain cells and drains into the CSF or is absorbed into the blood through terminal capillaries. The entire reservoir of CSF is about 90 to 150 mL in the normal adult, of which approximately 75 mL is intracranial, and 40 to 60 mL in the newborn. This amount is completely replaced several times a day. The rate of formation is related to factors such as the osmotic and hydrostatic pressures of the blood and variations in venous pressure. The rate of formation is independent of the CSF pressure, so that even when there is a high volume and increased pressure of CSF within the ventricular system due to obstruction or lack of resorption, the pace of production is unaffected. The enzyme carbonic anhydrase is involved in the production of CSF. Carbonic anhydrase inhibitors, such as acetazolamide, decrease the production of CSF.

The fluid resembles an ultrafiltrate of plasma but with some differences. The CSF contains a small amount of protein, a little more than half the concentration of glucose as in plasma, a few cells, and various ions (Table 50.1). The ions are present in the CSF at concentrations different from plasma, and the pH is lower.

The CSF lies in the subarachnoid space, between the arachnoid and the pia mater. Within the subarachnoid space, web-like strands of arachnoid extend between the arachnoid and pia. The pia closely invests the surface of the brain and spinal cord, dipping into the fissures and sulci. The arachnoid bridges the fissures and sulci. The blood vessels that penetrate the brain go through the subarachnoid space and become invested with two layers of arachnoid; these arachnoid coats, which accompany the vessels for varying distances into the brain, are known as the perivascular (Virchow-Robin) spaces (Figure 2.4). The CSF flows into the perivascular spaces and is carried for a certain distance into the

TABLE 50.1 Normal Characteristics and Composition of the CSF

Appearance	Clear and Colorless
Cells	<6 lymphocytes or mononuclear cells
Total protein	15–50 mg/dL
IgG	<8.4 mg/dL
Gamma globulin	6%–13% of total protein
Oligoclonal bands	0–1 band
Myelin basic protein	0–4 ng/mL
CSF IgG index	0–0.77
CSF IgG synthesis rate	0–8 mg/24 h
Glucose	45–80 mg/dL, 60%–80% of blood sugar

CSF, cerebrospinal fluid; IgG, immunoglobulin G.

substance of the brain and spinal cord. The subarachnoid space, containing CSF, also extends outward for varying distances in periradicular and perineural spaces along exiting nerve roots and cranial nerves (CNs). In the spinal canal, a large subarachnoid space extends from the termination of the spinal cord to about the second sacral vertebra. This terminal sac contains the cauda equina and is the usual site for performing lumbar puncture (LP).

CEREBROSPINAL FLUID CIRCULATION

The CSF percolates from the lateral ventricles, through the foramen of Monro, into the third ventricle, and then down the cerebral aqueduct into the fourth ventricle. From the fourth, a small amount enters the central canal of the spinal cord while the majority is discharged through the foramina of Luschka and Magendie into the subarachnoid cisterns surrounding the brainstem and cerebellum. There is continuous circulation between these basal cisterns and the spinal subarachnoid space all the way to the lumbosacral region. Eventually, CSF migrates into the subarachnoid space over the convexities of the hemispheres alongside the superior sagittal sinus. Harvey Cushing referred to the flow of CSF as the "third circulation."

The arachnoid villi (pacchionian granulations) are small, convoluted projections of the subarachnoid space and arachnoid that penetrate into the venous sinuses. The arachnoid villi are the site where the CSF is reabsorbed into the venous blood. The CSF in the arachnoid granulations is separated from the venous blood in the dural sinuses by only a layer of mesothelial arachnoid cells and a layer of vascular endothelium (Figure 2.3). Villi are most numerous in the superior sagittal sinus but are also found in the other sinuses and along the spinal cord. The arachnoid villi function as one-way valves, allowing the passage of CSF into the venous blood, but no reverse flow. Some of the CSF is absorbed into the venous system from the periradicular and perineural spaces along the spinal roots and CNs, and from the perivenous spaces. There is also some absorption through gap junctions in the ventricular ependyma. The gap junctions permit the exchange of fluid between the CSF and the ISF. This route of absorption becomes more prominent when CSF flow is obstructed and the intraventricular CSF is under increased pressure.

CEREBROSPINAL FLUID FUNCTIONS

The CSF has many functions. One of its most important is mechanical, serving as a water jacket for the brain and spinal cord, bathing and protecting them. It helps support the weight of the brain and has a cushioning effect against displacement. Suspended in CSF, the brain weighs only a fraction of what it otherwise would. The CSF serves as a lubricant between the brain and the spinal cord on one side and the skull and spinal column on the other. It acts to dissipate the force of a blow to the head. It serves as a space-compensating mechanism for regulating the contents of the cranium and aids in keeping the intracranial pressure (ICP) relatively constant: If there is an increase in arterial pressure, blood content, or brain volume, there is a decrease in the amount of CSF, and if there is a decrease in the amount of brain tissue due to atrophy or degeneration, there is an increase in the amount of CSF.

The CSF is important in homeostasis, helping to maintain a constant external milieu for the brain. It is in equilibrium with the extracellular fluid of the brain. The CSF serves as a medium for the transfer of substances from within the brain and spinal cord to the bloodstream; it receives metabolic waste products and aids in eliminating them; it is important for the removal of pathologic products in disease and for the circulation of drugs in therapy. The CSF acts as a "sink" for the extracellular fluid of the brain. Solutes and products of metabolism diffuse from the extracellular fluid and flow into the CSF sink and then are carried away to be removed by the bulk flow resorption of the CSF into the venous system.

BLOOD-BRAIN BARRIER

Early investigators noticed that when an animal's circulatory system was injected with various dyes, all the body organs became stained except the brain. They postulated a blood-brain barrier (BBB) to explain this finding. Later investigators amply demonstrated the accuracy of the observation. The site of the BBB is at the level of the pial-glial membranes and the cerebral capillaries. The capillaries in the brain are distinguished by having tight endothelial cell junctions, unlike those of capillaries elsewhere in the body. Tight junction proteins, occludin and claudin, glue the endothelial cells together. Such tight junctions are also a feature of the epithelial cells of the choroid plexus, creating a blood-CSF barrier. They restrict the passive movement of macromolecular substances across the cellular barrier. In addition to the tight junctions between endothelial cells, brain capillaries are also encased by foot processes of astrocytes and have a higher number of mitochondria than do capillaries elsewhere in the body.

Specialized transport systems that regulate selective transport of certain substances also form part of the BBB. Neurons, astrocytes, and pericytes make up the neurovascular unit. Pericytes are a combination of smooth muscle and macrophage enclosed by a basal lamina. Astrocyte foot processes surround the basal lamina of the capillary and connect to the neurons, the third component of the neurovascular unit.

The ability of solutes to cross the BBB depends on their size and solubility. Small molecules enter the central nervous system (CNS) more easily than do large molecules, and very large molecules are excluded. Substances that are highly lipid soluble, such as oxygen, carbon dioxide, and volatile anesthetics, enter more easily than do those with low lipid solubility. Alcohol and nicotine are highly lipid soluble and easily transported into the brain. Substances highly bound to serum proteins are unable to penetrate the BBB. Some substances (e.g., glucose and amino acids) cross the BBB by active transport. Water has an anomalous structure that allows it to pass rapidly through endothelial cells. Many antibiotics cannot gain access to the CNS unless the meninges and the BBB are damaged by inflammation. Parkinson's disease is treated with L-DOPA because the BBB excludes dopamine, the compound really needed. Some areas of the CNS lack a BBB, including the following: the chemoreceptor trigger zone in the area postrema in the floor of the fourth ventricle, subfornical organ in the anterior wall of the third ventricle, the median eminence of the hypothalamus, choroid plexus, organum vasculosum lamina terminalis, and the pineal and posterior pituitary glands. These areas are collectively known as the circumventricular organs; their capillaries have fenestrations instead of tight junctions. Many drugs produce nausea and vomiting as a prominent side effect because the lack of a BBB allows unfettered access directly from the bloodstream to the area postrema and chemoreceptor trigger zone. The permeability of the BBB may be altered by various disease states.

LUMBAR PUNCTURE

Although not done as often as in the past, LP remains an important part of the neurologic workup for many patients. The use of atraumatic, noncutting, pencil-point (Sprotte) needles significantly reduces the incidence of post-LP complications, particularly headache, in comparison to traditional, cutting-tip (Quincke) needles, and is increasingly becoming the standard.

There are two essential bits of information obtained from LP: the CSF pressure and the CSF composition. The opening pressure (OP) measurement is a vital part of the LP and should never be omitted. Traditionally, normal has been considered up to 180 mm of CSF, values of 180 to 200 considered borderline, and pressures above 200 abnormal unless the patient is obese, where there is evidence to suggest the normal OP may be as high as 250. Some authors contend pressures as high as 250 should be considered normal even in nonobese adults. Spuriously elevated pressure readings may be caused by poor relaxation. Transmitted venous pulsations cause small fluctuations in the manometric pressure; respiration causes larger fluctuations. The OP is the most reliable indicator of the ICP. In some circumstances, the only LP abnormality is an elevated OP, as in idiopathic intracranial hypertension (IIH, pseudotumor cerebri). In other conditions, an elevation of the OP may be an important clue to the presence of intracranial pathology. It may be difficult to measure the CSF pressure in children, and counting the number of drops of CSF over a specified time is a simple, rapid method for estimating CSF pressure.

Once the OP has been determined, fluid is withdrawn for analysis. The studies done on the CSF depend on the clinical circumstances. In the majority of cases, the minimum amount of information requested includes cell count, differential, protein, and glucose. Normal CSF may contain up to five lymphocytes, but no neutrophils. Normal CSF glucose is one-half to two-thirds of the blood glucose. Normal CSF protein varies with location; intraventricular CSF protein is much lower than the protein from the lumbar theca. The CSF protein from LP is generally less than 40. Hayward and Shapiro studied a series of 555 consecutive cases, finding that additional CSF tests were useful in only 0.9% of patients when OP, cell count, and protein were normal. It requires about 2 hours for the blood sugar to equilibrate with the CSF sugar. For accurate CSF glucose determinations, the blood sample should be drawn 2 hours prior to LP, or the LP done in a fasting state. In addition to basic tests such as Gram stain, cultures, and cytology, an ever increasing number of sophisticated tests are possible on spinal fluid, including polymerase chain reaction (PCR) testing for various organisms, immunologic studies, aquaporin antibodies, 14-3-3 protein for prion disease, beta amyloid, tau, heavy and light neurofilaments, serologic tests for carcinoembryonic antigen, alpha-fetoprotein, antinuclear antibodies, angiotensin-converting enzyme, antineuronal antibodies, anti-Purkinje cell antibodies, Lyme disease antibodies, tumor markers, and many others. Rarely, substances are injected into the CSF, such as an isotope for cisternography.

There are several commonly encountered patterns of CSF abnormality: normal, acute bacterial infection, the aseptic meningeal pattern, and the albuminocytologic dissociation pattern. With acute bacterial infection, there is a markedly increased cell count, with the cells consisting primarily of polymorphonuclear lymphocytes, an elevated protein, and a decreased sugar. Glucose levels may be very low, often less than 10 mg/dL and sometimes zero. The "aseptic" pattern consists of an elevated cell count with predominantly mononuclear cells, elevated protein, and a normal sugar. The term aseptic in this context merely means the pattern is not that of acute bacterial infection. Viral infections, tuberculosis, fungal infection, partially treated bacterial meningitis, parameningeal infection, neoplastic meningitis, and parasitic infection may all produce an aseptic pattern. Occasionally, an aseptic pattern with slightly to moderately decreased glucose levels occurs with some viral infections, tuberculosis, and fungal or neoplastic meningitis. The pattern of albuminocytologic dissociation is seen most often in Guillain-Barré syndrome and consists of an elevated protein, sometimes extremely elevated, in the absence of an increased cell count or other abnormalities.

Special investigations may detect abnormalities in CSF that is normal on routine studies, particularly in patients with evidence of demyelinating disease, primarily multiple sclerosis (MS). When dysimmune processes involve the nervous system, the CSF may contain an abnormal level of immunoglobulins. Synthesis of immunoglobulin within the nervous system causes an elevation of immunoglobulin G (IgG) in the spinal fluid. For accuracy, the IgG level must be compared with the albumin level, because the presence of protein from some other process could cause the IgG level to be elevated on an absolute basis, but not in proportion to the albumin. It is always necessary to have the results of serum protein electrophoresis in order to properly interpret CSF immunoglobulin studies. The key abnormality is an increase in the IgG/albumin ratio or an abnormal IgG index ([CSF IgG/serum IgG]/[CSF albumin/serum albumin]). Increased CSF IgG with a normal index indicates leakage across the BBB; an elevated IgG index indicates the CNS is the source. It is also possible to calculate the IgG synthesis rate in the nervous system, which is frequently abnormal in MS. The immunoglobulins present are sometimes derived from limited clones of immunocompetent cells that manufacture the same protein and produce narrow, "oligoclonal" bands of immunoglobulin on electrophoresis. When necrosis and inflammation are active in the nervous system, it is often possible to detect an elevation of myelin basic protein. The battery of tests often used to look for evidence of demyelinating disease consists of IgG/albumin ratio, IgG index, IgG synthesis rate, oligoclonal bands, and myelin basic protein. Abnormal immunoglobulin studies in the spinal fluid can occur in conditions other than MS, such as neurosyphilis and other chronic infectious and inflammatory conditions. Systemic elevation of immunoglobulins, as with multiple myeloma, can also alter the IgG/albumin ratio.

INCREASED INTRACRANIAL PRESSURE

The intracranial cavity is a closed space. Three compartments occupy this space: blood, brain, and CSF. Normally, the volumes of the three compartments are in equilibrium. Brain volume is normally approximately 1,400 mL, intracranial CSF volume approximately 75 mL, and intracranial vascular volume about 75 mL. Because the cranium cannot expand, and the brain cannot be significantly compressed, when the volume of one of the compartments increases, the volume in the other compartments must undergo a compensatory decrease (Monro-Kellie hypothesis). Compensation is more effective for slowly evolving processes than for acute illnesses. If compensation fails, ICP increases. When ICP increases, plateau waves often occur. These are periodic further acute increases in ICP in the range of 600 to 1,300 mm H_2O that last 5 to 20 minutes and may occur several times per hour. Plateau waves may occur with suctioning and other manipulations. When ICP increases, there are two major deleterious consequences. The first is herniation of brain structures out of their normal location, causing crowding and compression in other locations. Plateau waves are associated with an increase in the risk of herniation. Some of the important herniation syndromes include central transtentorial, lateral transtentorial (uncal), and foramen magnum (see Chapter 51). The second is a decrease in cerebral perfusion pressure (CPP). Normally, arterial pressure is higher than ICP, allowing the brain to be perfused. The CPP is the difference between mean arterial blood pressure and ICP; normal ICP is 5 to 15 mm Hg. Because of autoregulatory mechanisms, cerebral blood flow can usually be maintained until the CPP decreases below 40 to 60 mm Hg; below this level, cerebral perfusion suffers and the brain is at risk of secondary ischemic damage (brain tamponade). The Cushing response is a reflex increase in arterial blood pressure to maintain CPP. Common causes of increased ICP include hydrocephalus, an increase in the volume of CSF, cerebral edema, an increase in the volume of brain, and intracranial space occupying mass lesions.

Hydrocephalus

Hydrocephalus is dilatation of the ventricular system. It may occur because of obstruction of CSF flow, impaired resorption, or as a compensatory mechanism for loss of brain volume (hydrocephalus ex vacuo). Obstructive, or noncommunicating, hydrocephalus is due to blockage of the CSF circulation within the ventricular system. Tumors may form in the region of the foramen of Monro, most commonly a colloid cyst of the third ventricle, and obstruct CSF flow, causing hydrocephalus and positional headache. Stenosis of the cerebral aqueduct may cause dilatation of the third and lateral ventricles with a normal-sized fourth ventricle. Obstructive hydrocephalus may develop when the outlet foramina of the fourth ventricle are occluded. When the outlet foramina fail to develop normally, the fourth ventricle becomes massively dilated, creating a cystic structure in the posterior fossa (Dandy-Walker syndrome). Very rarely, hydrocephalus is caused by overproduction of CSF, such as by a papilloma of the choroid plexus.

Communicating hydrocephalus is due to impaired circulation of the CSF after it leaves the ventricular system, such as from fibrosis and scarring of the basal cisterns because of meningitis, or impaired function of the arachnoid granulations from scarring due to previous subarachnoid hemorrhage. The impaired CSF circulation or decreased absorption transmits increased back pressure into the system, causing compensatory ventricular dilatation. Idiopathic normal pressure hydrocephalus (NPH) is a form of communicating hydrocephalus with ventricular enlargement but normal OP on LP that occurs spontaneously, without any identifiable antecedent event that may have caused meningeal scarring. It accounts for about one-third of the cases of adult-onset communicating hydrocephalus. NPH classically causes a triad of dementia, gait disturbance, and urinary incontinence (see **Video Link 50.1**). The original hope was that NPH was a cause of dementia treatable by ventriculoperitoneal shunt. However, considerable controversy still surrounds the diagnosis of NPH and the selection of patients for shunt. In a study of 10 patients with an antemortem diagnosis of idiopathic NPH (8 were shunted and 7 benefited), 1 had Alzheimer's disease, 1 had corticobasal degeneration, and in the remainder, various vascular lesions were seen at the final neuropathologic investigation.

Cerebral Edema

Cerebral edema is swelling of the brain, with an increase in brain volume due to an increased water content. Cerebral edema occurs under a variety of circumstances. Four types are recognized: vasogenic, cytotoxic, osmotic, and interstitial. In vasogenic edema, there is a disruption of the tight junctions that make up the BBB, causing an increase in extracellular fluid volume due to an increase in capillary permeability. The fluid contains protein and collects primarily in the white matter, often sending finger-like extensions along white matter tracts. This is the normal trajectory of ISF flow toward the ventricles for absorption. Vasogenic edema occurs primarily with a focal mass lesion in the brain, such as neoplasm or abscess. In cytotoxic edema, there is an increase in the intracellular fluid volume due to a failure of the energy-dependent mechanisms that normally keep water from entering the cell. The BBB remains intact. Neurons, glia, and capillary endothelial cells in both gray and white matter imbibe water and swell. This swelling compresses the extracellular space. It is the restricted diffusion of intracellular water that creates abnormalities on diffusion-weighted magnetic resonance imaging. Cytotoxic (cellular) edema occurs when the brain suffers damage due to hypoxia, ischemia, or other metabolic abnormalities such as uremia or diabetic ketoacidosis. Cytotoxic edema may be focal or diffuse. Osmotic edema occurs when there is hemodilution, as in inappropriate antidiuretic hormone secretion or rapid reduction of blood glucose in the hyperosmolar, hyperglycemic state. Brain osmolality then exceeds serum osmolality, and water flows into the brain along the abnormal pressure gradient, causing edema. Interstitial edema is an increase in extracellular fluid volume that occurs in the periventricular white matter because of transependymal transudation of CSF through the ventricular wall when the intraventricular pressure is increased. Both vasogenic and interstitial edema primarily affect the white matter. The fluid content in interstitial edema varies from that seen in vasogenic edema, containing very little protein.

An injury cascade affecting cells and blood vessels may follow a variety of insults, such as trauma, ischemia, hypoxia, or a mass lesion. With cytotoxic edema, there is release of the excitotoxin glutamate into the extracellular space. Glutamate opens Ca^{++} channels on cell membranes and Ca^{++} enters the cell. Extrusion of one Ca^{++} requires entry of three Na^{+} molecules, so Na^{+} accumulates intracellularly, creating an osmotic gradient that draws water into the cell, causing swelling. Excess intracellular Ca^{++} also activates cytotoxic processes that lead to cell death. Free radicals also contribute to the damage, especially after hypoxia, ischemia, and trauma.

Cytotoxic edema after stroke occurs 24 to 72 hours after the event. Reperfusion injury causes particularly aggressive cerebral edema and a risk of hemorrhagic conversion. Brain trauma causes a mixture of cytotoxic and vasogenic edema. Vasogenic edema after capillary damage leads to disruption of the BBB. The BBB may be breached when endothelial cell tight junctions fail, allowing proteases and free radicals to attack the capillaries. Inflammation may damage the BBB through production of cytokines and chemokines. Cerebrovascular disease is the major cause of cerebral edema in the adult. Other causes of cerebral edema include trauma, toxins, acute hepatic failure, hypertensive encephalopathy, rapid changes in serum osmolality, high-altitude cerebral edema, and mass lesions.

Clinical Manifestations of Increased Intracranial Pressure

The clinical manifestations of increased ICP vary with the nature of the underlying process, and whether it is acute or chronic. Headache is a common symptom. Headache due to increased ICP is thought to be due to traction on pain-sensitive structures and tends to be exacerbated by coughing, straining, or changes in position. Headache due to increased ICP is often worse at night. Pressure on the autonomic centers in the brainstem causes a variety of manifestations, including nausea, vomiting, increased blood pressure, changes in respiration, and bradycardia. Altered consciousness is common. Papilledema is often present. If the increase in ICP occurs before the cranial sutures have fused, there may be separation of suture lines, bulging of the anterior fontanelle, or head enlargement. Abducens nerve palsy is a common nonspecific manifestation of increased ICP. The Cushing reflex or Cushing's triad consists of hypertension, bradycardia, and slowing of respiration due to brainstem compromise.

Percussion of the skull may disclose dullness on the side of a tumor or subdural hematoma or a tympanitic percussion note in hydrocephalus and increased ICP. In infants and children with hydrocephalus, skull percussion may produce a more resonant sound than is normal (Macewen's sign, or "cracked pot" resonance).

IIH (benign intracranial hypertension, pseudotumor cerebri) is a common, fairly stereotyped syndrome of headache and papilledema without focal neurologic signs, with normal CSF and no evidence of a mass lesion or enlarged ventricles on imaging studies. The condition is most often idiopathic and without known causes. It may occur after occlusion of the superior sagittal or lateral sinus. A number of drugs may cause the syndrome, including vitamin A, tetracycline, corticosteroids (or the withdrawal from corticosteroids), and quinolone antibiotics. IIH is particularly common in overweight young women, classically with menstrual irregularities. Headache and papilledema are the cardinal manifestations, but patients may also have transient visual obscurations, pulsatile tinnitus, and diplopia due to CN VI palsy (false localizing sign). The papilledema may be severe and can lead to visual loss. Imaging studies are normal or show slit-like ventricles; an empty sella may occur. The pathogenesis remains uncertain. The incidence of IIH increased significantly in Olmsted County, Minnesota between 1990 and 2014, which paralleled the increase in obesity during the same period.

Intracranial hypotension may occur when there is a leakage of CSF, most commonly through the track left by an LP needle. There is also a "spontaneous" form, in which rents in the dura occur for various reasons. Such low CSF pressure syndromes are characterized by a headache that is strikingly postural, much worse when the patient is erect and relieved by recumbency. When severe, there may be signs of meningeal irritation.

Video Links

Video Link 50.1. Gait in NPH. http://neurosigns.org/wiki/Gait_of_normal_pressure_hydrocephalus

BIBLIOGRAPHY

Benarroch EE, Daube JR, Cutsforth-Gregory JK, et al. *Mayo Clinic Medical Neurosciences: Organized by Neurologic Systems and Levels*. 6th ed. Rochester; New York: Mayo Clinic Scientific Press; Oxford University Press, 2018.

Carmelo A, Ficola A, Fravolini ML, et al. ICP and CBF regulation: a new hypothesis to explain the "windkessel" phenomenon. *Acta Neurochir Suppl* 2002;81:112–116.

Carson D, Serpell M. Choosing the best needle for diagnostic lumbar puncture. *Neurology* 1996;47:33–37.

Chohan G, Pennington C, MacKenzie JM, et al. The role of cerebrospinal fluid 14-3-3 and other proteins in the diagnosis of sporadic Creutzfeldt-Jakob disease in the UK: a 10-year review. *J Neurol Neurosurg Psychiatry* 2010;81:1243–1248.

Corbett JJ, Mehta MP. Cerebrospinal fluid pressure in normal obese subjects and patients with pseudotumor cerebri. *Neurology* 1983;33:1386–1388.

DeBiasi RL, Kleinschmidt-DeMasters BK, Weinberg A, et al. Use of PCR for the diagnosis of herpes virus infections of the central nervous system. *J Clin Virol* 2002;25(Suppl 1):S5–S11.

Dodick D. Headache as a symptom of ominous disease. What are the warning signals? *Postgrad Med* 1997;101:46–64.

Eide PK, Brean A. Lumbar cerebrospinal fluid pressure waves versus intracranial pressure waves in idiopathic normal pressure hydrocephalus. *Br J Neurosurg* 2006;20:407–414.

Ellis RW III, Strauss LC, Wiley JM, et al. A simple method of estimating cerebrospinal fluid pressure during lumbar puncture. *Pediatrics* 1992;89:895–897.

Fraser C, Plant GT. The syndrome of pseudotumour cerebri and idiopathic intracranial hypertension. *Curr Opin Neurol* 2011;24:12–17.

Gilman S. *Clinical Examination of the Nervous System*. New York: McGraw-Hill, 2000.

Gilman S, Newman SW. *Manter and Gatz's Essentials of Clinical Neuroanatomy and Neurophysiology*. 10th ed. Philadelphia: FA Davis, 2003.

Grady PA, Blaumanis OR. Physiologic parameters of the Cushing reflex. *Surg Neurol* 1988;29:454–461.

Hoffmann J. Impaired cerebrospinal fluid pressure. *Handb Clin Neurol* 2017;146:171–185.

Jerrard DA, Hanna JR, Schindelheim GL. Cerebrospinal fluid. *J Emerg Med* 2001;21:171–178.

Kester MI, Scheffer PG, Koel-Simmelink MJ, et al. Serial CSF sampling in Alzheimer's disease: specific versus non-specific markers. *Neurobiol Aging* 2012;33:1591–1598.

Kilgore KP, Lee MS, Leavitt JA, et al. Re-evaluating the incidence of idiopathic intracranial hypertension in an era of increasing obesity. *Ophthalmology* 2017;124:697–700.

Klinge P, Marmarou A, Bergsneider M, et al. Outcome of shunting in idiopathic normal-pressure hydrocephalus and the value of outcome assessment in shunted patients. *Neurosurgery* 2005;57(3 Suppl):S40–S52.

Leinonen V, Koivisto AM, Savolainen S, et al. Post-mortem findings in 10 patients with presumed normal-pressure hydrocephalus and review of the literature. *Neuropathol Appl Neurobiol* 2012;38:72–86.

Lee SC, Lueck CJ. Cerebrospinal fluid pressure in adults. *J Neuroophthalmol* 2014;34:278–283.

Lin JJ, Harn HJ, Hsu YD, et al. Rapid diagnosis of tuberculous meningitis by polymerase chain reaction assay of cerebrospinal fluid. *J Neurol* 1995;242:147–152.

Marinac JS. Drug- and chemical-induced aseptic meningitis: a review of the literature. *Ann Pharmacother* 1992;26:813–822.

Mollan SP, Ali F, Hassan-Smith G, et al. Evolving evidence in adult idiopathic intracranial hypertension: pathophysiology and management. *J Neurol Neurosurg Psychiatry* 2016;87:982–992.

Mokri B. The Monro-Kellie hypothesis: applications in CSF volume depletion. *Neurology* 2001;56:1746–1748.

Muller B, Adelt K, Reichmann H, et al. Atraumatic needle reduces the incidence of post-lumbar puncture syndrome. *J Neurol* 1994;241:376–380.

Negrini B, Kelleher KJ, Wald ER. Cerebrospinal fluid findings in aseptic versus bacterial meningitis. *Pediatrics* 2000;105:316–319.

Olsson T. Multiple sclerosis: cerebrospinal fluid. *Ann Neurol* 1994;36(Suppl):S100–S102.

Perkins AT, Ondo W. When to worry about headache. Head pain as a clue to intracranial disease. *Postgrad Med* 1995;98:197–198.

Relkin N, Marmarou A, Klinge P, et al. Diagnosing idiopathic normal-pressure hydrocephalus. *Neurosurgery* 2005;57(3 Suppl):S4–S16.

Seehusen DA, Reeves MM, Fomin DA. Cerebrospinal fluid analysis. *Am Fam Physician* 2003;68:1103–1108.

Sindic CJ, Van Antwerpen MP, Goffette S. Clinical relevance of polymerase chain reaction (PCR) assays and antigen-driven immunoblots for the diagnosis of neurological infectious diseases. *Brain Res Bull* 2003;61:299–308.

Strupp M, Schueler O, Straube A, et al. "Atraumatic" Sprotte needle reduces the incidence of post-lumbar puncture headaches. *Neurology* 2001;57:2310–2312.

Ropper AH, Samuels MA, Klein J. *Adams and Victor's principles of neurology*. 10th ed. New York: McGraw-Hill Education Medical, 2014.

Virhammar J, Cesarini KG, Laurell K. The CSF tap test in normal pressure hydrocephalus: evaluation time, reliability and the influence of pain. *Eur J Neurol* 2012;19:271–276.

Walker RW. Idiopathic intracranial hypertension: any light on the mechanism of the raised pressure? *J Neurol Neurosurg Psychiatry* 2001;71:1–5.

Wall M. Update on Idiopathic Intracranial Hypertension. *Neurol Clin* 2017;35:45–57.

Weibers DO, Dale AJD, Kokmen E, et al., eds. *Mayo Clinic Examinations in Neurology*. 7th ed. St. Louis: Mosby, 1998.

Zidan AH, Girvin JP. Effect on the Cushing response of different rates of expansion of a supratentorial mass. *J Neurosurg* 1978;49:61–70.

CHAPTER 51

The Examination in Coma

Workup of the patient with coma or altered mental status (AMS) is often complex and always urgent. The neurologic examination is only one of several diagnostic methods that can be brought to bear in coma, and imaging, cerebrospinal fluid (CSF), and laboratory investigations play a vital role. However, the findings on examination often determine the early management and the urgency with which imaging and CSF studies are obtained. Coma is a complicated topic, and this discussion focuses on what can be learned from the examination.

Consciousness has two dimensions: arousal and cognition. Arousal is a primitive function sustained by deep brainstem and medial thalamic structures. Cognitive functions require an intact cerebral cortex and major subcortical nuclei. In coma, stupor, and hypersomnia, there is a lowering of consciousness; in confusion and delirium, there is a clouding of consciousness.

THE ANATOMY OF CONSCIOUSNESS

The ascending reticular activating system (RAS) is a system of fibers that arises from the reticular formation of the brainstem, primarily the paramedian tegmentum of the upper pons and midbrain, and projects to the paramedian, parafascicular, centromedian, and intralaminar nuclei of the thalamus. Neurons in the reticular formation also receive collaterals from the ascending spinothalamic pathways and send projections diffusely to the entire cerebral cortex so that sensory stimuli are involved not only with sensory perception but also—through their connections with the RAS—with the maintenance of consciousness. The fibers in the RAS are cholinergic, adrenergic, dopaminergic, serotonergic, and histaminergic. Experimentally, stimulation of the RAS produces arousal, and destruction of the RAS produces coma. The hypothalamus is also important for consciousness; arousal can be produced by stimulation of the posterior hypothalamic region. The RAS runs through the core of the brainstem. The nuclei and pathways controlling eye movements occupy the same regions, and eye movement assessment is an integral part of the evaluation of patients with altered consciousness.

Processes producing coma can be characterized as either structural or metabolic. Although restricted, focal lesions of the RAS can produce profound alterations in consciousness; hemispheric lesions cause coma only when extensive and bilateral, such as with traumatic brain injury (TBI), meningitis, encephalitis, or bilateral cerebral infarction. The degree of alteration in consciousness is roughly proportional to the volume of brain tissue involved in the process. There has been some conjecture that focal lesions of the left hemisphere are more likely to produce alterations of consciousness than lesions of the right hemisphere, and the left hemisphere has been said by some to be "dominant" for consciousness. Still, focal lesions restricted to either hemisphere rarely produce significant alterations of consciousness. Metabolic processes produce coma by diffusely affecting the cerebral hemispheres or depressing the activity in the RAS, or both.

INITIAL MANAGEMENT OF COMA

Because of the dire consequences to the brain of lack of substrate, the initial management of coma, unless the cause is immediately apparent, is directed toward correction of possible deficiencies in glucose, oxygenation, and blood pressure; these emergency measures are necessary, even before a detailed history and examination. After initial determination of vital signs, attention should first be directed toward ensuring an adequate airway and oxygenation, blood pressure, and intravenous access. After obtaining emergency blood samples, 50 cc of 50% glucose should be given, followed quickly by 100 mg of thiamine IV in case the patient is alcoholic (Wernicke's encephalopathy can be precipitated by IV glucose). Naloxone and flumazenil are often given empirically in case there has been an opiate or benzodiazepine overdose. A "coma cocktail," consisting of dextrose, flumazenil, naloxone, and thiamine, is sometimes used in the initial management of the comatose patient. Because the rapid reagent test strips used for glucose determination are not infallible, and because the correlation between the level of consciousness and the glucose level in hypoglycemia is poor, studies favor empirical administration of dextrose and thiamine to patients with altered consciousness. But naloxone should probably be reserved for patients with signs and symptoms of opioid intoxication and flumazenil best left for reversal of therapeutic conscious sedation and rare select cases of benzodiazepine overdose. Preparations for intubation, respiratory support, and use of pressor agents must be made, should they become necessary. Always assume a cervical spine injury may be present and immobilize the neck until a fracture can be ruled out.

DIAGNOSTIC ASSESSMENT

After ensuring adequate oxygenation and substrate for the central nervous system (CNS), a rapid neurologic examination should be performed to search for obvious signs, such as a dilated pupil, that may require urgent imaging and neurosurgical intervention. Otherwise, the initial emergent management should be followed by a history and general physical and neurologic examinations.

History

Though often difficult and sometimes impossible to obtain, historical information is extremely important and well worth pursuing vigorously. In the absence of family, a phone call to the neighbor, landlord, or companion may yield valuable details about the sequence of events leading to coma, the patient's past health and illnesses, and current medications. A history of known seizure disorder, diabetes mellitus, hypertension, substance abuse, depression, or suicide attempts may emerge. Check the wallet or purse for medication lists, a doctor's card or phone number, medical alert card, or other pertinent information. Talk with police or ambulance drivers if they are involved.

If possible, it would be useful to determine the time course of the loss of consciousness. Abrupt coma might occur from subarachnoid hemorrhage or seizure, a more gradual or fluctuating onset might suggest a mass lesion, especially subdural hematoma, or metabolic encephalopathy. Focal signs preceding the loss of consciousness suggest a structural lesion rather than a metabolic process. Premonitory transient symptoms might suggest vertebrobasilar ischemia. Recent fever suggests an infectious process; recent falls, an intracranial hematoma; and recent confusion, a metabolic or toxic etiology.

General Physical Examination

Findings on the general physical examination may be extremely helpful in elucidating the cause of altered consciousness (Table 51.1). The patient should always be examined carefully for bruises and hematomas, lacerations, fractures, and other signs of injury, especially about the head. It is essential to remember that two conditions may occur together (e.g., trauma and alcoholic intoxication). Simple vital signs may provide important clues. An elevated temperature suggests infection or serious intracranial disease. Fever with dry skin suggests anticholinergic intoxication or heat stroke. Hypothermia suggests sepsis, hypoglycemia, intoxication, or myxedema. Extremely elevated blood pressure suggests hypertensive encephalopathy, subarachnoid hemorrhage, intracranial hematomas, or a reversible posterior leukoencephalopathy syndrome. Hypotension suggests impaired CNS

TABLE 51.1 Findings on General Physical Examination That May Provide a Clue to the Etiology of Coma or Altered Mental Status

System	Finding	Possible Implications
Blood pressure	Hypotension	Hypovolemia, MI, intoxication (especially ETOH and barbiturates), Wernicke's encephalopathy, sepsis
	Hypertension	Stroke, intracranial hemorrhage, increased ICP, hypertensive encephalopathy, renal disease
Heart rate	Bradycardia	Heart disease, intoxication, increased ICP
	Tachycardia	Hypovolemia, cocaine overdose, infection
Respiration	Breath odor	Acetone (DKA), ETOH (intoxication), fetor hepaticus, uriniferous (uremia), garlic odor (arsenic poisoning), household gas (carbon monoxide)
	Hyperventilation	Hypoxia, hypercapnia, acidosis, fever, liver disease, sepsis, pulmonary emboli, toxins of drugs producing metabolic acidosis, central neurogenic hyperventilation, salicylism
	Hypoventilation	Overdose, myxedema
	Cheyne-Stokes	Bilateral cerebral disease, impending transtentorial herniation, upper brainstem lesions, metabolic encephalopathy, CHF
	Cluster breathing	Increased ICP, posterior fossa lesion
	Apneustic breathing	Pontine lesion, transtentorial herniation, metabolic coma
	Ataxic breathing	Medullary lesion
	Ondine's curse	Medullary lesion
Temperature	Fever	Infection, inflammation, neoplasms (rare), anticholinergics, SAH, hypothalamic lesion, heatstroke, thyroid storm malignant hyperthermia
	Hypothermia	Exposure, sepsis, shock, myxedema coma, Wernicke's encephalopathy, drug intoxication (especially barbiturates), hypothalamic lesion, hypoglycemia
Head and neck	Scalp laceration or edema, Battle's sign, raccoon eyes	Trauma
	Stiff neck	Meningitis, SAH, cerebellar tonsillar herniation
	Unilateral, fixed dilated pupil	Uncal herniation, aneurysm
	Small, reactive pupils	Metabolic coma, early transtentorial herniation
	Bilateral, large, fixed pupils	Midbrain or pretectal lesion (tectal pupils)
	Midposition, fixed pupils	Midbrain stage of transtentorial herniation
	Pinpoint pupils	Pontine hemorrhage or infarct, opiate overdose
	Fundus exam	Papilledema (increased ICP), hypertensive or diabetic retinopathy, subhyaloid hemorrhages, Roth spots
Skin	Needle tracks	Drug overdose
	Cyanosis	Hypoxia, cardiac disease, cyanide
	Cherry red	Carbon monoxide intoxication
	Jaundice	Hepatic encephalopathy, hemolysis
	Pallor	Anemia, hemorrhage, shock, vasomotor syncope
	Petechiae	DIC, TTP, meningococcemia, drugs, fat embolism
	Purpuric rash	Meningococcemia, RMSF, and others
	Maculopapular rash	Toxic shock syndrome, SBE, SLE, and others
	Bruises	Trauma, coagulopathy
	Bullous lesions	Drug overdose, especially barbiturates
	Sweating	Fever, hypoglycemia
	Flushing, erythema	Polycythemia, fever, alcohol intoxication
Heart	Arrhythmia	Cerebral embolism
	Murmur	SBE, embolism
Lungs	Pulmonary edema	Neurogenic pulmonary edema, CHF, anoxic encephalopathy
GI	Fecal incontinence + stool blood	Seizure with postictal coma
		Hepatic encephalopathy, GI hemorrhage
GU	Urinary incontinence	Seizure with postictal coma
	Hematuria	Cerebral embolism
Extremities	Subtle twitching	Subclinical status epilepticus

CHF, congestive heart failure; DIC, disseminated intravascular coagulation; DKA, diabetic ketoacidosis; ETOH, ethanol; GI, gastrointestinal; GU, genitourinary; ICP, intracranial pressure; MI, myocardial infarction; RMSF, Rocky Mountain spotted fever; SAH, subarachnoid hemorrhage; SBE, subacute bacterial endocarditis; SLE, systemic lupus erythematosus; TTP, thrombotic thrombocytopenic purpura.

perfusion because of some systemic process, such as hemorrhage or myocardial disease. Hypotension rarely occurs because of primary CNS disease, except in the terminal phase. Either tachycardia or bradycardia may impair CNS perfusion. The combination of hypertension and bradycardia suggests brainstem dysfunction, often because of increased intracranial pressure (the Cushing reflex).

Abnormalities of respiration are important in the evaluation of patients with depressed consciousness. Abnormal respiratory patterns because of neurologic disease include Cheyne-Stokes respirations (CSR), central neurogenic hyperventilation, ataxic breathing, and apneustic breathing. In CSR, periods of hyperpnea alternate with periods of hypopnea. Respirations increase in depth and volume up to a peak and then decline until there is a period of apnea, after which the cycle repeats. In posthyperventilation apnea, a brief period of hyperventilation is followed by apnea lasting 15 to 30 seconds or longer. Demonstration of posthyperventilation apnea requires the active cooperation of the patient. The mechanisms underlying CSR and posthyperventilation apnea are likely similar. CSR may be due to bilateral hemisphere lesions or bilateral thalamic lesions, as well as to increased intracranial pressure and cardiopulmonary dysfunction. CSR commonly induce a rhythmic pupillary dilatation during hyperpnea and constriction during apnea. The patient's eyelids may open, and she may become more rousable during hyperpnea. In respiratory ataxia, the pattern of breathing is irregular, with erratic shallow and deep respiratory movements. Ataxic breathing occurs with dysfunction of the medullary respiratory centers and may signify impending agonal respirations and apnea. Central neurogenic hyperventilation refers to sustained, rapid, and regular hyperpnea. It is primarily associated with disease affecting the paramedian reticular formation in the low midbrain and upper pons, but it may also occur with lesions in other brainstem locations, either intra-axial or extra-axial. Apneustic breathing, which is rare, causes a prolonged inspiratory phase, and occurs in pontine lesions just rostral to the trigeminal motor nuclei, or cervicomedullary compression. Abnormal respiratory patterns may occur because of systemic disease, such as diabetic ketoacidosis (Table 51.1). Slow, regular respirations are noted with a variety of substance or drug intoxications and in severe myxedema.

Note the patient's appearance and behavior, apparent age, grooming, and signs of acute or chronic illnesses such as fever, cyanosis, jaundice, pallor, and signs of dehydration and loss of weight. Assess responses to noises, verbal commands, visual stimuli, threats, and tactile and painful stimulation, and whether there has been incontinence. Note whether the patient, even in coma, appears to be comfortable and natural or assumes unnatural positions. Carefully observe spontaneous movements, and the reaction to various stimuli. Note general activity (immobile, underactive, restless, or hyperkinetic), tone (limp, relaxed, rigid, or tense), and the presence of abnormal movements (tremors, twitches, tics, grimaces, and spasms). Carphology (floccillation) is an involuntary tugging at the sheets and picking of imaginary objects from the bedclothes, and jactitation is a tossing to and fro on the bed; these may be seen in acute disease, high fevers, and exhaustion. Motor unrest and excessive activity are seen in both organic and psychogenic states. If there is seizure activity, note the distribution and pattern of spread of the convulsive movements and any associated manifestations such as the degree of impairment of consciousness, frothing at the mouth, tongue biting, and incontinence.

The behavior of the patient should be observed closely and as often as necessary until the diagnosis is established. Note the patient's reactions to physicians, nurses, and relatives. Do the eyes follow people? Is there some awareness of what is happening in the immediate environment? The conduct may be constant or may vary from time to time. For instance, the patient may appear to be completely unconscious and fail to respond to any type of stimulation while the observer is in the room, yet when not aware of being watched, may open the eyes, make furtive glances, and move around.

After the general physical exam, a focused neurologic exam may help characterize the pathologic process. Specific attention should be paid to the level of responsiveness, pupils, eye movements, and motor responses.

Neurologic Examination

The details of the neurologic examination in the various states of disordered consciousness necessarily vary with the degree of impairment and depth of coma. As a minimum, the following must be assessed: level of consciousness, pupils, eye movements (including reflex movements), fundoscopic, motor status, reflexes, and meningeal signs. Other portions of the examination then follow as necessary. Coma is most often due to a metabolic process. With rare exception, metabolic encephalopathies are characterized by reactive pupils and a symmetric neurologic examination. Any asymmetry in motor or sensory responses and any pupillary or eye movement abnormality should prompt an immediate, vigorous search for structural disease.

Level of Responsiveness

Coma is a state of complete loss of consciousness from which the patient cannot be aroused by ordinary stimuli. There is complete unresponsiveness to self and the environment. The patient in coma has no awareness of herself, makes no voluntary movements, and has no sleep-wake cycles. Stupor is a state of partial or relative loss of response to the environment in which the patient's consciousness may be impaired to varying degrees. The patient is difficult to arouse, and although brief stimulation may be possible, responses are slow and inadequate. The patient is otherwise oblivious to what is happening in the environment and promptly falls back into the stuporous state. The lethargic patient can usually be aroused or awakened and may then appear to be in complete possession of her senses, but promptly falls asleep when left alone. In confusional states, patients may appear alert but are confused and disoriented.

Terminologic description of the differences between various states of impaired altered consciousness is at best ambiguous. Because of imprecision and inconsistency in usage, such terms as semicoma and semistupor, all describing changes across a spectrum of altered awareness are best avoided. It is preferable to describe the patient's state of responsiveness or use an objective and well-defined scheme, such as the Glasgow Coma Scale (GCS), which has gained wide acceptance in the evaluation of patients with impaired consciousness, particularly in head injury. In the GCS, scores are obtained for ocular, verbal, and motor functions (Table 51.2). An alert person with normal eye and motor responses would score 15 points; a patient in profound coma would score three points. The FOUR (Full Outline of UnResponsiveness) score has four components (eye, motor, brainstem, and respiration); each component has a maximal score of four. It may address some shortcomings of the GCS, especially in ventilated patients. It can detect locked-in syndrome and is superior to the GCS because of the evaluation of brainstem reflexes, breathing patterns, and the ability to recognize different stages of herniation.

TABLE 51.2 The Glasgow Coma Scale

Eye opening	
Open spontaneously	4
Open only to verbal stimuli	3
Open only to pain	2
Never open	1
Best verbal response	
Oriented and converses	5
Converses, but disoriented, confused	4
Uses inappropriate words	3
Makes incomprehensible sounds	2
No verbal response	1
Best motor response	
Obeys commands	6
Localizes pain	5
Exhibits flexion withdrawal	4
Decorticate rigidity	3
Decerebrate rigidity	2
No motor response	1

Other coma scales are available, including the following: the Innsbruck, Glasgow-Liege, reaction level, coma recovery, ACDU (Alert, Confused, Drowsy, Unresponsive), and AVPU (Alert, responds to Voice, responds to Pain, Unresponsive). Although useful for grading the severity of coma, none of these scales are useful in differential diagnosis. Coma must be distinguished from the persistent vegetative state (PVS), locked-in syndrome, and mutism (see below).

The term AMS is often used to describe a variety of abnormalities of cerebral function. It is used haphazardly to describe patients who have impaired alertness, impaired cognition, or a deficit of higher cortical function. Strictly speaking, the term AMS should imply a change in the level of consciousness, somewhere on a continuum between confusion and coma. It should not be used to describe patients who have impaired cognition with a clear sensorium—those patients have dementia; patients who have focal deficits of higher cortical function, such as aphasia; or used to describe patients who have psychiatric disorders, such as psychosis or mania. Neurologically naive clinicians may lump all these conditions together under the rubric AMS. They are in fact distinctly different conditions, with different etiologies and treatments, and especially with different prognostic implications. Patients with Wernicke's aphasia are often thought to have AMS or an acute confusional state.

It is necessary to make reasonable attempts to arouse the patient, and this usually includes assessing the response to a painful stimulus. Commonly used painful stimuli are supraorbital pressure, trapezius squeeze, sternal rub, and nail bed pressure. The stimulus must be adequate but remain humane and considerate. Avoid leaving bruises or other marks on the patient; the reason for these may be misinterpreted by family members and ancillary personnel. An effective and stealthy painful stimulus is to forcibly twist a key or the handle of a reflex hammer between two fingers or toes squeezed tightly together.

Cranial Nerves

Although cranial nerve (CN) examination cannot be carried out in any detail in a patient with altered consciousness, examination of the pupils and extraocular movements is critical in evaluation of the comatose patient. The pupils are critical in the evaluation of altered consciousness. The size, shape, position, equality, and reactivity are all important. Bilateral pinpoint pupils occur with opiate toxicity and with lesions of the pons, such as pontine hemorrhage or thrombosis of the basilar artery. The bilateral miosis seen in large pontine lesions is probably due to dysfunction of the descending sympathetic pathways bilaterally. The light reaction is preserved with lesions involving the descending sympathetic system but may be very difficult to see without magnification when the pupils are extremely small. Focusing on a tiny pupil with the ophthalmoscope and turning the light off and then back on may reveal the residual light reactivity. Hypothermia can cause small, unreactive pupils. Bilateral large pupils in coma are usually an ominous sign, especially when unreactive to light. They occur as a terminal condition in many patients. Bilateral mydriasis may also occur in botulism or anticholinergic intoxication. Atropinic agents given during cardiopulmonary resuscitation may enlarge and fixate the pupils. Pilocarpine solution helps distinguish such pharmacologic blockade from mydriasis due to structural disease. Bilateral large, unreactive pupils that display hippos or dilate with neck scratching (ciliospinal reflex) suggest a tectal or pretectal lesion. Midposition (3 to 6 mm) unreactive pupils result from lesions affecting both sympathetic and parasympathetic pathways. They occur commonly as a feature of central transtentorial herniation. Abnormally shaped, for example, oval or elliptical, or misplaced ("ectopic") pupils suggest midbrain disease (see Chapter 14).

Pupillary asymmetry usually indicates structural disease. A unilaterally dilated pupil, especially if unreactive to light, is most often a sign of third nerve palsy and in the setting of coma usually indicates uncal herniation (Hutchinson's pupil). Because of the peripheral location of the pupillary fibers in the third nerve, they are especially susceptible to pressure, and pupillary dilation often occurs prior to any eye movement abnormality. Rarely, paradoxical unilateral dilation of the pupil on the side opposite the lesion occurs as a false localizing sign, especially with subdural or intraparenchymal hemorrhage. Coma with a unilaterally dilated pupil could also result from subarachnoid hemorrhage because of a posterior communicating artery aneurysm. Lateral medullary syndrome may cause anisocoria due to Horner's syndrome, along with evidence of brainstem dysfunction, but rarely causes coma. Horner's syndrome may also occur with lesions involving the hypothalamus or thalamus (particularly hemorrhage). Ipsilateral Horner's syndrome may occur because of carotid artery disease, especially occlusion, but is likely due to hypothalamic ischemia rather than dysfunction of the pericarotid sympathetic plexus. Rarely, seizures may cause transient anisocoria.

Pupillary reactivity is a key sign in distinguishing structural from metabolic coma. Normally, reactive pupils in the setting of coma suggest metabolic encephalopathy, which typically affects consciousness and respiration earlier than pupillary function. Loss of pupillary reactivity is more consistent with structural disease or anoxia. Structural lesions of the brainstem usually cause abnormal pupillary responses, and in brain death, pupillary responses are absent. Pupillary reactivity is usually preserved in drug-induced coma, except when so severe the patient requires ventilatory support. Certain agents may cause earlier pupillary unreactivity. Glutethimide may cause asymmetric and poorly reactive pupils but is rarely seen. Other agents that may fix the pupils include barbiturates, certain anticonvulsants, lidocaine, phenothiazines, and aminoglycosides. A notable exception to the rule that normally reactive pupils indicate metabolic encephalopathy is that posterior fossa mass effect exerted primarily on the mid and lower brainstem, such as cerebellar infarction or hemorrhage, may initially spare the pupils.

Pupillary light reaction is a key prognostic sign. Loss of reactivity portends a poor outcome. Brain injury patients, even those with a GCS of 3, if the pupils remain reactive, may survive. Loss of pupillary reactivity for more than a few minutes after an anoxic insult carries a poor prognosis. In a series of patients undergoing craniotomy for traumatic hematomas, 25% of those with fixed pupils for less than 6 hours made a functional recovery. The ciliospinal reflex is another test of pupil reactivity, but it involves pathways caudal to the foramen magnum.

Eye movements have been discussed in detail in Chapter 14, and the oculocephalic and oculovestibular reflexes in Chapter 17. Note the position of the eyes at rest, whether there is any nystagmus, and whether the range of ocular movement is full in both directions to passive head movement or oculovestibular stimulation. If there is any possibility of trauma, a cervical spine series should precede neck manipulation for eye movement examination. Roving eye movements indicate that brainstem function is intact. The roving eye movements of early coma cannot be mimicked, and their presence excludes psychogenic unresponsiveness. With deepening of coma, first to disappear are roving eye movements, then the oculocephalic response, and then the oculovestibular reflex. Conjugate eye deviation away from the paralyzed extremities is seen in destructive frontal lobe lesions; conjugate deviation in the direction of the paralyzed extremities indicates a brainstem lesion (Chapter 14). Conjugate gaze deviation, sometimes with accompanying nystagmoid jerking, may also occur because of seizure activity in the frontal eye fields on the side the patient is looking away from. Thalamic hemorrhage can cause "wrong-way eyes," with gaze deviation toward the hemiparesis. Vertical gaze deviations suggest brainstem disease; the most common is sustained downgaze with an upgaze deficit because of a lesion involving the upper midbrain or caudal thalamus. Hepatic encephalopathy can cause down-gaze deviation.

Reflex movements elicited by turning the head from side to side (doll's eye movements, oculocephalic reflex) or by the injection of ice water into the external auditory canal (caloric test, oculovestibular reflex) may reveal isolated weakness of particular extraocular muscles, gaze paresis, or other eye movement abnormalities (Figure 51.1). Supratentorial lesions and metabolic processes usually do not affect the oculocephalic reflex. Wernicke's encephalopathy is one metabolic encephalopathy that may affect eye movements; it is not limited to alcoholics. Caloric testing assesses the same brainstem reflexes as the doll's eye maneuver and is used if the oculocephalic reflex is not intact. After ensuring the external auditory canal is clear, the head is flexed to a 30-degree angle above horizontal, and 10 to 20 cc of ice water is instilled into the canal. If no response is obtained, larger volumes are used. After 15 to 60 seconds, eye deviation begins and may last several minutes. The expected response in coma is tonic deviation of the eyes toward the side of the irrigated ear. Warm water causes the opposite response. Testing of the other side may be done after about 5 minutes. Brainstem lesions affecting the pathways and nuclei subserving the

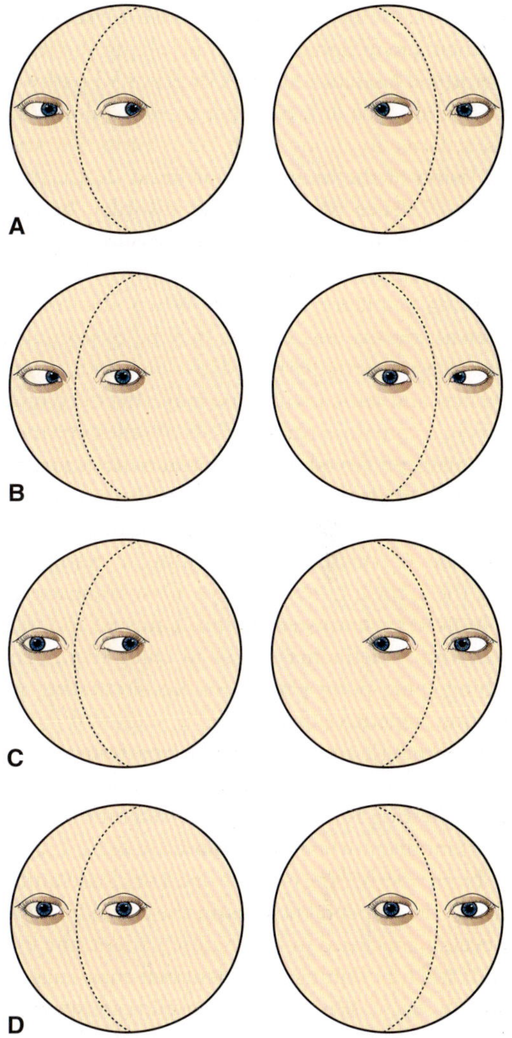

FIGURE 51.1 Examples of oculocephalic responses that may be seen in comatose patients. When the brainstem is intact, the eyes move in the opposite direction from head rotation. **A.** Normal response, the usual response in a patient with metabolic encephalopathy. **B.** Bilateral sixth nerve palsies. **C.** Right third nerve palsy or internuclear ophthalmoplegia. **D.** Absent response, seen when the reflex pathways are impaired.

reflex may cause an abnormal response. Dysconjugate movements may signal a lesion involving the medial longitudinal fasciculus or the CN III or VI pathways. In coma, absence of a response to cold calorics suggests sedative-hypnotic drug intoxication, a structural lesion of the brainstem, or brain death, unless there is evidence of a vestibular disorder, or exposure to vestibular-suppressant drugs. Some causes of metabolic coma may fix the eye movements while preserving pupillary reactivity. When the response is present, the eye movements may be dysconjugate. Some drugs, particularly sedative-hypnotic agents, tricyclics, and anticonvulsants, may affect eye movements in a comatose patient. Loss of reflex eye movements with preserved pupillary reactivity is virtually diagnostic of drug toxicity. Vertically dysconjugate gaze at rest may indicate skew deviation. The oculocephalic or bilateral oculovestibular testing can assess the vertical gaze pathways. Dysconjugacy usually indicates a brainstem lesion. Unusual spontaneous eye movements may occur in coma (e.g., ocular bobbing, ping-pong gaze, periodic alternating gaze deviation, repetitive divergence, nystagmoid jerking, ocular dipping), and the particular pattern often has localizing significance. If the patient is responsive enough, testing for optokinetic nystagmus may give important diagnostic information.

Note whether the eyes are open or closed and the width of the palpebral fissures on the two sides. When the eyelids are closed in a comatose patient, the lower pons is still functioning. Eyelids at half-mast suggest it is not. In "eyes-open" coma, the eyelids are spastically retracted because of failure of levator inhibition with a lesion in the pons. Spontaneous blinking requires an intact pontine reticular formation. Asymmetry of the palpebral fissures may indicate either upper facial weakness on the side of the wider fissure or ptosis on the side of the narrower fissure. If the eyes are partially or completely closed, the examiner may try to open them by gently raising the upper lids and then noting the speed with which the eyes close again. Unilateral orbicularis weakness may produce more leisurely closure on the affected side. In deep coma, the eyes may be open and a glassy stare evident. In profound illness, the patient often lies with the eyes only partially closed, even in sleep, so that a narrow portion of the cornea is visible between the upper and lower lids. In psychogenic unresponsiveness, the patient may keep the eyes tightly closed and resist attempts to open them, yet open the eyes and glance around when unaware that someone is observing the action. Note whether there is any blinking, flickering, or tremor of the eyelids at rest or in response to a bright light or sudden noise. The corneal reflexes may be absent in coma; any asymmetry of the response may be significant.

In some patients, it is possible to obtain facial movement by painful stimulation, such as supraorbital pressure, sternal rub, or pinprick stimulation of the face. The area of the upper nasolabial fold at the junction with the nose is particularly sensitive and a response to pinprick in this region can sometimes be obtained when there is no response over other parts of the face. It is important when examining facial sensation not to traumatize the face and leave pinprick marks, particularly in elderly patients with thin, fragile skin. Firm manual pressure over the supraorbital notch, at the point of emergence of the supraorbital nerve, will often produce facial grimacing. When facial movement does occur, compare the two sides for symmetry of the response. Elicitation of a blink response to loud noise provides a crude assessment of auditory function. The mouth may be either open or closed. In nonorganic unresponsiveness, the patient may resist attempts to passively open the mouth. A gag reflex may or may not be present. If present, the palate should rise in the midline.

No neurologic evaluation of coma, stupor, or disordered consciousness is complete without an ophthalmoscopic examination. The presence of papilledema is, of course, indicative of some process causing increased intracranial pressure. Papilledema takes a period of time to develop and may be absent in acute conditions. Normal spontaneous venous pulsations are a strong indicator of normal intracranial pressure, but absence of venous pulsations does not prove that intracranial pressure is increased. Subarachnoid hemorrhage may produce subhyaloid hemorrhages in the retina. The ophthalmoscopic examination is also important in detecting systemic diseases responsible for altered consciousness (e.g., diabetes, hypertension, or endocarditis). It is not possible to test either visual acuity or the visual fields reliably if significant impairment of consciousness is present. If the patient is responsive enough, it may be possible to determine if the patient follows objects, or blinks to threat.

Examination of Motor Status

The motor examination in disorders of consciousness requires skilled observation. It may be difficult to recognize the presence of a hemiplegia in a comatose patient. If the hemiplegia has been of sudden onset, the paralyzed side of the body is usually flaccid. The width of the palpebral fissure is increased, the nasolabial fold is shallow, and the angle of the mouth droops on that side. There may be drooling of saliva and puffing out and retraction of the cheek on expiration and inspiration.

If both arms are lifted, or placed with the elbows resting on the bed and the forearms at right angles to the arms, then released by the examiner, the affected extremity falls more rapidly and in a flail-like manner, whereas the normal arm drops slowly or may even remain upright for a brief period before falling. If the lower extremities are lifted from the bed and then released, the affected extremity falls rapidly, whereas the normal limb drops more gradually to the bed. If the lower extremities are passively flexed with heels resting on the bed and then released, the paretic limb rapidly falls to an extended position with the hip in external rotation, whereas the unaffected limb maintains the posture for a few moments and then gradually returns to its original position. If the depression of consciousness is not too deep, there may be some response to painful stimulation. Pinching the skin on the normal side is followed by withdrawal of the part stimulated. In contrast, a painful stimulus on the paralyzed side causes no local movement, although grimacing or movements of the opposite side of the body may indicate that some sensation is retained. It is important to appraise muscle tone, or resistance to passive movement, and to observe carefully for any abnormal movements. Generalized flaccidity may occur with critical illness polyneuropathy or myopathy. Flaccidity of both arms with normal tone in the legs may occur with border zone ischemia (man-in-the-barrel syndrome). Multifocal myoclonus, with widespread brief, random, asynchronous jerks, strongly suggests a metabolic or toxic etiology, especially hypoxic-ischemic encephalopathy. More subtle twitches, random or sustained, suggest nonconvulsive status epilepticus. Such twitches may be restricted to the facial muscles, fingers, or even the tongue.

Occasionally, spasticity instead of flaccidity develops after acute cerebral lesions. A previous spastic hemiplegia or extrapyramidal syndrome may have caused an alteration in tone that persists even in coma, and arthropathies and skeletal abnormalities may also interfere with joint movements. In catatonia, there may be a waxy resistance resembling that of extrapyramidal disease. Patients with AMS may have asterixis.

The motor responses to stimuli are probably the most important factor in gauging the depth of coma and prognosis. The highest level response is when the patient obeys simple commands (GCS 6). If there is no response to verbal commands, a painful stimulus is delivered. There are five possible outcomes. The patient may localize the painful stimulus and make appropriate movements to attempt to remove it (GCS 5). She may exhibit flexion withdrawal without localizing the stimulus (GCS 4). There may be abnormal flexor responses (decorticate rigidity, GCS 3), or, as the lowest level of response, an extensor response (decerebrate rigidity, GCS 2). The worst possible outcome is no response whatsoever (GCS 1).

Abnormal flexor and extensor responses are referred to as posturing. Abnormal posturing may occur spontaneously, as well as in response to stimuli. It is not uncommon for posturing to be different on the two sides of the body. When there is difficulty distinguishing purposeful withdrawal from decorticate posturing, a painful stimulus to the inner arm is useful. Abduction of the arm away from the stimulus is a high-level avoidance response; adduction into the stimulus is a low-level reflex response. Posturing usually indicates structural disease of the nervous system and is particularly common after head injury. Posturing can also occur with severe metabolic encephalopathy, particularly sedative-hypnotic drug intoxication. Posturing in metabolic encephalopathy is usually symmetric; posturing in structural CNS disease is frequently asymmetric.

Decerebrate and decorticate rigidity are discussed in Chapters 28 and 41. In brief, decorticate posturing includes upper-extremity adduction and flexion and lower-extremity extension. In decerebrate posturing, there is extension of both upper and lower extremities. Decerebration is traditionally thought to indicate a lesion below the red nucleus but above the lateral vestibulospinal tracts. These neuroanatomic correlates do not seem to apply as well in humans as experimental animals. Decerebrate posturing occurs in patients with bilateral cerebral lesions, well above the red nucleus. The distinction is useful prognostically; patients with decorticate posturing in response to pain tend to have a better prognosis than those with decerebrate posturing.

Sensory Examination

Depending on the level of coma, the patient may not perceive even the most painful stimulus or may respond to painful stimuli by wincing and withdrawing the part of the body stimulated. Often, the examination must be limited to comparing responses to painful stimulation on the two sides of the body. Sensory stimuli may be delivered by pinching the skin, pricking with a sharp object, pressing over the supraorbital notch, and squeezing the muscle masses and tendons, particularly the Achilles tendon.

Reflexes

At a minimum, the principal deep tendon reflexes (DTRs) and the plantar responses should be tested. Frontal release signs (forced grasping, palmomental, and suck or snout responses) and paratonic rigidity may be present with AMS of either structural or metabolic origin. Asymmetry of responses may have some localizing value. Similarly, extensor plantar responses may occur with either structural or metabolic coma.

Meningeal Signs

The examiner should attempt to elicit signs of meningeal involvement by flexing the neck passively and rotating it from side to side in order to detect nuchal rigidity. The Kernig, Brudzinski, and related signs may be absent in some cases of deep coma despite the presence of meningeal irritation. In subarachnoid hemorrhage, it requires some hours for meningeal signs to develop, and they may be absent at the time of presentation. Meningeal signs are discussed more fully in Chapter 52.

DIFFERENTIAL DIAGNOSIS OF COMA

There are three possible etiologies for acute coma: (a) primary CNS disease, (b) depression of the CNS by a systemic metabolic process or drug intoxication, and (c) psychogenic unresponsiveness. Statistically, the most likely etiology is involvement of the CNS by a systemic metabolic process or drug intoxication. Patients with metabolic encephalopathy characteristically have a symmetrical examination, devoid of lateralizing or focal abnormalities, intact reflex eye movements, and reactive pupils.

Structural Lesions

There are three mechanisms whereby structural lesions may cause coma: (a) a lateralized hemispheric mass lesion causes increased intracranial pressure, herniation, and compression or hemorrhage into the upper midbrain with secondary impairment of the RAS; (b) a brainstem lesion, such as hemorrhage or infarction, damages the RAS directly; and (c) a disease process affects both cerebral hemispheres or both hemispheres and the RAS. The findings with a hemispheric mass lesion depend upon the stage of evolution of the process. In the early stages, there are usually lateralizing findings and asymmetries on examination consistent with a focal process. These include hemiparesis, focal seizures, aphasia, hemianopia, apraxia, and other signs of hemispheric dysfunction. As the lesion expands and intracranial pressure increases, the other hemisphere becomes involved, herniation develops, and the focal nature of the process becomes complicated by findings due to herniation. Asymmetric motor responses and abnormal eye movements usually persist until the terminal stages. Herniation syndromes are due to shifting of brain structures caused by increased intracranial pressure. They are evidence of severe disease and are life-threatening. A number of different herniation syndromes have been recognized. The more common and important are central transtentorial, lateral transtentorial (uncal), and tonsillar (foramen magnum) herniation (Figure 51.2; Table 51.3).

Central transtentorial herniation is due to symmetric downward displacement of the hemispheres

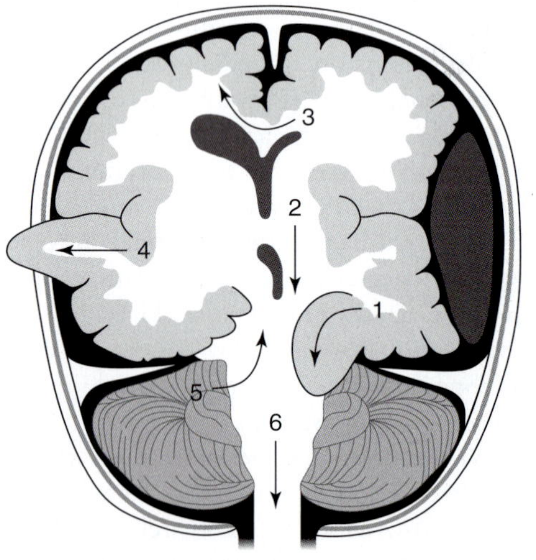

FIGURE 51.2 Types of brain herniation. *1*, uncal: ipsilateral CN III palsy and contralateral hemiplegia or posturing; *2*, central transtentorial: coma with bilateral small pupils and progression of posturing from decorticate to decerebrate with loss of brainstem reflexes; *3*, subfalcine: coma and contralateral weakness to posturing; *4*, extracranial (when craniectomy is present): deficits from herniated territory; *5*, upward cerebellar: cerebellar symptoms to coma and bilateral posturing; *6*, tonsillar (downward cerebellar): decreased arousal, pyramidal signs, respiratory insufficiency, coma. (Reprinted with permission from Sims KB, Peters JM, Musolino PL, Elibol MZ. Handbook of Pediatric Neurology. Philadelphia: Wolters Kluwer; 2014. Originally adapted with permission from Westover MB, Choi E, Awad KM. et al., eds. *Pocket Neurology*. Philadelphia: Lippincott Williams & Wilkins, 2010:46–47.)

TABLE 51.3 Clinical Manifestations of Common Herniation Syndromes

Herniation Syndrome	Clinical Manifestations
Central transtentorial	Impaired consciousness, abnormal respirations, symmetric small or midposition fixed or minimally reactive pupils, decorticate evolving to decerebrate posturing, rostrocaudal deterioration
Lateral transtentorial (uncal)	Impaired consciousness, abnormal respirations, third nerve palsy (unilaterally dilated pupil), hemiparesis (may be false localizing), rostrocaudal deterioration
Cerebellar tonsillar (foramen magnum)	Impaired consciousness, neck rigidity, opisthotonos, decerebrate rigidity, vomiting, irregular respirations, apnea, bradycardia
Upward	Prominent brainstem signs, downward gaze deviation, upgaze palsy, decerebrate posturing (usually because of a cerebellar mass lesion)

causing impaction of the diencephalon and midbrain into the tentorial notch. Pressure effects on the diencephalon and midbrain often cause small hemorrhages in the upper midbrain (Duret hemorrhages). Uncal herniation occurs when the temporal lobe and uncus shift medially into the tentorial notch, causing compression of the third CN and adjacent midbrain. Tentorial herniation, unless reversed, evolves into an orderly progression of neurologic dysfunction referred to as rostrocaudal deterioration.

During rostrocaudal deterioration, neurologic dysfunction becomes progressively more dramatic. Clinical stages occur as if the brain had been transversely sectioned at a particular level (diencephalon, midbrain, pons, or medulla). Respirations become progressively more abnormal, evolving from a Cheyne-Stokes pattern early to ataxic respirations to eventual apnea. Pupils become progressively more abnormal and eventually become fixed and unreactive. Reflex eye movements are eventually lost. Motor responses evolve from localizing to nonlocalizing to decorticate to decerebrate to flaccid. The end result of unchecked rostrocaudal deterioration is death.

Herniation of the cerebellar tonsils downward into the foramen magnum compresses the medulla and upper spinal cord and can result in rapid failure of vital functions. A dreaded complication of lumbar puncture is herniation, especially cerebellar tonsillar herniation, because of removal of spinal fluid.

A primary lesion involving the brainstem (e.g., pontine hemorrhage or infarction) produces coma that is abrupt in onset and causes focal or multifocal abnormalities, abnormal eye movements, pupillary abnormalities, pathologic reflexes, quadriparesis, abnormal posturing, and other objective neurologic signs. Brainstem stroke may also cause terminal hyperthermia without evidence of infection. In a series of patients with brainstem stroke, those who were not in coma had a small and unilateral lesion of the tegmentum or damage outside the tegmentum. In comatose patients, the lesions in the tegmentum were usually bilateral and were either restricted to the pons or in the upper pons and the midbrain. Most brainstem lesions causing coma involve infarction or hemorrhage. Tumor, osmotic demyelination syndrome (central pontine myelinolysis), and brainstem encephalitis are rare causes.

Disorders that cause bilateral hemispheric dysfunction or produce diffuse CNS involvement include bilateral subdural hematomas, bilateral cerebral infarction due to emboli, thrombotic thrombocytopenic purpura, and other processes that may cause multifocal lesions. In addition, some processes affect the CNS in a more diffuse or widespread manner and cause coma by dysfunction of the cerebral hemispheres bilaterally or the cerebral hemispheres as well as the RAS. Such conditions include meningitis, encephalitis, subarachnoid hemorrhage, and hypertensive encephalopathy. These cause variable focality on examination, depending on the specifics of the process, and occasionally cause very little in the way of focal or lateralizing signs. There typically are objective neurologic signs in the form of reflex abnormality, pathologic reflexes, evidence of meningeal irritation, and abnormalities on fundoscopic examination. In addition, there may be fever or other evidence of systemic disease. Such multifocal structural processes may simulate metabolic encephalopathy.

Metabolic Encephalopathy

Metabolic encephalopathies are conditions that typically produce no focal or lateralizing signs on neurologic examination, preserve pupil reactivity, and usually do not affect eye movements or cause other signs of brainstem dysfunction. Metabolic encephalopathy often begins with a period of confusion or delirium, which gradually evolves into stupor, then coma. There are three common etiologies: (a) intoxication, (b) severe systemic metabolic disturbance, and (c) systemic infection. Intoxication is usually due to alcohol, opiates, or sedative-hypnotic drugs. These conditions sometimes produce other abnormalities on physical examination that may be a clue as to etiology, such as pinpoint pupils, respiratory depression, or skin lesions. Various instruments have been used for the bedside evaluation of delirium. A systematic review of the accuracy of bedside instruments in diagnosing the presence of delirium in adults concluded that the Confusion Assessment Method had the best available supportive data as a bedside delirium instrument. Having a score of less than 24 on the Mini-Mental State Exam (see Chapter 8) was the least useful for identifying a patient with delirium.

The most common systemic metabolic disturbance to cause coma is the hypoxic-ischemic encephalopathy that follows cardiac arrest. Other examples include hypoglycemia, diabetic ketoacidosis, nonketotic hyperosmolar state, hyperammonemia, hypercalcemia, and hypercarbia. Many of these conditions occur under obvious clinical circumstances, such as known diabetes, end-stage alcoholism with cirrhosis, or severe pulmonary disease with hypercarbia, and the etiology is often revealed by routine blood chemistries. Severe infections and septicemia occasionally cause AMS (septic encephalopathy).

Although metabolic encephalopathies in general produce a uniform clinical picture of a symmetric examination with reactive pupils and intact brainstem eye movement reflexes, in some conditions, there may be deviations from this scheme. Occasionally, certain clinical features may provide clues as to etiology. In hypoglycemia, there may be lateralized deficits, extensor posturing, hypothermia, and seizures. In hepatic encephalopathy, there may be clinical evidence of alcoholism and end-stage liver disease, including ascites, jaundice, spider angiomas, palmar erythema, and gynecomastia. It is usually preceded by asterixis and confusion. There may be focal deficits, as well as abnormal posturing, and occasionally unusual eye findings, including ocular bobbing and gaze deviations. The encephalopathy of uremia is often associated with tremor, asterixis, myoclonus, seizures, and occasionally evidence of tetany. There may be mild focal deficits, but brainstem functions remain intact. Distinguishing features of the encephalopathy of hypercarbia include papilledema, asterixis, tremor, and myoclonus. Focal signs occur occasionally in hyponatremia, hypernatremia, and hyperosmolar coma. Sedative-hypnotic drug intoxication often affects eye movements, whereas pupillary light reactions remain unaffected. Abnormal posturing may also occur. This unusual combination of reactive pupils in the face of abnormal reflex eye movements and posturing is characteristic of sedative-hypnotic drug effects but can also occur with posterior fossa mass lesions causing pressure on the lower and mid-brainstem with relative preservation of the midbrain. This picture can also occur with upward transtentorial herniation.

In a review of 11 studies (1,914 patients) on the accuracy of the clinical examination in prognosis of post–cardiac arrest coma in adults, five clinical signs were found to strongly predict death or poor neurologic outcome: absent corneal reflexes at 24 hours, absent pupillary response at 24 hours, absent withdrawal response to pain at 24 hours, no motor response at 24 hours, and no motor response at 72 hours. In 75 patients at day 1 of post–cardiac arrest coma, 2 of 18 patients with absent pupillary reflexes, 2 of 32 with absent corneal reflexes, and 0 of 15 with absent oculovestibular reflexes recovered awareness. Purposeful movements were associated with a high probability of recovery.

Seizure Disorders

A seizure is a transient episode of uncontrollable motor activity, focal or generalized, usually accompanied by clouding or loss of consciousness. In addition to alteration of consciousness during the ictus, seizure disorders may also cause AMS because of postictal unresponsiveness, absence status, psychomotor status, and subclinical status epilepticus. In the postictal period, there is often depression of consciousness, a desire to sleep, confusion, and disorientation. Coma or stupor may be a sequel of a recent seizure, although it may not be possible to obtain a history of either a recent convulsion or previous attacks. The patient may show evidence of tongue biting, frothing at the mouth, bloody sputum, incontinence, and lacerations or other injuries to the body. Old scars may be found on the tongue. The postictal stupor is usually brief but may be followed by either profound sleep or confusion and irrational behavior. A prolonged postictal encephalopathy may last many hours, rarely days. Postictal stupor occurs most commonly with generalized tonic-clonic seizures but may follow other seizure types. In the absence of a history of seizure disorder, it may be difficult to differentiate between the postictal state and cerebral trauma.

In status epilepticus, there is prolonged seizure activity or repeated convulsions with failure to regain consciousness between them. Status epilepticus may cause a state of altered consciousness that may be confused with AMS or coma. In absence (petit mal) status, there is lowering and clouding of consciousness, and the patient may appear to be in a trance-like stupor, suggesting drug abuse or a psychiatric disorder. Patients in complex partial status epilepticus are commonly confused or lethargic. Subclinical status epilepticus, or seizures with subtle motor manifestations, may cause a coma-like state. Subclinical status may continue in patients when the motor manifestations have been suppressed with antiepileptic drugs. Patients with pseudoperiodic lateralized epileptiform discharges are often comatose because of a hemispheric process, such as large infarction or subdural hematoma, and the electroencephalogram (EEG) demonstrates characteristic discharges. The presence of myoclonus usually indicates that coma is of metabolic origin. Spontaneous, multifocal myoclonic jerking is common, particularly in uremia and hypercarbia. Massive generalized myoclonic jerks often occur as an aftermath of cardiac arrest and cerebral anoxia and are an extremely poor prognostic sign.

Locked-in Syndrome

In the locked-in syndrome, ventral brainstem destruction sparing the RAS renders the patient mute and quadriplegic but not comatose. There is complete paralysis of all four extremities and the lower CNs but no associated impairment of consciousness. Patients with locked-in syndrome have quadriplegia and anarthria, but variable preservation of consciousness and intellect. The patient is awake but speechless and motionless, with little response to stimuli. The lesion usually involves the midpons and results in paralysis of facial movement and horizontal gaze. If the supranuclear vertical gaze pathways, which pass rostral to the other corticobulbar and corticospinal pathways, are spared, there is preservation of vertical eye movements, and the patient may be able to blink. With effort, communication may be established using eye movement or blink signals. Sensory pathways, hearing, and vision are largely spared, and the patient is effectively "de-efferented." Other findings vary with the particulars of the lesion. A fulminant neuropathy, such as Guillain-Barré syndrome, can result in a clinical state resembling brain death through diffuse de-efferentation. A severe upper spinal cord lesion, myopathy, or neuromuscular junction disorder may also mimic the locked-in syndrome.

Jean-Dominique Bauby (deceased) bequeathed an eloquent and poignant description of the locked-in state from the victim's point of view in *The Diving Bell and the Butterfly: A Memoir of Life in Death* (Vintage Books, 1998). Bauby dictated his book by blinking one eyelid. The principal cause of locked-in syndrome is brainstem stroke (86%), but it may also occur after trauma (14%). The locked-in state is frequently mistaken for coma. Appreciation that the patient is not comatose or vegetative but locked-in does not usually occur for 2 to 3 months (mean 79 days), and average survival for patients in the locked in state is 71 months.

The Vegetative State

The pathology in patients with the vegetative state invariably entails massive bilateral hemispheric damage with a spared and intact brainstem. Preservation of the RAS permits behavioral arousal and sleep-wake cycles, but existence is devoid of cognition. Positron emission tomography (PET) has demonstrated cerebral metabolic rates for glucose far too low to sustain consciousness. The vegetative state may develop as a sequel to acute insults, typically following a temporary period of coma, or as the end stage of a progressive neurologic illness, such as Alzheimer's disease. The vegetative state is deemed persistent (PVS) after 3 months if the etiology was medical, after 12 months if traumatic.

In PVS, patients are awake but unaware. Despite a seemingly alert demeanor, they display no speech, comprehension, or purposeful movement. Reflex eye movements and orientation to noise—brainstem level functions—may persist. Yawning, sneezing, bruxism, and occasional meaningless smiles may occur. Impaired motor function with spasticity, posturing, or contractures is common. Painful stimuli evoke nonspecific erratic reactions without discrete motor responses or localization. All patients are incontinent of stool and urine. In PVS, patients exist in eyes-open permanent unconsciousness, with intact sleep-wake cycles but no awareness of self or environment, and without voluntary action or behavior of any kind. Though seemingly awake, they display no interactive behavior and no ability to express emotion or engage another person on any level. Extended observation forms the primary and most important basis for the diagnosis of PVS. Such patients show no behavioral responses whatsoever over a prolonged period of time. PVS must be differentiated from catatonia and from the locked-in syndrome.

A number of other terms have been used to describe states of altered awareness that are similar, if not identical, to PVS (e.g., akinetic mutism, abulia, apallic state, coma vigil, and pseudocoma). Much of the nomenclature is outdated and perplexing, the distinctions vague and of marginal clinical utility. The term PVS has come under justifiable fire for its pejorative and negative connotations. Persistent unresponsiveness and unresponsive wakefulness syndrome have been suggested as alternatives. The minimally conscious state (MCS) refers to a subgroup of patients with severe alteration in consciousness who do not meet diagnostic criteria for coma or PVS. These patients demonstrate "inconsistent but discernible evidence" of consciousness with intermittent, behavioral evidence of awareness of self or environment; diagnostic criteria have been provided. The rate of misdiagnosis between PVS and MCS has been estimated at 40%.

Brain magnetic resonance imaging (MRI), MR spectroscopy, PET, functional MRI (fMRI), EEG, and evoked potential studies are changing the understanding of patients in these states of disordered consciousness. There is increasing evidence of residual cognitive processing in some patients who do not clinically respond to commands. fMRI has shown evidence of preserved consciousness even in patients in apparent coma. In one apparently comatose patient, fMRI revealed robust cortical responses to visual, auditory, and tactile stimulation.

Numerous reports indicate that late recovery from PVS or MCS can occur, particularly after TBI. A series of 50 patients with PVS were followed for up to 4 years (mean 25.7 months). Ten patients (20% of the total sample) showed late (14 to 28 months) recovery of responsiveness. Six patients recovered consciousness. Young age and retained pupillary light reactivity predicted late recovery more than etiology of the PVS. Most such patients remain severely disabled, but recovery to independent living, including work and university studies, was reported in one young man after 19 months in a vegetative state after a TBI. Although some vegetative patients eventually become minimally conscious and some minimally conscious patients gain increased awareness, the overall prognosis for meaningful recovery remains poor.

Psychogenic Unresponsiveness

In psychogenic unresponsiveness (functional coma), usually because of either conversion disorder or malingering, the loss of consciousness is typically not deep, but the condition may occasionally simulate real coma. The patient often responds to painful stimuli, unless there is associated nonorganic sensory loss, and the reflexes are normal, with no pathologic responses. The temperature, pulse, respirations, and blood pressure are normal. The eyelids may flutter or the eyes may be closed tightly with the patient resisting attempts to open them. The vigorous eye closure may interfere with testing the corneal and pupillary reflexes, which are normal. When the eyelids are opened and then released by the examiner, they close gradually in the patient with real coma but quickly in the patient with factitious coma. The patient may resist other procedures and glance around when unaware she is being watched. When a hand is raised and allowed to drop toward the face, the patient with psychogenic unresponsiveness will usually avoid hitting herself, but this rule is not infallible. In true coma, the hand will hit the face. Caloric testing either arouses the patient or produces nystagmus, which never occurs in real coma.

An episode of psychogenic unresponsiveness is usually precipitated by emotional stress, and the onset is often dramatic. The patient may appear to be in a trance, or coma may alternate with weeping and thrashing movements. The performance is appropriately staged and occurs when observers are in the vicinity. Movements, if present, are not stereotyped but appear to be coordinated and purposive. The patient may struggle, clutch at objects or parts of the body, or attempt to tear off clothes. Although the patient appears to be unconscious, some response to external stimuli may be evident. If there is muscle hypertonicity, it is usually of a rigid type, and there may be opisthotonos with the arc de cercle. If the patient can be persuaded to talk, the responses may be of the type seen in Ganser's syndrome, with evasiveness and approximate but consistently inaccurate replies.

In psychotic states, there is rarely complete loss of consciousness. Severe depression, schizophrenia, and organic psychoses may cause mutism, in which the patient is either completely withdrawn from the environment or refuses to speak. Negativism, either passive or active, may be a symptom of various psychoses, but especially of schizophrenia. In severe depression, the patient may show psychomotor retardation that may simulate AMS. In catatonic stupor, there is apathy, mutism, and negativism, often with waxy rigidity of the extremities causing the patient to hold her limbs or entire body in bizarre and seemingly uncomfortable positions for long periods of time. Food may be held in the mouth. Catatonic stupor may resolve after lorazepam administration.

Brain Death

To meet clinical criteria for brain death, a high degree of certainty regarding the etiology of the brain death picture is imperative. Common causes include cerebral anoxia, cerebral hemorrhage, aneurysmal subarachnoid hemorrhage, and TBI. The patient must have no evidence of cerebral or brainstem activity, although segmental reflex activity mediated at the spinal cord level may persist. Preserved spinal cord reflex activity may lead to dramatic movements, such as the "Lazarus reflex" (see Chapter 24). Complex spinal automatisms may occur in as many as 40% of brain dead patients, usually within the first 24 hours. There may even be respiratory-like movements, with shoulder elevation and adduction, back arching, and intercostal expansion, but without significant tidal volumes. DTRs, superficial reflexes, and the Babinski sign may be present and do not countermand a diagnosis of brain death. Except for segmental reflexes, motor responses are absent. The pupils are fixed, and oculocephalic and oculovestibular reflexes are absent, even with large volume ice water caloric testing. There must be no evidence of sedative drug effects or any systemic metabolic abnormality severe enough to produce the clinical picture of brain death. There must be no significant hypothermia, as hypothermia can mimic brain death. The presence of neuromuscular blocking agents obviously precludes evaluation of motor status. If the patient meets these clinical criteria, an apnea test is performed, and if there is no respiratory effort with an arterial PCO_2 of 60 mm Hg or more, the diagnosis of brain death can be made. The apnea test is not without danger. Dramatic spontaneous movements are most likely to occur during the apnea test when the patient becomes hypoxic. These clinical conditions should persist for some time, the exact interval depending on the specific circumstances. A repetition of the evaluation is often done to confirm the findings; there is no decreed interval, but 6 hours is reasonable. These criteria apply to adults and may have to be modified for children, especially neonates.

Table 51.4 summarizes the 1995 practice parameter on determining brain death in adults prepared by the Quality Standards Subcommittee of the American Academy of Neurology (AAN), updated in 2010. Despite the availability of these guidelines, major differences exist in brain death guidelines among the leading neurologic hospitals in the United States. Although brain-death mimics have been reported, including fulminant Guillain-Barré syndrome, organophosphate intoxication, high cervical spinal cord injury, lidocaine toxicity, baclofen overdose, and delayed vecuronium clearance, there have been no reports in peer-reviewed medical journals of recovery of brain function after a determination of brain death using the 1995 AAN practice parameter.

TABLE 51.4 Summary of the Guidance for the Clinical Diagnosis of Brain Death in Adults from the American Academy of Neurology

I. Prerequisites
   A. Establish irreversible and proximate cause of coma
      1. The cause of coma can usually be established by history, examination, neuroimaging, and laboratory tests.
      2. Exclude the presence of complicating medical conditions such as a CNS-depressant drugs, neuromuscular blocking agents, severe electrolyte, acid-base, or endocrine disturbance.
   B. Achieve normal core temperature. In most patients, a warming blanket is needed to raise the body temperature and maintain a normal or near-normal temperature (>36°C).
   C. Achieve normal systolic blood pressure. Neurologic examination is usually reliable with a systolic blood pressure ≥100 mm Hg.
   D. Perform one neurologic examination (sufficient to pronounce brain death in most US states) if a certain period of time has passed since the onset of the brain insult to exclude the possibility of recovery.

(continued)

TABLE 51.4 Summary of the Guidance for the Clinical Diagnosis of Brain Death in Adults from the American Academy of Neurology *(Continued)*

II. Neurologic assessment
- A. Coma. Patients must lack all evidence of responsiveness. The clinical differentiation of spinal responses from retained motor responses associated with brain activity requires expertise.
- B. Absence of brainstem reflexes
  1. Absence of pupillary response
  2. Absence of ocular movements using oculocephalic testing and oculovestibular reflex testing
  3. Absence of corneal reflex
  4. Absence of facial muscle movement to a noxious stimulus
  5. Absence of the pharyngeal and tracheal reflexes
- C. Apnea. Absence of a breathing drive is tested with a CO_2 challenge
  1. Prerequisites: normotension, normothermia, euvolemia, eucapnia ($PaCO_2$ 35–45 mm Hg), absence of hypoxia, and no prior evidence of CO_2 retention.
  2. Procedure:
     - Adjust vasopressors to a systolic blood pressure $\geq$100 mm Hg.
     - Preoxygenate for at least 10 min with 100% oxygen to a PaO_2 > 200 mm Hg.
     - Reduce ventilation frequency to 10 breaths per minute to eucapnia.
     - Reduce positive end-expiratory pressure (PEEP) to 5 cm H_2O (oxygen desaturation with decreasing PEEP may suggest difficulty with apnea testing).
     - If pulse oximetry oxygen saturation remains >95%, obtain a baseline blood gas (partial pressure of oxygen [PaO_2], $PaCO_2$, pH, bicarbonate, base excess).
     - Disconnect the patient from the ventilator.
     - Preserve oxygenation (e.g., place an insufflation catheter through the endotracheal tube and close to the level of the carina and deliver 100% O_2 at 6 L/min).
     - Look closely for respiratory movements for 8–10 min. Respiration is defined as abdominal or chest excursions and may include a brief gasp.
     - Abort if systolic blood pressure decreases to <90 mm Hg.
     - Abort if oxygen saturation measured by pulse oximetry is <85% for >30 seconds. Retry procedure with T-piece, continuous positive airway pressure (CPAP) 10 cm H_2O, and 100% O_2 12 L/min.
     - If no respiratory drive is observed, repeat blood gas (PaO_2, $PaCO_2$, pH, bicarbonate, base excess) after approximately 8 min.
     - If respiratory movements are absent and arterial PCO_2 is $\geq$60 mm Hg (or 20 mm Hg increase in arterial PCO_2 over a baseline normal arterial PCO_2), the apnea test result is positive (i.e., supports the clinical diagnosis of brain death).
     - If the test is inconclusive but the patient is hemodynamically stable during the procedure, it may be repeated for a longer period of time (10–15 min) after the patient is again adequately preoxygenated.

III. Ancillary tests

Ancillary tests are not necessary or sufficient for the declaration of brain death. Ancillary tests can be used when uncertainty exists about the reliability of parts of the neurologic examination or when the apnea test cannot be performed. In clinical practice, EEG, cerebral angiography, nuclear scan, and transcranial Doppler are currently used ancillary tests in adults.

IV. Documentation

The time of brain death is documented in the medical records. Time of death is the time the arterial PCO_2 reached the target value. In patients with an aborted apnea test, the time of death is when the ancillary test has been officially interpreted. Federal and state law requires the physician to contact an organ procurement organization following determination of brain death.

Reprinted from Wijdicks EG, Valerlas PN, Gronseth GS, et al. Evidence-based guideline update: determining brain death in adults. Report of the Quality Standards Subcommittee of the American Academy of Neurology. *Neurology* 2010;74(23):1911–1918, with permission.

BIBLIOGRAPHY

AMA Council on Scientific Affairs, AMA Council on Ethical and Judicial Affairs. Persistent vegetative state and the decision to withdraw or withhold life support. *JAMA* 1990;263:426–430.

Adams ZM, Fins JJ. The historical origins of the vegetative state: Received wisdom and the utility of the text. *J Hist Neurosci* 2017;26:140–153.

Angel MJ, Chen R, Bryan Young G. Metabolic encephalopathies. *Handb Clin Neurol* 2008;90:115–166.

Angel MJ, Young GB. Metabolic encephalopathies. *Neurol Clin* 2011;29:837–882.

Balestreri M, Czosnyka M, Chatfield DA, et al. Predictive value of Glasgow Coma Scale after brain trauma: change in trend over the past ten years. *J Neurol Neurosurg Psychiatry* 2004;75:161–162.

Banasiak KJ, Lister G. Brain death in children. *Curr Opin Pediatr* 2003;15:288–293.

Baricich A, de Sire A, Antoniono E, et al. Recovery from vegetative state of patients with a severe brain injury: a 4-year real-practice prospective cohort study. *Funct Neurol* 2017;32:131–136.

Beleza P, Rocha J, Pinho J. Diagnosis, etiology, and treatment of nonconvulsive status epilepticus, a semiological oriented review. *Neurologist* 2015;19:160–167.

Booth CM, Boone RH, Tomlinson G, et al. Is this patient dead, vegetative, or severely neurologically impaired? Assessing outcome for comatose survivors of cardiac arrest. *JAMA* 2004;291:870–879.

Bruno MA, Gosseries O, Ledoux D, et al. Assessment of consciousness with electrophysiological and neurological imaging techniques. *Curr Opin Crit Care* 2011;17:146–151.

Chisholm N, Gillett G. The patient's journey: living with locked-in syndrome. *BMJ* 2005;331:94–97.

Cruse D, Gantner I, Soddu A, et al. Lies, damned lies and diagnoses: estimating the clinical utility of assessments of covert awareness in the vegetative state. *Brain Inj* 2014;28:1197–1201.

De Tanti A, Saviola D, Basagni B, et al. Recovery of consciousness after 7 years in vegetative state of non-traumatic origin: A single case study. *Brain Inj* 2016;30:1029–1034.

Edlow JA, Rabinstein A, Traub SJ, et al. Diagnosis of reversible causes of coma. *Lancet* 2014;384:2064–2076.

Eickhoff SB, Dafotakis M, Grefkes C, et al. fMRI reveals cognitive and emotional processing in a long-term comatose patient. *Exp Neurol* 2008;214:240–246.

Estraneo A, Moretta P, Loreto V, et al. Late recovery after traumatic, anoxic, or hemorrhagic long-lasting vegetative state. *Neurology* 2010;75:239–245.

Faran S, Vatine JJ, Lazary A, et al. Late recovery from permanent traumatic vegetative state heralded by event-related potentials. *J Neurol Neurosurg Psychiatry* 2006;77:998–1000.

Faugeras F, Rohaut B, Valente M, et al. Survival and consciousness recovery are better in the minimally conscious state than in the vegetative state. *Brain Inj* 2018;32:72–77.

Fins JJ, Schiff ND, Foley KM. Late recovery from the minimally conscious state: ethical and policy implications. *Neurology* 2007;68:304–307.

Fisher CM. The neurological examination of the comatose patient. *Acta Neurol Scand* 1969;45(Suppl 36):1–56.

Formisano R, Pistoia F, Sara M. Disorders of consciousness: a taxonomy to be changed? *Brain Inj* 2011;25:638–639.

Friedman Y, Lee L, Wherrett JR, et al. Simulation of brain death from fulminant de-efferentation. *Can J Neurol Sci* 2003;30:397–404.

Frontera JA. Metabolic encephalopathies in the critical care unit. *Continuum (Minneap Minn)* 2012;18:611–639.

Garrett WT, Chang CW, Bleck TP. Altered mental status in thrombotic thrombocytopenic purpura is secondary to nonconvulsive status epilepticus. *Ann Neurol* 1996;40:245–246.

Giacino JT, Ashwal S, Childs N, et al. The minimally conscious state: definition and diagnostic criteria. *Neurology* 2002;58:349–353.

Gill MR, Reiley DG, Green SM. Interrater reliability of Glasgow Coma Scale scores in the emergency department. *Ann Emerg Med* 2004;43:215–223.

Gonyea EF. The abnormal pupil in Cheyne-Stokes respiration. Case report. *J Neurosurg* 1990;72:810–812.

Gosseries O, Bruno MA, Chatelle C, et al. Disorders of consciousness: what's in a name? *NeuroRehabilitation* 2011;28:3–14.

Gray K, Anne KT, Wegner DM. More dead than dead: Perceptions of persons in the persistent vegetative state. *Cognition* 2011;121:275–280.

Greer DM, Varelas PN, Haque S, et al. Variability of brain death determination guidelines in leading US neurologic institutions. *Neurology* 2008;70:284–289.

Heiss WD. PET in coma and in vegetative state. *Eur J Neurol* 2012;19:207–211.

Hoffman JR, Schriger DL, Luo JS. The empiric use of naloxone in patients with altered mental status: a reappraisal. *Ann Emerg Med* 1991;20:246–252.

Hoffman RS, Goldfrank LR. The poisoned patient with altered consciousness. Controversies in the use of a 'coma cocktail'. *JAMA* 1995;274:562–569.

Hurwitz TA. Psychogenic unresponsiveness. *Neurol Clin* 2011;29:995–1006.

Iyer VN, Mandrekar JN, Danielson RD, et al. Validity of the FOUR score coma scale in the medical intensive care unit. *Mayo Clin Proc* 2009;84:694–701.

Jang S, Kim S, Lee H. Recovery from vegetative state to minimally conscious state: a case report. *Am J Phys Med Rehabil* 2016;95:e63–e66.

Kanich W, Brady WJ, Huff JS, et al. Altered mental status: evaluation and etiology in the ED. *Am J Emerg Med* 2002;20:613–617.

Kondziella D. Roald Dahl and the complete locked-in syndrome: "Cold dead body, living brain". *J Neurol Sci* 2017;379:276–278.

Laureys S, Celesia GG, Cohadon F, et al. Unresponsive wakefulness syndrome: a new name for the vegetative state or apallic syndrome. *BMC Med* 2010;8:68.

Levy, DE, Caronna JJ, Singer BH, et al. Predicting outcome from hypoxic-ischemic coma. *JAMA* 1985;253:1420–1426.

Liberati G, Hünefeldt T, Olivetti Belardinelli M. Questioning the dichotomy between vegetative state and minimally conscious state: a review of the statistical evidence. *Front Hum Neurosci* 2014;8:865.

Lieberman JD, Pasquale MD, Garcia R, et al. Use of admission Glasgow Coma Score, pupil size, and pupil reactivity to determine outcome for trauma patients. *J Trauma* 2003;55:437–442.

Luce JM. Chronic disorders of consciousness following coma: Part one: medical issues. *Chest* 2013;144:1381–1387.

Ludwig L, McWhirter L, Williams S, et al. Functional coma. *Handb Clin Neurol* 2016;139:313–327.

Maiser S, Kabir A, Sabsevitz D, et al. Locked-in syndrome #303. *J Palliat Med* 2016;19:460–461.

Malik K, Hess DC. Evaluating the comatose patient. Rapid neurologic assessment is key to appropriate management. *Postgrad Med* 2002;111:38–46, 49–50.

McNarry AF, Goldhill DR. Simple bedside assessment of level of consciousness: comparison of two simple assessment scales with the Glasgow Coma Scale. *Anaesthesia* 2004;59:34–37.

Naro A, Calabrò RS, Pollicino P, et al. Unexpected recovery from a vegetative state or misdiagnosis? Lesson learned from a case report. *NeuroRehabilitation* 2017;41:735–738.

O'Keefe KP, Sanson TG. Elderly patients with altered mental status. *Emerg Med Clin North Am* 1998;16:701–715.

Parvizi J, Damasio AR. Neuroanatomical correlates of brainstem coma. *Brain* 2003;126(Pt 7):1524–1536.

Posner JB, Plum F. *Plum and Posner's Diagnosis of Stupor and Coma.* 4th ed. Oxford; New York: Oxford University Press, 2007.

Posner JB. Clinical evaluation of the unconscious patient. *Clin Neurosurg* 1975;22:281–301.

Poston JN, Dorer R, Aboulafia DM. The diving bell and the butterfly revisited: a fatal case of locked-in syndrome in a man with Epstein-Barr virus-positive diffuse large B-cell lymphoma, not otherwise specified. *Clin Med Insights Blood Disord* 2018;11:1179545X18762799.

Practice parameters for determining brain death in adults (summary statement). The Quality Standards Subcommittee of the American Academy of Neurology. *Neurology* 1995;45:1012–1014.

Ragosta K. Miller Fisher syndrome, a brainstem encephalitis, mimics brain death. *Clin Pediatr (Phila)* 1993;32:685–687.

Razvi SS, Bone I. Neurological consultations in the medical intensive care unit. *J Neurol Neurosurg Psychiatry* 2003;74(Suppl 3):iii16–iii23.

Ropper AH, Samuels MA, Klein J. *Adams and Victor's Principles of Neurology*. 10th ed. New York: McGraw-Hill Education Medical, 2014.

Sancisi E, Battistini A, Di SC, et al. Late recovery from posttraumatic vegetative state. *Brain Inj* 2009;23:163–166.

Sprung CL. Changing attitudes and practices in forgoing life sustaining treatments. *JAMA* 1990;263:2211–2215.

Sutter R, Semmlack S, Kaplan PW. Nonconvulsive status epilepticus in adults—insights into the invisible. *Nat Rev Neurol* 2016;12:281–293.

Towne AR, Waterhouse EJ, Boggs JG, et al. Prevalence of nonconvulsive status epilepticus in comatose patients. *Neurology* 2000;54:340–345.

Truog RD, Robinson WM. The diagnosis of brain death. *N Engl J Med* 2001;345:617–618.

van Erp WS, Lavrijsen JC, van de Laar FA, et al. The vegetative state/unresponsive wakefulness syndrome: a systematic review of prevalence studies. *Eur J Neurol* 2014;21:1361–1368.

van Erp WS, Lavrijsen JC, Vos PE, et al. The vegetative state: prevalence, misdiagnosis, and treatment limitations. *J Am Med Dir Assoc* 2015;16:85.e9–85.e14.

Varelas PN, Lewis A. Modern approach to brain death. *Semin Neurol* 2016;36:625–630.

Wade DT, Johnston C. The permanent vegetative state: practical guidance on diagnosis and management. *BMJ* 1999;319:841–844.

Wade DT. How often is the diagnosis of the permanent vegetative state incorrect? A review of the evidence. *Eur J Neurol* 2018;25:619–625.

Wang HH, Varelas PN, Henderson GV, et al. Improving uniformity in brain death determination policies over time. *Neurology* 2017;88:562–568.

Wei LA, Fearing MA, Sternberg EJ, et al. The confusion assessment method: a systematic review of current usage. *J Am Geriatr Soc* 2008;56:823–830.

Weibers DO, Dale AJD, Kokmen E, et al. *Mayo Clinic Examinations in Neurology*. 7th ed. St. Louis: Mosby, 1998.

Wijdicks EF. Determining brain death in adults. *Neurology* 1995;45:1003–1011.

Wijdicks EF. The diagnosis of brain death. *N Engl J Med* 2001;344:1215–1221.

Wijdicks EF, Bamlet WR, Maramattom BV, et al. Validation of a new coma scale: the FOUR score. *Ann Neurol* 2005;58:585–593.

Wijdicks EF, Cranford RE. Clinical diagnosis of prolonged states of impaired consciousness in adults. *Mayo Clin Proc* 2005;80:1037–1046.

Wijdicks EF, Varelas PN, Gronseth GS, et al. American Academy of Neurology. Evidence-based guideline update: determining brain death in adults: report of the Quality Standards Subcommittee of the American Academy of Neurology. *Neurology* 2010;74:1911–1918.

Wijdicks EF. The case against confirmatory tests for determining brain death in adults. *Neurology* 2010;75:77–83.

Wijdicks EFM. Metabolic encephalopathy: behind the name. *Neurocrit Care* 2018.

Willmott L, White B. Persistent vegetative state and minimally conscious state: ethical, legal and practical dilemmas. *J Med Ethics* 2017;43:425–426.

Wong CL, Holroyd-Leduc J, Simel DL, et al. Does this patient have delirium?: value of bedside instruments. *JAMA* 2010;304:779–786.

Young GB, Doig G, Ragazzoni A. Anoxic-ischemic encephalopathy: clinical and electro-physiological associations with outcome. *Neurocrit Care* 2005;2:159–164.

Zamperetti N, Bellomo R, Defanti CA, et al. Irreversible apnoeic coma 35 years later. Towards a more rigorous definition of brain death? *Intensive Care Med* 2004;30:1715–1722.

Zeman A. Persistent vegetative state. *Lancet* 1997;350:795–799.

CHAPTER 52

Miscellaneous Neurologic Signs

Miscellaneous neurologic signs—some of them reflexes, some closely related to the defense and postural reflex mechanisms, and others more varied in nature—are elicited in certain diseases of the nervous system. Some of these are quite important, especially the signs of meningeal irritation; others are arcane and primarily of historical interest.

SIGNS OF MENINGEAL IRRITATION

Meningeal signs are elicited most frequently when the meninges are inflamed—from infection (e.g., bacterial meningitis) or from the presence of a foreign material (e.g., blood in the subarachnoid space). Meningismus is a term that refers to the presence of nuchal rigidity and other clinical signs of meningeal inflammation. Meningism is sometimes used synonymously with meningismus, but it is also used to refer to a syndrome characterized by neck stiffness without meningeal inflammation, seen in patients with systemic infections, particularly young children.

The clinical manifestations of meningeal irritation are varied and depend on the severity of the process. Accompaniments depend on etiology but commonly include headache, pain, and stiffness of the neck; irritability; photophobia; nausea and vomiting; and other manifestations of infection, such as fever and chills. The various maneuvers used to elicit meningeal signs produce tension on inflamed and hypersensitive spinal nerve roots, and the resulting signs are postures, protective muscle contractions, or other movements that minimize the stretch and distortion of the meninges and roots.

In a rational clinical examination article on the early recognition of acute meningitis, only 10 of 139 papers adequately addressed the utility of the clinical examination in confirmed cases of meningitis. In suspicious circumstances, the absence of fever, neck stiffness, and altered mental status effectively eliminates meningitis (sensitivity, 99% to 100% for the presence of one of these findings). Of the classic signs of meningeal irritation, only one study has assessed Kernig's sign, and no studies subsequent to the original report have evaluated Brudzinski's sign (see below). Forgie reviewed the current relevance of the classic eponymous signs of meningitis because more recent studies have suggested lower sensitivities and specificities compared to the original descriptions. These changes in sensitivity and specificity may be related to differences in examination technique, changes in the epidemiology and demographics of meningitis, an evolution in the pathogens causing meningitis, and changes in management.

Nuchal (Cervical) Rigidity

Nuchal rigidity is the most widely recognized and frequently encountered sign of meningeal irritation, and the diagnosis of meningitis is rarely made in its absence. It is characterized by stiffness and spasm of the neck muscles, with pain on attempted voluntary movement as well as resistance to passive movement. The degree of rigidity varies. There may be only slight resistance to passive flexion, or marked spasm of all the neck muscles. Nuchal rigidity primarily affects the extensor muscles, and the most prominent early finding in meningeal irritation is resistance to passive neck flexion. The physician is unable to place the patient's chin on his chest, but the neck can be hyperextended without difficulty; rotatory and lateral movements may also be preserved. With more severe nuchal rigidity, there may be resistance to extension and rotatory movements as well. Extreme rigidity causes retraction of the neck into a position of opisthotonos, the body assuming a wrestler's bridge or arc de cercle position, with the head thrust back and the

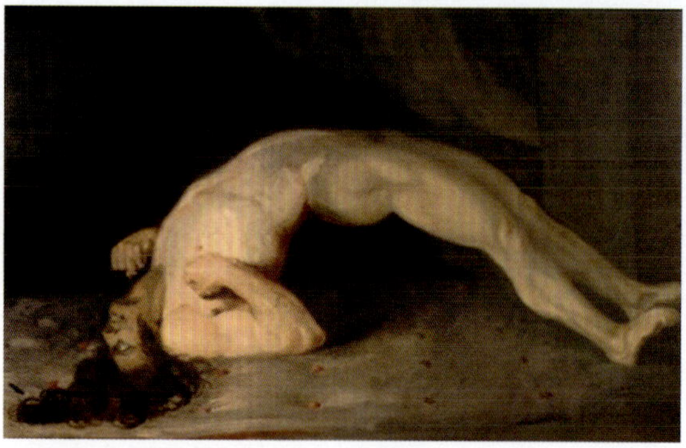

FIGURE 52.1 Opisthotonos in a patient suffering from tetanus; painting by Sir Charles Bell, 1809. Dr. Bell was a noted artist as well as physician (see Chapter 16).

trunk arched forward (Figure 52.1). Rigidity may be absent in meningitis when the disease is fulminating or terminal, when the patient is in coma, or in infants.

Stiffness and rigidity of the neck may occur in other conditions. A common problem is to distinguish restricted neck motion due to cervical spondylosis or osteoarthritis from nuchal rigidity. Patients with osteoarthritis typically have difficulty with rotation and lateral bending of the neck; these motions are usually preserved in patients who have meningismus, unless the meningeal irritation is extremely severe. Restricted neck motion may also occur with retropharyngeal abscess, cervical lymphadenopathy, neck trauma and as a nonspecific manifestation in severe systemic infections. Extrapyramidal disorders, particularly progressive supranuclear palsy, may also cause diffuse rigidity of the neck muscles. Meningeal signs may occur with increased spinal fluid pressure, and nuchal rigidity may be a manifestation of cerebellar tonsillar (foramen magnum) herniation. Meningeal irritation may also cause resistance to movement of the legs and back, with the patient lying with legs drawn up and resisting passive extension.

Kernig's Sign

There is some variability in the descriptions of how to elicit a Kernig's sign. Kernig described an involuntary flexion at the knee when the examiner attempted to flex the hip with the knee extended. The more common method is to flex the hip and knee to right angles and then attempt to passively extend the knee; this movement produces pain, resistance, and inability to fully extend the knee.

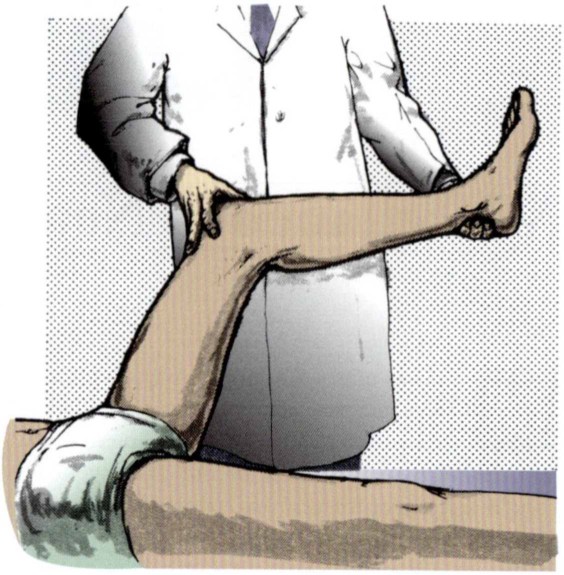

FIGURE 52.2 Method of eliciting Kernig's sign.

Another definition of Kernig's sign is inability to extend the knee to over 135 degrees while the hip is flexed (Figure 52.2). There is some overlap between Kernig's sign and Lasègue's (straight leg raising) sign. The technique is similar, but Lasègue's sign is used to check for root irritation in lumbosacral radiculopathy (see Chapter 47). Both Kernig's sign and straight leg raising are positive in meningitis because of diffuse inflammation of the nerve roots and meninges, and positive with acute lumbosacral radiculopathy because of focal inflammation of the affected root. In radiculopathy, the signs are usually unilateral, but in meningitis they are bilateral.

Brudzinski's Neck Sign

Placing one hand under the patient's head and flexing the neck while holding down the chest with the other hand causes flexion of the hips and knees bilaterally (Figure 52.3). With severe meningismus, it may not be possible to hold the chest down, and the patient may be pulled into a sitting position with only the examiner's hand behind the head. Occasionally, there may be extension of the hallux and fanning of the toes, and sometimes arm flexion. The leg may fail to flex on one side when meningeal irritation and hemiplegia coexist. The three tests, straight leg raise, Kernig's, and Brudzinski's, can quickly be done in that order.

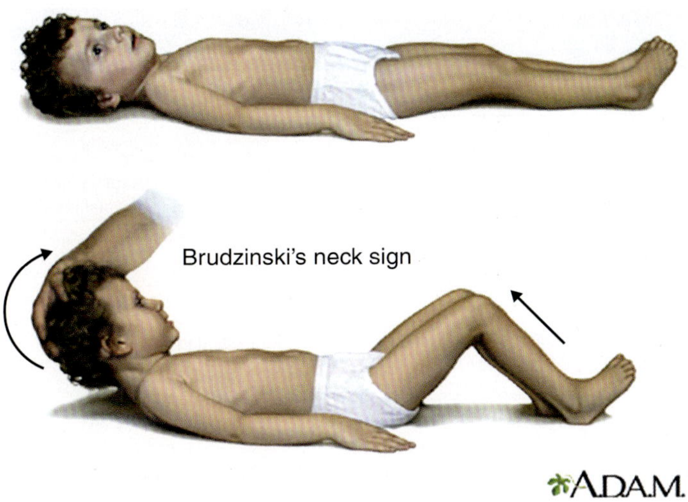

FIGURE 52.3 Brudzinski's sign. Flexing the neck causes the knees to flex.

Other Meningeal Signs

Jolt accentuation refers to an exacerbation of headache induced by quick, horizontal head rotations at two or three times per second. The 1999 rational clinical examination review concluded that in patients with fever and headache, jolt accentuation is a useful adjunct, with a sensitivity of 100%, specificity of 54%, positive likelihood ratio of 2.2, and negative likelihood ratio of 0 for the diagnosis of meningitis, but subsequent investigations have been less enthusiastic.

To avoid spinal flexion, the patient with meningitis may sit in bed with the hands placed far behind, the head thrown back, the hips and knees flexed, and the back arched (Amoss's, Hoyne's, or tripod sign). Other meningeal signs are summarized in Table 52.1. Brudzinski described several signs of meningeal inflammation in patients with tuberculous meningitis that likely reflected involvement of the parenchyma more than the meninges.

SIGNS OF TETANY

The clinical manifestations of tetany include spasm and tonic contractions of the skeletal muscles, principally the distal muscles of the extremities. There may be carpopedal spasm, with tonic contraction of the muscles of the wrists, hands, fingers, feet, and toes (see Chapter 30). There is hyperexcitability of the entire peripheral nervous system, as well as the musculature, to even minimal stimuli. Sensory nerve involvement may cause paresthesias in the hands, feet, and perioral region. Tetany is related to hypocalcemia, hypomagnesemia, or alkalosis. Either hypocalcemia or alkalosis causes a decrease in the ionized calcium level. Certain neurologic signs may be present that aid in making a diagnosis on the basis of the clinical examination alone. They are more easily obtained if the patient first hyperventilates for a few minutes (latent tetany). Severe tetany may cause seizures, laryngospasm, stridor, and respiratory arrest.

Chvostek's Sign

Tapping over the facial nerve causes a twitch, spasm, or tetanic, cramp-like contraction of some or all of the ipsilateral facial muscles (Table 16.2). Two points of stimulation have been described: just below the zygomatic process of the temporal bone, in front of the ear (Chvostek's sign), and midway between the zygomatic arch and the angle of the mouth (Schultz's sign). Sometimes, the response may be elicited merely by stroking the skin in front of the ear. The sign is minimal if only a slight twitch of the upper lip or the angle of the mouth results, moderate if there is movement of the ala nasi and the entire corner of the mouth, and maximal if the muscles of the forehead, eyelid, and cheek also contract (see **Video Link 52.1**). When the response is marked, even muscles supplied by the trigeminal nerve may respond. Chvostek's sign is the result of a hyperexcitability of the motor nerves, in this instance the facial nerve, to mechanical stimulation. It is an important sign in tetany but may occur in other conditions in which there is hyperreflexia, such as in lesions of the corticospinal tract, and in

TABLE 52.1 Miscellaneous Neurologic Signs

Sign	Technique	Finding	Significance
Bikele sign	With elbow flexed, shoulder abducted, elevated, and externally rotated, examiner attempts to passively extend the elbow	Resistance to elbow extension	Similar to Kernig's sign in that it stretches irritated nerve roots; positive in meningeal inflammation and in brachial plexitis
Brudzinski's contralateral leg sign	Passive flexion of one hip, especially with the knee extended, or passive knee extension after the hip has been flexed to a right angle	Flexion of the opposite hip and knee	Meningeal inflammation
Brudzinski's reciprocal contralateral leg sign	One knee and hip are flexed with the other leg extended; then the flexed limb is lowered	Contralateral extended leg goes into flexion	Meningeal inflammation
Brudzinski's cheek sign	Pressure against the cheeks on or just below the zygoma	Flexion at the elbows with an upward jerking of the arms	Meningeal inflammation
Brudzinski's symphysis sign	Pressure on the symphysis pubis	Flexion of both lower extremities	Meningeal inflammation
Guilland's sign	Pinching the skin over the quadriceps femoris muscle or squeezing the muscle on one side	Flexion of contralateral hip and knee	Meningeal inflammation
Edelmann great toe phenomenon	Flexion of the hip with the knee extended	Extension of the great toe	Meningeal inflammation
Tonic plantar reflex	Stroking sole of foot	Slow flexion and adduction of toes and distal part of the foot that persists for a minute or two	Prefrontal and extrapyramidal involvement; may be contralateral, ipsilateral, or bilateral with respect to the lesion
Soderbergh pressure reflex	Firm stroking of certain bony prominences	Slow muscular contraction (e.g., stroking the ulna causing flexion of the medial three fingers, stroking the radius causing thumb flexion)	Pyramidal and extrapyramidal disorders
Schrijver-Bernhard reflex	Percussing anterior surface of the leg or tapping over tibia or anterior leg muscles just below the knee	Plantar flexion of toes	Pyramidal and extrapyramidal disorders; a distant toe flexor reflex
Lomadtse sign	Pressure over anterior aspect of tibia	Plantar flexion of toes	Pyramidal and extrapyramidal disorders; a distant toe flexor reflex

children with epilepsy. It is present in a majority of neonates and disappears during childhood.

Chvostek's sign is elicited by percussing over the pes anserinus. The motor Tinel's sign has been reported as evidence of abnormal mechanosensitivity in entrapment neuropathies but may also occur in normals. Both Chvostek's sign and the Lust peroneal phenomenon (Table 52.2) are probably examples of a motor Tinel's sign.

Trousseau's Sign

Ischemia of the peripheral nerve trunks increases nerve excitability and causes spontaneous discharges. Compression of the arm by manual pressure, a tourniquet, or a sphygmomanometer cuff is followed first by distal paresthesias that progress centripetally, then by twitching of the fingers, and finally by cramping and contraction of the muscles of the fingers and hand with the thumb strongly adducted and the fingers stiffened, slightly flexed at the metacarpophalangeal joints, and forming a cone clustered about the thumb (obstetrician's or accoucheur's hand, *main d'accoucheur*, Figure 52.4, see **Video Link 52.2**). There may be a latent period of 1/2 to 4 minutes. Similar pressure around the leg or thigh will cause pedal spasm. A modification is to keep a moderately inflated sphygmomanometer cuff on one arm for about 10 minutes and then remove it and have the patient hyperventilate; typical tetanic spasm occurs

TABLE 52.2 Other Signs of Tetany

Sign	Technique	Finding
Pool-Schlesinger's	Forceful abduction and elevation of the arm to produce tension on the brachial plexus; or forceful flexion of the thigh on the trunk while the leg is extended to stretch the sciatic nerve	Tetanic spasm of the muscles of the forearm, hand, and fingers; or spasm of the muscles of the leg and foot
Schultze's	Mechanical stimulation of protruded tongue (e.g., by tapping with a percussion hammer)	Transient depression or dimpling at the site of stimulation (similar response may occur in myotonia or myotonic dystrophy)
Kashida thermic	Application of either hot or cold irritants	Hyperesthesias and spasms
Escherich's	Percussion of the inner surface of the lips or percussion of the tongue	Contractions of the lips, masseters, and tongue
Hochsinger's	Pressure on inner aspect of biceps muscle	Spasm and contraction of the hand (may be a variation of Trousseau sign)
Peroneal (Lust phenomenon)	Tapping over the common peroneal nerve as it winds around the neck of the fibula	Dorsiflexion and eversion of the foot

earlier in the previously ischemic arm. Trousseau's sign is more specific than Chvostek's sign for latent tetany. As many as 4% of healthy controls may have a positive Trousseau's sign; its sensitivity is unknown, but it can be absent in patients with definite hypocalcemia.

Other signs of tetany are reviewed in Table 52.2.

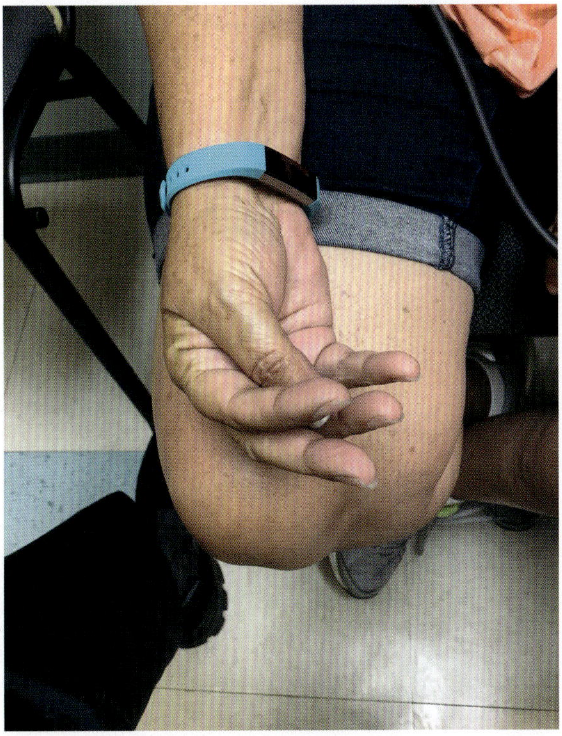

FIGURE 52.4 Trousseau's sign in hypocalcemia. The wrist and metacarpophalangeal joints are flexed, the interphalangeal joints are hyperextended, and the thumb is opposed.

Video Links

Video Link 52.1. Chvostek's sign. https://www.youtube.com/watch?v=kvmwsTU0InQ

Video Link 52.2. Trousseau's sign. https://www.youtube.com/watch?v=kvmwsTU0InQ

BIBLIOGRAPHY

Afhami S, Dehghan Manshadi SA, Rezahosseini O. Jolt accentuation of headache: can this maneuver rule out acute meningitis? *BMC Res Notes* 2017;10:540.

Agarwal KS, Baijal N, Tiwari L, et al. Swan-neck sign of the big toe–association with hypocalcaemia. *Trop Doct* 2007;37:238–239.

Athappan G, Ariyamuthu VK. Images in clinical medicine. Chvostek's sign and carpopedal spasm. *N Engl J Med* 2009;360:e24.

Attia J, Hatala R, Cook DJ, et al. The rational clinical examination. Does this adult patient have acute meningitis? *JAMA* 1999;282:175–181.

Forgie SE. The history and current relevance of the eponymous signs of meningitis. *Pediatr Infect Dis J* 2016;35:749–751.

Kamalanathan S, Balachandran K, Parthan G, et al. Chvostek's sign: a video demonstration. *BMJ Case Rep* 2012;2012. pii: bcr2012007098.

Méneret A, Guey S, Degos B. Chvostek sign, frequently found in healthy subjects, is not a useful clinical sign. *Neurology* 2013;80:1067.

Montagna P, Liguori R. The motor Tinel sign: a useful sign in entrapment neuropathy? *Muscle Nerve* 2000;23:976–978.

Nakao JH, Jafri FN, Shah K, et al. Jolt accentuation of headache and other clinical signs: poor predictors of meningitis in adults. *Am J Emerg Med* 2014;32:24–28.

Narayan SK, Sivaprasad P, Sahoo RN, et al. Teaching video NeuroImage: Chvostek sign with Fahr syndrome in a patient with hypoparathyroidism. *Neurology* 2008;71:e79.

Rehman HU, Wunder S. Trousseau sign in hypocalcemia. *CMAJ* 2011;183:E498.

Uchihara T, Tsukagoshi H. Jolt accentuation of headache: the most sensitive sign of CSF pleocytosis. *Headache* 1991;31:167–171.

SECTION **M** Diagnosis and Localization of Neurologic Disease

CHAPTER 53

Diagnostic Reasoning and Neurologic Differential Diagnosis

Epistemological research into the science of clinical diagnostic reasoning has identified three strategies: probabilistic, causal, and deterministic. Probabilistic reasoning depends on the statistical likelihood of clinical factors and is particularly useful for formulating diagnostic hypotheses and determining the significance of clinical findings. Differential diagnosis is commonly considered in order of probability. Occam's razor, or the principle of parsimony, states that the most likely solution is the simplest. In terms of medical diagnosis, it means that the least complex diagnosis is most likely to be correct, or never make two diagnoses when one will do. The precepts of Bayes' theorem, which takes into account the prevalence of a disease in the population and the results of prior tests, are often considered intuitively if not formally in probabilistic reasoning. When the prevalence of a disease is low, a positive test result is likely to be a false positive unless the test has very high specificity.

Causal reasoning relies on a pathophysiologic model and determines the consistency of the clinical findings in relation to the model. Causal reasoning is particularly important in testing diagnostic hypotheses. Deterministic reasoning employs rules, primarily of an "if-then" character, often depicted as flow charts or other graphic displays. "Fisher's rules" are clinical maxims collected by Caplan from his observations of C. Miller Fisher, a clinician of legendary diagnostic acumen. Some of these axioms are particularly helpful to bear in mind (Table 53.1).

Errors in clinical reasoning can lead to a variety of adverse consequences. A common error in diagnostic reasoning is accepting a diagnosis before it is fully verified (premature closure). Kassirer and Kopelman, in a study of diagnostic errors caused by faulty clinical cognition, found that the two most common sources of error lay in faulty triggering (failure to recognize a possible diagnostic hypothesis) and in faulty information gathering and processing. In the latter category, the most common errors related to faulty estimation of disease prevalence (the dictates of Bayes' theorem) and faulty data interpretation.

In a study of common errors in daily practice among neurology residents, the overall rate of diagnostic error and the frequency of diagnostic inaccuracy in various disease entities showed that the initial bedside diagnosis was correct in 67% of patients. The highest rates of inaccuracy were found in the diagnosis of subdural hematoma, myasthenia gravis (MG), subarachnoid hemorrhage (SAH), and Guillain-Barré syndrome (GBS). The common causes of diagnostic inaccuracy were errors of reasoning, an inadequate patient database, and an inadequate fund of knowledge. In a prospective study of the accuracy of bedside diagnoses on a neurology service, patients were evaluated independently by a junior resident, a senior resident, and a staff neurologist. Each individual was

TABLE 53.1 Fisher's Rules: A Selection of Axioms Relevant to Clinical Reasoning and Diagnostic Principles

- In arriving at a clinical diagnosis, think of the five most common findings (historical, physical findings, or laboratory) found in a given disorder. If at least three of these five are not present in a given patient, the diagnosis is likely to be wrong.
- Resist the temptation to prematurely place a case or disorder into a diagnostic cubbyhole that fits poorly. Allowing it to remain unknown stimulates continuing activity and thought.
- The details of a case are important; their analysis distinguishes the expert from the journeyman.
- Pay particular attention to the specifics of the patient with a known diagnosis; it will be helpful later when similar phenomena occur in an unknown case.
- Fully accept what you have heard or read only when you have verified it yourself.
- Maintain a lively interest in patients as people.

required to make an anatomical and etiologic diagnosis based solely on the history and physical examination. In 40 patients with laboratory-confirmed final diagnoses, the clinical diagnoses of the junior residents, senior residents, and staff neurologists were correct in 65%, 75%, and 77%, respectively. The errors by the junior residents, <senior residents>, and (staff) were attributed to incomplete history and examination in 4 <1> (0), inadequate fund of knowledge in 4 <3> (3), and poor diagnostic reasoning in 6 <6> (6). Thus, experience beyond a certain level is not necessarily a cure for faulty reasoning. Vickery et al. presented five common sources of cognitive diagnostic error: framing effects, anchoring, the availability heuristic, pattern misrecognition, and blind obedience and overreliance on test results without considering sensitivity and specificity.

In *Thinking Fast and Slow*, Daniel Kahneman, popularized the notion of System 1 and System 2 thinking. System 1 is quick and intuitive; System 2 is slow and deliberate. Medical educators have written about System 1, or Type 1, and System 2, or Type 2, as applied to medical diagnosis. The repetitive application of System 2 through accumulated experience, reading and study leads to the increasing use of System 1 diagnostic processes. This is a repackaging of the notion of pattern recognition. The idea that as skill and experience accumulate, clinicians evolve toward a pattern recognition approach is nothing new. The medical, and the medicolegal, literature, make it abundantly clear how common diagnostic errors are. The writing about System 1 and System 2, thinking fast and slow, point toward a potentially helpful countermeasure: slow down and think.

NEUROLOGIC DIFFERENTIAL DIAGNOSIS

Pathologic processes behave in certain ways depending on their location in the nervous system and in certain other ways related to their inherent natures. Neurologists deal in two basic clinical exercises: where is the lesion in the nervous system and what is the lesion in the nervous system or differential diagnosis by location and differential diagnosis by pathophysiology or etiology. The anatomic diagnosis and the etiologic diagnosis aid and support each other. In general, the neurologic examination aids primarily in establishing the anatomic or localization diagnosis and the history aids in the etiologic diagnosis, but there is overlap. The examination also serves to indicate the severity of the abnormality. A dependence on neuroimaging and other tests as the primary approach to diagnosis causes many errors. Defining the patient's illness first in terms of anatomy and likely etiology helps insure the appropriate use of neurodiagnostic studies.

Pathophysiologically, disease of the nervous system may cause manifestations because of destruction, release, "irritation," and partial assumption of function by healthy tissues. Symptoms and signs of destruction result from a transient or permanent loss of function similar to the manifestations of disease commonly found in other body systems. Peripheral nerve injury causes weakness, sensory loss, and areflexia in the distribution of the nerve. Destruction of the cerebral cortex may cause paresis, hypesthesia, blindness, or intellectual loss. Symptoms related to release of function occur when there is disease of a portion of the nervous system that has an inhibitory function. Some responses may be exaggerated because of disinhibition and the release of intact centers from higher control. A lesion of the corticospinal system is often followed by increased muscle tone, increased reflexes, and the presence of certain pathologic reflexes. These are positive rather than negative signs of disturbed function. Positive signs are apparent in a different manner in the presence of overactivity, excitation, or "irritation" of a part of the nervous system. Characteristic examples are the pain and muscle spasm that follow disease of a peripheral nerve and convulsions causing increased motor activity. Partial assumption of function by healthy tissues may compensate for loss of function because of disease in another part. There is a certain amount of overlapping and duplication of function in the nervous system; an intact center, nerve, or muscle may assume some of the physiologic activity of a diseased part. In some parts of the nervous system, large lesions may cause a paucity of signs and symptoms because of a minimum of physiologic activity of the part, duplication of function, or compensation elsewhere.

ANATOMICAL DIAGNOSIS

The patterns of abnormality help to localize a disease process to a particular part of the nervous system. Clinical features that are particularly helpful in neurologic differential diagnosis include the distribution of any weakness; the presence or absence of sensory symptoms; the presence or absence of pain; the presence or absence of cranial nerve abnormalities and whether they are ipsilateral or contralateral to the other abnormalities on examination; the status of the reflexes; the presence of pathologic reflexes; involvement of bowel and bladder function; and the presence or absence of symptoms that clearly indicate cortical involvement, such as seizures, aphasia, or altered mental status (AMS). Weakness may be unilateral or bilateral, symmetric or asymmetric, primarily proximal or primarily distal; each of these patterns has differential diagnostic significance. The pattern of sensory abnormalities also provides significant information.

It may be helpful to organize the nervous system anatomically by considering sequentially more peripheral or central structures, beginning either at the cerebral cortex or the muscle. Consider each level where disease tends to have a characteristic and reproducible clinical profile. At each major level, disease processes tend to have characteristic clinical features, although with some degree of overlap. For example, disease involving the muscle, neuromuscular junction (NMJ), peripheral nervous system (PNS), nerve roots, spinal cord, brainstem, and hemispheres each tend to produce a characteristic clinical picture. These are discussed in the following sections. Most of these levels can be further subdivided to narrow the differential diagnosis. Some diseases cause multifocal or diffuse abnormalities, and these are often particularly challenging. By trying to localize the disease process to one or two likely levels, such as muscle or NMJ, one can think more systematically about the etiologic possibilities. Manifestations of disease in different locations can sometimes be similar, causing confusion. Extraocular muscle dysfunction due to MG can simulate an internuclear ophthalmoplegia. Deafferentation due to peripheral nerve or posterior column disease can cause sensory ataxia difficult to distinguish from cerebellar disease. Distinguishing early GBS from early transverse myelopathy can be difficult.

Assuming the process under consideration is indeed neurologic, the first major attempt at localization should be to decide if the pathologic process likely lies in the PNS or the central nervous system (CNS). For purposes of this discussion, the PNS includes the NMJ and the muscle. Clinical features helpful in distinguishing PNS disease from CNS disease are summarized in Table 53.2. Some neurologic signs and symptoms occur very commonly in both CNS and PNS diseases, and arriving at the correct diagnosis sometimes depends more on analyzing the associated findings than the presenting manifestation. Some of the abnormalities that occur commonly in both peripheral and central disease include abnormal pupils, ptosis, diplopia, dysphagia, dysarthria, weakness, sensory loss, and difficulty walking.

CLINICAL MANIFESTATIONS OF DISEASE

The following paragraphs provide a brief summary of the clinical manifestations of disease at different levels of the nervous system, from muscle to cerebral cortex.

Myopathy

Myopathies are those conditions in which there is a primary dysfunction of skeletal muscle. Ten clinical patterns of presentation have been recognized (Table 53.3). Most patients with muscle disease usually have symmetric, proximal weakness, also referred to as the limb-girdle pattern of weakness (MP1 pattern, Table 53.3). Patients with muscle disease usually have symmetric, proximal weakness. They have trouble getting up from a chair, difficulty getting out of a car, and difficulty raising their arms overhead. Patients often have difficulty with everyday grooming activities, such as shaving or handling hair and makeup. Early on, patients with acquired muscle disease switch from tub baths to showers because they cannot get out of the tub. The examination typically reveals proximal weakness reflecting the clinical complaint. Reflexes are usually preserved unless the muscle weakness is very severe. There are no pathologic reflexes. There is

TABLE 53.2 Clinical Features That Suggest Central (Brain and Spinal Cord) versus Peripheral (Roots, Plexi, Peripheral Nerves, Neuromuscular Junctions, and Muscle) Nervous System Disease

Central Nervous System Disease	Peripheral Nervous System Disease
Lack of pain	Pain
Hemidistribution weakness	Symmetric, generalized weakness; very focal weakness (e.g., peripheral nerve distribution)
Hemidistribution sensory loss	Stocking-glove sensory loss
Crossed or dissociated sensory loss (e.g., Brown-Séquard syndrome)	Dermatomal or peripheral nerve distribution sensory loss
Hyperreflexia or clonus	Hyporeflexia
Muscle spasticity or hypertonia	Fluctuating weakness
Babinski's sign	Myotonia
Lhermitte's sign	Significant muscle atrophy
Abnormal involuntary movements (e.g., chorea)	Increased CK
Seizures	Abnormal EMG
Bowel, bladder, or sexual dysfunction	
Headache	
Meningeal signs	
Visual loss	
Abnormal pupils	
Crossed signs	
Cerebellar signs	
Presence of a bruit	
Altered mental status	
Dementia	
Focal cortical signs (aphasia, apraxia, etc.)	
Abnormal head or spine MRI	
Abnormal EEG	
Abnormal evoked potentials	

CK, creatine kinase; EEG, electroencephalogram; EMG, electromyogram; MRI, magnetic resonance imaging.

no sensory loss; bowel and bladder dysfunction generally do not occur; and there are no defects in coordination, mentation, or higher cortical function. The gait in myopathy is often abnormal, characteristically with a waddling character **(Video 44.1)**. Atrophy is not prominent unless the process is severe, as in some dystrophies. Pseudohypertrophy may occur in dystrophies, particularly dystrophinopathies (Figure 29.7). Patients may or may not have muscle pain, tenderness, or soreness, but usually they do not. Some muscle disorders are accompanied by myotonia. Many muscle diseases can cause rhabdomyolysis and myoglobinuria.

Although most myopathies cause symmetric proximal weakness, some conditions cause weakness with other patterns (Table 53.3). The distal myopathies are a group of conditions, mostly hereditary, that produces primarily distal weakness. The most common distal myopathy is myotonic dystrophy (MP2 pattern). A pattern of weakness involving the proximal upper extremities, particularly the periscapular region, and distal lower extremities is the scapuloperoneal pattern (MP3 pattern), and when the facial muscles are also weak, the most likely diagnosis is facioscapulohumeral muscular dystrophy. Weakness of the proximal lower extremities, particularly the quadriceps, and the distal upper extremities, particularly the wrist and finger flexors, occurs in inclusion body myositis (MP4 pattern). Other myopathies can have ptosis and ophthalmoplegia, neck weakness, and pharyngeal, tongue, or diaphragm weakness (MP5, MP6, MP7).

Myopathies can be divided into those that are inherited and those that occur sporadically, as this is often the initial step in clinical differential diagnostic thinking. A partial list of etiologies includes inflammatory myopathies, muscular dystrophies, congenital

TABLE 53.3 Clinical Patterns of Muscle Disorders

Pattern	Weakness				Episodic	Trigger	Diagnosis
	Proximal	Distal	Asymmetric	Symmetric			
MP1 Limb-girdle	+	–	–	+	–	–	Most myopathies, hereditary and acquired
MP2* Distal	–	+	–	+	+		Distal myopathies (also neuropathies)
MP3 Proximal arm/distal leg scapuloperoneal	+ Arm	+ Leg	+ (FSH)	+ (Others)	–	–	FSH, Emery-Dreifuss, acid maltase, congenital scapuloperoneal
MP4 Distal arm/proximal leg	+ Leg	+ Arm	+	–	–	–	IBM Myotonic dystrophy
MP5 Ptosis/ophthalmoplegia	+	–	+ (MG)	+ (Others)	–	–	OPMD, MG, myotonic dystrophy, mitochondria
MP6* Symmetric sensory loss and upper motor neuron signs	+	–	–	+	+	+	INEM, MG (also ALS)
MP7* Symmetric weakness without sensory loss	+	–	–	+	–	–	MG, LEMS, OPMD (also ALS)
MP8 Episodic weakness/pain/Rhabdomyolysis + trigger	+	–	–	+	+	+	McArdle, CPT, drugs, toxins
MP9 Episodic weakness Delayed or unrelated to exercise	+	–	–	+	+	+/–	Primary periodic paralysis Channelopathies Na^{++} Ca^{++} Secondary periodic paralysis
MP10—Stiffness/inability to relax	–	–	–	–	+	+/–	Myotonic dystrophy, Channelopathies, PROMM, rippling (also stiff-person, neuromyotonia)

*Overlap patterns with neuropathy/motor neuron disease.
ALS, amyotrophic lateral sclerosis; CPT, carnitine palmityl transferase; FSH, facioscapulohumeral muscular dystrophy; LEMS, Lambert-Eaton myasthenic syndrome; MG, myasthenia gravis; OPMD, oculopharyngeal muscular dystrophy; PROMM, proximal myotonic myopathy.

myopathies, metabolic and mitochondrial myopathies, toxic myopathies, and myopathies arising as a complication of many different systemic disorders. The causes of myopathy are legion (Table 53.4).

Neuromuscular Junction Disorders

The cardinal manifestation of diseases involving the NMJ is weakness because of impaired neuromuscular transmission (NMT). The character and distribution of the weakness and associated manifestations vary among the different conditions. The most common conditions encountered clinically are MG and the Lambert-Eaton myasthenic syndrome (LEMS). However, the most common condition by far is MG. Table 53.5 summarizes the clinical characteristics of these two conditions. Other rare disorders that can cause clinically significant NMT disorders include botulism, hypermagnesemia, and exposure to some toxins.

The most common initial pattern of presentation for NMJ disorders is ocular (MP5). Patients with NMJ disorders can also have symmetric, proximal muscle weakness (MP1 pattern), neck weakness (MP6 pattern), and bulbar or respiratory weakness (MP7 pattern). Ocular involvement produces weakness of eye movement causing diplopia and ptosis of one or both eyelids. Bulbar involvement produces dysphagia and dysarthria, with a tendency to nasal regurgitation of fluids. The weakness typically varies and fluctuates with the level of activity and with the time of day (MP9 pattern). Often weakness grows worse as the day progresses. There is no pain or sensory loss. Deep tendon reflexes (DTRs) remain

TABLE 53.4 Common Primary Muscle Diseases

I. Inherited diseases
  A. Dystrophies
    1. Dystrophinopathies (Duchenne's muscular dystrophy, Becker's muscular dystrophy, others)
    2. Myotonic dystrophy
    3. Facioscapulohumeral dystrophy
    4. Limb-girdle dystrophy
    5. Congenital dystrophies (Fukuyama, etc.)
  B. Metabolic
    1. Mitochondriopathies (ragged red fiber diseases [Kearns-Sayre syndrome, MELAS, MERRF, etc.])
    2. Glycogenoses (McArdle's disease, phosphofructokinase deficiency)
    3. Lipid myopathies (carnitine deficiency, carnitine palmitoyltransferase deficiency)
  C. Congenital myopathies
    1. Nemaline myopathy
    2. Central core disease
    3. Myotubular myopathy
    4. Congenital fiber type disproportion
  D. Channelopathies
    1. Myotonia congenita
    2. Periodic paralysis
    3. Malignant hyperthermia
II. Acquired diseases
  A. Inflammatory myopathies
    1. Polymyositis, dermatomyositis
    2. Inclusion body myositis
    3. Myopathies related to infection (HIV, HTLV-1, parasites)
  B. Myopathies complicating systemic illness
    1. Endocrine myopathies
    2. Sarcoidosis
    3. Critical illness myopathy
  C. Toxic myopathies
  D. Rhabdomyolysis

HTLV-1, human T-cell lymphotropic virus type 1; MELAS, mitochondrial encephalomyopathy, lactate acidosis, and stroke-like episodes; MERRF, myoclonic epilepsy with ragged red fiber disease.

normal in MG but may be depressed in LEMS and other presynaptic disorders. There are no pathologic reflexes.

Ptosis not present at rest can often be elicited by sustained upgaze, which fatigues the eyelid levators. Diplopia can be elicited at the bedside by prolonged gaze to the right or left or up or down. When involvement is limited to the extraocular muscles, eyelids, and orbicularis oculi, the condition is termed ocular or purely ocular myasthenia. With some patients, the disease may never progress beyond this point. In most, generalized myasthenia develops, usually within a year or 2, with eye symptoms remaining prominent. The differential diagnosis of MG includes other disorders that produce ocular and limb weakness such as thyroid eye disease, brainstem disease, mitochondrial myopathy, inflammatory myopathy, oculopharyngeal dystrophy, motor neuron disease, and cranial nerve compressive lesions.

Peripheral Neuropathy

Peripheral neuropathies are conditions that affect peripheral nerve axons, their myelin sheaths, or both. The cardinal manifestations of peripheral neuropathy are weakness, alterations in sensation, and reflex changes. Common causes of peripheral neuropathy include diabetes mellitus, alcoholism, and GBS. In many cases, the cause remains unknown, and these are referred to as idiopathic or cryptogenic. The term cryptogenic sensory polyneuropathy (CSPN, NP2 pattern, Table 53.6) is used for patients with a predominantly

TABLE 53.5 Comparison Between Myasthenia Gravis (MG) and Lambert-Eaton Syndrome

	MG	Lambert-Eaton Syndrome
Onset	2/3 of women before 40 y	After 40 y
Sex	Women:men, 4:3	Men:women, 5:1
Symptoms	Diplopia; ptosis; dysphagia; limb weakness and fatigability	Weakness and fatigability in legs; difficulty raising arms; dry mouth
Signs	Oculobulbar abnormality common; proximal limb weakness	Weakness of proximal legs; oculobulbar abnormality rare
Reflexes	Normal	Hypoactive or absent, obtainable after brief exercise or repeated taps
Brief exercise	Strength fatigable	Strength initially improves and later declines
Neoplasm	Thymoma in 15%	Small cell carcinoma of lung in 75%
Tensilon test	Definitely positive	Negative or mildly positive in some

Modified from Oh SJ. *Electromyography: Neuromuscular Transmission Studies*. Baltimore: Williams & Wilkins, 1988.

TABLE 53.6 Clinical Patterns of Peripheral Neuropathy

	Weakness								
Pattern	**Proximal**	**Dis**	**Asymm**	**Symm**	**Sensory Symptoms**	**Severe Proprioceptive Loss**	**UMN Signs**	**Autonomic Symps/Signs**	**Diagnosis**
NP1—Symmetric prox and distal weakness w/sensory loss	+	+		+	+				GBS/CIDP
NP2—Distal sensory loss with/without weakness		+		+	+				CSPN, metabolic, drugs, hereditary
NP3—Distal weakness with sensory loss		+	+		+				Multiple—Vasculitis, HNPP, MADSAM, infection Single—Mononeuropathy, radiculopathy
NP4—Asymmetric prox and distal weakness w/sensory loss	+	+	+		+				Polyradiculopathy, plexopathy
NP5—Asymmetric distal weakness w/out sensory loss		+	+				+/–		+ UMN – ALS Pure UMN – PLS – UMN – MMN, PMA, MAMA, BAD, LAD
NP6—Symmetric sensory loss and upper motor neuron signs		+		+	+	+	+		B_{12} deficiency; Copper deficiency, Friedreich's, adrenomyeloneuropathy
NP7*—Symmetric weakness without sensory loss	+/–	+		+					*Prox & Distal* SMA *Distal* Hereditary motor neuropathy
NP8*—Focal midline proximal symmetric weakness	+ Neck/extensor + Bulbar			+ +			+ +		ALS
NP9—Asymmetric proprioceptive loss w/out weakness			+		+	+			Sensory neuronopathy (ganglionopathy)
NP10—Autonomic dysfunction								+	HSAN, diabetes, GBS, amyloid, porphyria, Fabry's

ALS, amyotrophic lateral sclerosis; BAD, brachial amyotrophic diplegia; CIDP, chronic inflammatory demyelinating polyneuropathy; CSPN, cryptogenic sensory polyneuropathy; GBS, Guillain-Barré syndrome; HNPP, hereditary neuropathy with liability to pressure palsy; HSAN, hereditary sensory and autonomic neuropathy; LAD, leg amyotrophic diplegia; MADSAM, multifocal acquired demyelinating sensory and motor; MAMA, multifocal acquired motor axonopathy; MMN, multifocal motor neuropathy; PMA, progressive muscular atrophy; SMA, spinal muscular atrophy; UMN, upper motor neuron.

sensory neuropathy with no identifiable cause. Patients with generalized polyneuropathy have symmetric, predominantly distal weakness, sensory loss, depressed or absent DTRs, no pathologic reflexes, and no bowel or bladder dysfunction. Pain is a common accompaniment and often a major clinical feature. Although it is a good general rule that muscle disease causes proximal weakness and generalized peripheral nerve disease causes distal weakness, there are exceptions. For instance, myotonic dystrophy is a common muscular dystrophy that produces distal weakness, and GBS is a common peripheral nerve disease that frequently produces proximal weakness. A pattern recognition approach to peripheral neuropathies can be used similar to the myopathy approach (Table 53.3). Proximal weakness in demyelinating neuropathies is presumably due to demyelination involving both long and short nerve fibers (NP1); neuropathies with only distal weakness are usually due to an axonal process (NP2).

Peripheral nerve diseases are divided into polyneuropathies (all the nerves are affected) and mononeuropathies. In multiple mononeuropathy (mononeuritis multiplex NP3 pattern), more than one nerve is affected but not all. With a mononeuropathy (NP3 pattern), symptoms and signs are specifically related to the affected nerve (see Chapter 46). Table 53.7 lists some of the etiologies of peripheral nerve disease but is far from exhaustive.

Nerve fibers react to injury through two primary mechanisms: axonal degeneration and demyelination. In axonal neuropathies, the primary pathology is degeneration of the axonal cytoplasm. Wallerian degeneration specifically refers to the axonal degeneration distal to a traumatic nerve injury. In demyelinating neuropathies, the primary insult is to the myelin sheath or the Schwann cell. The ultimate goal in neuropathy evaluations is to establish a precise etiologic diagnosis in order to guide treatment, if any is available. The most important exercise is to distinguish demyelinating neuropathy from axonopathy (Table 53.8). In compression neuropathies, the demyelination is focal and involves only a discrete segment of nerve (segmental demyelination, e.g., carpal tunnel syndrome).

TABLE 53.7 Some Causes of Peripheral Neuropathy

Inflammatory demyelinating neuropathy
Acute inflammatory demyelinating polyradiculoneuropathy (Guillain-Barré syndrome)
Chronic inflammatory demyelinating polyradiculoneuropathy
Infectious and granulomatous neuropathy
Leprosy
Sarcoid
HIV related
Hepatitis B/C
Lyme disease
Neuropathy associated with systemic disease
Diabetes
Chronic renal disease
Alcoholism
Paraproteinemia
Dysimmune neuropathies
Hypothyroidism
Vitamin deficiency
Paraneoplastic neuropathy
Amyloidosis
Connective tissue disease
Critical illness polyneuropathy
Ischemic neuropathy
Peripheral vascular disease
Vasculitis
Metabolic neuropathy
Porphyria
Leukodystrophy
Lipidosis
Bassen-Kornzweig disease
Tangier disease
Refsum's disease
Fabry's disease
Hereditary neuropathy
Hereditary motor sensory neuropathies (HMSN, Charcot-Marie-Tooth disease and variants)
Hereditary sensory autonomic neuropathies (HSAN)
Hereditary neuropathy with liability to pressure palsies (tomaculous neuropathy)
Toxins
Pharmaceuticals
Environmental toxins

Modified from Campbell WW. *Essentials of Electrodiagnostic Medicine*. Philadelphia: Lippincott Williams & Wilkins, 1999.

Plexopathy

Diseases involving the brachial plexus are much more common than those involving the lumbosacral plexus. Patients with plexus disorders have clinical deficits that mirror the involved structures, so a knowledge of plexus anatomy is vital to deciphering the deficit. There is typically both weakness and sensory loss involving all or part of an extremity (NP4 pattern, Table 53.6), accompanied by depressed or absent DTRs in the involved area, no pathologic reflexes, and no bowel or bladder dysfunction. Other neurologic functions are intact. The most common cause of plexopathy is neuralgia amyotrophy, but diabetes and neoplastic are also common. Plexopathy is discussed in more detail in Chapter 46.

TABLE 53.8 Clinical Features That Help Distinguish Axonopathy from Myelinopathy

Axonopathy	Myelinopathy
• Insidious onset • Slow progression • Slow recovery • Evidence of length dependency • Loss of ankle jerks with presence of other reflexes • Stocking distribution sensory loss • Weakness limited to distal muscles • Symmetry • Normal CSF protein	• More rapid onset • More rapid recovery • Mild asymmetry • Global loss of reflexes • Proximal or diffuse weakness • Cranial nerve involvement • Motor > sensory dysfunction • Increased CSF protein

CSF, cerebrospinal fluid.
Modified from Campbell WW. *Essentials of Electrodiagnostic Medicine.* Philadelphia: Lippincott Williams & Wilkins, 1999.

Radiculopathy

Most radiculopathies are due to disc herniations or spondylosis. When severe, there are both motor and sensory deficits and a depressed DTR in the distribution of the involved root(s). Pain is common and often severe, usually accompanied by pain and limitation of motion of either the neck or lower back, along with signs of root irritability, such as a positive straight leg raising test. There are no pathologic reflexes and no bowel or bladder dysfunction. The presence of these findings suggests that there is concomitant spinal cord compression. Radiculopathy is discussed in more detail in Chapter 47.

Neuronopathy

Neuronopathies are disorders of the motor or sensory cell body. Motor neuronopathies are more common and are also referred to as motor neuron diseases. Amyotrophic lateral sclerosis (ALS) is the most common. ALS is an acquired disorder that most commonly affects both upper and lower motor neurons and usually presents with distal asymmetric weakness (NP5) or bulbar weakness (NP8). Both spinal muscular atrophy (SMA), an autosomal recessive condition with symmetric, proximal and distal weakness (NP7) and X-linked spinobulbar atrophy (NP8), primarily involve lower motor neurons. Sensory neuronopathies, also known as dorsal root ganglionopathies, cause asymmetric pure sensory loss and limb ataxia (NP9). The etiology is usually paraneoplastic.

Myelopathy

Spinal cord disorders often produce characteristic patterns of clinical abnormalities, with motor and sensory deficits in a certain distribution. Commonly seen patterns include transverse myelopathy, the Brown-Séquard (hemicord) syndrome, anterior cord syndrome, central cord syndrome, a syringomyelic pattern, posterolateral sclerosis or combined system disease, and an anterior horn syndrome (see Chapter 24). With transverse myelopathy, there is symmetric involvement causing bilateral weakness below a particular level, producing either paraparesis or quadriparesis. In addition to weakness below the level of the lesion, patients with spinal cord lesions may also have paresthesias, numbness, tingling, and sensory loss with a discrete sensory level, usually on the trunk. Common patterns of sensory loss are summarized in Table 53.9. The pattern of weakness is typically more localizing than sensory abnormalities in lesions of the cervical spinal cord, whereas the demonstration of a sensory level on the trunk is more helpful in localizing lesions of the thoracic cord. Bowel, bladder, and sexual dysfunction is common, often early and frequently severe. A false localizing sensory level can occur in compressive cervical myelopathies because the leg fibers are more superficial in the ascending spinothalamic tracts and more prone to compression.

Common causes of myelopathy include compression, trauma, and acute transverse myelitis. Spinal cord mass lesions are most commonly due to tumor, most often metastatic, abscess, or disc herniation. The lesion may be intramedullary, within the cord substance, or extramedullary, compressing the spinal cord or its blood supply. An extramedullary lesion may be intradural or extradural. Extradural tumors are generally malignant and the intradural tumors benign. A long duration of symptoms is more consistent with an intradural lesion. Other important causes of myelopathy include retroviral infection—HIV and human

TABLE 53.9 Findings on Sensory Examination That Are Strongly Suggestive of a Lesion of the Spinal Cord or Cauda Equina

Loss of position and vibratory sensation in the feet with preserved ankle jerks (dorsal cord syndrome)
Bilateral loss of position and vibratory sensation in the feet with a definite level of pinprick loss on the abdomen or chest (thoracic cord lesion)
Bilateral segmental sensory loss (i.e., sensory loss in the hands and forearms), not in a peripheral nerve distribution, with normal sensation in the legs and trunk and in the upper arms and neck (central cord syndrome, syringomyelia)
Loss of pinprick sensation on one side of the body with loss of position and vibration sensation on the other (Brown-Séquard syndrome)
Loss of pinprick sensation over the legs and trunk with normal sensation in the perianal area (intramedullary lesion or anterior extramedullary compression)
Loss of pinprick sensation in the perianal area and in the upper part of both posterior thighs (conus medullaris or L5-S1 cauda equina lesion)
Loss of pinprick sensation on the legs and trunk with normal position and vibration sense in the toes and fingers (anterior cord syndrome)

Modified from Woolsey RM, Young RR. The clinical diagnosis of disorders of the spinal cord. *Neurol Clin* 1991;9:573–583.

T-cell lymphotropic virus (HTLV) type 1—as well as B_{12} deficiency, connective tissue disorders, mucopolysaccharidosis, neurosarcoidosis, and radiation therapy.

Brainstem Disease

The classic distinguishing feature of brainstem pathology is that deficits are "crossed," with cranial nerve dysfunction on one side and a motor or sensory deficit on the opposite side. Common causes of brainstem disease include stroke, MS, and neoplasm. There are often symptoms reflecting dysfunction of other posterior fossa structures, such as vertigo, ataxia, dysphagia, nausea and vomiting, and abnormal eye movements. Unless the process has impaired the reticular activating system, patients are normal mentally, awake, alert, able to converse (though perhaps dysarthric), not confused, and not aphasic. The DTRs are usually hyperactive with accompanying pathologic reflexes in the involved extremities; pain is rare, and sphincter dysfunction occurs only if there is bilateral involvement. Brainstem disorders are discussed further in Chapter 21.

Cranial Neuropathy

Disease may selectively involve one, or occasionally more than one, cranial nerve. The long tract abnormalities, vertigo, ataxia, and similar symptoms and findings that are otherwise characteristic of intrinsic brainstem disease are lacking. Common cranial neuropathies include optic neuropathy due to MS, third nerve palsy due to aneurysm, and Bell's palsy. Involvement of more than one nerve occurs in conditions such as Lyme disease, sarcoidosis, and lesions involving the cavernous sinus. Cranial neuropathies are discussed further in Chapters 12 to 21.

Cerebellar Disease

Patients with cerebellar dysfunction suffer from various combinations of tremor, incoordination, difficulty walking, dysarthria, and nystagmus, depending on the parts of the cerebellum involved. There is no weakness, sensory loss, pain, hyperreflexia, pathologic reflexes, sphincter dyscontrol, or abnormalities of higher cortical function. When cerebellar abnormalities result from dysfunction of the cerebellar connections in the brainstem, there are usually other brainstem signs. Cerebellar disorders are discussed further in Chapter 43.

Basal Ganglia Disorders

Diseases of the basal ganglia cause movement disorders such as Parkinson's disease (PD) or Huntington's disease (HD). Movement disorders may be hypokinetic or hyperkinetic, referring to whether movement is in general decreased or increased. PD causes bradykinesia and rigidity. HD, in contrast, causes increased movements, which are involuntary and beyond the patient's control (chorea). Tremor is a frequent accompaniment of basal ganglia disease. Basal ganglia disorders are discussed further in Chapters 26 and 30.

Cerebral Hemisphere Disorders

Characteristic of unilateral hemispheric pathology is a "hemi" deficit: hemisensory loss, hemiparesis, hemianopsia, or perhaps hemiseizures. Other common manifestations include hyperreflexia and pathologic reflexes. Pain is not a feature unless the thalamus is involved, and there is no difficulty with sphincter control unless both hemispheres are involved. Within this framework, disease affecting the cerebral cortex behaves differently from disease of subcortical structures. Patients with cortical involvement may have aphasia, apraxia, astereognosis, impaired two-point discrimination, memory loss, cognitive defects, focal seizures, or other abnormalities that reflect the essential integrative role of the cortex. Processes affecting the dominant hemisphere often cause language dysfunction in the form of aphasia, alexia, or agraphia. With disease of the nondominant hemisphere, the patient may have higher cortical function disturbances involving functions other than language, such as apraxia. If the disease affects subcortical structures, the clinical picture includes the hemidistribution of dysfunction but lacks those elements that are typically cortical (e.g., language disturbance, apraxia, seizures, dementia). Certain processes involve wide areas of the cerebrum, causing diffuse dysfunction. In addition, some disorders may produce increased intracranial pressure, which creates additional abnormalities because of edema and pressure superimposed on the clinical manifestations related to the underlying pathology.

Multifocal/Diffuse Disorders

Some disease processes are diffuse or multifocal, producing dysfunction at more than one location, or involve a "system." For example, neuromyelitis optica (NMO) characteristically affects both the spinal cord and the optic nerves (i.e., it is multifocal). ALS is a system disorder causing diffuse dysfunction of the entire motor system from the spinal cord to the cerebral cortex, sparing sensation and higher cortical function.

Disorders of the Meninges, Ventricular System, and Intracranial Pressure

Many conditions can affect the meninges, including infections, neoplasia, sarcoidosis, and others. The most common disorders are infectious and present with evidence of infection and increased intracranial pressure. Some meningeal infections may be extremely indolent and lack the classical signs associated with infection. Chronic meningitis can also present as dementia or AMS. Abnormalities of the ventricular system can occur due to congenital anomalies, such as aqueductal stenosis, or acquired conditions, such as normal pressure hydrocephalus. Dilatation of the ventricular system may cause head enlargement in children. In adults, such conditions usually present with evidence of increased intracranial pressure or with dementia, AMS, gait problems, or difficulty with bladder control.

Disorders of the Skull and Vertebral Column

Disorders of the skull and vertebral column range from the minor and minimally significant, such as spina bifida occulta, to the severe, such as disfiguring craniosynostosis syndromes. The most common conditions are due to trauma, such as skull or spinal fractures. Occasional patients with bony tumors may present with localized pain. Sometimes bony lesions are picked up as incidental findings on radiographic studies done for other reasons. Congenital and developmental skeletal disorders may be immediately obvious at birth, such as myelomeningocele, or present well into adulthood, such as occult spinal dysraphism. Conditions may be limited to a bony abnormality, such as a linear skull fracture or spondylolysis, or involve neural structures as well, such as a depressed skull fracture or diastematomyelia. In the absence of trauma, the challenge is to remember to consider the possibility of a congenital or developmental skull or spinal disorder, even in the adult patient.

Disorders of the Vascular System

Diseases affecting the vascular system typically present as an ischemic or hemorrhagic event, single or multiple. The usual clue to a vasculopathy is multiple events involving different parts of the nervous system. Other presentations, such as dementia, can occur as well. Rare but important nonatherosclerotic conditions include vasculitis, moyamoya angiopathy, arterial trauma and dissections, fibromuscular dysplasia, migraine, cerebral autosomal dominant arteriopathy with subcortical infarcts and leukoencephalopathy, amyloid angiopathy, and complications of radiation therapy. Cerebrovascular disease may complicate systemic conditions such as collagen vascular disease and hypertensive encephalopathy. Hematologic disorders such as sickle cell disease, thrombotic thrombocytopenic purpura (TTP), polycythemia, intravascular lymphoma, and antiphospholipid syndrome may cause stroke. Coagulopathies may cause bleeding, as from anticoagulant effects or disseminated intravascular coagulation. The most common condition causing hypercoagulability-related stroke is activated protein C resistance. Vasculitis may complicate infections such as meningitis, meningovascular syphilis, or herpes zoster. Cerebral vasculitis may complicate systemic vasculitis, such as in systemic lupus, polyarteritis, Wegener's granulomatosis, and Churg-Strauss syndrome. Isolated angiitis of the brain may cause both infarct and hemorrhage. Other vasculitic disorders include Behçet's disease, Susac's syndrome, and Sneddon's syndrome.

DIFFERENTIAL DIAGNOSIS BY ETIOLOGY

From a differential diagnostic standpoint, it is usually most helpful to think first about the localization of the disease process in the nervous system, and secondarily about the etiology. Localization limits the etiologic differential diagnosis because certain disease processes typically involve or spare particular structures. If the clinical manifestations suggest cerebellar disease, then muscular dystrophy, MG, and GBS are not diagnostic considerations. Knowing the likely location of the pathology generally places the condition into a broad etiologic differential diagnostic category. Occasionally, the etiology is very obvious, such as stroke or CNS trauma, and the diagnostic exercise focuses mostly on the localization.

Categories and etiologic classifications of neurologic disease are necessarily somewhat arbitrary, as is the category in which to place a given entity. For instance, subacute combined degeneration of the spinal cord could be seen as a metabolic disorder, a nutritional deficiency, or as a complication of a systemic illness, pernicious anemia. Any classification scheme is stressed in an age in which we recognize entities as diverse as high-altitude cerebral edema (HACE), ciguatera intoxication, critical illness myopathy, sleep apnea, mitochondriopathies, Whipple's disease, intracranial hypotension, Susac's syndrome, NMDA encephalitis, Hashimoto's encephalopathy, and the jumping Frenchmen of Maine as conditions neurologists should be familiar with. Porphyria is one example of many conditions that are both metabolic and genetic disorders. The etiologic classifications used here are neoplasm, vascular disease, infection, inflammatory and autoimmune disorders, trauma, pharmaceuticals and other chemical agents, substance-related disorders, toxins, metabolic disorders, demyelinating disease, congenital and developmental abnormalities, genetic disorders, degenerative conditions, disorders due to physical agents, environmental related conditions, mitochondriopathies, channelopathies, paroxysmal disorders (seizures, headache and sleep), complications of systemic conditions, and nonorganic and psychiatric disease. Conditions such as epilepsy and migraine have important clinical manifestations far beyond the individual seizure or headache. The following paragraphs briefly summarize the features of some of these etiologic categories.

Neoplasms

The most common types of adult primary brain tumors are meningiomas and high-grade gliomas, but metastatic tumors are more common than primary brain tumors. Primary intracranial neoplasms may be divided into those that are intra-axial, arising within the brain or spinal cord substance, and those that are extra-axial, involving the meninges, cranial nerves, and other surrounding structures. Tumors are named according to their resemblance to cells that are found in the normal mature and developing nervous system. Intra-axial tumors are composed of cells of neuroectodermal origin. Examples of common intra-axial tumors include astrocytomas, oligodendrogliomas, ependymomas, medulloblastomas, and primary brain lymphoma. All are malignant because they invade the substance of the brain, but some more so than others. Common extra-axial tumors include pituitary adenoma, acoustic neuroma, and meningioma. Extra-axial tumors are more likely to be histologically benign and amenable to excision. They produce neurologic dysfunction primarily by exerting pressure rather than by invading. The symptoms and signs of intracranial tumors depend on their location, mass effect, pathologic characteristics, as well as their tendency to cause an increase in intracranial pressure. Focal manifestations of intracranial tumors include irritative phenomena such as seizures and symptoms related to progressively severe dysfunction of the structures involved. Clinical manifestations frequently result from vasogenic edema caused by the tumor. Hemiparesis, aphasia, and memory loss are common.

Of the primary intracranial neoplasms, approximately 50% belong to the glioma group. Astrocytoma is the most common primary intracerebral neoplasm. Meningiomas make up about 15% of all intracranial neoplasms. Most are supratentorial and produce symptoms and signs by pressure on the brain. An acoustic neuroma (schwannoma, neurinoma, neurilemmoma) is a tumor that usually arises from the vestibular portion of the eighth cranial nerve; it is by far the most common tumor to involve cranial nerves. Pituitary adenomas are relatively common and may cause both endocrine disturbances as well as neurologic dysfunction because of mass effect. Craniopharyngiomas are tumors of congenital origin that arise from cell rests in the region of the pituitary. They usually become manifest in childhood or young adult life.

Metastatic tumors are the most common type of intracranial neoplasm. The most common solid tumors to produce brain metastases are breast, lung, colon, and melanoma. Lung cancer, both non-small and small cell type, is the most common tumor overall to metastasize to the brain. Breast cancer is the most common cause the brain metastases in women. Although much less common, malignant melanoma carries a high risk of brain metastasis. Metastatic lesions often present in a subacute fashion but may present acutely because of intratumoral hemorrhage, which is particularly likely to occur with melanoma, renal cell, lung, and choriocarcinoma.

Malignancies can produce a host of nonmetastatic, paraneoplastic neurologic syndromes. The neurologic syndrome may precede the malignancy by months or years, occur simultaneously with presentation of the tumor, or develop in patients with known cancer. The paraneoplastic syndromes include but are not limited to progressive cerebellar ataxia, peripheral neuropathy, Lambert-Eaton syndrome, opsoclonus-myoclonus syndrome, "limbic encephalitis" (memory and emotional disturbances), and sensory ataxia due to dorsal root ganglion cell degeneration. One of the most common paraneoplastic syndromes is paraneoplastic cerebellar degeneration, which is usually associated with lymphoma or lung, breast, or gynecological cancer. Anti-Hu/Yo/Ri are the most frequently seen antineuronal antibodies.

Vascular Disease

Stroke remains the fourth leading cause of death in the United States. Recognized risk factors are increasing age, hypertension, diabetes mellitus, dyslipidemia, history of transient ischemic attack (TIA), cigarette smoking, carotid artery stenosis, and heart disease. Generally, cerebrovascular disease can be broadly divided into ischemic and hemorrhagic types (Table 53.10). It can be classified in a number of other clinically relevant ways: anterior circulation (carotid) versus posterior circulation (vertebrobasilar), large vessel (atherosclerotic) versus small vessel (hypertensive, diabetic, lacunar), and thrombotic versus embolic. Patients may present with many varieties of stroke related to these variables, as well as to the particular location of the event in the brain. About 70% to 80% of intracranial vascular events are ischemic, 15% are primary intracerebral hemorrhage (ICH), and about 5% are SAH. The majority of initial ischemic strokes are atherothrombotic infarctions; cardiac embolism produces about 15% to 30% of cases, small vessel lacunar disease about 15% to 30%, and other types, such as vasculitis or arterial dissection, 3%. The precise cause eludes identification in 30% to 40% of ischemic infarctions. Magnetic resonance imaging (MRI) and computed tomography (CT) frequently detect infarcts, primarily lacunes, for which there is no corresponding clinical history. Such subclinical infarcts are approximately five times more common than clinically evident strokes, and they may be associated with significant neurologic disability.

TABLE 53.10 A Classification Scheme for Stroke

- Ischemic stroke
  - Thrombotic
    - Occlusion of large extracranial or intracranial artery
    - Occlusion of small penetrating artery (lacunar syndrome)
  - Embolic
    - Central embolic source (heart or aortic arch)
    - Carotid bifurcation
    - Paradoxical embolism
  - Watershed stroke related to global hypoperfusion
- Hemorrhagic stroke (hemorrhagic conversion of an ischemic infarct)
- Spontaneous intracranial hemorrhage
  - Intracerebral hemorrhage
  - Subarachnoid hemorrhage

Reprinted from Campbell WW, Pridgeon RP. *Practical Primer of Clinical Neurology.* Philadelphia: Lippincott Williams & Wilkins, 2002, with permission.

Ischemic disease tends to present with an acute focal deficit in an alert patient. Intracranial hemorrhage is more likely to have an apocalyptic onset with coma and a poor outcome. Ischemic cerebrovascular disorders can be further subdivided into those due to thrombotic occlusion of a vessel, those due to embolic occlusion from distant sources such as the heart or the great vessels in the neck and chest, watershed infarcts occurring at border zones of perfusion when there is a general decrease in cerebral perfusion, lacunar infarcts (less than 2 cm in diameter and usually deep, the result of occlusion of perforating "end" arteries), and TIA. The onset of symptoms with all of these is usually abrupt, although the symptoms of thrombosis occasionally appear more gradually than those of either hemorrhage or embolism. It is important to identify precise time of onset, because this determines eligibility for treatment with tissue plasminogen activator, which must usually be given within 3 hours of symptom onset.

Stenosis or occlusion of extracerebral and even extracranial arteries is responsible for a large proportion of cerebrovascular disease. Affected vessels may be in the neck or chest and include the common and internal carotids, the vertebrals, and the arch of the aorta. Small vessel disease involves deep, penetrating small arteries and arterioles and is frequently related to hypertension. Large vessel disease tends to present as TIA or cortical stroke, small vessel disease as a subcortical lacunar syndrome. Anterior circulation events typically produce hemispheric infarction causing hemiparesis and higher cortical function defects such as aphasia, whereas posterior circulation events cause brainstem or occipital lobe ischemia. Thrombotic events tend to have onset during sleep and cause less severe, more restricted deficits. Thrombotic strokes may also have a stuttering course because of fluctuating hypoperfusion and gradual occlusion. Embolic events classically occur during activity, are more devastating, and are more likely to have associated cardiac disease.

Patients with TIAs experience brief episodes of neurologic dysfunction, by traditional definition lasting less than 24 hours but in fact usually lasting only 10 to 30 minutes and rarely more than 1 hour. The attacks resolve to leave no detectable clinical deficit. The pathology, not the duration of symptoms, is most important. As many as 50% of patients with transient deficits of less than 24-hour duration have evidence of infarction on imaging. Three basic forms are recognized: carotid distribution TIA (brief hemispheric spells), vertebrobasilar TIA (brainstem ischemia or visual field deficits), and amaurosis fugax (transient monocular visual disturbances because of ischemia in the ophthalmic artery distribution). TIAs presage major stroke in about 25% to 30% of patients. In a patient with TIA, the stroke risk is about 5% to 6% per year for the first 5 years and is greatest in the first year. Stroke occurs in up to 5% of patients within 48 hours of the TIA and in 10% within 90 days. Risk is higher in older patients, diabetics, those with hemiparesis or aphasia, or after an attack lasting longer than 10 minutes. The ABCD2 score was developed to capture these variables. It includes age, blood pressure, clinical features of the TIA, duration of symptoms, and history of diabetes. A diabetic patient ≥60 years of age with a blood pressure ≥140/90 who had unilateral weakness lasting ≥60 minutes would achieve the maximal score of 7, predicting a 2-day stroke risk of 8.1% and a 90-day stroke risk of 17.8%. Of patients diagnosed with stroke in emergency departments, 20% or more actually have a stroke mimic, such as seizure, migraine, brain tumor, systemic infection, or toxic-metabolic encephalopathy.

In ischemic stroke, the deficit depends on the arterial territory involved. Anterior cerebral artery ischemia is characterized by disproportionate weakness and numbness of the contralateral leg. Areas of particular clinical importance perfused by the middle cerebral artery (MCA) include the frontal eye fields, Broca's area, Wernicke's area, and the cortical areas subserving motor and sensory function for the arm and face. Large infarctions involving the entire MCA territory of the dominant hemisphere typically cause contralateral hemiplegia, hemianesthesia, dense homonymous hemianopsia, and global aphasia. Complete MCA distribution lesions in the nondominant hemisphere produce hemiplegia, various forms of apraxia, a visual field deficit, and differing combinations of the peculiar syndrome of neglect of the left side of space, denial of disability, and sometimes total failure to recognize the paralyzed extremities as part of the body (anosognosia). Patients with posterior cerebral artery strokes typically have homonymous hemianopia as the predominant clinical manifestation and may have no significant weakness or sensory loss. Internal carotid artery (ICA) occlusion may cause infarction of the entire hemisphere with the exception of the thalamus, inferior portion of the temporal lobe, and medial portion of the occipital lobe. Large infarctions, such as those that occur with ICA or MCA occlusions, often cause significant cerebral edema. Of all fatal ischemic strokes, cerebral edema and increased intracranial pressure are the cause of death in about one-third. Brainstem strokes are characterized by "crossed" syndromes of cranial nerve dysfunction ipsilateral to the lesion and long motor or sensory tract dysfunction contralaterally.

Many strokes are due to lacunar infarction related to fibrinoid necrosis, or lipohyalinosis, of small arterioles throughout the body. Hypertension is responsible for about 80% to 90% of lacunar infarctions. Diabetes mellitus is another important predisposing condition. Lacunar infarcts primarily affect subcortical structures such as the basal ganglia, thalamus, internal capsule, subcortical white matter, cerebellum, and brainstem. They do not involve the cerebral cortex. Occlusion of these small end arteries produces infarction, and the small infarctions result in little cavities filled with fluid (Fr. lacune "lake"), from 2 to 15 mm in size. The symptoms that occur depend on the location, but diffusion-weighted MRI studies have shown that the same lacunar syndrome can result from a lesion in a variety of locations and that lesions in the same location can cause different lacunar syndromes.

There are four classical lacunar strokes: pure motor stroke (PMS), pure sensory stroke, dysarthria-clumsy hand syndrome, and ataxic hemiparesis. Many other lacunar syndromes have been recognized; the present count is over 20. PMS is the most common and clinically best characterized of the lacunar syndromes. It accounts for about 10% of patients with acute stroke, and 50% of patients with lacunar stroke. The lesion usually involves the posterior limb of the internal capsule, damaging the corticospinal tract fibers in isolation and causing a dense hemiparesis but no sensory loss, visual field deficit, speech disturbance, eye movement disorder, or other evidence of dysfunction of the cerebral cortex—a pure motor deficit. The other lacunar syndromes are much less common than PMS. Although lacunar infarction is classically associated with small vessel disease, up to 25% are due to large vessel disease or cardiac embolism.

In contrast to ischemic cerebrovascular disease, intracranial hemorrhage characteristically produces either severe headache or early impairment of consciousness, or both. Intracranial hemorrhage may occur into the parenchyma or into one of the spaces that surround the brain. Intraparenchymal bleeding may occur into the supratentorial compartment (intracerebral), the cerebellum, or the brainstem. Supratentorial hemorrhage is often further divided into basal ganglia (usually putaminal) hemorrhage, thalamic hemorrhage, and so-called lobar or subcortical hemorrhage, which involves the deep white matter in the corona radiata. Extraparenchymal hemorrhage may involve the subarachnoid, subdural, or epidural spaces. Most extraparenchymal hemorrhage is due to head trauma. Spontaneous intracranial, extraparenchymal hemorrhage is usually into the subarachnoid space.

Hypertensive ICH usually involves the basal ganglia, subcortical white matter, thalamus, pons, or cerebellum, with basal ganglia and thalamic bleeds accounting for the vast majority. Patients typically have apocalyptic events with dense deficits and rapid impairment of consciousness. Amyloid angiopathy is an important cause of lobar hemorrhage in elderly patients. Other causes of ICH include arteriovenous malformation, bleeding disorders, anticoagulation, trauma, tumors, cavernous angiomas, and illicit drug use.

Trauma is the most frequent cause of SAH. Nontraumatic SAH is most often due to ruptured saccular aneurysm, occasionally to arteriovenous malformation, and in 10% to 15% of the cases to no identifiable etiology. The major etiologies of aneurysms are congenital, atherosclerotic, mycotic, and dissecting. Most saccular (berry) aneurysms occur at branching sites of the major arteries of the circle of Willis. The etiology is a combination of congenital and acquired factors. About 80% of berry aneurysms involve the anterior circulation and about 20% are located in the vertebrobasilar system. The most common sites of intracranial berry aneurysms are the distal ICA, posterior communicating artery, anterior communicating artery, tip of the basilar artery, middle cerebral bifurcation, and the posterior inferior cerebellar artery. Posterior communicating artery aneurysms frequently compress the oculomotor nerve. With aneurysmal SAH, the onset is usually precipitous. The patient develops a sudden, severe headache, often occipital or nuchal (thunderclap headache), often accompanied by convulsions, obtundation, or coma. Other causes of intracranial hemorrhage include amyloid angiopathy, vasculitis, and mycotic aneurysm.

Most cerebrovascular disease is related to atherosclerosis and hypertension, but there are other important etiologies (see above). Occlusive disease of the cerebral veins and the venous sinuses may also occur. There are also disorders of cerebrovascular autoregulation, such as hypertensive encephalopathy, reversible cerebral vasoconstriction syndrome, and posterior reversible encephalopathy syndrome (PRES).

Intracranial Infections

Numerous pathogenic microorganisms can infect the CNS. Clinical manifestations depend on the nature of the infecting organism, adequacy of host defenses, and the CNS area predominately involved. The clinical course may range from hyperacute (meningococcal meningitis), to chronic (tuberculous meningitis), to extremely chronic (prion infection). Many infections once rare have become commonplace since the advent of AIDS.

In acute bacterial meningitis, the patient typically appears acutely ill and toxic with fever, headache, altered sensorium, and stiff neck. Low sugar and polymorphonuclear leukocytosis characterize the cerebrospinal fluid (CSF). The differential diagnosis depends greatly on age and circumstances. Between 20 and 60 years, most cases are due to *Streptococcus pneumoniae*, and the next most common etiology is *Neisseria meningitidis*; over the age of 60, the most common organisms are *S. pneumoniae* and *Listeria monocytogenes*. Occasionally, causative organisms include *Haemophilus influenza*, group b *Streptococcus*, *Staphylococcus aureus*, and gram-negative bacilli. The possibility of bacterial meningitis should be considered in any patient with headache or AMS accompanied by fever. Patients with viral aseptic meningitis present in much the same way as patients with bacterial meningitis, except they generally appear less sick. The CSF in viral meningitis contains a predominance of mononuclear cells, a normal sugar level, and variable protein elevation. Many different viruses can produce viral meningitis, including enteroviruses (coxsackie, ECHO, other nonpolio enteroviruses), herpes simplex virus (HSV) type 2, HIV, West Nile virus (WNV), VZV, mumps, and lymphocytic choriomeningitis virus.

Other causes of an aseptic meningeal syndrome include neoplastic invasion of the meninges, sarcoid, reaction to certain medications, chemically induced meningeal inflammation, and infection by organisms difficult to culture. Some organisms can produce an indolent form of meningitis. The term aseptic is sometimes applied to these forms of meningitis because routine bacteriologic cultures prove sterile, but aseptic is most often used synonymously with viral meningitis. Major considerations include tuberculosis, cryptococcosis and other fungi, Lyme disease, and sarcoidosis. The CSF sugar is frequently low but rarely as low as in bacterial meningitis. Protein elevations, sometimes striking, are the rule.

Viral encephalitis differs from viral meningitis by virtue of the involvement of the brain parenchyma, which may produce altered consciousness progressing to coma, seizures, or focal signs such as hemiparesis, visual field deficits, and aphasia. Meningoencephalitis refers to involvement of both the meninges and the parenchyma. The epidemic forms of viral encephalitis most often follow an arbovirus infection, carried by arthropods (mosquitoes and ticks) from some natural host (e.g., horses) to man. The arboviral encephalitides include eastern equine, Western equine, St. Louis, Japanese B, WNV, and California encephalitis. HSV encephalitis is the most common type of sporadic viral encephalitis and the most common cause overall. The typical patient is a young and previously healthy adult who suddenly develops alteration of consciousness, followed rapidly by the onset of seizures and a focal neurologic deficit. Herpes simplex causes an acute, focal, necrotizing encephalitis with inflammation and edema; MRI may show abnormalities in the medial and inferior temporal lobe on the involved side. WNV has been responsible for the majority of cases of arboviral meningitis and encephalitis in the United States since 2002.

Brain abscesses can arise either because of direct spread from a contiguous infected source, such as a mastoid, or because of hematogenous spread. The term *cerebritis* is used to describe a nonencapsulated brain abscess. Brain abscesses often occur in immunocompromised hosts and are caused less often by bacteria than by fungi and parasites, such as *Toxoplasma gondii*. In Central and South America, the most common cause of brain abscess is neurocysticercosis. Patients typically present with varying combinations of headache, progressive neurologic deficits, seizures, and evidence of infection. However, fever and leukocytosis are absent in about half of the patients harboring a brain abscess.

Neurosyphilis is a specific subtype of tertiary syphilis and occurs after a long latent period following the primary and secondary stages. Although the manifestations are protean, several specific syndromes are recognized: tabes dorsalis, general paresis, and meningovascular syphilis. Early Lyme disease may present as meningitis, cranial nerve palsies, and radiculoneuritis. The late phase may consist of encephalopathy, encephalomyelitis, and polyradiculoneuropathies. In addition to predisposing to a variety of other infections or conditions, the HIV virus can directly infect the CNS, producing meningitis or encephalitis. With well-established disease, AIDS patients may develop a number of different neurologic syndromes, including cerebral toxoplasmosis, cytomegalovirus encephalitis, cryptococcal meningitis, tuberculous meningitis, neurosyphilis, CNS lymphoma, dementia, myelopathy or myelitis, polyradiculopathy, neuropathy, and inflammatory myopathy. Progressive multifocal leukoencephalopathy (PML) occurs frequently, as does CNS lymphoma. Estimates are that up to 5% of AIDS patients will develop PML. Other important but uncommon neurologic infections include Creutzfeldt-Jakob disease, WNV, subacute sclerosing panencephalitis, rabies, and poliomyelitis. Some infections (e.g., botulism, tetanus, and diphtheria) and infestations cause neurologic manifestations by the elaboration of a toxin that affects the nervous system.

Inflammatory and Autoimmune Disorders

Some disorders are characterized by a pathologic picture of inflammation but are not known to be infectious. Examples include neurosarcoidosis, Behçet's disease, acute and chronic inflammatory demyelinating polyradiculoneuropathy, acute disseminated encephalomyelitis (ADEM), inflammatory myopathies, and transverse myelitis. Clinically obvious neurologic involvement occurs in 5% to 15% of patients with sarcoidosis. The most common neurologic manifestation of sarcoidosis is facial nerve palsy, which may be bilateral. Neurologic manifestations may occur in patients with known sarcoidosis, but in approximately 50% of patients with neurosarcoidosis, neurologic signs are the presenting manifestations of the disease. Behçet's disease is a disorder of obscure pathogenesis; most of its clinical manifestations are believed to be due to vasculitis. The primary manifestations are recurrent oral or genital ulcerations, ocular disease, primarily uveitis, and involvement of multiple organ systems. The most common neurologic complication is recurrent meningoencephalitis. Clinical and neuroimaging findings support two major forms of neuro-Behcet's syndrome: parenchymal involvement and an extraparenchymal form that presents with cerebral venous sinus thrombosis. Behçet's disease is primarily relevant in the differential diagnosis of MS. The nervous system may be secondarily involved in systemic autoimmune disorders such as systemic lupus erythematosus (SLE) and related conditions or when the autoimmune process is directed against blood vessels.

Trauma

The clinical effects of trauma to the head involve complex dynamics because one moving body, the brain, is traveling in relation to another moving body, the skull. With abrupt deceleration, the most frequent injury mechanism, the brain, suspended inside the skull can impact against the inner table and the rigid meningeal structures, causing coup and contrecoup injuries. The areas most frequently injured are the frontal and temporal tips and the subfrontal regions.

Closed, or nonpenetrating, head injuries are those in which no fracture or only a simple linear fracture occurs, without displacement of the fragments, rupture of the dura, or penetration or exposure of the brain substance. Penetrating, or open, head injuries are those with either compound or depressed fractures or penetrating wounds. The type of pathologic brain injury may reflect differing injury mechanisms (closed vs. penetrating, blast vs. blunt trauma). About 35% of patients have suffered significant extracranial injuries, which can exacerbate the traumatic brain injury (TBI) because of associated blood loss, hypoxia, and other complications. In diffuse axonal injury, there is widespread disruption of axons, which can produce very significant clinical deficits. Severity of injury correlates best with duration of loss of consciousness and length of anterograde amnesia. The Glasgow Coma Scale is commonly used in the evaluation and management of patients with craniocerebral trauma (see Chapter 51). Head injuries with Glasgow Coma Scale scores of greater than 12 are considered mild; 9 to 12, moderate; and less than 9, severe. Cerebral contusion is a more severe form of closed head injury in which there is superficial hemorrhage over the cortex. The most severe closed head injuries may produce ICH. Complications of compound and depressed skull fractures and of severe contusions and lacerations include cerebral edema, intracerebral hematoma, epidural or subdural fluid collections, SAH, posttraumatic meningitis and brain abscess, focal cerebral cicatrices, osteomyelitis of the skull, traumatic pneumocephalus, arteriovenous aneurysm, organic brain syndrome, and posttraumatic epilepsy.

Subdural hematomas (SDH) arise from torn veins bleeding into the subdural space. Acute SDH most often follow obvious head trauma. The rapidly expanding intracranial mass produces impairment of consciousness and focal signs. Chronic SDH develop more slowly and often follow minor head trauma, particularly in elderly patients. The intracranial mass effect develops slowly and typically produces impairment of consciousness with only minor focality on examination. Epidural hematomas most commonly follow fractures through the thin temporal squamosa of the skull that lacerate the middle meningeal artery. Patients may have a lucid interval following the injury, only to lapse into coma as the hematoma expands minutes to hours later.

Pharmaceuticals and Other Chemical Agents

Neurologic complications of pharmaceuticals and similar agents, such as vitamins and supplements, are a common problem. These range from the relatively common and innocuous, such as dizziness because of drug-induced orthostatic hypotension, or headaches because of a prescription medication, to the catastrophic, such as PML due to natalizumab. Drugs may cause neurologic effects because of intoxication, either accidental or purposeful, withdrawal or because of adverse reactions. Patients may become habituated or addicted to properly prescribed and administered drugs, as in opiates for chronic pain or sedative-hypnotics for sleep, so distinguishing between substance use and abuse becomes murky. This section deals with prescription medications, vitamins, and substances. Substance abuse is considered below.

Drugs may have similar efficacy and a similar side effect profile, termed class effects. The manifestations of intoxication related to drugs of a given class are referred to as toxidromes (Table 53.11). Drug effects and side effects may mimic naturally occurring neurologic disease. The possibility of drug intoxication or withdrawal should be raised in any patient with AMS, delirium, or confusion.

Headache is a frequent drug effect. Commonly used drugs causing headache are NSAIDs, calcium channel blockers, beta-blockers, H_2 antagonists, proton pump inhibitors, and vasodilators. Analgesic overuse and withdrawal are common problems in headache patients. NSAIDs may also cause aseptic meningitis. Drug intoxication and withdrawal may produce AMS or a confusional state; common offenders are tranquilizers and sedative-hypnotics; antidepressants, including selective serotonin reuptake inhibitors (SSRIs); antiparkinsonian drugs; psychotropics; anticholinergics; H_2 antagonists; and opioids. Drugs that may cause cognitive impairment and memory disturbance include anticholinergics, antidepressants, antiepileptics, sedative-hypnotics, beta-blockers, H_2 blockers, and others. Coma may result from deliberate or accidental overdose of sedative-hypnotics, antidepressants, analgesics, or drug combinations, often with alcohol in addition. Many drugs may disturb sleep by causing excessive sleepiness, insomnia, sleep-disordered breathing, or parasomnias. Toxic leukoencephalopathy may result from antineoplastics or immunosuppressants. The list of drugs that may impair taste and smell is long (see Chapter 12) as is the list causing tremor and other movement disorders, peripheral neuropathy, and impaired NMT. Dysautonomia is a common side effect of anticholinergics and antihypertensives. Myopathy is one of the major complications of lipid-lowering agents, especially statins, but can complicate the use of a wide range of drugs, from amiodarone to zidovudine.

TABLE 53.11 Toxidromes and Associated Drugs

	Clinical Features		
Toxidrome	**Neurologic Manifestations**	**Other Signs**	**Common Drugs**
Adrenergic	Agitation, mydriasis, seizures	Hypertension, hyperthermia, tachycardia, tachypnea, arrhythmias	Amphetamines, caffeine, cathinone derivatives, cocaine, ephedrine, pseudoephedrine, *Ephedra* sp., phenylpropanolamine, theophylline
Anticholinergic	Agitation, delirium, mydriasis, seizures	Hyperthermia, tachycardia, decreased or absent bowel sounds, dry flushed skin and mucous membranes, urinary retention	First-generation H_1 receptor antagonists (e.g., classic antihistamines), belladonna alkaloids (e.g., scopolamine, hyoscyamine), benztropine, cyclic antidepressants, dicyclomine, muscle relaxants (e.g., orphenadrine, cyclobenzaprine), trihexyphenidyl
Cholinomimetic	Agitation, delirium, miosis, fasciculations, coma, seizures	Bradycardia, bronchorrhea, bronchospasm, diaphoresis, lacrimation, urination, diarrhea, vomiting	Carbamates, cholinesterase inhibitors (e.g., physostigmine, neostigmine, edrophonium)
Opiate, opioid	CNS depression, hypotonia, miosis	Bradycardia, bradypnea or apnea, hypothermia	Codeine, fentanyl, designer fentanyls, heroin, opioids (e.g., hydrocodone, oxycodone, meperidine, morphine), propoxyphene, central α_2-agonists (e.g., clonidine, imidazolines)
Sedative-hypnotic	Ataxia, CNS depression, hyporeflexia, slurred speech, stupor, or coma	Bradypnea or apnea, hypotension, hypothermia	Barbiturates, benzodiazepines, bromides, chloral hydrate, ethanol, ethchlorvynol, etomidate, glutethimide, meprobamate, methaqualone, methyprylon, propofol, zolpidem

Modified from Ford MD. Acute poisoning. In: Goldman L, Schafer AI, eds. *Goldman's Cecil Medicine*. 24th ed. Philadelphia: Elsevier/Saunders, 2012.

Some drug adverse side effects are particularly noteworthy, as they may be severe and life threatening. Examples include malignant hyperthermia (MH), neuroleptic malignant syndrome (NMS), and serotonin syndrome (SS). MH follows treatment with inhalational anesthetics or succinylcholine. NMS typically begins within 2 weeks of starting or increasing any neuroleptic but particularly phenothiazines. SS is related to the use or inadvertent interaction of serotonergic agents particularly SSRIs, but involving a range of drugs including opioids and triptans. Common to all is fever, diaphoresis, autonomic hyperactivity, AMS, and muscular rigidity. NMS and SS also cause myoclonus and tremor. The tyramine cheese reaction and anticholinergic toxicity share many features.

Certain drugs may cause a disorder that continues after the drug is discontinued. Examples include the induction of porphyria by sedative-hypnotics, autoimmune necrotizing myopathy due to statins, and MG due to penicillamine.

Neurologic syndromes related to vitamin deficiency are well known, but some vitamins also have important toxic effects. Vitamin A toxicity causes idiopathic intracranial hypertension. Excess vitamin A may result from the use of supplements or ingestion of carotenes in the diet. Many vegetables are rich in vitamin A, but so is liver. So-called liver lover's headache may result from excess ingestion, and vitamin A toxicity from eating polar bear liver may have caused the deaths of some early Arctic explorers. Pyridoxine may cause a sensory ganglionopathy because of acute high-level or chronic low-level exposure. Prolonged consumption of more than 200 mg/d may cause neuropathy; health food stores sell B_6 in formulations as high as 500 mg. Excess ingestion of zinc (to "boost immunity") may depress copper levels and cause a host of complications including a severe myelopathy. Ingestion of supplements to enhance athletic performance is probably not without risk. After a number of high-profile cases, ephedra was removed from the U.S. market. Supplements have been implicated in cases of heat injury and exertional rhabdomyolysis.

Substance Abuse Disorders

Side effects and complications can occur from the abuse of prescription drugs and from the abuse of illicit or "recreational" drugs, alcohol, and other substances. Patients may suffer from the effects and complications of these agents. Psychiatric comorbidities occur frequently. Clinical manifestations may occur because of intoxication, withdrawal, or substance-related complications, for example, rhabdomyolysis or heroin myelopathy. The key to the diagnosis of a substance-related neurologic syndrome is recognition of the possibility. The substance use history from the patient may or may not be reliable.

The neurologic complications of alcohol abuse and dependence are protean. The most common complications are seizures and peripheral neuropathy, but this is only the beginning. Some of the important complications of chronic alcoholism to recognize, either because they are common or because they are treatable if recognized, include alcohol-related seizures, peripheral neuropathy, Wernicke-Korsakoff disease, and alcoholic cerebellar degeneration. Alcohol withdrawal seizures are generalized tonic-clonic (GTC) convulsions that usually occur 12 to 48 hours after the cessation of drinking and are estimated to occur in 2% to 5% of alcoholics.

Neurologic complications of drug use are common. Like alcoholics, other substance abusers are rarely forthcoming about their ingestion habits. Commonly abused drugs include opioids, stimulants, sedative-hypnotics, marijuana, hallucinogens, anticholinergics, and inhalants or solvents. Patients may overuse and abuse prescription opioids, such as oxycodone, hydrocodone, codeine, meperidine, and fentanyl. Heroin is the usual street drug encountered. The desired effect is an intense euphoria or rush, but tolerance and dependence develop quickly. Neurologic complications, seen primarily with intravenous use of heroin, include coma with secondary rhabdomyolysis or nerve compression, vasculitis, endocarditis with mycotic aneurysm, embolic infarction, meningitis, and myelopathy. Meperidine intoxication may cause seizures.

The opioid epidemic in the United States developed because of multiple factors, including avaricious, unscrupulous drug companies that engaged in deceptive marketing of long acting opioids, inept government oversight, physician overprescribing, and a culture intolerant to pain and tolerant to drug use. Opioid prescriptions tripled over 20 years. There was a fourfold increase in overdose deaths from 1999 to 2008. The majority of drug overdoses are now from prescription opioids and heroin death rates now rival those of AIDS during the 1990s. One survey found that over 70% of people who abused prescription pain medications obtained them from friends or relatives; approximately 5% obtained them from a drug dealer. Newer opiates, such as fentanyl and carfentanil, are even more deadly than heroin. There is now a fentanyl epidemic superimposed on the opioid epidemic as drug dealers lace fentanyl, usually illicit, into either prescription opiates or heroin. In the nation's largest cities, fentanyl-related overdose deaths increased nearly 600% from 2014 to 2016.

The psychostimulants include cocaine, amphetamines (particularly methamphetamine), ecstasy (MDMA, a methamphetamine derivative), ephedrine, methylphenidate, and phenylpropanolamine. All produce elation, increased alertness, and heightened energy. Prescription stimulants used for attention deficit hyperactivity disorder (ADHD), including methylphenidate (Ritalin) and mixed amphetamine salts (Adderall), are sometimes abused, both by ADHD patients and by others. The most common manner of prescription stimulant abuse is crushing pills and snorting. Crack cocaine is the most potent and addictive form of the drug, producing euphoria within seconds. The euphoria is brief and followed by a crash. Occasionally, sedatives, opiates or alcohol, are ingested concomitantly to soften the crash, sometimes with unfortunate results. Prolonged, excessive use of psychostimulants may cause tics, tremors, myoclonus, chorea, and acute dystonia (see Chapter 30). Neurologic complications include seizures, ICH, and rhabdomyolysis. Stroke may occur from stimulant abuse because of vasoconstriction, cerebral vasculitis, dissection, embolism, or mycotic aneurysm. Crack cocaine causes 50% of all drug-related strokes.

Barbiturates are the prototypical sedative-hypnotic/anxiolytics; more problematic currently are benzodiazepines and similar GABA potentiators of the imidazopyridine class, such as zolpidem. The intoxicating and withdrawal effects resemble those of alcohol, causing coma with overdose and a withdrawal syndrome with anxiety, agitation, tremors, and possibly seizures. Although benzodiazepines do not depress respiration as severely as barbiturates do, their effects are additive with those of other CNS depressants, such as alcohol. Accidental overdoses, occasionally with fatal outcomes, have become common.

Other GABA-related drugs, such as gamma hydroxybutyrate (GHB) and analogs ("date rape" drugs), are similar. Addicts commonly use these drugs to manage opiate withdrawal or to ameliorate excessive effects of stimulants. Conversely, they use stimulants, including cocaine, to treat the hangover from alcohol or sedative-hypnotics. GHB also potentiates the effects of opiates.

For millennia, people have used and abused hallucinogens. Currently popular are lysergic acid diethylamide (LSD), phencyclidine (PCP), MDMA, GHB, ketamine, mescaline, psilocybin (magic mushrooms), salvia divinorum, and inhalants. The desired effect in all is altered perception and euphoria. PCP, ketamine, salvia, and dextromethorphan are sometimes classified as dissociative drugs; they produce perceptual distortions without causing actual hallucinations. LSD is the most potent of the hallucinogenic drugs. Ketamine is one of the drugs that has been implicated in date rape. The most severe side effect of most of these, particularly PCP, is acute psychosis. PCP intoxication may also cause muscle rigidity, hyperreflexia, nystagmus, ataxia, seizures, and coma. Anticholinergics are used as recreational drugs because they may cause hallucinations and delirium. Habitual huffers of organic solvents run the risk of serious neurologic sequela. Dextromethorphan, an NMDA antagonist, produces effects similar to ketamine and PCP ("Robo tripping"). Some compounds may cause mild hallucinations or perceptual distortions but are not classified as hallucinogens, and these include marijuana, zolpidem, and diphenhydramine. One infamous patient enjoyed simultaneously smoking marijuana and inhaling gasoline, leaded gas specifically, because that combination caused him to hallucinate in color.

"Designer drugs" are illicit synthetic drugs that are often analogs of a parent compound that have greater potency. Designer modifications of fentanyl have increased the potency, and the lethality, of an already potent and dangerous drug. Illicit attempts to increase the potency of meperidine created MPTP, which caused irreversible PD in those who ingested it. Synthetic cannabinoids (Spice, K2) are more potent than marijuana and can lead to agitation, psychosis, seizures, and death. Cathinones ("bath salts") can lead to agitation, psychosis, hyperthermia, and death. Other new and emerging drugs of abuse include salvia, desomorphine, kratom, and several designer benzodiazepines.

Toxins

Examples of environmental toxins include heavy metals (e.g., lead), industrial agents used in the manufacture of goods (e.g., *n*-hexane), pesticides (e.g., organophosphates), gases to which a patient might be accidentally or deliberately exposed (e.g., carbon monoxide), and biologic toxins derived from plants (e.g., chickpeas), fish (e.g., ciguatera, tetrodotoxin), or bacteria (e.g., diphtheria). The diagnosis of a neurotoxicological syndrome is usually difficult. There should be documentation or reasonable suspicion of exposure, a compatible clinical syndrome, and other likely responsible conditions must be rigorously excluded. It is a good general rule that when exposure is eliminated, the neurotoxicological syndrome should stabilize or regress.

Toxins encountered in the environment that affect the nervous system include heavy metals, solvents and related compounds, and biologic toxins. Important heavy metals causing neurologic dysfunction include lead, arsenic, organic and inorganic mercury, thallium, manganese, aluminum, and bismuth. Lead intoxication has many effects. The majority of adult elevated blood lead levels comes from workplace exposures but a crises of lead exposure from contaminated water developed in the United States in 2014. Moonshine is a frequent source of lead exposure in some parts of the United States. In adults, the primary neurologic complication is a peripheral neuropathy. Lead exposure has diverse purported consequences in children, which are quite different from adults. Arsenic and thallium toxicity primarily cause peripheral neuropathy. A generalized sensorimotor polyneuropathy is one of the major manifestations of arsenic poisoning and can develop 1 to 3 weeks after acute poisoning or insidiously because of chronic exposure. Acute arsenical neuropathy can closely simulate GBS. The elemental, inorganic and organic forms of mercury are all potentially toxic, and the form of exposure determines the toxic manifestation. Severe neurologic toxicity can result from the ingestion of organic mercury. Consumption of food contaminated with methylmercury caused epidemics of severe neurologic disease in Minamata, Japan, in the 1940s and in Iraq in 1971. There is no evidence to support an association of mercury toxicity with dementia.

There are many other environmental agents that may cause neurologic toxicity, including organic solvents, hexacarbon solvents (methyl butyl ketone and *n*-hexane), carbon disulfide, carbon monoxide, cyanide, nitrous oxide, ethylene oxide, organophosphate insecticides, and acrylamide. Exposure may occur in the workplace, as with hexacarbon solvents, through attempted homicide or suicide, a common cause of arsenic intoxication or carbon monoxide exposure, or because of substance abuse, as in nitrous oxide myelopathy (Layzer's syndrome) in dentists or those who inhale from whipped cream dispensers (whippets or nossies). Many of these compounds, such as cyanide or organophosphates, are the agents of chemical warfare.

Neurologic complications due to biologic toxins occur in botulism, tetanus, diphtheria, tick paralysis, ergotism, snake and spider envenomation, and other conditions. Botulism, tetanus, and diphtheria are considered with infections. Marine toxins are usually ingested, but divers and others working in a marine environment may be the victim of envenomation. Ciguatera toxin (ciguatoxin) accumulates in reef fish high in the food chain, such as barracuda. In some locations, ciguatera intoxication has caused public health authorities to ban consumption of barracuda. Ciguatoxin is a potent sodium channel blocker. The disorder begins with an acute gastrointestinal illness, followed by a primarily sensory neurologic syndrome with paresthesias and bizarre sensations such as temperature reversals. An exacerbation of chronic ciguatera symptoms can occur after exposure to foods containing alcohol or serotonin. Exposure to tetrodotoxin usually occurs because of the deliberate ingestion of puffer fish, considered a delicacy in some parts of Asia. Symptoms begin with paresthesias but may progress to neuromuscular, including respiratory, paralysis. Neurotoxic shellfish poisoning is due to brevetoxins, such as saxitoxin, and has manifestations similar to tetrodotoxin.

Some venomous snakes, such as coral snakes, cobras, and adders, inject a toxin that causes NMT defects that may lead to paralysis and death. Spiders and scorpions also elaborate neurotoxins. Attachment of some varieties of tick may cause the syndrome of tick paralysis, with progressive weakness resembling GBS. Chickpeas are drought resistant and may be the only food source during famine. They contain a toxin that when ingested in excess causes neurolathyrism, a progressive degeneration of the pyramidal tracts leading to irreversible, spastic paraparesis. The disease is presently restricted to India, Bangladesh, and Ethiopia. Konzo is similar but related to ingestion of cassava. The clinical manifestations of neurolathyrism and konzo are similar to HTLV-1 myelopathy/tropical spastic paraparesis. A third dietary neurotoxic disorder is tropical ataxic neuropathy, due to cyanide exposure.

Metabolic Disorders

Metabolic neurologic disorders include a wide variety of conditions, both acquired and inherited. Imbalances in key metabolic constituents, including gases, electrolytes, vitamins, and hormones, can produce dramatic systemic and neurologic consequences. Neurologic complications may arise because of the metabolic derangements that accompany many systemic disorders such as diabetes mellitus. In addition to oxygen and glucose, the brain depends on numerous compounds to serve as enzymes and cofactors in its metabolic reactions. Deficiency of even minute amounts of some of these can produce neurologic devastation. With electrolytes and hormones, deleterious effects can be seen with either excess or deficiency.

These metabolic disturbances tend to have fairly characteristic and typical clinical features depending on the element. Patients with vitamin B_{12} deficiency may develop several neurologic syndromes, including spinal cord disease (subacute combined degeneration), peripheral neuropathy, optic neuropathy, and dementia. Hematologic abnormalities are rarely present even in severe neurologic B_{12} deficiency, and the serum B_{12} level may be normal. Other neurologically important vitamin deficiency syndromes include thiamine (Wernicke's and Wernicke-Korsakoff syndrome), niacin ("dementia" and neuropsychiatric disturbances), pyridoxine (peripheral neuropathy in adults, seizures in infants), vitamin D (osteomalacic myopathy), and vitamin E (spinocerebellar degeneration, myelopathy, retinopathy, and neuropathy). Copper deficiency causes a myelopathy resembling that caused by vitamin B_{12} deficiency, and copper and vitamin B_{12} deficiency may coexist.

Patients with endocrine diseases often have neurologic complications. Hypoglycemia is one of the metabolic encephalopathies that may cause focal deficits, such as hemiparesis or aphasia, that resolve with glucose infusion. The neurologic manifestations correlate poorly with glucose concentrations. Seizures may occur, especially after sudden changes in the glucose level. The hyperosmolar hyperglycemic state (HHS) may cause seizures, often focal, and other focal signs such as hemiparesis. Both HHS and diabetic ketoacidosis (DKA) may produce progressive obtundation and coma. Stupor and coma are more common and occur earlier in HHS than DKA.

Some patients with HHS have hemichorea-hemiballismus. Hypothyroidism can present as progressive cerebellar ataxia, dementia, myopathy, or peripheral neuropathy. Hyperthyroidism can present as AMS, coma, myopathy, ophthalmopathy, or a movement disorder. Hyperparathyroidism can cause a neuromuscular disease simulating myopathy. Hyper- and hypoadrenalism can both have prominent neurologic manifestations.

The metabolic disturbances that occur with organ failure may be accompanied by pronounced neurologic abnormalities. One of the most common types of metabolic encephalopathy encountered clinically is ischemic-hypoxic encephalopathy because of cardiorespiratory arrest. The patient's baseline neurologic status and the duration and severity of the hypoxic insult determine the severity of the neurologic injury, with deficits ranging from subtle memory loss to coma. In survivors, common findings include anterograde and retrograde amnesia, confusion, cortical blindness, myoclonus, seizures, and bilateral arm weakness because of watershed-territory infarctions (man in a barrel syndrome). In comatose patients, preserved pupillary light reflexes and conjugate or orienting eye movements on initial examination suggest a better prognosis.

Acute hepatic encephalopathy occurs in patients with acute hepatic failure; chronic hepatic encephalopathy occurs in patients with chronic liver disease and portosystemic shunting of blood. Acute hepatic encephalopathy causes cerebral edema in 80% of patients. Hepatic (portal-systemic) encephalopathy may cause a constellation of neurologic alterations and symptoms, including AMS, tremors, asterixis, rigidity, and coma. The diagnosis of hepatic encephalopathy is primarily clinical; elevated ammonia concentrations are common, but a normal ammonia level does not exclude the diagnosis. Uremia may cause AMS, hallucinations, rambling speech, convulsions, tremor, myoclonus, asterixis, and other abnormal movements. PRES has been reported due to uremic encephalopathy. Encephalopathy can develop after dialysis is initiated due to dialysis disequilibrium syndrome. A severe metabolic encephalopathy may also develop with systemic infection, sepsis, burns, and multiple organ failure. Neurologic complications following organ transplantation are common.

There are many neurologic diseases in which the pathologic alterations and clinical manifestations are the result of an inborn error of metabolism. These conditions usually present in infancy or childhood. Some of the conditions that may present in adulthood include metachromatic leukodystrophy, adrenoleukodystrophy, Kufs' disease, Wilson's disease, Leigh's disease, Gaucher's disease, and Niemann-Pick disease. Storage diseases, with intracellular accumulation of abnormal material, include the lipidoses (e.g., gangliosidosis, Gaucher's disease, Niemann-Pick disease, and mucopolysaccharidosis), leukodystrophies (metachromatic leukodystrophy, Krabbe's disease, Pelizaeus-Merzbacher syndrome, and other variants), and neuronal ceroid-lipofuscinoses. The abnormal material is stored in lysosomes, and these disorders are also referred to as lysosomal diseases. The glycogenoses produce abnormal glycogen accumulation; there are numerous subtypes.

Wilson's disease is an autosomal recessive disorder of copper metabolism that causes accumulation of copper in the brain, liver, cornea, and other organs (see Chapter 30). The neurologic manifestations of Wilson's disease are many, and patients may present in a number of ways. Kayser-Fleischer rings are present in 98% of patients with neurologic involvement. In patients with hepatic involvement, the neurologic manifestations may be mistaken for hepatic encephalopathy. Common signs of CNS involvement include dysarthria, gait disturbances, ataxia, dystonia, tremor, and parkinsonism.

The porphyrias are a group of disorders due to enzyme defects involving the heme pathways in which there is excessive formation and excretion of porphyrins. The most important from a neurologic point of view is acute intermittent porphyria, which causes recurring attacks consisting of abdominal pain, hypertension, polyneuropathy, mental changes, convulsions, and the excretion of burgundy-red urine. It is an autosomal dominant disorder with low penetrance that results in a partial deficiency of porphobilinogen deaminase; symptoms develop due to a variety of exacerbating factors. When weakness develops, the pattern is unusual. It typically begins in the proximal upper extremities, then progresses to the lower extremities, and distally. Porphyric neuropathy can mimic GBS, and the absence of abdominal pain does not exclude the possibility.

There are many other inborn metabolic errors that involve amino acids and other organic acids. There is increasing recognition that inborn errors of metabolism may present in adulthood. Examples include metachromatic leukodystrophy, X-linked adrenoleukodystrophy, acid maltase deficiency and other glycogen storage disorders, ornithine transcarbamylase deficiency, homocystinuria, and mitochondriopathies. Even Lesch-Nyhan syndrome can present in adults as athetosis without cognitive impairment or behavioral abnormalities. One of us (WWC) has seen cerebrotendinous xanthomatosis present in an adult masquerading as vertebrobasilar insufficiency.

Demyelinating Disorders

Demyelinating diseases affect the myelin of the CNS. Most demyelinating disease is immunologically mediated; MS is the most common example. More rarely, myelin is involved in infectious processes (e.g., PML) or fails to develop normally (e.g., leukodystrophy).

The manifestations of MS are protean; among the most common are optic neuritis, transverse myelitis, cerebellar ataxia, brainstem syndromes, sensory disturbances, and internuclear ophthalmoplegia. The disease generally begins between 20 and 40 years of age with recurrent attacks followed by recovery, the relapsing and remitting form. MS begins as a relapsing remitting disease in more than 80% of patients. Some patients with long-standing relapsing-remitting disease develop nonfluctuating inexorably downhill disease (secondarily progressive MS). About 10% of patients began with nonfluctuating, gradually progressive disease (primary progressive MS). Classically, MS produces white matter lesions with relative sparing of axons.

A clinically isolated syndrome (CIS) is a single attack likely because of CNS demyelination where a formal diagnosis of MS cannot be made because of the lack of dissemination of lesions in time and space. Ultimately, most CIS patients develop MS. The diagnosis of MS requires dissemination of disease in time and space. Conditions to consider in the differential diagnosis of demyelinating disease are summarized in Table 53.12. Red flags include such things as arthritis, skin rash, pulmonary or GI symptoms, hearing loss, peripheral neuropathy, or atypical time of onset, either early childhood or over age 50.

NMO (Devic's disease) is an inflammatory disorder that causes both necrosis and demyelination and produces attacks of both optic neuritis and longitudinally extensive transverse myelitis that may be but are not necessarily concurrent. NMO was once thought to represent a subtype of MS but is now recognized to be a distinct disorder associated in most cases with autoantibodies to the aquaporin 4 channel in astrocytes. NMO is much less common than MS and presents clinically as an acute attack of optic neuritis and/or transverse myelitis.

TABLE 53.12 Some Conditions to Be Considered in the Differential Diagnosis of Demyelinating Disease

Multiple sclerosis
Neuromyelitis optica
Acute disseminated encephalomyelitis
Idiopathic transverse myelitis, idiopathic optic neuritis
CNS vasculitis, Susac's syndrome, correct CNS lymphoma
Cervical spondylosis
HTLV-1 myelopathy
PML, Lyme disease, tertiary syphilis, Whipple's disease
CADASIL
Connective tissue disorders, especially SLE and Sjögren's syndrome
Behçet's disease, Wilson's disease
Sarcoidosis
Vitamin B_{12}, vitamin E or copper deficiency
Leukodystrophies
Degenerative disorders

CNS, central nervous system; HTLV-1, human T-cell lymphotrophic virus type 1; PML, progressive multifocal leukoencephalopathy; SLE, systemic lupus erythematosus.

Reprinted from Campbell WW, Pridgeon RP. *Practical Primer of Clinical Neurology.* Philadelphia: Lippincott Williams & Wilkins, 2002, with permission.

Transverse myelitis is caused by inflammation and demyelination of the spinal cord and presents with the abrupt or subacute onset of motor and sensory loss below a specific spinal level, usually with loss of bowel and bladder control. Many cases are idiopathic, and some are the initial manifestation of MS. Other causes must be excluded, particularly compressive myelopathy and treatable infection. Longitudinally extensive disease raises the possibility of NMO.

As with transverse myelitis, an attack of optic neuritis may be idiopathic or the first manifestation of MS or NMO. Other potential etiologies include sarcoidosis and collagen vascular disease. Optic neuritis occurs sometime during the course of MS in 70% of patients and is the presenting feature in 25%. Optic neuritis is discussed more fully in Chapter 13.

ADEM typically follows a viral infection or immunization. It occurs primarily in children but may occur in adults. Similar postinfectious/postvaccinal dysimmune attacks can involve the optic nerve (optic neuritis) and the spinal cord (transverse myelitis), but in ADEM, the lesions are more widespread, and the patients typically have multifocal deficits, often with alteration of consciousness and sometimes with seizures.

Congenital and Developmental Disorders

The nervous system may fail to develop normally during intrauterine life or may be injured or damaged at the time of birth. One of the most common developmental disorders that presents in adulthood is type I Chiari malformation, a congenital defect that involves the brainstem and cerebellar tonsils (see Chapter 21). Other examples include aqueductal stenosis, occult spinal dysraphism, porencephaly, arachnoid cyst, Klippel-Feil syndrome, platybasia, and basilar impression.

Abnormalities of brain maturation during embryonic and fetal life may lead to microcephaly, macrocephaly, cerebral dysplasia and dysgenesis, congenital absence of structures (e.g., the corpus callosum), lissencephaly and other abnormalities of the gyri and convolutions, heterotopias, encephalocele, porencephalic cysts, hydranencephaly, congenital hydrocephalus, and many other conditions. Intellectual disability (ID), or mental retardation, refers to subnormal intellectual functioning that originates during the developmental period. ID occurs in 2% to 3% of the population; mild forms are much more common than severe forms. There are many potential causes. Approximately 75% of cases are due to genetic syndromes, perinatal asphyxia, cerebral dysgenesis, severe psychosocial deprivation, or toxin exposure. Down's syndrome and fragile X syndrome are the most common chromosomal disorders leading to ID.

Genetic Disorders

Many neurologic syndromes of formerly obscure pathogenesis have proven to be genetic. Recent advances have clarified the modes of inheritance and chromosomes involved in many of these. In a few, investigators have identified the abnormal gene and the protein or enzyme defect. Some well-recognized genetic conditions include HD (see Chapter 30), the hereditary ataxias (see Chapter 43), muscular dystrophies, SMA, the neurocutaneous syndromes, and many others. In other conditions, the genotype likely influences the clinical manifestations of a disorder in ways that are just being understood. A study in 2015 found that a monogenic neurologic disorder affected 1 in 1,100 individuals in Northern England, looking only at inherited muscle disease, hereditary neuropathies, hereditary ataxias, movement disorders, hereditary optic neuropathy, hereditary spastic paraparesis, and mitochondrial disease.

Portions of the nervous system share a common ectodermal embryologic origin with the skin. As a result, some conditions produce abnormalities of both skin and nervous system: the neurocutaneous syndromes or phakomatoses. Most, but not all, of these conditions are hereditary. The recognition of the skin lesions permits prediction of the neuropathology and in turn the prognosis and the pattern of inheritance. The term phako (Gr. mother-spot) refers to the skin (or eye) lesions that are the usual initial clue to the presence of a neurocutaneous syndrome. Typical neurologic accompaniments are seizures and ID, but other abnormalities can occur as well.

The most common neurocutaneous syndrome is neurofibromatosis type I (NF1, von Recklinghausen's disease), an autosomal dominant disorder characterized by multiple neurofibromas involving nerves throughout the body. Café au lait spots are also characteristic. The diagnostic criteria for NF1 are summarized in Table 53.13. The typical order of appearance of clinical manifestations is café au lait spots, axillary and/or inguinal freckling, Lisch nodules (Figure 13.13), and neurofibromas. Although NF1 is autosomal dominant, approximately half the cases are due to de novo mutations. Penetrance in an affected individual is complete, but expression is highly variable. Tuberous sclerosis (tuberous sclerosis complex, Bourneville's disease) is an autosomal dominant condition that causes seizures, ID, and various characteristic skin lesions. About 80% of cases are due to de novo mutations, and expression is highly variable. Patients may develop a variety of benign tumors in multiple organs, including the brain, heart, kidney, and liver. von Hippel-Lindau disease is characterized by the association of hemangioblastomas involving the retina and various portions of the CNS, especially the cerebellum. Patients are also at risk for developing other tumors, including renal cell carcinoma and pheochromocytoma. Sturge-Weber disease (encephalotrigeminal angiomatosis) describes the association between a vascular nevus of the face (port wine stain) and a vascular malformation involving the ipsilateral cerebral cortex. Unlike most other neurocutaneous syndromes, Sturge-Weber is sporadic, due to somatic mosaic mutations in the GNAQ gene. Common neurologic features include ID, seizures, visual field defects, and other focal neurologic deficits.

TABLE 53.13 Diagnostic Criteria for Neurofibromatosis Type 1

- Six or more café au lait spots 1.5 cm or larger in postpubertal individuals, 0.5 cm or larger in prepubertal individuals
- Two or more neurofibromas of any type or one or more plexiform neurofibromas
- Freckling in the axilla or groin
- Optic glioma
- Two or more Lisch nodules
- A distinctive bony lesion, for example, dysplasia of the sphenoid bone
- A first-degree relative with NF1

Degenerative Diseases

Degenerative diseases are those for which no clear etiologic basis is known. They are characterized by degeneration of functionally related populations of neurons, and the resulting clinical picture depends on which neurons are affected. With advancing knowledge, some conditions are removed from this category as their etiologic basis is clarified. The most common clinical conditions included under the rubric of neurodegenerative disorders are sporadic Alzheimer's disease (AD) and other dementias, PD and related syndromes, and ALS. Some of the other conditions often classified as neurodegenerative include corticobasal degeneration (CBD), dementia with Lewy bodies (DLB), multiple system atrophy (MSA), and progressive supranuclear palsy (PSP).

Dementia refers to loss of mental capacity and can occur either as a primary degenerative condition or as a secondary complication of some other disease, such as hypothyroidism or CNS infection. The thrust of a dementia workup is exclusion of a treatable cause (Table 53.14). It is important to be sure that the patient is not taking a medication known to interfere with memory, such as a beta-blocker, benzodiazepine, or anticholinergic. Four conditions account for the vast majority of the cases of dementia, three neurodegenerative conditions—AD, DLB, and frontotemporal dementia (FTD)—and vascular (multi-infarct) dementia (see Chapter 8). The incidence and prevalence of dementia are strikingly age dependent. In the population of 75 to 85, the prevalence may approach 30% to 50%. AD, either in isolation or in combination with some other process, such as cerebrovascular disease, accounts for about 60% to 80% of the cases of dementia. Less common etiologies include PD with dementia, alcohol-related dementia, chronic traumatic encephalopathy, and CJD. The early course of AD is dominated by difficulty with anterograde

TABLE 53.14 Some Treatable Causes of Dementia

Depression ("depressive pseudodementia")
Hypothyroidism
Vitamin B_{12} deficiency
Normal pressure hydrocephalus
Cerebral vasculitis
Cerebrovascular disease
Neurosyphilis
HIV infection
Cerebral mass lesion (e.g., subdural hematoma, olfactory meningioma)
Chronic meningitis (e.g., tuberculosis, cryptococcosis)
Drug intoxication

Reprinted from Campbell WW, Pridgeon RP. *Practical Primer of Clinical Neurology*. Philadelphia: Lippincott Williams & Wilkins, 2002, with permission.

memory, but patients with dementia do not usually present complaining of memory loss. More often the spouse or other family members bring the problem to attention. Informant-reported memory loss is a better predictor of the likelihood of cognitive impairment than patient-reported memory impairment. Depressed patients are more likely to complain about memory loss than those with dementia. Using CSF, positron emission tomography (PET), and MRI biomarkers has shown AD in cognitively normal individuals, suggesting a long incubation process and a spectrum of manifestations from preclinical, to mild cognitive impairment (MCI), to full-blown dementia. These investigations have shown that AD has an extended preclinical phase characterized by sequential changes in imaging and CSF biomarkers and subtle memory decline beginning more than a decade before the emergence of symptomatic memory loss heralding the beginning of the MCI stage. The apolipoprotein E ε4 allele is a prevalent and potent risk factor for AD.

The syndrome of MCI causes similar symptoms but does not meet the criteria for dementia and does not interfere with activities of daily living; MCI lies in the gray zone between dementia and the cognitive changes of normal aging. There are two subtypes: amnestic, in which the primary manifestation is memory impairment, and nonamnestic, in which there is either relatively isolated impairment in a single nonmemory domain, such as executive functioning, language or visuospatial skills or impairment in multiple domains with relative sparing of memory. Patients with MCI are at risk for developing dementia, primarily AD, at a rate of 10% to 15% per year. The prevalence increases with age, from 6.7% at age 60 to 64 to 25.2% at age 80 to 84. Disease evolution causes progressive cognitive deterioration and behavioral changes. When fully developed, deficits in multiple cognitive domains, including language, praxis, and visuospatial, affect activities of daily living. In contrast to FTD, major personality changes do not occur until late in the course.

The non-AD degenerative conditions can be divided into those with an abnormality of TDP-43 or tau protein (tauopathies)—such as PSP, CBD, and FTD—and those with an abnormality of α-synuclein, such as PD, MSA, and DLB. The tauopathies share as a common pathologic feature the accumulation of abnormal intracellular filaments of tau protein. In primary tauopathies, there is a disassociation between tau (a microtubule-associated protein) and microtubules as a result of tau hyperphosphorylation. Recent evidence suggests that aggregated tau may exhibit properties similar to those of prions. Clinical features may overlap, and definitive diagnosis is often challenging. The FTD syndromes are pathologically characterized by severe, circumscribed "knife-edge" atrophy that primarily involves the frontal and temporal poles. The FTD syndromes may present as a behavioral dementia syndrome (see Chapter 8) or as aphasia (see Chapter 9) parkinsonian and motor neuron symptoms may also occur, either initially or as the disease progresses. Patients with the behavioral variant of FTD are often thought to have early AD or a late-onset psychiatric disorder. The disinhibition, euphoria and poor judgment can mimic mania; the eating disturbance and apathy can mimic depression.

Like tau, α-synuclein proteins can undergo pathologic misfolding and aggregation and possibly exhibit prion-like spread. Lewy bodies are composed of aggregates of α-synuclein and other proteins. α-Synuclein pathology is traditionally associated with PD, MSA, and DLB and tau pathology with AD, PSP, CBD, and FTD. However, there is significant overlap and co-occurrence of α-synuclein and tau pathologies in a spectrum of neurodegenerative diseases, and α-synuclein and tau may interact to promote misfolding and aggregation of each other, suggesting important relationships between these two proteins, a "molecular conspiracy." There is now in vitro and in vivo evidence that α-synuclein behaves as a prion in MSA patients.

Some patients with depression have prominent complaints of memory difficulty (pseudodementia).

Multi-infarct dementia, or vascular dementia, results from multiple cerebral infarctions. Normal pressure hydrocephalus refers to a spontaneously occurring form of communicating hydrocephalus featuring a clinical triad of dementia, gait difficulties, and urinary incontinence. HIV dementia is more likely to occur in a younger patient and present with memory loss, which progresses over months. It may be the initial presentation of AIDS. ALS is due to degeneration of motor neurons in the spinal cord, brainstem, and cerebral cortex, which causes progressive weakness, atrophy, spasticity, hyperreflexia, dysphagia, dysarthria, and fasciculations (see Chapters 22 and 29). A combination of upper motor neuron and lower motor neuron abnormalities, particularly in the same limb, is characteristic. Failure to recognize early ALS is common; it may mimic radiculopathy, myelopathy, mononeuropathy, or arthropathy. A study found that 13% of a series of patients had undergone a surgical procedure for symptoms that in retrospect were due to ALS.

Disorders Due to Physical Agents

Therapeutic irradiation (XRT), while effective for many neoplasms, may have serious neurologic complications. During and up to a month after XRT, a steroid-responsive encephalopathy with increased intracranial pressure may develop, causing AMS, impaired memory, headaches, and cerebral edema and contrast enhancement on MRI. This syndrome is mediated by breakdown of the blood-brain barrier. A similar encephalopathy may develop 1 to 4 months after XRT related to injury to oligodendroglia and vasogenic edema.

Most complications of XRT develop months to years after treatment. The risk is related to the total dose and the size of the fractionated doses. A total dose of less than 5,500 Gy carries a 5% likelihood of complications; risk increases with concurrent chemotherapy. In the brain, cerebral atrophy, focal radiation necrosis, demyelination, and vasculopathy may occur, causing cognitive impairment, personality change, and gait disturbance. Distinguishing radionecrosis from recurrent tumor remains challenging; PET showing hypometabolism is more consistent with radionecrosis.

A transient radiation myelopathy related to demyelination may develop within the first 6 months after XRT and is typically self-limited. A more severe, chronic, progressive radiation myelopathy develops more than 1 year, often several years, after XRT, and is mediated by vasculopathy. Radiation may affect the brachial or lumbosacral plexus and is often difficult to distinguish from recurrent tumor. Myokymia on electromyography (EMG) and hypometabolism on PET favor radiation plexopathy. Likely mechanisms are small vessel damage and fibrosis. Peripheral nerves and roots are relatively resistant to XRT. Radiation to the neck may cause accelerated carotid atherosclerosis.

Electrical injury to the nervous system occurs because of lightning strikes or shocks delivered by electrical equipment. Immediate and delayed effects occur, which may be transient, permanent, or progressive. Lightning may cause a characteristic, almost pathognomonic, immediate transient syndrome of paraplegia with preserved sphincter function, accompanied by vasoconstriction with limb coolness, lividity, and cyanosis that resolves over hours or days (Charcot's paralysis). Delayed, sometimes for years, progressive sequela of electrical injury most commonly involve motor neurons, basal ganglia, or the spinal cord. An ALS-like syndrome has been reported.

Other physical injuries to the nervous system may result from thermal or atmospheric pressure injuries or exposure to altitude (see below).

Environmental Neurology

These disorders encompass a wide spectrum of conditions, ranging from a repetitive motion injury causing carpal tunnel syndrome (see Chapter 46) to back and neck pain (see Chapter 47), to exposure to a toxin in the workplace or in nature (see above). Heat injuries result from exposure to high environmental temperature, with or without an exertional component. A spectrum of injury may occur. Minor heat-related manifestations include fatigue, syncope, and muscle cramps. Serious heat injury includes heat exhaustion and heat stroke. Symptoms of heat exhaustion include fatigue, headache, and dizziness. With heat stroke, the individual loses thermoregulatory ability, stops sweating, and develops AMS progressing to coma, and the core temperature rises to 40°C or higher. When core temperature exceeds 41°C, neurologic manifestations such as seizures and impairment of consciousness may become prominent features of heat stroke. Approximately 20% of patients may have persistent neurologic deficits. Other manifestations of organ compromise develop, such as hepatopathy, kidney injury, and rhabdomyolysis. Classic heat stroke occurs in the very young and very old, often during heat waves. Exertional heat stroke occurs in young, otherwise healthy, individuals who have done strenuous exercise in conditions of high heat and humidity; rhabdomyolysis and lactic acidosis are common complications.

Hypothermia is defined as a core temperature less than 35°C and severe hypothermia as less than 28°C. Hypothermia may be primary, caused by cold exposure, or secondary to a disease causing impaired thermoregulation. Most hypothermia is accidental; therapeutic hypothermia is used as a medical intervention in conditions such as TBI, after neurosurgical procedures and following cardiac arrest. Mild hypothermia causes confusion, incoordination, and slowed reflexes. Severe hypothermia causes rigidity, areflexia, and impaired consciousness progressing to coma. At temperatures less than 20°C, hypothermia can simulate death clinically and electrophysiologically. The lowest known survival from accidental hypothermia in an adult was from a temperature of 9°C. In addition to environmental exposure, a number of medical conditions may result in hypothermia, including hypothyroidism, adrenal insufficiency, sepsis, malnutrition, hypoglycemia, and ethanol abuse. Peripheral cold injuries result from cold alone (frostbite) or from cold and wet conditions (trench foot); permanent peripheral nerve injury may occur.

Both high and low ambient pressures may cause clinical symptoms, but only decreased pressure is prone to cause neurologic injury, primarily by allowing the release of gases from solution. An interplay occurs between the effects of pressure changes and the gases involved, primarily oxygen, nitrogen, and carbon dioxide. The effects of low pressure are often combined with hypoxia, as in altitude sickness. The effects of high pressure are often modified by the effects of nitrogen or oxygen toxicity (nitrogen narcosis).

Decompression sickness (DCS, the *bends*) most often occurs after ascent from diving, occasionally from flying or driving in mountainous terrain after diving, and rarely from sudden decompression at altitude in an aircraft. Type I DCS causes limb and joint pain. Type II DCS causes CNS dysfunction, including impaired consciousness, weakness, headache, and gait disturbance. Severe DCS may cause coma or death; about 100 DCS-related deaths occur annually in the United States. Sudden decompression, as in very rapid ascent, may cause pulmonary barotrauma and air embolism with a resultant focal neurologic syndrome as occurs from any type of vessel occlusion. DCS may also cause an acute myelopathy.

Acute mountain sickness is the most common altitude-related syndrome, occurring in 50% of individuals who ascend above 15,000 ft without acclimating. Common symptoms include fatigue, headache, dizziness, nausea, and insomnia. HACE, a much more severe illness, occurring in 1% to 2% of individuals at such altitude, is often associated with high-altitude pulmonary edema. The arterial pO_2 at 18,000 ft is approximately 50 mm Hg. HACE often begins with severe headache, and without immediate descent or treatment, patients go on to develop ataxia, cognitive impairment, hallucinations, papilledema, focal signs such as cranial nerve palsies or hemiparesis, seizures, and impaired consciousness evolving from drowsiness to coma. Imaging studies may show cerebral edema, PRES, and changes in the splenium of the corpus callosum. Sudden, severe HACE may develop in apparently well-acclimated climbers at altitudes above 20,000 ft (Mt. Everest is 29,029 ft).

Mitochondriopathies

Mitochondrial disorders are a heterogeneous group of conditions that have diverse manifestations. Mitochondriopathies have a predilection for organ systems that rely heavily on aerobic metabolism and nervous system involvement is common. Neuromuscular features predominate, but there is often multisystem involvement. Examples include subacute necrotizing encephalomyelopathy (Leigh's disease); myoclonic epilepsy with ragged red fiber disease (MERRF); mitochondrial encephalomyopathy, lactate acidosis, and stroke-like episodes (MELAS); mitochondrial neurogastrointestinal encephalopathy (MNGIE); neuropathy, ataxia, and retinitis pigmentosa (NARP); Kearns-Sayre syndrome; Leber's hereditary optic neuropathy; and many others. Mitochondrial disorders due to mutations of nuclear DNA include carnitine deficiency, pyruvate dehydrogenase deficiency, Friedreich's ataxia, and others. Leigh's syndrome and MELAS are two of the most common mitochondrial disorders. The mitochondrial DNA depletion syndromes are conditions in which a decrease in mitochondrial DNA affects multiple tissues. There are several major types, including myopathic, encephalomyopathic, hepatocerebral, and neurogastrointestinal.

Channelopathies

Channelopathies are disorders due to ion channel dysfunction; most are neurologic conditions. The many ion channels involved produce a spectrum of clinical conditions with significant heterogeneity, but a common feature is paroxysmal dysfunction. Channelopathies may be genetic or autoimmune acquired and may affect the PNS or CNS. Examples of genetic channelopathies include periodic paralysis, myotonia congenita, paramyotonia, the congenital myasthenia syndromes, MH, familial hemiplegic migraine, familial episodic ataxia, and the idiopathic generalized epilepsies. Some epilepsies, previously classified as idiopathic, have been shown to be channelopathies. Benign familial neonatal convulsions and generalized epilepsy with febrile seizures are due to K^+ and Na^+ channelopathies. Acquired autoimmune channelopathies include MG, Lambert-Eaton syndrome, neuromyotonia, and paraneoplastic cerebellar degeneration. Some of the toxic effects of pharmaceuticals are mediated by their effects on ion channels. Activation of Na, K, and Cl ion co-transporters may play a role in cerebral edema in ischemia, trauma, and ammonia neurotoxicity. Nonneurologic ion channel diseases include cystic fibrosis and the congenital long Q-T syndrome.

Paroxysmal Disorders

Some disorders occur episodically in patients who are otherwise well and have no abnormalities on neurologic examination between attacks. Two of the most common paroxysmal disorders are migraine and seizures. Less common conditions that may occur as paroxysmal attacks include the episodic ataxias, certain movement disorders, narcolepsy, and periodic paralysis.

Seizure Disorders

Seizures are very common; about 10% of the population will suffer at least one seizure over an 80-year life span. The manifestations of a seizure depend on where the discharge begins in the brain and how it spreads. Seizures can be divided into those that start in a specific part of one hemisphere (focal, partial, or localization-related seizures) and those that begin simultaneously in both hemispheres (generalized seizures). Simple partial seizures, or focal seizures with retained awareness, are focal events that do not cause impairment of consciousness; the seizure discharge remains limited to a focal area of cortex. Complex partial seizures, or focal seizures with impaired awareness, are those that do impair consciousness.

Seizure discharges that begin focally produce focal symptoms and signs. If the discharge remains focal, the clinical manifestations remain focal and depend on what part of the cortex is involved. A seizure that affects the motor cortex causes contralateral focal motor seizures, an occipital lobe discharge causes visual phenomena, and a parietal seizure causes sensory symptoms. Spread of a discharge across the cortex may produce a Jacksonian march of seizure activity. If the discharge spreads down to deep midline structures, it frequently is then projected or propagated throughout the brain, resulting in loss of consciousness (secondary generalization). Seizures that affect either the entire brain or the deep midline structures that immediately project the discharge diffusely and bilaterally are referred to as primary generalized seizures.

Focal seizures that rapidly become secondarily generalized can be difficult to distinguish from primary generalized seizures. The importance of the distinction lies in the different likely etiologies of primary generalized seizures (idiopathic, familial, benign) as opposed to focal seizures with secondary generalization (focal cerebral lesions, e.g., tumor, abscess, or scar because of old stroke or trauma). The perception of the focal seizure activity that precedes secondary generalization is termed an aura. The nature of the aura helps localize the site of origin of the epileptic discharge. Seizures discharges in or near the uncus of the medial temporal lobe often produce an olfactory aura, referred to as an uncinate fit. About 60% of patients with focal epilepsy experience some sort of aura. Postictal focal neurologic dysfunction, such as weakness (Todd's paralysis) or sensory loss lasting minutes to hours, can also help localize the seizure focus. As a focal seizure evolves into a secondarily generalized seizure, the contralateral arm may extend as the ipsilateral arm flexes at the elbow, forming a "figure-four sign," which is useful for localizing the seizure focus.

Epilepsy is by definition characterized by recurrent seizures. Patients who have had an isolated seizure may or may not have epilepsy. There are many etiologies for seizures in addition to epilepsy, including metabolic abnormalities, drugs, or medical illnesses. The differential diagnosis of seizures is strikingly age dependent (Table 53.15). Common causes of acute symptomatic seizures in adults include acute ischemic or hemorrhagic stroke, particularly lobar hemorrhage, SAH, subdural hematoma, TBI, hypoxic-ischemic encephalopathy, meningitis or encephalitis, drug intoxication, alcohol and other withdrawal states, and metabolic derangements such

TABLE 53.15 Likely Causes of Recurrent Seizures in Different Age Groups

Neonatal and infancy	Birth injury or anoxia, metabolic disorders, congenital malformations, metabolic disorders, infantile spasms
Childhood	Febrile seizures, infantile spasms, perinatal anoxia or birth injury, idiopathic
Adolescence	Idiopathic, trauma
Early adulthood	Idiopathic, trauma, drug or alcohol use or withdrawal, neoplasm
Middle age	Neoplasm, alcohol or drug use or withdrawal, vascular disease, trauma
Elderly	Vascular disease, neoplasm, trauma, degenerative disease

Reprinted from Campbell WW, Pridgeon RP. *Practical Primer of Clinical Neurology*. Philadelphia: Lippincott Williams & Wilkins, 2002, with permission.

as hypoglycemia, hyperglycemia, hyperosmolar state, hyponatremia, and uremia.

GTC (grand mal, major motor) seizures involve a bilateral seizure discharge with loss of consciousness, generalized stiffness followed by bilaterally synchronous extremity movements, and often urinary and/or fecal incontinence and tongue biting. The GTC phase rarely lasts longer than 2 minutes. Following cessation of the clonic movements, the patient sleeps for time, then gradually awakens. Postictal lethargy and confusion are common. In addition to oral trauma, complications include shoulder dislocation, vertebral compression fractures, and aspiration pneumonia. Patients with severe seizures, particularly frequent GTC events are at risk for sudden unexplained death in epilepsy (SUDEP).

Generalized absence (petit mal, minor motor) seizures occur most often in children between 4 and 12 years of age and produce transient staring spells with unresponsiveness, often mistaken for daydreaming. Absence events lasting more than 20 seconds may be associated with automatisms, such as eye blinking and lip smacking. These seizures can often be provoked by hyperventilation. Myoclonic seizures are recurrent, quick, momentary muscle jerks unaccompanied by loss of consciousness. Atonic seizures cause an abrupt loss of muscle tone and may result in falls. Complex partial ("temporal lobe," psychomotor) seizures are characterized by loss of awareness of the environment without actual loss of consciousness, accompanied by various automatisms such as lip smacking, chewing, or idly picking at the clothing with one hand. The degree of impairment of consciousness can range from minimal to marked. These events usually last less than 3 minutes. The seizure focus most often lies in the temporal lobe, occasionally in the frontal lobe or elsewhere. Temporal lobe epilepsy is the most common seizure type in adults, accounting for about 40% of epilepsy cases and is usually caused by mesial temporal sclerosis. Alcohol-related (withdrawal) seizures are very common. The abstinence syndrome results in a tendency to have one (rarely several) generalized seizures within the first 6 to 48 hours. Alcohol withdrawal seizures are nonfocal, usually self-limited, and associated with a normal interictal electroencephalogram. The neurologic examination is normal, as are imaging studies. Febrile seizures occur in about 3% to 5% of children younger than 5 years. Most occur between 6 months and 4 years of age. Typically, these seizures are brief and generalized and occur with a rapidly rising fever, which peaks at 103°F or higher. About 30% of children have more than one episode. There are no long-term consequences for most affected individuals. Those who have prolonged or focal febrile seizures, or a family history of nonfebrile seizures, have a somewhat increased risk of developing epilepsy later in life.

Posttraumatic seizures are very common. The likelihood of developing seizures is directly related to the severity of the injury. The risk following a penetrating injury is 600 times that in the general population. About 20% of patients with severe closed head injuries develop epilepsy.

Psychogenic nonepileptic seizures (PNES, pseudoseizures) are psychogenic events that may resemble a seizure. Some patients with PNES also have epilepsy. Of patients evaluated in inpatient epilepsy monitoring units for intractable seizures, 25% to 40% prove to have PNES. Conversion disorders and dissociative disorders are felt to underlie most cases of PNES: factitious disorders and malingering are rare. Some features that might suggest PNES include an episode duration longer than 2 minutes, ictal eye closure, pelvic thrusting, waxing and waning motor activity, asynchronous movements, vocalization during the event, lack of incontinence and lack of postictal stupor, and confusion. Forced eye closure in particular suggests PNES. Definitive diagnosis requires video-EEG. PNES is more common in females, and about 80% have been victims of abuse. One of the subtypes of premotor frontal lobe epilepsy is referred to as hypermotor seizures. These events can produce dramatic, wild, asynchronous movements that are often confused with PNES and have even been termed pseudo—pseudoseizures.

Status epilepticus (SE) refers to prolonged seizures or seizures occurring back to back without the patient regaining consciousness in between. SE is a neurologic emergency with a mortality rate in adults in the 10% to 30% range. Some of the more common causes in adults include acute structural brain lesion (stroke, SAH, cerebral anoxia, meningitis, encephalitis); remote structural brain lesion (previous TBI, neurosurgery); noncompliance or discontinuation of antiepileptic drugs in patients with known epilepsy; withdrawal syndromes (alcohol, barbiturates, benzodiazepines); metabolic abnormalities (hypoglycemia, hyperglycemia, hyperosmolar state); and exposure to one of the many drugs that lower the seizure threshold. NORSE refers to a new entity characterized by the new onset of severe generalized seizures and refractory SE without a clear acute or active structural, toxic or metabolic cause, occurring in a patient without active epilepsy or other known preexisting neurologic disorder, often in the setting of a prodromal illness suggesting viral encephalitis. An autoimmune or paraneoplastic encephalitis may be found in up to 40% of these patients. Febrile infection-related epilepsy syndrome (FIRES) is a subcategory of NORSE characterized by a prodromal febrile infection preceding the onset of the refractory SE.

Nonconvulsive status epilepticus (NCSE) has many variants, including absence SE and complex partial SE. Most relevant here are patients in coma or with a prolonged confusional state without obvious seizure activity. In some patients, motor manifestations are subtle but present, and close observation may disclose jerking of the thumb, corner of the mouth, or tongue. Reports indicate electroencephalogram (EEG) monitoring may detect NCSE in 8% to 20% of comatose patients, even in the absence of clinical seizure activity. In one study, NCSE or electrographic seizures were detected in 21% of 170 subjects. Subtle clinical findings such as twitching of oral or ocular muscles and eye deviations were present in 50% of the group. Some patients with convulsive SE continue to have ictal EEG activity after control of movements with treatment. The etiologies for NCSE following convulsive SE are similar to the causes of convulsive SE. Common causes of NCSE in critically ill patients include stroke, SAH, CNS infection, TBI, intracranial tumor, anoxia, and toxic-metabolic encephalopathy. A number of drugs may cause NCSE, including beta-lactam antibiotics, fluoroquinolones, and cisplatin. In some cases, NCSE occurs as a manifestation of drug-induced PRES because of cyclosporine, tacrolimus, or other agents.

Episodic loss of consciousness or falling occur for many reasons besides seizures, and distinguishing these other causes (e.g., vasovagal syncope, micturition syncope, Stokes-Adams attacks, drop attacks, cataplexy) is a regular clinical exercise. Causes of syncope are many and range from simple faint or vasovagal syncope to life-threatening cardiac arrhythmias. Although neurologists see many patients with syncope, rarely is the cause actually neurologic. The most important consideration is to exclude serious underlying cardiac disease. There is a substantial risk of sudden death in older patients with cardiogenic syncope.

Headache

Most headaches are benign, but occasionally, headache will be the presenting complaint in a patient with serious and even life-threatening conditions (e.g., hemorrhage, mass lesion, CNS infection). Table 53.16 lists some clues in the presentation that may indicate potentially serious pathology. The following are some of the commonly seen headache syndromes.

Migraine is a very common cause of recurrent headaches. It is generally divided into two large categories: with aura (classic migraine) and without aura

TABLE 53.16 Clinical Features of Headache That Suggest a Serious Pathologic Condition

Age at onset	Childhood, >age 50
History	Abrupt onset; first, worst, or atypical headache; worse at night or first thing in the morning; associated with loss of consciousness, visual disturbance, change in behavior or personality, fever, or vomiting without nausea; occipitonuchal or interscapular pain; associated with focal neurologic complaints, altered mental status (AMS), or history of recent head trauma (no matter how trivial); progressively severe pain; immunocompromised state; family history or personal history of conditions associated with subarachnoid hemorrhage/aneurysm (autosomal dominant polycystic kidney disease, Marfan's syndrome, Ehlers-Danlos syndrome, fibromuscular dysplasia, pseudoxanthoma elasticum, neurofibromatosis type I)
Physical exam findings	Meningismus, fever, focal neurologic abnormalities, soft neurologic signs (pronator drift, asymmetric nasolabial fold, or plantar responses), clumsiness, drowsiness, AMS, papilledema

Reprinted from Campbell WW, Pridgeon RP. *Practical Primer of Clinical Neurology*. Philadelphia: Lippincott Williams & Wilkins, 2002, with permission.

(common migraine). About 75% of the patients have migraine without aura. These patients have unilateral or holocephalic, usually throbbing head pain, with accompanying nausea, vomiting, photophobia, and phonophobia. In migraine with aura, patients experience a well-defined aura preceding or accompanying the headache. The aura most often involves visual phenomena (scintillating scotomata, fortification spectra, flashing lights, wavy lines) but may consist of somatosensory dysfunction (heminumbness or hemitingling), hemiparesis, or other focal cortical aberrations such as aphasia. Sometimes the neurologic symptomatology occurs in relative isolation, with little or no headache (acephalgic migraine, migraine without head pain, migraine equivalents). When the neurologic dysfunction (with or without headache) is unusually severe or prolonged, becoming the most prominent part of the migraine episode, the condition is referred to as complicated migraine. Examples of complicated migraine include hemiplegic migraine, ophthalmoplegic migraine, and basilar artery migraine. Status migrainosus refers to a migraine attack that lasts longer than 72 hours despite treatment.

The traditional vascular theory of migraine, which held that the aura was due to vasoconstriction and the headache to vasodilation is no longer considered valid. Current concepts are that the pathophysiology of migraine involves cortical spreading depression, activation of the trigeminovascular system, neurogenic inflammation, and both peripheral and central sensitization. Magnetic resonance angiography studies have shown that migraine pain is not accompanied by extracranial arterial dilatation.

In cluster headache (one of the trigeminal autonomic cephalalgias), the pain is intense, steady, boring, aching, and relentless (not pulsatile) and located in a periorbital or retroorbital distribution. Cluster attacks are frequently associated with tearing or redness of the eye or stuffiness of the nose on the side of the headache. Horner's syndrome may occur with the attacks and occasionally will persist between attacks but intensify during attacks. The attacks are usually brief (about 30 to 60 minutes) and typically occur on a daily basis (sometimes several times a day) for a finite period of time (several weeks or several months). The patient may then enjoy long symptom-free intervals, lasting months and sometimes years. On average, clusters last 6 to 12 weeks and remissions last up to 12 months. In contrast to patients in the throes of a migraine, who prefer to remain still and quiet, patients with cluster are restless and prefer to move, pace around, sit and rock, and have even been known to go for a jog.

The other trigeminal autonomic cephalalgias are paroxysmal hemicrania, short-lasting unilateral neuralgiform headache with conjunctival injection and tearing (SUNCT), short-lasting unilateral neuralgiform headache attacks with cranial autonomic symptoms (SUNA), and hemicrania continua. These have common features but differ in attack duration and frequency and in response to therapy. The trigeminal autonomic cephalalgias are thought to involve synchronized abnormal activity in the hypothalamus, the trigeminovascular system, and the autonomic nervous system. There appears to be activation of the trigeminal-autonomic reflex, a reflex pathway consisting of a brainstem connection between the trigeminal nerve and facial nerve parasympathetic outflow.

Tension (TTH, tension-type, muscle contraction) headache is a term used most often to describe head pain judged nonmigrainous in origin. The typical TTH is mild to moderate in intensity, bilateral, nonpulsatile, and without other associated features. TTHs do not cause nausea and are not made worse by physical activity. The precise mechanisms of TTH are uncertain, and the pathogenesis is probably multifactorial, but the traditional notion of sustained contraction of pericranial muscles is no longer considered valid.

Sleep Disorders

The commonly seen sleep disorders are narcolepsy and sleep apnea. The full syndrome of narcolepsy includes attacks of excessive daytime sleepiness, cataplexy (sudden collapse without loss of consciousness produced by laughing or other strong emotion), sleep paralysis (episodes of inability to move during sleep-wake transitions), and hypnagogic or hypnopompic hallucinations (extremely vivid dreams during sleep-wake transitions). Patients with sleep apnea suffer from chronic sleep deprivation because of innumerable awakenings because of apneic episodes occurring through the course of a night's sleep. Patients are seldom aware of these awakenings and present complaining of excessive daytime sleepiness and fatigue. Two forms of sleep apnea are recognized: obstructive and central. Other important sleep disorders include restless legs syndrome, periodic limb movements, parasomnias, and rapid eye movement sleep behavior disorder.

Complications of Systemic Conditions

Large textbooks are devoted to this vast topic, and not more than passing mention of some of the major areas is possible here. Neurologic complications of endocrinopathy include many neuromuscular syndromes due to diabetes, thyroid disease, adrenal disease, and acromegaly. Coma and seizures may occur from hypo- or hyperglycemia, hyponatremia, or hypercalcemia. Hematologic diseases such as hemoglobinopathies, TTP, and coagulopathies may cause stroke; paraproteinemias are associated with neuropathy, and the neurologic complications of cancer, including paraneoplastic syndromes, are protean. Liver disease may cause encephalopathy, and there are many neurologic complications of liver transplantation. Cardiovascular diseases ranging from atherosclerosis and hypertension to embolism from atrial fibrillation or mural thrombus are major causes of stroke; textbooks are devoted to neurocardiology. The primary complications of renal disease are encephalopathy and neuropathy and the many disorders related to transplantation. Neurologists and pulmonologists share many patients with respiratory failure and coma. Some of the many rheumatologic disorders of interest to the neurologist include SLE, Sjögren's syndrome, and vasculitis. Neurologists and rheumatologists share an interest in muscle disease, particularly inflammatory myopathy.

Neurologists are frequent consultants in intensive care units, and patients with primarily neurologic problems commonly require intensive care. Critical care neurology has become an area of subspecialty interest, and certification and textbooks address the topic. The many neurologic aspects of obstetrics and gynecology include the management of the pregnant epileptic or MS patient and the many neurologic complications of pregnancy, including eclampsia, stroke, venous thrombosis, and femoral nerve palsy. Textbooks are devoted to the neurology of pregnancy alone. Many surgical and procedural complications are neurologic, ranging from post-CABG ulnar neuropathy to myelopathy from aortic aneurysm repair.

Nonorganic and Psychiatric Disease

The psychiatric disorders most often of neurologic concern are depression, conversion disorder, malingering, and somatic symptom disorder (formerly termed hypochondriasis). Neurologic findings because of conversion disorder or malingering are referred to as nonorganic or functional neurologic disorders (FND). Even the terminology used to describe such symptoms is unsatisfactory. Certainly, the term hysteria/hysterical is pejorative and outdated, but whether it is best for the consulting neurologist to state the findings are nonorganic, functional, psychogenic, psychosomatic, medically unexplained, nonphysiologic, conversion disorder, supratentorial, or stress-related is far from clear, and many physicians use a personally preferred code or state there is no evidence of neurologic disease. The diagnosis of nonorganic disease can be treacherous. Signs on physical examination are often extremely misleading. Functional neurologic deficits have been dubbed "neurologic nonsense" because of the complex and confusing presentation.

Formerly, there were three elements in reaching a diagnosis of FND: excluding neurologic disease, demonstrating positive signs of nonorganicity, and establishing the presence of psychopathology severe enough to explain the symptomatology. DSM-5 removed the last requirement. Nevertheless, patients who have a psychiatric condition severe enough to produce a symptomatic neurologic deficit deserve a psychiatric evaluation.

Organic and functional deficits may coexist—the problem of functional or psychogenic overlay. Some patients embellish by nature, others may exaggerate a real deficit for fear the physician may not take them seriously. The dilemma lies in performing an adequate workup to exclude organic disease versus overtesting or overtreatment of a functional disorder, which may reinforce and entrench the symptoms.

Functional disorders fall into the categories of somatoform disorder (somatic symptom disorder in DSM-5), where the physical symptoms are produced unconsciously, and factitious disorder or malingering, where there is an intent to deceive. Reliably distinguishing deficits produced unconsciously from those knowingly feigned is practically impossible. DSM-5 has renamed conversion disorder as conversion disorder (functional neurologic symptom disorder).

When confronted with an enigmatic patient, physicians, particularly when young and un-scarred, are often quick to conclude the problem is nonorganic. Unfortunately this attitude can be especially common if the patient is young, female, or has a history or depression or anxiety. Homosexual men and patients with a history of psychiatric disease are also likely to be unjustly stigmatized. But many diseases, particularly neurologic ones, may present with puzzling manifestations. With MS presenting as nonspecific sensory symptoms, the majority of misdiagnoses in women are psychiatric, and in men orthopedic, suggesting a gender-dependent bias in the way physicians interpret sensory complaints.

Mistakenly concluding an illness is nonorganic can have serious consequences. Examples abound of malpractice litigation, sometimes with psychiatrists as co-defendants, involving patients diagnosed as psychogenic who proved to have very real neurologic conditions. Less common is a suit because of subjecting a patient with a functional deficit to risky diagnostic procedures or treatments, such as TPA.

A large study of neurology outpatients concluded that 5.4% had a primary diagnosis of FND. All investigators agree the most common FND is PNES, making up about half the cases. The error rate has declined with modern neuroimaging, but misdiagnoses continue to occur with regularity. Studies from the 1960s suggested that on follow-up more than half the patients with a diagnosis of a functional deficit ultimately developed clearly explanatory neurologic or psychiatric conditions. Influential papers by Slater in 1965 cautioned about the misdiagnosis of "hysteria." More recent studies, "Slater revisited," suggest that an organic neurologic diagnosis does not often subsequently emerge for medically unexplained symptoms. In a study with 6-year follow-up, 3 of 64 patients (4.7%) developed a neurologic disorder that explained the original symptoms. In a 12-year longitudinal study, only 1 of 42 patients (2.4%) developed a neurologic disorder that explained the original presentation. But in a similar study with 10-year follow-up, in 11 of 73 patients (15%) thought to have conversion disorder causing pseudoneurologic symptoms, a clear neurologic diagnosis was subsequently made for the original symptom. A study of 4,470 neurologic inpatient admissions concluded that only 9% had a purely functional disorder, and these patients were accumulated prior to or at the dawn of the MRI era.

Before drawing conclusions, we must recognize the clinical acumen of clinicians of Slater's era and the limitations of neuroimaging. Mistakes are made with regularity because the wrong part of the neuraxis is scanned, contrast is not given, the scan is misread, or the distinction not made between central and peripheral nervous system disease. Spinal cord disease is a particularly difficult and diagnostically treacherous area with subtle clinical and radiologic findings that require a high level of expertise.

Major neurologic illnesses often initially diagnosed as conversion disorder, malingering, depression, anxiety, neurasthenia, or some other nonorganic disorder include MG, MS, porphyria, GBS, dystonia, and botulism. The average patient with MG sees 5 to 7 physicians before the correct diagnosis is made. Similar difficulties with diagnosis occur with MS. In a 2003 study of 50 consecutive MS patients, 58% had initially been given 41 wrong diagnoses, the patients had been referred to 2.2 ± 1.3 specialists before seeing a neurologist, and learned about their disease 3.5 years after the onset of symptoms. The majority of women were thought to have an FND. It is axiomatic that the patient with acute intermittent porphyria sees, in sequence, the surgeon, the psychiatrist, and then the neurologist. Patients with GBS have died while the physicians caring for them continued to presume the shortness of breath and paresthesias represented hyperventilation, and many patients with GBS are sent out from the emergency department one or more times before the diagnosis is made. In one cooperative study on plasmapheresis in GBS, young women with the illness were diagnosed as "hysterical" four times more frequently than men or older women. One of the leading misdiagnoses in botulism is a functional neurological deficit. Movement disorders are often mislabeled as nonorganic, particularly dystonia.

The issue of positive signs of nonorganicity is problematic. Many authors emphasize that the diagnosis of a functional deficit requires the presence of positive evidence of nonorgancity rather than simply the absence of evidence of organic disease. Techniques to "prove" a deficit is nonorganic have held a cherished place in neurology since the days of Charcot. But nearly all the examination techniques touted as proof of nonorganicity are fallible, particularly for sensory findings (see Chapter 36). Many of the history and examination findings purported as helpful in separating functional and organic deficits are unreliable. The attitude of *la belle indifference* may be misleading. Some patients, especially with nondominant hemisphere lesions, have neglect syndromes, and others are stoic. It is not of value in discriminating real from nonorganic disease. Things such as apparent secondary gain, nonanatomic deficits and variability of findings on examination have either not been studied or investigations have shown they are neither sensitive nor specific for functional disorders. Gould et al. examined 30 consecutive neurology service admissions with acute structural nervous system damage for the presence of seven of the most accepted features of nonorganicity: history of hypochondriasis, secondary gain, la belle indifference, nonanatomical sensory loss, midline splitting of pain or vibration, changing boundaries of hypalgesia, and give-away weakness. All subjects showed at least one of these findings and most had three or four. The authors concluded that the presence of these "positive" findings of nonorganicity in patients with acute structural brain disease invalidates their use as pathognomonic evidence of a functional deficit. Movement disorders and paralysis were most often mislabeled as nonorganic. Women, homosexual men, those with psychiatric comorbidities, and patients with a seemingly plausible psychogenic explanation for the deficit were most at risk for misdiagnosis. Even the seemingly ironclad finding of spontaneous movement of an extremity in sleep that does not move as well during wakefulness could occur because of motor neglect (see Chapter 10). As summarized by McGee, in studies of patients with known organic disorders, 8% have midline sensory splitting, 85% feel vibration in numb areas, 48% have sensory findings that change between examinations or do not make anatomical sense, and 33% have collapsing weakness. The long held but erroneous belief that functional motor and sensory symptoms, such as weakness, tremor and numbness, are more common on the left side of the body than the right has been convincingly disproven in a systematic review of 1,139 patients.

Conversely, somatoform disorders, causing physical symptoms suggesting an organic illness, are common. The prevalence of somatic symptom disorder (hysteria, Briquet's syndrome) has been estimated at 1.1% of the young adult population, with a female-to-male ratio of 5:1. It begins before the age of 30 and causes multiple, recurrent complaints, often including pain and pseudoneurologic symptoms. Factitious disorders and malingering may also simulate neurologic disease.

In addition to depression, conversion disorder, malingering, and somatic symptom disorder, certain other neurologic conditions and psychiatric conditions, may be confused with each other, and there may be some overlap. For example, patients with some degenerative diseases, such as DLB, AD, and end-stage PD, may develop prominent hallucinations. Determining whether the elderly patient with new-onset hallucinations suffers from a neurologic disorder or a psychiatric disorder is often difficult. Patients with disease in certain brain regions, notably the frontal and temporal lobes, may have symptoms resembling those seen in patients with primary psychiatric disease, including obsessiveness, compulsiveness, strange personalities, and hallucinations.

BIBLIOGRAPHY

Ahmad O, Ahmad KE. Functional neurological disorders in outpatient practice: an Australian cohort. *J Clin Neurosci* 2016;28:93–96.

Al Qahtani DA, Rotgans JI, Mamede S, et al. Does time pressure have a negative effect on diagnostic accuracy? *Acad Med* 2016;91:710–716.

Alonso AD, Beharry C, Corbo CP, et al. Molecular mechanism of prion-like tau-induced neurodegeneration. *Alzheimers Dement* 2016;12:1090–1097.

Amin FM, Asghar MS, Hougaard A, et al. Magnetic resonance angiography of intracranial and extracranial arteries in patients with spontaneous migraine without aura: a cross-sectional study. *Lancet Neurol* 2013;12:454–461.

Arboix A, Marti-Vilalta JL. New concepts in lacunar stroke etiology: the constellation of small-vessel arterial disease. *Cerebrovasc Dis* 2004;17(Suppl 1):58–62.

Arocha JF, Patel VL, Patel YC. Hypothesis generation and the coordination of theory and evidence in novice diagnostic reasoning. *Med Decis Making* 1993;13:198–211.

Bakradze E, Liberman AL. Diagnostic error in stroke-reasons and proposed solutions. *Curr Atheroscler Rep* 2018;20:11.

Barrows HS, Bennett K. The diagnostic (problem solving) skill of the neurologist. Experimental studies and their implications for neurological training. *Arch Neurol* 1972;26:273–277.

Bekelis K, Singer RJ, Maria BL. Intellectual disability. In: Roos RP, ed. *MedLink Neurology*. San Diego: MedLink Corporation. Available at www.medlink.com. Last updated: September 12, 2016.

Benatar M. How neurologists and neuro-ophthalmologists think. *J Neuroophthalmol* 2016;36:4–5.

Betjemann JP, Lowenstein DH. Status epilepticus in adults. *Lancet Neurol* 2015;14:615–624.

Boffeli TJ, Guze SB. The simulation of neurologic disease. *Psychiatr Clin North Am* 1992;15:301–310.

Booij HA, Hamburger HL, Jöbsis GJ, et al. Stroke mimicking conversion disorder: two young women who put our feet back on the ground. *Pract Neurol* 2012;12:179–181.

Bright GM. Abuse of medications employed for the treatment of ADHD: results from a large-scale community survey. *Medscape J Med* 2008;10:111.

Caplan LR. Fisher's rules. *Arch Neurol* 1982;39:389–390.

Charles A. Vasodilation out of the picture as a cause of migraine headache. *Lancet Neurol* 2013;12:419–420.

Charles A. Migraine. *N Engl J Med* 2017;377:553–561.

Chimowitz MI, Logigian EL, Caplan LR. The accuracy of bedside neurological diagnoses. *Ann Neurol* 1990;28:78–85.

Clark BW, Derakhshan A, Desai SV. Diagnostic errors and the bedside clinical examination. *Med Clin North Am* 2018;102: 453–464.

Clarke C, Howard R, Rossor M, et al., eds. *Neurology: A Queen Square Textbook*. 2nd ed. Chichester, West Sussex, UK/ Hoboken: John Wiley & Sons, Inc., 2016.

Coutts SB. Diagnosis and management of transient ischemic attack. *Continuum (Minneap Minn)* 2017;23:82–92.

Crimlisk HL, Bhatia K, Cope H, et al. Slater revisited: 6 year follow up study of patients with medically unexplained motor symptoms. *BMJ* 1998;316:582–586.

Darnell RB. Paraneoplastic neurologic disorders: windows into neuronal function and tumor immunity. *Arch Neurol* 2004; 61:30–32.

Davison JE, Rahman S. Recognition, investigation and management of mitochondrial disease. *Arch Dis Child* 2017; 102:1082–1090.

De Shazo RD, Johnson M, Eriator I, et al. Backstories on the US opioid epidemic. Good intentions gone bad, an industry gone rogue, and watch dogs gone to sleep. *Am J Med* 2018; 131:595–601.

Diaz GJ. Diagnostic reasoning in neurology. An analysis of the more frequent errors. *Neurologia* 2003;18(Suppl 2):3–10.

Duca A, Jagoda A. Transient ischemic attacks: advances in diagnosis and management in the emergency department. *Emerg Med Clin North Am* 2016;34:811–835.

Espay AJ, Aybek S, Carson A, et al. Current concepts in diagnosis and treatment of functional neurological disorders. *JAMA Neurol* 2018;75(9):1132–1141.

Fanciulli A, Wenning GK. Multiple-system atrophy. *N Engl J Med* 2015;372:249–263.

Ford, MD. Acute poisoning. In: Goldman L, Schafer AI, eds. *Goldman's Cecil Medicine*. 24th ed. Philadelphia: Elsevier/Saunders, 2012.

Friedman JH, LaFrance WC Jr. Psychogenic disorders: the need to speak plainly. *Arch Neurol* 2010;67:753–755.

Galasko D, Marder K. Picking away at frontotemporal dementia. *Neurology* 2002;58:1585–1586.

Gaspard N, Foreman BP, Alvarez V, et al. New-onset refractory status epilepticus: etiology, clinical features, and outcome. *Neurology* 2015;85:1604–1613.

Gifford DR, Mittman BS, Vickrey BG. Diagnostic reasoning in neurology. *Neurol Clin* 1996;14:223–238.

Goadsby PJ, Cittadini E, Cohen AS. Trigeminal autonomic cephalalgias: paroxysmal hemicrania, SUNCT/SUNA, and hemicrania continua. *Semin Neurol* 2010;30:186–191.

Goedert M, Masuda-Suzukake M, Falcon B. Like prions: the propagation of aggregated tau and α-synuclein in neurodegeneration. *Brain* 2017;140:266–278.

Goldman AM. Mechanisms of sudden unexplained death in epilepsy. *Curr Opin Neurol* 2015;28:166–174.

Gould R, Miller BL, Goldberg MA, et al. The validity of hysterical signs and symptoms. *J Nerv Ment Dis* 1986;174:593–597.

Graddy R, Buresh ME, Rastegar DA. New and emerging illicit psychoactive substances. *Med Clin North Am* 2018;102: 697–714.

Gray RG, Preece MA, Green SH, et al. Inborn errors of metabolism as a cause of neurological disease in adults: an approach to investigation. *J Neurol Neurosurg Psychiatry* 2000;69:5–12.

Groopman J. *How Doctors Think*. Boston: Houghton Mifflin Company, 2007.

Grossman H, Bergmann C, Parker S. Dementia: a brief review. *Mt Sinai J Med* 2006;73:985–992.

Groves M, O'Rourke P, Alexander H. The clinical reasoning characteristics of diagnostic experts. *Med Teach* 2003;25:308–313.

Hadjivassiliou M. Immune-mediated acquired ataxias. *Handb Clin Neurol* 2011;103:189–199.

Hankey GJ. The ability of the ABCD2 score to predict stroke 1 year after TIA or minor stroke was assessed. *Ann Intern Med* 2016;165:JC23.

Hentati F, El-Euch G, Bouhlal Y, et al. Ataxia with vitamin E deficiency and abetalipoproteinemia. *Handb Clin Neurol* 2011;103:295–305.

Hirsch LJ, Gaspard N, van Baalen A, et al. Proposed consensus definitions for new-onset refractory status epilepticus (NORSE), febrile infection-related epilepsy syndrome (FIRES), and related conditions. *Epilepsia* 2018;59:739–744.

Hoffmann J, May A. Diagnosis, pathophysiology, and management of cluster headache. *Lancet Neurol* 2018;17:75–83.

Hussein AS, Shafran SD. Acute bacterial meningitis in adults. A 12-year review. *Medicine (Baltimore)* 2000;79:360–368.

Ibitoye RT, Wilkins A, Scolding NJ. Neurosarcoidosis: a clinical approach to diagnosis and management. *J Neurol* 2017;264:1023–1028.

Iwafuchi Y, Okamoto K, Oyama Y, et al. Posterior reversible encephalopathy syndrome in a patient with severe uremia without hypertension. *Intern Med* 2016;55:63–68.

Jain KK. Ion channels and neurologic disorders. In: Roos RP, ed. *MedLink Neurology*. San Diego: MedLink Corporation. Available at www.medlink.com. Last updated: July 21, 2017.

Josephs KA. Current understanding of neurodegenerative diseases associated with the protein Tau. *Mayo Clin Proc* 2017;92: 1291–1303.

Kahneman D. *Thinking, Fast and Slow*. New York: Farrar, Straus and Giroux, 2011.

Kanwar P, Kowdley KV. Metal storage disorders: Wilson disease and hemochromatosis. *Med Clin North Am* 2014;98:87–102.

Kassirer JP. Diagnostic reasoning. *Ann Intern Med* 1989; 110:893–900.

Kassirer JP, Kopelman RI. Cognitive errors in diagnosis: instantiation, classification, and consequences. *Am J Med* 1989; 86:433–441.

Kemp AM, Clark MS, Dobbs T, et al. Top 10 facts you need to know about synthetic cannabinoids: not so nice spice. *Am J Med* 2016;129:240–244.e1.

Kempainen RR, Migeon MB, Wolf FM. Understanding our mistakes: a primer on errors in clinical reasoning. *Med Teach* 2003;25:177–181.

Kennedy PG. Viral encephalitis: causes, differential diagnosis, and management. *J Neurol Neurosurg Psychiatry* 2004;75(Suppl 1): i10–i15.

Kennedy PGE, Quan PL, Lipkin WI. Viral encephalitis of unknown cause: current perspective and recent advances. *Viruses* 2017;9(6). pii: E138.

Kinney MO, Craig JJ, Kaplan PW. Non-convulsive status epilepticus: mimics and chameleons. *Pract Neurol* 2018;18:291–305.

Klockgether T. Sporadic adult-onset ataxia of unknown etiology. *Handb Clin Neurol* 2011;103:253–262.

Knopman DS. Alzheimer's disease and other dementias. In: Goldman L, Schafer AI, eds. *Goldman's Cecil Medicine*. 24th ed. Philadelphia: Elsevier/Saunders, 2012.

Langa KM, Levine DA. The diagnosis and management of mild cognitive impairment: a clinical review. *JAMA* 2014;312:2551–2561.

Lanska, DJ. Functional weakness and sensory loss. *Semin Neurol* 2006;26:297–309.

Laureno R. Nutritional cerebellar degeneration, with comments on its relationship to Wernicke disease and alcoholism. *Handb Clin Neurol* 2011;103:175–187.

Lebouvier T, Pasquier F, Buée L. Update on tauopathies. *Curr Opin Neurol* 2017;30:589–598.

Lee PH, Oh SH, Bang OY, et al. Infarct patterns in atherosclerotic middle cerebral artery versus internal carotid artery disease. *Neurology* 2004;62:1291–1296.

Lempert T, Dieterich M, Huppert D, et al. Psychogenic disorders in neurology: frequency and clinical spectrum. *Acta Neurol Scand* 1990;82:335–340.

Levin N, Mor M, Ben Hur T. Patterns of misdiagnosis of multiple sclerosis. *Isr Med Assoc J* 2003;5:489–490.

Lorincz MT. Neurologic Wilson's disease. *Ann N Y Acad Sci* 2010;1184:173–187.

Louis ED, Mayer SA, Rowland LP, eds. *Merritt's Neurology*. 13th ed. Philadelphia: Wolters-Kluwer, 2016.

Mace, CJ, Trimble, MR. Ten-year prognosis of conversion disorder. *Br J Psychiatry* 1996;169:282–288.

MacKenzie JM. Intracerebral haemorrhage. *J Clin Pathol* 1996; 49:360–364.

Maguire MJ, Jackson CF, Marson AG, et al. Treatments for the prevention of Sudden Unexpected Death in Epilepsy (SUDEP). *Cochrane Database Syst Rev* 2016;(7):CD011792.

Malouf R, Brust JC. Hypoglycemia: causes, neurological manifestations, and outcome. *Ann Neurol* 1985;17:421–430.

Mascalchi M, Vella A. Magnetic resonance and nuclear medicine imaging in ataxias. *Handb Clin Neurol* 2011;103:85–110.

Mathew PG, Garza I. Headache. *Semin Neurol* 2011;31:5–17.

Mayer AR, Quinn DK, Master CL. The spectrum of mild traumatic brain injury: a review. *Neurology* 2017;89:623–632.

McGee S. *Evidence Based Physical Diagnosis*. 3rd ed. Philadelphia: Elsevier/Saunders, 2012.

McGill F, Griffiths MJ, Solomon T. Viral meningitis: current issues in diagnosis and treatment. *Curr Opin Infect Dis* 2017; 30:248–256.

Meola G, Hanna MG, Fontaine B. Diagnosis and new treatment in muscle channelopathies. *J Neurol Neurosurg Psychiatry* 2009; 80:360–365.

Meuth SG, Kleinschnitz C. Multifocal motor neuropathy: update on clinical characteristics, pathophysiological concepts and therapeutic options. *Eur Neurol* 2010;63:193–204.

Moene FC, Landberg EH, Hoogduin KA, et al. Organic syndromes diagnosed as conversion disorder: identification and frequency in a study of 85 patients. *J Psychosom Res* 2000;49:7–12.

Morris MC, Brockman J, Schneider JA, et al. Association of seafood consumption, brain mercury level, and APOE ε4 status with brain neuropathology in older adults. *JAMA* 2016; 315:489–497.

Newman LC. Trigeminal autonomic cephalalgias. *Continuum (Minneap Minn)* 2015;21(4 Headache):1041–1057.

Nicholson TR, Stone J, Kanaan RA. Conversion disorder: a problematic diagnosis. *J Neurol Neurosurg Psychiatry* 2011;82:1267–1273.

Nigrovic LE. Aseptic meningitis. *Handb Clin Neurol* 2013;112: 1153–1156.

Norman GR, Eva KW. Diagnostic error and clinical reasoning. *Med Educ* 2010;44:94–100.

Norman G, Sherbino J, Dore K, et al. The etiology of diagnostic errors: a controlled trial of system 1 versus system 2 reasoning. *Acad Med* 2014;89:277–284.

O'Malley GF. The blood of my veins—mercury, Minamata and the soul of Japan. *Clin Toxicol (Phila)* 2017;55:934–938.

Ostling PS, Davidson KS, Anyama BO, et al. America's opioid epidemic: a comprehensive review and look into the rising crisis. *Curr Pain Headache Rep* 2018;22:32.

Pandolfo M. Friedreich ataxia. *Handb Clin Neurol* 2011;103: 275–294.

Perlman SL. Spinocerebellar degenerations. *Handb Clin Neurol* 2011;100:113–140.

Puig JG, Torres RJ, Mateos FA, et al. The spectrum of HGPRT deficiency. Clinical experience based on 20 patients from 16 Spanish families. *Adv Exp Med Biol* 1998;431:25–29.

Rech MA, Donahey E, Cappiello Dziedzic JM, et al. New drugs of abuse. *Pharmacotherapy* 2015;35:189–197.

Ropper AH, Samuels MA, Klein J. *Adams and Victor's Principles of Neurology*. 10th ed. New York: McGraw-Hill Education Medical, 2014.

Rosenberg NR, Portegies P, de Visser M, et al. Diagnostic investigation of patients with chronic polyneuropathy: evaluation of a clinical guideline. *J Neurol Neurosurg Psychiatry* 2001; 71:205–209.

Rossetti AO, Lowenstein DH. Management of refractory status epilepticus in adults: still more questions than answers. *Lancet Neurol* 2011;10:922–930.

Rozenberg F. Acute viral encephalitis. *Handb Clin Neurol* 2013; 112:1171–1181.

Rudick RA, Schiffer RB, Schwetz KM, et al. Multiple sclerosis. The problem of incorrect diagnosis. *Arch Neurol* 1986;43: 578–583.

Saudubray JM, Mochel F. The phenotype of adult versus pediatric patients with inborn errors of metabolism. *J Inherit Metab Dis* 2018;41:753–756.

Schutte CM, van der Meyden CH, van Niekerk L, et al. Severe porphyric neuropathy—importance of screening for porphyria in Guillain-Barré syndrome. *S Afr Med J* 2015;106:44–47.

Selhorst JB, Waybright EA, Jennings S, et al. Liver lover's headache: pseudotumor cerebri and vitamin A intoxication. *JAMA* 1984;252:3365.

Slater E. Diagnosis of "hysteria". *Br Med J* 1965;1:1395–1399.

Slater ET, Glithero E. A follow-up of patients diagnosed as suffering from "hysteria". *J Psychosom Res* 1965;9:9–13.

Stein SC, Georgoff P, Meghan S, et al. 150 years of treating severe traumatic brain injury: a systematic review of progress in mortality. *J Neurotrauma* 2010;27:1343–1353.

Steiner I, Budka H, Chaudhuri A, et al. Viral meningoencephalitis: a review of diagnostic methods and guidelines for management. *Eur J Neurol* 2010;17:999–e57.

Steiner JA, Quansah E, Brundin P. The concept of alpha-synuclein as a prion-like protein: ten years after. *Cell Tissue Res* 2018;373:161–173.

Stone J, Sharpe M, Carson A, et al. Are functional motor and sensory symptoms really more frequent on the left? A systematic review. *J Neurol Neurosurg Psychiatry* 2002a;73:578–581.

Stone J, Zeman A, Sharpe M. Functional weakness and sensory disturbance. *J Neurol Neurosurg Psychiatry* 2002b;73:241–245.

Stone J, Sharpe M, Rothwell PM, et al. The 12 year prognosis of unilateral functional weakness and sensory disturbance. *J Neurol Neurosurg Psychiatry* 2003;74:591–596.

Stone J, Smyth R, Carson A, et al. La belle indifference in conversion symptoms and hysteria: systematic review. *Br J Psychiatry* 2006;188:204–209.

Sutter R. Are we prepared to detect subtle and nonconvulsive status epilepticus in critically ill patients? *J Clin Neurophysiol* 2016;33:25–31.

Tatsumoto N, Fujisaki K, Nagae H, et al. Reversible posterior leukoencephalopathy syndrome in a patient with severe uremic encephalopathy. *Clin Nephrol* 2010;74:154–158.

Thrift AG, Dewey HM, Macdonell RA, et al. Incidence of the major stroke subtypes: initial findings from the North East Melbourne stroke incidence study (NEMESIS). *Stroke* 2001;32: 1732–1738.

Transverse Myelitis Consortium Working Group. Proposed diagnostic criteria and nosology of acute transverse myelitis. *Neurology* 2002;59(4):499–505.

Traynor BJ, Codd MB, Corr B, et al. Amyotrophic lateral sclerosis mimic syndromes: a population-based study. *Arch Neurol* 2000;57:109–113.

Uygunoğlu U, Siva A. Behçet's syndrome and nervous system involvement. *Curr Neurol Neurosci Rep* 2018;18:35.

Vallat JM, Sommer C, Magy L. Chronic inflammatory demyelinating polyradiculoneuropathy: diagnostic and therapeutic challenges for a treatable condition. *Lancet Neurol* 2010;9: 402–412.

van Gijn J, Rinkel GJ. Subarachnoid haemorrhage: diagnosis, causes and management. *Brain* 2001;124:249–278.

Vickrey BG, Samuels MA, Ropper AH. How neurologists think: a cognitive psychology perspective on missed diagnoses. *Ann Neurol* 2010;67:425–433.

Vincent A, Palace J, Hilton-Jones D. Myasthenia gravis. *Lancet* 2001;357:2122–2128.

Waespe W, Niesper J, Imhof HG, et al. Lower cranial nerve palsies due to internal carotid dissection. *Stroke* 1988;19: 1561–1564.

Ward TN. Migraine diagnosis and pathophysiology. *Continuum (Minneap Minn)* 2012;18:753–763.

Warlow C, Sudlow C, Dennis M, et al. Stroke. *Lancet* 2003;362:1211–1224.

Weissk RD. Drug abuse and dependence. In: Goldman L, Schafer AI, eds. *Goldman's Cecil Medicine*. 24th ed. Philadelphia: Elsevier/Saunders, 2012.

Welch KM. Contemporary concepts of migraine pathogenesis. *Neurology* 2003;61(8 Suppl 4):S2–S8.

Whitley RJ. Herpes simplex encephalitis: adolescents and adults. *Antiviral Res* 2006;71:141–148.

Wijdicks EF. Hepatic encephalopathy. *N Engl J Med* 2016; 375:1660–1670.

Wilder-Smith EP, Lim EC, Teoh HL, et al. The NORSE (new-onset refractory status epilepticus) syndrome: defining a disease entity. *Ann Acad Med Singapore* 2005;34:417–420.

Williams VC, Lucas J, Babcock MA, et al. Neurofibromatosis type 1 revisited. *Pediatrics* 2009;123:124–133.

Woolsey RM, Young RR. The clinical diagnosis of disorders of the spinal cord. *Neurol Clin* 1991;9:573–583.

Yan X, Uronen RL, Huttunen HJ. The interaction of α-synuclein and Tau: a molecular conspiracy in neurodegeneration? *Semin Cell Dev Biol* 2018. pii: S1084-9521(17)30389-0. [Epub ahead of print]

Yang M, Li Z, Zhao Y, et al. Outcome and risk factors associated with extent of central nervous system injury due to exertional heat stroke. *Medicine (Baltimore)* 2017;96:e8417.

INDEX

Note: Page numbers followed by *f* indicate figures; those followed by *t* indicate table.

B

C

E

M

O

Q

R

S

T

U

V

W

X

Y

Z